Experimental Study Designs

Nontraditional Research Designs

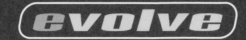

⋮ *To access your Student Resources, visit the web address below:*

http://evolve.elsevier.com/burns/practice/

Evolve Learning Resources for **The Practice of Nursing Research: Appraisal, Synthesis, and Generation of Evidence, 6th edition,** offer the following features:

- **Free access to Mosby's Index**
  A robust research tool that indexes more than 2,500 journals. Allows you to search articles for evidence-based practice or for an in-depth review of the literature.

- **Interactive Review Questions**
  More than 400 questions, with feedback for both correct and incorrect responses.

- **Data Sets with Data Set Activities**
  Qualitative and quantitative data sets with activities that provide practice in working with actual research data.

- **Reference Appendixes**
  Nine appendixes that serve as valuable resources for beginning nurse researchers.

- **Author Index**
  A searchable index of all authors cited in the text.

- **Sample Research Proposals**
  Five sample proposals that serve as excellent models for beginning researchers.

CONGRATULATIONS!

You now have access to Mosby's Index FREE for 6 months.

MOSBY'S
Index

Each **new** copy of **Burns & Grove's** *The Practice of Nursing Research: Appraisal, Synthesis, and Generation of Evidence,* **6th Edition,** includes a free 6-month subscription to **Mosby's Index.** Brought to you by Elsevier, Mosby's Index is a robust nursing and health professions journal abstracts and indexing database.

With a **user-friendly interface** and **powerful search capabilities,** Mosby's Index **saves research time and effort.** Based on the EMTREE thesaurus (Elsevier's leading Life Science thesaurus enhanced for nursing), Mosby's Index **encompasses more than 2,500 active nursing and health professions journals.**

To activate your FREE 6-month access to Mosby's Index, go to http://www.mosbysindex.com/promotion?campaign=BurnsGrovePractice6eOffer and complete the short registration form. Be sure to have your passcode available because you will need to provide it at the time of registration.

If the passcode card is removed or if the passcode has been used for subscription activation, this book cannot be returned. If you purchased a used copy of this book, you are not entitled to this free 6-month subscription, and the passcode may no longer be valid.

Passcode

MBMNV-6ZRQW

The
PRACTICE *of* NURSING RESEARCH

APPRAISAL, SYNTHESIS, and GENERATION of EVIDENCE

SIXTH EDITION

NANCY BURNS, PhD, RN, FCN, FAAN
Professor Emeritus
School of Nursing
The University of Texas at Arlington
Arlington, Texas;
Faith Community Nurse
St. Matthew Cumberland Presbyterian Church
Burleson, Texas

SUSAN K. GROVE, PhD, RN, ANP-BC, GNP-BC
Professor
School of Nursing
The University of Texas at Arlington
Arlington, Texas;
Adult Nurse Practitioner
Family Practice
Grand Prairie, Texas

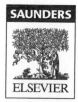

SAUNDERS

ELSEVIER

SAUNDERS
ELSEVIER

11830 Westline Industrial Drive
St. Louis, Missouri 63146

THE PRACTICE OF NURSING RESEARCH: APPRAISAL, SYNTHESIS,
AND GENERATION OF EVIDENCE, SIXTH EDITION   978-1-4160-5468-9

Previous editions copyrighted 2005, 2001, 1997, 1993, 1987

Library of Congress Cataloging-in-Publication Data

Burns, Nancy, Ph. D.
   The practice of nursing research: appraisal, synthesis, and generation of evidence / Nancy Burns,
Susan K. Grove. — 6th ed.
   p. ; cm.
   Includes bibliographical references and index.
   ISBN 978-1-4160-5468-9 (hardcover : alk. paper) 1. Nursing—Research—Methodology. 2. Evidence-based
nursing. I. Grove, Susan K. II. Title.
   [DNLM: 1. Nursing Research. 2. Evidence-Based Medicine.
WY 20.5 B967pa 2009]
   RT81.5.B86 2009
   610.73072—dc22   2008020034

Senior Editor: Lee Henderson
Senior Developmental Editor: Rae Robertson
Publishing Services Manager: Deborah Vogel
Project Manager: Brandilyn Tidwell
Designer: Paula Catalano

Printed in the United States of America
Last digit is the print number: 9 8 7 6 5 4 3 2 1

To our readers and researchers, nationally and internationally, who will provide the science to develop an evidence-based practice for nursing.

To our family members for their constant input, support, and love, especially our husbands

Jerry Burns

and

Jay Suggs.

Nancy and Susan

REVIEWERS

Phyllis S. Brenner, PhD, RN, CNAA, BC
Professor of Nursing
Madonna University
Livonia, Michigan

Dona Rinaldi Carpenter, EdD, RN
Professor of Nursing
University of Scranton
Scranton, Pennsylvania

Tracy B. Chamblee, MS, RN, CNS
CNS Coordinator
Wegmans School of Nursing
St. John Fisher College
Rochester, New York

Esther H. Condon, PhD, RN
Professor
School of Nursing
Hampton University
Hampton, Virginia

Maureen C. Creegan, EdD, RN
Professor and Director
Division of Nursing
Dominican College
Orangeburg, New York

Janet Berube Douglass, DNSc, MS, RN
Faculty at a Distance
St. Joseph's College of Maine
Standish, Maine

Sandra A. Faux, PhD, RN
Associate Professor
College of Nursing
Rush University
Chicago, Illinois

Susanne W. Gibbons, PhD, C-ANP, C-GNP
Graduate School of Nursing
Uniformed Services University of the Health
    Sciences
Bethesda, Maryland

Teresa Tarnowski Goodell, PhD, RN, CNS, CCRN, APRN-BC
Assistant Professor
School of Nursing
Oregon Health & Science University
Portland, Oregon

Jeanette C. Hartshorn, PhD, RN, FAAN
Dean
School of Nursing
University of Houston—Victoria
Victoria, Texas

Valera A. Hascup, PhD(c), MSN, RN-C, CTN, CCES
Assistant Professor
Director of Transcultural Nursing Institute
College of Natural, Applied and Health Sciences,
    Department of Nursing
Kean University
Union, New Jersey

Margaret J. Hegge, EdD, RN
Distinguished Professor
College of Nursing
South Dakota State University
Sioux Falls, South Dakota

Vallire D. Hooper, PhDc, MSN, RN, CPAN
Assistant Professor
School of Nursing
Medical College of Georgia
Augusta, Georgia

Helen Hough, MLS
Health Science/Central Library Science Librarian
Central Library
The University of Texas at Arlington
Arlington, Texas

Paula Karnick, PhD, ANP-C, CPNP
Assistant Professor of Nursing
School of Nursing
North Park University
Chicago, Illinois

Mary K. Kirkpatrick, EdD, MSN, RN
Professor and International Coordinator
College of Nursing
East Carolina University
Greenville, North Carolina

Joanne E. Layton, MS, RN, CCRN, ANP
Senior Teaching Associate
School of Nursing
University of Rochester
Rochester, New York

Nancy J. MacMullen, PhD, APM/CNS
Associate Professor and Program Coordinator
Nursing
Governors State University
University Park, Illinois

Carla Mueller, PhD, RN
Professor
Department of Nursing
University of Saint Francis
Fort Wayne, Indiana

Lynn Wemett Nichols, PhD, RN
Associate Professor
Wegmans School of Nursing
St. John Fisher College
Rochester, New York

Marsha Snyder, PhD, APRN-BC
Clinical Assistant Professor
College of Nursing
University of Illinois at Chicago
Chicago, Illinois

Martha B. Sparks, PhD, APRN-BC, FNGNA
Professor
College of Nursing and Health Professions
University of Southern Indiana
Evansville, Indiana

Amy Y. Spurlock, PhD, RN
Associate Professor
School of Nursing
Troy University
Troy, Alabama

Karen Anne Stevens, PhD, RN
Department of Nursing
Bowie State University
Bowie, Maryland

Kathleen A. Sullivan, PhD, RN
Professor of Nursing
La Roche College
Pittsburgh, Pennsylvania

Joan Tilghman, PhD, CRNP
Associate Dean, Masters in Nursing
Helene Fuld School of Nursing
Coppin State University
Baltimore, Maryland

Renee Samples Twibell, RN, DNS, CNE
Associate Professor
School of Nursing
Ball State University;
Ball Memorial Hospital
Muncie, Indiana

Paulette L. Williams, DrPH, MSN, RN
Assistant Professor
School of Nursing and Dental Hygiene
University of Hawaii—Manoa
Honolulu, Hawaii

Nan Russell Yancey, PhD, RN
Professor/Graduate Director
College of Nursing and Health Professions
Lewis University
Romeoville, Illinois

Deborah Zbegner, DNSc, CRNP, RN-C
Associate Professor, Nursing
Wilkes University
Wilkes-Barre, Pennsylvania

PREFACE

Research is a major force in the nursing profession that is used to change practice, education, and health policy. Our aim in developing the sixth edition of *The Practice of Nursing Research: Appraisal, Synthesis, and Generation of Evidence* is to increase excitement about research and to facilitate the development of evidence-based practice for nursing. It is critically important that all nurses, especially those in advanced-practice roles (nurse practitioners, clinical nurse specialists, nurse anesthetists, and nurse midwives), have an understanding of research and its link to the development of evidence-based practice. Nurses will have a significant role in providing evidence-based care and promoting quality, cost-effective healthcare outcomes for patients and families. Doctoral students might use this text to facilitate their development of research evidence through their dissertations.

The depth and breadth of content presented in this edition reflect the increase in research activities and the growth in research knowledge since the previous edition. Nursing research is introduced at the baccalaureate level and becomes an integral part of graduate education (master's and doctoral) and clinical practice. We hope that this new edition might increase the number of nurses at all levels involved in research activities such as critically appraising studies; using evidence-based guidelines in practice; and conducting quantitative, qualitative, outcome, and intervention research.

NEW CONTENT

The sixth edition provides comprehensive coverage of nursing research and is focused on the learning needs and styles of today's nursing student and practicing nurse. Several exciting, new areas of content are included in the sixth edition:

- Chapter 1, Discovering the World of Nursing Research, includes major revisions, with a model of the elements of evidence-based practice (EBP). This EBP model is linked to the framework for the textbook and stresses the significance of research in developing EBP.
- Chapter 2, The Evolution of Evidence-Based Practice in Nursing, is retitled and focused on building an EBP for nursing. This chapter includes the historical development of EBP in health care

and methodologies for developing an EBP in nursing. In addition, the reader is introduced to the best research evidence for practice that is provided by systematic reviews, meta-analyses, integrative reviews, metasummaries, and metasyntheses. The chapter includes a table that presents the purposes of these syntheses, the types of research included in these syntheses (the "sampling frame"), and the analysis for achieving the different types of syntheses. A model of the continuum of the levels of research evidence, from strongest to weakest evidence, is now provided.

- Chapter 4, Introduction to Qualitative Research, includes an introduction to and the philosophical bases for the following types of qualitative research: (1) phenomenology, (2) grounded theory, (3) ethnography, (4) historical research, (5) philosophical inquiry, and (6) critical social theory research, including feminist research.
- Chapter 6, Review of Relevant Literature, includes an expanded discussion of the processes for searching the literature for relevant sources. Details are provided for using state-of-the-art resources for conducting systematic reviews, integrative reviews, meta-analyses, and metasyntheses to determine the best research evidence for practice.
- Chapter 9, Ethics in Research, features updated coverage of (1) the Health Insurance Portability and Accountability Act (HIPAA), (2) U.S. Department of Health and Human Services (DHHS) regulations for protection of human subjects in research, and (3) Food and Drug Administration (FDA) regulations for protection of human research subjects. The chapter also discusses how changes in the laws have affected nursing research, with an expanded focus on the ethics of conducting qualitative studies and the processes for protecting participants in these studies.
- Chapter 11, Selecting a Quantitative Research Design, includes many currently used designs that are not covered in other leading texts but that are important to understand.
- Chapter 12, Outcomes Research, a unique feature of our text, was significantly rewritten to promote understanding of the history, significance, and impact of outcomes research on nursing

and health care, for both students and nurses in clinical practice. New content is included on nursing-sensitive patient outcomes, advanced-practice nursing outcomes, and practice-based research networks. In addition, the methodologies for conducting outcomes research have been expanded.

- Chapter 13, Intervention Research, reflects the increasing number of intervention studies being done in nursing and is also a unique feature of our text.
- Chapter 14, Sampling, now includes extensive coverage of sampling methods and sample sizes for qualitative research. New content in this chapter includes the formulas for calculating the acceptance and refusal rates for potential subjects and the retention and attrition rates for subjects participating in a study. Additional content is included to assist researchers in recruiting and retaining subjects for their studies.
- Chapter 15, Measurement Concepts, features detailed coverage of measurement in conducting qualitative studies and measuring outcomes of healthcare. New content included in this chapter is the use of sensitivity, specificity, and likelihood ratios to determine the quality of diagnostic tests. Understanding these concepts is important in delivering EBP.
- Chapter 16, Measurement Methods Used in Developing Evidence for Practice, provides more detail on the use of physiological measurement methods in research. An increasing number of nursing studies are focused on the measurement of the outcomes from interventions using physiological measurement methods, and this chapter equips the reader to understand and take part in those studies.
- Chapter 17, Collecting and Managing Data, now covers the importance of intervention fidelity and quality measurement in conducting the high-quality quasi-experimental and experimental studies needed to generate research evidence about the effectiveness of nursing interventions for practice.
- Chapter 23, Qualitative Research Methodology, has been completely reorganized to facilitate understanding of the conduct of qualitative research. The chapter features a marked increase in the examples from current qualitative studies.
- Chapter 25, Disseminating Research Findings, features expanded and updated content on communicating study findings through presentation and publication.

- Chapter 26, Critical Appraisal of Nursing Studies, now includes the concept of critical appraisal instead of critique. The critical appraisal processes for quantitative and qualitative studies to build an EBP for nursing are detailed.
- Chapter 27, Strategies for Promoting Evidence-Based Nursing Practice, has undergone extensive revision to achieve a completely new focus on evidence-based practice. The chapter now includes a discussion of the strengths and concerns related to evidence-based practice, guidelines for critically appraising systematic reviews, guidelines for critically appraising and conducting meta-analyses, and guidelines for critically appraising and conducting integrative reviews. Stetler's Model of Research Utilization to Facilitate Evidence-Based Practice and the Iowa Model of Evidence-Based Practice to Promote Quality of Care are presented to direct nurses in making evidence-based changes in their practice. The Grove Model for implementing national standardized guidelines in practice is described with the JNC VII used as an example for treating hypertension. Internet sites that include best research evidence for practice are identified. Finally, Evidence-Based Practice Centers and their contributions to evidence-based practice are described.

The sixth edition is written and organized to facilitate ease in reading, understanding, and implementing the research process. The major strengths of this text include the following:

- State-of-the-art coverage of EBP—a topic of vital and growing importance in a health care arena focused on quality and cost-effectiveness of patient care.
- A clear, concise writing style that is consistent among the chapters to facilitate student learning.
- Comprehensive coverage of quantitative, qualitative, outcomes, and intervention research techniques.
- A balanced coverage of qualitative and quantitative research methodologies.
- Electronic references and websites that direct the student to an extensive array of information that is important for conducting studies and using research findings in practice.
- Rich and frequent illustration of major points and concepts from the most current nursing research literature from a variety of clinical practices areas.
- A strong conceptual framework that links nursing research with EBP, theory, knowledge, and philosophy.

Our text provides a comprehensive introduction to nursing research for graduate and practicing nurses. At the master's and doctoral level, the text provides not only substantive content related to research but also practical applications based on the authors' experiences in conducting various types of nursing research, familiarity with the research literature, and experience in teaching nursing research at various educational levels.

The sixth edition of this text is organized into 4 units and 29 chapters. Unit One introduces the reader to the world of nursing research. The content and presentation of this unit have been designed to introduce EBP and to assist the reader in overcoming the barriers frequently experienced in understanding the language used in nursing research.

Unit Two provides an in-depth presentation of the research process for both quantitative and qualitative research. As with previous editions, this text provides extensive coverage of the many types of quantitative and qualitative research.

Unit Three addresses the implications of research for the discipline and profession of nursing. Content is provided to direct the student in conducting critical appraisals of both quantitative and qualitative research. A detailed discussion of EBP is provided, with models to direct nurses in providing evidence-based health care. Nursing and medical practice guidelines are included and provide essential direction for implementing evidence-based advanced nursing practice roles, such as nurse practitioner, clinical nurse specialist, nurse anesthetist, and nurse midwife.

Unit Four addresses seeking support for research. Readers are given direction for developing quantitative and qualitative research proposals and seeking funding for their research.

The changes in the sixth edition of this text reflect the advances in nursing research and also incorporate comments from outside reviewers, colleagues, and students. Our desire to promote the continuing development of the profession of nursing was the incentive for investing the time and energy required to develop this new edition.

STUDENT ANCILLARIES

An **Evolve Learning Resources website** is available at *http://evolve.elsevier.com/Burns/practice/* and features a wealth of assets, including the following:

Approximately 400 Interactive Review Questions
Data Sets and Data Set Activities
An Author Index
Sample Qualitative and Quantitative Research Proposals, and a Sample Funded Proposal

Nine Appendixes
Applied Nursing Research Discount Subscription Offer

A printed **Study Guide** accompanies this edition of *The Practice of Nursing Research*. This study guide is keyed chapter-by-chapter to the text. It includes the following:

- *Relevant Terms* activities that help students understand and apply the language of nursing research
- *Key Ideas* exercises that reinforce essential concepts
- *Making Connections* activities that give students practice in the higher-level skills of comprehension and content synthesis
- Puzzles that serve not only as a clever learning activity but also as a welcome "fun" activity for busy adult learners
- *Exercises in Critical Appraisal* that provide experiences for students and practicing nurses to critically evaluate both quantitative and qualitative studies
- *Going Beyond* activities that provide suggestions for further study
- An Answer Key that offers immediate feedback to reinforce learning
- A Published Studies appendix

INSTRUCTOR ANCILLARIES

The **Instructor's Resources** are available on Evolve at http://evolve.elsevier.com/Burns/practice/. Instructors also have access to the online student resources. The Instructor Resources includes an Instructor's Manual with Data Set Activities and syllabi, an expanded Test Bank including 600 questions (some in the NCLEX® Examination alternate format), PowerPoint Presentations totaling over 700 slides, and an Image Collection consisting of most images from the text.

The **Evolve Course Management System**, provided free for instructors, is an interactive learning environment that works in coordination with *The Practice of Nursing Research*, Sixth Edition, to provide online course management tools you can use not only to manage your course but also enhance classroom and home learning experiences. You can use Evolve to do the following:

- Publish your class syllabus, outline, and lecture notes.
- Set up "virtual office hours" and e-mail communication.
- Share important dates and information through the online class *Calendar*.
- Encourage student participation through *Chat Rooms* and *Discussion Boards*.

ACKNOWLEDGMENTS

Writing the sixth edition of this textbook has allowed us the opportunity to examine and revise the content of the previous edition based on input from the literature, a number of scholarly colleagues, and our graduate and undergraduate students. A textbook such as this requires synthesizing the ideas of many people and resources. We have attempted to extract from the nursing literature the essence of nursing knowledge related to the conduct of nursing research. Thus we would like to thank those nursing scholars who shared their knowledge with the rest of us in nursing and who made this knowledge accessible for inclusion in this textbook.

The ideas from the literature were synthesized and discussed with our colleagues and students to determine the revisions needed for the sixth edition. We would like to express our appreciation to Dean Elizabeth Poster, Associate Dean of Research; Dr. Carolyn Cason, Associate Dean of Doctoral Studies; Dr. Jennifer Gray; and faculty members of the School of Nursing at the University of Texas at Arlington, for their support during the long and sometimes

arduous experiences that are inevitable in developing a book of this magnitude. We would like to extend a special thanks to Helen Hough for her scholarly input regarding the literature review chapter. We would also like to thank Dr. Margarete Sandelowski for her suggestions regarding the qualitative research content in this text. We particularly value the questions raised by our students regarding the content of this text, which allow us a peek at the learner's perception.

We would also like to recognize the excellent reviews of the colleagues who helped us make important revisions in this text.

We want to thank the people at Elsevier, who have been extremely helpful to us in producing a scholarly, attractive, and appealing text. We extend a special thank you to the people most instrumental in the development and production of this book: Lee Henderson, Senior Editor, and Rae Robertson, Senior Developmental Editor. We also want to thank others involved with the production and marketing of this book—Brandi Tidwell, Project Manager; Julia Dummitt, Designer; and Susan Adkisson, Marketing Manager.

Nancy Burns, PhD, RN, FAAN

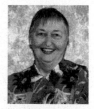

Susan K. Grove, PhD, RN, ANP-BC, GNP-BC

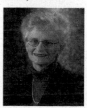

CONTENTS

UNIT ONE

Introduction to Nursing Research

CHAPTER 1
Discovering the World of Nursing Research

Welcome to the world of nursing research. You might think it is strange to consider research a "world," but research is truly a new way of experiencing reality. Entering a new world requires learning a unique language, incorporating new rules, and using new experiences to learn how to interact effectively within that world. As you become a part of this new world, your perceptions and methods of reasoning will be modified and expanded. Understanding the world of nursing research is critical to providing evidence-based care to your patients. Since the 1990s, there has been a growing emphasis for nurses, especially advanced practice nurses (APNs), administrators, educators, and nurse researchers, to promote an evidence-based practice in nursing (Brown, 1999; Craig & Smyth, 2007; Malloch & Porter-O'Grady, 2006; Melnyk & Fineout-Overholt, 2005; Nursing Executive Center, 2005; Pearson, Field, & Jordan, 2007). Evidence-based practice in nursing requires a strong body of research knowledge that nurses must synthesize and use to promote quality care for their patients. We developed this text to facilitate your understanding of nursing research and its contribution to the delivery of evidenced-based nursing practice.

This chapter explains broadly the world of research. We begin with a definition of nursing research, followed by the framework for this text that connects nursing research to the world of nursing. The chapter concludes with a discussion of the significance of research in developing an evidence-based practice for nursing.

DEFINITION OF NURSING RESEARCH

The root meaning of the word *research* is "search again" or "examine carefully." More specifically, research is the diligent, systematic inquiry or investigation to validate and refine existing knowledge and generate new knowledge. The concepts *systematic* and *diligent* are critical to the meaning of research because they imply planning, organization, and persistence. Many disciplines conduct research, so what distinguishes nursing research from research in other disciplines? In some ways there are no differences, because the knowledge and skills required to conduct research are similar from one discipline to another. However, in looking at other dimensions of research within a discipline, it is clear that research in nursing must also be unique to address the questions relevant to the profession. Nurse researchers need to implement the most effective research methodologies to develop a unique body of knowledge for nursing practice.

In 2003, the American Nurses Association (ANA) developed the following definition of nursing to clarify this unique body of knowledge:

Nursing is the protection, promotion, and optimization of health and abilities, prevention of illness and injury, alleviation of suffering through the diagnosis and treatment of human response, and advocacy in the care of individuals, families, communities, and populations. (ANA, 2003, p. 6)

Based on this definition, nursing studies need to focus on understanding human responses and determining the best interventions to promote health, prevent illness, and manage illness. Since the 1960s, the holistic perspective has also influenced the development and implementation of nursing studies and the interpretation of the findings (ANA, 2003; Riley, Beal, Levi,

& McCausland, 2002). Many nurses hold the view that nursing research should focus on acquiring knowledge that can be directly applied to clinical practice (Pearson et al., 2007). However, another view is that nursing research should include studies of nursing education, nursing administration, health services, and nurses' characteristics and roles, as well as clinical situations. Riley et al. (2002) support this view and believe nursing scholarship should include education, practice, and service. The research conducted in these areas will either directly or indirectly influence the development of an evidence-based practice for nursing. Research is needed to identify teaching-learning strategies to promote nurses' understanding and management of practice. Studies of nursing administration, health services, and nursing roles are necessary to promote quality in the health care system.

Therefore, nursing research generates knowledge that will directly and indirectly influence nursing practice. In this text, **nursing research** is defined as a scientific process that validates and refines existing knowledge and generates new knowledge that directly and indirectly influences the delivery of evidence-based nursing practice.

FRAMEWORK LINKING NURSING RESEARCH TO THE WORLD OF NURSING

To best explore nursing research, we have developed a framework to help establish connections between research and the various elements of nursing. The framework presented in the following pages links nursing research to the world of nursing and is used as an organizing model for this textbook. In the framework model (see Figure 1-1), nursing research is not an entity disconnected from the rest of nursing but rather is influenced by and influences all other nursing elements. The concepts in this model are pictured on a continuum from concrete to abstract. The discussion introduces this continuum and progresses from the concrete concept of the empirical world of nursing practice to the most abstract concept of nursing philosophy. The use of two-way arrows in the model indicates the dynamic interaction among the concepts.

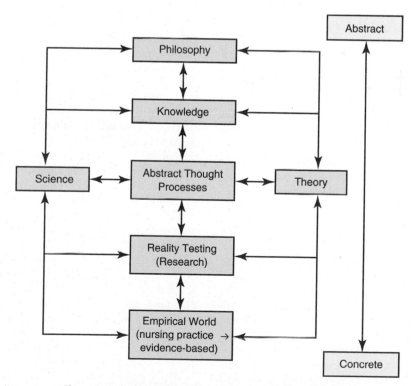

Figure 1-1 Framework linking nursing research to the world of nursing.

Concrete-Abstract Continuum

Figure 1-1 presents the components of nursing on a concrete-abstract continuum. This continuum demonstrates that nursing thought flows both from concrete to abstract thinking and from abstract to concrete thinking. Concrete thinking is oriented toward and limited by tangible things or by events that we observe and experience in reality. Thus, the focus of concrete thinking is immediate events that are limited by time and space. Most nurses believe they are concrete thinkers because they focus on the specific actions in nursing practice. Abstract thinking is oriented toward the development of an idea without application to, or association with, a particular instance. Abstract thinkers tend to look for meaning, patterns, relationships, and philosophical implications. This type of thinking is independent of time and space. Currently, graduate nursing education fosters abstract thinking, because it is an essential skill for developing theory and creating an idea for study. Nurses assuming advanced roles need to use both abstract and concrete thinking. For example, a nurse practitioner must explore the best research evidence about a practice problem (abstract thinking) before using his or her clinical expertise to diagnose and manage an individual patient's health problem (concrete thinking).

Nursing research requires skills in both concrete and abstract thinking. Abstract thought is required to identify researchable problems, design studies, and interpret findings. Concrete thought is necessary in both planning and implementing the detailed steps of data collection and analysis. This back-and-forth flow between abstract and concrete thought may be one reason why nursing research seems complex and challenging.

Empirical World

The empirical world is what we experience through our senses and is the concrete portion of our existence. It is what we often call *reality*, and "doing" kinds of activities are part of this world. There is a sense of certainty about the empirical or real world; it seems understandable, predictable, controllable. Concrete thinking focuses on the empirical world; words associated with this thinking include "practical," "down-to-earth," "solid," and "factual." Concrete thinkers want facts. They want to be able to apply whatever they know to the current situation.

The practice of nursing takes place in the empirical world, as demonstrated in Figure 1-1. The scope of nursing practice varies for the registered nurse (RN) and the APN. RNs provide care to and coordinate care for patients, families, and communities in a variety of settings. They initiate interventions and carry out treatments authorized by other health care providers. APNs (nurse practitioners, nurse anesthetists, nurse midwives, and clinical nurse specialists) have an expanded practice. Their knowledge, skills, and expertise promote role autonomy and overlap with medical practice. APNs usually concentrate their clinical practice in a specialty area, such as acute care, pediatrics, gerontology, adult, family, psychiatric-mental health, and women's health (ANA, 2003, 2004). The nursing profession is working toward an evidence-based practice for all types of nurses. The aspects of evidence-based practice and the significance of research in developing evidence-based practice are covered later in this chapter.

Reality Testing

People tend to *validate* or test the reality of their existence through their senses. In everyday activities, they constantly check out the messages received from their senses. For example, they might ask, "Am I really seeing what I think I am seeing?" Sometimes their senses can play tricks on them. This is why instruments have been developed to record sensory experiences more accurately. For example, does the patient just feel hot or actually have a fever? Thermometers were developed to test this sensory perception accurately. Through research, the most accurate and precise measures have been developed to assess the temperature of patients based on age and health status. Thus, research is a way to test reality and generate the best evidence to guide nursing practice.

Abstract Thought Processes

Abstract thought processes influence every element of the nursing world. In a sense, they link all the elements together. Without skills in abstract thought, we are trapped in a flat existence; we can experience the empirical world, we cannot explain or understand it (Abbott, 1952). Through abstract thinking, however, we can test our theories (which explain the nursing world) and then include them in the body of scientific knowledge. Abstract thinking also allows scientific findings to be developed into theories. Abstract thought enables both science and theories to be blended into a cohesive body of knowledge, guided by a philosophical framework, and applied in clinical practice (see Figure 1-1). Thus, abstract thought processes are essential for synthesizing research evidence and knowing when and how to use this knowledge in practice.

Three major abstract thought processes—introspection, intuition, and reasoning—are important in nursing

(Silva, 1977). These thought processes are used in critically appraising and applying best research evidence in practice, planning and implementing research, and developing and evaluating theory.

Introspection

Introspection is the process of turning your attention inward toward your own thoughts. It occurs at two levels. At the more superficial level, you are aware of the thoughts you are experiencing. You have a greater awareness of the flow and interplay of feelings and ideas that occur in constantly changing patterns. These thoughts or ideas can rapidly fade from view and disappear if you do not quickly write them down. When you allow introspection to occur in more depth, you examine your thoughts more critically and in detail. Patterns or links between thoughts and ideas emerge, and you may recognize fallacies or weaknesses in your thinking. You may question what brought you to this point and find yourself really enjoying the experience.

Imagine the following clinical situation. You have just left John Brown's home. John has a colostomy and has been receiving home health care for several weeks. Although John is caring for his colostomy, he is still reluctant to leave home for any length of time. You are irritated and frustrated with this situation. You begin to review your nursing actions and to recall other patients who reacted in similar ways. What were the patterns of their behavior?

You have an idea: Perhaps the patient's behavior is linked to the level of family support. You feel unsure about your ability to help the patient and family deal with this situation effectively. You recall other nurses describing similar reactions in their patients, and you wonder how many patients with colostomies have this problem. Your thoughts jump to reviewing the charts of other patients with colostomies and reading relevant ideas discussed in the literature. Some research has been conducted on this topic recently, and you could critically appraise these findings to determine the level of evidence for possible use in practice. If the findings are inadequate, perhaps other nurses would be interested in studying this situation with you.

Intuition

Intuition is an insight or understanding of a situation or event as a whole that usually cannot be logically explained (Rew & Barrow, 1987). Because intuition is a type of knowing that seems to come unbidden, it may also be described as a "gut feeling" or a "hunch." Because intuition cannot be explained with ease scientifically, many people are uncomfortable with it. Some

even say that it does not exist. Sometimes, therefore, the feeling or sense is suppressed, ignored, or dismissed as silly. However, intuition is not the lack of knowing; rather, it is a result of deep knowledge—tacit knowing or personal knowledge (Benner, 1984; Polanyi, 1962, 1966). The knowledge is incorporated so deeply within that it is difficult to bring it consciously to the surface and express it in a logical manner (Beveridge, 1950; Kaplan, 1964).

Intuition is generally considered unscientific and unacceptable for use in research. In some instances, that consideration is valid. For example, a hunch that there is a significant difference between one set of scores and another set of scores is not particularly useful as an analytical technique. However, even though intuition is often unexplainable, it has some important scientific uses. Researchers do not always need to be able to explain something in order to use it. A burst of intuition may identify a problem for study, indicate important variables to measure, or link two ideas together in interpreting the findings. The trick is to recognize the feeling, value it, and hang on to the idea long enough to consider it. Some researchers keep a journal to capture elusive thoughts and hunches as they think about their phenomenon of interest. These intuitive hunches often become important later as they conduct their studies.

Imagine the following situation. You have been working in an outpatient cardiac rehabilitation center for the past 3 years. You and two other nurses working on the unit have been meeting with the clinical nurse specialist to plan a study to determine which factors are important for promoting positive patient outcomes in the rehabilitation program. The group has met several times with a nursing professor at the university, who is collaborating with the group to develop the study. At present, the group is concerned with identifying the factors that need to be measured and how to measure them.

You have had a busy morning. Mr. Green, a patient, stops by to chat on his way out of the clinic. You listen, but not attentively at first. You then become more acutely aware of what he is saying and begin to have a feeling about one variable that should be studied. While he didn't specifically mention fear of breaking the news about having cancer to his children, you sense that he is anxious about conveying bad news to his loved ones. Although you cannot really explain the origin of this feeling, something in the flow of Mr. Green's words has stimulated a burst of intuition. You suspect other patients newly diagnosed with cancer face similar fear and hesitation about informing their family members about bad news. You believe the variable "fear of breaking bad news to loved ones" needs to be studied. You feel both excited and uncertain. What will the other nurses think? If the variable has not been studied, is it really significant? Somehow, you feel that it is important to consider.

Reasoning

Reasoning is the processing and organizing of ideas in order to reach conclusions. Through reasoning, people are able to make sense of their thoughts and experiences. This type of thinking is often evident in the verbal presentation of a logical argument in which each part is linked together to reach a logical conclusion. Patterns of reasoning are used to develop theories and to plan and implement research. Barnum (1998) identified four patterns of reasoning as being essential to nursing: (1) problematic, (2) operational, (3) dialectic, and (4) logistic. An individual uses all four types of reasoning, but frequently one type of reasoning is more dominant than the others. Reasoning is also classified by the discipline of logic into inductive and deductive modes (Chinn & Kramer, 2008; Omery, Kasper, & Page, 1995).

Problematic Reasoning. Problematic reasoning involves (1) identifying a problem and the factors influencing it, (2) selecting solutions to the problem, and (3) resolving the problem. For example, nurses use problematic reasoning in the nursing process to identify diagnoses and to implement nursing interventions to resolve these problems. Problematic reasoning is also evident when one identifies a research problem and successfully develops a methodology to examine it.

Operational Reasoning. Operational reasoning involves the identification of and discrimination among many alternatives and viewpoints. It focuses on the process (debating alternatives) rather than on the resolution (Barnum, 1998). Nurses use operational reasoning to develop realistic, measurable health goals with patients and families. Nurse practitioners use operational reasoning to debate which pharmacological and nonpharmacological treatments to use in managing patient illnesses. In research, operationalizing a treatment for implementation and debating which measurement methods or data analysis techniques to use in a study require operational thought (Kerlinger & Lee, 2000; Omery et al., 1995).

Dialectic Reasoning. Dialectic reasoning involves looking at situations in a holistic way. A dialectic thinker believes that the whole is greater than the sum of the parts and that the whole organizes the parts (Barnum, 1998). For example,

a nurse using dialectic reasoning would view a patient as a person with strengths and weaknesses who is experiencing an illness, and not just as the "stroke in room 219." Dialectic reasoning also involves examining factors that are opposites and making sense of them by merging them into a single unit or idea that is greater than either alone. For example, analyzing studies with conflicting findings and summarizing these findings to determine the current knowledge base for a research problem require dialectic reasoning.

Logistic Reasoning. Logic is a science that involves valid ways of relating ideas to promote understanding. The aim of logic is to determine truth or to explain and predict phenomena. The science of logic deals with thought processes, such as concrete and abstract thinking, and methods of reasoning, such as logistic, inductive, and deductive.

Logistic reasoning is used to break the whole into parts that can be carefully examined, as can the relationships among the parts. In some ways, logistic reasoning is the opposite of dialectic reasoning. A logistic reasoner assumes that the whole is the sum of the parts and that the parts organize the whole. For example, a patient states that she is cold. You logically examine the following parts of the situation and their relationships: (1) room temperature, (2) patient's temperature, (3) patient's clothing, and (4) patient's activity. The room temperature is 65°F, the patient's temperature is 98.6°F, and the patient is wearing lightweight pajamas and drinking ice water. You conclude that the patient is cold because of external environmental factors (room temperature, lightweight pajamas, and drinking ice water). Logistic reasoning is used frequently in research to develop a study design, plan and implement data collection, and conduct statistical analyses.

Inductive and Deductive Reasoning. The science of logic also includes inductive and deductive reasoning. People use these modes of reasoning constantly, although the choice of types of reasoning may not always be conscious (Kaplan, 1964). Inductive reasoning moves from the specific to the general, whereby particular instances are observed and then combined into a larger whole or general statement (Chinn & Kramer, 2008). An example of inductive reasoning follows:

A headache is an altered level of health that is stressful.

A fractured bone is an altered level of health that is stressful.

A terminal illness is an altered level of health that is stressful.

Therefore, all altered levels of health are stressful.

In this example, inductive reasoning is used to move from the specific instances of altered levels of health that are stressful to the general belief that all altered levels of health are stressful. By testing many different altered levels of health through research to determine whether they are stressful, one can confirm the general statement that all types of altered health are stressful.

Deductive reasoning moves from the general to the specific or from a general premise to a particular situation or conclusion. A premise or hypothesis is a statement of the proposed relationship between two or more variables. An example of deductive reasoning follows:

Premises

All human beings experience loss.
All adolescents are human beings.

Conclusion

All adolescents experience loss.

In this example, deductive reasoning is used to move from the two general premises about human beings experiencing loss and adolescents being human beings to the specific conclusion, "All adolescents experience loss." However, the conclusions generated from deductive reasoning are valid only if they are based on valid premises. Consider the following example:

Premises

All health professionals are caring.
All nurses are health professionals.

Conclusion

All nurses are caring.

The premise that all health professionals are caring is not necessarily valid or an accurate reflection of reality. Research is a means to test and confirm or refute a premise so that valid premises can be used as a basis for reasoning in nursing practice.

Science

Science is a coherent body of knowledge composed of research findings and tested theories for a specific discipline. Science is both a product (end point) and a process (mechanism to reach an end point) (Silva & Rothbart, 1984). An example from the discipline of physics is Newton's law of gravity, which was developed through extensive research. The knowledge of gravity (product) is a part of the science of physics that evolved through formulating and testing theoretical ideas (process). The ultimate goal of science is to explain the empirical world and thus to have greater control over it. To accomplish this goal, scientists must discover new knowledge, expand existing knowledge, and reaffirm previously held knowledge in a discipline (Greene, 1979; Toulmin, 1960). Health professionals integrate this evidence-based knowledge to control the

delivery of care and thereby improve patient outcomes (evidence-based practice).

The science of a field determines the accepted process for obtaining knowledge within that field. Research is an important process for obtaining scientific knowledge in nursing. Some sciences rigidly limit the types of research that can be used to obtain knowledge. A valued method for developing a science is the traditional research process, or quantitative research. According to this process, the information gained from one study is not sufficient for its inclusion in the body of science. A study must be replicated several times and must yield similar results each time before that information can be considered to be sound empirical evidence (Kerlinger & Lee, 2000; Toulmin, 1960).

Consider the research on the relationships between smoking and lung damage and cancer. Numerous studies conducted on animals and humans over the past few decades indicate relationships between smoking and lung damage and smoking and lung cancer. Everyone who smokes experiences lung damage; and although not everyone who smokes gets lung cancer, smokers are at a much higher risk for cancer. Extensive, quality quantitative research has been conducted to generate empirical evidence about the health hazards of smoking, and this evidence guides the actions of nurses in practice. We provide education, support, and new drugs like chantix (varenicline) to assist individuals to stop smoking.

Findings from studies are systematically related to one another in a way that seems to best explain the empirical world. Abstract thought processes are used to make these linkages. The linkages are called *laws, principles,* or *axioms,* depending on the certainty of the facts and relationships within the linkage. Laws express the most certain relationships and provide the best research evidence for use in practice. The certainty depends on the amount of research conducted to test a relationship and, to some extent, on the skills in abstract thought processes to link the research findings to form meaningful evidence. The truths or explanations of the empirical world reflected by these laws, principles, and axioms are never absolutely certain and may be disproved by further research.

Nursing science has been developed through the use of predominantly quantitative research methods. However, since 1980, a strong qualitative research tradition has evolved in nursing. Qualitative research is based on a philosophical orientation toward reality that is different from that of quantitative research (Kikuchi & Simmons, 1994; Marshall & Rossman, 2006; Munhall, 2001). Within the qualitative research tradition, many of the long-held tenets about science and ways of obtaining knowledge are questioned. The philosophical orientation of qualitative research is holistic, and the purpose of this research is to examine the whole rather than the parts. Qualitative researchers are more interested in understanding complex phenomena than in determining cause-and-effect relationships among specific variables. Both quantitative and qualitative research methods are important to the development of nursing knowledge (Craig & Smyth, 2007; Munhall, 2001; Pearson et al., 2007), and some researchers effectively combine these two methods to address selected problems in nursing (Foss & Ellefsen, 2002).

Medicine, health care agencies, and now nursing are focusing on the outcomes of patient care. Outcomes research is an important scientific methodology that has evolved to examine the end results of patient care and the outcomes for health care providers (nurse practitioners, nurse anesthetists, nurse midwives, and physicians) and health care agencies (Jones & Burney, 2002). Nurses are also engaged in intervention research, a new methodology for investigating the effectiveness of nursing interventions in achieving the desired outcomes in natural settings (Sidani & Braden, 1998). Nursing is in the beginning stages of developing a science for the profession, and additional original and replication studies are needed to develop the knowledge necessary for practice (Fahs, Morgan, & Kalman, 2003; Pearson et al., 2007).

Theory

A theory is a creative and rigorous structuring of ideas used to describe, explain, predict, or control a particular phenomenon or segment of the empirical world (Chinn & Kramer, 2008; Dubin, 1978). A theory consists of a set of concepts that are defined and interrelated to present a systematic view of a phenomenon. For example, Selye (1976) developed a theory about stress that continues to be useful in describing a person's response to life events. Extensive research has been conducted to detail the types, number, and severity of stressors experienced in life and the effective interventions to manage these stressful situations.

A theory is developed from a combination of personal experiences, research findings, and abstract thought processes. The theorist may use findings from research as a starting point and then organize the findings to best explain the empirical world. This is the process Selye used to develop his theory of stress. Alternatively, the theorist may use abstract thought processes, personal knowledge, and intuition to develop a theory of a phenomenon. This theory then requires testing through research to determine if it is an accurate reflection of reality. Thus, research has a

major role in theory development, testing, and refinement. Qualitative research often focuses on developing or generating theory. Types of quantitative research, outcomes research, and intervention research are often implemented to test the accuracy of theory and to refine aspects of the theory (Chinn & Kramer, 2008; Fawcett & Downs, 1999).

Knowledge

Knowledge is a complex, multifaceted concept. For example, you may say that you *know* your friend John, *know* that the earth rotates around the sun, *know* how to give an injection, and *know* pharmacology. These are examples of knowing—being familiar with a person, comprehending facts, acquiring a psychomotor skill, and mastering a subject. There are differences in types of knowing, yet there are also similarities. Knowing presupposes order or imposes order on thoughts and ideas (Engelhardt, 1980). People have a desire to know what to expect (Russell, 1948). There is a need for certainty in the world, and individuals seek it by trying to decrease uncertainty through knowledge (Ayer, 1966). Think of the questions you ask a person who has presented some bit of knowledge: "Is it true?" "Are you sure?" "How do you know?" Thus, the knowledge that we acquire is expected to be an accurate reflection of reality.

Ways of Acquiring Nursing Knowledge

We acquire knowledge in a variety of ways and expect it to be an accurate reflection of the real world (White, 1982). Nurses have historically acquired knowledge through (1) traditions, (2) authority, (3) borrowing, (4) trial and error, (5) personal experience, (6) role-modeling and mentorship, (7) intuition, (8) reasoning, and (9) research. Intuition, reasoning, and research were discussed earlier in this chapter; the other ways of acquiring knowledge are briefly described in this section.

Traditions. Traditions consist of "truths" or beliefs that are based on customs and past trends. Nursing traditions from the past have been transferred to the present by written and verbal communication and role-modeling and continue to influence the present practice of nursing. For example, some of the policies and procedures in hospitals and other health care facilities contain traditional ideas. In addition, some nursing interventions are transmitted verbally from one nurse to another over the years or by observation of experienced nurses. For example, the idea of providing a patient with a clean, safe, well-ventilated environment originated with Florence Nightingale (1859).

However, traditions can also narrow and limit the knowledge sought for nursing practice. For example, tradition has established the time and pattern for providing baths, evaluating vital signs, and allowing patient visitation on many hospital units. The nurses on these units quickly inform new staff members about the accepted or traditional behaviors for the unit. Traditions are difficult to change because they have existed for long periods of time and are frequently supported by people with power and authority. Many traditions have not been tested for accuracy or efficiency. The body of knowledge for nursing needs to have an empirical rather than a traditional base. Through the use of evidence-based interventions, nurses can exert a powerful, positive impact on the health care system and patient outcomes.

Authority. An authority is a person with expertise and power who is able to influence opinion and behavior. A person is thought of as an authority because she or he knows more in a given area than others do. Knowledge acquired from authority is illustrated when one person credits another person as the source of information. Nurses who publish articles and books or develop theories are frequently considered authorities. Students usually view their instructors as authorities, and clinical nursing experts are considered authorities within their clinical settings. However, persons viewed as authorities in one field are not necessarily authorities in other fields. An expert is an authority only when addressing his or her area of expertise. Like tradition, the knowledge acquired from authorities sometimes has not been validated through research and is not considered the best evidence for practice.

Borrowing. As some nursing leaders have noted, knowledge in the nursing practice is partly made up of information that has been borrowed from disciplines such as medicine, psychology, physiology, and education (Andreoli & Thompson, 1977; McMurrey, 1982). Borrowing in nursing involves the appropriation and use of knowledge from other fields or disciplines to guide nursing practice.

Nursing practice has borrowed knowledge in two ways. For years, some nurses have taken information from other disciplines and applied it directly to nursing practice. This information was not integrated within the unique focus of nursing. For example, some nurses have used the medical model to guide their nursing practice, thus focusing on the diagnosis and treatment of physiological diseases with limited attention to the patient's holistic nature. This type of borrowing continues today as nurses use technological advances to focus on the detection and treatment of disease, to the exclusion of health promotion and illness prevention.

Another way of borrowing, which is more useful in nursing, is the integration of information from other disciplines within the focus of nursing. Because disciplines share knowledge, it is sometimes difficult to know where the boundaries exist between nursing's knowledge base and those of other disciplines. Boundaries blur as the knowledge bases of disciplines evolve (McMurrey, 1982). For example, information about self-esteem as a characteristic of the human personality is associated with psychology, but this knowledge also directs the nurse in assessing the psychological needs of patients and families. However, borrowed knowledge has not been adequate for answering many questions generated in nursing practice.

Trial and Error. Trial and error is an approach with unknown outcomes that is used in a situation of uncertainty, when other sources of knowledge are unavailable. The profession evolved through a great deal of trial and error before knowledge of effective practices was codified in textbooks and journals. Because each patient responds uniquely to a situation, there is uncertainty in nursing practice. Because of this uncertainty, nurses must use trial and error in providing care. However, with trial and error, there is frequently no formal documentation of effective and ineffective nursing actions. When this strategy is used, the knowledge a practitioner gains from experience often is not shared with others. The trial-and-error way of acquiring knowledge can also be time-consuming, because multiple interventions might be implemented before one is found to be effective. There is also a risk of implementing nursing actions that are detrimental to a patient's health.

Personal Experience. Personal experience is the knowledge that comes from being personally involved in an event, situation, or circumstance. In nursing, personal experience enables one to gain skills and expertise by providing care to patients and families in clinical settings. The nurse not only learns but is able to cluster ideas into a meaningful whole. For example, students may be told how to give an injection in a classroom setting, but they do not *know* how to give an injection until they observe other nurses giving injections to patients and actually give several injections themselves.

The amount of personal experience you have will affect the complexity of your knowledge base as a nurse. Benner (1984) described five levels of experience in the development of clinical knowledge and expertise: (1) novice, (2) advanced beginner, (3) competent,

(4) proficient, and (5) expert. *Novice nurses* have no personal experience in the work that they are to perform, but they have preconceived notions and expectations about clinical practice that are challenged, refined, confirmed, or contradicted by personal experience in a clinical setting. The *advanced beginner* has just enough experience to recognize and intervene in recurrent situations. For example, the advanced beginner nurse is able to recognize and intervene to meet patients' needs for pain management.

Competent nurses frequently have been on the job for 2 or 3 years, and their personal experiences enable them to generate and achieve long-range goals and plans. Through experience, the competent nurse is able to use personal knowledge to take conscious, deliberate actions that are efficient and organized. From a more complex knowledge base, the *proficient nurse* views the patient as a whole and as a member of a family and community. The proficient nurse recognizes that each patient and family have specific values and needs that lead them to respond differently to illness and health.

The *expert nurse* has had extensive experience and is able to identify accurately and intervene skillfully in a situation. Personal experience increases an expert nurse's ability to grasp a situation intuitively with accuracy and speed. The clinical expertise of the nurse is a critical component of evidence-based practice. It is the expert nurse who has the greatest skill and ability to implement the best research evidence in practice to meet the unique values and needs of patients and families.

Role-Modeling and Mentorship. Role-modeling is learning by imitating the behaviors of an exemplar. An exemplar or role model knows the appropriate and rewarded roles for a profession, and these roles reflect the attitudes and include the standards and norms of behavior for that profession (Bidwell & Brasler, 1989). In nursing, role-modeling enables the novice nurse to learn from interacting with expert nurses or following their examples. Examples of role models are "admired teachers, practitioners, researchers, or illustrious individuals who inspire students through their examples" (Werley & Newcomb, 1983, p. 206).

An intense form of role-modeling is mentorship. In a mentorship, the expert nurse, or mentor, serves as a teacher, sponsor, guide, exemplar, and counselor for the novice nurse (or mentee). Both the mentor and the mentee or protégé invest time and effort, which often results in a close, personal mentor-mentee relationship. This relationship promotes a mutual exchange of ideas and aspirations relative to the mentee's career plans. The mentee assumes the values, attitudes, and

behaviors of the mentor while gaining intuitive knowledge and personal experience. Mentorship is essential for building research competence in nursing (Byrne & Keefe, 2002).

To summarize, in nursing, a body of knowledge must be acquired (learned), incorporated, and assimilated by each member of the profession and collectively by the profession as a whole. This body of knowledge guides the thinking and behavior of the profession and individual practitioners. It also directs further development and influences how science and theory are interpreted within the discipline. This knowledge base is necessary in order for health professionals, consumers, and society to recognize nursing as a science.

Philosophy

Philosophy provides a broad, global explanation of the world. It is the most abstract and most all-encompassing concept in the model (see Figure 1-1). Philosophy gives unity and meaning to the world of nursing and provides a framework within which thinking, knowing, and doing occur (Kikuchi & Simmons, 1994). Nursing's philosophical position influences its knowledge base. How nurses use science and theories to explain the empirical world depends on their philosophy. Ideas about truth and reality, as well as beliefs, values, and attitudes, are part of philosophy. Philosophy asks questions such as, "Is there an absolute truth, or is truth relative?" "Is there one reality, or is reality different for each individual?"

Everyone's world is modified by her or his philosophy, as a pair of eyeglasses would modify vision. Perceptions are influenced first by philosophy and then by knowledge. For example, if what you see is not within your ideas of truth or reality, if it does not fit your belief system, you may not see it. Your mind may reject it altogether or may modify it to fit your philosophy (Scheffler, 1967). As you start to discover the world of nursing research, it is important for you to keep an open mind to the value of research and your future role in the development or use of research evidence in practice.

Philosophical positions commonly held within the nursing profession include the view that human beings are holistic, rational, and responsible. Nurses believe that people desire health, and health is considered to be better than illness. Quality of life is as important as quantity of life. Good nursing care facilitates improved patterns of health and quality of life (ANA, 2003, 2004). In nursing, truth is relative, and reality tends to vary with perception (Kikuchi, Simmons, Romyn, 1996; Silva, 1977). For example, because nurses believe that reality varies with perception and that truth is relative, they would not try to impose their views of truth and reality on patients. Rather, they would accept patients' views of the world and help them seek health from within those worldviews, which is a critical component of evidence-based practice. This chapter concludes with a discussion of the significance of research in developing an evidence-based practice for nursing.

SIGNIFICANCE OF RESEARCH IN BUILDING AN EVIDENCE-BASED PRACTICE FOR NURSING

The ultimate goal of nursing is to provide evidence-based care that promotes quality outcomes for patients, families, health care providers, and the health care system (Craig & Smyth, 2007; Pearson et al., 2007). Evidence-based practice (EBP) evolves from the integration of the best research evidence with clinical expertise and patient needs and values (Institute of Medicine, 2001; Sackett, Straus, Richardson, Rosenberg, & Haynes, 2000). Figure 1-2 demonstrates the major contribution of the best research evidence to the delivery of EBP. The best research evidence is the empirical knowledge generated from the synthesis of quality study findings to address a practice problem. A discussion of the levels of best research evidence and the sources for this evidence are presented in Chapter 2. A team of expert researchers, health care professionals, policy makers, and consumers often synthesizes the best research evidence for developing standardized guidelines for clinical practice.

For example, research related to the chronic health problem of hypertension (HTN) has been conducted, critically appraised, and synthesized by experts to develop a practice guideline for implementation by APNs (such as nurse practitioners and clinical specialists) and physicians to ensure that patients with HTN receive quality, cost-effective care (Chobanian et al., 2003). The most current guidelines for the treatment of HTN, "The Seventh Report of the Joint National Committee on Prevention, Detection, Evaluation, and Treatment of High Blood Pressure: The JNC 7 Report," were published in 2003 in the *Journal of the American Medical Association* (Chobanian et al., 2003) and are available online at www.nhlbi.nih.gov/guidelines/hypertension. Many national standardized guidelines are available through the Agency for Healthcare Research and Quality (AHRQ), which is discussed in more detail in Chapters 2 and 27 of this text.

Clinical expertise is the knowledge and skills of the health care professional providing care. A nurse's clinical expertise is determined by his or her years of practice, current knowledge of the research and clinical literature, and educational preparation. The stronger the nurse's clinical expertise, the better his or her clinical judgment in the delivery of quality care (Craig & Smyth, 2007; Sackett et al., 2000). The patient's need(s) might focus on health promotion, illness prevention, acute or chronic illness management, or rehabilitation (see Figure 1-2). In addition, patients bring values or unique preferences, expectations, concerns, and cultural beliefs to the clinical encounter. With EBP, patients and their families are encouraged to take an active role in managing their health care

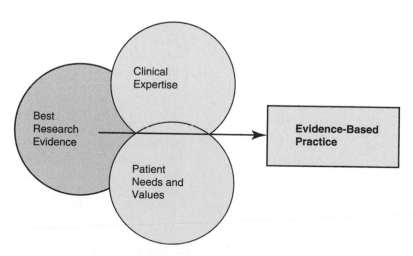

Figure 1-2 Model of evidence-based practice

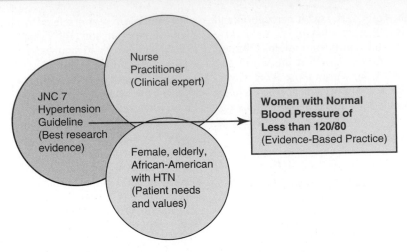

Figure **1-3** Evidence-based practice for elderly African-American women with hypertension (HTN).

(Pearson et al., 2007). In summary, expert clinicians use the best research evidence available to deliver quality, cost-effective care to a patients and families with specific health needs and values to achieve EBP (see Figure 1-2) (Brown, 1999; Craig & Smyth, 2007; Sackett et al., 2000).

Figure 1-3 provides an example of the delivery of evidence-based care to women with HTN. In this example, the best research evidence on HTN is the JNC 7 National Standardized Guideline (Chobanian et al., 2003). This guideline is translated by an expert nurse practitioner to meet the needs (chronic illness management) and values of elderly African-American women with HTN. In this case, the outcome of EBP is women with a normal blood pressure of less than 120/80 (see Figure 1-3). A detailed discussion of how to locate, critically appraise, and use national standardized guidelines (such as the JNC 7) in practice is presented in Chapter 27.

In nursing, the research evidence must focus on the description, explanation, prediction, and control of phenomena important to practice. The following sections address the types of knowledge that need to be generated in these four areas as nursing moves toward EBP.

Description

Description involves identifying and understanding the nature of nursing phenomena and, sometimes, the relationships among them (Chinn & Kramer, 2008). Through research, nurses are able to (1) describe what exists in nursing practice, (2) discover new information, (3) promote understanding of situations, and (4) classify information for use in the discipline. Some examples of clinically important research

evidence developed from research focused on description include the following:

- Identification of the responses of individuals to a variety of health conditions
- Description of the health promotion and illness prevention strategies used by various populations
- Determination of the incidence of a disease locally, nationally, and internationally.
- Identification of the cluster of symptoms for a particular disease
- Description of the effects and side effects of selected pharmacological agents in a variety of populations

For example, Ryan et al. (2007) conducted a study to determine the cluster of symptoms that represent an acute myocardial infarction (AMI). These researchers synthesized their findings as follows:

Symptoms of AMI occur in clusters, and these clusters vary among persons. None of the clusters identified in this study included all of the symptoms that are included typically as symptoms of AMI (chest discomfort, diaphoresis, shortness of breath, nausea, and lightheadedness). These AMI symptom clusters must be communicated clearly to the public in a way that will assist them in assessing their symptoms more efficiently and will guide their treatment-seeking behavior. Symptom clusters for AMI must also be communicated to the professional community in a way that will facilitate assessment and rapid intervention for AMI. (Ryan et al., 2007, p. 72)

The findings from this study provide insights into the varying symptom clusters of patients experiencing an

AMI. This type of research, focused on description, is essential groundwork for studies that will help to explain, predict, and control nursing phenomena.

Explanation

Explanation clarifies the relationships among phenomena and clarifies why certain events occur. Research focused on explanation provides the following types of evidence essential for practice:

- Determination of the assessment data (both subjective data from the health history and objective data from physical exam) needed to address a patient's health need
- Link of assessment data to determine a diagnosis (both nursing and medical)
- Link of causative risk factors or etiologies to illness, morbidity, and mortality
- Determine the relationships among health risks, health status, and health care costs

For example, Pronk Goodman, O'Connor, and Martinson (1999) studied the relationships between modifiable health risks (physical inactivity, obesity, and smoking) and health care charges and found that adverse health risks translate into significantly higher health care charges. Thus, managed health care systems, nurse providers, and consumers seeking to improve societal health and reduce health care costs need to promote the modification of health risks. Explanatory research continues to link sedentary behaviors to obesity and diabetes in adults (Hu, Li, Colditz, Willett, & Manson, 2003) and to link the prenatal environment and cumulated social risk factors in the overweight adolescent (Salsberry & Reagan, 2007). These studies illustrate how explanatory research can identify relationships among nursing phenomena that are the basis for research focused on prediction and control.

Prediction

Through prediction, one can estimate the probability of a specific outcome in a given situation (Chinn & Kramer, 2008). However, predicting an outcome does not necessarily enable one to modify or control the outcome. It is through prediction that the risk of illness is identified and linked to possible screening methods that will identify the illness. Knowledge generated from research focused on prediction is critical for EBP and includes the following:

- Prediction of the risk for a disease in different populations
- Prediction of the accuracy and precision of a screening instrument, such as mammogram, to detect a disease

- Prediction of the prognosis once an illness is identified in a variety of populations
- Prediction of behaviors that promote health and prevent illness
- Prediction of the health care required based on a patient's need and values

For example, Scheetz and Kolassa (2007, p. 399) examined "crash scene variables to predict the need for trauma center care in older persons." The researchers analyzed 26 crash scene variables and developed triage decision rules for managing persons with severe and moderate injuries. Further research is needed to determine whether the triage decision rules improve the health outcomes of the elderly following trauma. Predictive studies isolate independent variables that require additional research to ensure that their manipulation or control results in successful outcomes for patients, health care professionals, and health care agencies (Kerlinger & Lee, 2000; Omery et al., 1995).

Control

If one can predict the outcome of a situation, the next step is to control or manipulate the situation to produce the desired outcome. Dickoff, James, and Wiedenbach (1968) described control as the ability to write a prescription to produce the desired results. Using the best research evidence, nurses could prescribe specific interventions to meet the needs of patients and their families. This is the type of research evidence that nurses need in order to provide EBP (see Figure 1-2). Research in the following areas is important for generating an evidence-based practice in nursing:

- Testing interventions to improve the health status of individuals, families, and communities
- Testing interventions to improve health care delivery
- Determining the quality and cost-effectiveness of interventions
- Implementing an evidence-based intervention to determine if it is effective in managing a patient's health need (health promotion, illness prevention, acute and chronic illness management, and rehabilitation) and producing quality outcomes

Lusk, Ronis, Kazanis, Eakin, Hong, and Raymond (2003) conducted a study that implemented a prescribed, tailored intervention to increase the use of hearing protection devices (HPDs) by factory workers. They found that significantly more workers used HPDs in the intervention group than in the other groups. Thus, this intervention manipulated or controlled the situation to produce the positive outcome of HPD use in a noisy work environment.

Only a limited number of studies have been conducted to generate the research evidence in the areas of prediction and control that is needed for EBP in nursing (Pearson et al., 2007). Thus, there is a great need for additional research in nursing and many opportunities for you to be involved in the world of nursing research.

This chapter introduced you to the world of nursing research and the significance of research in developing an evidence-based practice for nursing. The following chapters will expand your ability to critically appraise studies, synthesize research findings, and use the best research evidence available in clinical practice. The text also provides you with a background for conducting research in collaboration with expert nurse researchers. We think you will find that nursing research is an exciting adventure that holds much promise for the future practice of nursing.

SUMMARY

- This chapter introduces you to the world of nursing research.
- Nursing research is defined as a scientific process that validates and refines existing knowledge and generates new knowledge that directly and indirectly influences the delivery of evidence-based nursing practice.
- This chapter presents a framework that links nursing research to the world of nursing and organizes the content presented in this textbook (see Figure 1-1). The concepts in this framework range from concrete to abstract and include concrete and abstract thinking, the empirical world (evidence-based nursing practice), reality testing (research), abstract thought processes, science, theory, knowledge, and philosophy.
- The goal of nurses and other health care professionals is to deliver evidence-based health care to patients and their families.
- Evidence-based practice (EBP) evolves from the integration of best research evidence with clinical expertise and patient needs and values (see Figure 1-2).
- The best research evidence is the empirical knowledge generated from the synthesis of quality studies to address a practice problem.
- The clinical expertise of a nurse is determined by his or her years of clinical experience, current knowledge of the research and clinical literature, and educational preparation.
- The patient brings values—such as unique preferences, expectations, concerns, and cultural beliefs, and health needs—to the clinical encounter.

- The knowledge generated through research is essential for describing, explaining, predicting, and controlling nursing phenomena.
- Reliance on tradition, authority, trial and error, and personal experience is no longer an adequate basis for sound nursing practice.
- Nursing practice based on synthesized research findings can have a powerful, positive impact on patient outcomes and the health care system.

REFERENCES

Abbott, E. A. (1952). *Flatland*. New York: Dover.

American Nurses Association. (2003). *Nursing's social policy statement* (2nd ed.). Washington, DC: Author.

American Nurses Association. (2004). *Nursing: Scope and standards of practice*. Washington, DC: Author.

Andreoli, K. G., & Thompson, C. E. (1977). The nature of science in nursing. *Image: Journal of Nursing Scholarship, 9*(2), 32–37.

Ayer, A. J. (1966). *The problem of knowledge*. Baltimore: Penguin.

Barnum, B. S. (1998). *Nursing theory: Analysis, application, evaluation* (5th ed.). Philadelphia: Lippincott Williams & Wilkins.

Benner, P. (1984). *From novice to expert: Excellence and power in clinical nursing practice*. Menlo Park, CA: Addison-Wesley.

Beveridge, W. I. B. (1950). *The art of scientific investigation*. New York: Vintage Books.

Bidwell, A. S., & Brasler, M. L. (1989). Role modeling versus mentoring in nursing education. *Image: Journal of Nursing Scholarship, 21*(1), 23–25.

Brown, S. J. (1999). *Knowledge for health care practice: A guide to using research evidence*. Philadelphia: Saunders.

Byrne, M. W., & Keefe, M. R. (2002). Building research competence in nursing through mentoring. *Journal of Nursing Scholarship, 34*(4), 391–396.

Chinn, P. L., & Kramer, M. K. (2008). *Theory and nursing: Integrated knowledge development* (6th ed.). St. Louis: Mosby.

Chobanian, A. V., Bakris, G. L., Black, H. R., Cushman, W. C., Green, L. A., Izzo, J. L., et al. (2003). The seventh report of the Joint National Committee on prevention, detection, evaluation, and treatment of high blood pressure: The JNC 7 report. *Journal of the American Medical Association, 289*(19), 2560–2572.

Craig, J. V., & Smyth, R. L. (2007). *The evidence-based practice manual for nurses* (2nd ed.). Edinburgh: Churchill Livingstone.

Dickoff, J., James, P., & Wiedenbach, E. (1968). Theory in a practice discipline: Practice oriented theory (Part I). *Nursing Research, 17*(5), 415–435.

Dubin, R. (1978). *Theory building* (Rev. ed.). New York: Free Press.

Engelhardt, H. T., Jr. (1980). Knowing and valuing: Looking for common roots. In H. T. Engelhardt, & D. Callahan (Eds.), *Knowing and valuing: The search for common roots* (Vol. 4, pp. 1–17). New York: Hastings Center.

Fahs, P. S., Morgan, L. L., & Kalman, M. (2003). A call for replication. *Journal of Nursing Scholarship, 35*(1), 67–71.

Fawcett, J., & Downs, F. S. (1999). *The relationship of theory and research* (3rd ed.). Norwalk, CT: Appleton-Century-Crofts.

Foss, C., & Ellefsen, B. (2002). Methodological issues in nursing research: The value of combining qualitative and quantitative approaches in nursing research by means of method triangulation. *Journal of Advanced Nursing, 40*(2), 242–248.

Greene, J. A. (1979). Science, nursing and nursing science: A conceptual analysis. *Advances in Nursing Science, 2*(1), 57–64.

Hu, F. B., Li, T. Y., Colditz, G. A., Willett, W. C., & Manson, J. E. (2003). Television watching and other sedentary behaviors in relation to risk of obesity and type 2 diabetes mellitus in women. *Journal of the American Medical Association, 289*(14), 1785–1791.

Institute of Medicine. (2001). *Crossing the quality chasm: A new health system for the 21st century*. Washington, DC: National Academy Press.

Jones, K. R., & Burney, R. E. (2002). Outcomes research: An interdisciplinary perspective. *Outcomes Management, 6*(3), 103–109.

Kaplan, A. (1964). *The conduct of inquiry*. New York: Harper & Row.

Kerlinger, F. N., & Lee, H. B. (2000). *Foundations of behavioral research* (4th ed.). Fort Worth, TX: Harcourt College Publishers.

Kikuchi, J. F., & Simmons, H. (1994). *Developing a philosophy of nursing*. Thousand Oaks, CA: Sage.

Kikuchi, J. F., Simmons, H., & Romyn, D. (1996). *Truth in nursing inquiry*. Thousand Oaks, CA: Sage.

Lusk, S. L., Ronis, D. L., Kazanis, A. S., Eakin, B. L., Hong, O., & Raymond, D. M. (2003). Effectiveness of a tailored intervention to increase factory workers' use of hearing protection. *Nursing Research, 52*(5), 289–295.

Malloch, K., & Porter-O'Grady, T. (2006). *Introduction to evidence-based practice in nursing and health care*. Sudbury, MA: Jones & Barlett.

Marshall, C., & Rossman, G. B. (2006). *Designing qualitative research* (4th ed.). Thousand Oaks, CA: Sage.

McMurrey, P. H. (1982). Toward a unique knowledge base in nursing. *Image: Journal of Nursing Scholarship, 14*(1), 12–15.

Melnyk, B. M., & Fineout Overholt, E. (2005). *Evidence-based practice in nursing & healthcare: A guide to best practice*. Philadelphia: Lippincott Williams & Wilkins.

Munhall, P. L. (2001). *Nursing research: A qualitative perspective* (3rd ed.). Sudbury, MA: Jones & Bartlett.

Nightingale, F. (1859). *Notes on nursing: What it is, and what it is not*. Philadelphia: Lippincott.

Nursing Executive Center. (2005). *Evidence-based nursing practice: Instilling rigor into clinical practice*. Washington, DC: The Advisor Board Company.

Omery, A., Kasper, C. E., & Page, G. G. (1995). *In search of nursing science*. Thousand Oaks, CA: Sage.

Pearson, A., Field, J., & Jordan, Z. (2007). *Evidence-based clinical practice in nursing and health care: Assimilating research, experience, and expertise*. Oxford: Blackwell.

Polanyi, M. (1962). *Personal knowledge*. Chicago: University of Chicago Press.

Polanyi, M. (1966). *The tacit dimension*. New York: Doubleday.

Pronk, N. P., Goodman, M. J., O'Connor, P. J., & Martinson, B. C. (1999). Relationship between modifiable health risks and short-term health care charges. *Journal of the American Medical Association, 282*(23), 2235–2239.

Rew, L., & Barrow, E. M. (1987). Intuition: A neglected hallmark of nursing knowledge. *Advances in Nursing Science, 10*(1), 49–62.

Riley, J. M., Beal, J., Levi, P., & McCausland, M. P. (2002). Revisioning nursing scholarship. *Journal of Nursing Scholarship, 34*(4), 383–389.

Russell, B. (1948). *Human knowledge, its scope and limits*. Brooklyn, NY: Simon & Schuster.

Ryan, C. J., DeVon, H. A., Horne, R., King, K. B., Milner, K., Moser, D. K., et al. (2007). Symptom clusters in acute myocardial infarction: A secondary data analysis. *Nursing Research, 56*(2), 72–81.

Sackett, D. L., Straus, S. E., Richardson, W. S., Rosenberg, W., & Haynes, R. B. (2000). *Evidence-based medicine: How to practice & teach EBM* (2nd ed.). London: Churchill Livingstone.

Salsberry, P. J., & Reagan, P. B. (2007). Taking the long view: The prenatal environment and early adolescent overweight. *Research in Nursing & Health, 30*(3), 297–307.

Scheetz, L. J., & Kolassa, J. E. (2007). Using crash scene variables to predict the need for trauma center care in older persons. *Research in Nursing & Health, 30*(4), 399–412.

Scheffler, I. (1967). *Science and subjectivity*. Indianapolis: Bobbs-Merrill.

Selye, H. (1976). *The stress of life*. New York: McGraw-Hill.

Sidani, S., & Braden, C. P. (1998). *Evaluating nursing interventions: A theory-driven approach*. Thousand Oaks, CA: Sage.

Silva, M. C. (1977). Philosophy, science, theory: Interrelationships and implications for nursing research. *Image: Journal of Nursing Scholarship, 9*(3), 59–63.

Silva, M. C., & Rothbart, D. (1984). An analysis of changing trends in philosophies of science on nursing theory development and testing. *Advances in Nursing Science, 6*(2), 1–13.

Toulmin, S. (1960). *The philosophy of science*. New York: Harper & Row.

Werley, H. H., & Newcomb, B. J. (1983). The research mentor: A missing element in nursing? In N. L. Chaska (Ed.): *The nursing profession: A time to speak* (pp. 202–215). New York: McGraw-Hill.

White, A. R. (1982). *The nature of knowledge*. Totowa, NJ: Rowman & Littlefield.

CHAPTER 2
The Evolution of Evidence-Based Practice in Nursing

Initially, nursing research evolved slowly, from Florence Nightingale's investigations in the nineteenth century to the studies of nursing education in the 1930s and 1940s and the research of nurses and nursing roles in the 1950s and 1960s. However, in the late 1970s and 1980s, numerous studies focused on improving nursing practice. This emphasis continued in the 1990s with research focused on testing the effectiveness of nursing interventions and examining patient outcomes. The goal in the new millennium is the development of an evidence-based practice for nursing, with the current best research evidence being used to deliver patient care.

Evidence-based practice (EBP) is the conscientious integration of best research evidence with clinical expertise and patient values and needs in the delivery of quality, cost-effective health care. Chapter 1 presents a model depicting the elements of evidence-based practice (see Figure 1-2). You probably have many questions about evidence-based practice, because this is a relative new and evolving concept for the profession of nursing. What does best research evidence mean? How is this research evidence developed? Are there levels of quality in the types of research evidence? How is the best research evidence implemented in nursing practice? This chapter will increase your understanding of how nursing research has evolved over the past 150 years and the current movement of the profession toward evidence-based practice. The chapter describes the historical events relevant to nursing research in building an evidence-based practice for nursing, identifies the methodologies used

in nursing to develop research evidence, and concludes with a discussion of the best research evidence needed to build an EBP.

HISTORICAL DEVELOPMENT OF RESEARCH IN NURSING

Some people think that research is relatively new to nursing, but Florence Nightingale initiated nursing research more than 150 years ago (Nightingale, 1859). Following Nightingale's work (1850–1910), research received minimal attention until the mid-1900s. In the 1960s, nurses gradually recognized the value of research, but few had the educational background to conduct studies until the 1970s. However, in the 1980s and 1990s, research became a major force in developing a scientific knowledge base for the nursing practice. Today, nurses obtain federal and corporate funding for their research, conduct complex studies in multiple settings, and generate sound research evidence for practice. Table 2-1 identifies some of the key historical events that have influenced the development of nursing research and the movement toward EBP in nursing. These events are discussed in the following section.

Florence Nightingale

Nightingale has been described as a reformer, reactionary, and researcher who has influenced nursing specifically and health care in general. Nightingale's book, *Notes on Nursing* (1859), described her initial

TABLE 2-1	Historical Events Influencing Nursing Research

Year	Historical Event
1850	Florence Nightingale is the first nurse researcher.
1859	*Nightingale's Notes on Nursing* is published.
1900	*American Journal of Nursing* is first published.
1923	Teacher's College at Columbia University offers the first educational doctoral program for nurses.
1929	First master of nursing degree is offered at Yale University.
1932	Association of Collegiate Schools of Nursing is organized.
1950	American Nurses Association (ANA) publishes study of nursing functions and activities.
1952	*Nursing Research* is first published.
1953	Institute of Research and Service in Nursing Education is established.
1955	American Nurses Foundation is established to fund nursing research.
1963	*International Journal of Nursing Studies* is first published.
1965	ANA sponsors first nursing research conferences.
1967	*Image* (Sigma Theta Tau publication) is first published.
	Stetler/Marram Model for Application of Research Findings to Practice is first published.
1970	ANA Commission on Nursing Research is established.
1972	Professor Archie Cochrane, a Scottish epidemiologist, publishes his book *Effectiveness and Efficiency: Random Reflections on Health Services*, which promotes the acceptance of the concepts behind evidence-based practice.
	ANA Council of Nurse Researchers is established.
1973	First Nursing Diagnosis Conference is held.
1978	*Research in Nursing & Health* is first published. *Advances in Nursing Science* is first published.
	Western Interstate Commission for Higher Education (WICHE) Project focused on research utilization is published.
1979	*Western Journal of Nursing Research* is first published.
1980s–1990s	David Sackett and his research team develop methodologies to determine "best evidence" for practice.
1982–1983	*Conduct and Utilization of Research in Nursing (CURN) Project* is published.
1983	*Annual Review of Nursing Research* is first published.
1985	National Center for Nursing Research (NCNR) is established within the National Institutes of Health.
1987	*Scholarly Inquiry for Nursing Practice* is first published.
1988	*Applied Nursing Research* is first published.
	Nursing Science Quarterly is first published.
1989	Agency for Health Care Policy and Research (AHCPR) is established.
	AHCPR first publishes clinical practice guidelines.
1992	U.S. Department of Health and Human Services publishes the *Healthy People 2000* document.
	Cochrane Center, rooted on the evidence-based practice efforts of Dr. Cochrane, is launched.
	Clinical Nursing Research is first published.
1993	NCNR is renamed the National Institute of Nursing Research (NINR).
	Cochrane Collaboration is initiated providing systematic reviews and evidence-based guidelines for practice (www.cochrane.org).
1994	*Qualitative Health Research* is first published.
1999	AHCPR is renamed Agency for Healthcare Research and Quality (AHRQ).
	American Association of Colleges of Nursing publishes its Position Statement on Nursing Research.
	Institute of Medicine Study is published, which focuses on quality care issues and emphasizes the need for evidence-based practice.
2000	The U.S. Department of Health and Human Services publishes the *Healthy People 2010* document.
	Biological Research for Nursing is first published.
2001	Stetler publishes her model "Steps of Research Utilization to Facilitate Evidence-Based Practice."
2002	Joint Commission revises accreditation policies, emphasizing patient care quality through the use of the most current research evidence in practice.
2004	*Worldviews on Evidence-Based Nursing* is first published.
2007	NINR identifies mission and funding themes for the future (www.nih.gov/ninr).
2007	AHRQ identifies mission and goals for the future (www.ahrq.gov).

research activities, which focused on the importance of a healthy environment in promoting the patient's physical and mental well-being. She identified the need to gather data on the environment, such as ventilation, cleanliness, temperature, purity of water, and diet, to determine their influence on the patient's health (Herbert, 1981).

Nightingale is most noted for her data collection and statistical analyses during the Crimean War. She gathered data on soldier morbidity and mortality rates and the factors influencing them and presented her results in tables and pie charts, a sophisticated type of data presentation for the period (Palmer, 1977). Nightingale's research enabled her to instigate attitudinal, organizational, and social changes. She changed the attitudes of the military and society toward the care of the sick. The military began to view the sick as having the right to adequate food, suitable quarters, and appropriate medical treatment. These interventions drastically reduced the mortality rate from 43% to 2% in the Crimean War (Cook, 1913). Nightingale improved the organization of army administration, hospital management, and hospital construction. Because of Nightingale's research evidence and influence, society began to accept responsibility for testing public water, improving sanitation, preventing starvation, and decreasing morbidity and mortality rates (Palmer, 1977).

Early 1900s

From 1900 to 1950, research activities in nursing were limited, but a few studies advanced nursing education. These studies included the Nutting Report, 1912; Goldmark Report, 1923; and Burgess Report, 1926 (Abdellah, 1972; Johnson, 1977). On the basis of recommendations of the Goldmark Report, more schools of nursing were established in university settings. The baccalaureate degree in nursing provided a basis for graduate nursing education, with the first master of nursing degree offered by Yale University in 1929. Teachers College at Columbia University offered the first doctoral program for nurses in 1923 and granted a degree in education (Ed.D.) to prepare teachers for the profession. The Association of Collegiate Schools of Nursing, organized in 1932, promoted the conduct of research to improve education and practice. This organization also sponsored the publication of the first research journal in nursing, *Nursing Research*, in 1952 (Fitzpatrick, 1978).

A research trend that started in the 1940s and continued in the 1950s focused on the organization and delivery of nursing services. Studies were conducted on the numbers and kinds of nursing personnel, staffing patterns, patient classification systems, patient and personnel satisfaction, and unit arrangement. Types of care such as comprehensive care, home care, and progressive patient care were evaluated. These evaluations of care laid the foundation for the development of self-study manuals, which are similar to the quality assurance manuals of today (Gortner & Nahm, 1977).

Nursing Research in the 1950s and 1960s

In 1950, the American Nurses Association (ANA) initiated a 5-year study on nursing functions and activities. The findings were reported in *Twenty Thousand Nurses Tell Their Story*, and this study enabled the ANA to develop statements on functions, standards, and qualifications for professional nurses in 1959. Also during this time, clinical research began expanding as specialty groups, such as community health, psychiatric, medical-surgical, pediatrics, and obstetrics, developed standards of care. The research conducted by ANA and the specialty groups provided the basis for the nursing practice standards that currently guide professional nursing practice (Gortner & Nahm, 1977).

Educational studies were conducted in the 1950s and 1960s to determine the most effective educational preparation for the registered nurse. A nurse educator, Mildred Montag, developed and evaluated the 2-year nursing preparation (associate degree) in the junior colleges. Student characteristics, such as admission and retention patterns and the elements that promoted success in nursing education and practice, were studied for both associate- and baccalaureate degree–prepared nurses (Downs & Fleming, 1979).

In 1953, an Institute for Research and Service in Nursing Education was established at Teacher's College, Columbia University, which provided research-learning experiences for doctoral students (Werley, 1977). The American Nurse's Foundation, chartered in 1955, was responsible for receiving and administering research funds, conducting research programs, consulting with nursing students, and engaging in research. In 1956, a Committee on Research and Studies was established to guide ANA research (See, 1977).

A Department of Nursing Research was established in the Walter Reed Army Institute of Research in 1957. This was the first nursing unit in a research institution that emphasized clinical nursing research (Werley, 1977). Also in 1957, the Southern Regional Educational Board (SREB), the Western Interstate Commission on Higher Education (WICHE), and the New England Board of Higher Education (NEBHE) were developed. These organizations are actively involved in promoting research and disseminating the findings. The ANA sponsored the first of a series of research conferences in 1965, and the conference sponsors required that the studies presented be relevant to nursing and conducted by a nurse researcher (See, 1977). These ANA conferences continue to be an important means of disseminating nursing research findings.

In the 1960s, a growing number of clinical studies focused on quality care and the development of criteria to measure patient outcomes. Intensive care units were being developed, which promoted the investigation of nursing interventions, staffing patterns, and cost-effectiveness of care (Gortner & Nahm, 1977).

Nursing Research in the 1970s

In the 1970s, the nursing process became the focus of many studies, with the investigations of assessment techniques and guidelines, goal-setting methods, and specific nursing interventions. In 1973, the first Nursing Diagnosis Conference was held; these conferences continue to be held every 2 to 3 years. Studies have focused on identifying appropriate diagnoses for nursing and generating an effective diagnostic process (Carlson-Catalano & Lunney, 1995). Many of the studies conducted in the 1970s were not being used in practice, so Stetler and Marram (1976) developed a model to promote the communication and use of research findings in practice.

The educational studies of the 1970s evaluated teaching methods and student learning experiences. A number of studies were conducted to differentiate the practices of nurses with baccalaureate and associate degrees. These studies, which primarily measured abilities to perform technical skills, were ineffective in differentiating between the two levels of education.

In the service setting, primary nursing care, which involves the delivery of patient care predominantly by registered nurse, was the trend of the 1970s. Studies were conducted to examine the implementation and outcomes of primary nursing care delivery models. The number of nurse practitioners (NPs) and clinical nurse specialists (CNSs) with master's degrees increased rapidly during the 1970s. Limited research has been conducted on the CNS role; however, the NP and nurse midwifery roles have been researched extensively to determine their positive impact on productivity, quality, and cost of health care (Brown & Grimes, 1995; Mundinger et al., 2000). In addition, those clinicians with master's degrees were provided the background to conduct research and to use research findings in practice.

In the 1970s, nursing scholars began developing models, conceptual frameworks, and theories to guide nursing practice. The works of these nursing theorists also directed future nursing research. In 1978, a new journal, *Advances in Nursing Science*, began publishing the works of nursing theorists and the research related to their theories. The number of doctoral programs in nursing and the number of nurses prepared at the doctoral level greatly expanded in the 1970s (Jacox, 1980). Some of the nurses with doctoral degrees increased the conduct and complexity of nursing research; however, many doctorally prepared nurses did not become actively involved in research. In 1970, the ANA Commission on Nursing Research was established; in turn, this commission established the Council of Nurse Researchers in 1972 to advance research activities, provide an exchange of ideas, and recognize excellence in research. The commission also prepared position papers on subjects' rights in research and on federal guidelines concerning research and human subjects, and it sponsored research programs nationally and internationally (See, 1977).

Federal funds for nursing research increased significantly, with a total of slightly more than $39 million awarded for research in nursing from 1955 to 1976. Even though federal funding for nursing studies rose, the funding was not comparable to the $493 million in federal research funds received by those doing medical research in 1974 alone (de Tornyay, 1977).

The dissemination of research findings was a major focus in the 1970s. Sigma Theta Tau, the International Honor Society for Nursing, sponsored national and international research conferences, and the chapters of this organization sponsored many local conferences to promote the dissemination of research findings. *Image*, a journal initially published in 1967 by Sigma Theta Tau, contains many nursing studies and articles about research methodology. A major goal of Sigma Theta Tau is to advance scholarship in nursing by promoting the conduct, communication, and utilization of research in nursing. The addition of two new research journals in the 1970s, *Research in Nursing & Health* in 1978 and *Western Journal of Nursing Research* in 1979, also increased the communication of nursing research findings.

Professor Archie Cochrane originated the concepts of evidence-based practice with a book he published in 1972 titled *Effectiveness and Efficiency: Random Reflections on Health Services*. Cochrane advocated the provision of health care based on research to improve the quality of care and patient outcomes. To facilitate the use of research evidence in practice, the Cochrane Center was established in 1992 and the Cochrane Collaboration in 1993. The Cochrane

Collaboration and Library house numerous resources to promote EBP, such as systematic reviews of research and evidence-based guidelines for practice (discussed later in this chapter) (see the Cochrane Collaboration at www.cochrane.org).

Nursing Research in the 1980s and 1990s

The conduct of clinical nursing research was the focus in the 1980s and 1990s. A variety of clinical journals (*Cancer Nursing; Cardiovascular Nursing; Dimensions of Critical Care Nursing; Heart & Lung; Journal of Obstetric, Gynecologic, and Neonate Nursing; Journal of Neurosurgical Nursing; Oncology Nursing Forum; Pediatric Nursing;* and *Rehabilitation Nursing*) published an increasing number of studies. One new research journal was published in 1987, *Scholarly Inquiry for Nursing Practice*, and two in 1988, *Applied Nursing Research* and *Nursing Science Quarterly*.

Even though the body of empirical knowledge generated through clinical research grew rapidly in the 1970s and 1980s, little of this knowledge was used in practice. Two major projects were launched to promote the use of research-based nursing interventions in practice: the Western Interstate Commission for Higher Education (WICHE) Regional Nursing Research Development Project and the Conduct and Utilization of Research in Nursing (CURN) Project. In these projects, nurse researchers, with the assistance of federal funding, designed and implemented strategies for using research findings in practice. The WICHE Project participants selected a research-based intervention for use in practice and then functioned as change agents to implement the selected intervention in a clinical agency. Because of the limited amount of research that had been conducted, the project staff and participants had difficulty identifying adequate clinical studies with findings ready for use in practice (Krueger, Nelson, & Wolanin, 1978).

The CURN Project was a 5-year venture (1975–1980) directed by Horsley, Crane, Crabtree, and Wood (1983) to increase the utilization of research findings by (1) disseminating findings, (2) facilitating organizational modifications necessary for implementation, and (3) encouraging collaborative research that was directly transferable to clinical practice. Research utilization was seen as a process to be implemented by an organization rather than by an individual practitioner. Activities of the research utilization included (1) identification and synthesis of multiple studies in a common conceptual area (research base), (2) transformation of the knowledge derived from a research base

into a solution or clinical protocol, (3) transformation of the clinical protocol into specific nursing actions (innovations) that are administered to patients, and (4) clinical evaluation of the new practice to ascertain whether it produced the predicted result (Horsley et al., 1983). The clinical protocols developed during the project were published to encourage nurses in other health care agencies to use these research-based intervention protocols in their practice (CURN Project, 1981–1982).

To ensure that the studies were incorporated into nursing practice, the findings needed to be synthesized for different topics. In 1983, the first volume of the *Annual Review of Nursing Research* was published (Werley & Fitzpatrick, 1983). This annual publication contains experts' reviews of research in selected areas of nursing practice, nursing care delivery, nursing education, and the profession of nursing. The *Annual Review of Nursing Research* continues to be published each year to (1) expand the synthesis and dissemination of research findings, (2) promote the use of research findings in practice, and (3) identify directions for future research.

Many nurses obtained master's and doctoral degrees during the 1980s and 1990s, and postdoctoral education was encouraged for nurse researchers. The ANA Cabinet on Nursing Research identified the research participation for various levels of educational preparation. As indicated in Figure 2-1, nurses at all levels of education have a role in research (ANA, 1989). The nursing educational

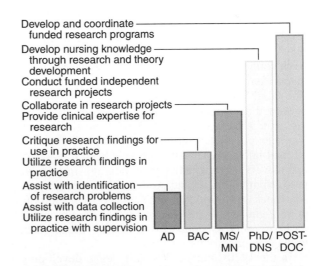

Figure 2-1 Nurses at various levels of education participate in research.

preparation provides a background for nurses at the following levels:

- The nurse with an associate degree to assist with problem identification and data collection
- The nurse with a baccalaureate degree to use research findings in practice
- The nurse with a master's degree to collaborate in research projects
- The nurse with a doctoral degree to conduct independent, funded research projects
- The nurse with a postdoctoral degree to implement a funded program of research

These research expectations for each level of nursing education were supported by the American Association of Colleges of Nursing's (AACN's) 1999 position statement on nursing research (AACN, 1999).

Another priority of the 1980s and 1990s was to obtain greater funding for nursing research. Most of the federal funds in the 1980s were designated for studies involving the diagnosis and cure of diseases. Therefore, nursing received a small percentage of the federal research and development (R&D) funds (approximately 2% to 3%) compared with medicine (approximately 90%), even though nursing personnel greatly outnumber medical personnel (Larson, 1984). However, the ANA achieved a major political victory for nursing research with the creation of the National Center for Nursing Research (NCNR) in 1985. This center was created after years of work and two presidential vetoes (Bauknecht, 1986). The purpose of the NCNR was to support the conduct of basic and clinical nursing research and the dissemination of findings. The NCNR was established under the National Institutes of Health (NIH) and provided visibility for nursing research at the federal level. In 1993, during the tenure of its first director, Dr. Ada Sue Hinshaw, the NCNR became the National Institute of Nursing Research (NINR). This change in title enhanced the recognition of nursing as a research discipline and expanded the funding for nursing research.

Outcomes research emerged as an important methodology for documenting the effectiveness of health care services in the 1980s and 1990s. This type of research evolved from the quality assessment and quality assurance functions that originated with the professional standards review organizations (PSROs) in 1972. During the 1980s, William Roper, the director of the Health Care Finance Administration (HCFA), promoted outcomes research for determining the quality and cost-effectiveness of patient care (Johnson, 1993). In 1989, the Agency for Health Care Policy and Research (AHCPR) was established to facilitate the conduct of outcomes research (Rettig, 1991).

The AHCPR also had an active role in communicating research findings to health care practitioners and was responsible for publishing the first clinical practice guidelines in 1989. Several of these guidelines, including the latest research findings with directives for practice, were published in the 1990s. The Healthcare Research and Quality Act of 1999 reauthorized the AHCPR, changing its name to the Agency for Healthcare Research and Quality (AHRQ). This significant change positioned the AHRQ as a scientific partner with the public and private sectors to improve the quality and safety of patient care by promoting the use of the best research evidence available in practice (see www.ahcpr.gov).

Building on the process of research utilization, physicians, nurses, and other health care professions focused on the development of EBP for health care during the 1990s. A research group led by Dr. David Sackett at McMaster University in Canada developed explicit research methodologies to determine the "best evidence" for practice. The term *evidence based* was first used by David Eddy in 1990 with the focus on providing EBP for medicine (Craig & Smyth, 2007; Sackett, Straus, Richardson, Rosenberg, & Haynes, 2000). In 2002, the Joint Commission on Accreditation of Healthcare Organizations (JCAHO) revised the accreditation policies for hospitals to support the implementation of evidence-based health care. To facilitate the movement of nursing toward EBP, Stetler (2001) develop the "Research Utilization to Facilitate EBP" model (see Chapter 27 for a description of this model).

Nursing Research in the Twenty-First Century

The vision for nursing in the twenty-first century includes conducting quality studies, synthesizing the study findings into the best research evidence available, and using that research evidence effectively in practice (Brown, 1999; Craig & Smyth, 2007; Malloch & Porter-O'Grady, 2006; Melnyk & Fineout-Overholt, 2005; Pearson, Field, & Jordan, 2007). This vision is consistent with the mission of the NINR, which is to support the conduct of biological and clinical research and facilitate the communication of this research to promote an EBP for nursing (NINR, 2007, at www.nih.gov/ninr). With the conduct of biological research a priority for the NINR, the journal *Biological Research for Nursing* was initiated in 2000. The focus on EBP in nursing was supported with the initiation of the *Worldviews on Evidence-Base Nursing* journal in 2004.

The AHRQ has been designated the lead agency supporting research designed to improve the quality of health care, reduce its cost, improve patient safety, decrease medical errors, and broaden access to essential services. The AHRQ sponsors and conducts research that provides evidence-based information on health care outcomes, quality, cost, use, and access. This research information promotes effective health care decision making by patients, clinicians, health system executives, and policy makers. The three future goals of the AHRQ are to (1) support improvements in health outcomes; (2) strengthen quality measurements and improvements; and (3) identify strategies to improve access, foster appropriate use of health care resources, and reduce unnecessary expenditures (AHRQ, 2007, www.ahrq.gov). Currently, the AHRQ and NINR work collaboratively to promote funding for nursing studies. These agencies often jointly call for proposals for studies of high priority to both agencies.

The focus of health care research and funding is expanding from the treatment of illness to include health promotion and illness prevention interventions. *Healthy People 2000* and *Healthy People 2010*, government documents published by the U.S. Department of Health and Human Services (1992, 2000), have increased the visibility of and identified priorities for health promotion research. In the twenty-first century, nurses can have a major role in the development of interventions to promote health and prevent illness in individuals, families, and communities.

To ensure an effective research enterprise in nursing, the discipline must do the following:

1. Create a research culture.
2. Provide quality educational (baccalaureate, master's, doctoral, and postdoctoral) programs to prepare a workforce of nurse scientists.
3. Develop a sound research infrastructure.
4. Obtain sufficient funding for essential research (AACN, 1999).

METHODOLOGIES FOR DEVELOPING RESEARCH EVIDENCE IN NURSING

Scientific method incorporates all procedures that scientists have used, currently use, or may use in the future to pursue knowledge (Kaplan, 1964). This broad definition dispels the belief that there is one way to conduct research and embraces the use of both quantitative and qualitative research methodologies in developing research evidence for practice.

Since the 1930s, many researchers have narrowly defined scientific method to include only quantitative research. This research method is based in the philosophy of logical empiricism or positivism (Norbeck, 1987; Scheffler, 1967). Therefore, scientific knowledge is generated through an application of logical principles and reasoning, whereby the researcher adopts a distant and noninteractive posture with the research subject to prevent bias (Silva & Rothbart, 1984). Quantitative research is a formal, objective, systematic process in which numerical data are used to obtain information about the world. This research method is used to describe variables, examine relationships among variables, and determine cause-and-effect interactions between variables. Currently, the predominantly used method of scientific investigation in nursing is quantitative research.

Qualitative research is a systematic, interactive, subjective approach used to describe life experiences and give them meaning (Marshall & Rossman, 2006; Munhall, 2001). Qualitative research is not a new idea in the social and behavioral sciences (Baumrind, 1980; Glaser & Strauss, 1967). This type of research is conducted to describe and promote our understanding of human experiences such as pain, caring, and comfort.

Comparison of Quantitative and Qualitative Research

The quantitative and qualitative types of research complement each other because they generate different kinds of knowledge that are useful in nursing practice. The problem and purpose to be studied determines the type of research to be conducted, and the researcher's knowledge of both types of research promotes accurate selection of the methodology for the problem identified (McPherson & Leydon, 2002). Quantitative and qualitative research methodologies have some similarities, because both require researcher expertise, involve rigor in implementation, and result in the generation of scientific knowledge for nursing practice. Some of the differences between the two methodologies are presented in Table 2-2.

Philosophical Origin of Quantitative and Qualitative Research

The quantitative approach to scientific inquiry emerged from a branch of philosophy called logical positivism, which operates on strict rules of logic, truth, laws, axioms, and predictions. Quantitative researchers hold the position that truth is absolute and that there is a single reality that one could define by careful measurement. To find truth as a quantitative researcher, you must be completely objective, meaning that values, feelings, and personal perceptions cannot enter into the measurement of reality. Quantitative researchers believe that all human behavior is objective, purposeful, and measurable. The researcher needs only to find or develop the "right" instrument or tool to measure the behavior.

TABLE 2-2 Quantitative and Qualitative Research Characteristics		
Characteristic	**Quantitative Research**	**Qualitative Research**
Philosophical origin	Logical positivism	Naturalistic, interpretive, humanistic
Focus	Concise, objective, reductionistic	Broad, subjective, holistic
Reasoning	Logistic, deductive	Dialectic, inductive
Basis of knowing	Cause-and-effect relationships	Meaning, discovery, understanding
Theoretical focus	Tests theory	Develops theory
Researcher involvement	Control	Shared interpretation
Methods of measurement	Structured interviews, questionnaires, observations, scales, or physiological instruments	Unstructured interviews and observations
Data	Numbers	Words
Analysis	Statistical analysis	Individual interpretation
Findings	Generalization, accept or reject theoretical propositions	Uniqueness, dynamic, understanding of phenomena, and new theory

Today, however, many nurse researchers base their quantitative studies on more of a postpositivist philosophy (Clark, 1998). This philosophy evolved from positivism but focuses on the discovery of reality that is characterized by patterns and trends that can be used to describe, explain, and predict phenomena. With postpositivism, "truth can be discovered only imperfectly and in a probabilistic sense, in contrast to the positivist ideal of establishing cause-and-effect explanations of immutable facts" (Ford-Gilboe, Campbell, & Berman, 1995, p. 16). The postpositivist approach also rejects the idea that the researcher is completely objective about what is to be discovered but continues to emphasize the need to control environmental influences (Newman, 1992).

Qualitative research is an interpretive methodological approach that is thought to produce more of a subjective science than quantitative research. Qualitative research evolved from the behavioral and social sciences as a method of understanding the unique, dynamic, holistic nature of human beings. The philosophical base of qualitative research is interpretive, humanistic, and naturalistic and is concerned with helping those involved to understand the meaning of their social interactions. Qualitative researchers believe that truth is both complex and dynamic and can be found only by studying persons as they interact with and within their sociohistorical settings (Marshall & Rossman, 2006; Munhall, 2001).

Focus of Quantitative and Qualitative Research

The focus or perspective for quantitative research is usually concise and reductionistic. Reductionism involves breaking the whole into parts so that the parts can be examined. Quantitative researchers remain detached from the study and try not to influence it with their values (objectivity). Researcher involvement in the study is thought to bias or sway the study toward the perceptions and values of the researcher, and biasing a study is considered poor scientific technique (Kerlinger & Lee, 2000).

The focus of qualitative research is usually broad, and the intent is to give meaning to the whole (holistic). The qualitative researcher has an active part in the study, and the researcher's values and perceptions influence the findings. Thus, this research approach is subjective, but the approach assumes that subjectivity is essential for the understanding of human experiences (Marshall & Rossman, 2006; Munhall, 2001).

Uniqueness of Conducting Quantitative and Qualitative Research

Quantitative research describes and examines relationships and determines causality among variables. Thus, this method is useful for testing a theory by testing the validity of the relationships that compose the theory. Quantitative research incorporates logistic, deductive reasoning as the researcher examines particulars to make generalizations about the universe.

Qualitative research generates knowledge about meaning and discovery. Inductive and dialectic reasoning are predominant in these studies. For example, the qualitative researcher studies the whole person's response to pain by examining premises about human pain and determining the meaning that pain has for a particular person. Because qualitative research is concerned with meaning and understanding, the findings from these studies can be used to identify the relationships among the variables, and these relational statements are used to develop theories.

Quantitative research requires control (see Table 2-2). The investigator uses control to identify and limit the problem to be researched and attempts to limit the effects of extraneous or outside variables that are not the focus of the study. For example, as a quantitative researcher, you might study the effects of nutritional education on serum lipid levels (total serum cholesterol, low-density lipoprotein [LDL], and high-density lipoprotein [HDL]). You would control the educational program by manipulating the type of education provided, the teaching methods, the length of the program, the setting for the program, and the instructor. You could also control other extraneous variables, such as participant's age, history of cardiovascular disease, and exercise level, because they might affect the serum lipid levels. The intent of this control is to more precisely examine the effects of nutritional education on serum lipid levels.

Quantitative research also requires the use of (1) structured interviews, questionnaires, or observations; (2) scales; or (3) physiological instruments that generate numerical data. Statistical analyses are conducted to reduce and organize data, determine significant relationships, and identify differences among groups. Control, instruments, and statistical analyses are used to ensure that the research findings accurately reflect reality so that the study findings can be generalized. Generalization involves the application of trends or general tendencies (which are identified by studying a sample) to the population from which the research sample was drawn. Researchers must be cautious in making generalizations, because a sound generalization requires the support of many studies with a variety of samples.

Qualitative researchers use unstructured observations and interviews to gather data. The data include the shared interpretations of the researcher and the subjects, and no attempts are made to control the interaction. For example, the researcher and subjects might share their experiences of powerlessness in the health care system. The data are subjective and incorporate the perceptions and beliefs of the researcher and the subjects (Munhall, 2001).

Qualitative data take the form of words and are analyzed in terms of individual responses, descriptive summaries, or both. The researcher identifies categories for sorting and organizing the data (Miles & Huberman, 1994). The intent of the analysis is to organize the data into a meaningful, individualized interpretation, framework, or theory that describes the phenomenon studied. The findings from a qualitative study are unique to that study, and it is not the researcher's intent to generalize the findings

to a larger population. However, understanding the meaning of a phenomenon in a particular situation is useful for understanding similar phenomena in similar situations.

Classification for the Research Methodologies Presented in This Text

Research methods used frequently in nursing have been classified in different ways, so a classification system was developed for this text and is presented in Table 2-3. The quantitative research methods are classified into four categories: (1) descriptive, (2) correlational, (3) quasi-experimental, and (4) experimental. Types of quantitative research are used to test theories and generate and refine knowledge for nursing practice. Quantitative research methods are introduced in this section and described in more detail in Chapter 3.

The qualitative research methods included in this textbook are (1) phenomenological research, (2) grounded theory research, (3) ethnographic research, (4) historical research, (5) philosophical inquiry, and (6) critical social theory. These approaches, all methodologies for discovering knowledge, are introduced in this section and described in depth in Chapters 4 and 23. Unit Two of this textbook focuses on understanding the research process and includes discussions of both quantitative and qualitative research.

TABLE 2-3   Classification System of Nursing Research Methods for This Textbook
Types of Quantitative Research
Descriptive research
Correlational research
Quasi-experimental research
Experimental research
Types of Qualitative Research
Phenomenological research
Grounded theory research
Ethnographic research
Historical research
Philosophical inquiry:
• Foundational inquiry
• Philosophical analysis
• Ethical analysis
Critical social theory methodology
Outcomes Research
Intervention Research

Quantitative Research Methods

Descriptive Research. Descriptive research provides an accurate portrayal or account of characteristics of a particular individual, situation, or group (Kerlinger & Lee, 2000). Descriptive studies offer researchers a way to (1) discover new meaning, (2) describe what exists, (3) determine the frequency with which something occurs, and (4) categorize information. Descriptive studies are usually conducted when little is known about a phenomenon and provide the basis for the conduct of correlational, quasi-experimental, and experimental studies.

Correlational Research. Correlational research involves the systematic investigation of relationships between or among two or more variables that have been identified in theories, observed in practice, or both. If the relationships exist, the researcher determines the type (positive or negative) and the degree or strength of the relationships. The primary intent of correlational studies is to explain the nature of relationships, not to determine cause and effect. However, correlational studies are the means for generating hypotheses to guide quasi-experimental and experimental studies that focus on examining cause-and-effect interactions.

Quasi-Experimental Research. The purposes of quasi-experimental research are (1) to identify causal relationships, (2) to examine the significance of causal relationships, (3) to clarify why certain events happened, or (4) a combination of these objectives (Cook & Campbell, 1979). These studies test the effectiveness of nursing interventions that can then be implemented to control the patient and family outcomes in nursing practice.

Quasi-experimental studies are less powerful than experimental studies because they involve a lower level of control in at least one of three areas: (1) manipulation of the treatment or independent variable, (2) manipulation of the setting, and (3) selection of subjects. When studying human behavior, especially in clinical areas, researchers are commonly unable to manipulate or control certain variables. Also, subjects are not randomly selected but are selected on the basis of convenience. Thus, as a nurse researcher you will probably conduct more quasi-experimental than experimental studies.

Experimental Research. Experimental research is an objective, systematic, controlled investigation conducted for the purpose of predicting and controlling phenomena. This type of research examines causality (Kerlinger & Lee, 2000). Experimental research is considered the most powerful quantitative method because of the rigorous control of variables. Experimental studies have three main characteristics: (1) a controlled manipulation of at least one treatment variable (independent variable),

(2) administration of the treatment to some of the subjects in the study (experimental group) and not to others (control group), and (3) random selection of subjects or random assignment of subjects to groups, or both. Experimental studies usually have highly controlled settings in laboratories or research units in clinical agencies. A randomized controlled trial (RCT) is a type of experimental research that produces the strongest research evidence for practice.

Qualitative Research Methods

Phenomenological Research. Phenomenological research is a humanistic study of phenomena that is conducted in a variety of ways according to the philosophy of the researcher. The aim of phenomenology is to explore an experience as it is lived by the study participants and interpreted by the researcher. During the study, the researcher's experiences, reflections, and interpretations influence the data collected from the study participants (Munhall, 2001). Thus, the participants' lived experiences are expressed through the researcher's interpretations and based on the underlying philosophy of the phenomenological study. Phenomenological research is an effective methodology to discover the meaning of a complex experience as it is lived by a person, such as the lived experience of health or dealing with chronic illness.

Grounded Theory Research. Grounded theory research is an inductive research method initially described by Glaser and Strauss (1967). This research approach is useful for discovering what problems exist in a social setting and the process people use to handle them. Grounded theory methodology emphasizes observation and the development of practice-based intuitive relationships among variables. Throughout the study, the researcher formulates, tests, and redevelops propositions until a theory evolves. The theory developed is "grounded," or has its roots in, the data from which it was derived.

Ethnographic Research. Ethnographic research was developed by anthropologists to investigate cultures through an in-depth study of the members of the culture. This type of research attempts to tell the story of people's daily lives while describing the culture in which they live. The ethnographic research process is the systematic collection, description, and analysis of data to develop a theory of cultural behavior. The researcher (ethnographer) actually lives in or becomes a part of the cultural setting to gather the data. Through the use of ethnographic research, different cultures are described, compared, and contrasted to add to our understanding of the impact of culture on human behavior and health (Germain, 2001).

Historical Research. Historical research is a narrative description or analysis of events that occurred in the remote or recent past. Data are obtained from records, artifacts, or verbal reports. Through historical research, nursing has a way of understanding itself and interpreting the discipline and its contributions to others. The mistakes of the past can be examined to help nurses understand and respond to present situations affecting nurses and nursing practice. In addition, historical research has the potential to provide a foundation for and to direct the future movements of the profession (Fitzpatrick, 2001).

Philosophical Inquiry. Philosophical inquiry uses intellectual analyses to (1) clarify meanings, (2) make values manifest, (3) identify ethics, and (4) study the nature of knowledge (Ellis, 1983). As a philosophical researcher, you would consider an idea or issue from all perspectives by extensively exploring the literature, examining conceptual meaning, raising questions, proposing answers, and suggesting the implications of those answers. The research is guided by philosophical questions that have been posed.

This textbook covers three categories of philosophical inquiry: foundational inquiry, philosophical analysis, and ethical inquiry. Foundational inquiry involves the analysis of the structure of a science and the process of thinking about and valuing certain phenomena held in common by members of a scientific discipline. Philosophical analysis examines meaning and develops theories of meaning through concept analysis or linguistic analysis. Ethical inquiry, another type of philosophical inquiry, involves the intellectual analysis of problems of ethics related to obligation, rights, duty, right and wrong, conscience, justice, choice, intention, and responsibility. Ethical inquiry is a means of striving for rational ends when other people are involved.

Critical Social Theory. Critical social theory provides the basis for research that focuses on understanding how people communicate and develop symbolic meanings in a society. Many of the meanings occur in a world where certain facts of the society are taken for granted rather than being discussed or disputed. The established political, social, and cultural orders are perceived as closed to change and are not questioned. Critical social theory provides a philosophical basis for multiple research methods to generate knowledge that might promote empowerment and political change (Ford-Gilboe et al., 1995). Nurses need to be aware of constraints and power imbalances in society that affect areas such as access to care, care of the chronically ill and elderly, and pain management of the terminally ill. The health needs of patients and families and the health care system developed to meet these needs are continuously influenced by the social system that surrounds them.

Outcomes Research

The spiraling cost of health care has generated many questions about the quality and effectiveness of health care services and the patient outcomes. Consumers want to know what services they are buying and whether these services will improve their health. Health care policy makers want to know whether the care is cost-effective and high quality. These concerns have promoted the development of outcomes research, which examines the results of care and measures the changes in health status of patients (AHRQ, 2007; Doran, 2003). Key ideas related to outcomes research are addressed throughout the text, and Chapter 12 contains a detailed discussion of this methodology.

Intervention Research

Intervention research investigates the effectiveness of a nursing intervention in achieving the desired outcome or outcomes in a natural setting. "Interventions are defined as treatments, therapies, procedures, or actions implemented by health professionals to and with clients, in a particular situation, to move the clients' condition toward desired health outcomes that are beneficial to the clients" (Sidani & Braden, 1998, p. 8). An intervention can be a specific treatment implemented to manage a well-defined patient problem or a program. A program intervention, such as a cardiac rehabilitation program, consists of multiple nursing actions that are implemented as a package to improve the health conditions of the participants (Brown, 2002). The goal of intervention research is to generate sound scientific knowledge for actions that nurses can use to provide evidence-based nursing care. The details of intervention research are presented in Chapter 13. In summary, nurse researchers conduct a variety of research methodologies (quantitative, qualitative, outcomes, and intervention research) to develop the research evidence needed for practice.

INTRODUCTION TO BEST RESEARCH EVIDENCE FOR PRACTICE

Evidence-based practice (EBP) involves the use of best research evidence to support clinical decisions in practice. As a nurse, you make numerous clinical decisions each day that impact the health outcomes of your patients and families. By using the best research evidence available, you can make quality clinical decisions that will improve the health outcomes for patients, families, and communities. This section introduces you to the concept of best research evidence for practice by providing the following: (1) a definition of the term *best research evidence*, (2) a model of the levels of research evidence available, and (3) a link of the best research evidence to evidence-based guidelines for practice.

Definition of Best Research Evidence

Best research evidence is a summary of the highest quality, current empirical knowledge in a specific area of health care that is developed from a synthesis of quality studies (quantitative, qualitative, outcomes, and intervention) in that area. The synthesis of study findings is a complex, highly structured process that is best conducted by at least two or even a team of expert researchers and health care providers. There are various types of research synthesis, and the type of synthesis conducted varies based on the quality and types of research evidence available.

The quality of the research evidence available in an area depends on the number and strength of the studies. Replicating or repeating of studies with

similar methodology adds to the quality of the research evidence. The strengths and weaknesses of the studies are determined by critically appraising the validity or credibility of the study outcomes (see Chapter 26). The types of research commonly conducted in nursing were identified earlier in this chapter as quantitative, qualitative, outcomes, and intervention. The research synthesis process used to summarize knowledge varies for quantitative and qualitative research. In building the best research evidence for practice, the quantitative experimental study, such as a randomized controlled trial (RCT), has been identified as producing the strongest research evidence for practice (Craig & Smyth, 2007; Institute of Medicine, 2001; Malloch & Porter-O'Grady, 2006; Melnyk & Fineout-Overholt, 2005; Pearson et al., 2007; Sackett et al., 2000).

Research evidence in nursing and health care is synthesized by using the following processes: (1) systematic review, (2) meta-analysis, (3) integrative review, (4) metasummary, and (5) methasynthesis. Depending on the research findings available, the best

---

TABLE 2-4 ■ Processes Used to Synthesize Research Evidence

Synthesis Process	Purpose of Synthesis	Types of Research Included in the Synthesis (Sampling Frame)	Analysis for Achieving Synthesis
Systematic review	Use of specific, systematic methods to identify, select, critically appraise, and synthesized research evidence to address a particular problem in practice (Craig & Smyth, 2007).	Quantitative studies with similar methodology usually randomized controlled trials (RCT); also includes meta-analyses focused on the selected practice problem	Narrative and statistical
Meta-analysis	Synthesis or pooling of the results from several previous studies using statistical analysis to determine the effect of an intervention or the strength of relationships.	Uses quantitative studies with similar methodology, such as quasi-experimental and experimental studies focused on the effect of an intervention or correlational studies focused on relationships	Statistical
Integrative review	Synthesis of the findings from a variety of independent studies to determine the current knowledge in an area.	Summarizes a variety of quantitative and qualitative studies; review often includes theoretical literature	Narrative
Metasummary	Quantity-oriented aggregation or synthesis of qualitative research findings to sum the findings across reports in a target area (Sandelowski & Barroso, 2007).	Summarizes existing qualitative studies and provides basis for metasynthesis	Narrative
Metasynthesis	Integration of qualitative study findings that offers a "novel interpretation of findings that are the result of interpretive transformations far removed from these findings as given in the research reports" (Sandelowski & Barroso, 2007, p. 18).	Uses original qualitative studies and metasummaries to produce synthesis	Narrative

Table adapted from: Craig, J. V., & Smyth, R. L. (2007). *The evidence-based practice manual for nurses.* Edinburgh: Churchill Livingstone, Elsevier. Sandelowski, M., & Barroso, J. (2007). *Handbook for synthesizing qualitative research.* New York: Springer Publishing Company. Whittemore, R. (2005). Combining evidence in nursing research: Methods and implications. *Nursing Research, 54*(1), 56–62.

research evidence might be synthesized by one or more of these five processes. Table 2-4 identifies the processes used in research evidence synthesis, the purpose of each synthesis process, the types of research included in the synthesis (sampling frame), and the analysis techniques used to achieve the synthesis of research evidence (Whittemore, 2005). A systematic review is a structured, comprehensive synthesis of quantitative studies in a particular health care area to determine the best research evidence available for expert clinicians to use to promote an EBP. Systematic reviews are conducted to synthesize research evidence from numerous, high-quality quantitative studies with similar methodologies (Craig & Smyth, 2007). These reviews are often conducted by teams or panels of expert researchers and clinicians, who use the results of these reviews to produce the national and international standardized guidelines for managing health care problems such as hypertension (Chobanian et al., 2003). These standardized guidelines are made available online, published in articles and books, and presented at conferences and professional meetings. Some of the common sources for these standardized guidelines are presented at the end of this chapter.

Meta-analysis is a type of study that statistically pools the results from previous, similar studies into a single quantitative analysis that provides one of the highest levels of evidence for an intervention's efficacy (Conn & Rantz, 2003). The studies synthesized are usually quasi-experimental or experimental types of studies. In addition, a meta-analysis can be performed on correlational studies to determine the type (positive or negative) or strength of relationships among selected variables (see Table 2-4). Because meta-analyses involve statistical analysis to combine study findings, it is possible to be objective rather than subjective in synthesizing research evidence. Some of the strongest evidence for using an intervention in practice is generated from a meta-analysis of multiple, controlled quasi-experimental and experimental studies. Thus, many systematic reviews conducted to generate evidence-based guidelines include meta-analyses. The process for conducting a meta-analysis is presented in Chapter 27.

An integrative review of research identifies, analyzes, and synthesizes research findings from independent quantitative and qualitative studies to determine the current knowledge (what is known and not known) in a particular area. Most of the studies synthesized in an integrative review are quantitative (descriptive, correlational, quasi-experimental, and experimental), but some reviews also include important findings from qualitative studies and theoretical literature (see Table 2-4). Integrative reviews of research direct future studies and are sometimes included in systematic reviews. The value of an integrative review depends on the standards used to the conduct the review, which is similar to the standards of clarity, rigor, and replication required for conducting primary research. The process for conducting an integrative review of research is presented in Chapter 27.

Qualitative research synthesis is the process and product of systematically reviewing and formally integrating the findings from qualitative studies (Sandelowski & Barroso, 2007). Qualitative research synthesis includes two categories: qualitative metasummary and qualitative metasynthesis (see Table 2-4). Qualitative metasummary is the synthesis or summing of the findings across qualitative reports to determine the current knowledge in an area. Metasummary can be an end in itself to identify current knowledge or can provide a foundation for conducting qualitative metasynthesis. Qualitative metasynthesis provides a fully integrated, novel description or explanation of a target event or experience verses a summary view of that event or experience. Metasynthesis requires more complex, integrative thought in developing a new perspective or theory based of the findings of previous qualitative studies. These qualitative research synthesis processes have been used to generate research evidence that contributes to the knowledge needed for EBP. Sandelowski and Barroso (2007) have developed a book that focuses on the synthesis of qualitative research, and their processes for conducting metasummary and metasynthesis are addressed in Chapter 27.

Levels of Research Evidence

The strength or validity of the best research evidence in an area depends on the quality and quantity of the studies conducted in the area. Quantitative studies, especially experimental studies like the RCT, are thought to provide the strongest research evidence. Also the replication or repetition of studies with similar methodology increases the strength of the research evidence generated. The levels of the research evidence can be thought of as a continuum with the highest quality of research evidence at one end and weakest research evidence at the other (see Figure 2-2) (Craig & Smyth, 2007; Malloch & Porter-O'Grady, 2006; Melnyk & Fineout-Overholt, 2005; Pearson et al., 2007). The systematic research reviews and meta-analyses of high-quality experimental studies provide the strongest or best research evidence for use by expert clinicians in practice. Meta-analyses and integrative

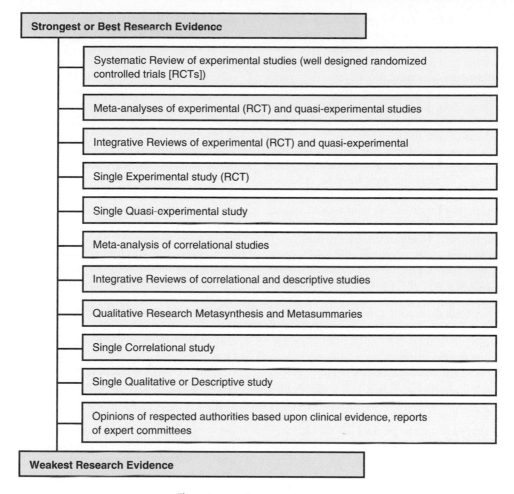

Figure 2-2 Levels of research evidence.

reviews of quasi-experimental and experimental studies also provide strong research evidence for managing practice problems. Correlational, descriptive, and qualitative studies direct further research and provide some useful findings for practice (see Figure 2-2). The weakest evidence comes from expert opinions, which can include expert clinicians' opinions or the opinions expressed in committee reports. When making a decision in your clinical practice, be sure to base that decision on the best research evidence available.

The levels of research evidence identified in Figure 2-2 will help nurses to determine the quality and validity of the evidence that is available for them to use in practice. Advance practice nurses must seek out the best research knowledge available in an area to ensure that they manage patients' acute and chronic illnesses with a high quality of care (Kania-Lachance, Best, McDonah, & Ghosh, 2006). This best research evidence generated from systematic reviews, meta-analyses, and integrative reviews is used most often to develop standardized or evidence-based guidelines for practice.

Introduction to Evidence-Based Guidelines

Evidence-based practice guidelines are rigorous, explicit clinical guidelines that are based on the best research evidence available in that area. These guidelines are usually developed by a team or panel of expert researchers; expert clinicians (physicians, nurses, pharmacists, and other health professionals); and sometimes consumers, policy makers, and economists. The expert panel seeks consensus on the content of the guideline to provide clinicians with the best information for making clinical decisions in practice. There has been a dramatic growth in the production of evidence-based guidelines to assist health care providers in building an EBP and in improving health care outcomes for patients, families, providers, and health care agencies.

Every year, new guidelines are developed, and some of the existing guidelines are revised based on new research evidence. These guidelines have become the gold standard (or standard of excellence) for patient care, and nurses and other health care providers are encouraged to incorporate these standardized guidelines into their practice. Many of these evidence-based guidelines have been made available online by expert national and international government agencies, professional organizations, and centers of excellence. When selecting a guideline for practice, be sure that a credible agency or organization developed the guideline and that the reference list reflects the synthesis of extensive research evidence.

An extremely important source for evidence-based guidelines in the United States is the National Guideline Clearinghouse (NGC), which was initiated in 1998 by the Agency for Healthcare Research and Quality (AHRQ). The NGC started with 200 guidelines and has expanded to more than 1000 evidence-based guidelines (see www.guideline.gov). Another excellent source of systematic reviews and evidence-based guidelines is the Cochrane Collaboration and Library in the United Kingdom, which can be accessed at www.cochrane.org. Professional nursing organizations, such as the Oncology Nursing Society (www.ons.org) and the National Association of Neonatal Nurses (www.nann.org), have also developed evidence-based guidelines for nursing practice. These websites will introduce you to some of evidence-based guidelines that exist nationally and internationally. Chapter 27 will help you to critically appraise the quality of an evidence-based guideline and implement that guideline in your practice.

and master's degrees. In the 1970s and 1980s, the major focus was on the conduct of clinical research to improve nursing practice.

- Outcomes research emerged as an important methodology for documenting the effectiveness of health care service in the 1980s and 1990s. In 1989, the Agency for Health Care Policy and Research (AHCPR) was established to facilitate the conduct of outcomes research.
- The vision for nursing in the twenty-first century is the development of a scientific knowledge base that enables nurses to implement an evidence-based practice (EBP).
- Nursing research incorporates both quantitative and qualitative research and two relatively new methodologies, outcomes research and intervention research.
- Quantitative research is classified into four types for this textbook: descriptive, correlational, quasi-experimental, and experimental.
- Qualitative research is classified into six types for this textbook: phenomenological research, grounded theory research, ethnographic research, historical research, philosophical inquiry, and critical social theory.
- Outcomes research focuses on determining the end results of care or a measure of the change in health status of the patient and family.
- Intervention research involves the investigation of the effectiveness of a nursing intervention in achieving the desired outcomes in a natural setting.
- Best research evidence is a summary of the highest quality, current empirical knowledge in a specific area of health care that is developed from a synthesis of high-quality studies (quantitative, qualitative, outcomes, and intervention) in that area. Research evidence in nursing and health care is synthesized using the following processes: (1) systematic review, (2) meta-analysis, (3) integrative review, (4) meta-summary, and (5) methasynthesis.
- The levels of the research evidence can be thought of as a continuum with the highest quality of research evidence at one end and the weakest at the other. The best research evidence is synthesized by a team or panel of experts to develop evidence-based guidelines for clinicians in practice.

SUMMARY

- Florence Nightingale initiated nursing research more than 150 years ago; this was followed by years of limited research until the 1950s. During the 1950s and 1960s, research became a higher priority, with the development of graduate programs in nursing that increased the number of nurses with doctorates

REFERENCES

Abdellah, F. G. (1972). Evolution of nursing as a profession. *International Nursing Review, 19*(3), 219–235.

Agency for Healthcare Research and Quality (AHRQ). (2007). Agency for Healthcare Research and Quality homepage. Retrieved November 23, 2007, from www.ahrq.gov.

American Association of Colleges of Nursing (AACN). (1999). Position statement on nursing research. *Journal of Professional Nursing, 15*(4), 253–257.

American Nurses Association (ANA). (1950). *Twenty thousand nurses tell their story.* Kansas City: Author.

American Nurses Association (ANA). (1989). *Education for participation in nursing research.* Kansas City: Author.

Bauknecht, V. L. (1986). Congress overrides veto, nursing gets center for research. *American Nurse, 18*(1), 24.

Baumrind, D. (1980). New directions in socialization research. *American Psychologist, 35*(7), 639–652.

Brown, S. A., & Grimes, D. E. (1995). A meta-analysis of nurse practitioners and nurse midwives in primary care. *Nursing Research, 44*(5), 332–339.

Brown, S. J. (1999). *Knowledge for healthcare practice: A guide to using research evidence.* Philadelphia: W.B. Saunders.

Brown, S. J. (2002). Focus on research methods. Nursing intervention studies: A descriptive analysis of issues important to clinicians. *Research in Nursing & Health, 25*(4), 317–327.

Carlson-Catalano, J., & Lunney, M. (1995). Quantitative methods for clinical validation of nursing diagnoses. *Clinical Nurse Specialist, 9*(6), 306–311.

Chobanian, A. V., Bakris, G. L., Black, H. R., Cushman, W. C, Green, L. A., Izzo, J. L., et al. (2003). The seventh report of the Joint National Committee on prevention, detection, evaluation, and treatment of high blood pressure: The JNC 7 report. *Journal of the American Medical Association, 289*(19). 2560–2572.

Clark, A. M. (1998). The qualitative-quantitative debate: Moving from positivism and confrontation to post-positivism and reconciliation. *Journal of Advanced Nursing, 27I*(6), 1242–1249.

Conduct and Utilization of Research in Nursing (CURN) Project. (1981–1982). *Using research to improve nursing practice.* New York: Grune & Stratton.

Conn, V. S., & Rantz, M. J. (2003). Research methods: Managing primary study quality in meta-analyses. *Research in Nursing & Health, 26*(4), 322–333.

Cook, Sir E. (1913). *The life of Florence Nightingale* (Vol. 1). London: Macmillan.

Cook, T. D., & Campbell, D. T. (1979). *Quasi- experimentation: Design and analysis issues for field settings.* Chicago: Rand McNally.

Craig, J. V., & Smyth, R. L. (2007). *The evidence-based practice manual for nurses* (2nd ed.). Edinburgh: Churchill Livingstone.

de Tornyay, R. (1977). Nursing research: The road ahead. *Nursing Research, 26*(6), 404–407.

Doran, D. M. (2003) *Nursing sensitive outcomes: State of the science.* Boston: Jones & Bartlett.

Downs, F. S., & Fleming, W. J. (1979). *Issues in nursing research.* New York: Appleton-Century-Crofts.

Ellis, R. (1983). Philosophic inquiry. In H. H. Werley & J. J. Fitzpatrick (Eds.), *Annual review of nursing research* (Vol. 1, pp. 211–228). New York: Springer.

Fitzpatrick, M. L. (1978). *Historical studies in nursing.* New York: Teachers College Press.

Fitzpatrick, M. L. (2001). Historical research: The method. In P. L. Munhall (Ed.), *Nursing research: A qualitative perspective* (3rd ed., pp. 403–415). Sudbury, MA: Jones & Bartlett.

Ford-Gilboe, M., Campbell, J., & Berman, H. (1995). Stories and numbers: Coexistence without compromise. *Advances in Nursing Science, 18*(1), 14–26.

Germain, C. P. (2001). Ethnography: The method. In P. L. Munhall (Ed.), *Nursing research: A qualitative perspective* (3rd ed., pp. 277–306). New York: National League for Nursing.

Glaser, B. G., & Strauss, A. L. (1967). *The discovery of grounded theory: Strategies for qualitative research.* Chicago: Aldine.

Gortner, S. R., & Nahm, H. (1977). An overview of nursing research in the United States. *Nursing Research, 26*(1), 10–33.

Herbert, R. G. (1981). *Florence Nightingale: Saint, reformer or rebel?* Malabar, FL: Robert E. Krieger.

Horsley, J. A., Crane, J., Crabtree, M. K., & Wood, D. J. (1983). *Using research to improve nursing practice: A guide; CURN Project.* New York: Grune & Stratton.

Institute of Medicine. (2001). *Crossing the quality chasm: A new health system for the 21st century.* Washington, DC: National Academy Press.

Jacox, A. (1980). Strategies to promote nursing research. *Nursing Research, 29*(4), 213–218.

Johnson, J. E. (1993). Outcomes research and health care reform: Opportunities for nurses. *Nursing Connections, 6*(4), 1–3.

Johnson, W. L. (1977). Research programs of the National League for Nursing. *Nursing Research, 26*(3), 172–176.

Kania-Lachance, D. M., Best, P. J., McDonah, M. R., & Ghosh, A. K. (2006). Evidence-based practice and the nurse practitioner. *The Nurse Practitioner, 31*(10), 46–53.

Kaplan, A. (1964). *The conduct of inquiry: Methodology for behavioral science.* New York: Chandler.

Kerlinger, F. N., & Lee, H. B. (2000). *Foundations of behavioral research* (4th ed.). Fort Worth, TX: Harcourt.

Krueger, J. C., Nelson, A. H., & Wolanin, M. A. (1978). *Nursing research: Development, collaboration, and utilization.* Germantown, MD: Aspen.

Larson, E. (1984). Health policy and NIH: Implications for nursing research. *Nursing Research, 33*(6), 352–356.

Malloch, K., & Porter-O'Grady, T. (2006). *Introduction to evidence-based practice in nursing and health care.* Sudbury, MA: Jones & Barlett.

Marshall, C., & Rossman, G. B. (2006). *Designing qualitative research* (4th ed.). Thousand Oaks, CA: Sage.

McPherson, K., & Leydon, G. (2002). Quantitative and qualitative methods in UK health research: Then, now and …? *European Journal of Cancer Care 11(3)*, 225–231.

Melnyk, B. M., & Fineout-Overholt, E. (2005). *Evidence-based practice in nursing & healthcare: A guide to best practice.* Philadelphia: Lippincott Williams & Wilkins.

Miles, M. B., & Huberman, A. M. (1994). *Qualitative data analysis: A sourcebook of new methods* (2nd ed.). Beverly Hills, CA: Sage.

Mundinger, M. O., Kane, R. L., Lenz, E. R., Totten, A. M., Tsai, W., Cleary, P. D., et al. (2000). Primary care outcomes in patients treated by nurse practitioners or physicians: A randomized trial. *Journal of the American Medical Association, 283*(1), 59–68.

Munhall, P. L. (2001). *Research methods: A qualitative perspective* (3rd ed.). Sudbury, MA: Jones & Bartlett.

National Institute of Nursing Research (2007). National Institute of Nursing Research mission and research agenda. Retrieved November 23, 2007, from www.nih.gov/ninr.

Newman, M.A. (1992). Prevailing paradigms in nursing. *Nursing Outlook, 40*(1), 10–13, 32.

Nightingale, F. (1859). *Notes on nursing: What it is, and what it is not.* Philadelphia: Lippincott.

Norbeck, J. S. (1987). In defense of empiricism. *Image: Journal of Nursing Scholarship, 19*(1), 28–30.

Palmer, I. S. (1977). Florence Nightingale: Reformer, reactionary, researcher. *Nursing Research, 26*(2), 84–89.

Pearson, A., Field, J., & Jordan, Z. (2007). *Evidence-based clinical practice in nursing and health care: Assimilating research, experience, and expertise*. Oxford: Blackwell.

Rettig, R. (1991). History, development, and importance to nursing of outcomes research. *Journal of Nursing Quality Assurance, 5*(2), 13–17.

Sackett, D. L., Straus, S. E., Richardson, W. S., Rosenberg, W., & Haynes, R. B. (2000). *Evidence-based medicine: How to practice & teach EBM* (2nd ed.). London: Churchill Livingstone.

Sandelowski, M., & Barroso, J. (2007). *Handbook for synthesizing qualitative research*. New York: Springer.

Scheffler, I. (1967). *Science and subjectivity*. Indianapolis: Bobbs-Merrill.

See, E. M. (1977). The ANA and research in nursing. *Nursing Research, 26*(3), 165–171.

Sidani, S., & Braden, C. P. (1998). *Evaluating nursing interventions: A theory-driven approach*. Thousand Oaks, CA: Sage.

Silva, M. C., & Rothbart, D. (1984). An analysis of changing trends in philosophies of science on nursing theory development and testing. *Advances in Nursing Science, 6*(2), 1–13.

Stetler, C. B. (2001). Updating the Stetler model of research utilization to facilitate evidence-based practice. *Nursing Outlook, 49*(6), 272–279.

Stetler, C. B., & Marram, G. (1976). Evaluating research findings for applicability in practice. *Nursing Outlook, 24*(9), 559–563.

U.S. Department of Health and Human Services. (1992). *Healthy people 2000*. Washington, DC: Author.

U.S. Department of Health and Human Services. (2000). *Healthy people 2010*. Washington, DC: Author.

Werley, H. H. (1977). Nursing research in perspective. *International Nursing Review, 24*(3), 75–83.

Werley, H. H., & Fitzpatrick, J. J. (Eds.). (1983). *Annual review of nursing research* (Vol. 1). New York: Springer.

Whittemore, R. (2005). Combining evidence in nursing research: Methods and implications. *Nursing Research, 54*(1), 56–62.

CHAPTER 3
Introduction to Quantitative Research

What do you think of when you hear the word *research*? Frequently, the word *experiment* comes to mind. One might equate experiments with randomizing subjects into groups, collecting data, and conducting statistical analyses. Many people believe that an experiment is conducted to "prove" something, such as that one pain medicine is more effective than another. These common notions are associated with the classic experimental design originated by Sir Ronald Fisher (1935). Fisher is noted for adding structure to the steps of the research process with ideas such as the null hypothesis, research design, and statistical analysis.

Fisher's experimentation provided the groundwork for what is now known as experimental research. Throughout the years, other quantitative approaches have been developed. Campbell and Stanley (1963) developed quasi-experimental approaches. Karl Pearson developed statistical approaches for examining relationships among variables, which increased the conduct of correlational research. The fields of sociology, education, and psychology are noted for their development and expansion of strategies for conducting descriptive research. The steps of the research process used in these different types of quantitative study are the same, but the philosophy and strategies for implementing these steps vary with the approach.

Many quantitative research approaches are essential to develop the body of knowledge needed for evidence-based practice. Thus, quantitative research is a major focus throughout this textbook. This chapter provides an overview of quantitative research by (1) discussing concepts relevant to quantitative research, (2) identifying the steps of the quantitative research process, and (3) providing examples of different types of quantitative studies.

CONCEPTS RELEVANT TO QUANTITATIVE RESEARCH

Some concepts relevant to quantitative research are basic research, applied research, rigor, and control. These concepts are defined, and major points are reinforced with examples from quantitative studies.

Basic Research

Basic, or pure, research is a scientific investigation that involves the pursuit of "knowledge for knowledge's sake," or for the pleasure of learning and finding truth (Nagel, 1961). The purpose of basic research is to generate and refine theory and build constructs; thus, frequently the findings are not directly useful in practice. However, because the findings are more theoretical in nature, they can be generalized to various settings (Wysocki, 1983).

Basic research also examines the underlying mechanisms of actions of an intervention or outcome (Wallenstein, 1987). For example, cachexia in cancer patients clinically presents with anorexia, weight loss, and wasting of skeletal muscles that decrease patients' functioning and quality of life. What are the pathological mechanisms of cancer cachexia with resulting skeletal muscle wasting? What interventions might be implemented to preserve skeletal muscle mass in patients with cancer? Because little is known about the pathology of cancer cachexia with skeletal muscle wasting and possible treatments for these clinical problems, basic research on animals is needed to generate knowledge in these areas. Graves, Hitt, Pariza, Cook, and McCarthy (2005) conducted basic research to examine the effect of a diet supplemented with 0.5% conjugated linoleic acid (CLA) on muscle wasting in mice with cancer. In this laboratory study, the tumor-bearing mice were experiencing cancer cachexia with progressive weight loss, skeletal muscle wasting, fatigue, and anorexia. CLA was the independent variable or treatment implemented to determine its effect on the dependent or outcome variable of the gastrocnemius muscle mass in mice with and without cancer.

Laboratories with animals often implement basic research to examine the effect of newly proposed interventions. Researchers identified CLA as a potential treatment for cachexia with skeletal muscle wasting and implemented it as a dietary supplement for tumor-bearing mice. Basic research usually precedes or is the basis for applied research. Thus, Graves et al.'s (2005) basic study provides a basis for studying the effects of the CLA dietary supplement on weight loss and skeletal muscle wasting on cancer patients. Graves et al. (2005) found that CLA seems to preserve muscle mass in tumor-bearing mice by reducing the catabolic effects of the tumor necrosis factor (TNF) on skeletal muscle. This study increases our understanding of the pathology of cancer cachexia and contributes to the development of dietary treatments to reduce the loss of skeletal muscle mass with cancer. Additional applied research is needed to determine if the CLA dietary supplement preserves muscle mass and maintains weight of cancer patients.

Applied Research

Applied, or practical, research is a scientific investigation conducted to generate knowledge that will directly influence or improve clinical practice. The purpose of applied research is to solve problems, to make decisions, or to predict or control outcomes in real-life practice situations. Because applied research focuses on specific problems, the findings are less generalizable than those from basic research. Applied research is also used to test theory and validate its usefulness in clinical practice. Often, the new knowledge discovered through basic research is examined for usefulness in practice by applied research, making these approaches complementary (Bond & Heitkemper, 1987).

Artinian et al. (2007) conducted an applied study to determine the effectiveness of a nurse-managed telemonitoring (TM) program on the blood pressure (BP) of urban African Americans. The TM program (1) provided BP equipment for patients to monitor their BP at home, (2) improved access to care by

sending patients' BP readings over the phone to health care agencies, and (3) increased monitoring of the patients' BP by a care provider with immediate feedback to the patient. The treatment group received the nurse-managed TM intervention or treatment, and the comparison group received usual care (UC). The TM treatment group had a significant reduction in systolic BP when compared to the UC group, and their diastolic BP was greatly reduced but was not statistically significant from the comparison group at 12 months. Thus, the TM intervention did have a positive impact on the BPs of African Americans, and additional research is needed to determine if the intervention has a long-term effect on BPs and improves hypertension control in this population. The findings from this applied study do have implications for practice because this nurse-managed TM intervention significantly affected BP in a population with a high incidence of hypertension (Artinian et al., 2007). We will use this quasi-experimental study as an example to reinforce key points throughout this chapter.

Many nurse researchers have conducted applied studies to produce findings that directly affect clinical practice. Usually applied studies focus on developing and testing the effectiveness of nursing interventions in the treatment of patient and family health problems. In addition, most federal funding has been granted for applied research. However, additional basic research is needed to expand our understanding of several pathophysiological variables, such as impaired oxygenation and perfusion, fluid and electrolyte imbalance, altered neurological function, impaired immune system, nutritional disorders, and sleep disturbance. Because the future of any profession rests on its research base, both basic and applied studies are needed to develop knowledge for evidence-based practice in nursing.

Rigor in Quantitative Research

Rigor is the strive for excellence in research and involves discipline, scrupulous adherence to detail, and strict accuracy. A rigorous quantitative researcher constantly strives for more precise measurement methods, structured treatments, representative samples, and tightly controlled study designs. Characteristics valued in these researchers include (1) critical examination of reasoning and (2) attention to precision.

Logistic reasoning and deductive reasoning are essential to the development of quantitative research. The research process consists of specific steps that are developed with meticulous detail and logically linked together. These steps are critically examined and reexamined for errors and weaknesses in areas such as design, treatment implementation, measurement, sampling, statistical analysis, and generalization. Reducing these errors and weaknesses is essential to ensure that the research findings are an accurate reflection of reality.

Another aspect of rigor is precision, which encompasses accuracy, detail, and order. Precision is evident in the concise statement of the research purpose, the detailed development of the study design, and the formulation of explicit treatment protocols. The most explicit use of precision, however, is evident in the measurement of the study variables. Measurement involves objectively experiencing the real world through the senses: sight, hearing, touch, taste, and smell. The researcher continually searches for new and more precise ways to measure elements and events of the world (Kaplan, 1964).

Control in Quantitative Research

Control occurs when the researcher imposes "rules" to decrease the possibility of error and thus increase the probability that the study's findings are an accurate reflection of reality. The rules used to achieve control are referred to as design. Through control, the researcher can reduce the influence or confounding effect of extraneous variables on the study variables. For example, if a study focused on the effect of relaxation therapy on the perception of incisional pain, the extraneous variables, such as type of surgical incision and the timing, amount, and type of pain medicine administered after surgery, would have to be controlled to prevent them from influencing the patient's perception of pain.

Controlling extraneous variables enables the researcher to identify relationships among the study variables accurately and examine the effects of one variable on another. Researchers can control extraneous variables by randomly selecting a certain type of subject, such as only those individuals who are having abdominal surgery or those with a certain medical diagnosis. The selection of subjects is controlled with sample criteria and sampling method. The setting can also be structured to control extraneous variables such as temperature, noise, and interactions with other people. The data collection process can be sequenced to control extraneous variables such as fatigue and discomfort.

Quantitative research requires varying degrees of control, ranging from minimal control to highly controlled, depending on the type of study (Table 3-1). Descriptive studies are usually conducted with minimal control of the study design, because subjects are examined as they exist in their natural setting, such as home, work, or school. However, the researcher still

TABLE 3-1 ■ Control in Quantitative Research	
Type of Research	Control in Development of the Research Design
Descriptive research	Minimal or partial control
Correlational research	Minimal or partial control
Quasi-experimental research	Moderate control
Experimental research	High control

hopes to achieve the most precise measurement of the research variables as possible. Experimental studies are highly controlled and often conducted on animals in laboratory settings to determine the underlying mechanisms for and effectiveness of a treatment. Some common areas in which control might be enhanced in quantitative research are (1) selection of subjects (sampling), (2) selection of the research setting, (3) development and implementation of a treatment or intervention, (4) measurement of study variables, and (5) subjects' knowledge of the study.

Sampling

Sampling is a process of selecting subjects, events, behaviors, or elements for participation in a study. In performing quantitative research, you will use both random and nonrandom sampling methods to obtain study samples. Random sampling methods usually provide a sample that is representative of a population, because each member of the population has a probability greater than zero of being selected for a study. Thus, random or probability sampling methods require greater researcher control and rigor than nonrandom or nonprobability sampling methods (see Chapter 14).

Research Settings

There are three common settings for conducting research: natural, partially controlled, and highly controlled. Natural settings are uncontrolled, real-life settings where studies are conducted (Kerlinger & Lee, 2000). Descriptive and correlational types of quantitative research are often conducted in natural settings. A partially controlled setting is an environment that the researcher manipulates or modifies in some way. An increasing number of quasi-experimental studies are being conducted to test the effectiveness of nursing interventions, and these studies are often conducted in partially controlled settings. Highly controlled settings are artificially constructed environments that are developed for the sole purpose of conducting research. Laboratories, research or experimental centers, and test units are highly controlled settings often used for the conduct of experimental research. Chapter 14 discusses the process for selecting a setting for the conduct of quantitative and qualitative research.

Development and Implementation of Study Interventions or Treatments

Quasi-experimental and experimental studies examine the effect of an independent variable or intervention on a dependent variable or outcome. More intervention studies are being conducted in nursing to establish an evidence-based practice (Melnyk & Fineout-Overholt, 2005). Controlling the development and implementation of a study intervention increases the validity of the study design and the credibility of the findings (Ryan & Lauver, 2002). A study intervention must be (1) clearly and precisely developed, (2) consistently implemented with protocol, and (3) examined for effectiveness through quality measurement of the dependent variables (Santacroce, Maccarelli, & Grey, 2004; Sidani & Braden, 1998). Artinian et al. (2007) provided the following detailed description of the implementation of the nurse-managed TM (telemonitoring) intervention to improve the BPs of African-American subjects:

> Participants in the TM group received UC [usual care] plus nurse-managed TM. Specially trained registered nurses delivered the intervention. During a prescheduled appointment, the intervention nurse delivered the BP monitor and TM link device (device that links BP monitor to the telephone) to the participant's home. At the time of the home visit, an intervention nurse taught participants how to self-monitor BP in accordance with The Seventh Report of the Joint National Committee on Prevention, Detection, Evaluation, and Treatment of High Blood Pressure (JNC VII) guidelines (Chobanian et al., 2003), set up the home TM system, demonstrated the system, had participants practice using the BP monitor, and answered questions. Given the memory in the BP monitor and that all BPs recorded by the monitor were telephonically sent to care providers and the principal investigator, participants received verbal and written reminders that the BP monitor was exclusively for their use ... LifeLink Monitoring, Inc. (Bearsville, NY) provided TM services for this study.... Telemonitoring participants were also asked to telephonically send their BP readings to the intervention nurse and their care providers.... Once the intervention nurses received the BP reports, they telephoned each participant to provide feedback in relation to the target goals and to provide telecounseling about lifestyle modification and medication adherence in accordance with JNC-VII guidelines (Chobanian et al., 2003). (Artinian, 2007, p. 315)

Measurement of Study Variables

When you are conducting a quantitative study, you will attempt to use the most precise instruments available to measure the study variables. Using a variety of quality measurement methods promotes an accurate and comprehensive understanding of the study variables. In addition, researchers want to rigorously control the process for measuring study variables to improve the design validity and quality of the study findings. Artinian et al. (2007) described their precise measurement of the dependent variable, BP, with a valid, nationally standardized device:

> The outcome measure of the BP was measured with electronic BP monitor (Omron HEM-737 Intellisense, Omron Healthcare, Inc., Vernon Hills, IL) that has been validated in accordance with the criteria of the British Hypertension Society and the Association of the Advancement of Medical Instrumentations (Dabl Educational Trust, 2005). (Artinian et al., 2007, p. 316)

Measurement concepts, process, and strategies are the foci of Chapters 15 and 16.

Subjects' Knowledge of a Study

Subjects' knowledge of a study could influence their behavior and possibly alter the research outcomes. This threatens the validity or accuracy of the study design. An example of this type of threat to design validity is the Hawthorne effect, which was identified during the classic experiments at the Hawthorne plant of the Western Electric Company during the late 1920s and early 1930s. The employees at this plant exhibited a particular psychological response when they became research subjects: They changed their behavior simply because they were subjects in a study, not because of the research treatment. In these studies, the researcher manipulated the working conditions (altered the lighting, decreased work hours, changed payment, and increased rest periods) to examine the effects on worker productivity (Homans, 1965).

The subjects in both the treatment group (whose work conditions were changed) and the control group (whose work conditions were not changed) increased their productivity. The subjects seemed to change their behaviors (increase their productivity) solely in response to being part of a study. In the study by Artinian et al. (2007, p. 321), both the treatment and the comparison groups experienced decreases in their blood pressures and the researchers indicated "the Hawthorne effect may have been a factor, with participants paying more attention to their BP and hypertension self-care behaviors because they were aware of their participation in the study."

There are several ways to strengthen a study by decreasing the threats to design validity and selecting the strongest design for the proposed study. Chapter 10 addresses design validity, and Chapter 11 focuses on the process for selecting an appropriate study design. Your understanding of rigor and control provide the basis for the implementation of the steps of the quantitative research process, which are precisely executed in descriptive, correlational, quasi-experimental, and experimental research.

STEPS OF THE QUANTITATIVE RESEARCH PROCESS

The quantitative research process involves conceptualizing a research project, planning and implementing that project, and communicating the findings. Figure 3-1 identifies the steps of the quantitative research process and shows the logical flow of this process as each step progressively builds on the previous steps. This research process is also flexible and fluid, with a flow back and forth among the steps as the researcher strives to clarify the steps and strengthen the proposed study. This flow back and forth among the steps is indicated in the figure by the two-way arrows connecting the steps of the process. Figure 3-1 also contains a feedback arrow, which indicates that the research process is cyclical, for each study provides a basis for generating further research in the development of knowledge for evidence-based practice.

In this chapter, we briefly introduce you to the steps of the quantitative research process, and we present them in detail in Unit Two, The Research Process (Chapter 5 through 22, 24, and 25). The descriptive correlational study conducted by Hulme and Grove (1994), on the symptoms of female survivors of child sexual abuse, is used as an example for introducing the steps of the research process; quotations from and descriptions of this study appear throughout this section.

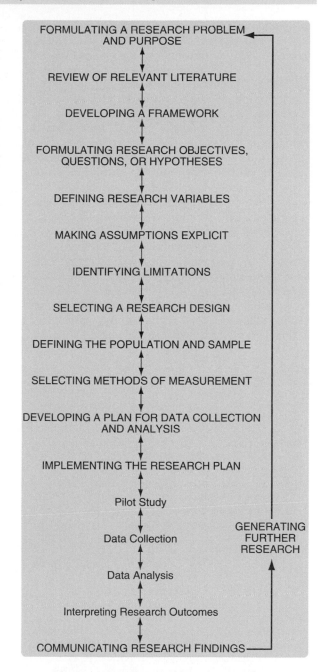

Figure **3-1** Steps of the quantitative research process.

Formulating a Research Problem and Purpose

A **research problem** is an area of concern where there is a gap in the knowledge base needed for nursing practice. The problem identifies an area of concern for a particular population and often indicates the concepts to be studied. The major sources for nursing research problems include nursing practice, researcher and peer interactions, literature review, theory, and research priorities. As a researcher, you will use deductive reasoning to generate a research problem from a research topic or a broad problem area of personal interest that is relevant to nursing.

The research purpose is generated from the problem and identifies the specific goal or aim of the study. The goal of a study might be to identify, describe, explain, or predict a solution to a situation. The purpose often indicates the type of study to be conducted (descriptive, correlational, quasi-experimental, or experimental) and usually includes the variables, population, and setting for the study.

As the clarity and conciseness of a research problem and purpose improve, you will be able to determine the feasibility of conducting the study. Chapter 5 provides a background for formulating a research problem and purpose. Hulme and Grove (1994) identified the following problem and purpose for their study of female survivors of child sexual abuse.

■ PROBLEM

The actual prevalence of child sexual abuse is unknown but is thought to be high. Bagley and King (1990) were able to generalize from compiled research that at least 20% of all women in the samples surveyed had been victims of serious sexual abuse involving unwanted or coerced sexual contact up to the age of 17 years. Evidence indicates that the prevalence is greater for women born after 1960 than before (Bagley, 1990).

The impact of child sexual abuse on the lives of the girl victims and the women they become has only lately received the attention it deserves.… The knowledge generated from research and theory has slowly forced the recognition of the long-term effects of child sexual abuse on both the survivors and society as a whole.… Brown and Garrison (1990) developed the Adult Survivors of Incest (ASI) Questionnaire to identify the patterns of symptoms and the factors contributing to the severity of these symptoms in survivors of childhood sexual abuse. This tool requires additional testing to determine its usefulness in identifying symptoms and contributing factors of adult survivors of incest and other types of child sexual abuse. (Hulme & Grove, 1994, pp. 519–520)

■ PURPOSE

The purpose of this study was twofold: (a) to describe the patterns of physical and psychosocial symptoms in female sexual abuse survivors using the ASI Questionnaire, and (b) to examine relationships among the symptoms and identified contributing factors. (Hulme & Grove, 1994, p. 520)

The research purpose clearly indicates that the focus of this study is both descriptive and correlational.

Review of Relevant Literature

A review of relevant literature is conducted to generate an understanding of what is known about a particular situation or phenomenon and the knowledge gaps that exist. Relevant literature refers to those sources that are pertinent or highly important in providing the in-depth knowledge needed to study a selected problem. This background enables you as a researcher to build on the works of others. The concepts and interrelationships of the concepts in the problem will guide your selection of relevant theories and studies for review. We review theories to clarify the definitions of concepts and to develop and refine the study framework.

By reviewing relevant studies, you will be able to clarify (1) which problems have been investigated, (2) which require further investigation or replication, and (3) which have not been investigated. In addition, the literature review can direct you in designing the study and interpreting the outcomes (see Chapter 6). Hulme and Grove's (1994) review of the literature covered relevant theories and studies related to child sexual abuse and its contributing factors and long-term effects, as shown in the following extracts:

Theorists indicated that … the act of child sexual abuse can be explained as an abuse of power by a trusted parent figure, usually male, on a dependent child, violating the child's body, mind, and spirit. The family, which normally functions to nurture and protect the child from harm, is viewed as not fulfilling this function, leaving the child to feel further betrayed and powerless. Acceptance of the immediate psychological trauma of child sexual abuse has given impetus for acknowledging the long-term effects.

Studies of both nonclinical and clinical populations have lent support to these theoretical developments. When compared with control groups consisting of women who had not been sexually abused as children, survivors of child sexual abuse consistently have higher incidence of depression and lower self-esteem. Other psychosocial long-term effects encountered include suicidal plans, anxiety, distorted body image, decreased sexual satisfaction, poor general social adjustment, lower positive affect, negative personality characteristics, and feeling different from significant others.... The physical long-term effects suggested by research include gastrointestinal problems such as ulcers, spastic colitis, irritable bowel syndrome, and chronic abdominal pain; gynecological disorders; chronic headache; obesity; and increased lifetime surgeries.

Studies of contributing factors that may affect the traumatic impact of child sexual abuse are less in number and less conclusive than those which identify long-term effects. However, poor family functioning, increased age difference between the victim and perpetrator, threat or use of force or violence, multiple abusers, parent or primary caretaker as perpetrator, prolonged or intrusive abuse, and strong emotional bond to the perpetrator with betrayal of trust may all contribute to the increased severity of the long-term effects. (Hulme & Grove, 1994, pp. 521–522)

Developing a Framework

A framework is the abstract, logical structure of meaning that will guide the development of your study and enable you as the researcher to link the findings to the body of knowledge used in nursing practice. In quantitative research, the framework is often a testable midrange theory that has been developed in nursing or in another discipline, such as psychology, physiology, or sociology. The framework may also be developed inductively from clinical observations.

The terms related to frameworks are *concept, relational statement, theory,* and *framework map.* A concept is a term to which abstract meaning is attached. A relational statement or proposition declares that a relationship of some kind exists between two or more concepts. A theory consists of an integrated set of defined concepts and propositions that present a view of a phenomenon and can be used to describe, explain, predict, or control the phenomenon. The propositions or relationship statements of the theory, not the theory itself, are tested through research.

A study framework can be expressed as a map or a diagram of the relationships that provide the basis for a study or can be presented in narrative format. The steps for developing a framework are described in Chapter 7. The framework for Hulme and Grove's (1994) study, described in the following quotation, is based on Browne and Finkelhor's (1986) theory of traumagenic dynamics in the impact of child sexual abuse.

■ *FRAMEWORK*

As shown in [Figure 3-2], child sexual abuse is at the center of the adult survivor's existence. Arising from the abuse are four trauma-causing dynamics: traumatic sexualization, betrayal, powerlessness, and stigmatization. These traumagenic dynamics lead to behavioral manifestations and collectively indicate a history of child sexual abuse. The behavioral manifestations were operationalized as physical and psychosocial symptoms for the purposes of this study. Piercing the adult survivor are the contributing factors, which are characteristics of the child sexual abuse or other factors occurring later in the survivor's life, that affect the severity of behavioral manifestations (Follette, Alexander, & Follette, 1991). The contributing factors examined in this study were age when the abuse began, duration of the abuse, and other victimizations. Other victimizations included past or present physical and emotional abuse, rape, control by others, and prostitution. (Hulme & Grove, 1994, pp. 522–523)

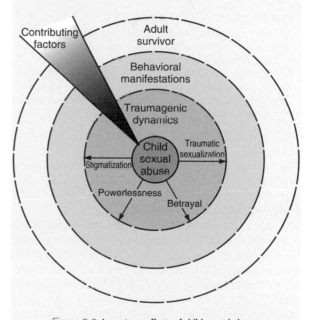

Figure 3-2 Long-term effects of child sexual abuse.

Formulating Research Objectives, Questions, or Hypotheses

Research objectives, questions, and hypotheses bridge the gap between the more abstractly stated research problem and purpose and the study design and plan for data collection and analysis. Objectives, questions, and hypotheses are narrower in focus than the research purpose and often (1) specify only one or two research variables, (2) identify the relationship between the variables, and (3) indicate the population to be studied.

Some quantitative studies do not include objectives, questions, or hypotheses; the development of such a study is directed by the research purpose. Many descriptive studies include only a research purpose, and other descriptive studies include a purpose and objectives or questions. Some correlational studies include a purpose and specific questions or hypotheses. Quasi-experimental and experimental studies often use hypotheses to direct the development and implementation of the studies and the interpretation of findings. Chapter 8 examines the development of research objectives, questions, and hypotheses. Hulme and Grove (1994) developed the following research questions to direct their descriptive-correlational study.

■ *RESEARCH QUESTIONS*
1. What patterns of physical and psychosocial symptoms are present in women 18 to 40 years of age who have experienced child sexual abuse?
2. Are there relationships among the number of physical and psychosocial symptoms, the age when the abuse began, the duration of abuse, and number of other victimizations? (Hulme & Grove, 1994, p. 523)

The focus of question 1 is description and that of question 2 is correlation, or examination of relationships.

Defining Research Variables

The research purpose and the objectives, questions, or hypotheses identify the variables you will be examining in your study. Research **variables** are concepts of various levels of abstraction that are measured, manipulated, or controlled in a study. The more concrete concepts, such as temperature, weight, and blood pressure, are referred to as "variables." The more abstract concepts, such as creativity, empathy, and social support, are sometimes referred to as "research concepts."

The variables or concepts in a study are operationalized when they are conceptually and operationally defined. A **conceptual definition** provides a variable or concept with theoretical meaning (Fawcett, 1999) and either is derived from a theorist's definition of the concept or is developed through concept analysis. An **operational definition** allows the variable to be measured or manipulated in a study. The knowledge

you gain from studying the variable will increase your understanding of the theoretical concept that the variable represents (see Chapter 8).

Hulme and Grove (1994) provided conceptual and operational definitions of the study variables identified in their purpose and research questions: physical and psychosocial symptoms, age when abuse began, duration of abuse, and multiple victimizations. Only the definitions for physical symptoms and multiple victimizations are presented as examples here.

■ *PHYSICAL SYMPTOMS*

Conceptual Definition
Physical symptoms are "behavioral manifestations that result directly from the traumagenic dynamics of child sexual abuse." (Hulme & Grove, 1994, p. 522)

Operational Definition
The ASI Questionnaire was used to measure physical symptoms.

■ *MULTIPLE VICTIMIZATIONS*

Conceptual Definition
Adult survivor who has experienced multiple forms of abuse, including "past and present physical and emotional abuse, rape, control by others, and prostitution." (Hulme & Grove, 1994, p. 523)

Operational Definition
The ASI Questionnaire was used to measure victimizations.

Making Assumptions Explicit

Assumptions are statements that are taken for granted or are considered true, even though they have not been scientifically tested (Silva, 1981). Assumptions are often embedded (unrecognized) in thinking and behavior, and uncovering them requires introspection. Sources of assumptions include universally accepted truths (e.g., all humans are rational beings), theories, previous research, and nursing practice (Myers, 1982).

In studies, assumptions are embedded in the philosophical base of the framework, study design, and interpretation of findings. Theories and instruments are developed on the basis of assumptions that the researcher may or may not recognize. These assumptions influence the development and implementation of the research process. Being able to recognize assumptions is a strength, not a weakness. Assumptions influence the logic of the study, so their recognition leads to more rigorous study development.

Williams (1980) reviewed published nursing studies and other health care literature to identify commonly embedded assumptions, which include the following:

1. People want to assume control of their own health problems.
2. Stress should be avoided.
3. People are aware of the experiences that most affect their life choices.
4. Health is a priority for most people.
5. People in underserved areas feel underserved.
6. Most measurable attitudes are held strongly enough to direct behavior.
7. Health professionals view health care in a different manner than do lay persons.
8. People operate on the basis of cognitive information.
9. Increased knowledge about an event lowers anxiety about the event.
10. Receipt of health care at home is preferable to receipt of care in an institution. (Williams, 1980, p. 48)

Hulme and Grove (1994) did not identify assumptions for their study, but the following assumptions seem to provide a basis for it: (1) the child victim bears no responsibility for the sexual contact, (2) some survivors remember and are willing to report their past child sexual abuse, and (3) physical and psychological signs and symptoms indicate lack of optimal health and functioning.

Identifying Limitations

Limitations are restrictions or problems in a study that may decrease the generalizability of the findings. The two types of limitations are theoretical and methodological.

Theoretical limitations are weaknesses in a study framework and conceptual and operational definitions of variables that restrict the abstract generalization of the findings. Theoretical limitations include the following:

1. A concept might not be clearly defined in the theory used to develop the study framework.
2. The relationships among some concepts might not be identified or are unclear in the theorist's work.
3. A study variable might not be clearly linked to a concept in the framework.
4. An objective, question, or hypothesis might not be clearly linked to a relationship or proposition in the study framework.

Methodological limitations are weaknesses in the study design that can limit the credibility of the findings and restrict the population to which the findings

can be generalized. Methodological limitations result from factors such as unrepresentative samples, weak designs, single setting, limited control over treatment (intervention) implementation, instruments with limited reliability and validity, limited control over data collection, and improper use of statistical analyses. Limitations regarding design (see Chapter 10), sampling (see Chapter 14), measurement (see Chapter 15), and data collection (see Chapter 17) are discussed later in this text. Some theoretical and methodological limitations are identified before the conduct of the study, and researchers minimize these limitations as much as possible. However, some limitations are not identified until the study is conducted and are identified in the discussion section of the study report with implications of how they might have influenced the study findings. Hulme and Grove (1994) identified the following methodological limitation.

■ *METHODOLOGICAL LIMITATION*
This study has limited generalizability due to the relatively small nonprobability sample.... Additional replications drawing from various social classes and age groups are needed to improve the generalizability of Brown and Garrison's (1990) findings and establish reliability and validity of their tool. (Hulme & Grove, 1994, pp. 528–529)

Selecting a Research Design
A research design is a blueprint for maximizing control over factors that could interfere with a study's desired outcome. The type of design directs the selection of a population, sampling procedure, methods of measurement, and a plan for data collection and analysis. The choice of research design depends on the researcher's expertise, the problem and purpose for the study, and the desire to generalize the findings.

Designs have been developed to meet unique research needs as they emerge; thus, a variety of descriptive, correlational, quasi-experimental, and experimental designs have been generated over time. In descriptive and correlational studies, no treatment is administered, so the study design centers on improving the precision of measurement. Quasi-experimental and experimental study designs usually involve treatment and control groups and focus on achieving high levels of control, as well as precision in measurement (Cook & Campbell, 1963, Kerlinger & Lee, 2000). Chapter 10 covers the purpose of a design and the threats to design validity. Chapter 11 presents models and descriptions of several types of descriptive, correlational, quasi-experimental, and experimental designs.

MEASUREMENT OF VARIABLES

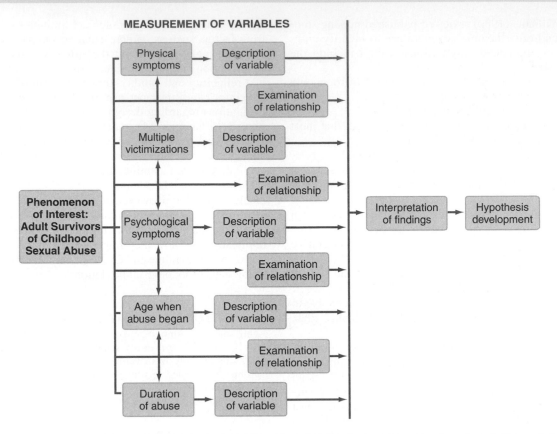

Figure 3-3 Proposed descriptive correlational design for the Hulme and Grove (1994) study of symptoms of female survivors of child sexual abuse.

Hulme and Grove (1994) used a descriptive correlational design to direct their study. A diagram of the design, presented in Figure 3-3, identifies the phenomenon of interest (adult survivors of childhood sexual abuse); variables measured and described (physical symptoms, multiple victimization, psychological symptoms, age when abuse began, and duration of abuse); and the relationships examined among variables. The findings generated from descriptive-correlational research provide a basis for generating hypotheses for testing in future research.

Defining the Population and Sample

The population is all the elements (individuals, objects, or substances) that meet certain criteria for inclusion in a given universe (Kaplan, 1964; Kerlinger & Lee, 2000). For example, suppose you wanted to conduct a study to describe patients' responses to nurse practitioners as their primary care providers. You could define the population in different ways: It could include all patients being seen for the first time in (1) a single clinic, (2) all clinics in a specific network in one city, or (3) all clinics in that network nationwide. Your definition of the population would depend on the sample criteria and the similarity of subjects in these various settings. The researcher must determine which population is accessible and can be best represented by the study sample.

A sample is a subset of the population that is selected for a particular study, and sampling defines the process for selecting a group of people, events, behaviors, or other elements with which to conduct a study. Nursing studies use both probability (random) and nonprobability (nonrandom) sampling methods (see Chapter 14). The following quotation identifies the sampling method, setting, sample size, population, sample criteria, and sample characteristics for the study conducted by Hulme and Grove (1994).

■ SAMPLE

The convenience sample [nonrandom sampling method] was obtained by advertising for subjects at three state universities in the southwest [setting]. Despite the sensitive nature of the study, 22 [sample size] usable interviews were obtained. The sample included women [population] between the ages of 18 and 39 years (mean = 28 years, SD = 6.5 years) who were identified as survivors of child sexual abuse [sample criteria]. The majority of these women were white (91%) and students (82%). A little more than half (54%) were single, seven (32%) were divorced, and three (14%) were married. Most (64%) had no children. A small percentage (14%) was on some form of public assistance and only 14% had been arrested. Although 27% of the subjects had stepfamily members, the parents of 14 subjects (64%) were still married. Half the fathers were working class or self-employed; the rest were professionals. Mothers were either working class or self-employed (50%), homemakers (27%), or professionals (11%). Most subjects (95%) had siblings, and 36% knew or suspected their siblings also had been abused [sample characteristics]. (Hulme & Grove, 1994, pp. 523–524)

Selecting Methods of Measurement

Measurement is the process of assigning "numbers to objects (or events or situations) in accord with some rule" (Kaplan, 1964, p.177). A component of measurement is instrumentation, which is the application of specific rules to the development of a measurement device or instrument. An instrument is selected to examine a specific variable in a study. Data generated with an instrument are at the nominal, ordinal, interval, or ratio level of measurement. The level of measurement, with nominal being the lowest form of measurement and ratio being the highest, determines the type of statistical analyses that you can perform on the data.

Selection of an instrument requires extensive examination of its reliability and validity. Reliability assesses how consistently the measurement technique measures a concept. The validity of an instrument is the extent to which it actually reflects the abstract concept being examined. Chapter 15 introduces the concepts of measurement and explains the different types of reliability and validity for instruments. Chapter 16 provides a background for selecting measurement methods for a study. Hulme and Grove (1994) provided the following description of the ASI Questionnaire that was used to measure their study variables.

■ MEASUREMENT METHODS

The ASI Questionnaire contains 10 sections: demographics; family origin; educational history, occupational history and public assistance; legal history; characteristics of the child sexual abuse (duration, perpetrator, pregnancy, type, and threats); past and present other victimizations; past and present physical symptoms; past and present psychosocial symptoms; and relationship with own children. Each section is followed by a response set that includes space for "other." Content validity was established by Brown and Garrison (1990) using an in-depth review of 132 clinical records.... For this descriptive correlational study, content validity of the ASI questionnaire was examined by asking an open-ended question: Is there additional information you would like to share or think is important for describing your experience? (Hulme & Grove, 1994, p. 524)

Developing a Plan for Data Collection and Analysis

Data collection is the precise, systematic gathering of information relevant to the research purpose or the specific objectives, questions, or hypotheses of a study. The data collected in quantitative studies are usually numerical. Planning data collection will enable you to anticipate problems that are likely to occur and to explore possible solutions. Usually, detailed procedures for implementing a treatment and collecting data are developed, with a schedule that identifies the initiation and termination of the process (see Chapter 17).

Planning data analysis is the final step before the study is implemented. The analysis plan is based on (1) the research objectives, questions, or hypotheses; (2) the data to be collected; (3) research design; (4) researcher expertise; and (5) availability of computer resources.

Several statistical analysis techniques are available to describe the sample, examine relationships, or determine significant differences within studies. Most researchers consult a statistician for assistance in developing an analysis plan.

Implementing the Research Plan

Implementing the research plan involves treatment or intervention implementation, data collection, data analysis, interpretation of research findings, and, sometimes, a pilot study.

Pilot Study

A pilot study is commonly defined as a smaller version of a proposed study conducted to refine the methodology (Van Ort, 1981). It is developed much like the proposed study, using similar subjects, the same setting, the same treatment, and the same data collection and analysis techniques. However, you could use a pilot study to develop various steps in the research process (Prescott & Soeken, 1989). For example, you could conduct a pilot study to develop and refine an intervention or treatment, a measurement method, a data collection tool, or the data collection process. Thus, a pilot study could be used to develop a research plan rather than to test an already developed plan.

Some of the reasons for conducting pilot studies are as follows (Prescott & Soeken, 1989; Van Ort, 1981):

1. To determine whether the proposed study is feasible (e.g., are the subjects available, does the researcher have the time and money to do the study?).
2. To develop or refine a research treatment or intervention.
3. To develop a protocol for the implementation of a treatment.
4. To identify problems with a study design.
5. To determine whether the sample is representative of the population or whether the sampling technique is effective.
6. To examine the reliability and validity of the research instruments.
7. To develop or refine data collection instruments.
8. To refine the data collection and analysis plan.
9. To give the researcher experience with the subjects, setting, methodology, and methods of measurement.
10. To try out data analysis techniques.

Hayward et al. (2007) believed that conducting a pilot study improved the strength of their study design and directed their development of a quality proposal for a large multisite trial that received external grant support. Thus, as a researcher you conduct pilot studies to improve the development and implementation of your future major studies.

Data Collection

In quantitative research, data collection involves obtaining numerical data to address the research objectives, questions, or hypotheses. To collect data, you must obtain consent or permission from the setting or agency where the study is to be conducted and from potential subjects. Frequently, the subjects are asked to sign a consent form, which describes the study, promises the subjects confidentiality, and indicates that the subjects can stop participation at any time (see Chapter 9).

During data collection, the study variables are measured through a variety of techniques, such as observation, interview, questionnaires, scales, and physiological measurement methods. In a growing number of studies, nurses measure physiological variables with high-technology equipment. The data are collected and recorded systematically for each subject and are organized to facilitate computer entry. Hulme and Grove (1994) identified the following procedure for data collection:

> Although the tool can be self-reporting, it was administered by personal interview to allow for elaboration of "other" responses. The interviews lasted about one hour and were conducted in a private room provided by The University of Texas at Arlington. Each interview started with a discussion of the study benefits and risks and included signing a consent form. Risks included possible painful memories and embarrassment during the interview as well as emotional and physical discomfort after the interview. Sources of public and private counseling were provided to assist subjects with any difficulties experienced related to the study. (Hulme & Grove, 1994, pp. 524–525)

Data Analysis

Data analysis reduces, organizes, and gives meaning to the data. The analysis of data from quantitative research involves the use of (1) descriptive and exploratory procedures (see Chapter 19) to describe study variables and the sample, (2) statistical techniques to test proposed relationships (see Chapter 20), (3) techniques to make predictions (see Chapter 21), and (4) analysis techniques to examine causality (see Chapter 22). Computers are used to perform most analyses, so Chapter 18 provides a background for using computers in research.

The choice of analysis techniques implemented is determined primarily by the research objectives, questions, or hypotheses; the research design; and the level of measurement achieved by the research instruments. Hulme and Grove (1994) chose frequencies, percentages, means, standard deviations, and Pearson correlations to answer their research questions.

■ RESULTS

The first research question focused on description of the patterns of physical and psychosocial symptoms. Six physical symptoms occurred in 50% or more of the subjects: insomnia, sexual dysfunction, overeating, drug abuse, severe headache, and two or more major surgeries.... Eleven psychosocial symptoms occurred in 75% or more of the subjects: depression, guilt, low self-esteem, inability to trust others, mood swings, suicidal thoughts, difficulty in relationships, confusion, flashbacks of the abuse, extreme anger, and memory lapse.... Self-injurious behavior was reported by eight subjects (33%). (Hulme & Grove, 1994, pp. 527–528)

The second research question focused on the relationships among the number of physical and psychosocial symptoms and three contributing factors (age abuse began, duration of abuse, and multiple victimizations). There were five significant correlations among study variables: physical symptoms with multiple victimizations ($r = 0.59$, $p = 0.002$), physical symptoms with psychosocial symptoms ($r = 0.56$, $p = 0.003$), age abuse began with duration of abuse ($r = 0.50$, $p = 0.009$), psychosocial symptoms with multiple victimizations ($r = 0.40$, $p = 0.033$), and duration of abuse with psychosocial symptoms ($r = 0.40$, $p = 0.034$). (Hulme & Grove, 1994, p. 528)

Interpreting Research Outcomes

The results obtained from data analysis require interpretation to be meaningful. Interpretation of research outcomes involves (1) examining the results from data analysis, (2) exploring the significance of the findings, (3) forming conclusions, (4) generalizing the findings, (5) considering the implications for nursing, and (6) suggesting further studies. Data analysis yields five types of results: significant as predicted by the researcher, nonsignificant, significant but not predicted by the researcher, mixed findings, and unexpected findings. The study results are then translated and interpreted to become findings, and these findings are synthesized to form conclusions. The conclusions provide a basis for identifying nursing implications, generalizing findings, and suggesting further studies (see Chapter 24). In the excerpts that follow, Hulme and Grove (1994) discuss their findings, with implications for nursing and suggestions for further study.

■ DISCUSSION

While this study may have limited generalizability due to the relatively small nonprobability sample, the findings do support previous research.... In addition, the findings support Browne and Finkelhor's (1986) framework that a wide range of behavioral manifestations (physical and psychosocial symptoms) comprise the long-term effects of child sexual abuse. (Hulme & Grove, 1994, p. 528)

Brown and Garrison's (1990) ASI Questionnaire was effective in identifying patterns of physical and psychosocial symptoms in women with a history of child sexual abuse.... As data on the behavioral manifestations (physical and psychosocial symptoms) and the effect of each of the contributing factors accumulate, hypotheses need to be formulated to further test Browne and Finkelhor's (1986) framework explaining the long-term effects of child sexual abuse.... With additional research, the ASI Questionnaire might be adapted for use in clinical situations. This questionnaire might facilitate identification and delivery of appropriate treatment to female survivors of child sexual abuse in clinical settings. (Hulme & Grove, 1994, pp. 529–530)

Communicating Research Findings

Research is not considered complete until the findings have been communicated. Communicating research findings involves developing and disseminating a research report to appropriate audiences; the research report is disseminated through presentations and publication (see Chapter 25). The Hulme and Grove (1994) study was presented at a national nurse practitioner conference and published in the *Issues in Mental Health Nursing* journal.

TYPES OF QUANTITATIVE RESEARCH

This text describes four types of quantitative research: (1) descriptive, (2) correlational, (3) quasi-experimental, and (4) experimental. The level of existing knowledge for the research problem influences the type of research planned. When little knowledge is available, descriptive studies are often conducted. As the knowledge level increases, correlational, quasi-experimental, and experimental studies are implemented. This section identifies the purpose of each quantitative research approach and presents an example of the steps of the research process from a published quasi-experimental study.

Descriptive Research

The purpose of descriptive research is to explore and describe phenomena in real-life situations. This approach is used to generate new knowledge about concepts or topics about which limited or no research has been conducted. Through descriptive research, concepts are described and relationships are identified that provide a basis for further quantitative research and theory testing. The study by Hulme and Grove

(1994) on the symptoms of female survivors of child sexual abuse, which we used earlier in the chapter to illustrate the basic discussion of the steps of the quantitative research process, is a combined descriptive and correlational study. The descriptive aspects of this study can be clearly identified in its purpose, research questions, design, data analysis, and findings.

Correlational Research

Correlational research examines linear relationships between two or more variables and determines the type (positive or negative) and degree (strength) of the relationship. The strength of a relationship varies from −1 (perfect negative correlation) to +1 (perfect positive correlation), with 0 indicating no relationship. The positive relationship indicates that the variables vary together—that is, the two variables either increase or decrease together. The negative or inverse relationship indicates that the variables vary in opposite directions; thus, as one variable increases, the other decreases. The descriptive correlational study conducted by Hulme and Grove (1994), presented earlier in this chapter, provides an example of the steps of the quantitative research process for correlational research.

Quasi-Experimental Research

The purpose of quasi-experimental research is to examine cause-and-effect relationships among selected independent and dependent variables. Quasi-experimental studies in nursing are conducted to determine the effects of nursing interventions or treatments (independent variables) on patient outcomes (dependent variables) (Cook & Campbell, 1979). Artinian et al. (2007) conducted a quasi-experimental study to determine the effects of nurse-managed telemonitoring (TM) on the BP of African-Americans. The steps for this study, which were introduced earlier in this chapter, are described here and illustrated with extracts from the study.

STEPS OF THE RESEARCH PROCESS IN A QUASI-EXPERIMENTAL STUDY

■ 1: RESEARCH PROBLEM

Nearly one in three, or approximately 65 million adults in the United States have hypertension, defined as (a) having systolic blood pressure (SBP) of 140 mm Hg or higher or diastolic blood pressure (DBP) of at least 90 mm Hg or higher, (b) taking antihypertensive medication, or (c) being told at least twice by a physician or other health professional about having high blood pressure (BP) (American Heart Association [AHA], 2004; AHA Statistics Committee & Stroke Statistics Subcommittee [AHASC], 2006; Fields et al., 2004).... Estimated direct and indirect costs associated with hypertension total $63.5 billion (AHA, 2004).... The crisis of high BP (HBP) is particularly apparent among African Americans; their prevalence of HBP is among the highest in the world.... Unless healthcare professionals can improve care for individuals with hypertension, approximately two thirds of the population will continue to have uncontrolled BP and face other major health risks (Chobanian et al., 2003).... There is a need to test alternative treatment strategies. (Artinian et al., 2007, pp. 312–313)

■ 2: RESEARCH PURPOSE

The purpose of this randomized controlled trial with urban African Americans was to compare usual care (UC) only with BP telemonitoring (TM) plus UC to determine which leads to greater reduction in BP from baseline over 12 months of follow-up, with assessments at 3, 6, and 12 months postbaseline. (Artinian et al., 2007, p. 313)

■ 3: REVIEW OF LITERATURE

The literature review for this study included relevant, current studies that summarized what is known about the impact of TM on BP. The sources were current and ranged in publication dates from 1998 to 2005, with the majority of the studies published in the last 5 years. The study was accepted for publication on May 31, 2007 and published in the September/October 2007 issue of *Nursing Research*. Artinian et al. (2007, p. 314) summarized the current knowledge about the effect of TM on BP by stating "Although promising, the effects of TM on BP have been tested in small, sometimes nonrandomized, samples, with one study suggesting that patients may not always adhere to measuring their BP at home. The influence of TM on BP control warrants further study."

■ 4: FRAMEWORK

Artinian et al. (2007) developed a model that identified the theoretical basis for their study. The model is presented in Figure 3-4 and indicates that nurse-managed TM is an innovative strategy that may offer hope to hypertensive African Americans who have difficulty accessing care for frequent BP checks.... In other words, TM may lead to a reduction in opportunity costs or barriers for obtaining follow-up care by minimizing the contextual risk factors that interfere with frequent healthcare visits.... Combined with information about how to control hypertension, TM may both help individuals gain conscious control over their HBP and contribute to feelings

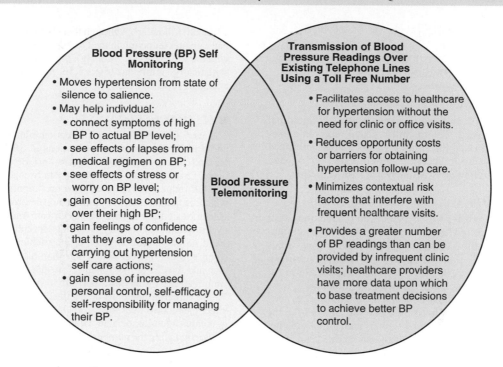

Figure 3-4 Theoretical basis for the effects of telemonitoring on blood pressure.

of confidence for carrying out hypertension self-care actions... Home TM appeared to contribute to individuals' increased personal control and self-responsibility for managing their BP, which ultimately led to improved BP control (Artinian et al., 2004; Artinian, Washington, & Templin, 2001). (Artinian et al., 2007, pp. 313–314) The framework for this study was based on tentative theory that was developed from the findings of previous research by Artinian et al. (2004; 2001) and other investigators. This framework provides a basis for interpreting the study findings and giving them meaning.

■ 5: HYPOTHESIS TESTING

H1: Individuals who participate in UC plus nurse-managed TM will have a greater reduction in BP from baseline at 3-, 6-, and 12-month follow-up than would individuals who receive UC only. (Artinian et al., 2007, p. 317)

■ 6: VARIABLES

The independent variable was TM Program and the dependent variables were SBP and DBP. Only the TM Program and SBP conceptual and operational definitions are presented as examples. The conceptual definitions are derived from the study framework and the operational

definitions are often found in the methods section under measurement methods and intervention headings.

Independent Variable: TM Program
Conceptual Definition

TM program is an innovative strategy that may offer hope to hypertensive African Americans to reduce their opportunity costs and barriers for obtaining follow-up care for BP management (Artinian et al., 2007).

Operational Definition

TM "refers to individuals self-monitoring their BP at home, then transmitting the BP readings over existing telephone lines using a toll-free number" (Artinian et al., 2007, p. 313). The readings were reviewed by the care providers with immediate feedback provided to the patients about their treatment plan.

Independent Variable: SBP
Conceptual Definition

SBP is an indication of the patient's blood pressure control and ultimately the management of his or her hypertension.

Operational Definition

The outcome of SBP was measured with the electronic BP monitor (Omron HEM-737 Intellisense, Omron Health Care, Inc.). (Artinian et al., 2007)

■ 7: DESIGN

A randomized, two-group, experimental, longitudinal design was used. The treatment group received nurse-managed TM and the control group received enhanced UC. Data were collected at baseline and 3-, 6-, and 12-month follow-ups. (Artinian et al., 2007, p. 314)

■ 8: SAMPLE

African Americans with hypertension [population] were recruited through free BP screenings offered at community centers, thrift stores, drug stores, and grocery stores located on the east side of Detroit [natural settings]. (Artinian et al., 2007, p. 315) The sample criteria for including and excluding subjects from the study were detailed and provided a means of identifying patients with hypertension. The sample size was 387 (194 in the TM group and 193 in the UC group) with a 13% attrition or loss of subjects over the 12-month study.

■ 9: PROCEDURES

Artinian et al. (2007) detailed the nurse-managed TM intervention that was presented earlier in this chapter and provided in entirety on pages 315–316 in the research article. The BP was measured with the electronic Omron BP monitor after a 5-minute rest period; at least two BPs were measured, and the average of all was used for analyses. Participants wore unrestrictive clothing and sat next to the interviewer's table, their feet on the floor; their back supported; and their arm abducted, slightly flexed, and supported at heart level by the smooth, firm surface of a table. (Artinian et al., 2007, pp. 316–317)

Most of the data were collected during 2-hour structured face-to-face interviews and brief physical exams, which were conducted by trained interviewers in a private room at one of the project-affiliated neighborhood community centers. Mailed postcards provided interview appointment reminders 1 week before the scheduled interview; telephone call reminders were made the evening before the interview.... Participants were compensated $25.00 after the completion of each interview. (Artinian et al., 2007, p. 316) The study was approved by the Wayne State University Human Investigation Committee and all participants signed consent forms indicating their willingness to be subjects in the study.

■ 10: RESULTS

The hypothesis was supported partially by the data. Overall, the TM intervention group had a greater reduction in SBP (13.0 mm Hg) than the UC group did (7.5 mm Hg; $t = -2.09$, $p = 0.04$) from baseline to the 12-month follow-up. Although the TM intervention group had a greater reduction in the DBP (6.3 mm Hg) compared with the UC group (4.1 mm Hg), the differences were not statistically significant ($t = -1.56$, $p = 0.12$). (Artinian et al., 2007, pp. 317–318)

■ 11: DISCUSSION

The nurse-managed TM group experienced both clinically and statistically significant reductions in SBP (13.0 mm Hg) and clinically significant reductions in DBP (6.3 mm Hg) over a 12-month monitoring period [study conclusions]....
The BP reductions achieved here are important results, which, if maintained over time, could improve care and outcomes significantly for urban African Americans with hypertension.... This may mean that an individual could avoid starting a drug regimen or may achieve BP control using a one-drug regimen rather than a two-drug regimen and thus be at risk for fewer medication side effects [implications of the findings for nursing practice]....
Future research needs to determine if this intervention effect maintained over time leads to reducing the number of complications associated with uncontrolled BP and if it leads to reducing the number of drugs necessary to achieve BP control. (Artinian et al., 2007, pp. 320–321)

Experimental Research

The purpose of experimental research is to examine cause-and-effect relationships between independent and dependent variables under highly controlled conditions (Campbell & Stanley, 1963). The researcher exerts high control over the planning and implementation of experimental studies, and often these studies are conducted in a laboratory setting on animals or objects. The Graves et al. (2005) study introduced earlier in this chapter is an experimental study of the effect of a diet supplemented with 0.5% conjugated linoleic acid (CLA) on muscle mass in mice with cancer that was conducted in a laboratory setting. To improve your understanding of the steps of the research process, read this study and identify the steps of quantitative research process outlined in this chapter.

SUMMARY

- Nurses use a broad range of quantitative approaches—including descriptive, correlational, quasi-experimental, and experimental—to develop nursing knowledge.
- Some of the concepts relevant to quantitative research are (1) basic and applied research, (2) rigor, and (3) control.

- Basic, or pure, research is a scientific investigation that involves the pursuit of "knowledge for knowledge's sake" or for the pleasure of learning and finding truth.
- Applied, or practical, research is a scientific investigation conducted to generate knowledge that will directly influence or improve clinical practice.
- Rigor involves discipline, scrupulous adherence to detail, and strict accuracy.
- Control involves the imposing of "rules" by the researcher to decrease the possibility of error and thus increase the probability that the study's findings are an accurate reflection of reality.
- The quantitative research process involves conceptualizing a research project, planning and implementing that project, and communicating the findings.
- The steps of the quantitative research process are as follows:
  1. *Formulating a research problem and purpose* identifies an area of concern and the specific goal or aim of the study.
  2. *Reviewing relevant literature* allows the researcher to build a picture of what is known about a particular situation or phenomenon and identify the knowledge gaps that exist.
  3. *Developing a framework* guides the development of the study and enables the researcher to link the findings to the body of knowledge in nursing.
  4. *Formulating research objectives, questions, or hypotheses* allows the researcher to bridge the gap between the more abstractly stated research problem and purpose and the study design and plan for data collection and analysis.
  5. *Operationalizing research variables* involves developing a conceptual definition and operational definition for each variable.
  6. *Identifying theoretical and methodological limitations* involves determining the restrictions in a study that may decrease the generalizability of the findings.
  7. *Selecting a research design* directs the selection of a population, sampling procedure, methods of measurement, and a plan for data collection and analysis.
  8. *Defining the population and sample* determines who will participate in the study.
  9. *Selecting methods of measurement* involves determining the best method(s) to measure each study variable.
  10. *Developing a plan for data collection and analysis* directs the precise, systematic gathering of information relevant to the research purpose or the specific objectives, questions, or hypotheses of a study and involves the selection of appropriate statistical techniques to analyze the study data.
  11. *Implementing the research plan* involves treatment implementation, data collection, data analysis, and interpretation of research outcomes.
  12. *Communicating findings* includes the development and dissemination of a research report to appropriate audiences through presentations and publication.
- This chapter introduces four types of quantitative research: descriptive, correlational, quasi-experimental, and experimental. Examples from published studies are used to illustrate the steps of the quantitative research process.

REFERENCES

American Heart Association. (2004). *Heart disease and stroke statistics: 2005 update*. Dallas, TX: Author.

American Health Association Statistics Committee and Stroke Statistics Subcommittee. (2006). Heart disease and stroke statistics: 2006 update. *Circulation, 113*(6), e85–e152.

Artinian, N. T., Flack, J. M., Nordstrom, C. K., Hockman, E. M., Washington, O. G. M., Jen, K. C., et al. (2007). Effects of nurse-managed telemonitoring on blood pressure at 12-month follow-up among urban African Americans. *Nursing Research, 56*(5), 312–322.

Artinian, N. T., Washington, O. G., Klymko, K. W., Marbury, C. M., Miller, W. M., & Powell, J. L. (2004). What you need to know about home blood pressure telemonitoring, but may not know to ask. *Home Healthcare Nurse, 22*(10), 680–686.

Artinian, N. T., Washington, O. G., & Templin, T. N. (2001). Effects of home telemonitoring and community-based monitoring on blood pressure control in urban African Americans: A pilot study. *Heart & Lung, 30*(3), 191–199.

Bagley, C. (1990). Development of a measure of unwanted sexual contact in childhood, for use in community health surveys. *Psychology Reports, 66*(2), 401–402.

Bagley, C., & King, K. K. (1990). *Child sexual abuse: The search for healing*. New York: Travistock/Routledge.

Bond, E. F., & Heitkemper, M. M. (1987). Importance of basic physiologic research in nursing science. *Heart & Lung, 16*(4), 347–349.

Brown, B. E., & Garrison, C. J. (1990). Patterns of symptomatology of adult women incest survivors. *Western Journal of Nursing Research, 12*(5), 587–600.

Browne, A., & Finkelhor, D. (1986). Initial and long-term effects: A review of the research. In D. Finkelhor (Ed.): *A source book on child sexual abuse* (pp. 143–179). Beverly Hills, CA: Sage Publications.

Campbell, D. T., & Stanley, J. C. (1963). *Experimental and quasi-experimental designs for research*. Chicago: Rand McNally.

Chobanian, A., Bakris, G., Black, H., Cushman, W., Green, L., Izzo, J., Jr., et al. (2003). Seventh report of the Joint National Committee on Prevention, Detection, Evaluation, and Treatment of High Blood Pressure. *Hypertension, 42*(6), 1206–1252.

Cook, T. D., & Campbell, D. T. (1979). *Quasi-experimentation: Design and analysis issues for field settings.* Chicago: Rand McNally.

Dabl Educational Trust. (2005). *Device table: Upper arm devices for self-measurement of blood pressure.* Retrieved October 2, 2007, from www.dableducational.com/sphygmomanometers.html.

Fawcett, J. (1999). *The relationship of theory and research* (3rd ed.). Philadelphia: F.A. Davis.

Fields, L., Burt, V., Cutler, J., Hughers, J., Roccella, E., & Sorlie, P. (2004). The burden of adult hypertension in the United States 1999–2000: A rising tide. *Hypertension, 44*(4), 398–404.

Fisher, Sir R. A. (1935). *The designs of experiments.* New York: Hafner.

Follette, N. M., Alexander, P. C., & Follette, W. C. (1991). Individual predictors of outcome in group treatment for incest survivors. *Journal of Consulting and Clinical Psychology, 59*(1), 150–155.

Graves, E., Hitt, A., Pariza, M. W., Cook, M. E., & McCarthy, D. O. (2005). Conjugated linoleic acid preserves gastrocnemius muscle mass in mice bearing the colon-26 adenocarcinoma. *Nursing Research & Health, 28*(1), 48–55.

Hayward, K., Campbell-Yeo, M., Price, S., Morrison, D., Whyte, R., Cake, H. et al. (2007). Cobedding twins: How pilot study findings guided improvements in planning a larger multicenter trial. *Nursing Research, 56*(2), 137–143.

Homans, G. (1965). Group factors in worker productivity. In H. Proshansky & B. Seidenberg (Eds.), *Basic studies in social psychology* (pp. 592–604). New York: Holt, Rinehart & Winston.

Hulme, P. A., & Grove, S. K. (1994). Symptoms of female survivors of child sexual abuse. *Issues in Mental Health Nursing, 15*(5), 519–532.

Kaplan, A. (1964). The conduct of inquiry: *Methodology for behavioral science.* New York: Chandler.

Kerlinger, F. N., & Lee, H. B. (2000). *Foundations of behavioral research* (4th ed.). New York: Harcourt Brace.

Melnyk, B. M., & Fineout-Overholt, E. (2005). *Evidence-based practice in nursing & healthcare: A guide to best practice.* Philadelphia: Lippincott Williams & Wilkins.

Myers, S. T. (1982). The search for assumptions. *Western Journal of Nursing Research, 4*(1), 91–98.

Nagel, E. (1961). *The structure of science: Problems in the logic of scientific explanation.* New York: Harcourt, Brace & World.

Prescott, P. A., & Soeken, K. L. (1989). Methodology corner: The potential uses of pilot work. *Nursing Research, 38*(1), 60–62.

Ryan, P., & Lauver, D. R. (2002). The efficacy of tailored interventions. *Journal of Nursing Scholarship, 34*(4), 331–337.

Santacroce, S. J., Maccarelli, L. M., & Grey, M. (2004). Methods: Intervention fidelity. *Nursing Research, 53*(1), 63–66.

Sidani, S., & Braden, C. J. (1998). *Evaluating nursing interventions: A theory-driven approach.* Thousand Oaks, CA: Sage.

Silva, M. C. (1981). Selection of a theoretical framework. In S. D. Krampitz & N. Pavlovich (Eds.), *Readings for nursing research* (pp. 17–28). St. Louis: C.V. Mosby.

Van Ort, S. (1981). Research design: Pilot study. In S. D. Krampitz & N. Pavlovich (Eds.), *Readings for nursing research* (pp. 49–53). St. Louis: C.V. Mosby.

Wallenstein, S. L. (1987). Issues in pain research. Research perspectives: A response. *Journal of Pain and Symptom Management, 2*(2), 103–106.

Williams, M. A. (1980). Assumptions in research [Editorial]. *Research in Nursing & Health, 3*(2), 47–48.

Wysocki, A. B. (1983). Basic versus applied research: Intrinsic and extrinsic considerations. *Western Journal of Nursing Research, 5*(3), 217–224.

CHAPTER **4**

Introduction to Qualitative Research

Qualitative research is a systematic, subjective approach used to describe life experiences and give them significance. It is a way to gain insights through discovering meanings. These insights are obtained not through establishing causality but through improving our comprehension of the whole. Within a holistic framework, qualitative research allows us to explore the depth, richness, and complexity inherent in phenomena. The insights from this process can guide nursing practice and aid in the important process of theory development for building nursing knowledge (Anfara & Martz, 2006; Flinders & Mills, 1993). Although qualitative research is flexible and evolving, it is a systematic and precise process that requires high skill in conceptualization, imaginative reasoning, and elegant expression.

To critically appraise studies in publications, use the findings in practice, and develop the skills needed to conduct qualitative research, you must comprehend qualitative research methodologies. Nurse researchers conducting qualitative studies are contributing important information to our body of knowledge that cannot be obtained by quantitative means. The terminology used in qualitative research and the methods of reasoning are different from those of quantitative research and are reflections of the philosophical orientations of qualitative research. The specific philosophical orientation differs with each qualitative approach and directs the methodology and interpretation of data. Although each qualitative approach is unique, there are many commonalities. To help you comprehend these methodologies, in this chapter we explore the logic underlying the qualitative approach, using gestalt change as a model. The chapter presents a general overview of the following qualitative approaches: phenomenological research, grounded theory research, ethnographic research, historical research, philosophical inquiry, and critical social theory.

THE LOGIC OF QUALITATIVE RESEARCH

The qualitative approaches are based on a holistic worldview that has the following beliefs:
1. There is not a single reality.
2. Reality, based on perceptions, is different for each person and changes over time.
3. What we know has meaning only within a given situation or context.

The reasoning process used in qualitative research involves perceptually putting pieces together to make wholes. From this process, meaning is produced. Because perception varies with the individual, many meanings are possible. You can understand this reasoning process by exploring the formation of gestalts.

GESTALTS

The concept of gestalt is closely related to holism and proposes that knowledge about a particular phenomenon is organized into a cluster of linked ideas, a gestalt. A theory is a form of gestalt. If we are trying to understand something new and are offered a theory that explains it, our reaction may be "Now that makes sense" or "Oh, I see." The concept has "come together" for us.

One disadvantage of this process is that once we understand a phenomenon through the interpretation of a particular theory, it is difficult for us to "see" the phenomenon outside the meaning given it by that particular theory. Therefore, in addition to giving meaning, a theory can limit meaning. "Seeing" the phenomenon from the perspective of one point of view may limit our ability to see it from another point of view. For example, because Selye's theory of stress is so familiar to us as nurses, it would be difficult to examine the phenomenon of stress without using Selye's perception.

Experiencing Gestalt Change

One qualitative researcher, Ihde (1977), has explained the process of (1) forming a gestalt, (2) "getting outside" that gestalt, and (3) developing a new gestalt in such a way that you can experience the process. Experiencing the process is the best way to understand it.

Ihde (1977) conducted his extensive research in the area of vision. He has studied how our eyes and brain perceive an image—for example, how our eyes sometimes see one line as shorter or longer than another when the lines are actually equal in length. Ihde associated the vision of the eye with the way we "see" mentally. Consider the concrete thinking behind sayings such as "seeing makes it real," "seeing is believing," and "I saw it with my own eyes." It is easy to generalize from seeing to the other senses (hearing, touching, smelling, tasting), or empirical ways of knowing, and from there to perception. In fact, we often use phrases such as "I see" or "I hear you" to mean "I understand."

Ihde (1977) proposed that we have an initial way of perceiving (or seeing) a phenomenon that is naive and inflexible but that we believe is the one and only way of seeing the phenomenon that is real. "Seeing" occurs, however, within a specific context of beliefs, which Ihde called a natural or sedimented view. In other words, we see things from the perspective of a specific frame of reference, worldview, or theory. This is our reality, which gives us a sense of certainty, security, and control. Ihde used line drawings to demonstrate this sedimented view. Examine the following line drawing:

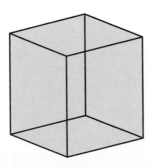

Most people who passively view this figure see a cube. If you continue to gaze at it, however, you will find that the cube reverses itself. The figure actually seems to move. It "jumps" and then becomes fixed again in your view. With practice, you can see first one view and then the other, and then reverse the cube again.

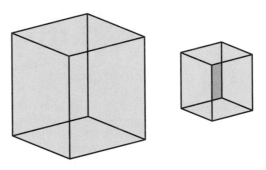

Ihde (1977) developed five alternative ways to view the following drawing and suggested that there are more. He referred to the smaller cube on the right as the "guide picture":

Suppose, now, that the cube drawing is not a cube at all, but is an insect in a hexagonal opening.... Suppose I tell you that the cube is not a cube at all, but is a very oddly cut gem. The central facet (the shaded area of the guide picture) is nearest you, and all the other facets are sloping downwards and away from it.... Now, suppose I tell you that the gem is also reversible. Suppose you are now inside the gem, looking upwards, so that the central facet (the shaded area of the guide picture) is the one farthest away from you, and the oddly cut side facets are sloping down towards you. (Idhe, 1977, pp. 96–98)

Ihde proposed that to see an alternative view of the drawing, you must first deconstruct your original sedimented view. You must then reconstruct another view. This activity involves the use of intuition. He regarded this process as jumping from one gestalt to another.

Try examining the line drawing shown here. What is your sedimented view? Can you reconstruct another gestalt or view?

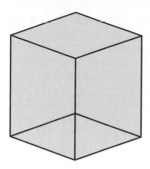

Ihde (1977) found that one important strategy for switching from one view of a drawing to another was to change one's focus. Try focusing on a different point of the drawing or looking at it as two-dimensional rather than as three-dimensional. If you concentrate and gaze for a long enough time, you can experience the change in gestalt. Ihde cautioned that a new reconstruction tends to be considered odd at first and unnatural but attains stability and naturalness after a while.

Once you have accomplished this "jump," you are no longer naive; you cannot go back to the idea that the phenomenon you have observed can be seen in only one way. You have become more open and receptive to experiencing the phenomenon; you can explore deeper layers of the phenomenon. Viewing these deeper layers requires a second-order deconstruction and an additional increase in openness. Ihde (1977) referred to this increase as ascendance to an open context. It allows you to see more depth and complexity within the phenomenon you examine; you have enlarged your capacity for insight. Ihde suggested that ascendance to the open context gives you multistability and greater control than the sedimented view.

Changing Gestalts in Nursing

Nursing has a strong traditional base. With this tradition comes a sedimented view of phenomena such as patients, illness situations, health, and nursing care and its effects. We are introduced to these sedimented views early in our nursing experiences. Now, in this era of nursing research, we are beginning to question many of these long-held ideas, and the insights gained are changing nursing practice.

For example, for many years, nurses perceived the patient as being passive, dependent, and unable to take responsibility for his or her care. Now, nurses more often view patients as participating in their care and being responsible for their health. Ascendance to the open context requires more than just switching from

one sedimented view to another. The nurse functioning within an open context would be able to view the patient from a variety of perspectives, regarding him or her as passive and dependent in some ways, participating with health care providers in other ways, and directing his or her care in yet other ways.

Qualitative research provides a process through which we can examine a phenomenon outside the sedimented view. The earliest and perhaps most dramatic demonstration of the influence that qualitative research can have on nursing practice was the 4-year study conducted by Glaser and Strauss (1965, 1968, 1971), who used a qualitative approach referred to as *grounded theory*. This study was reported in three books titled *Awareness of Dying, Time for Dying*, and *Status Passage*. These books described the social environment of dying patients in hospitals. At that time, the gestalt commonly held was that people could not cope with knowing that they were dying and must be protected from that knowledge. The environment of care was designed to keep from a dying patient the knowledge that he or she was dying.

Glaser and Strauss examined the meanings this social environment had to the patient. The study changed our gestalt. We now saw that instead of protecting the patient, traditional care of the dying was creating loneliness and isolation. We began to "see" the patient in a new light, and our care began to change. Kubler-Ross (1969), perhaps influenced by the work of Glaser and Strauss, then began her studies of the dying using an approach similar to that of phenomenology. From this new orientation of caring for the dying, hospice care emerged, and now, the environment of care for the dying has changed.

PHILOSOPHY AND QUALITATIVE RESEARCH

Each type of qualitative research is guided by a particular philosophical stance considered a paradigm. The philosophy directs the questions we ask, the observations we make, and how we interpret the data (Munhall, 2001). The researcher does not always clearly state the philosophical stance on which the study is based; however, one can identify the stance by carefully reading the literature review, observing how the problem is presented, and examining the researcher's methods (Sandelowski, 1993). These philosophical bases and their methodologies, developed outside nursing, will likely undergo evolutionary changes within nursing. The works of Parse (1987, 1995, 1999, 2001), Leininger (1985), Chenitz and Swanson (1986), and Artinian (1988), discussed later in the chapter, are examples of these evolutionary changes.

RIGOR IN QUALITATIVE RESEARCH

Scientific rigor is valued because it is associated with the worth of research outcomes, and studies are critically appraised as a means of judging rigor. Rigor is defined differently for qualitative research because the desired outcome is different (Burns, 1989; Dzurec, 1989; Morse, 1989; Sandelowski, 1986). In qualitative research, rigor is associated with openness, relevance (including clarity of the research question and its significance to nursing), epistemological and methodological congruence, scrupulous adherence to a philosophical perspective (methodological rigor), thoroughness in collecting data, and consideration of all the data in the analysis process, and the researcher's self-understandings. The researcher's self-understandings are important because qualitative research is an interactive process shaped by the researcher's personal history, biography, gender, social class, race and ethnicity, as well as those of the study participants.

To be rigorous in conducting qualitative research, the researcher must ascend to an open context and be willing to continue to let go of sedimented views (referred to as deconstructing the sedimented views). Maintaining openness requires discipline. The researcher will be examining many dimensions of the area being studied and forming new ideas (referred to as reconstructing new ideas or views) while continuing to recognize that the present reconstruction is only one of many possible ways of organizing ideas. Critical appraisal of the rigor of qualitative studies is discussed in more detail in Chapter 26.

APPROACHES TO QUALITATIVE RESEARCH

Six approaches to qualitative research being used in nursing are presented here: phenomenological research, grounded theory research, ethnographic research, historical research, philosophical inquiry, and critical social theory. In some ways, these approaches are very different. Ethnography and historical research are broad and are the accepted methodologies for a discipline. Critical social theory is narrow in focus and controversial in its philosophical perspective. The worldview of phenomenology is also controversial. However, in each method, the purpose is to examine meaning.

Although the data are gathered through the use of an open context, this fact does not mean that the interpretation is value-free. Each approach is based on a philosophical orientation that influences the interpretation of the data. Thus, it is critical to understand the philosophy on which the method is based. In selecting a qualitative method, the researcher should consider the following questions: "What is the most appropriate methodology and why? Which method of data collection will produce the richest set of data? How should the data be analyzed? What checks should be undertaken to maximize the accuracy of the findings?" (Cutcliffe, 1997, p. 969). Each approach is discussed in relation to the philosophical orientation and nursing knowledge.

Phenomenological Research

Phenomenology is both a philosophy and a research method. The purpose of phenomenological research is to describe experiences (or phenomena) as they are lived—in phenomenological terms, to capture the "lived experience" of study participants. The philosophers from whom phenomenology emerged include Husserl, Kierkegaard, Heidegger, Marcel, Sartre, and Merleau-Ponty. The philosophical positions taken by phenomenological researchers are very different from those common in the culture and research traditions of the nursing field.

Philosophical Orientation

Phenomenologists view the person as integral with the environment. The world is shaped by the self and also shapes the self. At this point, however, phenomenologists diverge in their beliefs, based on adherence to a particular phenomenological philosopher. Taylor (1995) provided an excellent description of her search for a compatible phenomenological perspective, discussing the methods of Langeveld (1978), Heidegger (1962), Husserl (1960, 1964, 1970, 1980), and Gadamer (1975). According to Taylor (1995):

> The search for the nature of a phenomenon begins with the people, in their place and time, and it leads to an explication of the aspects of a phenomenon. The nature of a phenomenon is a reflection of the nature of people as human beings, who find themselves within the context of a healthcare institution, who are living and making sense of their experiences. The language used by the people in the study not only illuminates the nature of the phenomenon of interest, but it also shows some of their own There-Being as human beings (full-text article available in the Cumulative Index to Nursing and Allied Health Literature database).

The two phenomenological philosophers most commonly adhered to in qualitative nursing research are

Heidegger and Husserl, whose views of the person and their world differ (Johnson, 2000). Heideggerian phenomenologists believe that the person is a self within a body. Thus, the person is referred to as embodied. "Our bodies provide the possibility for the concrete actions of self in the world" (Leonard, 1989, p. 48). The person has a world, which is "the meaningful set of relationships, practices, and language that we have by virtue of being born into a culture" (Leonard, 1989, p. 43). The person is situated as a consequence of being shaped by his or her world and thus is constrained in the ability to establish meanings through language, culture, history, purposes, and values. Therefore, the person has only *situated freedom,* not total freedom. A person's world is so pervasive that he or she usually does not notice it, unless some disruption occurs. Not only is the world of each person different, but each person's concerns are qualitatively different. The body, the world, and the concerns, unique to each person, are the context within which that person can be understood. Heideggerians believe that the person experiences being within the framework of time. This is referred to as being-in-time. The past and the future influence the now and thus are part of being-in-time (Leonard, 1989).

Husserl developed his ideas about phenomena in an effort to resolve the conflict in thought between human sciences (primarily psychology) and the basic sciences (such as physics). Phenomena are the world of experience. They cannot be explained by examining causal relations but need to be studied as the very things they are. Phenomena occur only when there is a person who experiences the phenomenon. Thus, the experience must be described, not studied using statistics. To describe it, the researcher must experience the phenomenon in a naive way (Kvigne, Gjengedal, & Kirkevold, 2002; Sadala & Adorno, 2002).

Husserlian phenomenologists believe that although self and world are mutually shaping, it is possible to bracket oneself from one's beliefs, to see the world firsthand in a naive way. Heideggerians do not agree, taking the position that bracketing is not possible.

All phenomenologists agree that there is not a single reality; each individual has his or her own reality. Reality is considered subjective; thus, an experience is considered unique to the individual. This is true even for the researcher's experiences in collecting data for a study and analyzing the data. "Truth is an interpretation of some phenomenon; the more shared that interpretation is, the more factual it seems to be, yet it remains temporal and cultural" (Munhall, 1989, p. 22). The researcher must invest considerable time

exploring the various philosophical stances within phenomenology to select one compatible with his or her perspective.

Sjöström and Dahlgrem (2002) described a perspective referred to as phenomenography, which has emerged from educational research. This approach assumes that individuals experience the world differently. The focus of phenomenography is to describe these differences. This approach to research is viewed as complementary to other research perspectives. In nursing research, the focus emphasizes "the differences between how different patients experience their states and needs. The clinical implications of such an emphasis on differences would mean that professionals in health care would be prepared to take different measures to fulfill the needs of different patients" (p. 340). Interviewing is the primary data-gathering method, with the researcher interpreting immediately what the respondent is saying so that the researcher can decide about the direction of further questioning or probing. Misunderstanding the participant can threaten the quality of the data for analysis. Analysis involves categorizing data and selecting particular sections or excerpts that "convey the most significant information" (p. 341).

Nursing Knowledge and Phenomenology

Phenomenology is the philosophical base for three nursing theories: Parse's (1999) human becoming theory, Paterson and Zderad's (1976) theory of humanistic nursing, and Watson's (1999) theory of caring. By virtue of the assumptions of her theory, Parse (1987, 1990) has stated that the only acceptable method of testing her theory is using qualitative research methods. She also holds that any qualitative method—phenomenological, ethnographic, exploratory, or case method—can be used because all of these methods are consistent with phenomenological theory (Parse, 1990). Parse (1999) also developed a human becoming research methodology, which "includes the processes of dialogical engagement (researcher-person dialogues), extraction-synthesis (transforming the data across levels of abstraction to the level of science), and heuristic interpretation (specifying the findings in the light of the man-living-health theory and integrating them into the language of the theory)" (p. 140).

A number of the published phenomenological nursing studies are based on the human becoming theory. Parse (1990) has regarded these studies as clarifying or substantiating her theory. The following abstract is from a study using Parse's method.

The experience of being listened to for older adults living in long-term care facilities was explored using a qualitative descriptive method outlined in Parse (2001), with the human becoming theory as the theoretical framework. The themes that emerged from this study—Nurturing Contentment, Vital Genuine Connections, and Deference Triumphs Mediocrity—affirmed the experience of being listened to as fundamental to the participants' quality of life. The findings expand nursing theory, provide enhanced understanding of the experience of being listened to, and offer ideas for future research. Through the voices of older adults participating in this study, the authors learn how critical listening is to quality care, and thus to excellence in nursing practice. (Jonas-Simpson, Mitchell, Fisher, Jones, & Linscott, 2006, p. 46)

Grounded Theory Research

Grounded theory research is an inductive research technique developed for health-related topics by Glaser and Strauss (1967). It emerged from the discipline of sociology. The term grounded means that the theory developed from the research is based on or has its roots in the data from which it was derived. As Artinian (1998, p. 5) indicated "grounded theory provides a way to transcend experience—to move it from a description of what is happening to understanding the process by which it happens."

Philosophical Orientation

Grounded theory is based on symbolic interaction theory, which holds many views in common with phenomenology. George Herbert Mead (1934), a social psychologist, was a leader in the development of symbolic interaction theory. Symbolic interaction theory explores how people define reality and how their beliefs are related to their actions. People create reality by attaching meanings to situations. Meaning is expressed in terms of symbols, such as words, religious objects, and clothing. These symbolic meanings are the basis for actions and interactions.

Symbolic meanings are different for each individual. We cannot completely know the symbolic meanings of another individual. In social life, groups share meanings. They communicate these shared meanings to new members through socialization processes. Group life is based on consensus and shared meanings. Interaction may lead to redefinition and new meanings and can result in the redefinition of self. Because of its theoretical importance, the interaction is the focus of observation in grounded theory research.

Grounded theory has been used most frequently to study areas in which little previous research has been conducted and to gain a new viewpoint in familiar areas of research. Because of the basic quality of theory generated through this methodology, however, further theory testing is not usually needed to enhance usefulness.

Nursing Knowledge and Grounded Theory

Artinian (1988) has identified four qualitative modes of nursing inquiry within grounded theory, each used for different purposes: descriptive mode, discovery mode, emergent fit mode, and intervention mode.

The descriptive mode provides rich detail and must precede all other modes. This mode, ideal for the beginning researcher, answers questions such as "What is going on?" "How are activities organized?" "What roles are evident?" "What are the steps in a process?" and "What does a patient do in a particular setting?"

The discovery mode allows you to identify patterns in life experiences of individuals and relates the patterns to one another. Through this mode, a theory of social process, referred to as substantive theory, is developed that explains a particular social world.

Use the emergent fit mode to extend or refine substantive theory after you have developed it. This mode will enable you to focus on a selected portion of the theory, to build on previous work, or to establish a research program around a particular social process.

The intervention mode tests the relationships in the substantive theory. The fundamental question for this mode is, "How can I make something happen in such a way as to bring about new and desired states of affairs?" This mode demands deep involvement on the part of the researcher or practitioner.

The following abstract is taken from a grounded theory study.

Objective: The objective of this study was to identify the facilitators and barriers associated with integrating nurse practitioners (NPs) into Canadian emergency departments (EDs) from the perspectives of NPs and ED staff.

Methods: We conducted 24 semi-structured interviews with key multidisciplinary stakeholders in 6 Ontario EDs to gain a broad range of perspectives on implementation issues. Data were analyzed using a grounded-theory approach.

Results: Qualitative analysis of the interview data revealed 3 major issues associated with NP implementation: organizational context, role clarity, and NP recruitment. Organizational context refers to the environment an NP enters and involves issues related to the ED culture, physician reimbursement system, and patient volume. Role clarity refers to understanding the NP's function in the ED. Recruitment issues are associated with attracting and retaining NPs to work in EDs. Examples of each issue using respondent's own words are provided.

Conclusion: Our study identified 3 issues that illustrate the complex issues involved when implementing NPs in EDs. The findings may inform policy makers and health care professionals in the future development of the role of NPs in Canadian EDs. (Thrasher & Purc-Stephenson, 2007, p. 275)

As you can see, grounded theory research examines a much broader scope of dimensions than is usually possible with quantitative research. The reader can intuitively verify these findings through her or his own experiences. The clear, cohesive description of the phenomenon allows greater understanding and thus more control of nursing practice.

Ethnographic Research

Ethnographic research provides a mechanism for studying our own culture and that of others. The word *ethnographic* means "portrait of a people." Although ethnography originated as the research methodology for the discipline of anthropology, it is now a part of the cultural research conducted by a number of other disciplines, including social psychology, sociology, political science, education, and nursing, and is also used in feminist research. Although all ethnography focuses on culture, not all cultural research is, or needs to be, ethnography. Ethnography describes and analyzes aspects of the ways of life of particular cultures, subcultures, or subculture groups. Ethnographic studies result in theories of culture. Ethnography has been associated with studies of primitive, foreign, or remote cultures. Such studies enabled the researcher to acquire new perspectives beyond his or her own ethnocentric perspective. Today, the emphasis has shifted to obtaining cultural knowledge within one's own society (Germain, 2001). Within nursing, one of the major contributions of ethnography may be to promote culturally specific care (Baillie, 1995).

Philosophical Orientation

Anthropology, which began about the same time as the nursing discipline did, in the mid-nineteenth century, seeks to understand people: their ways of living, ways of believing, and ways of adapting to changing environmental circumstances. The philosophical basis for anthropology has not been spelled out clearly, is evolving, and needs considerable refinement (Sanday, 1983). Culture is the most central concept. Leininger (1970, pp. 48–49), a nurse anthropologist, defined culture for nursing as "a way of life belonging to a

designated group of people ... a blueprint for living which guides a particular group's thoughts, actions, and sentiments ... all the accumulated ways a group of people solve problems, which are reflected in the people's language, dress, food, and a number of accumulated traditions and customs." The purpose of anthropological research is to describe a culture through examining these various cultural characteristics.

Anthropologists study the origin of people, their past ways of living, and their ways of surviving through time. These insights increase our ability to predict the future directions of cultures and the forces that guide their destiny or may provide opportunities to influence the direction of cultural development (Leininger, 1970). We must first understand the cultural aspects of our own society before we can address issues related to health.

Culture-sharing groups in American society may be found in rural and urban ethnic and/or racial enclaves; in nonethnic/nonracial groups such as those situated in prisons, bars, factories, or complex organizations; in the social institutions of education including academe; in the military and on military bases; in health care institutions such as assisted-living facilities, nursing homes, hospitals, or shelters for the homeless or the abused; in community-based groups of various types such as street gangs, motorcycle clubs, and volunteer organizations; in high-school groups such as jocks, skinheads, geeks, and nerds; in religious communities; and in professional disciplines such as nursing and medicine. Thus, for example, nursing is a professional culture, a hospital is a sociocultural institution, and a unit of a hospital can be viewed as a subculture. (Germain, 2001, p. 278)

A number of dimensions of culture are of interest within anthropology. Material culture consists of all hand-made objects associated with a given group. Ethnoscientific ethnography focuses on the ideas, beliefs, and knowledge that a group holds; they are expressed in language and may address aspects such as symbolic referents, the network of social relations, and the beliefs reflected in social and political institutions. Cultures also have ideals that the people hold as desirable, even though they do not always live up to these standards. A relatively new approach, referred to as cognitive anthropology, asserts that culture is an adaptive system that is in the minds of people and is expressed in the language or semantic system of the group. Studies from this perspective examine observable patterns of behavior, customs, and ways of life. Anthropologists seek to discover the many parts of a whole culture and how these parts are interrelated, so that a picture of the wholeness of the culture evolves. Ethnographic research is used in nursing not just to increase ethnic cultural awareness but also to enhance the provision of quality health care for all cultures (Germain, 2001; Laugharne, 1995; Leininger, 1970).

Nursing Knowledge and Ethnography

A group of nurse scientists have developed a strategy of ethnonursing research, which emerged from Leininger's theory of transcultural nursing (Leininger, 1985, 1990, 1991, 1997). Ethnonursing research "focuses mainly on observing and documenting interactions with people of how these daily life conditions and patterns are influencing human care, health, and nursing care practices" (Leininger, 1985, p. 238). The following abstract is taken from an ethnographic study.

The incidence of overweight and obese children, especially those from low-income and minority backgrounds, continues to rise. Multiple factors contribute to the rising rates. In order to gain an understanding of factors contributing to obesity in low-income families, a qualitative study was conducted with the purpose of gaining knowledge of low-income urban caretakers' understanding and attitudes regarding children's nutrition. A focused ethnography was used as a means of understanding behavior within the context of a person's cultural environment. The sample was 17 caretakers of children in the 1st–3rd grades. Four focus groups were conducted. Two themes emerged from caretakers' perceptions: knowing the right things children should eat and balancing healthy nutrition with unhealthy choices. Four categories emerged regarding influences on food choices: tradition, finances, time constraints, and role models. Lastly, five barriers and three facilitating factors emerged. Implications of the study findings for school nurses include the need, when implementing healthy eating programs for school children, to gain information from caretakers about their perceptions of childhood nutrition. (Kelly & Patterson, 2006, p. 345)

Studies such as this one provide insights that can be used in many clinical situations. Reading this type of study can lead the nurse to ask different questions about patients and their behavior.

Historical Research

Historiography examines events of the past. Many historians believe that the greatest value of historical knowledge is a greater self-understanding. Historical nursing research also increases nurses' understanding of their profession.

Philosophical Orientation

History is a very old science that dates back to the beginnings of humankind. The primary questions of history are "Where have we come from?" "Who are we?" and "Where are we going?" Although the questions do not change, the answers do.

The most ancient form of history is the myth. The myth explains origins and justifies the order of existence. In the myth, past, present, and future are not distinguishable. Myths, which are a form of storytelling, provide an image of and legitimize the existing order.

History moved beyond the myth to the chronicling of events such as great deeds, victories, and stories about people and citizens. These descriptions blurred the distinction between the real and the ideal. Historians then moved to comparing histories, selecting histories on the basis of values, and identifying patterns of regularity and change.

More recently, there has been a move to interpretive history, an effort to make sense out of it, to search for meaning. Interpretation may be accomplished by developing concepts, by explaining causality through theory development, and by generalizing to other events and other times. As Miller (1967, p. xxxi) suggested, "History is an estimate of the past from the standpoint of the present." Looking at history from the present, historians may see their role as that of patriots, as judges and censors of morals, or as detached observers. The values contained in each of these roles are reflected in the nature of the historical interpretation.

Philosophers found that understanding humankind as a historical phenomenon held out the promise of understanding the essence of humankind. To this extent, the development of a historical method was of interest to philosophy (Pflug, 1971). Voltaire developed the initial philosophy of history and an associated research methodology (Sakmann, 1971). His strategy was to look at general lines of development rather than to offer an indiscriminate presentation of details, the common practice of historians of his period. Using this strategy, Voltaire moved history from chronicling to critical analysis. He recognized that in history there can be no certainty, but he searched for criteria by which historical truth could be ascertained.

One of the assumptions of historical philosophy is that "there is nothing new under the sun." Because of this assumption, the historian can search throughout history for generalizations. For example, we may ask the question "What causes wars?" The historian could search throughout history for commonalities and develop a theoretical explanation of the causes of wars. The questions asked, the factors that the historian selects to look for throughout history, and the nature of the explanation are all based on a worldview (Heller, 1982).

Another assumption of historical philosophy is that we can learn from the past. The philosophy of history is a search for wisdom, with the historian examining what has been, what is, and what ought to be. Historical philosophers have attempted to identify a developmental scheme for history, to explain all events and structures as elements of the same social process. Heller (1982) identified three developmental schemes found in philosophies of history:

1. History reflects progression—the development from "lower" to "higher" stages.
2. History has a tendency to regress—development is from "higher" stages to "lower" stages; movement is toward a decrease in freedom and the self-destruction of our species.
3. History shows a repetition of developmental sequences in which patterns of progression and regression can be seen.

Fitzpatrick (2001, p. 405) made the following suggestion:

There is usually a tendency to justify historical research in professional fields like nursing from the standpoint of its helping to inform future decisions and to avoid repeating past mistakes. Such arguments have only slight merit because they serve a reductionist belief that historical facts can be distilled with a formula. History, although its goal is the establishment of fact that leads us to truth, cannot be reduced to statistical proof.

Nursing Knowledge and Historiography

Christy (1978, p. 9) asked, "How can we in nursing today possibly plan where we are going when we don't know where we have been nor how we got here?" One criterion of a profession is that there is a knowledge base of the history of the profession that is transmitted to those entering the profession. Until recently, historical nursing research has not been a valued activity, and few nurse researchers had the skills or desire to conduct it. Therefore, our knowledge of our past is sketchy. However, there is now a growing interest in the field of historical nursing research. Sarnecky (1990) suggested that the greater interest in historiography is related to the move from a total focus on logical positivism to a broader perspective that is fully supportive of the type of knowledge provided by historical research.

The following abstract is taken from a nursing historical study.

The medical experiments conducted on non-consenting prisoners of Nazi concentration camps during World War II necessitated the codification of principles to protect human subjects of research. Auschwitz was the largest and one of the most infamous of the camps and the site of numerous 'medical' experiments. This historical study uses primary source documents obtained from archives in England and Germany to describe one type of experiment carried out at Auschwitz—the sterilization experiments. The purpose of these experiments was to perfect a technique in which non-Aryans could be prevented from reproducing while still being able to work as slave laborers. These narratives regarding the sterilization experiments at Auschwitz are remarkable in that they contain previously undocumented information regarding the voluntary and involuntary involvement of nurses. Following these narratives, a discussion of ethics in relation to the Holocaust is presented with a specific focus on the work of Agamben. Implications of the Auschwitz narratives for the application of codes of ethical principles and contemporary nursing are discussed from a postmodernist perspective. (Benedict & Georges, 2006, p. 277)

Philosophical Inquiry

Philosophy is not generally thought of as a discipline within which one conducts research, because philosophy is not a science. Philosophy does, however, have strong links with science. Most important, philosophy guides the methods within any given science; it is the foundation of science. Furthermore, we can use philosophy to develop theories about science and to debate issues related to science. The purpose of philosophical inquiry is to perform research using intellectual analyses to clarify meanings, make values manifest, identify ethics, and study the nature of knowledge (Ellis, 1983).

Philosophical Orientation

The philosophical researcher considers an idea or issue from all perspectives by exploring the literature extensively, examining conceptual meaning, raising questions, proposing answers, and suggesting the implications of those answers. The research is guided by philosophical questions posed. As with other qualitative approaches, data collection in philosophical inquiry coincides with analysis and focuses on words. However, because philosophy attends to ideas, meaning, and abstractions, the content the researcher seeks may be implied rather than clearly stated in the literature. It may be necessary for the researcher to come to some conclusions about what the author meant in a specific text. During the analysis phase, researchers often join with colleagues to explore and debate ideas, questions, answers, and consequences.

The process is cyclical, with answers generating further questions, leading to further analysis. Therefore, the thoughtful posing of questions is considered more important than the answers.

To avoid bias in their analysis, philosophers cultivate detachment from any particular type of knowledge or method. Published reports of philosophical inquiries do not describe the methodology used but focus on discussing the conclusions of the analyses. There are three categories of philosophical inquiry: foundational inquiry, philosophical analysis, and ethical analysis.

Foundational Inquiry

The foundations of a science are its philosophical bases, concepts, and theories. A new science tends to borrow elements from the foundations of other sciences, although sometimes they are a poor fit. Even those developed within the science may have problems, such as logical inconsistencies. Foundational inquiries examine the foundations for a science. The studies include analyses of the structure of a science, as well as of the process of thinking about and valuing certain phenomena held in common by the science. They are important to perform before developing theories or programs of research. The debates related to qualitative and quantitative research methods and triangulation of methods emerge from foundational inquiries.

Nursing Knowledge and Foundational Inquiry. Philosophical analyses are expected to be carried out by scientists within a particular field, such as nursing, rather than by philosophers as such. The nurse scientist who desires to perform a philosophical study would do well to consult with a philosopher. An example of a foundational analysis is presented in Chapter 23.

Purposes. The purposes for a foundational study include the following:

1. Compare different philosophical bases, different theories, and different definitions of concepts.
2. Seek common meanings in radically different theories.
3. Critically examine operational definitions of concepts.
4. Explore the relationship between the concept and the science being examined.
5. Define the boundaries of a specific science by showing what phenomena belong to the field and what do not (boundary delineation).
6. Assist in the development of programs of research capable of shaping the empirical content of the field.
7. Draw attention to differences in ways of exploring, explaining, proving, and valuing.

8. Explain the rationale or thoughtful consequences of choosing various ways to investigate phenomena.
9. Analyze the reasoning that underlies the science.
10. Describe productive reasoning activities from which the science may develop methods for conducting foundational inquiries, as well as conceiving, planning, executing, and monitoring its programs of research.

Philosophical Analysis

Because philosophical questions are critical to the process of philosophical inquiry, it is important for nurse researchers to formulate questions that are of concern to the discipline. Ellis (1983, pp. 212, 224) identified the following questions that need to be addressed in nursing from the perspective of philosophical inquiry: "What does it mean to be human? What is the meaning of dignity? What does it mean to be compassionate, humane, and caring? What is nursing?... What views of humans are appropriate, for what purpose, and for what questions?"

Nursing Knowledge and Philosophical Analysis. The following scholars have posed philosophical questions addressing foundational issues related to various qualitative perspectives. Holmes (1996) questioned the fit between phenomenological philosophy and nursing philosophy. Paley (1998) challenged the position of "lived experience" researchers that their philosophical base is Heidegger, stating that "hermeneutic studies of 'lived experience' are incompatible with Heidegger's ontology, since they are thoroughly Cartesian in spirit" (p. 817).

> *It is an implicit assumption of LER [lived experience research] that people's experience, and their accounts of it, cannot be challenged. That is, their interpretations of the world, as lived in, cannot be wrong, misguided, distorted, or lopsided. How could they be?... A person's experience is her experience and, as such, cannot be "incorrect." To say anything else would be tantamount to denying that she had the experience, or claiming that it was not as she describes it. (Paley, 1998, p. 821)*

Crotty (1996) argued that phenomenological research being conducted by North American nurses is a subjective description of the phenomenon by a third person (the researcher) and is not consistent with European phenomenological research. Phenomenology, according to Crotty, is a critical methodology that allows researchers to revisit conscious experiences, opening themselves to the emergence of new meaning or renew present meanings. Nurse researchers, he said, use descriptive methods, not critical methods. Nurse researchers uncritically accept the participant's subjective account of the experience as the phenomenon, when it is not. He suggested that to uncritically accept what others tell us is not scholarly. He recognized that it was important for nurses to understand the subjective experiences of patients. However, in Crotty's view, this is not phenomenology (Barkway, 2001).

Ellis (1983) suggested that many of the "nursing theories" are actually philosophies of nursing, even though they were not developed through the use of philosophical analysis. These philosophies were developed to express the essence of nursing and its desired goals. They are statements of the way nursing ought to be. Concept analyses are strengthening our nursing theories and providing conceptual definitions for our research. An example of a concept analysis using the methods of philosophical analysis is presented in Chapter 23.

These arguments and the philosophical underpinnings on which they are based are hard to understand. However, it is important to grasp these ideas. As Van der Zalm & Bergum (2000) pointed out:

> Adherence by nurse researchers to a specific research tradition ultimately will determine the direction of knowledge development for nursing, and as a result, will impact on the knowledge available for utilization in practice. Thus, it is important to have an understanding of the philosophical assumptions fundamental to a research tradition, as well as an understanding of the implications that research traditions have for nursing practice. (full-text article available in CINAHL)

Ethical Inquiry

Ethics is the branch of philosophy that deals with morality. This discipline contains a set of propositions for the intellectual analysis of morality. The problems of ethics relate to obligation, rights, duty, right and wrong, conscience, justice, choice, intention, and responsibility. Ethics is a means of striving for rational ends when others are involved. The desirable rational ends are justice, generosity, trust, faithfulness, love, and friendship. These ends reflect respect for the other person. An ethical dilemma occurs when one must choose between conflicting values. In some cases, both

choices are good, and in other cases, neither choice is good but one must choose even so.

Nursing Knowledge and Ethics. Curtin (1979), a nurse ethicist, claimed that the goals of nursing are not scientific; the goals are moral and to seek good. To her, nursing is not a science; it is an art. Scientific knowledge is used as a tool in the artful practice of nursing (Curtin, 1990). As such, ethical inquiry is a research method required to clarify the means and ends of nursing practice. Much of the ethical analyses in the nursing literature address the following three issues: (1) combining the roles of nurse and scientist, (2) protecting human subjects, and (3) engaging in peer and institutional review. An example of a study using ethical inquiry is presented in Chapter 23.

Critical Social Theory

Another philosophy with a unique qualitative research methodology is critical social theory. Feminist research, which is receiving growing interest in nursing, uses critical social theory methods and could be considered a subset of critical social theory. Allen (1985, p. 62) believes that critical social theory is important to nursing because nurses need to "be as conscious as possible about the constraints operating on both nurse and client." She also has suggested that the way nurses define health, promote health, and define themselves as nurses is governed by factors explored within this philosophy (Allen, 1986).

The perspective of critical social theory has led to the development of a new approach to research called participatory research, in which representatives from the group that is being studied are included as members of the research team. This approach to research is described in Chapter 23. The intent of the research method is to give control of some aspects of the study—such as what is studied, how it is studied, and who is informed of the findings—to the participants. The study is designed to empower the participants to take control of their life situations.

Philosophical Orientation

Critical social theory contains the views of a number of philosophers, with its beginnings in Frankfurt, Germany, at the Institute for Social Research. In the 1920s and 1930s, critical social theory was influenced by the writings of Karl Marx. These philosophers, who contend that social phenomena must be examined within a historical context, believe that most societies function on the basis of closed systems of thought, which lead to patterns of domination and prevent personal growth of individuals within the society. In the late 1960s, a second generation of German philosophers, the most prominent being Habermas (1971), revised critical social theory, leading to a resurgence of interest in these ideas (Thompson, 1987):

From a critical perspective, knowledge is not something that stands alone or is produced in a vacuum by a sort of "pure" intellectual process. Instead, all knowledge is considered value laden and shaped by historic, social, political, gender, and economic conditions. Ideology— the taken-for-granted assumptions and values that usually remain hidden and unquestioned— creates a social structure that serves to oppress particular groups by limiting the options available to them. In today's social world, these are referred to as vulnerable or marginalized populations. A fundamental assumption among critical researchers is that knowledge ought not be generated for its own sake but should be used as a form of social or cultural criticism. Critical scholars hold that oppressive structures can be changed by exposing hidden power imbalances and by assisting individuals, groups, or communities to empower themselves to take action.... A critical agenda then focuses on creating knowledge that has the potential to produce change through personal or group empowerment, alterations in social systems, or a combination of these. Implicit in this view is a valuing of people as the experts in their own lives, who have an important stake in how issues are resolved. Critical scholars ... do not wish to control and predict, or to understand and describe, the world; they wish to change it. Hence, the type of knowledge sought must be capable of meeting this challenge. (Berman, Ford-Gilboe, & Campbell, 1998, p. 2)

To accomplish this goal, the researcher must construct a picture of society that exposes the prevailing system of domination, expresses the contradictions embedded in the domination, assesses society's potential for emancipatory change, and criticizes the system in order to promote that change (Stevens, 1989).

According to Berman et al. (1998, p. 3), a critical social theory study has the following aims:
1. The study addresses an issue that is of concern to a group that is disadvantaged, oppressed, or marginalized in some way.
2. The research process or results have the potential to benefit the group, immediately or longer term.

3. The researcher's assumptions, motivations, biases, and values are made explicit and their influence on the research process is examined.
4. Prior scholarship is critiqued in an attempt to elucidate the ways in which biases, especially those related to gender, race, and class, have distorted existing knowledge.
5. Interactions between the researcher and participants convey respect for the expertise of the participants.

An example of a study using critical social theory methods is presented in Chapter 23.

Friere's Theory of Cultural Action

Friere (1972), a Brazilian educator, used critical social theory methodology to develop a theory of cultural action through his experiences in attacking illiteracy in his country. Friere's theory is beginning to attract the interest of nurse researchers. In Friere's view, the world is not a static and closed order but a problem to be worked on and solved. It is his conviction that every human being, no matter how "ignorant" or submerged in the "culture of silence," is capable of looking critically at the world in a dialogical encounter with others. "Provided with the proper tools for such an encounter, he can gradually perceive his personal and social reality as well as the contradictions in it, become conscious of his own perception of that reality, and deal critically with it" (Shaull, 1972, p. 12).

"Dialogue cannot exist, however, in the absence of a profound love for the world and for men" (Friere, 1972, p. 77). Redefining the world is an act of creation and is not possible if it is not infused with love:

Love is an act of courage, not of fear, love is commitment to other men.... If I do not love the world—if I do not love life—if I do not love men—I cannot enter into dialogue. On the other hand, dialogue cannot exist without humility.... How can I dialogue if I always project ignorance onto others and never perceive my own? How can I dialogue if I regard myself as a case apart from other men?... Dialogue further requires an intense faith in man, faith in his power to make and remake, to create and re-create, faith in his vocation to be more fully human. (Friere, 1972, pp. 78–79)

Shaull (1972) pointed out that a peasant can facilitate this process for his or her neighbor more effectively than a teacher brought in from outside.

In his book *Pedagogy of the Oppressed*, Friere (1972) described the behavior of both the oppressed group and the oppressors. He described an act of oppression as any act that prevents a person from being more fully human. In his view, both the oppressed and the oppressor must be liberated. If not, the liberated oppressed will simply become oppressors, because both oppressors and oppressed fear freedom, autonomy, and responsibility. However, a person cannot be liberated by others but must liberate himself or herself. For Friere, the fight against oppression is an act of love.

Friere (1972) pointed out that education can be a tool of conformity to present social situations or an instrument of liberation. He has advocated working with groups, which leads to cultural synthesis, rather than trying to manipulate groups, which leads to cultural invasion. In a true educational experience, both teacher and student learn, and all grow as a consequence. This type of education is the practice of freedom. Friere's ideas are currently being applied to nursing situations.

Feminist Research

Feminist research is considered by some to emerge from critical social theory. According to Rafael (1997):

> Feminism is based on the premise that gender is a central construct in a society that privileges men and marginalizes women.... Feminist perspectives seek to equalize the power relations between men and women.... Critical social feminism emphasizes the social action required to bring about changes in social structures that are oppressive to women, whereas poststructural ... feminism seeks to expose patriarchal power relations in societal institutions, particularly those that generate knowledge. (p. 34)

Feminist researchers use a broad range of research methodologies, both qualitative and quantitative. Although some feminists see themselves as speaking for all women, others, such as Baber and Allen (1992, p. 19) have claimed that "there is no woman's voice, no woman's story, but rather a multitude of voices that sometimes speak together but often must speak separately." Glass and Davis (1998, p. 49) have held that "there is not one [philosophical] explanation for women's or nurses' oppression. Therefore, while general strategies aimed at transforming oppressive states may be appropriate in some contexts, consideration should always be given to individualized

and context-specific experiences and subsequent strategies."

Sigsworth (1995), basing ideas on those of Harding (1987), has suggested the following methodological conditions for feminist research:

1. Feminist research should be based on women's experiences, and the validity of women's perceptions as the "truth" for them should be recognized.
2. Artificial dichotomies and sharp boundaries are suspect in research involving women and other human beings. They should be carefully scrutinized as reflecting a logical positivist approach to research.
3. The context and relationship of phenomena, such as history and concurrent events, should always be considered in designing, conducting, and interpreting research.
4. Researchers should recognize that the questions asked are at least as important as the answers obtained.
5. Researchers should address questions that women want answered (i.e., the research should be for women).
6. The researcher's point of view (i.e., biases, background, and ethnic and social class) should be treated as part of the data. This involves ensuring that the researcher is on a plane with the person being researched. (Sigsworth, 1995, p. 897)

Nursing Knowledge and Critical Social Theory

Cody (1998), using a foundational analysis approach, expressed the following concern about the use of critical social theory in nursing research and practice:

> Critical theorists seek to inspire their readers to action, either instrumental or communicative, toward social change in the direction of freedom and justice. In recent years nurse scholars have explicated critical theory in relation to the practice of nursing, the role of the nurse in society, the fact that most nurses are women, and the relation between nurses and those who are oppressed.... For those espousing the use of critical theory in nursing, action on the part of the nurse should promote emancipation from oppressive sociocultural systems....
>
> I would like to invite nurses who have considered using critical theories to guide their practice to consider an alternative. Critical theory evolved from sociology, and the phenomena of concern to critical theorists are, in the main, sociological phenomena—the

dynamics of social systems, the rules that underpin stability and change in societies, and so on. Most scholars would concede that the goal of nursing and the goal of critical theory are different. The first plank of the American Nurses' Association Code for Nurses (1985) states in essence that the nurse provides care to any client without regard to individual or health-related characteristics that may offend the nurse. How does one, then, ethically, turn a critical eye on the reasoning, discourse, and practices of one's client? Much of the literature on critical theory that has appeared in nursing journals could be said to reflect the sociology of healthcare systems. Little or no literature on critical theory in nursing has linked critical theory to the theoretical discourse on self-care, interpersonal relations in nursing, goal attainment in nursing, the person as an adaptive biopsychosocial system, the conservation principles, humanistic nursology, cultural care, human-environment field patterning, human becoming, health as expanding consciousness, transpersonal caring, or nursing as caring. (Cody, 1998, pp. 44–45)

More on Qualitative Research Methods

Strategies prescribed for the design and implementation of each of the qualitative methods are described in Chapter 23. In addition, content related to qualitative research methods is provided in Chapter 5 (Research Problem and Purpose), Chapter 6 (Review of Relevant Literature), Chapter 7 (Frameworks), Chapter 8 (Objectives, Questions, and Hypotheses), Chapter 9 (Ethics in Research), Chapter 14 (Sampling), Chapter 15 (Measurement Concepts), Chapter 17 (Collecting and Managing Data), Chapter 25 (Disseminating Research Findings), Chapter 26 (Critical Appraisal of Nursing Studies), Chapter 27 (Strategies for Promoting an Evidence-Based Practice in Nursing), Chapter 28 (Writing Research Proposals), and Chapter 29 (Seeking Funding for Research). In addition, Chapter 12 (Outcomes Research) includes discussion of the use of qualitative studies, often triangulated with quantitative studies, to determine the outcomes of patient care. Chapter 13 (Intervention Research) describes a new method of designing and testing the effectiveness of nursing interventions using a combination of qualitative and quantitative methods.

SUMMARY

- The qualitative approach's concepts and methods of reasoning are very different from those of quantitative research.
- Some major concepts important to qualitative research are gestalt, sedimented view, and open context.
- Qualitative research requires the rigorous implementation of qualitative research techniques, such as openness, scrupulous adherence to a philosophical perspective, thoroughness in collecting data, and inclusion of all the data in the theory development phase.
- The goal of phenomenological research is to describe experiences as they are lived.
- Grounded theory is an approach for discovering what problems exist in a social scene and how the persons involved handle them.
- Ethnographic research is the investigation of cultures through an in-depth study of the members of the culture.
- Historical research is a narrative description or analysis of events that occurred in the remote or recent past.
- Philosophical inquiry consists of three types: foundational studies, philosophical analysis, and ethical analysis.
- Critical social theory involves analysis of systems of thought that lead to patterns of domination and prevent personal growth of individuals within a society.

REFERENCES

Allen, D. G. (1985). Nursing research and social control: Alternative models of science that emphasizes understanding and emancipation. *Image: The Journal of Nursing Scholarship, 17*(2), 58–64.

Allen, D. G. (1986). Using philosophical and historical methodologies to understand the concept of health. In P. L. Chinn (Ed.), *Nursing research methodology: Issues and implementation* (pp. 157–168). Rockville, MD: Aspen.

Anfara, V. A. Jr., & Mertz, N. T. (2006). *Theoretical frameworks in qualitative research*. Thousand Oaks, CA: Sage.

Artinian, B. M. (1988). Qualitative modes of inquiry. *Western Journal of Nursing Research, 10*(2), 138–149.

Artinian, B. M. (1998). Grounded theory research: Its value for nursing. *Nursing Science Quarterly, 11*(1), 5–6.

Baber, K. M., & Allen, K. R. (1992). *Women and families: Feminist reconstructions*. New York: Guilford Press.

Baillie, L. (1995). Ethnography and nursing research: A critical appraisal. *Nurse Researcher, 3*(2), 5–21.

Barkway, P. (2001). Michael Crotty and nursing phenomenology: Criticism or critique? *Nursing Inquiry, 8*(3), 191–195.

Benedict, S., & Georges, J. M. (2006). Nurses and the sterilization experiments of Auschwitz: A postmodernist perspective. *Nursing Inquiry, 13*(4), 277–288.

Berman, H., Ford-Gilboe, M., & Campbell, J. C. (1998). Combining stories and numbers: A methodologic approach for a critical nursing science. *Advances in Nursing Science, 21*(1), 1–15.

Burns, N. (1989). Standards for qualitative research. *Nursing Science Quarterly, 2*(1), 44–52.

Chenitz, W. C., & Swanson, J. M. (1984). Surfacing nursing process: A method for generating nursing theory from practice. *Journal of Advanced Nursing, 9*(7), 205–215.

Chenitz, W. C., & Swanson, J. M. (1986). *From practice to grounded theory: Qualitative research in nursing*. Menlo Park, CA: Addison-Wesley.

Christy, T. E. (1978). The hope of history. In M. L. Fitzpatrick (Ed.), *Historical studies in nursing* (pp. 3–11). New York: Teachers College.

Cody, W. K. (1998). Critical theory and nursing science: Freedom in theory and practice. *Nursing Science Quarterly, 11*(2), 44–46.

Crotty, M. (1996). *Phenomenology and nursing research*. Melbourne, Australia: Churchill Livingstone.

Curtin, L. L. (1979). The nurse as advocate: A philosophical foundation for nursing. *Advances in Nursing Science, 1*(3), 1–10.

Curtin, L. L. (1990). Integrating practice with philosophy, theory and methods of inquiry. *Proceedings: Symposium on knowledge development: I. Establishing the linkages between philosophy, theory, methods of inquiry and practice*, September 6–9, 1990. University of Rhode Island College of Nursing.

Cutcliffe, J. (1997). Qualitative research in nursing: A quest for quality. *British Journal of Nursing, 6*(17), 969.

Dzurec, L. C. (1989). The necessity and evolution of multiple paradigms for nursing research. *Advances in Nursing Science, 11*(4), 69–77.

Ellis, R. (1983). Philosophic inquiry. In H. H. Werley & J. J. Fitzpatrick (Eds.), *Annual review of nursing research* (Vol. I, pp. 211 228). New York: Springer.

Fitzpatrick, M. L. (2001). Historical research: The method. In P. Munhall (Ed.), *Nursing research: A qualitative perspective* (3rd ed., pp. 403–416). Sudbury, MA: Jones & Bartlett.

Flinders, D. J., & Mills, G. E. (Eds.) (1993). *Theory and concepts in qualitative research: Perceptions from the field*. New York: Teacher's College Press.

Friere, P. (1972). *Pedagogy of the oppressed* (M. B. Ramos, Trans.). New York: Herder & Herder.

Gadamer, H. G. (1975). *Truth and method* (G. Braden & J. Cumming, Trans.). New York: Seabury.

Germain, C. P. (2001). Ethnography: The method. In P. Munhall (Ed.), *Nursing research: A qualitative perspective* (3rd ed., pp. 277–306). Sudbury, MA: Jones & Bartlett.

Glaser, B. G., & Strauss, A. (1965). *Awareness of dying*. Chicago: Aldine.

Glaser, B. G., & Strauss, A. (1967). *The discovery of grounded theory: Strategies for qualitative research*. Chicago: Aldine.

Glaser, B. G., & Strauss, A. (1968). *Time for dying*. Chicago: Aldine.

Glaser, B. G., & Strauss, A. (1971). *Status passage*. London: Routledge & Kegan Paul.

Glass, N., & Davis, K. (1998). An emancipatory impulse: A feminist postmodern integrated turning point in nursing research. *Advances in Nursing Science, 21*(1), 43–52.

Habermas, J. (1971). *Knowledge and human interests* (J. J. Shapiro, Trans.). Boston: Beacon.

Harding, S. (1987). *Feminism and methodology*. Bloomington, IN: Open University Press.

Heidegger, M. (1962). *Being and time* (J. Macquarrie & E. Robinson, Trans.). New York: Harper & Row.

Heller, A. (1982). *A theory of history*. London: Routledge & Kegan Paul.

Holmes, C. A. (1996). The politics of phenomenological concepts in nursing. *Journal of Advanced Nursing, 24*(3), 579–587.

Husserl, E. (1960). *Cartesian meditations: An introduction to phenomenology* (D. Carins, Trans.). The Hague, Netherlands: Martinus Nijhoff.

Husserl, E. (1964). *The idea of phenomenology* (W P. Alston & G. Nakhnikian, Trans.). The Hague, Netherlands: Martinus Nijhoff.

Husserl, E. (1970). *The crisis of the European sciences and transcendental phenomenology*. Evanston, IL: Northwestern University Press.

Husserl, E. (1980). *Phenomenology and the foundations of the sciences* (T. E. Klein & W. E. Pohl, Trans.). The Hague, Netherlands: Martinus Nijhoff.

Ihde, D. (1977). *Experimental phenomenology: An introduction*. New York: Putnam.

Johnson, M. E. (2000). Heidegger and meaning: Implications for phenomenological research. *Nursing Philosophy, 1*(2), 134–146.

Jonas-Simpson, C., Mitchell, G. H., Fisher, A., Jones, G., & Linscott, J. (2006). The experience of being listened to: A qualitative study of older adults in long-term care settings. *Journal of Gerontological Nursing, 32*(1), 46–53.

Kelly, L. E., & Patterson, B. J. (2006). Childhood nutrition: Perceptions of caretakers in a low-income urban setting. *Journal of School Health, 22*(6), 345–351.

Kubler-Ross, E. (1969). *On death and dying*. New York: Macmillan.

Kvigne, K., Gjengedal, E., & Kirkevold, M. (2002). Gaining access to the life-world of women suffering from stroke: Methodological issues in empirical phenomenological studies. *Journal of Advanced Nursing, 40*(1), 61–68.

Langeveld, M. J. (1978). The stillness of the secret place. *Phenomenology and Pedagogy, 1*(1), 181–189.

Laugharne, C. (1995). Ethnography: Research method or philosophy? *Nurse Researcher, 3*(2), 54.

Leininger, M. M. (1970). *Nursing and anthropology: Two worlds to blend*. New York: Wiley.

Leininger, M. M. (1985). *Qualitative research methods in nursing*. Orlando: Grune & Stratton.

Leininger, M. M. (1990). Ethnomethods: The philosophic and epistemic bases to explicate transcultural nursing knowledge. *Journal of Transcultural Nursing, 1*(2), 40–51.

Leininger, M. M. (1991). *Ethnonursing: A research method with enablers to study the theory of culture care* (pp. 73–117). (NLN Publication #15–2402). New York: National League for Nursing.

Leininger, M. M. (1997). Transcultural nursing research to transform nursing education and practice: 40 years. *Image: The Journal of Nursing Scholarship, 29*(4), 341–347.

Leonard, V. W. (1989). A Heideggerian phenomenologic perspective on the concept of the person. *Advances in Nursing Science, 11*(4), 40–55.

Mead, G. H. (1934). *Mind, self and society.* Chicago: University of Chicago Press.

Miller, P. S. (1967). Introduction. In M. A. Fitzsimons, A. G. Pundt, & C. E. Nowell (Eds.), *The development of historiography* (pp. xxv–xxxii). Port Washington, NY: Kennikat.

Morse, J. M. (1989). Qualitative nursing research: A free-for all? In J. M. Morse (Ed.), *Qualitative nursing research: A contemporary dialogue* (pp. 14–22). Rockville, MD: Aspen.

Munhall, P. L. (1989). Philosophical ponderings on qualitative research methods in nursing. *Nursing Science Quarterly, 2*(1), 20–28.

Munhall, P. L. (2001). *Nursing research: A qualitative perspective* (3rd ed.). Sudbury, MA: Jones & Bartlett.

Paley, J. (1998). Misinterpretive phenomenology: Heidegger, ontology and nursing research. *Journal of Advanced Nursing, 27*(4), 817–824.

Parse, R. R. (1987). *Nursing science: Major paradigms, theories, and critiques.* Philadelphia: W.B. Saunders.

Parse, R. R. (1990). Health: A personal commitment. *Nursing Science Quarterly, 3*(3), 136–140.

Parse, R. R. (1995). *Illuminations: The human becoming theory in practice and research.* New York: National League for Nursing.

Parse, R. R. (1999). *Hope: An international human becoming perspective.* New York: National League for Nursing.

Parse, R. R. (2001). *Qualitative inquiry: The path of sciencing.* New York: National League for Nursing.

Paterson, J. G., & Zderad, L. T. (1976). *Humanistic nursing.* New York: Wiley.

Pflug, G. (1971). The development of historical method in the eighteenth century. In G. Pflug, P. Sakmann, & R. Unger (Eds.), *History and theory: Studies in the philosophy of history* (pp. 1–23). Middletown, CT: Wesleyan University Press.

Rafael, A. R. F. (1997). Advocacy oral history: A research methodology for social activism in nursing. *Advances in Nursing Science, 20*(2), 32–44.

Sadala, M. L. A., & Adorno, R. C. F. (2002). Phenomenology as a method to investigate the experience lived: A perspective from Husserl and Merleau Ponty's thought. *Journal of Advanced Nursing, 37*(3), 282–293.

Sakmann, P. (1971). The problems of historical method and of philosophy of history in Voltaire [1906]. In G. Pflug, P. Sakmann, & R. Unger (Eds.), *History and theory: Studies in the philosophy of history* (pp. 24–59). Middletown, CT: Wesleyan University Press.

Sanday, P. (1983). The ethnographic paradigm(s). In J. Van Maanen (Ed.), *Qualitative methodology* (pp. 19–36). Beverly Hills, CA: Sage. (Original work published 1979, in *Administrative Science Quarterly, 24,* 527–538.)

Sandelowski, M. (1986). The problem of rigor in qualitative research. *Advances in Nursing Science, 8*(3), 27–37.

Sandelowski, M. (1993). Theory unmasked: The uses and guises of theory in qualitative research. *Research in Nursing & Health, 16*(3), 213–218.

Sarnecky, M. T. (1990). Historiography: A legitimate research methodology for nursing. *Advances in Nursing Science, 12*(4), 1–10.

Sigsworth, J. (1995). Feminist research: Its relevance to nursing. *Journal of Advanced Nursing, 22*(5), 896–899.

Sjöström, B., & Dahlgrem, L. O. (2002). Applying phenomenography in nursing research. *Journal of Advanced Nursing, 40*(3), 339–345.

Stevens, P. E. (1989). A critical social reconceptualization of environment in nursing: Implications for methodology. *Advances in Nursing Science, 11*(4), 56–68.

Taylor, B. (1995). Interpreting phenomenology for nursing research. *Nurse Researcher, 3*(2), 66–79.

Thompson, J. L. (1987). Critical scholarship: The critique of domination in nursing. *Advances in Nursing Science, 10*(1), 27–38.

Thrasher, C., & Purc-Stephenson, R. J. (2007). Integrating nurse practitioners into Canadian emergency departments: A qualitative study of barriers and recommendations. *Journal of the Canadian Association of Emergency Physicians, 9*(4), 275–281.

Van der Zalm, J. E., & Bergum, V. (2000). Hermeneutic phenomenology: Providing living knowledge for nursing practice. *Journal of Advanced Nursing, 31*(1), 211.

Watson, J. (1999). *Nursing: Human science and human care: A theory of nursing.* Boston: Jones & Bartlett.

UNIT TWO

The Research Process

CHAPTER **5**

Research Problem and Purpose

We are constantly asking questions to better understand ourselves and the world around us. This human ability to wonder and ask creative questions about behaviors, experiences, and situations in the world provides a basis for identifying research topics and problems. Identifying a problem is the initial step, and one of the most significant, in conducting quantitative, qualitative, outcomes, and intervention research. The research purpose evolves from the problem and directs the subsequent steps of the research process.

Research topics are concepts or broad problem areas that researchers can focus on to enhance evidence-based nursing. Research topics contain numerous potential research problems, and each problem provides the basis for developing many research purposes. Thus, the identification of a relevant research topic and a challenging, significant problem can facilitate numerous study purposes to direct a lifetime program of research. However, the abundance of research topics and potential problems frequently are not apparent to an individual struggling to identify his or her first research problem.

This chapter differentiates a research problem from a purpose, identifies sources for research problems, and provides a background for formulating a problem and purpose for study. The criteria for determining the feasibility of a proposed study problem and purpose are described. The chapter concludes with examples of research topics, problems, and purposes from current quantitative, qualitative, outcomes, and intervention studies.

WHAT IS A RESEARCH PROBLEM AND PURPOSE?

A research problem is an area of concern where there is a gap in the knowledge base needed for nursing practice. Research is conducted to generate knowledge that addresses the practice concern, with the ultimate goal of providing evidence-based health care. A research problem can be identified by asking questions such as the following: What is wrong or is of concern in this clinical situation? What information do we need to improve this situation? Will a particular intervention work in a clinical situation? Would another intervention be more effective in producing the desired outcomes? What are the outcomes of the intervention? What changes must we make to improve this intervention based on the outcomes?

By questioning and reviewing the literature, the researcher will begin to recognize a specific area of concern and the knowledge gap that surrounds it. The knowledge gap, or what is not known about this clinical problem, determines the complexity and number of studies needed to generate essential knowledge for nursing practice (Wright, 1999). In addition to the area of concern, the research problem also identifies a population and often a setting for the study.

A research problem includes significance, background, and a problem statement. The significance of a problem indicates the importance of the problem to nursing and to the health of individuals, families, and communities; the background for a research problem briefly identifies what we know about the problem area; and the problem statement identifies the specific gap in the knowledge needed for practice. The following example research problem is from the study by Andrews, Felton, Wewers, Waller, and Tingen (2007), who examined the effects of a smoking cessation intervention on smoking cessation and abstinence in African-American women residing in public housing.

Tobacco use is the leading cause of preventable death among all individuals in the United States (U.S.), with widening gaps in health disparities occurring among ethnic minorities (U.S. Department of Health and Human Services, 1998). African American women residing in urban subsidized housing developments report prevalence rates of 40–60% in some communities, which is at least twice the rate of women in the general populations [problem significance].... African America women in subsidized housing developments indicate that cigarette smoking provides an alternate source of pleasure in the absence of other available resources, and that it is used to regulate mood and depression, manage stress, and cope with their living conditions (Andrews, et al., 2004; Jarvis & Wardle, 1999).... Pilot data findings suggest the CHWs [community health workers] who are ethnically, socioeconomically, and experientially indigenous to the community show promise in enhancing social support, building confidence in the ability to quit smoking, and in promoting spiritual well being among tobacco-dependent African American women in public housing (Andrews, et al., 2005) [problem background].... Because of the limited research that has targeted African American women of low socioeconomic status who smoke, no evidence is available of the effectiveness of gender- and ethnic/racial-specific smoking cessation interventions [problem statement]. (Andrews et al., 2007, pp. 45–46)

In this example, the research problem identifies an area of concern (tobacco use) for a particular population (African-American women) in a selected setting (public housing). The significance of the problem focuses on the health concerns with tobacco use and the high incidence of smoking among African-American women living in subsidized housing. The background research in this area identifies the reasons the women smoke and a community-based intervention that might encourage them to stop smoking. The last sentence in this example is the problem statement that identifies the gap in the knowledge needed for practice. In this study, there is limited research on specific interventions designed to encourage African-American women of low socioeconomic status to cease smoking.

The research problem in this example includes concepts or research topics such as tobacco use,

preventable death, health disparities, cigarette smoking, smoking cessation intervention, low socioeconomic status, and smoking cessation. Smoking cessation intervention is an abstract concept, and a variety of nursing actions could be implemented to determine their effectiveness in encouraging members of different populations to give up smoking. Thus, each problem may generate many research purposes. The knowledge gap regarding the effectiveness of interventions to promote smoking cessation among African-American women of low socioeconomic status provides clear direction for formulating the research purpose.

The research purpose is a clear, concise statement of the specific goal or aim of the study that is generated from the research problem. The purpose usually indicates the type of study (quantitative, qualitative, outcomes, or intervention) to be conducted and often includes the variables, population, and setting for the study. The goals of quantitative research include identifying and describing variables, examining relationships among variables, and determining the effectiveness of interventions in managing clinical problems. The goals of qualitative research include exploring a phenomenon, such as depression as it is experienced by pregnant women; developing theories to describe and manage clinical situations; examining the health practices of certain cultures; and describing the historical evolution of leaders in the profession and of health-related issues, events, and situations (Munhall, 2001; Munhall & Boyd, 1999). The focus of outcomes research is to identify, describe, and improve the outcomes or end results of patient care (Doran, 2003). Intervention research focuses on investigating the effectiveness of a nursing intervention in achieving the desired outcomes in a natural setting (Sidani & Braden, 1998). Regardless of the type of research, every study needs a clearly expressed purpose statement. Andrews et al. (2007) clearly and concisely stated the purpose of their study following the literature review section of their article:

The purpose of this research was to test the effectiveness of a community-partnered intervention to promote smoking cessation among African American women in subsidized housing developments. (Andrews et al., 2007, p. 46)

This research purpose indicates that Andrews et al. conducted a quantitative quasi-experimental study to determine the effectiveness of an independent or treatment variable (a community-partnered smoking cessation intervention) on a dependent or outcome variable (smoking cessation) in a population of African American women living in public housing (setting). The researchers also identified five hypotheses to direct their study, which included additional dependent variables of social support, smoking cessation self-efficacy, and spiritual well-being (see Chapter 8 for a discussion of hypotheses). The study results showed a 6-month continuous smoking abstinence of 27.5% in the intervention group and 5.7% in the comparison group. Andrews et al. (2007, p. 45) indicated "These findings support the use of a nurse/community health worker model to deliver culturally tailored behavioral interventions with marginalized communities." The findings from this study and other research provided evidence of the effectiveness of methods designed to manage smoking behaviors in marginalized populations.

SOURCES OF RESEARCH PROBLEMS

Research problems are developed from many sources, but you need to be curious, astute, and imaginative to identify problems from these sources. Moody, Vera, Blanks, and Visscher (1989) studied the source of research ideas and found that 87% came from clinical practice, 57% from the literature, 46% from interactions with colleagues, 28% from interactions with students, and 9% from funding priorities. These findings indicate that researchers often use more than one source to identify a research problem. The sources for research problems included in this text are (1) clinical practice, (2) researcher and peer interactions, (3) literature review, (4) theory, and (5) research priorities identified by funding agencies and specialty groups.

Clinical Practice

The practice of nursing must be based on knowledge or evidence generated through research. Thus, clinical practice is an extremely important source for research problems. Problems can evolve from clinical observations. For example, while watching the behavior of a patient and family in crisis, you may wonder how you as a nurse might intervene to improve the family's coping skills. A review of patient records, treatment plans, and procedure manuals might reveal concerns or raise questions about practice that could be the basis for research problems. For example, you may wonder what nursing intervention will open the lines of communication with a patient who has had a stroke? What is the impact of home visits on the level of function, readjustment to the home environment, and rehospitalization pattern of a child with a severe chronic illness? What is the most effective treatment

for acute and chronic pain? What is the best pharmacological agent or agents for treating hypertension in an elderly, African American, diabetic patient—β-blocker, angiotensin-converting enzyme inhibitor, angiotensin II receptor blocker, calcium channel blocker, α_1 antagonist, or diuretic, or a combination of these drugs? What are the most effective pharmacological and nonpharmacological treatments for a patient with a serious and persistent mental illness? These significant clinical questions could direct you to research that will generate essential evidence for use in practice.

Extensive patient data, such as diagnoses, treatments, and outcomes, are now computerized. Analyzing this information might generate research problems that are significant to a clinic, community, or nation. For example, you may ask, why has adolescent obesity increased so rapidly in the past 10 years and what treatments will be effective in managing this problem? What pharmacological and nonpharmacological treatments have been most effective in treating common acute illnesses such as otitis media, sinusitis, and bronchitis in your practice or nationwide? What are the outcomes (patient health status and costs) for treating such chronic illnesses as type 2 diabetes, hypertension, and dyslipidemia in your practice? Some students and nurses keep logs or journals that contain research ideas derived from their practice (Artinian & Anderson, 1980). They might record their experiences, thoughts, and the observations of others. These logs often reveal patterns and trends in a setting and help these nurses and students to identify patient care concerns such as the following: Do the priority needs perceived by the patient direct the care received? Why do patients frequently fail to follow the treatment plan provided by their nurse practitioner or physician? How are family members involved in patient care, and what impact does this have on the family unit?

Questions about the effectiveness of and the desire to improve certain interventions and health care programs have led to the development of intervention effectiveness research (Sidani & Braden, 1998). Studies have focused on interventions directed at alleviating well-defined clinical problems and on a research program that combines interventions that address various aspects of patient health and are focused on improving overall health outcomes.

Because health care is constantly changing in response to consumer needs and trends in society, the focus of current research varies based on these needs and trends. For example, research evidence is needed to improve practice outcomes for infants and new mothers, the elderly and residents in nursing homes, and persons from vulnerable and culturally diverse populations. Health care agencies would benefit from studies of varied health care delivery models. Society would benefit from interventions recognized to promote health and prevent illness. In summary, clinically focused research is essential if nurses are to develop the knowledge needed for evidence-based practice (Melnyk & Fineout-Overholt, 2005).

Researcher and Peer Interactions

Interactions with researchers and peers offer valuable opportunities for generating research problems. Experienced researchers serve as mentors and help novice researchers to identify research topics and formulate problems. Nursing educators assist students in selecting research problems for theses and dissertations. When possible, students conduct studies in the same area of research as the faculty. Faculty members can share their expertise regarding their research program, and the combined work of the faculty and students can build a knowledge base for a specific area of practice. This type of relationship could also be developed between an expert researcher and a nurse clinician. Building an evidence-based practice for nursing requires collaboration between nurse researchers and clinicians, as well as collaboration with researchers from other health-related disciplines.

Beveridge (1950) identified several reasons for discussing research ideas with others. Ideas are clarified and new ideas are generated when two or more people pool their thoughts. Interactions with others enable researchers to uncover errors in reasoning or information. These interactions are also a source of support in discouraging or difficult times. In addition, another person can provide a refreshing or unique viewpoint, which prevents conditioned thinking or following an established habit of thought. A workplace that encourages interaction can stimulate nurses to identify research problems. Nursing conferences and professional organization meetings also provide excellent opportunities for nurses to discuss their ideas and brainstorm to identify potential research problems.

The Internet has greatly extended the ability of researchers and clinicians around the world to share ideas and propose potential problems for research. Most schools of nursing have websites that identify faculty research interests and provide mechanisms for contacting individuals who are conducting research in your area of interest. Thus, interactions with others are essential to broaden your perspective and knowledge base and to support you in identifying significant research problems and purposes.

Literature Review

Reviewing research journals, such as *Advances in Nursing Science, Applied Nursing Research, Clinical Nursing Research, Evidence Based Nursing, International Journal of Psychiatric Nursing Research, Journal of Nursing Scholarship, Journal of Advanced Nursing, Journal of Research in Nursing, Nursing Research, Nursing Science Quarterly, Research in Nursing & Health, Scholarly Inquiry for Nursing Practice: An International Journal, Southern Online Journal of Nursing Research,* and *Western Journal of Nursing Research,* as well as theses and dissertations will acquaint novice researchers with studies conducted in an area of interest. The nursing specialty journals, such as *American Journal of Maternal Child Nursing, Archives of Psychiatric Nursing, Dimensions of Critical Care, Heart & Lung, Infant Behavior and Development, Journal of Pediatric Nursing,* and *Oncology Nursing Forum,* also place a high priority on publishing research findings. Reviewing research articles enables you to identify an area of interest and determine what is known and not known in this area. The gaps in the knowledge base provide direction for future research. (See Chapter 6 for the process of reviewing the literature.)

At the completion of a research project, an investigator often makes recommendations for further study. These recommendations provide opportunities for others to build on a researcher's work and strengthen the knowledge in a selected area. For example, the Andrews et al. (2007) study, introduced earlier in this chapter, examined the effect of a multicomponent smoking cessation intervention on the ability of African-American women to quit smoking and provided excellent recommendations for further research.

Research is needed to explore behavioral mediating factors that improve the health of low-income African American women, including spirituality.... Further research is needed to design and test protocols and instrumentation for spiritual interventions targeting smoking cessation and other lifestyle behaviors so that their effectiveness can be further evaluated.... Additional research is needed to explore different uses and levels of activities of CHWs [community health workers] with smoking cessation and other lifestyle behavior changes with low-income African America women. Further studies that evaluate the dosage and intensity of CHW interventions, as well as their potential cost effectiveness, are needed. (Andrews et al., 2007, pp. 57–58)

These researchers encouraged others to validate their findings through replication studies that varied the dosage and intensity of the CHW interventions. They also encouraged other researchers to generate new knowledge about the effects of spirituality interventions designed to improve the outcomes for study participants who sought to stop smoking and to make other lifestyle behavior changes.

Replication of Studies

Reviewing the literature is a way to identify a study to replicate. Replication involves reproducing or repeating a study to determine if similar findings will be obtained (Fahs, Morgan, & Kalman, 2003). Replication is essential for knowledge development because it (1) establishes the credibility of the findings, (2) extends the generalizability of the findings over a range of instances and contexts, (3) reduces the number of type I and type II errors, (4) corrects the limitations in studies' methodologies, (5) supports theory development, and (6) lessens the acceptance of erroneous results (Beck, 1994; Fahs et al., 2003). Some researchers replicate studies because they agree with the findings and wonder if the findings will hold up in different settings with different subjects over time. Others want to challenge the findings or interpretations of prior investigators. Some researchers develop research programs focused on expanding the knowledge needed for practice in an area. This program of research often includes replication studies that strengthen the evidence for practice.

Four different types of replication are important in generating sound scientific knowledge for nursing: (1) exact, (2) approximate, (3) concurrent, and (4) systematic extension (Beck, 1994; Haller & Reynolds, 1986). An exact (or identical) replication involves duplicating the initial researcher's study to confirm the original findings. All conditions of the original study must be maintained; thus, "there must be the same observer, the same subjects, the same procedure, the same measures, the same locale, and the same time" (Haller & Reynolds, 1986, p. 250). Exact replications might be thought of as ideal to confirm original study findings, but these are frequently not attainable. In addition, one would not want to replicate the errors in an original study, such as small sample size, weak design, or poor-quality measurement methods.

When conducting an approximate (or operational) replication, the subsequent researcher repeats the original study under similar conditions, following the methods as closely as possible (Beck, 1994). The intent is to determine whether the findings from the original study hold up despite minor changes in the research conditions. If the findings generated through replication are consistent with the findings of the original study, these data are more credible and have a greater probability of accurately reflecting the real world. If the replication fails to support the original findings, the designs and methods of both studies should be examined for limitations and weaknesses, and further research must be conducted. Conflicting findings might also generate additional theoretical insights and provide new directions for research.

For a concurrent (or internal) replication, the researcher collects data for the original study and the replication study simultaneously thereby checking the reliability of the original study (Beck, 1994; Brink & Wood, 1979). The confirmation, through replication of the original study findings, is part of the original study's design. For example, your research team might collect data simultaneously at two different hospitals and compare and contrast the findings. Consistency in the findings increases the credibility of the study and the likelihood that others will be able to generalize the findings. Some expert researchers obtain funding to conduct multiple concurrent replications, in which a number of individuals conduct of a single study, but with different samples in different settings. Clinical trials that examine the effectiveness of the pharmacological management of chronic illnesses, such as diabetes, hypertension, and dyslipidemia, are examples of concurrent replication studies. As each study is completed, the findings are compiled in a report that specifies the series of replications that were conducted to generate these findings. Some outcome studies involve concurrent replication to determine if the outcomes vary for different health care providers and health care settings across the United States.

A systematic (or constructive) replication is done under distinctly new conditions. The researchers conducting the replication do not follow the design or methods of the original researchers; rather, the second investigative team identifies a similar problem but formulates new methods to verify the first researchers' findings (Haller & Reynolds, 1986). The aim of this type of replication is to extend the findings of the original study and test the limits of the generalizability of such findings. Intervention research might use this type of replication to examine the effectiveness of various interventions devised to address a practice problem (Sidani & Braden, 1998).

Beck (1994) conducted a computerized and manual review of the nursing literature from 1983 through 1992 and found only 49 replication studies. Possibly, the number of replication studies is limited because (1) some view replication as less scholarly or less important than original research, (2) the discipline of nursing lacks resources for conducting replication studies, and (3) editors of journals limit the number of replication studies they publish (Beck, 1994; Fahs et al., 2003). However, the lack of replication studies severely limits the generation of sound research findings needed for evidence-based practice in nursing (Beck, 1994; Fahs et al., 2003; Martin, 1995; Reynolds & Haller, 1986). Thus, replicating a study should be respected as a legitimate scholarly activity for both expert and novice researchers. Funding from both private and federal sources is needed to support the conduct of replication studies, with a commitment from journal editors to publish these studies.

Replication provides an excellent learning opportunity for the novice researcher to conduct a significant study, validate findings from previous research, and generate new research evidence about different populations and settings. Students studying for their master's degree could be encouraged to replicate studies for their theses, possibly to replicate faculty studies. Expert researchers, with programs of research, implement replication studies to generate sound evidence for use in practice. When developing and publishing a replication study, it is important to designate the type of replication conducted and the contribution the study made to the existing body of knowledge.

Landmark studies are significant research projects that not only generate knowledge but influence a discipline and sometimes society. These studies are frequently replicated or are the basis for the generation of additional studies. For example, Williams (1972) studied factors that contribute to skin breakdown, and these findings provided the basis for numerous studies on the prevention and treatment of pressure ulcers. Many of these studies are summarized in the document *Pressure Ulcers in Adults: Prediction and Prevention* published by the Agency for Health Care Policy and Research (Panel for the Prediction and Prevention of Pressure Ulcers in Adults, 1992). Updates and revisions of this guideline can be found online at the Agency for Healthcare Research and Quality (AHRQ) (see www.ahrq.gov) and the National Guideline Clearinghouse (see www.guideline.gov).

Theory

Theories are an important source for generating research problems because they set forth ideas about events and situations in the real world that require testing (Chinn & Kramer, 2008). In examining a theory, one notes that it includes a number of propositions and that each proposition is a statement of the relationship of two or more concepts. A research problem and

purpose could be formulated to explore or describe a concept or to test a proposition from a theory. In qualitative research, the purpose of the study might be to generate a theory to describe a new event or situation (Marshall & Rossman, 2006; Munhall, 2001).

Some researchers combine ideas from different theories to develop maps or models for testing through research. The map serves as the framework for the study and includes key concepts and relationships from the theories that the researchers want to study. Frenn, Malin, and Bansal (2003, p. 38) conducted a quasi-experimental study to examine the effectiveness of a "4-session Health Promotion/transtheoretical Model-guided intervention in reducing percentage of fat in the diet and increasing physical activity among low- to middle-income culturally diverse middle school students." The intervention was based on the "components of two behaviorally based research models that have been well tested among adults—Health Promotion Model (Pender, 1996) and Transtheoretical Model (Prochaska, Norcross, Fowler, Follick, & Abrams, 1992)—but have not been tested regarding low-fat diet with middle school–aged children" (Frenn et al., 2003, p. 36). They developed a model of the study framework (Figure 5-1) and described the concepts and propositions from the model that guided the development of different aspects of their study.

A combined Health Promotion/Transtheoretical Model guided the intervention designed for this study [see Figure 5-1]. The first individual characteristic examined in this study was temptation (low self-efficacy), defined as the inability to overcome barriers in sustaining a low-fat diet … and an intervention helping adolescents develop behavioral control may enhance self-efficacy and improve health habits.

The second characteristic common to both the Health Promotion and Transtheoretical Models was benefits/barriers. In a study of fifth through seventh grade children, Baranowski and Simons-Morton (1990) found the most common barriers to reducing saturated fat in the diet were (a) giving up preferred foods, (b) meals outside the home that contained fat, (c) not knowing what foods were low in fat, and (d) not wanting to take the time to read labels.

The last individual characteristic used in this study was access to low-fat foods. This concept from the Health Promotion Model is important in a middle school–aged population, as they are, to some extent, dependent on others for the types of food available. (Frenn et al., 2003, pp. 37–38)

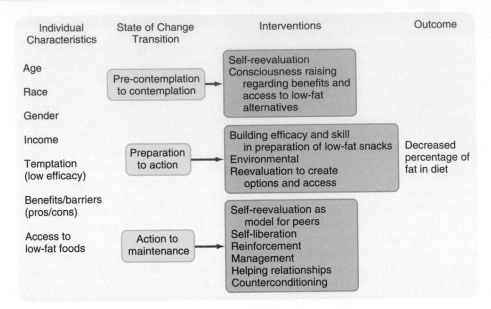

Figure **5-1** The health promotion stage of change model: A synthesis of health promotion and transtheoretical models guiding low-fat diet intervention for students in an urban middle school.

Frenn et al. (2003) used the Pender (1996) Health Promotion Model and the Transtheoretical Model (Prochaska et al., 1992) to develop the following research questions, which guided their study:

(a) Do demographic variables, access to low-fat foods, perceived self-efficacy, benefits/barriers, and stages of change predict percentage of fat reported in the diet by middle school–aged children? (b) Does the application of a Health Promotion/Transtheoretical Model intervention in 4 classroom sessions significantly improve adoption of a diet lower in fat and duration of physical activity as compared with a control group of students not engaged with the program? (Frenn et al., 2003, p. 39)

The findings from a study either support or do not support the relationships identified in the model. The study by Frenn et al. (2003) added support to the Health Promotion/Transtheoretical Model with their findings that the classroom intervention decreased dietary fat and increased physical activity for middle school–age adolescents. Further research is needed to determine if classroom interventions over time reduce body mass index, body weight, and the percentage of body fat of overweight and obese adolescents. As a graduate student, you could use this model as a framework and test some of the relationships in your clinical setting.

Research Priorities

Since 1975, expert researchers, specialty groups, professional organizations, and funding agencies have identified nursing research priorities. The research priorities for clinical practice were initially identified in a study by Lindeman (1975). Those original research priorities included nursing interventions related to stress, care of the aged, pain, and patient education. Developing evidence-based nursing interventions in these areas continues to be a priority.

Many professional nursing organizations use websites to communicate their current research priorities. For example, the American Association of Critical Care Nurses (AACN) determined initial research priorities for this specialty in the early 1980s (Lewandowski & Kositsky, 1983) and revised these priorities in 1993 (Lindquist et al., 1993) and 1999. The most current AACN (2006) research priorities are identified on this organization's website as (1) effective and appropriate use of technology to achieve optimal patient assessment, management, or outcomes; (2) creation of a healing, humane environment; (3) processes and systems that foster the optimal contribution of critical care nurses; (4) effective approaches to symptom management; and (5) prevention and management of complications. The AACN website is located at www.aacn.org (search for "research priorities"). If your specialty is critical care, this website might assist you in identifying a priority problem and purpose for study.

The American Organization of Nurse Executives (AONE, 2006) provides a discussion of their research priorities online at www.aone.org/aone/edandcareer/priorities.html. For 2007, AONE identified more than 25 research priorities in four strategic areas: (1) design of future patient care delivery systems, (2) healthful practice environments, (3) leadership, and (4) the positioning nurse leaders as valued health care executives and managers. To promote the design of future patient care delivery systems, AONE encourages research focused on new technology, patient safety, and the work environment that allows strategies for improvement crucial to the success of the delivery system. In the area of healthful practice environments, AONE encourages research focused on practice environments that attract and retain nurses and promote professional growth and continuous learning, including mentoring of staff nurses and nursing leaders. In the area of leadership, AONE encourages research focused on evidence-based leadership capacity, measurement of patient care quality outcomes, and technology to complement patient care. To promote the positioning of nurse leaders as valued health care executives and managers, AONE encourages research focused on patient safety and quality, disaster preparedness, and workforce shortages. AONE recognizes the importance of supporting education and research initiatives to create a healthy work environment, a quality health care system, and strong nurse executives. You can search online for the research priorities of other nursing organizations to assist you in identifying priority problems for study.

A significant funding agency for nursing research is the National Institute of Nursing Research (NINR). A major initiative of the NINR is the development of a national nursing research agenda that will involve identifying nursing research priorities, outlining a plan for implementing priority studies, and obtaining resources to support these priority projects. The NINR has an annual budget of more than $90 million with 74% of the budget used for extramural research project grants, 7% for predoctoral and postdoctoral training, 6% for research management and support, 5% for the centers program in specialized areas, 5% for other research including career development, 2% for the intramural program, and 1% for contracts and other expenses.

The NINR (2006) developed four strategies for building the science of nursing for 2006–2010: "(1) integrating biological and behavior science for better health; (2) adopting, adapting, and generating new technologies for better health care; (3) improving methods for future scientific discoveries; and (4) developing scientists for today and tomorrow." The areas of research emphasis for 2006–2010 include (1) promoting health and preventing disease, (2) improving quality of life, (3) eliminating health disparities, and (4) setting directions for end-of-life research (NINR, 2006). Specific research priorities were identified for each of these four areas of research emphasis and included in the NINR Strategic Plan for 2006–2010. These research priorities provide important information for nurses seeking funding from the NINR. Details about the NINR mission, strategic plan, and areas of funding are available on its website at www.nih.gov/ninr.

Another federal agency that is funding health care research is the Agency for Healthcare Research and Quality (AHRQ), formerly the Agency for Health Care Policy and Research (AHCPR). The purpose of the AHRQ is to enhance the quality, appropriateness, and effectiveness of health care services, and access to such services, by establishing a broad base of scientific research and promoting improvements in clinical practice and in the organization, financing, and delivery of health care services. Some of the current funding priorities are research focused on prevention; health information technology; patient safety; long-term care; pharmaceutical outcomes; system capacity and emergency preparedness; and the cost, organization, and socio-economics of health care. For a complete list of funding opportunities and grant announcements, see the AHRQ website at www.ahcpr.gov.

Nursing research priorities are also being identified in Europe, Africa, and Asia. Some European countries (United Kingdom, Denmark, and Finland) have been conducting nursing research for more than 30 years, but most of the countries have been involved in nursing research for less than a decade. The European countries have identified the following research topics as priorities: (1) promoting health and well-being across the life span, (2) managing symptoms, (3) caring for the elderly, (4) evaluating cost-effectiveness, (5) restructuring health care systems, (6) examining self-care and self-management of health and illness, and (7) developing knowledge for practice (Tierney, 1998). The two major priorities for nursing research in Africa are human immunodeficiency virus/acquired immunodeficiency syndrome (HIV/AIDS) and health behaviors. In Asia, limited nursing research is being conducted, with the priorities focused on health service research, including human resources and health outcomes (Henry & Chang, 1998).

The World Health Organization (WHO) is encouraging the identification of priorities for a common nursing research agenda among countries. A quality health care delivery system and improved patient and family health have become global goals. By 2020, the world's population is expected to increase by 94%, with the elderly population increasing by almost 240%.

Seven of every 10 deaths are expected to be caused by noncommunicable diseases, such as chronic conditions (heart disease, cancer, and depression) and injuries (unintentional and intentional). The priority areas for research identified by WHO are to (1) improve the health of the world's most marginalized populations; (2) study new diseases that threaten public health around the world; (3) conduct comparative analyses of supply and demand of the health workforce of different countries; (4) analyze the feasibility, effectiveness, and quality of education and practice of nurses; (5) conduct research on health care delivery modes; and (6) examine the outcomes for health care agencies, providers, and patients around the world (WHO, 2006). A discussion of WHO's mission, objectives, and research priorities can be found online at www.who.int/en.

Healthy People 2010 identifies and prioritizes the health objectives of all age groups over the next decade (U.S. Department of Health and Human Services, 2000). These health objectives direct future research in the areas of health promotion, illness prevention, illness management, and rehabilitation and can be accessed online at www.health.gov. Betz (2002, pp. 154–155) identified 123 objectives from *Healthy People 2010* that address the concerns of infants, children, adolescents, and young adults. Some of the top health objectives for children include the following:

> *(1) increasing the proportion of persons with health insurance; (2) increasing the proportion of persons appropriately counseled about health behaviors; (3) reducing hospitalization rates for three ambulatory-care-sensitive conditions—pediatric asthma, uncontrolled diabetes, and immunization-preventable pneumonia and influenza; (4) reducing the proportion of children and adolescents who are overweight or obese; and (5) reducing the number of cases of HIV infections among adolescents and young adults. (Betz, 2002, pp. 154–155)*

In summary, funding organizations, professional organizations, and governmental health care organizations nationally and internationally are sources for identifying priority research problems and offer opportunities for obtaining funding for future research.

FORMULATING A RESEARCH PROBLEM AND PURPOSE

Potential nursing research problems often emerge from real-world situations, such as those in nursing practice. A *situation* is a significant combination of circumstances that occur at a given time. Inexperienced researchers tend to want to study the entire situation, but it is far too complex for a single study. Multiple problems exist in a single situation, and each can be developed into a study. A researcher's perception of what problems exist in a situation depends on that individual's clinical expertise, theoretical base, intuition, interests, and goals. Some researchers spend years developing different problem statements and new studies from the same clinical situation.

The exact thought processes used to extract problems from a situation have not been clearly identified because of the abstractness and complexity of the reasoning involved. However, in formulating their study problems, researchers often implement the following steps: (1) examine a real-world situation, (2) identify research topics, (3) generate questions, and (4) ultimately clarify and refine a research problem. From the problem, the researcher develops a specific goal or research purpose for study. The flow of these steps is presented in Figure 5-2 and described in the following sections.

Research Topics

A nursing situation often includes a variety of research topics or concepts that identify broad problem areas requiring investigation. Nurses frequently investigate patient- and family-related topics such as stress, pain, coping patterns, the teaching and learning process, self-care deficits, health promotion, rehabilitation, prevention of illness, disease management, and social support. Other relevant research topics focus on the health care system and providers, such as cost-effective care, advanced practice nurse role (nurse practitioner, clinical nurse specialist, midwife, and nurse anesthetist), managed care, and redesign of the health care system. Outcomes research focuses on topics of health status, quality of life, cost-effectiveness, and quality of care. A specific outcome study might focus on a particular condition such as terminal cancer and examine outcomes such as nutrition, hygiene, skin integrity, and pain control with a variety of treatments (Doran, 2003).

Generating Questions

Situations encountered in nursing stimulate a constant flow of questions. The questions fit into three categories: (1) questions answered by existing knowledge, (2) questions answered with problem solving, and (3) research-generating questions. The first two types of questions are nonresearchable and do not facilitate the formulation of research problems that will generate knowledge for practice. Some of the questions

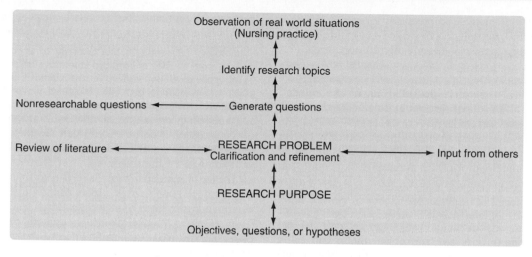

Figure 5-2 Formulating a research problem and purpose.

raised have a satisfactory answer within the nursing profession's existing body of knowledge, and these answers are available in the literature and online, from evidenced-based guidelines, or from experts in nursing or other disciplines. For example, suppose you have questions about performing some basic nursing skills, such as a protocol for taking a temperature or giving injections; you can find answers to questions such as these in the research literature and procedure manuals. However, suppose your questions focus on investigating new techniques to improve existing skills, patient responses to techniques, or ways to educate patients and families to perform techniques. Your efforts to answer these types of questions could add to knowledge needed for evidence-based practice.

Some of the questions raised can be answered using problem-solving or evaluation projects. The problem-solving process addresses a particular problem situation, and the goal of the research process is the generation of knowledge to be generalized to other similar situations. Many evaluation projects are conducted with minimal application of the rigor and control required with research. These projects do not fit the criteria of research, and the findings are relevant for a particular situation. For example, quality assurance is an evaluation of the patient care implemented by a specific health care agency; the results of this evaluation project are usually relevant only to the agency conducting the review.

The type of question that can initiate the research process is one that requires further knowledge to answer it. Some of the questions that come to mind about situations include the following: Is there a need

to explore or describe concepts, to know how they are related, or to be able to predict or control some event within the situation? What is known and what is not known about the concepts? What are the most urgent factors or outcomes to know? Is there a need to generate or test theory in an area important to practice? Which intervention is most effective in achieving quality patient outcomes? Research experts have found that asking the right question is frequently more valuable than finding the solution to a problem. The solution identified in a single study might not withstand the test of time or might be useful in only a few situations. However, one well-formulated question can generate numerous research problems, direct a lifetime of research activities, and significantly contribute to a discipline's body of knowledge.

Clarifying and Refining a Research Problem

Fantasy and creativity are part of formulating a research problem, so imagine prospective studies related to the situation. Imagine the difficulties likely to occur with each study, but avoid being too critical of potential research problems at this time. Which studies seem the most workable? Which ones appeal intuitively? Which problem is the most significant to nursing? Which study is of personal interest? Which problem has the greatest potential to provide a foundation for further research in the field? (See Campbell, Daft, & Hulin, 1982; Kahn, 1994; Wright, 1999.)

The problems investigated need to have professional significance and potential or actual significance for society. A research problem is significant when it has the potential to generate or refine knowledge to build an evidence-based practice for nursing (Melnyk & Fineout-Overholt, 2005). Moody et al. (1989) surveyed nurse researchers and identified the following criteria for significant research problems: They should be (1) focused on real-world concerns (57%), (2) methodologically sound (57%), (3) knowledge building (51%), (4) theory building (40%), and (5) focused on current or timely concerns (31%). The problems that are considered significant vary with time and the needs of society. The priorities identified earlier indicate some of the current, significant nursing research topics and problems.

Personal interest in a problem influences the quality of the problem formulated and the study conducted. A problem of personal interest is one that an individual has pondered for a long time or one that is especially important in the individual's nursing practice or personal life. For example, if you know someone who has had a mastectomy, you may be particularly interested in studying the emotional impact of a mastectomy or strategies for caring for mastectomy patients. This personal interest in the topic can become the driving force needed to conduct a quality study (Beveridge, 1950).

Answering these questions regarding significance and personal interest can often assist you in narrowing the number of problems. Without narrowing potential problems to only one idea, try some of the ideas out on colleagues. Let them play the devil's advocate and explore the strengths and weaknesses of each idea. Then begin some preliminary reading in the area of interest. Examine literature related to the situation, the variables within the situation, measurement of the variables, previous studies related to the situation, and supportive theories. The literature review often will enable you to refine the problem and clearly identify the gap in the knowledge base. Once you have identified the problem, you must frame it or ground it in past research, practice, and theory (Stone, 2002). The discussion of the problem must culminate in a problem statement that identifies the gap in the knowledge base that your proposed study will address. Thus, the refined problem has documented significance to nursing practice, is based on past research and theory, and identifies a gap in nursing knowledge that directs the development of the research purpose.

Research Purpose

The purpose is generated from the problem, identifies the goal or goals of the study, and directs the development of the study. In the research process, the purpose is usually stated after the problem, because the problem identifies the gap in knowledge in a selected area and the purpose clarifies the knowledge to be

generated by a study. The research purpose must be stated *objectively*, that is, in a way that does not reflect particular biases or values of the researcher. Investigators who do not recognize their values might include their biases in the research. This can lead them to generate the answers they want or believe to be true and might add inaccurate information to a discipline's body of knowledge (Kaplan, 1964). Therefore, based on your research purpose, you can develop specific research objectives, questions, or hypotheses to direct your study (see Chapter 8).

The purpose of an outcomes research project is usually complex and requires a team of multidisciplinary health care providers to accomplish it. Your research team members must be cautious in identifying a purpose that will make a significant contribution to the health care system and yet be feasible. Some possible purposes for outcomes research projects include the following:

> *(1) Comparing one treatment with another for effectiveness in the routine treatment of a particular condition; (2) describing in measurable terms the typical course of a chronic disease; (3) using variations in outcomes to identify opportunities for improving clinical process; and (4) developing decision support programs for use with individual patients when choosing among alternative treatment options. (Davies, Doyle, Lansky, Rutt, Stevic, & Doyle, 1994, p. 11)*

EXAMPLE OF PROBLEM AND PURPOSE DEVELOPMENT

You might have observed the women receiving treatment at a psychiatric facility and noted that many were withdrawn, depressed, and unable to discuss certain events in their lives. Their progress in therapy was usually slow, and they seemed to have similar physical and psychological symptoms. Often, after developing a rapport with a therapist, they would reveal that they were victims of sexual abuse as a child. This situation could lead you to identify research topics and generate searching questions. Research topics of interest include sexual abuse, childhood incest, physical and psychological symptoms of incest, history of incest, assessment of emotional problems, and therapeutic interventions to manage sexual abuse. Possible questions include the following: What are the physical and psychological symptoms demonstrated by someone who has experienced childhood sexual abuse? How would one assess the occurrence, frequency, and impact of rape or incest on a woman? What influences do age and duration of abuse have on the woman's current behavior? How frequently is childhood sexual abuse a problem in the mentally disturbed adult female? How does a health care provider assess and diagnose the emotional problems of adult survivors of child sexual abuse? What type of treatment is effective in an individual who has experienced child abuse? These are the types of questions that Brown and Garrison (1990) might have raised as they developed the following problem, purpose, and questions for their investigation.

■ *RESEARCH PROBLEM*

There is evidence that one in four girls and one in seven boys are sexually abused in some way prior to their 18th birthday…. The long-term consequences of child sexual abuse make it one of the most severe offenses against a child's dignity and sense of well-being…. Unreported, untreated child sexual abuse results in long-term dysfunctional behavior requiring therapy (Browne & Finkelhor, 1986). Gold (1986) suggested that histories of incest are not often obtained by a systematic interviewing protocol or by specifically trained interviewers. Thus, the need for a systematic assessment tool to identify childhood incest in this high-risk population is imperative. (Brown & Garrison, 1990, pp. 587–588)

Child sexual abuse is a significant health care topic because it occurs frequently and has a long-lasting impact on the victim's physical and emotional health. The problem statement that "a systematic assessment tool is needed to identify childhood incest in this high-risk population" is supported by past research, practice, and theory.

■ *RESEARCH PURPOSE*

The purpose of this study was to (a) identify physical and psychosocial patterns of symptomatology in adult women incest survivors, and (b) design a systematic assessment instrument to identify incest early in nonreporting adult women survivors. (Brown & Garrison, 1990, p. 588)

This purpose clearly develops from the problem and identifies the goals of the study, which are to ascertain patterns of symptoms and design an assessment instrument. The variables studied are physical and psychosocial symptoms and an assessment instrument in a population of adult women incest survivors.

■ *RESEARCH QUESTIONS*

1. What patterns of physical symptoms are present in adult women incest survivors?
2. What patterns of psychosocial symptoms are present in adult women incest survivors?
3. Is there a correlation between the frequency of multiple victimization and the number of reported physical and psychosocial symptoms?
4. Is there a correlation between the age when the sexual abuse began and its duration? (Brown & Garrison, 1990, p. 588)

These research questions are clearly developed from the first part of the purpose, "to identify physical and psychosocial patterns of symptomatology." However, there is no link of the research questions to the second part of the purpose that focused on designing an assessment instrument. This is a break in the logical flow of this study and could lead to problems in the development of the remaining steps of the research process.

FEASIBILITY OF A STUDY

As the research problem and purpose increase in clarity and conciseness, the researcher has greater direction in determining the feasibility of a study. The feasibility of a study is determined by examining the time and money commitment; the researcher's expertise; availability of subjects, facility, and equipment; cooperation of others; and the study's ethical considerations (Kerlinger & Lee, 2000; Rogers, 1987).

Time Commitment

Conducting research frequently takes longer than anticipated, which makes it difficult for any researcher, especially a novice, to estimate the time that will be involved. In estimating the time commitment, the researcher examines the purpose of the study; the more complex the purpose, the greater the time commitment. You can approximate the time needed to complete a study by assessing the following factors: (1) type and number of subjects needed, (2) number and complexity of the variables to be studied, (3) methods for measuring the variables (are instruments available to measure the variables or must they be developed?), (4) methods for collecting data, and (5) the data analysis process. Also, researchers often overlook the time commitment necessary to write the research report for presentation and publication. You must approximate the time needed to complete each step of the research process and determine whether the study is feasible.

Most researchers propose a designated period of time or set a specific deadline for their project. For example, an agency might set a 2-year deadline for studying the turnover rate of staff. The researcher must determine whether the identified purpose can be accomplished by the designated deadline; if not, the purpose could be narrowed or the deadline extended. Researchers are often cautious about extending deadlines because a project could continue for many years. The individual interested in conducting qualitative research frequently must make an extensive time commitment of 2 years or longer to allow for quality collection and analysis of data. Time is as important as money, and the cost of a study can be greatly affected by the time required to conduct it.

Money Commitment

The problem and purpose selected are influenced by the amount of money available to the researcher. Potential sources for funding should be considered at the time the problem and purpose are identified. For example, Andrews et al. (2007), who studied the effects of a smoking cessation intervention for African American women, obtained funding from the National Institute of Nursing Research (NINR) and the American Legacy Foundation to support their study. Federal and private sources of funding greatly strengthen the feasibility of conducting a research project.

The cost of a research project can range from a few dollars for a student's small study to hundreds of thousands of dollars for complex projects, such as multisite clinical trials and major qualitative studies. In estimating the cost of a research project, the following questions need to be considered as well as other areas of expense based on the study conducted:

1. *Literature:* What will the review of the literature —including computer searches, copying articles, and purchasing books—cost?
2. *Subjects:* How many subjects will need to be recruited for the study, and will the subjects have to be paid for their participation in the project?
3. *Equipment:* What will the equipment for the study cost? Can the equipment be borrowed, rented, bought, or obtained through donation? Is the equipment available, or will it need to be built? What type of maintenance will be required for the equipment during the study? What will the measurement instruments cost?
4. *Personnel:* Will assistants or consultants, or both, be hired to collect, computerize, and analyze the data and assist with the data interpretation? Will clerical help be needed to type and

distribute the report and prepare a manuscript for publication?
5. *Computer time:* Will computer time be required to analyze the data? If so, what will be the cost?
6. *Transportation:* What will be the transportation costs for conducting the study and presenting the findings?
7. *Supplies:* Will any supplies—such as envelopes, postage, pens, paper, or photocopies—be needed? Will a cell phone be needed to contact the researcher about potential subjects? Will long-distance phone calls or overnight mailing be needed?

Researcher Expertise

A research problem and purpose must be selected based on the ability of the investigator. Initially, you might work with another researcher (mentor) to learn the process and then investigate a familiar problem that fits your knowledge base or experience. Selecting a difficult, complex problem and purpose can only frustrate and confuse the novice researcher. However, all researchers need to identify problems and purposes that are challenging and collaborate with other researchers as necessary to build their research background.

When a team of researchers conducts a study, the team members often have a variety of research and clinical experiences that add to the quality of the study conducted. In the study conducted by Andrews et al. (2007), these investigators had research and clinical expertise in biobehavioral nursing, public health, biostatistics, and pediatric medicine. They were all doctorally prepared and seasoned faculty members of universities, usually indicating research expertise. On the first page of the article the types of positions and employment sites for the investigators were identified as follows: (1) Andrews was an assistant professor, Department of Biobehavioral Nursing, Medical College of Georgia; (2) Felton was a professor at the College of Nursing, University of South Carolina; (3) Wewers was a professor and associate dean for research, Department of Public Health, Ohio State University; (4) Waller was an associate professor, Department of Biostatistics, Medical College of Georgia; and (5) Tingen was an associate professor, Department of Pediatrics, Medical College of Georgia (Andrews et al., 2007). The researchers all appear to have strong backgrounds for conducting research in the discipline of nursing and health care. You can obtain more information about the authors by searching their name online.

Availability of Subjects

In selecting a research purpose, you must consider the type and number of subjects needed. Finding a sample might be difficult if the study involves investigating a unique or rare population, such as quadriplegic individuals who live alone and are currently attending college. The more specific the population selected for study, the more difficult it is to find subjects. The money and time available to the researcher will affect the subjects selected. With limited time and money, the researcher might want to investigate subjects who are accessible and do not require payment for participation. Even if you identify a population with a large number of potential subjects, those individuals may be unwilling to participate in the study because of the topic selected. For example, nurses could be asked to share their experiences with alcohol and drug use, but many might fear that sharing this information would jeopardize their jobs and licenses. Researchers need to be prepared to pursue the attainment of subjects at whatever depth is necessary. Having a representative sample of reasonable size is critical for generating quality research findings (Kahn, 1994). Andrews et al. (2007) selected settings where they could obtain the sample size that they needed for their study of the smoking cessation intervention as identified in the following quote:

> Two of 16 subsidized housing developments in Augusta-Richmond County, Georgia were selected based on similar number of residents, housing units, and household income from data supplied by the Augusta Housing Authority. These two low-income housing communities were 99.5% African American, with 95% living at or below the poverty level. Approximately 500 women resided in these two communities and an estimated 200 women were current smokers. (Andrews et al., 2007, p. 47)

Availability of Facilities and Equipment

Researchers need to determine whether their studies will require special facilities to implement. Will a special room be needed for an educational program, interview, or observations? If the study is conducted at a hospital, clinic, or school or college of nursing, will the agency provide the facilities that are needed? Setting up a highly specialized laboratory for the conduct of a study would be expensive and probably require external funding. Most nursing studies are done in natural settings such as a hospital room or unit, a clinic, or a patient's home. Andrews et al. (2007) conducted all their research activities in the community centers for two housing developments (natural settings). The NINR and the American Legacy Foundation funding assisted with the study costs.

Nursing studies frequently require a limited amount of equipment, such as a tape or video recorder for interviews or a physiological instrument, such as a scale or thermometer. Often you can borrow equipment from the facility where the study is conducted, or you can rent it. Some companies are willing to donate equipment if the study focuses on determining the effectiveness of the equipment and the findings are shared with the company. If specialized facilities or equipment are required for a study, you must be aware of the options available before actively pursuing the study.

Cooperation of Others

A study might appear feasible but, without the cooperation of others, it is not. Some studies are conducted in laboratory settings and require the minimal cooperation of others. However, most nursing studies involve human subjects and are conducted in hospitals, clinics, schools, offices, or homes. Having the cooperation of people in the research setting, the subjects, and the assistants involved in data collection is essential. People are frequently willing to cooperate with a study if they view the problem and purpose as significant or if they are personally interested. Andrews et al. (2007) gained the support of the managers for the housing developments and the women living in these developments, so that 103 women participated in the study. Having the cooperation of others can improve the subject participation and promote the successful completion of the study (see Chapter 17 for details on the data collection process).

Ethical Considerations

The purpose selected for investigation must be ethical, which means that the subjects' rights and the rights of others in the setting are protected. If your purpose appears to infringe on the rights of the subjects, you should reexamine that purpose and the investigation may have to be revised or abandoned. There are usually some risks in every study, but the value of the knowledge generated should outweigh the risks. Andrews et al. (2007) received Human Assurance Committee approval from two universities before the study started and informed consent from each of the study participants. By taking these steps, the researchers attempted to implement an ethical study that protected the rights of the African-American women who participated (see Chapter 9 for details on ethical conduct in research).

QUANTITATIVE, QUALITATIVE, OUTCOMES, AND INTERVENTION RESEARCH TOPICS, PROBLEMS, AND PURPOSES

Quantitative and qualitative research approaches enable nurses to investigate a variety of research problems and purposes. Examples of research topics, problems, and purposes for some of the different types of quantitative studies are presented in Table 5-1. The research purpose usually reflects the type of study that is to be conducted. The purposes of descriptive research are to describe variables, identify relationships among variables, or compare and contrast groups on selected variables. For example, Minnick, Mion, Johnson, Catrambone, and Leipzig (2007) described the prevalence and variation of physical restraint use in acute care settings in the United States. The research topics, problems, and purposes for this study are presented in Table 5-1.

The purpose of correlational research is to examine the type (positive or negative) and strength of relationships among variables. In their correlational study, Howell, Rice, Carmon, and Hauber (2007) examined the relationships among anxiety, anger, and blood pressure in children (see Table 5-1). Quasi-experimental studies are conducted to determine the effect of a treatment or independent variable on designated dependent or outcome variables. Berry, Savoye, Melkus, and Grey (2007) examined the effects of a coping skills training (CST) intervention on the body mass index (BMI) and body fat percentage (BFP) of obese multiethnic parents whose overweight children were attending a weight management program. The parents receiving the CST had significantly lower BMI and BFP than the parents in the comparison group (Berry et al., 2007).

Experimental studies are conducted in highly controlled settings and under highly controlled conditions to determine the effect of one or more independent variables on one or more dependent

TABLE 5-1	Quantitative Research: Topics, Problems, and Purposes	
Type of Research	**Research Topic**	**Research Problem and Purpose**
Descriptive research	Physical restraints, acute care hospitals, therapy disruption, patient safety	*Title of study:* "Prevalence and variation of physical restraint use in acute care settings in the U.S." (Minnick et al., 2007, p. 30). *Problem:* "Practitioners' use of physical restraints (PR) in health care settings is a controversial practice that occurs in developed countries worldwide (Choi & Song, 2003; Hamers & Huizing, 2005…). Although intended to protect patients, physical restraint use can have direct deleterious effects, e.g., pressure ulcers and death…. For the past 15 years, U.S. regulatory and accrediting agencies have launched major initiatives aimed at restraint reduction in hospitals (U.S. DHHS [Department of Health and Human Services], 1992, 1995…). Despite these regulatory pressures, little is known about the current extent of PR use" (Minnick et al., 2007, p. 30). *Purpose:* The purpose of this study was "to (a) describe U.S. hospital PR rates and patterns, and (b) explore how U.S. policy and research initiatives might be shaped by the findings" (Minnick et al., 2007, p. 30).
Correlational research	Hypertension, blood pressure, psychosocial factors, biological factors	*Title of study:* "The relationships among anxiety, anger, and blood pressure in children" (Howell et al., 2007, p. 17). *Problem:* "Hypertension affects over 50 million Americans aged 6 and over and is a recognized risk factor for the development of cardiovascular disease (American Heart Association, 2004). Although few children have hypertension or cardiovascular disease, biological and psychosocial risk factors for the development of hypertension in adulthood are estimated to be present in children by the age of 8 (Solomon & Matthews, 1999)…. Although the contribution of these factors to the development of hypertension has been investigated in adults and adolescents… much less research has been done with children (Hauber, Rice, Howell, & Carmon, 1998)" (Howell et al., 2007, p. 17). *Purpose:* "The purpose of this study was to determine the relationships between trait anxiety, trait anger, height, weight, patterns of anger expression, and blood pressure in a group of elementary school children" (Howell et al., 2007, p. 18).

Continued

variables. Rasmussen and Farr (2003) conducted an experimental study of the effects of morphine and time of day on pain and beta-endorphin (BE) in groups of mice in a laboratory setting. In this basic research, the investigators found that morphine abolishes the BE response to pain but does not inhibit pain equally at all times of the day. Thus, morphine doses should be titrated to maximize pain control with less medication. However, additional human research is needed before the findings will have implications for nursing practice.

The problems formulated for qualitative research identify an area of concern that requires investigation. The purpose of a qualitative study indicates the focus of the study and whether it is a subjective concept, an event, a phenomenon, experience, or a facet of a culture or society (Marshall & Rossman, 2006; Munhall, 2001). Examples of research topics, problems, and purposes from some different types of qualitative studies are presented in Table 5-2. Phenomenological research seeks an understanding of human experience from an individual researcher's perspective, such as the lived experience of adult survivors of childhood cancer conducted by Prouty, Ward-Smith, and Hutto (2006). Four themes emerged from this study: "(1) ongoing consequences for having had cancer, (2) living with uncertainty, (3) the cancer experience is embodied into one's present sense of self, and (4) support is valued" (Prouty et al., 2006, p. 143).

In grounded theory research, the problem identifies the area of concern and the purpose indicates the focus of the theory to be developed from the research

TABLE 5-1   Quantitative Research: Topics, Problems, and Purposes—Cont'd

Type of Research	Research Topic	Research Problem and Purpose
Quasi-experimental research	Obesity, overweight, coping skills, behavior control, stress management, multiethnic	*Title of study:* "An intervention for multiethnic obese parents and overweight children" (Berry et al., 2007). *Problem:* "Obesity is increasing at an alarming rate in the United States [U.S.]. The percentage of at risk for overweight or overweight children and overweight and obese adults has increased dramatically over the past 40 years, with Black, Hispanic, and native American families disproportionately affected (Jolliffe, 2004; U.S. Department of health and Human Services, 2001). Currently, 64% of adults are either overweight or obese, and 30% of the children.... Coping skills training (CST) is a form of a cognitive behavioral intervention and is based on social learning theory (Bandura, 1977), which is designed to improve self-efficacy outcomes.... Grey, Boland, Davidson, Li, and Tamborlane (2000) found that in female patients with type 1 diabetes, CST prevented weight gain and improved long-term metabolic and psychosocial outcomes... There are no data about interventions using CST to target multiethnic obese parents and their overweight children attending weight management programs" (Berry et al., 2007, pp. 63–64.) *Purpose:* "The purpose of this pilot study was to determine the effects of the addition of coping skills training for obese multiethnic parents whose overweight children were attending a weight management program" (Berry et al., 2007, 63).
Experimental research	Pain management, morphine, beta-endorphin, circadian rhythm, animals	*Title of study:* "Effects of morphine and time of day on pain and beta-endorphin" (Rasmussen & Farr, 2003). *Problem:* "Although narcotics have been used as analgesics for many years, clients still are experiencing pain.... Morphine is an important pharmacological modulator of pain and initiator of analgesia.... Circadian (approximately 24 hours) rhythms influence the expression of pain and the body's responsiveness to analgesic medications (Gagnon et al., 2001).... Endogenous opioids, such as morphine, activate the descending pain control system.... Currently, the timing of the administration of morphine is not based on its circadian effects. Both PLRL [paw-licking response latency in mice] and BE [beta-endorphin] are known to exhibit a circadian rhythm, or a rhythm that repeats once in a 24-hour period. Yet no well-controlled, time-based studies have been conducted to test the effects of morphine on pain response (PLRL) and plasma BE when administered at different times of day" (Rasmussen & Farr, 2003, pp. 105–107). *Purpose:* The purpose of the study was to "investigate whether there were time-of-day differences in the effects of morphine on the pain tolerance threshold and the circadian plasma BE response to pain" (Rasmussen & Farr, 2003, p. 107).

TABLE 5-2 ⬛ Qualitative Research: Topics, Problems, and Purposes

Type of Research	Research Topic	Research Problem and Purpose
Phenomenological research	Lived experience, childhood cancer, survivorship, phenomenology	*Title of study:* "The lived experience of adult survivors of childhood cancer" (Prouty et al., 2006, p. 143). *Problem:* "In the mid-1970s fewer than 65% of children diagnosed with cancer survived 5 years…. Today, as many as 78% of children diagnosed with and treated for cancer before age 20 survive 5 years, and as many as 70% of those survivors live to adulthood (American Cancer Society, 2000). By 2010, it is estimated that 1 in every 250 young adults will be a long-term survivor of childhood cancer…. Physical consequences of cancer and treatment are well documented in the literature, and psychosocial issues have also been addressed. However, little is known about the adult survivor's perspective of living with the consequences of having had and having been treated for cancer" (Prouty et al., 2006, pp. 143–144). *Purpose:* "The purpose of this phenomenological study was to examine the lived experience of 12 adults who survived childhood cancer" (Prouty et al., 2006).
Grounded theory research	Self-care, poverty, schizophrenia, diabetes mellitus	*Title of study:* "Doing my best: Poverty and self-care among individuals with schizophrenia and diabetes mellitus" (El-Mallakh, 2007, p. 49). *Problem:* "Mental health clinicians and researchers increasingly recognize that individuals with schizophrenia have a high risk of developing diabetes mellitus (DM) (Bushe & Holt, 2004…). Whereas rates of diabetes in the general populations range from 2% to 6%, prevalence rates of diabetes among individuals with schizophrenia range from 15% to 18%, and up to 30% have impaired glucose tolerance (Bushe & Holt, 2004; Schizophrenia and Diabetes Expert Consensus Group, 2004)…. The recent mental health literature has focused on the screening, diagnosis, and treatment of diabetes in this population, including discussions of the risks and benefits of atypical antipsychotic use…. However, few researchers have investigated the influence of social and demographic characteristics on diabetic self-care among individuals with schizophrenia and diabetes" (El-Mallakh, 2007, pp. 49–50). *Purpose:* "A grounded theory study was conducted to examine several aspects of diabetic self-care in individuals with schizophrenia and DM" (El-Mallakh, 2007, p. 50).
Ethnography research	Critical illness, mechanical ventilation, weaning, family presence	*Title of study:* "Family presence and surveillance during weaning from prolonged mechanical ventilation" (Happ et al., 2007, p. 47). *Problem:* "During critical illness, mechanical ventilation imposes physical and communication barriers between family members and their critically ill loved ones…. Most studies of family members in the intensive care unit (ICU) have focused on families' needs for information, access to the patient, and participation in decisions to withdraw or withhold life-sustaining treatment…. Although numerous studies have been conducted of patient experiences with short- and long-term mechanical ventilation (LTMV), research has not focused on family interactions with patients during weaning from mechanical ventilation. Moreover, the importance of family members' bedside presence and clinicians' interpretation of family behaviors at the bedside have not been critically examined" (Happ et al., 2007, pp. 47–48). *Purpose:* "With the use of data from an ethnographic study of the care and communication processes during weaning from LTMV, we sought to describe how family members interact with the patients and respond to the ventilator and associated ICU bedside equipment during LTMV weaning" (Happ et al., 2007, p. 48).
Historical research	Disclosure, terminal status, death, dying, historical analysis	*Title of study:* "An historical analysis of disclosure of terminal status" (Krisman-Scott, 2000). *Problem:* "In the last century the manner and place in which Americans experience death has changed. Sudden death has decreased and slow dying has increased…. Often, in response to both avoidance and denial, the dying pretend to be unaware. This cycle of pretense, instead of being helpful, robs a person of the opportunity to make appropriate end-of-life decisions and maintain power and control over what remains of life…. Nurses, for a variety of reasons, have for the most part avoided telling people they are close to death, even though secrecy creates serious problems in caring for the dying…. The amount of information given to patients about illness, treatment, and prognosis has changed over time. Movement toward greater disclosure of health information to patients has occurred in the past 60 years" (Krisman-Scott, 2000, p. 47).

Continued

Type of Research	Research Topic	Research Problem and Purpose

TABLE 5-2 Qualitative Research: Topics, Problems, and Purpose—*Cont'd*

Type of Research	Research Topic	Research Problem and Purpose
		Purpose: "The purpose of this study was to examine the concept of disclosure as it relates to terminal prognosis and trace its historical development and practice in the United States over the last 60 years" (Krisman-Scott, 2000, p. 47).
Philosophi-cal analysis research	Rights, human rights, patient rights, health care	*Title of study:* "Conceptual analysis of rights using a philosophic inquiry approach" (Reckling, 1994).
		Problem: "Nurses encounter the word right(s) in many aspects of their personal and professional lives. Patients' rights documents are displayed in healthcare institutions.... Yet the idea of rights often is not understood clearly. For instance, controversy exists regarding whether access to healthcare is a human right. Furthermore, individual rights are not always honored. Sometimes rights are in conflict, as when one individual's right to confidentiality conflicts with another's right to information" (Reckling, 1994, p. 309).
		Purpose: "Philosophers have analyzed the ontology and epistemology of rights: Do rights exist? If so, what constitutes them? How do we recognize one when we see it? Where do rights originate? What does having a right imply?" (Reckling, 1994, p. 311).
Critical social theory research	Oppressed group behaviors	*Title of study:* "A case study of oppressed group behavior in nurses" (Hedin, 1986).
		Problem: "The study of the behavior of others sometimes reflects our own behaviors."
		Purpose: "A study was carried out in the Federal Republic of Germany (FRG) to analyze the social, economic, and political factors affecting the nursing education system.... Theoretical constructs from the work of critical social theorist Jurgen Habermas and adult educator Paulo Freire were used to achieve a deeper understanding of the interrelations between the cultural context and the nursing education system as well as to provide direction for conceptualizing ways to transcend oppressive circumstances" (Hedin, 1986, p. 53).

(Munhall, 2001). For example, El-Mallakh (2007) investigated the poverty and self-care among individuals with schizophrenia and diabetes mellitus. Based on the findings from this grounded theory study, El-Mallakh (2007, p. 49) developed a "model, Evolving Self-Care, that describes the process by which respondents developed health beliefs about self-care of dual illnesses. One subcategory of the model, Doing My Best, was further analyzed to examine the social context of respondents' diabetic self-care."

In ethnographic research, the problem and purpose identify the culture and the specific attributes of the culture to be examined, described, analyzed, and interpreted. Happ, Swigart, Tate, Arnold, Sereika, and Hoffman (2007) conducted an ethnographic study of family presence and surveillance during weaning of their family member from a ventilator. These researchers concluded that "this study provided a potentially useful conceptual framework of family behaviors with long-term critically ill patients that could enhance the dialogue about family-centered care and guide future research on family presence in the intensive care unit" (Happ et al., 2007, p. 47).

The problem and purpose in historical research focus on a specific individual, a characteristic of society,

an event, or a situation in the past and identify the period in the past that will be examined. For example, Krisman-Scott (2000) conducted a historical study of disclosure of terminal status from 1930 to 1990 (see Table 5-2). The researcher concluded that disclosure of terminal status has slowly changed over time, from concealment in the 1930s to more general acceptance of disclosure today. The groundwork for the change took place in the 1950s and 1960s and culminated in the 1970s. This change is based on the expanding view of individual rights, perceptions of death, and the responsibilities of health care providers. The information from this study can assist nurses in knowing what and when to communicate to patients with terminal illness.

The problem and purpose in philosophical inquiry identify the focus of the analysis, whether it is to clarify meaning, make values manifest, identify ethics, or examine the nature of knowledge. Of the three types of philosophical inquiry (foundational inquiry, philosophical analysis, and ethical analysis), only an example of philosophical analysis is provided with an analysis of the concept of "rights" (Reckling, 1994). The problem and purpose in critical social theory identify a society and indicate the particular aspects

Type of Research	Research Topic	Research Problem and Purpose
TABLE 5-3 Outcomes Research: Topics, Problem, and Purpose		
Outcomes research	Patient outcomes, special care unit, intensive care unit, chronically critically ill	*Title of study:* "Patient outcomes for the chronically critically ill: Special care unit versus intensive care unit" (Rudy et al., 1995).
		Problem: "The original purpose of intensive care units (ICUs) was to locate groups of patients together who had similar needs for specialized monitoring and care so that highly trained health care personnel would be available to meet these specialized needs. As the success of ICUs has grown and expanded, the assumption that a typical ICU patient will require only a short length of stay in the unit during the most acute phase of an illness has given way to the recognition that stays of more than one month are not uncommon.... These long-stay ICU patients represent a challenge to the current system, not only because of costs, but also because of concern for patient outcomes.... While ample evidence confirms that this subpopulation of ICU patients represents a drain on hospital resources, few studies have attempted to evaluate the effects of a care delivery system outside the ICU setting on patient outcomes, costs, and nurse outcomes" (Rudy et al., 1995, p. 324).
		Purpose: "The purpose of this study was to compare the effects of a low-technology environment of care and a nurse case management care delivery system (specific care unit, SCU) with the traditional high-technology environment (ICU) and primary nursing care delivery system on the patient outcomes of length of stay, mortality, readmission, complications, satisfaction, and cost" (Rudy et al., 1995, p. 324).

of the society that will be examined to determine their influence on an event, a situation, or a system in that society. Hedin (1986) conducted critical social theory research in examining the oppressed group behaviors in nurses.

Outcomes research is conducted to examine the end results of care. Table 5-3 includes the topics, problem, and purpose from an outcomes study by Rudy, Daly, Douglas, Montenegro, Song, and Dyer (1995). This study was conducted to determine the patient outcomes for the chronically critically ill in the special care unit (SCU) versus the intensive care unit (ICU). The investigators examined common outcomes of cost, patient satisfaction, length of stay, complications, and readmissions to determine the impact of care from these two units on the patients and the health care system. The findings from this 4-year study demonstrated that nurse case managers in an SCU setting can produce patient outcomes equal to or better than those obtained in the traditional ICU environment for long-term, critically ill patients. In addition, the SCU group showed significant cost savings compared with the ICU group.

Intervention research determines the interventions that are most effective in managing clinical problems. Some interventions might focus on risk reduction, prevention, treatment, or resolution of health-related problems or symptoms; management of a problem or symptom; or prevention of complications associated with a practice problem. In intervention research, the interventions might have more than one purpose and multiple outcomes. For example, McCain et al. (2003) examined the effectiveness of two complex interventions, cognitive-behavioral stress management (CBSM) and social support, on the multiple outcomes of patients with HIV infection. Table 5-4 provides the topics, problem, and purpose from the study by McCain et al. (2003). The outcomes measured in this study were many physiological and psychological variables, which are commonly used to determine the health status of patients with HIV. The CBSM intervention was found to be the most effective in producing positive physical and psychological outcomes for patients with HIV infection.

SUMMARY

- A research problem is an area of concern where there is a gap in the knowledge base needed for nursing practice and includes significance, background, and problem statement.
- The major sources for nursing research problems include nursing practice, researcher and peer interactions, literature review, theory, and research priorities identified by individuals, specialty groups, professional organizations, and funding agencies.

TABLE 5-4 Intervention Research: Topics, Problem, and Purpose		
Type of Research	**Research Topic**	**Research Problem and Purpose**
Intervention research	Stress management, social support, nursing interventions, HIV/AIDS, psychoneuroimmunology (PNI), quality of life, coping, psychosocial functioning, immune status, somatic health, viral load	*Title of study:* "Effects of stress management on PNI-based outcomes in persons with HIV disease" (McCain et al., 2003, p. 102). *Problem:* "Although it remains potentially fatal, infection with the human immunodeficiency virus (HIV) has become eminently more treatable as a chronic illness with the advent of highly active antiretroviral therapies.... Insights as to the relationship of psychological and physiological health in HIV and other disease are emanating from research in psychoneuroimmunology (PNI).... A growing body of research with persons who have HIV disease, as well as those who have other chronic and potentially fatal illnesses such as cancer, indicates that not only can a variety of biobehavioral strategies for stress management mitigate psychological distress and improve coping skills, they also can enhance immune function through neuroendocrine–immune system modulation.... More recent work has continued to support the use of CBSM [cognitive-behavioral stress management] as an effective strategy in the management of distress associated with HIV disease.... Little comparative research has been done to determine the relative effect of these two types of interventions on either psychological or physiological status" (McCain et al., 2003, pp. 102–105). *Purpose:* "This study was undertaken to compare the effects of CBSM groups, social support groups (SSG), and a wait-listed control group on the outcomes of psychosocial functioning (perceived stress, coping patterns, social support, uncertainty, psychological distress), quality of life, neuroendocrine mediation (salivary cortisol, DHEA levels), and somatic health (disease progression; HIV-specific health status; viral load; immune status)" (McCain et al., 2003, p. 105).

- Replication is essential for the development of evidence-based knowledge for practice and includes four types: exact, approximate, concurrent, and systematic.
- The research purpose is a concise, clear statement of the specific goal or aim of the study and usually indicates the type of study (quantitative, qualitative, outcomes, or intervention research) to be conducted.
- The researcher examines the real-world situation, identifies research topics, generates questions, and ultimately clarifies and refines a research problem.
- From the problem, a specific goal or research purpose is developed that provides a clear focus for the study.
- Based on the research purpose, specific research objectives, questions, or hypotheses are developed to direct the study.
- The feasibility of the research problem and purpose are determined by examining the time and money commitments; researchers' expertise; availability of subjects, facility, and equipment; cooperation of others; and the study's ethical considerations.
- Quantitative, qualitative, outcomes, and intervention studies enable nurses to investigate a variety of research problems and purposes.

REFERENCES

American Association of Critical-Care Nurses (AACN), (2006). *AACN's research priority areas*. Retrieved October 3, 2007, from www.aacn.org.

American Cancer Society. (2000). *Cancer facts and figures 2000*. Atlanta, GA: Author.

American Heart Association. (2004). *Statistical supplement*. Retrieved August 10, 2004, from http://americanheart.org.

American Organization of Nurse Executives (AONE). (2006). *AONE 2007 education and research priorities*. Retrieved October 3, 2007, from www.aone.org/aone/edandcareer/priorities.html.

Andrews, J. O., Bunting, S., Felton, G., & Heath, J. (2004). *A grounded theory study of successful smoking cessation in African American women*. Unpublished manuscript.

Andrews, J. O., Felton, G., Wewers, M. E., Waller, J., & Humbles, P. (2005). Sister to sister: Assisting low-income women to quit smoking. *Southern Online Journal of Nursing Research, 6*(1), 2–23. Retrieved October 3, 2007, from www.snrs.org/publications/SOJNR_articles/iss01vol06.pdf.

Andrews, J. O., Felton, G., Wewers, M. E., Waller, J., & Tingen, M. (2007). The effect of a multi-component smoking cessation intervention in African American women residing in public housing. *Research in Nursing & Health, 30*(1), 45–60.

Artinian, B. M., & Anderson, N. (1980). Guidelines for the identification of researchable problems. *Journal of Nursing Education, 19*(4), 54–58.

Bandura, A. (1977). *Social learning theory.* Englewood Cliffs, NJ: Prentice-Hall.

Baranowski, T., & Simons-Morton, B. (1990). A center-based program for exercise change among Black-Americans. *Health Education Quarterly, 17*(3), 179–186.

Beck, C. T. (1994). Replication strategies for nursing research. *Image: Journal of Nursing Scholarship, 26*(3), 191–194.

Berry, D., Savoye, M., Melkus, G., & Grey, M. (2007). An intervention for multiethnic obese parents and overweight children. *Applied Nursing Research, 20*(2), 63–71.

Betz, C. L. (2002). Healthy children 2010: Implications for pediatric nursing practice [Editorial]. *Journal of Pediatric Nursing, 17*(3), 153–156.

Beveridge, W. I. B. (1950). *The art of scientific investigation.* New York: Vintage.

Brink, P. J., & Wood, M. J. (1979). Multiple concurrent replication. *Western Journal of Nursing Research, 1*(2), 117–118.

Brown, B. E., & Garrison, C. J. (1990). Patterns of symptomatology of adult women incest survivors. *Western Journal of Nursing Research, 12*(5), 587–600.

Browne, A., & Finkelhor, D. (1986). Impact of child sexual abuse: A review of the research. *Psychological Bulletin, 99*(1), 66–77.

Bushe, C., & Holt, R. (2004). Prevalence of diabetes and impaired glucose tolerance in patients with schizophrenia. *British Journal of Psychiatry, 184*(Suppl. 47), S67–S71.

Campbell, J. P., Daft, R. L., & Hulin, C. L. (1982). *What to study: Generating and developing research questions.* Beverly Hills, CA: Sage.

Chinn, P. L., & Kramer, M. K. (2008). *Integrated theory and knowledge development* (7th ed.). St. Louis: Mosby.

Choi, E., & Song, M. (2003). Physical restraint use in Korean ICU. *Journal of Clinical Nursing, 12*(5), 651–659.

Davies, A. R., Doyle, M. A. T., Lansky, D., Rutt, W., Stevic, M. O., & Doyle, J. B. (1994). Outcomes assessment in clinical settings: A consensus statement on principles and best practices in project management. *The Joint Commission Journal on Quality Improvement, 20*(1), 6–16.

Doran, D. (2003). *Nursing-sensitive outcomes: State of the science.* Sudbury, MA: Jones & Bartlett.

El-Mallakh, P. (2007). Doing my best: Poverty and self-care among individuals with schizophrenia and diabetes mellitus. *Archives of Psychiatric Nursing, 21*(1), 49–60.

Fahs, P. S., Morgan, L. L., & Kalman, M. (2003). A call for replication. *Journal of Nursing Scholarship, 35*(1), 67–71.

Frenn, M., Malin, S., & Bansal, N. K. (2003). Stage-based interventions for low-fat diet with middle school students. *Journal of Pediatric Nursing, 18*(1), 36–45.

Gagnon, B., Lawlor, P. C., Mancini, I. L., Pereira, J. L., Hanson, J., & Bruera, E. D. (2001). The impact of delirium on the circadian distribution of breakthrough analgesia in advanced cancer patients. *Journal of Pain Symptom Management, 22*(4), 826–833.

Gold, E. R. (1986). Long-term effects of sexual victimization in childhood: An attributional approach. *Journal of Consulting and Clinical Psychology, 54*(4), 471–475.

Grey, M., Boland, E. A., Davidson, M., Li, J., & Tamborlane, W. V. (2000). Coping skills training for youth with diabetes mellitus has long-lasting effect on metabolic control and quality of life. *Journal of Pediatrics, 137*(1), 107–113.

Haller, K. B., & Reynolds, M. A. (1986). Using research in practice: A case for replication in nursing: Part II. *Western Journal of Nursing Research, 8*(2), 249–252.

Hamers, J. P., & Huizing, A. R. (2005). Why do we use physical restraints with the elderly? *Zeitschrift fur Gerontologie and Geriatrie, 38*(1), 19–25.

Happ, M. B., Swigart, V. A., Tate, J. A., Arnold, R. M., Sereika, S. M., & Hoffman, L. A. (2007). Family presence and surveillance during weaning from prolonged mechanical ventilation. *Heart & Lung, 36*(1), 47–57.

Hauber, R. P., Rice, M. H., Howell, C. C., & Carmon, M. (1998). Anger and blood pressure readings in children. *Psychosomatic Medicine, 11*(1), 2–11.

Hedin, B. A. (1986). A case study of oppressed group behavior in nurses. *Image: Journal of Nursing Scholarship, 18*(2), 53–57.

Henry, B. M., & Chang, W. Y. (1998). Nursing research priorities in Africa, Asia, and Europe. *Image: Journal of Nursing Scholarship, 30*(2), 115–116.

Howell, C. C., Rice, M. H., Carmon, M., & Hauber, R. P. (2007). The relationships among anxiety, anger, and blood pressure in children. *Applied Nursing Research, 20*(1), 17–23.

Jarvis, M. J., & Wardle, J. (1999). Social patterning of individual health behaviors: The case of cigarette smoking. In M. Marmot & R. G. Wilkinson (Eds.), *Social determinates of health* (pp. 240–255). Oxford: Oxford University Press.

Jolliffe, D. (2004). Continuous and robust measures of the overweight epidemic: 1971–2000. *Demography, 41*(2), 303–314.

Kahn, C. R. (1994). Picking a research problem: The critical decision. *New England Journal of Medicine, 330*(21), 1530–1533.

Kaplan, B. A. (1964). *The conduct of inquiry: Methodology for behavioral science.* New York: Harper & Row.

Kerlinger, F. N., & Lee, H. B. (2000). *Foundations of behavioral research* (4th ed.). Fort Worth, TX: Harcourt College Publishers.

Krisman-Scott, M. A. (2000). An historical analysis of disclosure of terminal status. *Journal of Nursing Scholarship, 32*(1), 47–52.

Lewandowski, A., & Kositsky, A. M. (1983). Research priorities for critical care nursing: A study by the American Association of Critical Care Nurses. *Heart & Lung, 12*(1), 35–44.

Lindeman, C. A. (1975). Delphi survey of priorities in clinical nursing research. *Nursing Research, 24*(6), 434–441.

Lindquist, R., Banasik, J., Barnsteiner, J., Beecroft, P. C., Prevost, S., Riegel, B., et al. (1993). Determining AACN's research priorities for the 90s. *American Journal of Critical Care, 2*(2), 110–117.

Marshall, C., & Rossman, G. B. (2006). *Designing qualitative research.* Thousand Oaks, CA: Sage.

Martin, P. A. (1995). More replication studies needed. *Applied Nursing Research, 8*(2), 102–103.

McCain, N. L., Munjas, B. A., Munro, C. L., Elswick, R. K., Robins, J. L. W., Ferreira-Gonzales, A., et al. (2003). Effects of stress management on the PNI-based outcomes in persons with HIV disease. *Research in Nursing & Health, 26*(2), 102–117.

Melnyk, B. M., & Fineout-Overholt, E. (2005). *Evidence-based practice in nursing and healthcare: Guide to best practice.* Philadelphia: Lippincott Williams & Wilkins.

Minnick, A. F., Mion, L. C., Johnson, M. E., Catrambone, C., & Leipzig, R. (2007). Prevalence and variation of physical restraint use in acute care settings in the U.S. *Journal of Nursing Scholarship, 39*(1), 30–37.

Moody, L., Vera, H., Blanks, C., & Visscher, M. (1989). Developing questions of substance for nursing science. *Western Journal of Nursing Research, 11*(4), 393–404.

Munhall, P. L. (2001). *Nursing research: A qualitative perspective* (3rd ed.). Sudbury, MA: Jones & Bartlett.

Munhall, P. L., & Boyd, C. O. (1999). *Nursing research: A qualitative perspective* (2nd ed.). New York: National League for Nursing Press.

National Institute of Nursing Research (NINR). (2006). *Strategic plan National Institute of Nursing Research: Areas of research emphasis.* Retrieved October 3, 2007, from www.ninr.nih.gov/AboutNINR/NINRMissionandStrategicPlan.

Panel for the Prediction and Prevention of Pressure Ulcers in Adults. (1992). *Pressure ulcers in adults: Prediction and prevention. Clinical practice guideline.* AHCPR Pub. No. 92–0047. Rockville, MD: Agency for Health Care Policy and Research, Public Health Service, U.S. Department of Health and Human Services.

Pender, N. J. (1996). *Health promotion in nursing practice* (3rd ed.). Stamford, CT: Appleton & Lange.

Prochaska, J. O., Norcross, J. C., Fowler, J. L., Follick, M. J., & Abrams, D.B. (1992). Attendance and outcome in a work site weight control program: Processes and stages of change as process and predictor variables. *Addictive Behaviors, 17*(1), 35–45.

Prouty, D., Ward-Smith, P., & Hutto, C. J. (2006). The lived experience of adult survivors of childhood cancer. *Journal of Pediatric Oncology Nursing, 23*(3), 143–151.

Rasmussen, N. A., & Farr, L. A. (2003). Effects of morphine and time of day on pain and beta-endorphin. *Biological Research for Nursing, 5*(2), 105–116.

Reckling, J. B. (1994). Conceptual analysis of rights using a philosophic inquiry approach. *Image: Journal of Nursing Scholarship, 26*(4), 309–314.

Reynolds, M. A., & Haller, K. B. (1986). Using research in practice: A case for replication in nursing: Part I. *Western Journal of Nursing Research, 8*(1), 113–116.

Rogers, B. (1987). Is the research project feasible? *AAOHN Journal, 35*(7), 327–328.

Rudy, E. B., Daly, B. J., Douglas, S., Montenegro, H. D., Song, R., & Dyer, M. A. (1995). Patient outcomes for the chronically critically ill: Special care unit versus intensive care unit. *Nursing Research, 44*(6), 324–330.

Schizophrenia and Diabetes Expert Consensus Group. (2004). Consensus summary. *British Journal of Psychiatry, 47*(2), S112–S114.

Sidani, S., & Braden, C. P. (1998). *Evaluating nursing interventions: A theory-driven approach.* Thousand Oaks, CA: Sage.

Solomon, K., & Matthews, K. (1999, March). *Paper presented at the American Psychosomatic Society Annual Meeting.* Vancouver, British Columbia, Canada.

Stone, P. W. (2002). What is a systematic review? *Applied Nursing Research, 15*(1), 52–53.

Tierney, A. J. (1998). Nursing research in Europe. *International Nursing Review, 45*(1), 15–18.

U.S. Department of Health and Human Services. (1992). *FDA safety alert: Potential hazards with restraint devices.* Rockville, MD: Author.

U.S. Department of Health and Human Services. (1995). *FDA safety alert: Entrapment hazards with hospital bed side rails.* Rockville, MD: Author.

U.S. Department of Health and Human Services. (1998). Tobacco use among U.S. racial/ethnic minority groups. *A report of the surgeon general—1998.* Rockville, MD: Office on Smoking and Health.

U.S. Department of Health and Human Services. (2000). *Healthy people 2010.* Washington, DC: Author.

U.S. Department of Health and Human Services. (2001). *The surgeon general's call to action to prevent and decrease overweight and obesity 2001.* Washington, DC: U.S. Department of Health and Human Services, Public Health Service, Office of the Surgeon General, U.S. Government Printing Office.

Williams, A. (1972). A study of factors contributing to skin breakdown. *Nursing Research, 21*(3), 238–243.

World Health Organization (WHO). (2006). *Research for health: A position paper on WHO's role and responsibilities in health research.* Retrieved on October 5, 2007, from http://who.int/rpc/en.

Wright, D. J. (1999). Developing an effective research question. *Professional Nurse, 14*(11), 786–789.

CHAPTER **6**

Review of Relevant Literature

A wealth of information is available in the literature for students, practicing nurses, and researchers, and more appears every day. The number of nursing journals is increasing dramatically, and many full-text research reports are available in both electronic and print forms. Thus, conducting a literature review is more enlightening now than in the past. Reviewing the existing literature in an area of interest is a critical step in the writing process. As Becker (1986) put it:

None of us invent it all from scratch when we sit down to write. We depend on our predecessors. We couldn't do our work if we didn't use their methods, results, and ideas. Few people would be interested in our results if we didn't indicate some relationship between them and what others have said and done before us. (p. 140)

This chapter discusses the purposes of various literature reviews, describes quantitative and qualitative reviews, and guides you through the process of performing a Quantitative and qualitative literature review for research purposes. The literature review process is used for many purposes in research, such as developing the problem, purpose, significance, and framework of the study. However, the focus of this chapter will be the review of previous research studies relevant to a proposed study. The three major stages of literature reviews that are discussed are searching the literature, reading the literature, and writing the literature review. The chapter concludes with an explanation of integrative reviews, metasyntheses, and meta-analyses.

Purpose of the Literature Review in Writing Course Papers

For most course papers, your instructor will expect you to review published information on the topic of your paper. Thus, these papers will require literature reviews although the literature you search for may be different. The search should include both periodicals and monographs. For some topics, you may primarily find your material in periodicals, whereas for other topics, you will derive most information from monographs and find little in periodicals. You may find it fruitful to search the Internet for research on some topics. However, document the source and validity of the Internet content you find.

Purpose of the Literature Review in Examining the Strength of the Evidence

The purpose of the literature review designed to examine the strength of the evidence is to identify all studies that provide evidence of a particular intervention, to critique the quality of each study, and to synthesize all of the studies providing evidence of the effectiveness of a particular intervention. It is also important to locate and include previous evidence-based papers that have examined the evidence of a particular intervention, because the conclusions of these authors are highly relevant. This type of literature review is described in greater detail in Chapter 27, Strategies for Promoting Evidence-Based Nursing Practice.

Purpose of the Literature Review in Quantitative Research

The review of literature in quantitative research directs the development and implementation of a study. The major literature review is conducted at the beginning of the research process, and a limited review is conducted during the generalization phase of the research report to integrate knowledge from the literature with new knowledge obtained from the study. The purpose of the literature review is similar for the different types of quantitative studies (descriptive, correlational, quasi-experimental, and experimental). Relevant sources are cited throughout a quantitative research report in the introduction, methods, results, and discussion sections. The introduction section uses relevant sources to summarize the background and significance of the research problem. The review of literature section includes both theoretical and empirical sources that document the current knowledge of the problem. The framework section is developed from the theoretical literature and sometimes from empirical literature, depending on the focus of the study. The methods section describes the design, sample, measurement methods, treatment, and data collection process of the planned study and is based on previous research. Thus, previous studies may be cited in the methods section. In the results section, the data are analyzed with knowledge of the results of previous studies. These studies and their findings should be identified at this point and cited. The discussion section of the research report provides conclusions that are a synthesis of the cited findings from previous research and those from the present study.

Purpose of the Literature Review in Qualitative Research

In qualitative research, the purpose and timing of the literature review vary based on the type of study to be conducted. Some phenomenologists believe the literature should not be reviewed until after the data have been collected and analyzed so that the literature will not influence the researcher's openness (Munhall, 2006). For example, if a researcher decided to describe the phenomenon of dying, the review of literature would include Kubler-Ross's (1969) five stages of grieving. Knowing the details of these stages early on could influence the way the researcher views the phenomenon during data collection and analysis. However, after data analysis, the information from the literature can be compared with findings from the present study to determine similarities and differences. The findings can then be combined to reflect the current knowledge of the phenomenon.

In grounded theory research, a minimal review of relevant studies is done at the beginning of the research process. This review is only a means of making the researcher aware of what studies have been conducted, but the information from these studies is not used to direct data collection or theory development for the current study. The researcher primarily uses the literature to explain, support, and extend the theory generated in the study (Munhall, 2006).

Ethnographic research is reviewed in a manner similar to that used for quantitative research. The literature is reviewed early in the research process to provide a general understanding of the variables to be examined in a selected culture. The literature is usually theoretical because few studies have typically been conducted in the area of interest. From these sources, the researcher develops a framework for examining complex human situations in the selected culture (Munhall, 2006). The literature review also provides a background for conducting the study and interpreting the findings.

In historical research, an initial literature review is conducted to select a research topic and to develop research questions. Then the investigator develops an inventory of sources, locates these sources, and examines them; thus, the literature is a major source of data in historical research. Because historical research requires an extensive review of literature that is sometimes difficult to locate, the researcher can spend months and even years locating and examining sources. The investigator then analyzes and organizes the literature into a report that explains how an identified phenomenon has evolved over a particular time period (Munhall, 2006).

WHAT IS "THE LITERATURE"?

"The literature" consists of all written sources relevant to the topic you have selected. The amount of research information available continues to escalate, with the production of over 6000 new scientific articles a day. At this rate, published scientific knowledge is doubling every 1-2 years. Computerized bibliographic databases have made the process of searching for relevant empirical or theoretical literature easy. There are, however, more difficulties in locating all of the relevant sources for qualitative studies.

WHAT IS A LITERATURE REVIEW?

The purpose of the review is to convey to the reader what is currently known regarding the topic of interest. Thus the literature that is reviewed may include such material as written information in newspapers and popular magazines such as *U.S. News and World Report*, sources of statistical information provided by various departments of the government such as the Census Bureau, the

CDC (Centers for Disease Control and Prevention), the World Health Organization, information relevant to evidence-based practice, and the scholarly literature describing research that has been conducted in the topic of interest. Broadly, the literature searched will include literature for the problem, background, significance, theory, and literature review. A broad range of material may be used for the problem, background, and significance. For example, statistics from such sources as the Census Bureau and CDC may be important for your topic. Content related to health policy publications may be important. For some studies such as those related to problems of caring for the uninsured, news reports may be useful in documenting the significance of your proposed work. Primary sources should be used for theory and the framework. You should limit your material for the literature review section of the paper to relevant studies for which you can obtain full text content. An abstract or condensed version does not allow you sufficient information to adequately review the processes of the study.

The literature review is an organized written presentation of what has been published on a topic by scholars and includes a presentation of research conducted in your selected field of study. The review should be organized into sections that present themes or identify trends. The purpose is not to list all the material published, but rather to synthesize and evaluate it based on the focus of the review. The last section of this chapter, "Writing the Review of Literature," discusses strategies for writing the review of literature.

Literature reviews may be written for various purposes: Class assignments to examine literature related to an assigned topic, review of research to determining the strength of evidence on which to base clinical nursing practice, and reviews conducted to propose or guide the conduct of research. Your literature review should be designed to address the following questions (Asian Institute of Technology, 2000; Union Institute Research Engine, 1999):

- What is known about your topic?
- What is the chronology of the development of knowledge about your topic? Knowledge related to an empirical study includes theories and empirical studies.
- What research evidence is lacking, inconclusive, contradictory, or too limited
- Is there a consensus or significant debate on issues? What are the various positions?
- What directions for your study are indicated by the work of other researchers?
- What are the characteristics of the key concepts or variables in relevant theories or previous studies?

- What are the relationships among the key concepts or variables in relevant theories or previous studies?
- What are the existing theories in the field of study?
- Where are the inconsistencies or other shortcomings in the knowledge base?
- What views need to be (further) tested?
- Why should a problem be (further) studied?
- What contribution can the present paper be expected to make?
- What approaches, designs, or methods of previous studies seem unsatisfactory?

Time Frame for a Literature Review

The time required to review the literature is influenced by the problem studied, sources available, and goals of the reviewer. There is no set length of time for reviewing the literature, but there are guidelines for directing the review process. The narrower the focus of the topic, the less time will be required to review the literature. The difficulty you experience identifying and locating sources and the number of sources to be located also influence the time involved, as will the intensity of effort. Only through experience does one become knowledgeable about the time frame for a literature review. Novice reviewers will require more time to find the needed literature than an experienced searcher, and the novice frequently underestimates the time needed for the review. A time estimation device for novice searchers, as recommended by at least one librarian, is for the searcher to make a good "reasonable" time estimation and then multiply this number by four. This longer estimate is often more realistic. As both time judgment and searching skills are refined the need to use this expanded estimate reduces.

If researchers attempted to read every source that is somewhat related to a selected problem, they would be well read but would probably never complete their search. Some individuals, even after a thorough literature review, continue to believe that they do not know enough about their area of interest, so they persist in their review; however, this ultimately becomes an excuse for not progressing with their work. The opposite of this situation is the individual who wants to move rapidly through the review of literature to reach the "important part" of their work. In both situations, the person has not been able to set realistic goals for conducting the literature review.

Students repeatedly ask, "How many articles should I have? How far back in years should I go to find relevant information?" The answer to both those questions is an emphatic "It depends." Course faculty for masters courses commonly require that you obtain full text articles of all studies (covering all variables in the proposed study) for the previous ten years plus the classic studies conducted in the field of research. Doctoral students are expected to conduct a more extensive review for course papers. If you are writing a research proposal for a thesis or dissertation, the literature required will be extensive. You need to locate the key papers in the field of interest. If you are searching for research, you need to identify the landmark or seminal studies done. Seminal studies are the first studies that prompted the initiation of the field of research. Landmark studies mark an important stage of development or a turning point in the field of research. Beyea & Nicoll (1998) provide some good advice about knowing when you have sufficient sources:

> Many people ask, "How will I know when my literature search is complete?" On one hand, it never will be because new information constantly is being added to literature. Even so, it is important to know when to stop. From our experience, we found that research will reach an apparent saturation point. As you look at reference lists, you will realize that every article and every author is familiar to you. Or, you might see a pattern in the research and it will be evident when the search has reached its natural conclusion. (p. 879)

Sources Included in a Literature Review

Two types of literature are cited in the review of literature for research: theoretical and empirical. Theoretical literature consists of concept analyses, models, theories, and conceptual frameworks that support a selected research problem and purpose. Theoretical sources can be found in serials, periodicals, and monographs. Serials are published over time or may be in multiple volumes but do not necessarily have a predictable publication date. Periodicals are subsets of serials with predictable publication dates, such as journals, which are published over time and are numbered sequentially for the years published. This sequential numbering is seen in the year, volume, issue, and page numbering of a journal. Monographs, such as books, booklets of conference proceedings, or pamphlets, are usually written once and may be updated with a new edition. Periodicals and monographs are available in a variety of media, such as print, online, CD-ROM, or in downloadable form. Textbooks are good sources of theories in nursing. These textbooks are not primary sources but will enable you to identify appropriate theories and then locate and obtain the primary sources.

Empirical literature comprises relevant studies in journals and books, as well as unpublished studies, such as master's theses and doctoral dissertations. A thesis is a research project completed by a master's student as part of the requirements for a master's degree. A dissertation is an extensive, usually original research project that is completed as the final requirement for a doctoral degree. The word *empirical* is defined as knowledge derived from research. You need to acquire the entire published study rather than relying on summaries or abstracts of studies. The empirical literature reviewed depends on the study problem and the type of research conducted. Research problems that have been frequently studied or are currently being investigated have more extensive empirical literature than new or unique problems. All major variables to be included in the proposed study must be included in the research literature reviewed. Other types of published information, such as descriptions of clinical situations, educational literature, and position papers, may be included in the discussion of background and significance of the research topic but because of their subjectivity often are not cited in the review of literature (Marchette, 1985; Pinch, 1995).

The published literature contains primary and secondary sources. A primary source is written by the person who originated, or is responsible for generating, the ideas published. In research publications, a primary source is written by the person or people who conducted the research. A primary theoretical source is written by the theorist who developed the theory or conceptual content. A secondary source summarizes or quotes content from primary sources. Thus, authors of secondary sources paraphrase the works of researchers and theorists. The problem with a secondary source is that the author has interpreted the works of someone else, and this interpretation is influenced by that author's perception and bias. Sometimes errors and misinterpretations have been spread by authors using secondary sources rather than primary sources. You should use mostly primary sources to write literature reviews. Secondary sources are used only if primary sources cannot be located or if a secondary source contains creative ideas or a unique organization of information not found in a primary source. Citation is the act of quoting a source, using it as an example, or presenting it as support for a position taken.

SEARCHING THE LITERATURE

Before writing a literature review, you must first perform literature searches to identify sources relevant to your topic of interest. Auston, Cahn, and

Selden (1992) of the National Library of Medicine have defined a literature search as "a systematic and explicit approach to the identification, retrieval, and bibliographical management of independent studies (usually drawn from published sources) for the purpose of locating information on a topic, synthesizing conclusions, identifying areas for future study, and developing guidelines for clinical practice." As a student, practicing nurse, or nurse researcher, your goal is to develop a search strategy designed to retrieve as much of the relevant literature as possible given the time and financial constraints of your project.

Today, good libraries provide access to large numbers of electronic databases that supply a broad scope of the available literature internationally, enabling library users not only to identify relevant sources quickly but to print full-text versions of many of these sources immediately. Through the use of these databases, researchers can quickly locate a large volume of references. You can make photocopies from journals found in your local library, and you can obtain photocopies of other articles through interlibrary loan arrangements between your library and other libraries across the country. All libraries, public, private, college, and university, have interlibrary loan capabilities. Be aware, however, that research and publication trends vary over time. Material of interest could have been published before the advent of electronic databases. Based on the type of question you are posing in your research, you may need to search both electronic databases and print indexes. Also, given that no database covers everything in a particular discipline, you must consider multiple databases from a variety of related fields. Now, the most complex part of a literature review is identifying the material, not obtaining it. Increasingly, full-text copies of articles can be printed immediately from the Internet. These services—librarian consultations, database searching, interlibrary loan services, full-text article downloads, and more—are often available to faculty and student researchers, even those who live far from the university. We can link with the university library through the Internet, direct telecommunication connections, and e-mail. These resources are also available at many health care facilities and can be accessed by nurses employed there. Those without this access can purchase electronic facsimile (fax) copies of resources from some of the bibliographical search engines, although any library at which you have borrowing privileges can provide you with an interlibrary loan. Because of these resources, researchers can now spend more time reading and synthesizing and less time searching. The next section of the chapter guides you through the process of using these strategies to obtain the relevant literature for your study.

Develop a Search Strategy

Before you begin searching the literature, you must consider exactly what information you are seeking. By writing out your search strategy, you will save considerable time in this phase of your study. A written plan helps you to (1) avoid going back along paths you have already searched, (2) retrace your steps if need be, and (3) search new paths.

Your initial search should be based on the widest possible interpretation of your topic. This strategy enables you to envision the extent of the relevant literature. As you see the results of the initial searches and begin reading the material, you will refine your topic, and then you can narrow the focus of your searches. Consider consulting with an information professional, such as a subject specialist librarian, to develop a literature search approach. These consultations can be performed via e-mail, so that communication occurs at the convenience of both the researcher and information professional. Many university libraries provide this consultation service whether or not the library user is affiliated with the university.

Select Databases to Search

A bibliographical database is a compilation of citations. The database may consist of citations relevant to a specific discipline or may be a broad collection of citations from a variety of disciplines. Databases can be divided into the following three types:

1. Indexes and abstracts compile citations with subject headings and may include a paragraph or so about the citation. These may include or link to full-text materials.
2. Full-text reprint services may or may not include detailed subject analysis.
3. Citation search indexes link citations on the basis of the references at the end of articles.

The databases first used for literature searches were in printed form. They were card catalogs, abstract reviews, and indexes. In nursing, the most relevant print database is the Cumulative Index to Nursing and Allied Health Literature (CINAHL), which contains citations of nursing literature published after 1955. Nursing scholars fondly referred to the print version of CINAHL as "the Red Books" because all the editions were bound with red covers. The print version of CINAHL is still available in libraries, and you may find it useful when searching for citations published before 1982 or if computerized databases are not available. Another print database popular among nurse researchers is the Index Medicus (IM), which was first published in 1879 and is the oldest health-related index. The Index Medicus includes some citations of nursing publications, with the number of nursing journals cited growing; however, the CINAHL contains a more extensive listing of nursing publications and uses more nursing terminology as subject headings. The earliest printed nursing index is the Nursing Studies Index, developed by Virginia Henderson, which consists of citations of nursing literature published from 1890 to 1959. The National Library of Medicine provides free access to several databases, including MEDLINE, the online equivalent of the Index Medicus, with access through Internet Grateful Med and PubMed software (available at www.nlm.nih.gov/medlineplus).

Many government agencies that produce bibliographical databases, such as the National Library of Medicine, provide free access to them. However, vendors may distribute the same data, providing "value-added" enhancements with their search software.

Full-text databases of journal articles are now available for some journals. To have access to these databases, libraries must subscribe to the service. For a variety of reasons, including the cost of receipt and storage as well as convenience to library users, many libraries are discontinuing subscriptions to paper versions of journals and, instead, subscribe to services that provide access to electronic versions. This arrangement gives the user immediate access to articles that can be read online, printed, or saved as a computer file, often whenever and wherever an affiliated user is located. As a result of these innovations, users now have more immediate access to a wide range of literature, including international sources.

Although more and more literature is available immediately in full-text form, the integration of libraries' various bibliographical databases and full-text collections is not always seamless. Often the most useful database, in terms of ease of searching, content coverage, and terminology, may not include the text of the materials of interest. Be prepared to view the search process as one step and the literature thus identified as a second step. Even with the number of full-text digital collections, all researchers must keep in mind that not everything has been digitized, and print resources, including journals, may need to be consulted occasionally.

Select Keywords

Keywords are the major concepts or variables that must be included in your computer search. To determine keywords, identify the concepts relevant to your study.

TABLE 6-1 ■ Purposes of the Literature Review in Quantitative Research

Clarify the research topic
Clarify the research problem
Verify the significance of the research problem
Specify the purpose of the study
Describe relevant theories
Summarize current knowledge
Facilitate development of the framework
Specify research objectives, questions, or hypotheses
Develop definitions of major variables
Identify limitations and assumptions
Select a research design
Identify methods of measurement
Direct data collection and analysis
Interpret findings

Ascertain the populations that are of particular interest in your area of study, specific interventions, measurement methods, or outcomes that are relevant. In quantitative studies, information obtained from the review of literature influences the development of several steps in the research process; these steps are listed in Table 6-1. Search strategies should be designed to ensure that you obtain adequate information for each of the steps presented in Table 6-1. In most databases, subject headings and phrases can be used, as well as single terms. Your problem and purpose statements will guide in identifying relevant terms (see Chapter 5).

You should then think of alternative terms (synonyms) that authors might use for each concept or variable you have identified. You may need to express your search using the exact words the authors have used in the literature you seek. Many bibliographical databases, such as CINAHL, have an article-specific subject analysis and provide formal subject headings for each article. Studies have shown that most searchers rarely use these formal subject terms in the searching process (Lawrence & Levy, 2004; Meats, Brassey, Heneghan, & Glasziou, 2007; Shiri & Revic, 2006). Knowledge and use of this capability can improve your searches dramatically.

These databases have a thesaurus that the researcher, as well as anyone who reads the article, can use as keyword search terms. By logging on to the database, you can access the thesaurus to select relevant terms. The formal subject terms included in the thesaurus may encompass a number of the terms that you have identified and allow you to expand your search to obtain more references or to focus your search to be more specific to your interest. This expansion or focus occurs because someone who has already read the articles has grouped all citations with similar concepts according to similar terms or concepts. For example, depending on the database, the researcher may not have to worry whether *teens, teenagers, youth, adolescents*, or *adolescence* must be searched individually, because it is likely that a search for one term will identify all. A simple way to begin identifying a database's standardized subject terms is to display a few useful full records found by using keywords. The records are the descriptions of the articles, not the articles themselves. Examine the terminology used to describe these articles, and use the terms in additional refined searches. Frequently, word processing programs, dictionaries, and encyclopedias are helpful in identifying synonymous terms and subheadings. A combination of both keywords and formal subjects most often retrieves better search results. Some of the synonymous terms and subheadings for the research topic of postoperative experience are outlined in Table 6-2.

Truncating words can allow you to locate more citations related to that term. For example, authors might have used *intervene, intervenes, intervened, intervening, intervention*, or *intervenor*. To capture all of these terms, you can use a truncated term in your search (the form depends on the rule of the search engine being used), such as *interven, interven**, or *interven$*. Do not truncate words to fewer than four letters; you will get far too many unwanted citations.

Pay attention to variant spellings. You may need to know, for example, that *orthopedic* may also be spelled *orthopaedic*. Consider irregular plurals, such as *woman* and *women*.

If an author is cited frequently, you can perform a search using the author's name. In this case, you should identify the name as an author term, not a keyword term. Recognize that some databases list authors only under first and middle initials, whereas others use full first names. Identifying and using citations to seminal studies in various citation indexes or full-text databases can lead you to other, more current works that have also used the seminal studies as references. You may need to search using the full-text, free keyword, or cited references options if you are trying to locate more current references to a frequently referenced known work. Web of Knowledge, a database developed from the Science Citation Index and the Social Science Citation Index, focuses on the relationships based on these citations. Several other databases, depending on the vendor, may also have a Cited Search function. You may also know of or discover particular journals that are key to your field of research. If so, you may wish to use the journal title as a search term.

Add your selected search terms to your written search plan. As you search, add other terms that you discover from the references you locate. For each search, record (1) the name of the database you used, (2) the date you performed the search, (3) your exact search strategy, (4) the number of articles found, and (5) the percentage of relevant articles. You can develop a table to record this information from multiple search strategies, as shown in Table 6-3. Save the results of each search on your computer's hard disk, a memory stick (flash disk), or a CD-ROM for later reference; in your written search record, document the file name of the search results.

Systematically Record References

The bibliographical information on a source should be recorded in a systematic manner, according to the format that you will use in the reference list. Many

TABLE 6-2 ▪ Clarifying a Research Topic

Research Topic	Synonymous Terms	Subheadings
Postoperative experience	Postoperative care	Postoperative ambulation
	Postoperative recovery	Postoperative attitude
	Postsurgical experience	Postoperative complications
	Surgical care	Postoperative hospitalization
	Surgical recovery	Postoperative pain
		Postoperative teaching

TABLE 6-3 ▪ Written Search Record

Database Searched	Date of Search	Search Strategy	Number of Articles Found	Percentage of Articles Relevant
CINAHL				
MEDLINE				
Academic Search Premier				
Cochrane Library				

From Burns, N., & Grove, S. K. (2007). *Understanding nursing research* (4th ed.). Philadelphia: Saunders, p. 147.

journals and academic institutions use the format developed by the American Psychological Association (APA) (2001). The reference lists in this text are presented in APA format. Computerized lists of sources usually contain complete citations for references and should be saved electronically to access complete reference citations. The editors of the APA publication manual are currently reevaluating the APA format for electronic resources. Many technological changes have occurred since the manual was published in 2001. These changes, which include some nonobvious ones like the ability of a library to link from a citation in one database to the full-text article in a totally different database and the cessation of the print Dissertation Abstracts, have created a need for a technical revision in APA formatting of electronic references. A formal supplement to the manual has been released, and a revision may be considered.

Sources that will be cited in a paper or recorded in a reference list should be cross-checked two or three times to prevent errors. Damrosch and Damrosch (1996) have identified some of the common errors that authors make when applying the APA format, and they provide guidelines for how to avoid them. The sources cited in the reference list should follow the correct format for print and online full-text versions.

Print Version

Nichol, L. H. (2003). A practical way to create a library in a bibliography database manager: Using electronic sources to make it easy. *CIN: Computers, Informatics, Nursing, 21*(1), 48–54.

Online Full-Text Version

Retrieved May 28, 2004, from OVID database, CINAHL, item 22431086.

One problem still not resolved is directly quoting from online full-text articles. Typically, APA stipulates that at the end of a direct quote, the author, year, and page number(s) be cited, allowing the reader to easily find the citation in the original work. Identifying the page number is not possible with an online full-text article that is provided in search engines using hypertext markup language (HTML), because the page numbers are not the same as in the original text. It is possible if the text is provided in portable document format (PDF). APA (2001) has suggested several possibilities for addressing this problem, one of which is to count the number of paragraphs from the beginning of the article to the place of the direct quote. However, none of the proposed strategies has been commonly accepted as a standard. In this text, we have chosen

to list the author's (or authors') last name(s) and the year, omitting the page numbers. If the online text was retrieved from CINAHL, we have indicated this, allowing easy access to the cited article.

Use Reference Management Software

Reference management software can make tracking the references you have obtained through your searches considerably easier. You can use such software to conduct searches and to store the information on all search fields for each reference obtained in a search, including the abstract. Once you have done so, all of the needed citation information and the abstract are readily available to you electronically when you write the literature review. As you read the articles, you can also insert comments into the reference file about each one.

Reference management software has been developed to interface directly with the most commonly used word processing software to organize the reference information using whatever citation style you stipulate. You can insert citations into your paper with just a keystroke or two. The three most commonly used software packages, along with websites that contain information about them, are as follows:

- ProCite (www.procite.com)
- EndNote (www.endnoteweb.com) operates from the Web.
- RefWorks (www.refworks.com) operates from the Web and can be accessed free to some universities' affiliates depending on the license.

Locate Relevant Literature

Within each database, initiate your search of relevant literature by performing a separate search of each keyword you have identified. Search engines are unforgiving of misspellings, so watch your spelling carefully. Most databases allow you to indicate quickly where in the database records you wish to search for the term—in the article titles, journal names, keywords, formal subject headings, citation lists, or full texts of the articles. The most recent citations are usually listed first. You may examine the earliest citations first by changing the order of citations.

Most databases provide abstracts of the articles in which the term is cited, allowing you to get some sense of their content so you may judge whether the information is useful in relation to your selected topic. If you find the information to be an important reference, save it to a file.

At this point in the process, do not try to examine all of the citations listed. Look instead at the number of citations (or "hits") that the search found. In some

TABLE **6-4**	Search Terms and Total Number of Records Retrieved
CINAHL, Plus with Full Text Database, October 6, 2007	
Coping	16,168 records retrieved
Social support	6155 records retrieved
Coping AND social support	1253 records retrieved
Coping AND *social support*, limit Research Article	1069 records retrieved
Coping AND *social support*, limit Research Article, English	1036 records retrieved
Coping AND *social support*, limit Research Article, English, Date from 200401	290 records retrieved
Coping AND *social support*, limit Research Article, English, Date from 200401, Full Text	173 records retrieved

cases, you may have obtained several thousand hits—far too many to examine. For example, on October 6, 2007, a search of CINAHL using the keyword *coping* yielded 16,168 hits. The key term *social support* yielded 6155 hits (Table 6-4).

After you have performed a search, save it as a file, record the number of citations, and proceed to the next keyword. An easy way to do this is to print the search history. The search history usually has the database name noted somewhere, and the printout may have the date on it (Figure 6-1). When you have completed this activity, you will have some sense of the extent of available literature in your area of interest. At this point, you have the information you need to plan more complex searches.

Performing Complex Searches

A complex search of the literature combines two or more concepts or synonyms in one search. You can also select specified areas or fields of a database record, such as *cited references* or *instrumentation*, as a complex search. Determining which of the concepts or synonyms to combine may be based on the results of your previous searches or performed for theoretical reasons. The method of performing more complex searches varies with the bibliographical database, so when you use a particular database for the first time, look for instructions, examine the refine or advanced search options, and consider consulting with

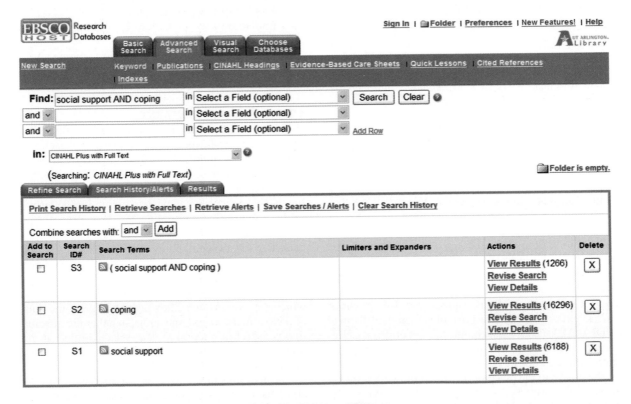

Figure **6-1** Example search history.

a librarian. Do a simple review of the database layout and features first. Once you have an idea of how useful a resource may be, then start refining and including additional concepts and use the features. It can be difficult to determine the cause of little or no results without systematic refinement of simple to more complex searches.

There are several ways to arrange terms in a database search phrase or phrases. The three most common ways are by using (1) Boolean, (2) locational (field labels), and (3) positional operators. Operators permit you to group ideas, select places to search in a database record, and show relationships within a database record, sentence, or paragraph. Examine the Help screen carefully to determine whether the operators you want to use are available and how they are used.

The Boolean operators are the three words AND, OR, and NOT. Often they must be capitalized. The Boolean operators AND and NOT are used with your identified concepts. Use AND when you want to search for the presence of two or more terms in the same citation. Use NOT when you want to search for one idea but not another in the same citation. NOT is rarely used because it is too easy to lose good citations. The Boolean operator OR is most useful with synonymous terms or concepts. Use OR when you want to search for the presence of any of a group of terms in the same search (Table 6-5).

Locational operators (field labels) identify terms in specific areas or fields of a record. These fields may be parts of the simple citation, such as the article title, author, and journal name, or they may be from

---

TABLE 6-5   Venn Diagrams of Boolean Operators Showing Inclusions and Exclusions

AND (more restrictive) [good for including different concepts] all records must contain the terms coping AND social support

OR (less restrictive) [good for including synonyms of a concept] all records must contain either the terms coping OR social support OR both

NOT (restrictive) [good for eliminating undesired concepts] [use with care] all records must contain the term coping but NOT the term social support

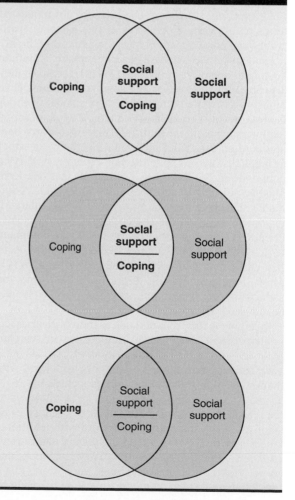

additional fields provided by the database, such as subject headings, abstracts, cited references, publication type notes, instruments used, and even the entire article. In some databases, these specific fields can be selected using a drop-down menu in the database input area. In other databases, specific coding can be used to do the same thing. Do not assume that the entire article is being searched when using the default search; the default is usually looking for your terms in the title, abstract, and/or subject fields. Common formats for locational searches use the database field codes. Each of the following examples shows two ways to perform the same type of search, depending on the specific database being used:

- Coping in ab or coping ab: Find the word coping in the abstract.
- Orem in rf or Orem rf: Find the name Orem in the cited references.
- ENABL in tx or ENABL tx: Find the program ENABL anywhere in the full text.

Positional operators are used to look for requested terms within certain distances of one another. Availability and phrasing of positional operators are highly dependent on the database search software. Common positional operators are NEAR, WITH, and ADJ; they also are often required to be capitalized and may have numbers associated with them. A positional operator is most useful in records with a large amount of information, such as those with full-text articles attached, and is often used with locational operators, in either an implied way or explicitly. For example, ADJ is an abbreviation for *adjacent*; it specifies that one term must be adjacent to another, in any order. ADJ2 commands that there must be no more than two intervening words between the search terms. NEAR usually defines the specific order of the terms; the command term1 NEAR1 term2 requires that the first term occur first and within two words of the second term. WITH often indicates that the terms must be within the same sentence, paragraph, or region (such as subject headings) of the record.

In highly textual records such as those with abstracts or entire articles, using truncation in keyword searches yields good results. Truncation symbols are also database defined and may have numbers associated with them. Common truncation symbols include !, +, $, *, ?, and #. They allow you to enter parts of words as the search phrase, so that the search engine locates all occurrences of that part of the word with additional letters attached. For example, *Catheter*$ can retrieve *catheter, catheters, catheterize, catheterization,* and so on. If the base of the term is very short, just a few letters, consider a limited truncation by using an associated number. For example: *Pet$1* can retrieve up to one character more, for example, *pet* and *pets* but not *petard*.

There is no standardization across database vendors for the format, or even the names of these operators and capabilities. For example, truncation symbols may be called *wildcards*. Most of these features are available in most databases but it can be difficult to determine the language, form, and style to be able to use them. Knowing that the features exist is the first step in locating the necessary help screens in the database you are using.

Many of these various operators are quickly accessible in front of the database software, but others may require further exploration of the Help screens. Different search engines (software) may require different means of structuring your terms so that the software will perform the search in the way you conceive of it. For example, in CINAHL and using EBSCO Host software, you can initiate a Boolean search by entering both terms in the same search. In July 2007, a search in CINAHL for *coping* and *social support* yielded 1223 hits.

In some bibliographical databases, the term AND is used to combine terms. In some databases, the word must be in uppercase. Sometimes quotation marks must be placed around the concepts—for example, "coping" and "social support." In others, just typing *coping* and *social support* will find the references you seek. Combining concepts in some databases is done by adding a plus sign (+) before each term you wish to include. The search terms would appear as follows: +*coping* +*social support*. There must be no space between the + and the term following it, but there must be a space after each term listed. These search methods find references in which both (all listed) terms appear in the same article.

In some databases, you can use the positional term NEAR to indicate that the two words you have selected must be near each other rather than just appear in the same article—for example, coping NEAR social support. The term OR can be used to expand a search. For example, you might wish to search with the phrase *intervention* OR *treatment*; in this case, if either term is used in an article or paper, it will be listed.

Searches for some topics may reveal that many hits are not useful because the search term you have selected also includes another term that is of no interest to you. For example, you may want to examine studies of coping but not those discussing coping in relation to support. To eliminate references with the term *support*, use *coping* NOT *support* as your search phrase.

A number of other complex operations can be used to search databases, but the search methods described here will get you started. Look for instructions about search options in the database you are using. Some databases provide an advanced search option in which separate boxes are available for including multiple terms. For example, you might wish to include an author's last name, one or more key terms, and a journal title in a single search.

Limiting Your Search

You can use several strategies to limit your search if, after performing Boolean searches, you continue to get too many hits. The limits you can impose vary with the database. In CINAHL, for example, you may limit your search to English-language articles. You can also limit the years of your search. For example, you might choose to limit the search to articles published in the past 10 years. Searches can be limited to find only papers that are research, are reviews, are published in consumer health journals, include abstracts, or are available in full text.

When the combined search for *coping* and *social support,* described in the previous section, was limited to research papers in English, there were 1036 hits. Limiting the search to research papers in English published between 2004 and 2007 yielded 290 hits. Limiting the search to research papers in English with full text available yielded 173 hits. Examining 1036 hits is possible but will require considerable time, and if you needed only the most recent studies, you might wish to examine only those. If your interest and time are limited, you might choose to obtain only the 173 hits available in full text (see Table 6-5). Use caution in making this decision; you may, in doing this, fail to obtain some of the most relevant papers on your topic. Exercising the limit to full-text option may result in access to only those items available in that particular database distributed by that particular vendor. Many libraries have a variety of databases distributed by different vendors. Limiting your search to full-text articles can eliminate links from one resource to full text in another (see Table 6-5). However, overall the number of full-text articles available increases yearly as more journals provide full text.

From the titles, you can select (by clicking the box to the left of the reference in the list of citations, OVID software) the hits that seem most relevant to your topic. You can then either print or save to a file the citations you have selected. Saving each citation to a file and then printing it with a word processing program takes considerably less paper than trying to print directly from the database. Consider including the database name, search strategy, and date of search as part of the printout as a record of what terms

were effective, where they were effective, and when they were effective. You may wish to select the full-text option for hits with full text available; you can then either print these papers or save them to files for printing or reading later on the computer screen.

Selecting Search Fields

Search fields indicate the various pieces of information provided about an article by the bibliographical database. The fields vary with the bibliographical database. In CINAHL, by selecting Search Fields at the top of the search page, you can indicate the search fields available in CINAHL you wish listed for the references you select. The following list explains the search fields available for CINAHL:

- *Accession Number.* The number assigned to the citation when it was entered into the CINAHL database.
- *Special Fields Contained.* A list of the special fields available for a particular citation. *Special fields* include abstracts and cited references.
- *Authors.* The names of the authors, last name first, then initials of first names. Author names are in blue and underlined. The underlining indicates that clicking on the name will result in a search listing all of the citations in the database in which that individual is an author. This option allows you to identify other publications of authors who are central to building the body of knowledge about the topic you have elected to study.
- *Institution.* The institution at which each author was affiliated at the time the article was published. This information might be useful if you wished to contact the author.
- *Title.* The title of the article.
- *Source.* The journal title, volume number, issue, page numbers, year, month, and number of references.
- *Abbreviated Source.* An abbreviated version of the journal title, volume number, issue, page numbers, year, month, and number of references.
- *Document Delivery.* The National Library of Medicine (NLM) serial identifier number. This number is useful if you plan to request delivery of the document by fax, e-mail, or postal delivery. In many cases, there is a rather large fee for this service. Contact a library for interlibrary loan arrangements, which may be free or have a nominal cost.
- *Journal Subset.* The categories to which the journal has been assigned. For example, the journal may be classified as a core nursing journal, a nursing journal, a peer-reviewed journal, or a U.S. journal.
- *Special Interest Category.* The categories of specialization to which the journal has been assigned.

For example, the journal may be classified in the category Oncologic Care.

- *CINAHL Subject Headings.* The keywords from the CINAHL thesaurus that have been assigned to the article. Professional indexers who have read the article have made these assignments. Examination of these subject headings in the references you have obtained in a search can suggest additional keywords for your keyword list.
- *Instrumentation.* A list of the measurement instruments used in the study.
- *Abstract.* An abstract of the study.
- *ISSN.* The International Standard Serial Number, an identifier number for the journal.
- *Publication Type.* The type of article, for example, Journal Article, Research Journal Article, Dissertation; also indicates the presence of tables, graphs, and charts.
- *Language.* The language in which the article is written. In many cases, articles that are not in English have English abstracts.
- *Entry Month.* The month in which the citation was entered in the CINAHL database.
- *Cited References.* A list of full references for all citations in the paper. These references can be valuable because you can use them to cross-check the completeness of your computer searches.

To accomplish a cross-check using the database's Cited References list, compare the list with the citations you have obtained from your searches. This is easy to do if you have used reference management software. In many cases, you will find "treasures" you would have missed if you had relied only on the computer search. Some of the references may not be journals or books listed in the databases that you have searched and may provide clues to other databases containing additional useful sources. These references may also suggest new keywords for another computer search in the databases you have been using.

Saved Searches and Alerts

If you are working on a research project in which the literature review may take months or are engaged in a field of study that will interest you for years, you might want to repeat the same search regularly. Many databases permit you to create an account where you can save your search strategy so you can redo the same search with just a few clicks and without having to manually enter the entire strategy again. You might want to have just the new updates of a search strategy sent to you automatically by e-mail without having to redo the entire search, even though this redo now entails just a few clicks. These *Saved Search* and *Alert* features may be available in your favorite databases. However, review your saved and alert strategies with some regularity to ensure you are obtaining what you really desire. Many journals also permit a table of contents to be sent to you automatically when new issues come out. Examine the database or journal home page help screens to determine how to create and use these features.

Searching Electronic Journals

A number of nursing journals are published only in electronic form. Because of the high costs of publishing and distributing a printed journal, a publishing company risks losing money unless there is a large market for the journal. Most of the electronic journals are targeted to relatively small specialty audiences. These journals may have more current information on your topic than you will find in traditional journals, because articles submitted by authors are reviewed and published within 3 to 4 months; for articles submitted to printed journals, the time from submission to publication is 1 to 2 years. Many electronic journals have been established at universities by faculty members interested in a particular specialty area. In some cases, you may have to subscribe to the online journal to gain access to the articles. Some electronic journals are listed in available bibliographical databases, and you can access full-text articles from an electronic journal through the database. However, many electronic journals are not yet in the bibliographical databases or may not be in the database you are using. Ingenta (www.ingenta.com) is a commercial website that allows you to search thousands of online journals from many disciplines.

To obtain relevant articles from an electronic journal, locate the journal on the Internet and scan the titles of articles published. Many libraries have contracts with vendors that enable their affiliated users to have off-campus access to some of these journals and databases. Some contracts specify that nonaffiliated users may use the resources only within the library. Other contracts require that all use of the resources must occur in the library, specified buildings, or specific computers. A list of the current electronic nursing journals is available at www.4nursingjournals.com.

Many libraries provide lists of the electronic journals available to their affiliated users. You should also examine the lists. If you are affiliated with the library, you may be able to obtain articles easily.

Searching the Internet/World Wide Web (www)

Although it is unlikely you will find studies relevant to your topic by searching the World Wide Web, you may find information relevant to the background, significance, framework, design, methods of measurement, and statistical procedures for your study. One advantage of information obtained from the Web is that it is likely to be more current than material you find in books. One disadvantage is that the information is uneven in terms of accuracy. There is no screening process for information placed on the Web. Thus, you find a considerable amount of misinformation, as well as some "gems" you might not find elsewhere. It is important to check the source of any information you obtain from the Web so that you can judge its validity. Use a protocol to evaluate a Web resource similar to that with which you would judge the validity of a journal article; consider who wrote the article and the author's qualifications, where was it published (a quality journal or .gov, .com, .org), when was it created or updated, the appropriate attribution of ideas and facts, and so on. Occasionally you might discover a significant resource on the Web that is available at a cost. Contact your library to see if the resource is available at your institution or may be obtained through Interlibrary Loan or other services at a much reduced or no cost to you.

Various search engines are available for conducting Web searches. Search engines vary in (1) the approach used to search the Web, (2) the extent of Web coverage (most do not cover the entire Web, so you may need to use more than one engine), (3) the frequency with which they update the websites indexed by the search engine, and (4) ease of use. New search engines appear on the scene almost daily, so identifying the "best" search engine in this text is not particularly useful. Many university libraries provide a list of good search engines for your use.

Complex searches may be performed with search engines. The search methods vary with the search engine. Check the instructions for the search engine you are using. These instructions are usually available on the Advanced Search or Help pages. Various engines use the following terms to conduct complex searches:

- Quotation marks
- Brackets
- NEAR (used to narrow the search to only those sites in which two words are close to each other on the page)
- NOT or –
- AND or +
- OR (used when quotation marks or brackets are not used)

Conceptually, techniques used in bibliographical database searching and Web searching do not differ a lot. Terminology and the specifics of ways to search may

be found on the appropriate Help screens. When you find a promising site, you can store its location in your Web browser (called "Favorites" in Internet Explorer). Remember, however, that if you use a website as a reference in your bibliography, you will need to note the date you retrieved it and the address (uniform resource locator [URL]) it had when you viewed it, which are required for proper citation. Storing a website's address in your browser allows you to return to the website easily to check information. Also, websites are frequently updated, and you can check for new information. Sometimes clicking on a link (underlined or highlighted name) on one website will send you to another website with helpful information. Following these links, referred to as surfing the Web, is an important part of a Web search. One problem you may encounter in surfing the Web is information overload; you may find too much information and will need to be selective about what you retrieve.

Although both Internet Explorer and Mozilla Firefox store a history of the websites you have visited as you move from one to another, it is wise to store their locations in your browser to avoid having to retrace your steps through the links. Also, websites are often changed or deleted, so you may wish to save a particularly useful Web page as a file. You may save the text, a graphic, or both from the Web.

Metasearchers offer relatively new approaches to searching the Web. These programs use multiple search engines to perform a search, enabling a single search to cover more of the Web. One disadvantage of metasearchers is that you cannot reliably use Boolean search methods with them. As of the writing of this chapter, our favorite metasearcher is Google, which can be found at www.google.com. Google uses an innovative strategy for searching that increases the number of hits on a topic and identifies documents from a variety of formats beyond html.

Finding Every Relevant Source: What It Takes

It is rarely, if ever, possible to identify every relevant source in the literature. The most extensive retrievals of literature are probably the funded literature review projects focused on defining evidence-based practice or developing clinical practice guidelines. In these projects, a literature review coordinator manages the literature review process. The project employs several full-time, experienced, professional librarians as literature searchers. For these projects, at least two preliminary computerized literature searches are performed; then a comprehensive search is conducted that may encompass material not included in electronic databases, including unpublished sources; finally, periodic searches are performed to update the material. The process requires at least 1 or 2 years of extensive work (Auston et al., 1992). When these extensive literature reviews are completed, the results are published so that you may have access to them and to the citations from the review, either on the World Wide Web (the Web) or in journal articles.

READING AND CRITIQUING SOURCES

Reading and critiquing sources promotes understanding of the current knowledge of a research problem. It involves skimming, comprehending, analyzing, and synthesizing content from sources. Skills in reading and critiquing sources are essential to the development of a high-quality literature review. Many projects require a review of the literature and a summary of current knowledge; examples are a project to use research findings in practice, a research proposal, and a research report. This section focuses mainly on reading skills, with a brief introduction to the critiquing process.

Skimming Sources

Skimming a source is quickly reviewing a source to gain a broad overview of its content. You would probably read the title, the author's name, and an abstract or introduction for the source. Then you would read the major headings and sometimes one or two sentences under each heading. Finally, you would review the conclusion or summary. Skimming enables you to make a preliminary judgment about the value of a source and to determine whether it is a primary or secondary source. Secondary sources are reviewed and used to locate cited primary sources, but they are seldom cited in a research proposal or report.

Comprehending Sources

Comprehending a source requires that you read all of it carefully. Focus on understanding major concepts and the logical flow of ideas within the source. Highlight the content you consider important; you might even want to record its ideas in the margins. Notes might be recorded on photocopies of articles, indicating where the information will be used in developing a research proposal. It is also relatively easy, with just a little practice, to copy and paste salient phrases from digital copies, as well as to record these same types of notes onto documents to accompany a photocopy or into your reference management software user notes.

The kind of information you highlight or note in the margins of a source depends on the type of study or source. The information highlighted on theoretical sources might include relevant concepts, definitions of those concepts, and relationships among them. The notes recorded in the margins of empirical literature might include relevant information about the researcher, such as (1) whether this is a critical or major researcher of a selected problem and (2) other studies this individual has conducted. For a research article, the research problem, purpose, framework, major variables, study design, sample size, data collection, analysis techniques, and findings are usually highlighted. You may wish to record quotations (including page numbers) that might be used in a review of literature section. The decision to paraphrase these quotes can be made later.

You might also record creative ideas about content that develop while you are reading a source. At this point, you will identify relevant categories for sorting and organizing sources. These categories will ultimately guide you in writing the review of literature section, and some may even be major headings in this section.

Analyzing Sources

Through *analysis*, you can determine the value of a source for a particular study. Analysis must take place in two stages. The first stage involves the critique of individual studies. The process of critiquing individual studies, including the steps of comprehension, comparison, analysis, evaluation, and conceptual clustering, is detailed in Chapter 26. During the critique, relevant content in sources is clearly identified, and sources are sorted into a sophisticated system of categories.

Pinch (1995) has developed a table format, which we have modified by adding two columns, that is useful in sorting information from studies into categories for analysis (Table 6-6). Conducting an analysis of sources to be used in a research proposal requires some knowledge of the subject to be critiqued, some knowledge of the research process, and the ability to exercise judgment in evaluation (Fleming & Hayter, 1974; Pinch, 1995). However, the critique of individual studies is only the first step in developing an adequate review of the literature. Any written literature review that simply critiques individual studies paragraph by paragraph is inadequate.

The second stage of analysis involves making comparisons among studies. This analysis allows you to critique the existing body of knowledge in relation to the research problem. You will be able to determine (1) theoretical formulations that have been used to explain how the variables in the problem influence one another, (2) what methodologies have been used

TABLE 6-6 ■ Example of Literature Review Summary Table

(Stress and Coping in CABG Patients and Family Members)

Source	Purpose/Problem	Sample	Framework	Concepts	Design	Instrument(s)	Results	Implications	Comments
Acorn (1995)	Developmental education/support program for families of head-injured patients	19 family members of head-injured patients	Not specified	Coping Self-esteem Well-being	Pretest–posttest Quasi-experimental	Jalowiec Coping Scale, Rosenberg's Self-esteem Scale Life Satisfaction Index	Practical/experimental effects but not statistically significant in coping	Community based Intervention does not necessarily lead to increase	Short time frame Small sample Head injury families
Jalowiec & Powers (1981)	Compare stress of groups, and ID coping strategies used	25 ER patients and 25 hypertensive patients	Lazarus	Stress Coping	Comparative/descriptive	Modified Rahe's Stressful Life Events Quest Jalowiec Coping Scale	Coping used: hope, control, problem-solving	Balance of strategies may be helpful	Not transplant Early Jalowiec patients
Twibell (1998)	Examine how family members used coping styles and effectiveness	59 family members	Not specified	Coping Needs	Exploratory/descriptive	Jalowiec Coping Scale	Effectiveness low Older used more than young	Interventions: discussion, flexible visiting; ID high-risk; diminish ineffective coping; share goals	ICU patients Family
Hanton (1988)	Examine stressors before heart transplantation via case study	1 child awaiting heart transplant	Lazarus & Folkman	Stress Appraisal Coping	Case study	Observation	Fatigue and financial concerns for parents	Evaluate and support family coping skills Recognize that needs change Involve team	Little data on coping Child with/heart
LaMontagne & Pawlak (1990)	ID parents' stressors and coping strategies	30 parents of children in PICU	Lazarus	Stress Coping	Descriptive/exploratory	Semistructured interview Ways of Coping Quest	Combo of problem-solving and emotional Seeking social support	Clinicians can offer assistance and emotional support	PICU patients Parents

Continued

TABLE 6-6 ■ Example of Literature Review Summary Table—*Cont'd*

(Stress and Coping in CABG Patients and Family Members)

Source	Purpose/Problem	Sample	Framework	Concepts	Design	Instrument(s)	Results	Implications	Comments
Voepel-Lewis, Ketefian, Starr, & White (1990)	ID stressors and coping strategies of family members of kidney transplant recipients after transplant	50 family members	Lazarus & Folkman	Stress Coping	Descriptive/ exploratory	Kidney Transplant Quest	More stressors, more coping strategies used Self-controlling and problem-solving coping highest	Teaching plans Team support	Kidneys Family
Collins, White-Williams, & Jalowiec (1996)	ID common stressors experienced by spouses of heart transplant candidates	85 heart transplant candidates	Lazarus & Folkman	Stress Appraisal	Comparative cross-sectional survey	Spouse Transplant Stressors Scale Jalowiec Coping Scale	High levels of spouse stress Fear of death worst	Could lead to interventions to reduce stress	Only spouses Heart transplant rather than liver Some patients not in ICU Coping scores not reported
Gilliss (1984)	Describe stressors of patient/spouses during/after CABG	41 couples	Not specified	Stress	Longitudinal descriptive	Semistructured interviews Impact of Event Scale	Need for info and emotional support	Develop educational program for families/ expectations	CABG Coping not studied Spouses
Porter, Krout, Parks, Gibbs, Luers, Gould, Cupples et al. (1992)	ID transplant patients' fears and concerns while waiting for organ	3 patients awaiting hearts	Not specified	Stress Coping	Retrospective case study	Interviews, open-ended and guided	Family and spiritual support important Denial, humor, meeting with post-transplant patients	Larger, broader studies needed	Heart Coping not focus Small study patients
Nolan, Cupples, Brown, Pierce, Lepley, & Ohler (1992)	Explore stress and coping strategies among families of pre-heart transplant patients	38 family members	T-Double ABCX Model of Family Adjustment	Stress Coping	Descriptive	Family Crisis Oriented Personal Scale, others	More coping strategies used than normal subjects Problem solving	Coping strategies seen as effective in reducing stress	Heart FCOPES Families

Source	Purpose/Problem	Sample	Framework	Concepts	Design	Instrument(s)	Results	Implications	Comments
Reider (1994)	Anxiety levels of family members and variables affecting them	75 family members	T-Double ABCX Model of Family Adjustment	Anxiety Stress	Descriptive	Brief Symptom Inventory FCOPES	Better coping = lower anxiety	ID coping patterns Give info Give family time with patient	General ICU patients Family
Molter (1979)	ID needs of families, and whether being met	40 relatives of patients in critical condition	Crisis theory	Needs	Exploratory/descriptive	Structured interviews with Molter	Hope, caring, info	Info giving Relatively well met	Needs survey Nontransplant Families
Daley (1984)	ID needs of family members of ICU patients and who can meet them	40 family members	Not specified (crisis noted)	Needs	Exploratory	Structured interview Molter survet	Relief of anxiety Need for info, visiting	Team of dr/RN Info	Molter Nontransplant Coping not addressed
Freichels (1991)	Compare family perceptions of needs over time	41 family members	Crisis theory: normaliza-tion theory	Needs longitudinal	Exploratory	Molter CCFNI	Hope, assurance high Hope decreases over time	Generally consistent over time but lesser degree	Family ICU patients Needs Molter
Kleinpell & Powers (1992)	ID needs of family members and whether being met	64 family members and 58 nurses	Family systems theory	Needs	Descriptive/comparative	Molter CCFNI	Info, hope, changes both important Staff variable more important to families	Better staff role info to families	Family Needs Molter Family
Leske (1986)	ID/compare reported needs of families of ICU patients	55 family members of ICU patients	Crisis intervention theory	Needs	Comparative/descriptive	Molter survey, revised: CCFNI	Emotional needs high Hope	Info and emotional support	Needs, continues Molter Families
Norris & Grove (1986)	ID perceptions of family and ICU nurses about family needs	20 family members, 20 nurses	Bertalanffy's general system theory	Needs	Descriptive	Molter survey, revised	Hope, caring, info needs high for families Nurses rate info over caring	Family focus for nursing interventions	Molter Psychosocial General ICU patients Not coping Family, nurses

Continued

TABLE 6-6 ■ Example of Literature Review Summary Table—Cont'd

(Stress and Coping in CABG Patients and Family Members)

Source	Purpose/Problem	Sample	Framework	Concepts	Design	Instrument(s)	Results	Implications	Comments
Davis-Martin (1994)	Compare needs of families of long vs. short ICU stays	26 family members	Not specified	Needs	Descriptive, ex post facto	Molter survey	Needs similar Info	Continue info and support strategies	SICU patients Family
Weichler (1993)	ID info needs/ concerns of caretakers of children after transplant	21 primary caretakers of children after transplant	Not specified	Stress Needs	Descriptive/ exploratory	Semistructured questionnaire	Knowledge key to families	Nurses anticipating needs may decrease stress and increase coping	Mostly Caucasian Children Post liver-renal transplant
Moser, Dracup, & Marsden (1993)	ID needs of patients and spouses following cardiac event	55 patient-spouse pairs	Not specified	Needs	Descriptive/ comparative	Needs assessment instrument	Info needs differed Needs for info unmet by doctors, nurses	Better teaching	Cardiac patients/ spouses
Carmody, Hickey, & Bookbinder (1991)	ID and rank the needs of families of patients undergoing oncology surgery	49 family members	Not specified	Needs	Exploratory/ descriptive	Perioperative Family Needs Quest	Info needs high priority	Info needs Keep informed about condition Designate info nurse	Oncology Coping not investigated Family
Kristensson-Hallström (1999)	Ways parents feel secure Degree of parental participation	224 parents of hospitalized children	Not specified	Security Participation	Nonrandom anonymous survey	Quest Developed for study	Parents wanted varied levels of participation	Role clarification might be helpful for parents	Parents of children, any illness Doesn't address coping specifically

Source	Purpose/Problem	Sample	Framework	Concepts	Design	Instrument(s)	Results	Implications	Comments
Nyamathi, Jacoby, Constancia, & Ruvevich (1992)	Examine relationship of six factors of emotional/ physical adjustment of spouses	100 spouses of critically ill adults	Comprehensive Health Seeking and Coping Paradigm	Adjustment Coping Personality Factors	Descriptive	Spousal Coping Instrument, revised	Emotional coping related to negative personality factor Problem coping with positive	Adjustment may be related to personality factors High-risk may be emotion-focused	Cardiac Spouses
Wainwright (1995)	Examine recovery/ experiences of liver transplant patients	10 liver transplant patients	Grounded theory	Transformation Adjustment	Focused interviews	Topic guide	Family support important	Active teaching needed Support groups helpful	Small sample Patients, not families Liver transplant
Mishel & Murdaugh (1987)	Explore processes for handling uncertainty among families of heart transplant patients	20 family members of heart transplant patients	Grounded theory	Uncertainty adaptation	Interviews	Open-ended question	Alteration in adaptation over time	High psychoso-cial needs of families	Heart transplant Little info on actual coping strategies Families

Modified by graduate student Molly O'Brien, from Pinch, W. J. (1995). Synthesis: Implement a complex process. *Nurse Educator, 20*(1): 34-40.

CABG, Coronary artery bypass grafting; *CCFNI*, critical care family needs inventory; *dr*, doctor; *ER*, emergency room; *eval*, evaluate; *ICU*, intensive care unit; *ID*, identify; *info*, information; *PICU*, pediatric intensive care unit; *Quest*, Questionnaire; *RN*, registered nurse; *SICU*, surgical intensive care unit.

Note: Example provided to illustrate structure of table references not included in reference list.

to study the problem, (3) the methodological flaws in previous studies, (4) what is known about the problem, and (5) what the most critical gaps in the knowledge base are. The information gathered by using the table format shown in Table 6-6 can be useful in making these comparisons. Various studies addressing a research problem have approached the examination of the problem from different perspectives. They may have organized the study from different theoretical perspectives, asked different questions related to the problem, selected different variables, or used different designs. As Galvan (1999, p. 3) so wisely pointed out:

> Due to the fact that empirical research provides only approximations and degrees of evidence on research problems that are necessarily limited in scope, creating a synthesis is like trying to put together a jigsaw puzzle, knowing in advance that most of the pieces are missing and that many of the available pieces are not fully formed.

Sometimes, findings from different studies conflict, leaving understanding in that area unclear and pointing to the need for further research with improved methodologies. As Galvan (1999, p. 3) has suggested, "You may soon find yourself acting like a juror, deliberating about which researchers seem to have the most cohesive and logical arguments, which ones have the strongest evidence and so on." O'Connor (1992) has developed a strategy for using graphing methods to visually indicate the linkage of studies. Lines are drawn from a study to all of the studies cited in it, using a time line to illustrate the development of ideas. This process is repeated until all the studies cited have been mapped.

Synthesizing Sources

Synthesis of sources involves clarifying the meaning obtained from the sources as a whole. Through synthesis, one can cluster and interrelate ideas from several sources to form a gestalt. Rather than using direct quotes from an author, you should paraphrase his or her ideas. Paraphrasing involves expressing the ideas clearly and in your own words. The meanings of these sources are then connected to the proposed study. Last, the meanings obtained from all sources are combined, or clustered, to determine the current knowledge of the research problem (Pinch, 1995). Synthesis is the basis for developing the review of literature section for a research proposal, report, or evidence-based project.

Becker (1986) has suggested that there is a drawback to reviewing the literature; it can "deform" the

position you wish to take about the research topic and the direction further research should take:

> Suppose there is real literature on your subject, the result of years of normal science or what, by extension, we could call normal scholarship. Everyone who works on the topic agrees on the kinds of questions to ask and the kinds of answers they will accept. If you want to write about the topic, or even use that subject matter as the material for a new topic, you will probably have to deal with the old way even though you think it quite foreign to your interests. If you take the old way too seriously, you can deform the argument you want to make, bend it out of shape in order to make it fit into the dominant approach. What I mean by bending your argument out of shape is this. What you want to say has a certain logic that flows from the chain of choices you made as you did the work. If the logic of your argument is the same as the logic of the dominant approach to the topic, you have no problem. But suppose it isn't. What you want to say starts from different premises, addresses different questions, recognizes a different kind of answer as appropriate. When you try to confront the dominant approach to this material, you start to translate your argument into its terms. Your argument will not make the kind of sense it made in its own terms; it will sound weak and disjointed and will appear ad hoc. It cannot look its best playing an opponent's game. And that phrasing puts the point badly, because what's involved is not a contest between approaches, after all, but a search for a good way to understand the world. The understanding you're trying to convey will lose its coherence if it is put in terms that grow out of a different understanding.
>
> If, on the other hand, you translate the dominant argument into your terms, you will not give it a fair shake, for much the same reasons. When you translate from one way of analyzing a problem into another, there is a good chance that the approaches are, as Kuhn (1962) suggested, incommensurable. Insofar as they address different questions, the approaches have very little to do with one another. There is nothing to translate. They are simply not talking about the same things.... A serious scholar ought routinely to inspect competing ways of talking about the same subject matter. The feeling that you can't say what you mean in the language you are using will warn you

that the literature is crowding you.... Use the literature, don't let it use you. (Becker, 1986, pp. 146–149)

WRITING THE REVIEW OF LITERATURE

A thorough, organized literature review facilitates the development of a research proposal. Students frequently ask how long the literature review should be. Unfortunately, there is no way for an instructor to answer this question. The length of the review varies considerably according to the extent of research that has been conducted in the area. In a relatively new area of research, you may find only two or three previous studies, whereas in an established field of research, such as that of coping and social support, a vast quantity of literature exists. You should have two or three studies that include information on each of your variables. These may be the same studies but in all likelihood will not be.

Sorting Your Sources

Relevant sources (theoretical and empirical) are organized for inclusion in the different chapters of the research proposal. The sources to be included in the review of literature chapter are organized to reflect the current knowledge about the research problem. Those sources that provide background and significance for the study are included in the introduction chapter. Certain theoretical sources establish the framework for the study. Other relevant sources become the basis for defining research variables and identifying assumptions and limitations. Content from methodologically strong studies is used to direct the development of the research design, guide the selection of instruments, influence data collection and analysis, and provide a basis for interpretation of findings. Usually, at this point, a researcher is beginning to get a complete picture of his or her study and is excited about its potential. The researcher commonly feels confident about his or her knowledge of the research problem and ability to make the study a reality.

Developing the Written Review

The purpose of the written literature review is to establish a context for your study. The literature review for a study has four major sections: (1) the introduction, (2) a discussion of theoretical literature, (3) a discussion of empirical literature, and (4) a summary.

Introduction

The introduction to the literature review indicates the focus or purpose of the study, identifies the purpose of the literature review, and presents the organizational structure of the review. You should make clear in this section what you will and will not be covering. If you are taking a particular position or developing a logical argument for a particular perspective on the basis of the literature, make this position clear in the introduction. This section should be brief and catch the interest of the reader (Galvan, 1999).

Discussion of Theoretical Literature

The theoretical literature section contains concept analyses, models, theories, and conceptual frameworks that support the research purpose. Concepts, definitions of concepts, relationships among concepts, and assumptions are presented and analyzed to build a theoretical knowledge base for the study. This section of the literature review is sometimes used to present the framework for the study and may include a conceptual map that synthesizes the theoretical literature (see Chapter 7 for more detail on developing frameworks).

Discussion of Empirical Literature

The presentation of empirical literature should be organized by concepts or organizing topics. Although in the past, for each study reviewed, the researcher was expected to present the purpose, sample size, design, and specific findings with a scholarly but brief critique of the study's strengths and weaknesses, this approach is expected less commonly now. Developing tables such as Table 6-7 and Table 6-8 can be a useful way for you to organize this information as preparation for writing your review.

Currently, literature reviews tend to focus on synthesis of studies, with a critique of the strengths and weaknesses of the overall body of knowledge rather than a detailed presentation and critique of each study. This synthesis may be organized by concepts or variables that are the focus of the study. The findings from the studies should logically build on each other so that the reader can see how the body of knowledge in the research area evolved.

Evidence from multiple studies is pooled to reveal the current state of knowledge in relation to a particular concept or study focus (topic area). Conflicting findings and areas of uncertainty are explored. Similarities and differences in the studies should be explored. Gaps and areas needing more research are discussed. A summary of findings in the topic area is presented, along with inferences, generalizations, and conclusions you have drawn from your review of the literature. A conclusion is a statement about the state of knowledge in relation to the topic area. This should include a discussion of the strength of evidence available for each conclusion.

TABLE 6-7 Synthesizing Studies to Generate a Review of Literature							
Author and Year	**Purpose**	**Framework**	**Sample**	**Measurement**	**Treatment**	**Results**	**Findings**
Allman (1991)							
Bergstrom, Braden, Laguzza, & Holman (1987)							
Berlowitz & Wilking (1989)							
Braden & Bergstrom (1987)							
Harrison, Wells, Fisher, & Prince (1996)							
Norton (1989)							
Norton, McLaren, & Exton-Smith (1975)							
Okamoto, Lamers, & Shurtleff (1983)							

From Burns N., & Grove, S. K. (2007). *Understanding Nursing Research* (4th ed.). Philadelphia: Saunders, p. 154.

TABLE 6-8 Comparison and Contrast Study Findings on the Prediction and Prevention of Pressure Ulcers			
Author and Year	**Finding 1**	**Finding 2**	**Finding 3**
Allman (1991)			
Bergstrom et al. (1987)			
Berlowitz & Wilking (1989)			
Braden & Bergstrom (1987)			
Harrison et al. (1996)			
Norton (1989)			
Norton et al. (1975)			
Okamoto et al. (1983)			

From Burns, N., & Grove, S. K. (2007). *Understanding Nursing Research* (4th ed.). Philadelphia: Saunders, p. 155.

Ethical issues must be considered in your presentation of sources. The content from sources should be presented honestly, not distorted to support the selected problem. Researchers frequently read a study and wish that the author had studied a slightly different problem or that the study had been designed or conducted differently. However, they must recognize their own opinions and must be objective in presenting information.

The defects of a study need to be addressed, but it is not necessary to be highly critical of another researcher's work. The criticisms must focus on the content that is in some way relevant to the proposed study and to be stated as possible or plausible explanations, so that they are more neutral and scholarly than negative and blaming.

Authors' works must be accurately documented so the authors receive credit for their publications. APA requires that the reference list contain only those sources that have been cited in the development of the proposal or report.

Summary
The summary consists of a concise presentation of the current knowledge base for the research problem. Other literature reviews conducted in relation to your field of research should be discussed. The gaps in the knowledge base are identified, with a discussion of how the proposed study will contribute to the development of knowledge in the defined field of research. A critique of the adequacy of methodologies used in the studies reviewed should be presented, along with

recommendations for improving the methodologies in future studies (Galvan, 1999). The summary concludes with a statement of how your study will contribute to the body of knowledge in this field of research.

Checking References

All references used in the literature review should be carefully checked for accuracy and completeness. Anyone reviewing the literature has at some time been frustrated by inaccurate references in publications. Foreman and Kirchhoff (1987) studied the accuracy of references in 17 nursing journals; 65 of the inaccurate references were from clinical journals and 47 were from nonclinical journals. The errors were classified as major (preventing retrieval of the source) or minor (not preventing retrieval). Errors occurred more frequently in clinical journals (38.4%) than in nonclinical journals (21.3%). Clinical references also had a 4.5% incidence of major errors, whereas the nonclinical references had no major errors.

To prevent these errors, check all the citations within the text of your literature review and each citation in your reference list. Typing or keyboarding errors may result in inaccurate information. You may omit some information, planning to complete the reference later, and then forget to do so. Downloading citations from a database directly into a reference management system and using the system's manuscript formatting functions reduces some errors but does not eliminate all of them. Use your knowledge and skills to enhance your technology use; relying on technology alone will not create a quality manuscript.

The following reference citation errors are common in research studies:

- No citation is listed for a direct quotation.
- The citation for a direct quotation has the author's name and year, but no page number.
- The author's name is spelled differently in the text and in the reference list.
- The year of a citation is different in the text and in the reference list.
- The citation in the reference list is incomplete.
- A study is cited in the text for which there is no citation in the reference list.
- A citation appears in the reference list for which there is no citation in the text.

In revising your text, you may rearrange or renumber citations, resulting in inaccuracies. Biancuzzo (1997) described this sort of problem in one of her publications:

My own article (Biancuzzo, 1991) said "… although epidural anesthesia affects sensory neurons, motor neurons are not completely blicked.[16]" After publication, I was horrified to see that citation #16 was entitled "Maternal positions for childbirth: A historical review of nursing care practices." The correct citation should have been #15 entitled, "The influence of continuous epidural bupivacaine analgesia on the second stage of labor and method of delivery in nulliparous women." (p. 1)

A similar problem can occur when you cite several publications written by the same author. In this case, it is easy to reference the right author but the wrong source.

To detect these easily made errors, check your references immediately before completing your paper. The most accurate check involves comparing each reference with the original journal article or online with CINAHL or other bibliographical databases.

EXAMPLE OF A LITERATURE REVIEW

A literature review from an actual published descriptive study is presented here to reinforce the points that were addressed in this chapter. The study focuses on "validation of oxygen saturation monitoring in neonates" (Shiao & Ou, 2007, pp. 168–178).

> The accurate measurement of oxygen saturation in neonates is dependent on the level of oxyhemoglobin after serum levels of carbon monoxide hemoglobin and methemoglobin and the effects of fetal hemoglobin have been accounted for (Harris, Sendak, Donham, & Duncan, 1988; Moyle, 1996; Shiao, 2002b). In healthy adults, levels of carbon monoxide hemoglobin and methemoglobin together are less than 2% for blood samples (Shiao, 2002b). In addition to carbon monoxide hemoglobin and methemoglobin, neonates have fetal hemoglobin, a variation of hemoglobin that has high affinity for oxygen (Bunn & Forger, 1986; Wimberly, Siggaard-Anderson, & Fogh-Anderson, 1990), therefore, the measurements from clinical oximeters should be used with caution because they cannot account for variations in type of hemoglobin (Barker, Tremper, & Hyatt, 1989; Blaisdell, Goodman, Clark, Casella, & Loughlin, 2000; Bunn and Forger, 1986; Carter, Carlin, Tibballs, Mead, Hochmann, & Osborne, 1998; Comber & Lopez, 1996; Hampson, 1998; Haney, Tait, & Tremper, 1994; Krzeminski, 1992; Pianosi, Charge, Esseltine, & Coates, 1993; Rausch-Madison, & Mohsenifar, 1997; Wimberly, Siggaard-Anderson, & Fogh-Anderson, 1990).
>
> Only one published study (O'Connor & Hall, 1994) provided complete information on the validation of Sao_2 and Svo_2 measurements in neonates; however, in that study the

proportion of fetal hemoglobin was not determined, and its effects were not adjusted for when oxygen saturation measurements were calculated. When fetal hemoglobin effects are not adjusted for on hemoximeter tests, measurements of carbon monoxide hemoglobin are artificially increased, which then widens the differences between oxygen saturation and oxyhemoglobin readings and leads to inaccurate oxygen saturation values (Harris, Sendak, Donham, Thomas, & Duncan, 1988; Moyle, 1996; Wimberly, 1993; Wimberly, Siggaard-Anderson, & Fogh-Anderson, 1990).

Newer models of hemoximeter (after 1993) adjust oxygen saturation or oxyhemoglobin readings for fetal hemoglobin levels (Krzeminski, 1992). However, a pulse oximeter can overestimate oxygen saturation by as much as 6% when fetal hemoglobin level is not calculated (Rajadurai, Walker, Yu, & Oates, 1992; Shiao, 2002a; Whyte, Jangaard, & Dooley, 1995; Wimberly, 1993; Wimberly, Siggaard-Anderson, & Fogh-Anderson, 1990), leading clinicians to miss significant desaturation events. This problem also occurs in adults with abnormal hemoglobin; for example, in cases of congenital anemia (Bunn & Forger, 1986), sickle cell or hemoglobin mutations (Rochette, Craig, & Thein, 1994; Vadolas, Wardan, Orford, Williamson, & Ioannou, 2004), malignant blood-related cancers (Bunn & Forger, 1986), diabetes (Koskinen, Lahtela, & Koivula, 1994), ketosis (Peters, Rohloff, Kohlmann, et al., 1998), pregnancy (Moore, Nahlen, Ofulla, et al, 1997; Samura, Peril, Sohda, et al., 2000), or smoke inhalation (Imai, Tientadakul, Opartkiattikul, et al., 2001).

Transfusion of adult blood to neonates may decrease the fetal hemoglobin content and increase the adult hemoglobin content, thereby increasing tissue oxygenation (James, Greenough, & Naik, 1997); however, such transfusion also can add a burden to neonates' cardiac function (Bunn & Forget, 1986; Nemeto, Aoki, Dehua, & Imai, 2000). To prevent oxygen poisoning following blood transfusions in neonates, oxygenation status should be monitored closely, as right-shifting oxyhemoglobin curves result in more oxygen being released to the tissues (James, Greenough, & Naik, 1997; DeHalleux, Truttmann, Gagnon, & Bard, 2002).

When Sao_2 and Svo_2 are monitored together they can offer insights into oxygen demand (White, 1985) and provide complete information on systemic oxygenation balance (White, 1985; Siggard-Anderson & Gothgen, 1995). During nursing care and interventions, decreases in Svo_2 occur sooner and in more obvious increments than do decreases in Sao_2 (Hirschl, Palmer, Heiss, Hulquist, Fazzalari, & Barlett, 1993; Nakanishi, Yoshioka, Okano, & Nishimura, 1993); the 2 measurements together provide a more complete assessment of oxygenation status than either alone (White, 1985; Siggard-Anderson & Gothgen, 1995). However, Svo_2 is rarely monitored or measured in neonates.

Previous studies (Poets, 1999; Poets & Southall, 1994) in neonates have indicated that the mean difference between Sao_2 displayed on the clinical monitor (monitor Sao_2) and Spo_2 is 2% without consideration of fetal hemoglobin. In adults, the difference between monitor Sao_2 and blood oxyhemoglobin is 3% (Smatlak, & Knebel, 1998). The mean differences between monitor Sao_2 and Spo_2 in neonates can be from 5% to 6% when desaturation occurs during mechanical ventilation (Shiao, 2002a). Widely spread Spo_2 readings have been reported with Pao_2 values, without provision of a reasonably precise oxyhemoglobin dissociation curve (Bucher, Fanconi, Beeckert, & Duc, 1989; Poets, Wilken, Seidenberg, Southall, & van der Hardt, 1993).

The accuracy of pulse oximetry is limited when the readings decrease below 80% (Blaisdell, Goodman, Clark, Casella, & Loughlin, 2000; Severinghaus, Naifeh, & Koh, 1989; Trivedi, Ghouri, Lai, Shah, & Barker, 1997; Trivedi, Ghouri, Shah, Lai, & Barker, 1997), particularly in neonates with fetal hemoglobin (Hohl, Sherburne, Feeley, Huisman, & Burns, 1998; Shiao, 2002a). The normal clinical range for Pao_2 is defined as 50 to 75 mm Hg for infants (Askin, 1997). In adults, an Spo_2 of 85% to 94% is associated with a Pao_2 of 50 to 75 mm Hg. (Grossbach, 1993; Yelderman, & New, 1985). Comparable ranges of oxygen saturation measurements that account for fetal hemoglobin must be established for neonates. A previous article (Shiao, 2005) focused on use of paired arterial and venous blood samples to obtain accurate measurements of oxygen saturation. In this article we extend those findings by including additional blood and monitor measurements to validate clinical safety limits for use in neonates.

Note: this example is more brief than proposals will be because of space limitations in a textbook. The critique of reviews is presented in Chapter 26.

INTEGRATIVE REVIEWS

Integrative reviews are a type of secondary source that may be important to a review of the literature. Integrative reviews are conducted to identify, analyze, and synthesize the results from independent studies to determine the current knowledge (what is known and not known) in a particular area (Beyea & Nicoll, 1998; Ganong, 1987; Smith & Stullenbarger, 1991). Such a review contains a comprehensive list of references and summarizes empirical literature for selected topics (Cooper, 1984). In some cases, an integrative review is built around one or more theories used in the field of research. Review articles are primary sources in terms of the author's synthesis of the literature; however, they are secondary sources in terms of the author's discussion of previous authors' works. To use this information, you need to turn to the primary source of each author's work. For some research problems, you will find policy papers, standards of practice, or proposed legislation that may be important to include as part of the literature review. Clinical papers may be important for addressing the background and significance of the problem, but they should not be included in the review of literature. Integrative reviews are particularly important for examining the strength of evidence available to guide clinical practice.

An example of a source that provides integrative reviews is the *Annual Review of Nursing Research*, first published in 1983 (Werley & Fitzpatrick). The volumes of this publication, which continue to be published annually, contain excellent and thorough integrative reviews of research in the areas of nursing practice, nursing care delivery, nursing education, and the profession of nursing. Integrative reviews have also been published in a variety of clinical and research journals.

Worldviews on Evidence-Based Nursing (at www. nursingsociety.org/Publications/Journals/Pages/ worldviews.aspx) is published by Sigma Theta Tau as both a print and an online publication. It is a quarterly, peer-reviewed, evidence-based nursing journal and information resource that provides knowledge synthesis articles with best practice applications and recommendations for clinical practice, and a forum that encourages readers to engage in an ongoing dialogue on critical issues and questions in evidence-based nursing. Subscription to the journal is required to access the online journal.

The Oncology Nursing Forum provides syntheses of oncology studies at ONS (Oncology Nursing Society) online at http://ons.metapress.com/home/main. mpx. The University of Texas Health Science Center at San Antonio School of Nursing has developed the Academic Center for Evidence Based Practice (ACE) at www.acestar.uthscsa.edu.

Metasynthesis

Integrative reviews of qualitative research, or metasyntheses, are beginning to appear in the literature and will provide an important dimension to the synthesis of knowledge. Sandelowski, Docherty, and Emden (1997, p. 366) defined metasynthesis as "the theories, grand narratives, generalizations, or interpretive translations produced from the integration or comparison of findings from qualitative studies." One difficulty is locating qualitative studies, which is more difficult than locating quantitative studies in the literature databases. Flemming and Briggs (2006) provided some strategies. Because metasynthesis is relatively new, systematic approaches to synthesizing qualitative studies is in early stages of development. A number of authors cite Noblit and Hare (1988) as the basis of

their methodology for metasynthesis. Other sources cited include Estabrooks, Field, and Morse (1994); Finfgeld (2003); Jensen and Allen (1996); Kearney (2001); Kirkevold (1997); McCormick, Rodney, and Varcoe (2003); Morse, (2001); Patterson and Thorne (2003); Patterson, Thorne, Canam, and Jillings (2001); Ritzer (1992); Sandelowski (2006); Sandelowski and Barroso (2003a, 2000b); Sandelowski et al. (1997); Sandelowski, Barroso, and Voils (2007); Sherwood (1999); Thorne (1998); Thorne and Paterson (2002); Thorne, Jensen, Kearney, Noblit, and Sandelowski (2004); and Zhao (1991). Some authors are pooling strategies recommended by several sources. Others are developing their own methods. A metasynthesis is given here to demonstrate the methods used.

Coffey (2006) described her metasynthesis as follows:

The purpose of this study was to create a comprehensive chronicle of the phenomena of parenting a child with a chronic illness. This accumulated body of knowledge is presented from the parents' point of view as they care for a child with a chronic illness.

Procedure. To begin the procedure, a review of the literature was done using the following resources, including online databases such as CINAHL, ERIC, Psyclit, Sociological Abstracts, PubMed, and Dissertation Abstracts. These databases were searched for the time period between 1960 and the present. Studies from all years were reviewed; however, the studies chosen were published between 1989 and 2000. The key words used in the search were chronic illness, pediatrics, parenting, and qualitative study. The key work choice narrowed the search and eliminated studies that did not mention mother and father in the findings. There were several qualitative studies found in the inquiry. In addition, the query produced numerous quantitative studies and topical articles, as well as two triangulated studies that had a descriptive phenomenological component.

Sample. The criteria for inclusion into the studies were (a) the focus of the study was parenting a child with chronic illness; (b) the studies included both mother and father and may have mentioned family life; however, that was not the focus of the criteria; and (c) the research design was qualitative or had a qualitative component.

Articles identified as qualitative research were reviewed. All methods of qualitative research were included in the study. Nine of the 11 designs were exclusively qualitative.

Two of the studies were triangulated. The qualitative studies represented several different methods. There were three grounded theory studies, three phenomenological studies, one secondary analysis, two triangulation, and two descriptive qualitative studies.

The literature search yielded 11 studies to be included in the metasynthesis. During the course of the search, it was noted that there is a plethora of quantitative studies and topical articles on parenting and chronic illness. The articles chosen were all from nursing journals, although three studies had second authors from disciplines that included child life, medicine, and human development....

The 11 studies chosen were conducted in four different countries. Five of the studies were conducted in the United States, one in Japan, one in Germany, and four in Canada. The studies involved 533 participants, with 140 of those clearly identified as fathers. The remainder of the participants were identified as mothers, with the exception of five families from one study with no indication of the parental role of the participants. The age of the children ranged from birth to 22 years of age. One study using older children was retrospective and asked the parents to reflect on parenting when the child was younger.

Data analysis. The approach used for this metasynthesis on parenting children with chronic illness was based on Noblit & Hare's method (1988) found in their book *Metaethnography: Synthesizing Qualitative Studies*. The approach consists of seven phases as listed below.

Getting started and deciding on a phenomenon of study. The researcher chose parenting of a child with chronic illness as the area of interest.

Deciding what qualitative studies are relevant to the initial interest. The researcher reviewed over 30 studies to narrow the selection based on inclusion criteria stated earlier.

Reading the qualitative studies. Each study was read and reread to identify key metaphors, themes, or concepts. Detailed notes were kept on these themes, concepts, and metaphors.

Determining how the studies are related to each other. In this phase, the synthesizer made a list of the key metaphors in each study and their relations to each other. The term "metaphor" referred to themes, concepts, or phrases.

Three different assumptions can be made about the relationships between the studies to be synthesized. These key assumptions are "(1) the accounts are directly comparable as reciprocal translations; (2) the accounts stand in relative opposition to each other and are essentially refutational; or (3) the studies taken together present a line of argument rather than a reciprocal or refutational translation" (Noblit & Hare, 1988, p. 27). In this metasynthesis, the synthesis took the form of reciprocal translations because the studies were about similar themes. With reciprocal translations, each study is translated into the metaphors of the others and vice versa.

Translating the studies into one another. As Noblit & Hare (1988) explained, "Translations are especially unique syntheses, because they protect the particular, respect holism, and enable comparison. An adequate translation maintains the central metaphors and/or concepts of each account in their relation to other key metaphors or concepts in that account." (p. 28).

Synthesizing translations. This involves creating a whole as something more than the individual parts imply. The translations as a group are one level of a metasynthesis. Next, the translations can be compared to decide if the same metaphors/themes or concepts can be encompassed into those of others. This is a second level of synthesis. At this point, the study was reviewed by an expert in qualitative research as a check in the analytic process.

Expressing the synthesis through the written word, plays, art, videos, or music. The preface to the book written by Noblit & Hare includes the following poignant quotation: "When we synthesize, we give meaning to the set of studies under consideration. We interpret them in a fashion similar to an ethnographer interpreting a culture" (1988, p. 7).

The qualitative researcher must enter this endeavour well aware of the responsibility to clearly synthesize the information and present it for the reader to make sense of the phenomena. In the metasynthesis, each parent's words coalesce to provide the practitioner insight into the life of parenting a child with chronic illness. (Coffey, 2006, pp. 51–53).

Table 6-9 shows the themes extracted during the analysis. Using this table, how would you synthesize the information?

TABLE 6-9 ■ Themes

Study	Living Worried	Staying in the Struggle	Carrying the Burden	Survival as a Family	Bridge to the Outside World	Critical Times	Taking Charge
Mothers' Experience Living Worried When Parenting Children with Spina Bifida	Worry about birth, future always present	Exhaustion, hopelessness, overwhelmed hope, defeat, refusal to give up, deep disappointment		Worried how siblings will shoulder responsibility of the ill child			
"They Don't Leave You on Your Own": A Qualitative Study of the Home Care of Chronically Ill Children		Helpless at discharge	Extremely burdened by care, carrying all responsibility	Home nurses give family time and integrate care into daily life	Mom unable to leave home and nurse is the bridge	Discharge from the hospital	Refusal of care from a new home care nurse
Mothers Perceptions of Parenting Children with Disabilities	Worry about the future, missing work	Self-pity, emotional detachment		Close bond of the disabled child with the family, we are a family first	Only other parents can grasp the heartache, find a support group	Meeting or not meeting milestones	Advocate, rise to the occasion, fight for services
Hazardous Secrets and Reluctantly Taking Charge: Parenting a Child with Repeated Hospitalizations	Worry about procedures, learning professionals	Recycling grief; exhaustion, planned breaks	Exhaustion for designated parent usually the mother		In the provider parent relationship information not always shared		Vigilance, gaps in information
Distress and Growth Outcomes in Mothers of Medically Fragile Infants			Mother as primary caregiver must be flexible	Adapting treatment to make it fit with family life			
Parents' Reports of "Tricks of the Trade" for Managing Childhood Chronic Illness		Tricks of the trade, adherence	Mothers have the tricks of the trade in their head every day				Develop tricks of the trade to manage illness

Continued

TABLE 6-9 ■ Themes—Cont'd

Study	Living Worried	Staying in the Struggle	Carrying the Burden	Survival as a Family	Bridge to the Outside World	Critical Times	Taking Charge
Long-Term Follow-Up of Cerebral Palsy Children and Coping Behavior of Parents	Anxiety of what happens at parents death	Weep for a week, could not think	Major burden carried by mother	Organize care and fit into family schedules	Initial isolation improves with clinic visits, support groups helpful	Diagnosis, infancy, turning age 5, 18, going to school or not, parents too old to give care	Control time and be organized, increase confidence, parents accept managing illness is a daily job
Parents' Experience of Coming to Know the Care of a Chronically Ill Child		Confusion, anger, turmoil, feel unprepared, overwhelmed		Multiple losses for the family, concern about sharing energy with all family members, pervasive influence in each member of the family	Isolation, being at odds with health care providers		
Parents' Perceptions of Caring for an Infant or Toddler with Diabetes	Anticipatory worry, future worry, stress	Immense responsibility, complex care, anger, fear, grief, guilt, overwhelmed	Mothers give up work, loss of ideal mom-child relationship, fathers rearrange schedules	Restriction of family activities, difficult to find time for siblings	Social isolation, accepting the lack of support from the family and friends, loss of support at discharge, trapped, vulnerable and afraid	Hospitalizations, diagnosis, Learning care, toddler, entering school, milestones	Taking charge of the situation, being assertive and advocating for the child
Caring for Chronically Ill Children at Home: Factors that Influence Parents' Coping	On guard constantly, perpetual demanding care		Mothers not able to work and carry the burden of caregiving				Parents walk a fine line between assertion and insulting the health care professional
Critical Times for Families with a Chronically Ill Child			Mothers are primary caregivers, mother centered patterns		Religion and spirituality a support	Diagnosis, first year after diagnosis, learning symptoms, calling MD, rehospitalization or relocation	

From Coffey, J. S. (2006). Parenting a child with chronic illness: A metasynthesis. *Pediatric Nursing, 32*(1): 55–56.

Meta-Analysis

Meta-analysis involves merging findings from many studies that have examined the same phenomenon. The design uses specific statistical analyses to determine the overall findings from a combined examination of reports of statistical findings of each study. The statistical values used include the means and standard deviations for each group in the study. One of the outcomes of a meta-analysis is the estimation of a population effect size for the topic under study. Because studies seldom have exactly the same focus, conclusions are never absolute but do give some sense of unity to knowledge within that area (O'Flynn, 1982).

One problem that researchers constantly encounter in meta-analyses is that the studies being examined are inconsistent in design quality. However, researchers conducting meta-analyses have not successfully identified a generally acceptable means to measure the research quality of studies. Brown (1991) proposed a research quality scoring method to accomplish this important task. Another problem with meta-analyses is that basic research information is often missing from research reports. Calculating effect sizes requires means and standard deviations in each study for both experimental and control groups. In addition, the beginning sample size must be reported, as well as the sample size at the time of the posttest. Often, the treatment has been poorly described, making it difficult to determine the most effective treatments (Brown, 1991).

Lee, Soeken, and Picot (2007) conducted a meta-analysis of the effectiveness of intervention in improving the mental health of informal stroke caregivers. The following describes the study:

In this meta-analysis, mental health was defined as a psychological state as measured by the Short Form Health Survey (SF-36).... The specific outcome was the difference in the SF-36 mental health score between the experimental group and the control group. The independent variable included any type of intervention that was implemented for informal stroke caregivers to improve their mental health.

Methods

Literature Search

Searches were performed using MEDLINE (1966–2005) and Cumulative Index for Nursing and Allied Health Literature (CINAHL, 1982–2005) computerized databases. The searches were limited to articles published in the English language using combinations of the keywords caregiving, stroke caregiver, stroke caregiving, control group, and interventions. For the keyword search, the author wanted to identify experimental studies with stroke caregivers. The database searches of MEDLINE and CINAHL revealed a total of 30 articles. A citation search of the Social Sciences Citation Index and Science Citation Index yielded one additional article for inclusion. In addition, the Cochrane library search to find additional studies resulted in the same finding as that found in the computerized database searches. Unpublished studies were not included in this meta-analysis because they have not undergone peer review.

Study Selection

Abstracts of the 31 studies identified through the search were independently reviewed by the first author for inclusion in this meta-analysis. The inclusion criteria were (a) sample included informal caregivers of stroke patients; (b) intervention for stroke caregivers to improve their mental health; (c) outcome variables include the SF-36; (d) quantitative study; and (e) use of a comparison group on the outcome measure. From the 31 abstracts, only 11 articles met the inclusion criteria.

Based on a review of the 11 studies, 7 articles were excluded for various reasons including: (a) using the SF-36 outcome, but not reporting the data (Dennis, O'Rourke, Slattery, Staniforth, & Warlow, 1997; Printz-Feddersen, 1990); (b) inadequate descriptive statistics (Grant, 1999); (c) not presenting caregivers' data in results section (Forster & Young, 1996; Lincoln, Francis, Lilley, Sharma, & Summerfield, 2003; Mayo et al., 2000); and (d) only reporting qualitative data (Stewart, Doble, Hart, Langille, & MacPherson, 1998). Finally, 4 studies were retained for this meta-analysis.

Data Collection Methods

After initially reviewing the four studies to be included in this meta-analysis, variables were selected for inclusion in the codebook. Coded were: first author, year, design, number of subjects in each group (experimental and control), intervention characteristics, theoretical background for the intervention, intervention period, setting, data collection period, attrition rate, and statistical results. The first author and a second coder independently extracted data from all four studies. Coder agreement was initially 95.8%. Coders then reviewed items for which there was lack of agreement. After discussion, consensus was reached on all items. The data extracted were entered into an EXCEL file.

TABLE 6-10   Summary of Sample Studies

First Author	Mean Age	Intervention	Interview Period
Grant, Elliott, Weaver, Bartolucci, & Giger (2002)	Men 58 ± 12 Women 56 ± 12	3 to 4 weeks poststroke, initial 3 hour meeting in home; thereafter weekly telephone sessions 2 to 4 weeks postdischarge, and biweekly weeks 6, 8, 10, and 12 postdischarge	Interviews were conducted 1 to 2 days predischarge, 5 to 9 weeks postdischarge, and 13 weeks postdischarge.
Van den Heuvel, Witte, Stewart, Schure, Sanderman, & Meyboom-de Jong (2002)	Group program 66.4 Home visits 63.2 Control 60.8	6 months to 3.5 (3.81) years post-stroke; group support consists of 8 weeks group program (eight meetings, 16 hours of education), or an 8- to 10-week home visit program (four visits, 8 hours of education)	Started within 4 weeks following the baseline interview, second interview was approximately 14 weeks postbaseline and final interview 6 months after second interview.

Continued

For the quality rating, several items were selected from a quality measure previously used by Soeken and colleagues (2003). These items assessed study aim, randomization, blinding, attrition, statistical testing, and discussion section. Using this quality rating scale, the range of total quality points is 0 to 16. Because all the studies used a randomized design, and treatment personnel conducted the interventions, the quality assessment scale specifically addressed blinding of caregivers, treatment personnel, or data collector. Studies with scores of 0 to 9 were considered low quality and those with scores 10 to 16 were considered high quality.

All studies were assessed for quality by two independent raters. The agreement rate between the two raters was 90%. Following discussion, the raters reached consensus for all items. Quality scores for four studies ranged from 9–13. One study was rated low quality because no one was blinded (Van den Heuval et al., 2002). The remaining three were rated high quality (Grant, Elliot, Warver, Bartolucci, & Giger, 2002; Mant, Carter, Wade, & Winner, 2000; Rodgers et al., 1999).

Statistical Methods

An effect size (d) was calculated for each of the individual studies converting the reported statistics into the standardized effect size. The raw effect sizes were weighted for study sample size because raw effect sizes from studies with small samples are prone to overestimate the population effect size (Shadish & Haddock, 1994). An overall mean weighted effect size for the four studies was calculated. Additionally, 95% confidence intervals were calculated for each effect size.

To assess sensitivity of the results, mean weighted effect sizes were computed by study quality rating. Subgroup analyses examined differences regarding types of intervention (education/support), presence of a theoretical background for creating the intervention (yes/no), and study setting (Europe/United States). Finally, potential publication bias was assessed using the fail-safe N.

Results

General Descriptions

The four study samples included 718 individuals with a large proportion of women (71.7%). The mean age of the subjects was 61.1 years. All of the studies used randomized controlled designs...

Pooled Results

Effect sizes and 95% confidence intervals for each individual study and for the overall mean weighted effect size (MWES) were calculated. Effect sizes ranged from 0 to 0.92. The four studies had varied effect with an overall MWES of 0.277 (p < 0.001) with a 95% CI from 0.118 to 0.435 (N = 718). Thus, across the four studies the results indicate that the intervention was effective in improving the mental health of informal stroke caregivers. (Lee, Soeken, & Picot, 2007, pp. 344–348)

Table 6-10 summarizes the sample studies in the Lee et al. (2007) study.

TABLE 6-10 ▪▪ Summary of Sample Studies—*Cont'd*

First Author	Mean Age	Intervention	Interview Period
Mant, Carter, Wade, & Winner (2000)	Family support 65.1 Control 63.7	Intervention began within 6 weeks of stroke; nature and frequency of interaction was based on the judgment of the family support organizer; included an average of one hospital visit, one home visit, and three telephone calls, and referral to one other service	Subjects were interviewed 6 months after stroke and intervention.
Rodgers, Atkinson, Bond, Suddes, Dobson, & Curless (1999)	Stroke Education Program 58 Control 60	One-hour inpatient small group educational session, followed by six hourly sessions postdischarge; a minimum of three session attendances required for completion	Participants were interviewed 6 months poststroke.

From Lee, J., Soeken, K., & Picot, S. J. (2007). A meta-analysis of interventions for informal stroke caregivers. *Western Journal of Nursing Research, 29*(3): 349.

SUMMARY

- Reviewing the existing literature related to your study is a critical step in the research process.
- The three major stages of a literature review delineated here are searching the literature, reading the literature, and writing the literature review.
- The literature consists of all written sources relevant to the topic you have selected.
- Two types of literature are predominantly used in the review of literature for research: theoretical and empirical.
- Theoretical literature includes concept analyses, models, theories, and conceptual frameworks that support a selected research problem and purpose.
- Empirical literature includes relevant studies in journals and books, as well as unpublished studies, such as master's theses and doctoral dissertations.
- Reading and critiquing sources promotes understanding of the current knowledge of a research problem and involves skimming, comprehending, analyzing, and synthesizing content from sources.
- A thorough, organized literature review facilitates the development of a research proposal.
- The literature review for a study has four major sections: the introduction, a discussion of theoretical literature, a discussion of empirical literature, and a summary.

REFERENCES

Acorn, S. (1995). Assisting families of head-injured survivors through a family support programme. *Journal of Advanced Nursing, 21*(5), 872–877.

Allman, R. M. (1991). *Pressure ulcers among bedridden hospitalized elderly.* Division of Gerontology/Geriatrics, University of Alabama at Birmingham. Unpublished data compiled.

American Psychological Association (APA). (2001). *Publication manual of the American Psychological Association* (5th ed.). Washington, DC: Author.

Asian Institute of Technology, Center for Language and Educational Technology. (2000). *Writing and research: The literature review.* Retrieved February 25, 2000, from www.languages.ait.ac.th/el21open.htm.

Askin, D. F. (1997). Interpretation of neonatal blood gases, part II: disorders of acid-base balance. *Neonatal Network, 16*(6), 23–29.

Auston, I., Cahn, M. A., & Selden, C. R. (1992). Literature search methods for the development of clinical practice guidelines. National Library of Medicine, Office of Health Services Research Information. Retrieved February 25, 2000, from www.nlm.nih.gov/nichsr/litsrch.html.

Barker, S. J., Tremper, K. K., & Hyatt, J. (1989). Effects of methemoglobinemia on pulse oximetry and mixed venous oximetry. *Anesthesiology, 70*(1), 112–117.

Becker, H. S. (1986). *Writing for social scientists: How to start and finish your thesis, book, or article.* Chicago: University of Chicago Press.

Bergstrom, N., Braden, B. J., Laguzza, A., & Holman, V. (1987). The Braden Scale for predicting pressure sore risk. *Nursing Research, 36*(4), 205–210.

Berlowitz, D. R., & Wilking, S. V. (1989). Risk factors for pressure sores: A comparison of cross-sectional and cohort-derived data. *Journal of the American Geriatric Society, 37*(11), 1043–1050.

Beyea, S., & Nicoll, L. H. (1998). Writing an integrative review. *AORN Journal, 67*(4), 877–880.

Biancuzzo, M. (1991). Does the hands-and-knees posture help to rotate the occiput posterior fetus? *Birth, 18*(1), 40–47.

Biancuzzo, M. (1997). Checking references: Tips for reviewers. *Nurse Author & Editor, 7*(3), 1–3.

Blaisdell, C. J., Goodman, S., Clark, K., Casella, J. F., & Loughlin, G. M. (2000). Pulse oximetry is a poor predictor of hypoxemia in stable children with sickle cell disease. *Archives of Pediatric Adolescent Medicine, 154*(9), 900–903.

Braden, B., & Bergstrom, N. (1987). A conceptual schema for the study of the etiology of pressure sores. *Rehabilitation Nursing, 12*(1), 8–12.

Brown, S. A. (1991). Measurement of quality of primary studies for meta-analysis. *Nursing Research, 40*(6), 352–355.

Bucher, H. U., Fanconi, S., Beeckert, P., & Duc, G. (1989). Hyperoxemia in newborn infants: detection by pulse oximetry. *Pediatrics, 84*(2) 226–230.

Bunn, H. F., & Forger, B. G. (1986). *Hemoglobin: Molecular, genetic and clinical aspects.* Philadelphia: W.B. Saunders.

Carmody, S., Hickey, P., & Bookbinder, M. (1991). Perioperative needs of families: Results of a survey. *AORN Journal, 54*(3), 561–567.

Carter, B. G., Carlin, J. B., Tibballs, J., Mead, H., Hichmann, M., & Osborne, A. (1998). Accuracy of two pulse oximeters at low arterial hemoglobin-oxygen saturation. *Critical Care Medicine, 26*(6),1128–1133.

Coffey, J. S. (2006). Parenting a child with chronic illness: A metasynthesis. *Pediatric Nursing, 32*(1), 51–59.

Collins, E. G., White-Williams, C., & Jalowiec, A. (1996). Spouse stressors while awaiting heart transplantation. *Heart & Lung: Journal of Acute & Critical Care, 25*(1), 4–13.

Comber, J. T., & Lopez, B. L. (1996). Evaluation of pulse oximetry in sickle cell anemia patients presenting to the emergency department in acute vasocclusive crisis. *American Journal of Emergency Medicine, 14*(1),16–18.

Cooper, H. M. (1984). *The integrative research review: A systematic approach.* Beverly Hills, CA: Sage.

Daley, L. (1984). The perceived immediate needs of families with relatives in the intensive care setting. *Heart & Lung, 13*(3), 231–237.

Damrosch, S., & Damrosch, G. D. (1996). Methodology corner. Avoiding common mistakes in APA style: The briefest of guidelines. *Nursing Research, 45*(6), 331–333.

Davis-Martin, S. (1994). Perceived needs of families of long-term critical care patients: A brief report. *Heart & Lung, 23*(6), 515–518.

Dehalleux, V., Truttmann, A., Gagnon, C., & Bard, H. (2002). The effect of blood transfusion on the hemoglobin oxygen dissociation curve of very early preterm infants during the first week of life. *Seminars in Perinatology, 26*(6), 411–415.

Dennis, M., O'Rourke, S., Slattery, J., Staniforth, T., & Warlow, C. (1977). Evaluation of a stroke family care worker: Results of a randomised controlled trial. *British Medical Journal, 314*(7087), 1071–1076.

Estabrooks, C. A., Field, P. A., & Morse, J. M. (1994). Aggregating qualitative findings: An approach to theory development. *Qualitative Health Research, 4*(4), 503–511.

Finfgeld, D. L. (2003). Metasynthesis: The state of the art-so far. *Qualitative Health Research, 13*(7), 893–904.

Fleming, J. W., & Hayter, J. (1974). Reading research reports critically. *Nursing Outlook, 22*(3), 172–175.

Flemming, K., & Briggs, M. (2006). Electronic searching to locate qualitative research: Evaluation of three strategies. *Journal of Advanced Nursing, 57*(1), 95–100.

Foreman, M. D., & Kirchhoff, K. T. (1987). Accuracy of references in nursing journals. *Research in Nursing & Health, 10*(3), 177–183.

Forster, A., & Young, J. (1996). Specialist nurse support for patients with stroke in the community: A randomised controlled trial. *British Medical Journal, 312*(7047), 1642–1646.

Freichels, T. A. (1991). Needs of family members of patients in the intensive care unit over time. *Critical Care Nursing Quarterly, 14*(3), 16–29.

Galvan, J. L. (1999). *Writing literature reviews.* Los Angeles: Pyrczak.

Ganong, L. H. (1987). Integrative reviews of nursing research. *Research in Nursing & Health, 10*(1), 1–11.

Gilliss, C. L. (1984). Reducing family stress during and after coronary artery bypass surgery… the patient-spouse pair. *Nursing Clinics of North America, 19*(1), 103–112.

Grant, J. S. (1999). Social problem-solving partnerships with family caregivers. *Rehabilitation Nursing, 24*(6), 254–260.

Grant, J. S., Elliott, T. R., Weaver, M., Bartolucci, A. A., & Giger, J. N. (2002). Telephone intervention with family caregivers of stroke survivors after rehabilitation. *Stroke, 33*(8), 2060–2065.

Grossbach, I. (1993). Case studies in pulse oximetry monitoring. *Critical Care Nurse, 13*(4), 63–65.

Hampson, N. B. (1998). Pulse oximetry in severe carbon monoxide poisoning. *Chest, 114*(4), 1036–1041.

Haney, M., Tait, A. R., & Tremper, K. K. (1994). Effect of carboxy-hemoglobin on the accuracy of mixed venous oximetry monitors in dogs. *Critical Care Medicine, 22*(7), 1181–1185.

Hanton, L. B. (1988). Caring for children awaiting heart transplantation: Psychosocial implications. *Pediatric Nursing, 24*(3), 214–218.

Harris, A. P., Sendak, M. J., Donham, R. T., Thomas, M., & Duncan, D. (1988). Absorption characteristics of human fetal hemoglobin at wavelengths used in pulse oximetry. *Journal of Clinical Monitoring, 4*(3), 175–177.

Harrison, M. B., Wells, G., Fisher, A., & Prince, M. (1996). Practice guidelines for the prediction and prevention of pressure ulcers: Evaluating the evidence. *Applied Nursing Research, 9*(1), 9–17.

Hirschl, R. B., Palmer, P., Heiss, K. F., Hultquist, K., Fazzalari, F., & Barlett, R. H. (1993). Evaluation of the right arterial venous oxygen saturation as a physiologic monitor in a neonatal model. *Journal of Pediatric Surgery, 28*(7), 901–905.

Hohl, R. J., Sherburne, A. R., Feeley, J. E., Huisman, T. H., & Burns, C. P. (1998). Low pulse oximeter-measured hemoglobin oxygen saturation with haemoglobin Cheverly. *American Journal of Haematology, 59*(3), 181–184.

Imai, K., Tientadakul, P., Opartkiattikul, N., Luenee, P., Winichagoon, P., Svasti, J., et al. (2001). Detection of haemoglobin variants and inference of their functional properties using complete oxygen dissociation curve measurements. *British Journal of Haematology, 112*(2), 483–487.

Jalowiec, A., & Powers, M. J. (1981). Stress and coping in hypertensive and emergency room patients. *Nursing Research, 30*(1), 10–15.

James, L., Greenough, A., & Naik, S. (1997). The effect of blood transfusion on oxygenation in premature ventilated neonates. *European Journal of Pediatrics, 156*(2), 139–141.

Jensen, L. A., & Allen, M. N. (1996). Metasynthesis of qualitative findings. *Qualitative Health Research, 6*(4), 553–560.

Kearney, M. H. (2001). New directions in grounded formal theory. In R. Schreiber & P. N. Stern (Eds.), *Using grounded theory in nursing* (pp. 227–246). New York: Springer.

Kirkevold, M. (1997). Integrative nursing research: An important strategy to further the development of nursing science and nursing practice. *Journal of Advanced Nursing, 25*(5), 977–984.

Kleinpell, R. M., & Powers, M. J. (1992). Needs of family members of intensive care unit patients. *Applied Nursing Research, 5*(1), 2–8.

Koskinen, L. K., Lahtela, J. T., & Koivula, T. A. (1994). Fetal hemoglobin in diabetic patients. *Diabetic Care, 17*(8), 828–831.

Kristensson-Hallström, I. (1999). Strategies for feeling secure influence parents' participation in care. *Journal of Clinical Nursing, 8*(5), 586–592.

Krzeminski, A. (1992). *How is fetal hemoglobin determined and corrected for in the OSM3, the ABL510, and the ABL 520?* Copenhagen, Denmark: Radiometer, Info No. 1992-4-1-4.

Kubler-Ross, E. (1969). *On death and dying.* New York: Macmillan.

Kuhn, T. (1962). *The structure of scientific revolutions* (2nd ed). Chicago: University of Chicago Press.

LaMontagne, I. L., & Pawlak, R. (1990). Stress and coping of parents of children in a pediatric intensive care unit. *Heart & Lung, 19*(4), 416–421.

Lawrence, J., & Levy, L. (2004). Comparing the self-described searching knowledge of first-year medical and dental students before and after a MEDLINE class. *Medical Reference Services Quarterly, 23*(1), 73–81.

Lee, J., Soeken, K., & Picot, S. J. (2007). A meta-analysis of interventions for informal stroke caregivers. *Western Journal of Nursing Research, 29*(3), 344–356.

Leske, J. S. (1986). Needs of relatives of critically ill patients: A follow-up. *Heart & Lung, 15*(2), 189–193.

Lincoln, M. B., Francis, V. M., Lilley, S. A., Sharma, J. C., & Summerfield, M. (2003). Evaluation of a stroke family support organiser: A randomized controlled trial. *Stroke, 34*(1), 116–121.

Mant, J., Carter, J., Wade, D. T., & Winner, S. (2000). Family support for stroke: A randomised controlled trial. *Lancet, 356*(9232), 808–813.

Marchette, L. (1985). Research: The literature review process. *Perioperative Nursing Quarterly, 1*(4), 69–76.

Mayo, N. E., Wood-Dauphinee, S., Cote, R., Gayton, D., Carlton, J., Buttery, J., et al. (2000). There's no place like home: An evaluation of early supported discharge for stroke. *Stroke, 31*(5), 1016–1023.

McCormick, J., Rodney, P., & Varcoe, C. (2003). Reinterpretations across studies: An approach to meta-analysis. *Qualitative Health Research, 13*(7), 933–944.

Meats, E., Brassey, J., Heneghan, C., & Glasziou, P. (2007). Using the Turning Research into Practice (TRIP) database: how do clinicians really search? *Journal of the Medical Library Association, 95*(2), 156–163.

Mishel, M. H., & Murdaugh, C. L. (1987). Family adjustment to heart transplantation: Redesigning the dream. *Nursing Research, 36*(6), 332–338.

Molter, N. C. (1979). Needs of relatives of critically ill patient. *Heart & Lung, 8*(2), 332–339.

Moore, J. M., Nahlenl, B., Ofulla, A. V., Caba, J., Ayisi, J., Oloo, A., et al. (1997). A simple perfusion technique for isolation of maternal intervillous blood mononuclear cells from human placentae. *Journal of Immunological Methods, 209*(1), 93–104.

Morse, J. M. (2001). Qualitative verification: Building evidence by extending basic findings. In J. Morse, J. Swanson, & A. Kuzel (Eds.), *The nature of qualitative evidence* (pp. 203–220), Thousand Oaks, CA: Sage.

Moser, D. K., Dracup, K. A., & Marsden, C. (1993). Needs of recovering cardiac patients and their spouses: Compared views. *International Journal of Nursing Studies, 30*(2), 105–114.

Moyle, J. T. (1996). Uses and abuses of pulse oximetry. *Archives of Diseases in Childhood, 74*(1): 77–80.

Munhall, P. L. (2006). *Nursing research: A qualitative perspective* (4th ed.). Sudbury, MA: Jones & Bartlett.

Nakanishi, M., Yoshioka, T., Okano, Y., & Nishimura, T. (1993). Continuous Fick cardiac output measurement during exercise by monitoring of mixed venous oxygen saturation and oxygen uptake. *Chest, 104*(2), 419–426.

Nemeto, S., Aoki, M., Dehua, C., & Imai, Y. (2000). Free haemoglobin impairs cardiac function in neonatal rabbit heart. *Annals of Thoracic Surgery, 69*(5), 1484–1489.

Noblit, G. W., & Hare, R. D. (1988). *Meta-ethnography: Synthesizing qualitative studies.* Newbury Park, CA: Sage.

Nolan, M. T., Cupples, S. A., Brown, M., Pierce, L., Lepley, D., & Ohler, L. (1992). Perceived stress and coping strategies among families of cardiac transplant candidates during the organ waiting period. *Heart & Lung, 21*(6), 540–547.

Norris, L., & Grove, S. K. (1986). Investigation of selected psychosocial needs of family members of critically ill adult patients. *Heart & Lung, 15*(2), 194–199.

Norton, D. (1989). Calculating the risk: Reflections on the Norton Scale. *Decubitus, 2*(3), 24–31.

Norton, D., McLaren, R., & Exton-Smith, A. N. (1975). *An investigation of geriatric nursing problems in hospital.* London: Churchill Livingstone.

Nyamathi, A., Jacoby, A., Constancia, P., & Ruvevich, S. (1992). Coping and adjustment of spouses of critically ill patients with cardiac disease. *Heart & Lung, 21*(2), 160–166.

O'Connor, S. E. (1992). Network theory: A systematic method for literature review. *Nurse Education Today, 12*(1), 44–50.

O'Connor, T. A., & Hall, R. T. (1994). Mixed venous oxygenation in critically ill neonates. *Critical Care Medicine, 22*(2), 343–346.

O'Flynn, A. I. (1982) Meta-analysis. *Nursing Research, 31*(5), 314–316.

Okamoto, G. A., Lamers, J. V., & Shurtleff, D. B. (1983). Skin breakdown in patients with myelomeningocele. *Archives of Physical Medicine Rehabilitation, 64*(1), 20–23.

Paterson, B. L., & Thorne, S. (2003). The potential of metasynthesis for nursing care effectiveness research. *Canadian Journal of Nursing Research, 35*(3), 39–43.

Paterson, B. L., Thorne, S. E., Canam, C., & Jillings, C. (2001). *Meta-study of qualitative health research. A practical guide to meta-analysis and meta-synthesis.* Thousand Oaks, CA: Sage.

Peters, A., Rohloff, D., Kohlmann, T., Renner, F., Jantschek, G., Kerner, W., et al. (1998). Fetal hemoglobin in starvation ketosis of young women. *Blood, 91*(2), 691–694.

Pianosi, P., Charge, T. D., Esseltine, D. W., & Coates, A. L. (1993). Pulse oximetry in sickle cell disease. *Archives of Disabled Children, 68*(6), 735–738.

Pinch, W. J. (1995). Synthesis: Implementing a complex process. *Nurse Educator, 20*(1), 34–40.

Poets, C. F. (1999). Assessing oxygenation in healthy infants. *Journal of Pediatrics, 135*(5), 541–543.

Poets, C. F., & Southall, D. P. (1994). Non-invasive monitoring of oxygenation in infants and children: practical considerations and areas of concern. *Pediatrics, 93*(5), 737–746.

Poets, C. F., Wilken, M., Seidenberg, J., Southhall, D. P., & van der Hardt, H. (1993). Reliability of a pulse oximeter in the detection of hyperoxemia. *Journal of Pediatrics, 122*(1), 87–90.

Porter, R., Krout, L., Parks, V., Gibbs, S., Luers, E., Gould, M., et al. (1992). Perceived stress and coping strategies among cardiac transplant patients during the organ waiting period. *Heart & Lung, 21*(3), 292.

Printz-Feddersen, V. (1990). Group process effect on caregiver burden. *Journal of Neuroscience Nursing, 22*(3), 164–168.

Rajadurai, V. S., Walker, A. M., Yu, V. Y., & Oates, A. (1992). Effect of fetal haemoglobin on the accuracy of pulse oximetry in preterm infants. *Journal of Paediatric Child Health, 28*(1), 43–46.

Rausch-Madison, S., & Mohsenifar, Z. (1997). Methodologic problems encountered with cooximetry in methemoglobinemia. *American Journal of Medical Science, 314*(3), 203–206.

Reider, J. A. (1994). Anxiety during critical illness of a family member. *DCCN: Dimensions of Critical Care Nursing, 13*(5), 272–279.

Ritzer, G. (1992). Metatheorizing in sociology: Explaining the coming of age. In G. Ritzer (Ed.), *Metatheorizing* (pp. 7–26). Newbury Park, CA: Sage.

Rochette, J., Craig, J. E., & Thein, S. L. (1994). Fetal haemoglobin levels in adults. *Blood Review, 8*(4), 213–224.

Rodgers, H., Atkinson, C., Bond, S., Suddes, M., Dobson, R., & Curless, R. (1999). Randomized controlled trial of a comprehensive stroke education program for patients and caregivers. *Stroke, 30*(12), 2585–2591.

Samura, O., Peril, B., Sohda, S., Johnson, K. L., Sekizawa, A., Falco, V. M., et al. (2000). Female fetal cells in maternal blood: Use of DNA polymorphism to prove origin. *Human Genetics, 107*(1), 28–32.

Sandelowski, M. (2006). "Meta-Jeopardy": The crisis of representation in qualitative metasynthesis. *Nursing Outlook, 54*(1), 10–16.

Sandelowski, M., & Barroso, J. (2003a). Classifying the findings in qualitative studies. *Qualitative Health Research, 13*(7), 905–923.

Sandelowski, M., & Barroso, J. (2003b). Creating meta-summaries of qualitative findings. *Nursing Research, 52*(4), 226–231.

Sandelowski, M., Barroso, J., & Voils, C. I. (2007). Using qualitative metasummary to synthesize qualitative and quantitative descriptive findings. *Research in Nursing & Health, 30*(1), 99–111.

Sandelowski, M., Docherty, S., & Emden, C. (1997). Focus on qualitative methods. Qualitative metasynthesis: Issues and techniques. *Research in Nursing & Health, 20*(4), 365–371.

Severinghaus, J. W., Naifeh, K. H., & Koh, S. O. (1989). Errors in 14 pulse oximeters during profound hypoxia. *Journal of Clinical Monitoring, 5*(2), 72–81.

Shadish, W. R., & Haddock, C. K. (1994). Combining estimates of effect size. In H. M. Cooper & L. V. Hedges (Eds.), *The handbook of research synthesis* (pp. xvi, 573). New York: Russell Sage Foundation.

Sherwood, G. D. (1999). Meta-synthesis: Merging qualitative studies to develop nursing knowledge. *International Journal for Human Caring, 3*(1), 37–42.

Shiao, S. P. K. (2002a). Desaturation events in neonates during mechanical ventilation. *Critical Care Nursing Quarterly, 24*(4), 14–29.

Shiao, S. P. K. (2002b). Functional versus fractional oxygen saturation readings: Bias and agreement using simulated solutions and adult blood. *Biological Research for Nursing, 2*(3), 210–221.

Shiao, S. P. K. (2005). Accurate measurements of oxygen saturation in neonates: Paired arterial and venous blood analyses. *Newborn Infant Nursing Review, 5*(4), 170–178.

Shiao, S. P. K. & Ou, C. N. (2007). Validation of oxygen saturation monitoring in neonates. *American Journal of Critical Care, 16*(2), 168–178.

Shiri, A., & Revie, C. (2006). Query expansion behavior within a thesaurus-enhanced search environment: A user-centered evaluation. *Journal of the American Society for Information Science & Technology, 57*(4), 462–478.

Siggaard-Anderson, O., & Gothgen, I. H. (1995). Oxygen and acid-base parameters of arterial and mixed venous blood, relevant versus redundant. *Acta Anaesthesiology* (Suppl. 107), 21–27.

Smatlak, P., & Knebel, A. R. (1998). Clinical evaluation of non-invasive monitoring of oxygen saturation in critically ill patients. *American Journal of Critical Care, 7*(5), 370–373.

Smith, M. C., & Stullenbarger, E. (1991). A prototype for integrative review and meta-analysis for nursing research. *Journal of Advanced Nursing, 16*(11), 1272–1283.

Soeken, K. L., & Sripusanapan, A. (2003). Assessing publication bias in meta-analysis. *Nursing Research, 52*(1), 57–60.

Stewart, M. J., Doble, S., Hart, G., Langille, L., & MacPherson, K. (1998). Peer visitor support for family caregivers of seniors with stroke. *Canadian Journal of Nursing Research, 30*(2), 87–117.

Thorne, S. (1998). Ethical and representational issues in qualitative secondary analysis. *Qualitative Health Research, 8*(4), 547–555.

Thorne, S., Jensen, L., Kearney, M. H., Noblit, G., & Sandelowski, M. (2004). Qualitative metasynthesis: Reflections on methodological orientation and ideological agenda. *Qualitative Health Research, 14*(10), 1342–1365.

Thorne, S., & Paterson, B. (2002). Two decades of insider research: What we know and don't know about chronic illness experience. *Annual Review of Nursing Research, 18*, 3–25.

Trivedi, N. S., Ghouri, A. F., Lai, E., Shah, N. K., & Barker, S. J. (1997). Pulse oximeter performance during desaturation and resaturation: A comparison of seven models. *Journal of Clinical Anesthesia, 9*(3), 184–188.

Trivedi, N. S., Ghouri, A. F., Shah, N. K., Lai, E., & Barker, S. J. (1997). Effects of motion, ambient light, and hypoperfusion on pulse oximeter function. *Journal of Clinical Anesthesia, 9*(3), 179–183.

Twibell, R. S. (1998). Family coping during critical illness. *Dimensions of Critical Care Nursing, 17*(2), 100–112.

Union Institute Research Engine. (1999). What is a literature review? Retrieved February 25, 2000, from www.tui.edu/current/phd/first/lr.asp.

Vadolas, J., Wardan, H., Orford, M., Williamson, R., & Ioannou, P. A. (2004). Cellular genomic reporter assays for screening and evaluation of inducers of fetal hemoglobin. *Human Molecular Genetics, 13*(2), 223–233.

Van den Heuvel, E. T., Witte, L. P., Stewart, R. E., Schure, L. M., Sanderman, R., & Meyboom-de Jong, B. (2002). Long-term effects of a group support program and an individual support program for informal caregivers of stroke patients: Which caregivers benefit the most? *Patient Education & Counseling, 47*(4), 291–299.

Voepel-Lewis, T., Ketefian, S., Starr, A., & White, M. J. (1990). Stress, coping, and quality of life in family members of kidney transplant recipients. *ANNA Journal, 17*(6), 427–431.

Wainwright, S. P. (1995). The transformational experience of liver transplantation. *Journal of Advanced Nursing, 22*(6), 1068–1076.

Weichler, N. K. (1993). Caretakers' informational needs after their children's renal or liver transplant. *ANNA Journal, 20*(2), 135–140, 146.

Werley, H., & Fitzpatrick, J.(1983). *Annual review of nursing research* (Vol. I). New York: Springer.

White, K. M. (1985). Completing the hemodynamic picture: Svo_2. *Heart & Lung, 14*(3), 272–280.

Whyte, R. K., Jangaard, K. A., & Dooley, K. C. (1995). From oxygen content to pulse oximetry: Completing the picture in the newborn. *Acta Anaesthesiology Scandinavia* (Suppl. 107), 95–100.

Wimberly, P. D. (1993). Oxygen monitoring in the newborn. *Scandinavian Journal of Clinical Laboratory Investigation* (Suppl. 214), 127–130.

Wimberly, P. D., Siggaard-Anderson, O., & Fogh-Anderson, N. (1990). Accurate measurement of haemoglobin oxygen saturation, and fraction of carboxyhemoglobin and methemoglobin in fetal blood using Radiometer OSM3: Corrections for fetal haemoglobin fraction and pH. *Scandinavian Journal of Clinical Laboratory Investigation* (Suppl. 203), 235–239.

Yelderman, M., & New, W. (1985). Evaluation of pulse oximetry, *Anesthesiology, 59*(4), 349–352.

Zhao, S. (1991). Metatheory, metamethod, meta-data-analysis: What, why, and how? *Sociological Perspectives, 34*(3), 377–390.

CHAPTER 7
Frameworks

A framework is an abstract, logical structure of meaning. It guides the development of the study and enables you to link the findings to the body of knowledge used in nursing. Frameworks are used in both quantitative and qualitative research. In quantitative studies, the framework is a testable theory that may emerge from a conceptual model or may develop inductively from published research or clinical observations. In qualitative research, the initial framework is a philosophy or worldview; a theory consistent with the philosophy may be developed as an outcome of the study.

Every quantitative study has a framework, even when that framework is not explicitly expressed. The framework should be well integrated with the methodology, carefully structured, and clearly presented. When you critically appraise studies to determine if you will apply them in clinical practice or to develop a study, you must be able to identify and evaluate the framework. Your ability to understand the meaning of study findings will depend on your ability to understand the logic within the framework and determines how you will use the findings. Thus, your ability to apply the findings of a study grows when you understand the framework and can relate it to the findings for use in your nursing practice. To help you build the knowledge and skills needed to develop a framework, this chapter explains relevant terms, describes how frameworks are constructed, and discusses the critical analysis of frameworks.

DEFINITION OF TERMS

The first step in understanding theories and frameworks is to familiarize yourself with the terms related to theoretical ideas and their application. These terms

and the ways they are used come from the philosophy of science, where the main concern is the nature of scientific knowledge. As nurses have studied philosophies of science, philosophies of nursing science are beginning to emerge.

In the following section, we explain terms such as *concept, relational statement, conceptual model, theory,* and *conceptual map*. Within philosophies of science, the term *theory* is used in a variety of ways that could include both theories and conceptual models (Suppe & Jacox, 1985). In philosophies of nursing science, however, theory tends to be defined narrowly and is different from the term conceptual model.

Concept

A concept is a term that abstractly describes and names an object, a phenomenon, or an idea, thus providing it with a separate identity or meaning. An example of a concept is the term *anxiety*. At high levels of abstraction, such as is found in conceptual models, concepts have general meanings and are sometimes referred to as constructs. For example, a construct associated with the concept of anxiety might be "emotional responses."

At a more concrete level, terms are referred to as variables and have narrow definitions. A variable is more specific than a concept and implies that the term is defined so that it is measurable. The word variable implies that the numerical values associated with the term vary from one instance to another. A variable related to anxiety might be "palmar sweating," which the researcher can measure by assigning numerical values to different amounts of sweat on the subject's palm. The links among constructs, concepts, and variables are illustrated here:

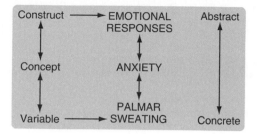

Defining concepts allows us to be consistent in the way we use a term in the discipline, apply it to a theory, and incorporate it in a field of study. A **conceptual definition** differs from the **denotative** (or dictionary) **definition** of a word. A conceptual definition (connotative meaning) is more comprehensive than a denotative definition because it includes associated meanings the word may have. For example, we may connotatively associate the term "fireplace" with images of hospitality and warm comfort, whereas the dictionary definition would be more concrete and narrower. A conceptual definition can be established through concept synthesis, concept derivation, or concept analysis.

Concept Synthesis

In nursing, many phenomena have not yet been identified as discrete entities. However, recognizing, naming, and describing these phenomena are often critical steps to understanding the process and outcomes of nursing practice. The process of describing and naming a previously unrecognized concept is **concept synthesis**. In the discipline of medicine, Selye (1976) performed concept synthesis to identify and define the concept of stress. Before his work, stress was not known as a phenomenon. Nursing studies often involve previously unrecognized and unnamed phenomena that must be named and carefully defined. Concept synthesis is also important in the development of nursing theory (Walker & Avant, 2004).

Concept Derivation

In some cases, the researcher may obtain conceptual definitions from theories in other disciplines. A conceptual definition obtained in this way will explain a phenomenon important to a non-nursing discipline. Therefore, it will need to be carefully evaluated to determine whether or not it has the same conceptual meaning within nursing. The conceptual definition may need to be modified so that it is meaningful within nursing and consistent with nursing thought (Walker & Avant, 2004). This process, referred to as **concept derivation**, may require a concept analysis that examines the use of the concept in nursing literature, compares the results with the existing conceptual definition, and, if the two are different, modifies the definition to be consistent with nursing usage.

Concept Analysis

Concept analysis is a strategy that identifies a set of characteristics essential to the connotative meaning of a concept. The procedure will require you to explore the various ways the term is used and to identify a set of characteristics that clarify the range of objects or ideas to which that concept may be applied. You will also use these characteristics to distinguish the concept from similar concepts. Several approaches to concept analysis have been described in the literature, and the authors of these strategies are listed in Table 7-1. In addition, a number of concept analyses have been published in the nursing literature, such as those listed in Table 7-2. Concept analysis is a type of philosophical inquiry, although not all concept analyses follow the philosophical format; an example of a philosophical concept analysis is provided in Chapter 23. Multiple concept analyses are often performed related to a selected concept until there is some degree of consensus within the discipline regarding the conceptual definition. Conceptual definition often leads to methods for measuring the concept and to theories as well.

Importance of a Conceptual Definition: An Example

Morse, Solberg, Neander, Bottorff, and Johnson (1990) illustrated the importance of a conceptual definition. They analyzed published definitions of the concept of caring in a project funded by the National Center for Nursing Research. In examining previous conceptual definitions of caring, Morse and colleagues found that authors had difficulty separating meanings for caring, care, and nursing care. Caring may be an action, such as "taking care of," or a concern, such as "caring about." On the other hand, caring may be viewed from the perspective of the nurse or of the patient. Each of these perspectives alters how *caring* is conceptually defined. How might a nurse practitioner define *caring*?

Morse et al. (1990) used content analysis to examine how 35 authors defined the term caring. The analysis included definitions of caring from three nursing theorists: Orem, Watson, and Leininger. The researchers identified five categories of caring: (1) caring as a human trait, (2) caring as a moral imperative, (3) caring as an affect, (4) caring as an interpersonal relationship, and (5) caring as a therapeutic intervention. In addition, they

TABLE 7-1 ■■ Publications on How to Conduct a Concept Analysis

Author	Date	Publication
Avant	2000	The Wilson method of concept analysis. In *Concept Development in Nursing: Foundations, Techniques, and Applications.*
Broome	2000	Integrated literature reviews in the development of concepts. In *Concept Development in Nursing: Foundations, Techniques, and Applications.*
Caron & Bowers	2000	Methods and applications of dimensional analysis: A contribution to concept and knowledge development in nursing. In *Concept Development in Nursing: Foundations, Techniques, and Applications.*
Chinn & Kramer	2007	*Integrated Theory and Knowledge Development in Nursing.*
Haase, Leidy, Coward, Britt, & Penn	2000	Simultaneous concept analysis: A strategy for developing multiple interrelated concepts. In *Concept Development in Nursing: Foundations, Techniques, and Applications.*
Lackey	2000	Concept clarification: Using the Norris method in clinical research. *Concept Development in Nursing: Foundations, Techniques, and Applications.*
Maas et al.	2000	Concept development of nursing-sensitive outcomes. In *Concept Development in Nursing: Foundations, Techniques, and Applications.*
Morse	2000	Exploring pragmatic utility: Concept analysis by critically appraising the literature. In *Concept Development in Nursing: Foundations, Techniques, and Applications.*
Rodgers	2000	Concept analysis: An evolutionary view. In *Concept Development in Nursing: Foundations, Techniques, and Applications.*
Sadler	2000	A multiphase approach to concept analysis and development. In *Concept Development in Nursing: Foundations, Techniques, and Applications.*
Schwartz-Barcott & Kim	2000	An expansion and elaboration of the hybrid model of concept development. In *Concept Development in Nursing: Foundations, Techniques, and Applications.*
Walker & Avant	2004	*Strategies for Theory Construction in Nursing.*
Wuest	2000	Concept development situated in the critical paradigm. In *Concept Development in Nursing: Foundations, Techniques, and Applications.*

TABLE 7-2 ■■ Recently Published Concept Analyses

Author	Date	Concept Analyzed
Chang	2007	Susceptibility
Easley	2007	Harmony
Gomes	2007	Relational aggression
Leh	2007	Preconceptions
Lorenz	2007	Protection
Schantz	2007	Compassion
Wilde & Garvin	2007	Self-monitoring

identified two outcomes of caring: (1) the subjective experience of the patient and (2) the physical response of the patient. The following questions emerged from the analysis:

1. "Is caring a constant and uniform characteristic, or may caring be present in various degrees within individuals?" (Morse et al., 1990, p. 9).
2. Is caring an emotional state that can be depleted?
3. "Can caring be nontherapeutic? Can a nurse care too much?" (Morse et al., 1990, p. 10).
4. Can cure occur without caring? Can a nurse engage in safe practice without caring?
5. "What difference does caring make to the patient?" (Morse et al., 1990, p. 11).

These researchers concluded that, at the time of their analysis, a clear conceptual definition of caring did not exist. Their careful analysis has stimulated curiosity within the nursing practice as nurse scholars continue to seek a better understand of the concept of caring as it is used in nursing. Since their study, theoretical work—including additional literature reviews and concept analyses on caring—has increased, not just in the United States but across the world (Table 7-3).

A number of scales have been developed worldwide to measure caring in nursing (Table 7-4), and a number of qualitative studies have been conducted to gain insight on caring (Table 7-5). This work is increasing our understanding of caring in nursing, and enabling us to further implement caring in our practice. How might caring be measured in the work of nurse practitioners? Might qualitative studies increase the insight on caring in the primary care role?

TABLE 7-3 ■ Concept Analyses of Caring

Year	Author	Title
1990	Marck	Therapeutic reciprocity: A caring phenomenon
1991	Roberts & Fitzgerald	Serenity: Caring with perspective
1992	Eriksson	The alleviation of suffering: The idea of caring
1992	Eriksson	Different forms of caring communion
1992	O'Berle & Davies	Support and caring: Exploring the concepts
1992	Pepin	Family caring and caring in nursing
1993	Jones & Alexander	The technology of caring: A synthesis of technology and caring for nursing administration
1995	Buchanan & Ross	A concept analysis of caring
1995	Fealy	Professional caring: The moral dimension
1995	Kyle	The concept of caring: A review of the literature
1995	Scott	Correlates of health promotion in elders
1995	Smith	An analysis of altruism: A concept of caring
1997	McCance, McKenna, & Boore	Caring: Dealing with a difficult concept
1997	Sherwood	Meta-synthesis of qualitative analyses of caring: Defining a therapeutic model of nursing
1997	Sourial	An analysis of caring
1997	Wilde	The caring connection in nursing: A concept analysis
1998	Kelly	Caring and cancer nursing: Framing the reality using selected social science theory
1998	Wilkes & Wallis	A model of professional nurse caring: Nursing students' experience
1998	Wilkinson	What it means to care
1999	Fredriksson	Modes of relating in a caring conversation: A research synthesis on presence, touch, and listening
1999	Patistea	Nurses' perceptions of caring as documented in theory and research
1999	Rodriquez	Medicine or caring science in ancient Greece [Spanish]
1999	Smith	Caring and the science of unitary human beings
1999	Swanson	What is known about caring in nursing science: A literary meta-analysis
1999	Swanson	Effects of caring, measurement, and time on miscarriage impact and women's well-being
2000	Priest	Focus: the use of narrative in the study of caring: A critique
2001	Kunyk & Olson	Clarification of conceptualizations of empathy
2001	Mattsson-Lidsle & Lindström	Consolation: A concept analysis [Swedish]
2001	McCance, McKenna, & Boore	Exploring caring using narrative methodology: An analysis of the approach
2003	Covington	Caring presence: Delineation of a concept for holistic nursing
2003	Duffy & Hoskins	The quality-caring model: Blending dual paradigms
2003	Lewis	Practice applications: Caring as being in nursing: Unique or ubiquitous?
2003	Lin & Chiou	Concept analysis of caring [Chinese]
2004	Coffey	Development of the concept of covenant between nurse and patient
2004	Pang et al.	Towards a Chinese definition of nursing
2004	Sadler	Descriptions of caring uncovered in student's baccalaureate program admission essays
2005	Brilowski & Wendler	An evolutionary concept analysis of caring
2005	Brunelli	A concept analysis: the grieving process for nurses
2005	Cowling & Taliaferro	Emergence of a healing-caring perspective: Contemporary conceptual and theoretical directions
2005	Niu	The philosophy of nursing management: A concept analysis [Chinese]
2006	Fridh & Bergbom	To watch: A study of the concept [Norwegian]
2006	Coffey	The nurse-patient relationship in cancer care as a shared covenant: A concept analysis
2006	Sadler	In response to Brilowski & Wendler (2005)
2006	Sumner	Concept analysis: The moral construct of caring in nursing as communicative action
2007	Anderberg, Lepp, M., Berglund, A.L., & Segesten	Preserving dignity in caring for older adults: A concept analysis
2007	Schantz	Compassion: A concept analysis
2007	Finfgeld-Connett	Concept comparison of caring and social support

TABLE 7-4 ■ Scales Developed to Measure Caring

Year	Author	Scale
1987	Larson	CARE-Q
1989	Nyberg	Nyberg Caring Attributes Scale CAS
1990	Duffy	Caring Assessment Tool CAT
1994	Wolf, Giardino, Osborne, & Ambrose	CBI
1997	Coates	The Caring Efficacy Scale
1997	Nahas	Nurse Caring Behavior Instrument
1997	Watson & Lea	The Caring Dimensions Inventory
1998	Lea, Watson, & Deary	Nursing Dimensions Inventory
1999a	Watson, Deary, & Lea	
1999b	Watson et al.	
2001	Watson, Deary, & Hoogbruin	
2002	Deary et al.	
1998	Arthur, Pang, & Wong	The Caring Attributes Questionnaire
1999	Arthur et al.	
2001	Arthur et al.	Caring Attributes, Professional Self and Technological Influences
2002	Noh, Arthur, & Sohng	
2004	Arthur, Chong, Rujkorakarn, Wong, & Wongpanarak	
1994	Wolf et al.	Wolf's Caring Behaviors Inventory
2000	Brunton & Beaman	
2000	Christopher & Hegedus	Respondents Perceptions of Caring Behaviour Scale
2004	Wolf et al.	Caring Behaviors Inventory for Elders
2005	Cossette, Pepin, Ricard, & Côté	The Caring Nurse-Patient Interaction Scale
2006	Cossette, Côté, Pepin, Ricard, & D'Aoust	
2007	Kuo, Turton, Lee-Hsieh, Tseng, & Hsu	Peer Caring Measurement
2007	Duffy, Hoskins, & Seifert	Caring Assessment Tool

TABLE 7-5 ■ Qualitative Studies of Caring

Year	Author	Title
1995	Fealy	Professional caring: The moral dimension
1998	Amendola	Toward a caring curriculum
1998	Fagerström, Eriksson, & Engberg	The patient's perceived caring needs as a message of suffering
1999	Fredriksson	Modes of relating in a caring conversation: A research synthesis on presence, touch and listening
1999	Joudrey & Gough	Caring and curing revisited: Student nurses' perceptions of nurses' and physicians' ethical stances
1999	Patistea	Nurses' perceptions of caring as documented in theory and research
1999	Rodriquez	Medicine or caring science in ancient Greece [Spanish]
1999	Smith	Caring and the science of unitary human beings
1999	Smith-Campbell	A case study on expanding the concept of caring from individuals to communities
2001	Henderson	Emotional labor and nursing: An under-appreciated aspect of caring work
2001	Johns	Reflective practice: Revealing the [he]art of caring
2001	Turkel, Ray & Malinski	Relational complexity: From grounded theory to instrument development and theoretical testing
2002	Barnhill	The perception of caring in labor and delivery: a phenomenological study
2002	Schoenhofer	Theoretical concerns: Philosophical underpinnings of an emergent methodology for nursing as caring inquiry

Continued

Relational Statements

A relational statement declares that a relationship of some kind exists between or among two or more concepts (Walker & Avant, 2004). Relational statements form the core of a framework. Skills in expressing statements are essential for constructing an integrated framework that will, in turn, lead to a well-designed study. The statements expressed in your framework will determine (1) your objective, question, or hypothesis; (2) your study's design; (3) the statistical analyses you will perform; and (4) the type of findings you can expect. Frameworks developed with inadequate expression of statements provide only a broad orientation for the study and do not guide the research process.

Understanding relational statements is essential also for appraising frameworks. Being able to evaluate the links among the hypotheses, the design, and the framework is also an essential part of determining the quality of a study. Judging whether the

TABLE 7-5	Qualitative Studies of Caring—Cont'd	
Year	**Author**	**Title**
2002	Yonge & Molzahn	Exceptional nontraditional caring practices of nurses
2003	Cortis & Kendrick	Nursing ethics, caring and culture
2003	Fredriksson & Eriksson	The ethics of the caring conversation
2003	Helin & Lindström	Sacrifice: An ethical dimension of caring that makes suffering meaningful
2003	McCance	Caring in nursing practice: The development of a conceptual framework
2003	Rogers	Nursing: An ethic of caring
2003	Söderlund	Qualitative research approaches of relevance for caring sciences [Swedish]
2004	Celich & Crossetti	Being with the carer: A dimension of the caring process [Portuguese]
2004	Clark	Human caring theory: Expansion and explication
2004	Coffman	Cultural caring in nursing practice: A meta-synthesis of qualitative research
2004	Cowling & Taliaferro	Emergence of a healing-caring perspective: Contemporary conceptual and theoretical directions
2004	Forbat	The care and abuse of minoritized ethnic groups: The role of statutory services
2004	Gramling	Ice chips and hope: The coach's story of caring art
2004	Gregg & Magilvy	Values in clinical nursing practice and caring
2004	Lake	Transformation: Student nurses' experiences in learning the caring process in nursing
2004	Lucena & Crossetti	The meaning of caring in the intensive care unit [Portuguese]
2004	McIntosh	Nurses' experiences with healing and spirituality
2005	Biley & Bauer	Bringing the heart back to nursing: Human caring practice and education in Germany and the UK
2005	Brand	The lived experiences of six women during adjuvant chemotherapy for stage l or ll breast cancer
2005	Budo & Saupe	Ways of care in rural communities: Culture permeating the nursing care [Portuguese]
2005	Schumacher	Caring behaviors of preceptors as perceived by new nursing graduate orientees
2005	Wannapornsiri, Sindhu, Phancharoenworakul, & Gasemgitvatana	Caring process of Thai women with breast cancer receiving chemotherapy
2006	Coelho	Caring gestures in nursing [Portuguese]
2006	Delmar	Caring-ethical phronetic research: Epistemological considerations
2006	Hupcey & Miller	Community dwelling adults' perception of interpersonal trust vs. trust in health care providers
2006	Jensen	To see with the heart's eye [Danish]
2006	Lindholm, Nieminen, Mäkelä, & Rantanen-Siljamäki	Clinical application research: A Hermeneutical approach to the appropriation of caring science
2006	Liu, Mok, & Wong	Caring in nursing: Investigating the meaning of caring from the perspective of cancer patients in Beijing, China
2006	Nåden & Saeteren	Cancer patients' perception of being or not being confirmed
2006	Perini et al.	The meaning of caring from the viewpoint of patients with wounds due to peripheral vascular disease [German]
2006	Sun, Long, Boore, & Tsao	Patients and nurses' perceptions of ward environmental factors and support systems in the care of suicidal patients

study was successful depends, in part, on identifying the statements in the framework and tracking their examination by the study.

Characteristics of Relational Statements

Relational statements describe the direction, shape, strength, symmetry, sequencing, probability of occurrence, necessity, and sufficiency of a relationship (Fawcett, 1999; Stember, 1986; Walker & Avant, 2004). One statement may have several of these characteristics; each characteristic is not exclusive of the others. Statements may be expressed in literary form (such as a sentence), in diagrammatic form (such as a conceptual map), or in mathematical form (such as an equation). Statements in nursing tend to be expressed in literary and diagrammatic forms.

Direction. The direction of a relationship may be positive, negative, or unknown. A positive linear relationship implies that as one concept changes (the value or amount of the concept increases or decreases), the second concept will also change in the *same* direction. For example, the literary statement "The risk of illness (A) increases as stress (B) increases" expresses a positive relationship. This positive relational statement could also be expressed as "The risk of illness decreases as stress decreases." This relationship could be diagramed as follows:

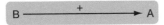

A negative linear relationship implies that as one concept changes, the other concept changes in the *opposite* direction. For example, the literary statement "As relaxation (A) increases, blood pressure (B) decreases" expresses a negative linear relationship. This relationship could be diagrammed as follows:

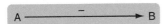

If a relationship is believed to exist but the nature of the relationship is unclear, the following diagram could be used to depict it:

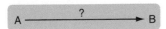

This last type of statement might be appropriate for discussing the relationship between coping and social support. We might say that although there is evidence that a relationship exists between these two concepts, the studies examining that relationship have conflicting

findings. For example, some researchers find coping to be positively related to social support—that is, as social support increases, coping increases. However, others may find a negative relationship—that is, as social support increases, coping decreases. Thus, the nature of the relationship between coping and social support is uncertain. It is possible that the conflicting findings may result from differences in how the two concepts have been defined and measured in various studies. But perhaps there is a confounding variable that has not been identified that changes the relationship between coping and social support.

Shape. Most relationships are assumed to be linear, and statistical tests are conducted to look for linear relationships. In a linear relationship, the relationship between the two concepts remains consistent regardless of the values of each of the concepts. For example, if the value of A increases by 1 point each time the value of B increases by 1 point, then the values continue to increase at the same rate whether the value is 2 or 200. The relationship can be illustrated by a straight line, as shown in Figure 7-1.

Relationships can also be curvilinear or form some other shape. In a curvilinear relationship, the relationship between two concepts varies according to the relative values of the concepts. The relationship between anxiety and learning is a good example of a curvilinear relationship. Very high or very low levels of anxiety are associated with low levels of learning, whereas moderate levels of anxiety are associated with high levels of learning (Fawcett, 1999). This type of relationship is illustrated by a curved line, as shown in Figure 7-2.

Strength. The strength of a relationship is the amount of variation explained by the relationship. Some of the variation in a concept, but not all, is associated with variation in another concept. In discussing the strength of a relationship, researchers sometimes use the term effect size. The effect size

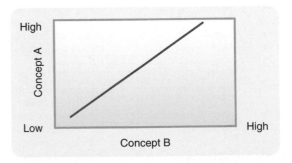

Figure **7-1** Example of a linear relationship.

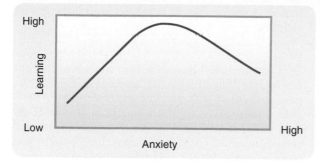

Figure 7-2 Example of a curvilinear relationship.

explains how much "effect" variation in one concept has on variation in a second concept.

In some cases, a large portion of the variation can be explained by the relationship; in others, only a moderate or a small portion of the variation can be explained by the relationship. For example, one might examine the strength of the relationship between coping and compliance. A portion of the variance in a measure of compliance is associated with the measure of a person's coping ability, but the remaining portion of this variation cannot be explained by how well a person copes. Conversely, only a portion of variation in a measure of a person's ability to cope can be explained by variation in a measure of his or her compliance. The portions of the two concepts that are associated are explained by the strength of the relationship.

Strength is usually determined by correlational analysis and is expressed mathematically by a correlation coefficient such as the following:

$$r = 0.35$$

The statistic r is the coefficient obtained by performing the statistical procedure known as Pearson's product moment correlation. A value of 0 indicates no strength, whereas a +1 or a −1 indicates the greatest strength, as signified in the following diagram:

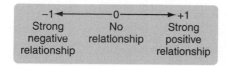

The + or − does not have an impact on strength. For example, r = −0.35 is as strong as r = +0.35. A weak relationship is usually considered one with an r value of 0.1 to 0.3; a moderate relationship is one with an r value of 0.31 to 0.5; and a strong relationship

is one with an r value greater than 0.5. The greater the strength of a relationship, the easier it is to detect relationships between the variables being studied. We explore this idea further in the chapters on sampling, measurement, and data analysis.

Symmetry. Relationships may be symmetrical or asymmetrical. In an **asymmetrical relationship**, if A occurs (or changes), then B will occur (or change); but there may be no indication that if B occurs (or changes), A will occur (or change) (Fawcett, 1999). A previously cited example showed that when changes in a person's relaxation level (A) occurred, changes in blood pressure (B) occurred. However, one cannot say that when changes in blood pressure occur, changes in relaxation levels occur. Therefore, the relationship is asymmetrical. An asymmetrical relationship may be diagrammed as follows:

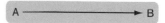

A **symmetrical relationship** is complex and contains two statements, such as if A occurs (or changes), B will occur (or change); if B occurs (or changes), A will occur (or change) (Fawcett, 1999). An example is the symmetrical relationship between the occurrences of cancer and impaired immunity. As the cancer increases, impaired immunity increases; as impaired immunity increases, cancer increases. A symmetrical relationship may be diagrammed as follows:

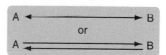

Sequencing. Time is the important factor in explaining the sequential nature of a relationship. If both concepts occur simultaneously, the relationship is **concurrent** (Fawcett, 1999). The relationship between relaxation (A) and blood pressure (B) may seem to be concurrent. If so, it would be expressed as follows:

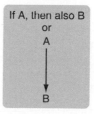

If one concept occurs later than the other, the relationship is **sequential**. If relaxation (A) was thought to occur first, and then blood pressure (B) decreased, the relationship is sequential. This relationship is expressed as follows:

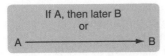

If A, then later B
or
A ————————→ B

Probability of Occurrence. A relationship can be deterministic or probabilistic depending on the degree of certainty that it will occur. Deterministic (or causal) relationships are statements of what always occurs in a particular situation. A scientific law is one example of a deterministic relationship (Fawcett, 1999). It is expressed as follows:

If A, then always B

Another deterministic relationship describes what always happens if no conditions interfere. This is referred to as a tendency statement. A tendency statement might propose that an immobilized patient lying in a typical hospital bed (A) will always develop pressure sores (B) after 6 weeks if there are no interfering conditions. A tendency statement would be expressed in the following form:

If A, then always B if there are no interfering conditions

A probability statement expresses the probability that something will happen in a given situation (Fawcett, 1999). This relationship is expressed as follows:

If A, then probably B

Probability statements are tested statistically to determine the extent of probability that B will occur in the event of A. For example, one could state that there is greater than a 50% probability that a patient who has an indwelling catheter for 1 week will experience a urinary bladder infection. This probability could be expressed mathematically as follows:

$$p > 0.50$$

The p is a symbol for probability. The > is a symbol for "greater than." This mathematical statement asserts that there is more than a 50% probability that the relationship will occur.

Necessity. In a necessary relationship, one concept must occur for the second concept to occur. For example, one could propose that if sufficient fluids are administered (A), and only if sufficient fluids are administered, then the unconscious patient will

remain hydrated (B). This relationship is expressed as follows:

If A, and only if A, then B

In a substitutable relationship, a similar concept can be substituted for the first concept and the second concept will still occur. For example, a substitutable relationship might propose that if tube feedings are administered (A_1), or if hyperalimentation is administered (A_2), the unconscious patient can remain nourished (B). This relationship is expressed as follows:

If A_1, or if A_2, then B

Sufficiency. A sufficient relationship states that when the first concept occurs, the second concept will occur, regardless of the presence or absence of other factors (Fawcett, 1999). A statement could propose that if a patient is immobilized in bed longer than a week, he or she will lose bone calcium, regardless of anything else. This relationship is expressed as follows:

If A, then B, regardless of anything else

A contingent relationship will occur only if a third concept is present. For example, a statement might claim that if a person experiences a stressor (A), the person will manage the stress (B), but only if she or he uses effective coping strategies (C). The third concept, in this case effective coping strategies, is referred to as an intervening (or mediating) variable. Intervening variables can affect the occurrence, strength, or direction of a relationship. A contingent relationship can be expressed as follows:

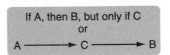

If A, then B, but only if C
or
A ——→ C ——————→ B

Statement Hierarchy

Statements about the same two conceptual ideas can be made at various levels of abstractness. The statements found in conceptual models (general propositions) are at a high level of abstraction. Statements found in theories (specific propositions) are at a moderate level of abstraction. Hypotheses, which are a form of statement, are at a low level of abstraction and are specific. As statements become less abstract, they become narrower in scope (Fawcett, 1999), as shown in the following diagram:

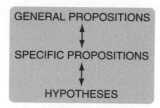

Statements at varying levels of abstraction that express relationships between or among the same conceptual ideas can be arranged in hierarchical form, from general to specific. This arrangement allows you to see (or evaluate) the logical links among the various levels of abstraction. Statement sets link the relationships expressed in the framework with the hypotheses, research questions, or objectives that guide the methodology of the study.

Roy and Roberts (1981) developed statement sets related to Roy's nursing model that could be used in frameworks for research, as shown in the following excerpts.

■ GENERAL PROPOSITION

"The magnitude of the internal and external stimuli will positively influence the magnitude of the physiological response of an intact system." (Roy & Roberts, 1981, p. 90)

■ SPECIFIC PROPOSITION

"The amount of mobility in the form of exercising positively influences the level of muscle integrity." (Roy & Roberts, 1981, p. 90)

■ HYPOTHESIS

"If the nurse helps the patient maintain muscle tone through proper exercising, the patient will experience fewer problems associated with immobility." (Roy & Roberts, 1981, p. 90)

Conceptual Models

A conceptual model is a set of highly abstract, related constructs. It broadly explains phenomena of interest, expresses assumptions, and reflects a philosophical stance. A number of conceptual models have been developed in nursing. For example, Roy's (1984, 1988, 1990) model describes adaptation as the primary phenomenon of interest to nursing. This model identifies the constructs she considers essential to adaptation and how these constructs interact to produce adaptation. Orem (2001) considered self-care to be the phenomenon central to nursing. Her model explains how nurses facilitate the self-care of clients. Rogers (1970,

1980, 1983, 1986, 1988) regarded human beings as the central phenomenon of interest to nursing, and her model is designed to explain the nature of human beings. A conceptual model may use the same or similar constructs as other models but define them in different ways. Thus, Roy, Orem, and Rogers may all use the construct health but define it in different ways.

Most disciplines have several conceptual models, each with a distinctive vocabulary. Table 7-6 lists some of the conceptual models or grand theories in nursing. These philosophical and theoretical statements of nursing vary in their level of abstraction and the breadth of phenomena they explain. However, each provides an overall picture, a gestalt of the phenomena they explain. It is not their purpose to provide detail or to be specific. Most are not directly testable through research and thus cannot be used alone as the framework for a study (Fawcett, 1999; Walker & Avant, 2004). However, a framework can include a combination of a more abstract conceptualization of nursing and a theory.

An organized program of research is important for building a body of knowledge related to the phenomena explained by a particular conceptual model. This program of research is referred to as a research tradition. To develop a research tradition for a particular model, a group of scholars must be willing to dedicate time and energy to this endeavor. Middle-range theories compatible with the model must be developed. The research tradition for the conceptual model must be defined. The definition must (1) identify acceptable strategies for developing and testing theory on the basis of the model, (2) define the phenomena to be studied, (3) establish priorities for testing theory statements, (4) develop research methods and measurement techniques, (5) describe data collection strategies, and (6) select acceptable approaches to data analyses (Fawcett, 1999). These research traditions should include the advanced practice roles in nursing and their phenomena.

Researchers conducting studies consistent with a particular tradition may be scattered across the country (or the world), but they often maintain a network of communication about their work. In some cases, they hold annual conferences that focus on the model. These gatherings give researchers the opportunity to share findings, discuss methods, explore theoretical ideas, identify priorities for future research, and maintain network contacts. The organizations of advanced practice nurses should interface with organizations that conduct studies according to a particular tradition; this type of interaction will facilitate studies relevant to advanced nursing practice.

TABLE 7-6 ■ Nursing Philosophies and Nursing Theories

Author	Name	Development Date	Classification according to Walker & Avant (2005)	Classification according to Marriner-Tomy & Alligood (2006)
Nightingale, Florence	Modern Nursing	1859	Representative Grand Nursing Theories	Philosophies
Watson, Jean	Philosophy and Science of Caring	1985		Philosophies
Ray, Marilyn Anne	Theory of Bureaucratic Caring	1981		Philosophies
Benner, Patricia	From Novice to Expert: Excellence and Power in Clinical Nursing Practice	1984		Philosophies
Martinsen, Kari	Philosophy of Caring	1990		Philosophies
Eriksson, Katie	Theory of Caritative Caring	1990		Philosophies
Henderson, Virginia	Definition of Nursing	1955	Representative Grand Nursing Theories	Philosophies (Historically Significant)
Abdellah. Faye Glenn	Twenty-One Nursing Problems	1960		Philosophies (Historically Significant)
Weidenbach, Ernestine	The Helping Art of Clinical Nursing	1964	Representative Grand Nursing Theories	Philosophies (Historically Significant)
Hall, Lynda	Core, Care, and Cure Model	1964	Representative Grand Nursing Theories	Philosophies (Historically Significant)
Levine, Myra Estrin	The Conservation Model	1967	Representative Grand Nursing Theories	Nursing Models
Rogers, Martha E.	Unitary Human Beings	1970	Representative Grand Nursing Theories	Nursing Models
Orem, Dorothea E.	Self-Care Deficit Theory of Nursing	1971	Representative Grand Nursing Theories	Nursing Models
King, Imogene	Interacting Systems Framework and Middle Range Theory of Goal Attainment	1971	Representative Grand Nursing Theories	Nursing Models
Neuman, Betty	Systems Model	1974	Representative Grand Nursing Theories	Nursing Models
Roy, Sister Callista	Adaptation Model	1976	Representative Grand Nursing Theories	Nursing Models
Johnson, Dorothy E.	Behavioral Systems Model	1980	Representative Grand Nursing Theories	Nursing Models
Boykin, Anne & Schoenhofer Savina O.	Nursing as Caring: A Model for Transforming Practice	1993	Representative Grand Nursing Theories	Nursing Models
Roper, Nancy, Logan, Winifred W., & Tierney, Alison J.	A Model for Nursing Based on a Model of Living	1980, 1985–1990	Representative Grand Nursing Theories	Nursing Models (Historically Significant)
Newman, Margaret A.	Theory Development in Nursing	1979	Representative Grand Nursing Theories	
Ujhely, Gertrud	Determinates of the Nurse-Patient Relationship	1968	Representative Grand Nursing Theories	

Orlando, Ida Jean (Pelletier)	Nursing Process Theory	1961	Representative Grand Nursing Theories	Nursing Theories
Pender, Nola J.	Health Promotion Model	1982, 2002		Nursing Theories
Leininger, Madeleine	Culture Care Theory of Diversity and Universality	1985	Representative Grand Nursing Theories	Nursing Theories
Newman, Margaret A.	Health as Expanding Consciousness	1986	Representative Grand Nursing Theories	Nursing Theories
Parse, Rosemarie Rizzo	Human Becoming	1981	Representative Grand Nursing Theories	Nursing Theories
Erickson, Helen C., Tomlin, Evelyn M., & Swain, Mary Ann P.	Modeling and Role-Modeling	1983	Representative Grand Nursing Theories	Nursing Theories
Husted, Gladys L. & Husted, James H.	Symphonological Bioethical Theory	1999		Nursing Theories
Peplau, Hildegrad E.	Theory of Interpersonal Relations	1952	Representative Grand Nursing Theories	Nursing Theories (Historically Significant)
Travelbee, Joyce	Human-to-Human Relationship Model	1966, 1971	Representative Grard Nursing Theories	Nursing Theories (Historically Significant)
Barnard, Kathryn E.	Child Health Assessment Interaction Model	1978		Nursing Theories (Historically Significant)
Adam, Evelyn	Conceptual Model for Nursing	1980		Nursing Theories (Historically Significant)
Mercer, Ramona T.	Maternal Role Attainment – Becoming a Mother	1985, 1995		Middle Range Theories
Mishel, Merle H.	Uncertainty in Illness Theory	1988		Middle Range Theories
Reed, Pamela G.	Self-Transcendence Theory	1991, 2003		Middle Range Theories
Wiener, Carolyn L. & Dodd, Marylin J.	Theory of Illness Trajectory	1993		Middle Range Theories
Eakes, Georgene Gaskill, Burke, Mary Lermann, & Hainsworth, Margaret A.	Theory of Chronic Sorrow	1998		Middle Range Theories
Barker, Phil	The Tidal Model of Mental Health Recovery	1995–1997		Middle Range Theories
Kolcaba, Katharine	Theory of Comfort	1994		Middle Range Theories
Beck, Cheryl Tatano	Postpartum Depression Theory	1993–2004		Middle Range Theories
Swanson, Kristen M.	Theory of Caring	1991, 1993–2001		Middle Range Theories
Ruland, Cornelia M. & Moore, Shirley M.	Peaceful End of Life Theory	1998		Middle Range Theories

One example of a conceptual nursing model with an emerging research tradition is Orem's model of self-care. Orem's (2001) model focuses on the domain of nursing practice and on what nurses actually do. She proposed that individuals generally know how to take care of themselves (self-care). If they are dependent in some way, as are children, the aged, or the handicapped, family members take on this responsibility (dependent care). If individuals are ill or have some health problem (such as diabetes or a colostomy), they or their family members acquire special skills to provide that care (therapeutic self-care). An individual's capacity to provide self-care is referred to as self-care agency. A self-care deficit occurs when self-care demand exceeds self-care agency (Hartweg & Orem, 1991).

An individual obtains nursing care only when there is a deficit in the self-care or dependent care that the individual and his or her family can provide (self-care deficit). In this case, the nurse or nurses develop a system to provide the needed care. This system involves prescribing, designing, and providing care. The goal of nursing care is to help the individual resume self-care independently or with family assistance. There are three types of nursing systems: wholly compensatory, partly compensatory, and supportive-educative. The system chosen is based on the person's capacity to perform self-care.

A research tradition related to the testing of propositions of the theory requires a commitment to develop valid and reliable scales to measure the concepts of the theory. Instruments based on Orem's model are shown in Table 7-7. Orem (2001) has developed three theories related to her model: the theory of self-care deficits, the theory of self-care, and the theory of nursing systems (also referred to

TABLE 7-7 ▪ Development of Instruments to Measure Concepts in Orem's Theories and Use in Studies

Year	Instrument	Authors
1979	Exercise of Self-Care Agency Scale (translated to Chinese)	Ailinger & Deer, 1993; Beatty, 1991; Beauchesne, 1989; Brown, 1996; Carroll, 1995; Folden, 1990; Kearney & Fleischer, 1979; Mapanga, 1994; McBride, 1987, 1991; Pressly, 1995; Riesch & Hauck, 1988; St. Onge, 1988; Wang & Laffrey, 2001
1980	Denyes Self-Care Agency Instrument–90	Baker, 1991; Campbell & Soeken, 1999; Canty, 1993; Denyes, 1980; Hurst, 1991; James, 1991; Jesek-Hale, 1994; McBride, 1991; Monsen, 1988; Robinson, 1995; Schott-Baer, 1993; Slusher, 1999
1982	Self-Care Agency in Adolescents	Denyes, 1982
1984	Self-Care Behavior Log	Dodd, 1984b, 1987
1984	Self-Care Behavior Questionnaire	Dodd 1984a, 1984b, 1987
1985	Perception of Self-Care Agency	Greenfeld, 1989; Hanson & Bickel, 1985; McBride, 1991; McDermott, 1989; Weaver, 1987
1987	ADL Self-Care Scale	Gulick, 1987, 1988, 1989; Mosher & Moore, 1998
1987	Appraisal of Self-Care Agency Scale (translated to Chinese, Dutch, Norwegian, and Danish) Turkish, 2004	Brown, 1996; Evers, Isenberg, Philipsen, Senten, & Brouns, 1993; Fok, Alexander, M.F., Wong, T.K., & McFayden, 2002; Hart, 1993; Hart & Foster, 1998; Isenberg, Evers, G., & Brouns, 1987; Lorensen, Holter, Evers, Isenberg, & van Achterberg, 1993; Nahcivan, 2004; Simmons, 1990; Soderhamn & Cliffordson, 2001; van Achterberg et al., 1991; Vannoy, 1989
1988	Nurse Performance Evaluation Tool	Kostopoulos, 1988
1988	Self-Care Agency Questionnaire	Bottorff, 1988; Koster, 1995; St. Onge, 1988
1988	Self-Care Questionnaire	Riley, 1988
1989	Denyes/Fildey Dependent-Care Agency Instrument	Haas, 1990; Moore & Gaffney, 1989; Moore & Mosher, 1997
1989	Mother's Performance of Self-Care Activities for Children	Moore & Gaffney, 1989
1990	Denyes Health Status Instrument	Frey & Fox, 1990
1990	Functional Status Instrument	Willard, 1990
1991	Conditioning Factor Profile	Cull, 1995; McCaleb, 1991
1991	Diabetes Self-Care Practices Instrument	Frey & Fox, 1990

Continued

as the general theory of nursing). Studies testing statements that have emerged from Orem's theories appear in the literature (Table 7-8). Research methodologies acceptable for testing Orem's theories have not been specified in the literature. Orem has suggested that researchers examine the qualitative characteristics of self-care, as well as its presence or absence. She also recommended studying the phases in which individuals (1) investigate the possibility of caring for themselves, (2) make the decision to do so, and (3) begin to engage in self-care behaviors. The focus of self-care in Orem's work should provide a basis for research by nurse practitioners who, in most cases, must depend on the client's self-care abilities to implement the instructions provided during primary care. Are there strategies that nurse practitioners could use to increase the self-care capabilities of their clients? Could the effectiveness of a new strategy be tested through research and published to guide other nurse practitioners?

Theory

A theory is more narrow and specific than a conceptual model and is directly testable. A theory consists of an integrated set of defined concepts, existence statements, and relational statements that can be used to describe, explain, predict, or control that phenomenon. Existence statements declare that a given concept exists or that a given relationship occurs. For example, an existence statement might claim that a condition referred to as stress exists and that there is a relationship between stress and health.

TABLE 7-7	Development of Instruments to Measure Concepts in Orem's Theories and Use in Studies—Cont'd	
Year	**Instrument**	**Authors**
1991	Self-as-Carer Inventory	Freeman, 1992; Geden & Taylor, 1991; Lukkarinen & Hentinen, 1997; Metcalfe, 1996; White, 2000
1991	Self-Care Agency Assessment	Gammon, 1991
1991	Cystic Fibrosis Self-Care Practice Instrument	Baker, 1991
1992	HIV-Specific Therapeutic Self-Care Demand Inventory	Freeman, 1992
1992	HIV-Related Self-Care Behaviors Checklist	Freeman, 1992
1993	Children's Self-Care Performance Questionnaire	Moore, 1993; Moore & Mosher, 1997
1993	Hart Prenatal Care Actions Scale	Hart, 1993
1993	Task Scale (measures dependent care)	Schott-Baer, 1993
1995	Bess's Measurement of Diabetes Self-Care Practices Scale	Bess, 1995
1995	Health Self-Determinism Index for Children	Koster, 1995
1995	Maieutic Dimensions of Self-Care Agency	O'Connor, 1995
1995	Self-Care of Older Persons Evaluation	Dellasega, 1995
1995	Self-Care Practices of Children and Adolescents	Moore, 1995
1996	Basic Conditioning Factors Form	Metcalfe, 1996
1996	COPD Self-Care Knowledge Questionnaire	Metcalfe, 1996
1996	COPD Self-Care Action Scale	Metcalfe, 1996
1996	Self-Care Needs Inventory (French)	Page & Ricard, 1996
1998	Self-Care Management and Life-Quality Amongst Elderly	Lorensen, 1998
2001	Characterization of therapeutic self-care needs of an individual submitted to bone marrow transplantation (Portuguese)	da Silva, 2001
2001	Heart Failure Self-Care Inventory	Ahrens, 2001
2002	Revised Heart Failure Self-Care Behavior Scale	Artinian, Magnan, Sloan, & Lange, 2002
2003	Facts on Osteoporosis Quiz – revised	Ailinger, Lasus, & Braun, 2003
2003	Psychiatric Patients Caregiver Burden Scale	Pipatananond & Hanucharurnkul, 2003
2004	Self-care scale for dysmenorrhic adolescents	Hsieh, Gau, Mao, & Li, 2004

TABLE 7-8 ■ Studies Testing Statements from Orem's Theories

Year	Number of Studies	Researchers
1988	2	Alexander, Younger, Cohen, & Crawford; Hartley
1989	2	Frey & Denyes; Hanucharurnkul
1990	1	Weintraub & Hagopian
1991	2	Baker; Hartweg
1993	8	Ailinger & Deer; Baker; Canty; Dodd & Dibble; Folden; Hart; Moore; Schott-Baer
1994	4	Dowd; Jesek-Hale; Mapanga; McCaleb & Edgil
1995	8	Bess; Carroll; Cull; Hart; Koster; Robinson; Schott-Baer, Fisher, & Gregory; Villarruel
1996	6	Aish & Isenberg; Dodd et al.; Gaffney & Moore; Hagopian; Metcalfe; Wang & Fenske
1997	4	Ailinger & Deer; Lukkarinen & Hentinen; Moore & Mosher; Wang
1998	2	Hart & Foster; Mosher & Moore
1999	5	Campbell & Soeken; Lee; Renker; Slusher; Torres, Davim, & da Nobrega
2000	3	Dodd & Miaskowski; Weber; White
2001	2	Cade; Wang & Laffrey
2002	3	Artinian, Magnan, Sloan, & Lange; Fialho, Pagliuca, & Soares; Monteiro, da Nobraga, & de Lima
2003	7	Callaghan; Dashiff; Fok & Daly; Fok & Wong; Phelan, Oliveria, Christos, Dusza, & Halpern; Sousa; Wattanawech, Srimoragot, Kasemkitwattana, & Kimpee
2004	3	Harris; Velsor-Friedrich, Pigott, & Louloudes et al.; Williams & Schreier
2005	6	Callaghan; Hurst, Montgomery, Davis, Killion, & Baker; Sousa & Zauszniewski; Velsor-Friedrich, Pigott, & Srof; Zrinyi & Rimar
2006	7	Ailinger, Moore, Nguyen, & Lasus; Callaghan; Kongsaktrakul et al.; Santos & da Silva; Su, Songwathana, & Naka; Wilson, Brown, & Stephens-Ferris
2007	1	Zrinyi & Zekanyne

Relational statements clarify the relationship that exists between or among concepts. For example, a relational statement might propose that high levels of stress are related to declining levels of health. It is the statements of a theory that are tested through research, not the theory itself. Thus, identifying statements within the theory is critical to the research endeavor and forms the basis of the study's framework. The types of theory discussed here are scientific, substantive, and tentative.

Middle-Range Theories

Middle-range theories present a partial view of nursing reality. Merton, a sociologist, developed middle-range theories, in 1968. These theories are less abstract and address more specific phenomena than grand theories do. They directly apply to practice and focus on explanation and implementation. Middle-range theories may emerge from grand theories or may develop inductively from research findings. Qualitative studies have been a good source of middle range theory. Some middle-range theories have been developed by combining nursing theories with theories from other disciplines. Recently, some middle-range theories have been developed from clinical practice guidelines.

Middle-range theories are useful in both research and practice. They often help the practitioner to understanding the client's behavior, enabling more effective interventions. Because of their usefulness in practice, some authors refer to middle-range theories as practice theories. Middle-range theories are used more commonly than grand theories as frameworks for research. As a researcher, it will be important for you to carefully consider what aspects of a particular middle-range theory are appropriate for before using it. Table 7-9 identifies some of the more frequently used middle-range theories.

Scientific Theory

The term scientific theory is restricted to a theory that has valid and reliable methods of measuring each concept and whose relational statements have been tested through research and demonstrated to be valid. Scientific theories have empirical generalizations, statements that have been repeatedly tested and have not been disproved. There are no scientific theories within nursing. Scientific theories from other disciplines are commonly used within the nursing practice. For example, most physiological theories are scientific in nature.

TABLE 7-9 ■ Middle Range Theories Commonly Used in Nursing

Author	Reference	Philosophy/Theory
Abdellah, Faye Glenn	Abdellah, F. G., Beland, I. L, Martin, A., & Matheney, R. V. (1960). *Patient-centered approaches in nursing.* New York: Macmillan.	Twenty-One Nursing Problems (1960)
Adam, Evelyn	Adam, E. (1980). *To be a nurse.* Toronto, Canada: W.B. Saunders	Conceptual Model for Nursing (1980)
Barker, Phil	Barker, P. (1998). *The Tidal Model: An integrative framework for caring within an interpersonal paradigm.* Newcastle: University of Newcastle.	The Tidal Model of Mental Health Recovery (1995–1997)
Barnard, Kathryn E.	Barnard, K. (1979). *Nursing child assessment satellite teaching manual.* Seattle: NCAST Publications	Child Health Assessment Interaction Model (1978)
Beck, Cheryl Tatano	Beck, C. T. (1993). Teetering on the edge: A substantive theory of postpartum depression. *Nursing Research, 42*(1): 42–48.	Postpartum Depression Theory (1993)
Benner, Patricia	Benner, P. (1984). *From novice to expert: Promoting excellence and power in clinical nursing practice.* Menlo Park, CA: Addison-Wesley	From Novice to Expert: Excellence and Power in Clinical Nursing Practice (1984)
Boykin, Anne & Schoenhofer, Savina O.	Boykin, A., & Schoenhofer, S. (1993) *Nursing as caring: A model for transforming practice.* New York: National League for Nursing	Nursing as Caring: A Model for Transforming Practice (1993)
Eakes, Georgene, Burke, Mary, & Hainsworth, Margaret	Eakes, G. G., Burke, M. L., & Hainsworth, M. A. (1993). Middle-range theory of chronic sorrow. *Image: Journal of Nursing Scholarship. 30*(2): 179–184.	Theory of Chronic Sorrow (1998)
Erickson, Helen, Tomlin, Evelyn, & Swain, Mary Ann	Erickson, H. C., Tomlin, E., & Swain, M. A. (1983). *Modeling and role-modeling: A theory and paradigm for nursing.* Englewood Cliffs, NJ: Prentice Hall.	Modeling and Role Modeling (1983)
Eriksson, Katie	Eriksson, K. (1990). Systematic and contextual caring science: A study of the basic motive of caring and context. *Scandinavian Journal of Caring Sciences, 4*(1), 3–5.	Theory of Caritative Caring (1990)
Hall, Lynda	Hall, L. E. (1964). Nursing: What is it? *The Canadian Nurse, 60,* 150–154.	Core, Care, and Cure Model (1964)
Henderson, Virginia	Henderson, V. (1966) *The nature of nursing.* New York: Macmillan.	Definition of Nursing (1955)
Husted, Gladys, & Husted, James	Husted, J. H., & Husted, G. L. (1999). Agreement: the origin of ethical action. *Critical Care Nursing Quarterly; 22*(3): 12–18.	Symphonological Bioethical Theory (1999)
Johnson, Dorothy	Johnson, D. E. (1980). The behavioral system model for nursing. In J. P. Riehl & C. Roy (Eds.), *Conceptual models for nursing practice* (pp. 207–216). New York: Appleton-Century-Crofts.	Behavioral Systems Model (1980)
King, Imogene	King, I. M. (1981). *A theory for nursing: Systems, concepts, process.* New York: John Wiley & Sons.	Interacting Systems Framework and Middle Range Theory of Goal Attainment (1971)
Kolcaba, Katharine	Kolcaba, K. Y. (1994). A theory of holistic comfort for nursing. *Journal of Advanced Nursing, 19*(6): 1178–1184.	Theory of Comfort (1994)

Continued

TABLE 7-9 ■ Middle Range Theories Commonly Used in Nursing—Cont'd

Author	Reference	Philosophy/Theory
Leininger, Madeleine	Leininger, M. M. (1985). Transcultural care diversity and universality: A theory of nursing. *Nursing and Health Care, 6*(4), 208–212.	Culture Care Theory of Diversity and Universality (1985)
Levine, Myra	Levine, M. E. (1967). The four conservation principles of nursing. *Nursing Forum, 6*(1): 45–59.	The Conservation Model (1967)
Martinsen, Kari	Martinsen, K. (1990). Moral practice and documentation in practical nursing. In T. K. Jensen (Ed.), *Foundational problems in nursing ethics, theories of science, leadership and society* [Norwegian]. Philosophia. Aarhus.	Philosophy of Caring (1990)
Mercer, Ramona	Mercer, R. (1986). *First-time motherhood: Experiences from teens to forties.* New York: Springer. Mercer, R. (1995). *Becoming a mother: Research on maternal identity from Rubin to the present.* New York: Springer.	Maternal Role Attainment—Becoming a Mother (1986, 1995)
Mishel, Merle	Mishel, M. (1988). The theory of uncertainty in illness. *Image, 20*(4), 225–232.	Uncertainty in Illness Theory (1988)
Neuman, Betty	Neuman, B. (1974). The Betty Neuman Health-Care Systems Model: A total person approach to patient problems. In J. P. Riehl & C. Roy (Eds.), *Conceptual models for nursing practice* (pp. 99–114). New York: Appleton-Century-Crofts.	Systems Model (1974)
Newman, Margaret	Newman, M. A. (1979). *Theory Development in Nursing,* Philadelphia: F.A. Davis. (see particularly Chapter 6)	Theory Development in Nursing (1979)
Newman, Margaret	Newman, M. A. (1986). *Health as expanding consciousness.* St. Louis: C.V. Mosby.	Health as Expanding Consciousness (1986)
Nightingale, Florence	Nightingale, F. (1957). *Notes on nursing.* Philadelphia: J.B. Lippincott. (Original publication in 1859)	Modern Nursing (1859)
Orem, Dorothea	Orem, D. E. (1971). *Nursing: Concepts of practice.* New York: McGraw-Hill	Self-Care Deficit Theory of Nursing (1971)
Orlando, Ida Jean (Pelletier)	Orlando, I. J. (1961). *The dynamic nurse-patient relationship: Function, process and principles.* New York: G.P. Putnam.	Nursing Process Theory (1961)
Parse, Rosemarie	Parse, R. R. (1981). *Man-living-health: A theory of nursing.* New York: Wiley.	Human Becoming (1981)
Pender, Nola	Pender, N. J. (1982). *Health promotion in nursing practice.* New York: Appleton-Century-Crofts. Most recent edition, 2005	Health Promotion Model (1982; 2005)
Peplau, Hildegard	Peplau, H. E. (1952). *Interpersonal relations in nursing.* New York: G.P. Putnam.	Theory of Interpersonal Relations (1952)
Ray, Marilyn	Ray, M. (1981). A philosophical analysis of caring within nursing. In M. Leininger (Ed.): *Caring: An essential human need* (pp. 25–36). Thorofare, NJ: Charles B. Slack.	Theory of Bureaucratic Caring (1981)

Theorist	Citation	Theory
Reed, Pamela	Reed, P. G. (1991). Toward a nursing theory of self-transcendence: Deductive reformulation using developmental theories. *Advances in Nursing Science 13*(4), 64–77.	Self-Transcendence Theory (1991; 2003)
Rogers, Martha	Rogers, M. E. (1970). *An introduction to the theoretical basis of nursing*. Philadelphia: F.A. Davis.	Unitary Human Beings (1970)
Roper, Nancy, Logan, Winifred, & Tierney, Alison	Roper, N., Logan, W., & Tierney. A. (1980, 1985, 1990, 1996). *Elements of Nursing*. Edinburgh: Churchill Livingstone. Roper, N, Logan, W., & Tierney, A. (1996) The Roper-Logan-Tierney Model: a model in nursing practice. The Roper-Logan-Tierney Model: a model in nursing practice. In P.H. Walker (Ed.), *Blueprint for use of nursing models: education, research, practice, and administration.* National League for Nursing, pp. 289–314.	A Model for Nursing Based on a Model of Living (1980, 1985, 1990)
Roy, Sister Callista	Roy, C. (1976). *Introduction to nursing: An adaptation model.* Englewood Cliffs, NJ: Prentice-Hall.	Adaptation Model (1976)
Ruland, Cornelia, & Moore, Shirley	Ruland, C. M., & Moore, S. M. (1998). Theory construction based on standards of care: a proposed theory of the peaceful end of life. *Nursing Outlook, 46*(4): 169–175.	Peaceful End of Life Theory (1998)
Swanson, Kristen	Swanson, K. M. (1991). Empirical development of a middle range theory of caring. *Nursing Research, 40*(3): 161–166.	Theory of Caring (1991)
Travelbee, Joyce	Travelbee, J. (1966). *Interpersonal aspects of nursing.* Philadelphia: F.A. Davis.	Human-to-Human Relationship Model (1966, 1971)
Ujhely, Gertrud	Ujhely, G. (1968). *Determinants of the nurse-patient relationship.* New York: Springer.	Determinants of the Nurse-Patient Relationship (1968)
Watson, Jean	Watson, J. (1985). *Nursing: Human science and human care.* New York: Appleton-Century-Crofts.	Philosophy and Science of Caring (1985)
Wiedenbach, Ernestine	Wiedenbach, E. (1964). *Clinical nursing: A helping art.* New York: Springer.	The Helping Art of Clinical Nursing (1964)
Wiener, Carolyn, & Dodd, Marylin	Wiener, C. L., & Dodd, M. J. (1993). Coping amid uncertainty: An illness trajectory perspective. *Scholarly Inquiry for Nursing Practice, 7*(1): 17–31.	Theory of Illness Trajectory (1993)

Developed by Helen Hough, Nursing Librarian, University of Texas at Arlington.

Substantive Theory

Substantive theory is useful for explaining important phenomena within the discipline. The knowledge you gain from a substantive theory may be valuable in practice settings. An example of a substantive theory is the theory of reasoned action (Ajzen & Fishbein, 1980; Fishbein & Ajzen, 1975), which proposes that a person's expectation that a particular behavior will lead to a given outcome increases his or her intention to perform the behavior. Research has shown that intention predicts behavior. Blue (1995) has reviewed studies that examine the capacity of this theory to predict a person's willingness to participate in exercise programs.

Substantive theories do not have the validity of a scientific theory. Some of the statements may have been tested and verified, but others have not. In some cases, the statements in the theory may not have been clearly identified by the theorist or by those using the theory.

Tentative Theory

A **tentative theory** is newly proposed, has had minimal critical appraisal, and has undergone little testing. Tentative theories propose an integrated set of relationships among concepts that have not been satisfactorily addressed in a substantive theory. Because tentative theories are newly emerging and untested, they tend to be less well developed than substantive theories. Many tentative theories have short lives, but others may eventually be more extensively developed and validated through multiple studies.

Tentative theories may be developed from clinical insights, from elements of existing theories not previously related, as outcomes of qualitative studies, or from conceptual models. One type of tentative theory of great importance in nursing today is intervention theories. These middle-range theories seek to explain the dynamics of a patient problem and exactly how a specific nursing intervention is expected to change patient outcomes. Currently, these new theories are tentative, but some will likely become substantive in the future. Intervention theories are discussed in detail in Chapter 13.

Tentative theories developed in nursing often contain concepts and relational statements derived from sociological, psychosocial, psychological, and physiological theories. In some cases, the framework may require that the nurse researcher merge concepts using theory from other sciences with concepts from nursing science theories. Tentative theories in nursing often emerge from questions related to identified nursing problems or from the clinical insight that a relationship exists between or among elements important to

desired outcomes. These situations tend to be concrete and require that the researcher express these concrete ideas in more abstract language. This issue is particularly difficult for the beginning researcher. The neophyte researcher's awareness of theoretical ideas related to the situation may be limited, or the researcher may perceive the situation in such concrete terms that even though the researcher knows the theories, he or she fails to link them to the situation.

For example, one nurse, a novice researcher who worked in a newborn intensive care unit, was convinced from her clinical experiences that a mother's frequent visits to the hospital were related to her infant's weight gain. The nurse's ideas could be diagrammed as follows:

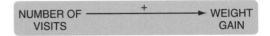

She wanted to study this relationship but was having difficulty expressing her ideas as a framework. Number of visits and weight gain are concrete ideas. From the perspective of research, these ideas are variables. However, to develop a framework, the researcher must express the variables in a more abstract and general way as concepts. This novice researcher lacked the knowledge and skills needed to accomplish this task. She was "stuck" at a concrete level of viewing her problem.

Many students recognize that they are concrete thinkers and believe that they are incapable of moving beyond that limited way of thinking. However, the capacity for abstract thinking is not an innate ability; it is a learned skill. Acquiring it simply requires that one invest the energy to obtain the knowledge and practice the skills.

Converting a concretely expressed term to a higher level of abstractness—from a variable to a concept—is a form of translation. Because the translation in this case is from a lower level of abstractness to a higher level (as shown in the following diagram), we can apply inductive reasoning:

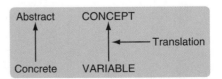

However, the researcher must know of equivalent terms at both the concrete and abstract levels in order to perform the translation. Conducting a literature search can be useful in identifying equivalent abstract terms. The search may be difficult if the novice researcher is blind to the theoretical ideas presented in the literature and picks up only the concrete ideas.

Sometimes, probing questions can help a researcher to move from concrete to more abstract thinking. For example, one could ask, "Why is it important that the mother visit?" "What happens when the mother visits?" Answering these questions may help the researcher to label what happens when the mother visits; existing theories have named this process bonding or attachment. The following diagram could be used to describe this process:

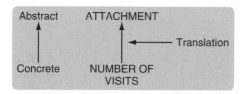

One can then ask, "What happens when the baby gains weight?" "Why is this important?" "How is it different from the baby who gains weight more slowly or fails to gain weight?" One name for this phenomenon is growth; another is thriving. There might be other ways to express the phenomenon. The following diagram could be used to describe this process:

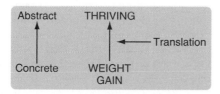

At this point, the novice nurse researcher is ready to search the literature more thoroughly. Theories related to bonding, attachment, growth, and thriving can be examined. The novice researcher may find literature that proposes a positive relationship between attachment and thriving. This relationship could be expressed as follows:

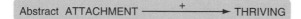

When the aforementioned ideas are linked, we have the beginning of a tentative theory. The diagram— really the beginning of a conceptual map—has the following appearance:

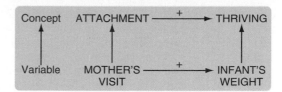

However, the ideas for a framework and a tentative theory are still incomplete. What other factors are important in influencing the relationship between mother's visits and infant's weight gain, between attachment and thriving? Again, the researcher can consult the literature. Researchers in this field have examined elements relevant to this question. What concepts did they include? What relationships did they find? Are their findings consistent with the emerging framework? Clinically, what other elements seem to be associated with this phenomenon? Do the newly found concepts need to be included in the framework? While pondering these questions, the researcher can obtain conceptual definitions for attachment and thriving and statements expressing the relationship between the two concepts from existing theories, from synthesis of the literature, or from qualitative data analysis.

As the framework expressing a tentative theory takes shape, it is time to consider moving to an even higher level of abstraction, that of conceptual models. Is there a possible fit between a conceptual model in nursing and the tentative theory expressed in the developing framework? Can the study concepts be translated to the even more abstract constructs of a conceptual model? Are the study statements linked in any way with the broad statements of a conceptual model? If a conceptual nursing model is included in the framework, the links between the conceptual model and the tentative theory must be made clear.

Conceptual Maps

One strategy for expressing a framework is a conceptual map that diagrams the interrelationships of the concepts and statements (Artinian, 1982; Fawcett, 1999; Moody, 1989; Newman, 1979, 1999; Silva, 1981). Figures 7-3 through 7-7 are examples of conceptual maps. A conceptual map summarizes and integrates what we know about a phenomenon more succinctly and clearly than a literary explanation and allows us to grasp the gestalt of a phenomenon. A conceptual map should be supported by references from the literature.

A conceptual map explains which concepts contribute to or partially cause an outcome. Conditions, both direct and indirect, that may produce the outcome are specified. A conceptual map illustrates the process in which factors must cumulatively interact over time in some sequence to have a causal effect. Conceptual maps vary in complexity and accuracy, depending on the available body of knowledge related to the phenomenon. Mapping can also identify gaps in the logic of the theory being used as a framework and reveals inconsistencies, incompleteness, and errors.

Conceptual maps are useful beyond the study for which they were developed. A conceptual map may suggest hypotheses that can be tested in future studies. In addition, through map development, the researcher may gain insight about different situations in which the same process may be occurring. Publication of the map may stimulate the interest of other researchers, who may then use it in their own studies. Thus, a well-developed conceptual map may help to build a body of knowledge related to a particular theory. In addition to conceptual maps included as the framework for a study, more maps are being published that are outcomes of extensive reviews of the literature expressed as tentative theories.

THE STEPS FOR CONSTRUCTING A STUDY FRAMEWORK

Developing a framework is one of the most important steps in the research process but, perhaps, also one of the most difficult. Examples of frameworks from the literature are helpful but not sufficient as a guide to framework development. The brief but impressive presentation of a framework in a published study belies the careful, thoughtful work required to arrive at that point. Yet, as a neophyte researcher you will need to learn how to perform that thoughtful work.

As the body of knowledge related to a phenomenon grows, it becomes easier for researchers to develop a framework to express that knowledge. Therefore, frameworks for quasi-experimental and experimental studies, which should have a background of descriptive and correlational studies and perhaps some substantive theory, should be more easily and fully developed than those for descriptive studies. Descriptive studies and qualitative studies often examine multiple factors to explore a phenomenon not previously well studied. Previous theoretical work related to the phenomenon may be tentative or nonexistent. Therefore, the framework may be less comprehensive. In qualitative studies, in which the framework development is an outcome of the study, even identifying concepts may not be clear at the beginning of the study, and statements will be synthesized from the data. The basis for developing qualitative studies is more philosophical than theoretical.

To illustrate the development of a framework, we will use a middle-range theory by Kamphuis, van Lenthe, Giskes, Brug, and Mackenback (2007) that explains socioeconomic inequalities in health behavior using constructs from the theory of planned behavior (Ajzen, 1991). As you read through the extracts from this study, however, keep in mind that the nicely turned phrases in a framework require much time, effort, thought, and reflection. They do not easily and miraculously appear in their present form. You are examining the finished framework and will not be able to see the process of thinking or the work involved as ideas develop.

The following steps introduce the reasoning used to develop a framework. The steps of the process are (1) selecting and defining concepts, (2) developing statements relating the concepts, (3) expressing the statements in hierarchical fashion, and (4) developing a conceptual map that expresses the framework. The steps are not usually performed in order. In reality, there is a flow of thought from one step to another, back and forth, as ideas are developed and refined.

Selecting and Defining Concepts

Concepts are selected for a framework on the basis of their relevance to the phenomenon you are studying. Thus, the problem statement, which describes the phenomenon, is a rich source of concepts for the framework. If you begin from a concrete clinical perspective, the ideas may be first identified as variables and then translated to concepts. Every major variable included in the study should reflect a concept included in the framework. You may modify the framework as you develop the rest of the study. As you gain additional insight into the phenomenon through a thorough search of theoretical, research, and clinical publications, you may identify additional relevant concepts or propose new relationships. While incorporating these new elements into the framework, consider their implications for the study design.

The framework presented here was developed by researchers from the public health field, not nursing, but it is imminently relevant for nursing research. As Kamphuis and colleagues indicated:

Poorer people experience worse health (Mackenbach et al., 2003; Van Herton, 2002) with higher rates of mortality and morbidity from cardiovascular diseases, obesity, type 2 diabetes and cancers (Choiniere et al., 2000; Kaplan &

Lynch, 1997; Van Lenthe & Mackenback, 2002). Fruit and vegetable consumption and physical activity play a protective role in the onset of these chronic diseases (Ness & Powles, 1997; US DHHS [U.S. Department of Health and Human Services], 1996; Van Duyn & Pivonka, 2000; Wannamethee et al., 2000). Low socioeconomic groups consume less fruits and vegetables (Smith & Brunner, 1997; James et al., 1997) and do less physical activity (Droomers et al., 1998; US DHHS, 1996) than people from higher socioeconomic backgrounds, which is considered one of the explanations for socioeconomic inequalities in health. (p. 493)

Their framework "specifies the pathways between socioeconomic status (SES), environmental factors, personal level factors (constructs from the Theory of Planned Behaviour: see Ajzen, 1991) and health behaviours" (p. 494).

Each concept included in a framework must be defined conceptually. When available and appropriate, use conceptual definitions from existing theoretical works, with definitions quoted and sources cited. If theories that define the concept are not available, you will need to develop the definition. Conceptual definitions may be available in the literature in the absence of theories that use the concept. For an example of the extraction of conceptual definitions from the literature, see Chapter 6 in *Understanding Nursing Research* (Burns & Grove, 2007).

One source of conceptual definitions is published concept analyses. Previous studies using the concept may also provide a conceptual definition. Another source of a conceptual definition is literature associated with instrument development related to the concept. Although the instrument itself is an operational definition of the concept, the author will often provide a conceptual definition on which the instrument development was based. The general literature can sometimes provide a conceptual definition. Although it may not have been as carefully thought out as the definitions in a theory or a concept analysis, this conceptual definition may reflect the only definition available in the discipline.

When acceptable conceptual definitions are not available, perform concept synthesis or concept analysis to develop the definition. You must present various definitions of the concept from the literature to validate the conceptual definition you selected for the study.

Kamphuis et al. (2007) provided the conceptual definitions in the following excerpts.

■ *ACCESSIBILITY AND AVAILABILITY*

Including financial, geographical and temporal accessibility of products and facilities that are needed for (un)healthy behaviour, and interventions to support behaviour change. (Kamphuis et al., 2007, p. 494)

■ *PSYCHOSOCIAL CONDITIONS*

Including social relationships, and psychosocial stress. (Kamphuis et al., 2007, p. 494)

■ *CULTURAL CONDITIONS*

Including culture-specific lifestyle patterns, childhood circumstances, general value orientations, and cultural participation. (Kamphuis et al., 2007, p. 494)

■ *MATERIAL CONDITIONS*

Including financial problems, material and social deprivation, and unfavourable working, housing and neighbourhood conditions. These may affect behaviour factors. For instance, a person's budgetary situation may partly determine one's access to products and facilities, or in what neighbourhood one can afford to live. (Kamphuis et al., 2007, p. 494)

Developing Relational Statements

The next step in framework development is to link all of the concepts through relational statements. Whenever possible, obtain relational statements from theoretical works and the sources cited. If such statements are unavailable, propose the relationships. Provide evidence from the literature for the validity of each relational statement whenever available. This support must include a discussion of previous quantitative or qualitative studies (or both) that have examined the proposed relationship and published observations from the clinical practice perspective.

As you develop the framework, you may have to extract statements that are embedded in the literary text of an existing theory, published research, or clinical literature. When you first begin extracting statements, the task can be overwhelming because every sentence in the text seems to be a relational statement. A little practice makes the task easier. The steps in the process of extracting statements are as follows:

1. Select a portion of a theory that discusses the relationships between or among two or three concepts.
2. Write down a single sentence from the theory that seems to be a relational statement.
3. Express it by using the statement diagrams presented earlier in the chapter.

4. Move to the next statement, and express it with diagrams.
5. Continue until all of the statements related to the selected concepts have been expressed using statement diagrams.
6. Examine the links among the diagrammatic statements you have developed. The logic of what the theorist is saying will gradually become clearer.

This process is illustrated in greater detail in Chapter 6 of *Understanding Nursing Research* (Burns & Grove, 2007).

If statements relating the concepts of interest are not available in the literature, **statement synthesis** is necessary. Develop statements that propose specific relationships among the concepts you are studying. You may gain the knowledge for your statement synthesis through clinical observation and integrative literature review (Walker & Avant, 2004).

In descriptive studies, theoretical statements related to the phenomenon may be sparse. In this case, developing a framework requires more synthesis and has a higher level of uncertainty. You may note in the statement that a relationship between A and B is proposed but the type of relationship is unknown. Follow this statement with a research question based on this relationship rather than a hypothesis. For example, ask, "What is the nature of the relationship between A and B?" An objective might be to examine the nature of the relationship between A and B.

Kamphuis et al. (2007) offered the relational statements shown in the following excerpts, each of which is followed by a diagram of the relationship.

1. Rates of physical activity is associated with neighbourhood attractiveness, accessibility and proximity of neighbourhood facilities and neighbourhood safety. (Kamphuis et al., 2007, p. 494)

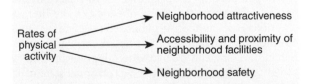

2. Participation in social activities is a strong predictor of socioeconomic differences in low leisure-time physical activity, which may be mediated by a higher extent of encouragement or peer pressure to participate in physical activities experienced by persons with high social participation. (Kamphuis et al., 2007, p. 494)

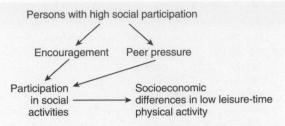

3. A range of possible mediating environmental factors between area deprivation and an unhealthy diet includes a lower prevalence of supermarkets, a higher prevalence of fast food restaurants and a relatively higher premium on the price of healthy compared to less healthy food in deprived areas. (Kamphuis et al., 2007, p. 494)

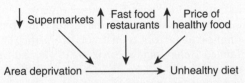

4. Social participation and social support may play a role in inequalities in fruit and vegetable consumption, as a lack of social participation might indicate a less extensive social network and less social support for adhering to a healthy diet. (Kamphuis et al., 2007, p. 494)

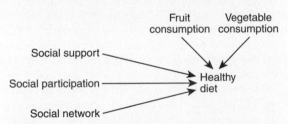

5. Cultural influences, such as traditional beliefs about appropriate or healthy diets may contribute to socioeconomic differences in fruit and vegetable consumption. (Kamphuis et al., 2007, p. 494)

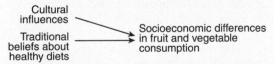

Developing Hierarchical Statement Sets

A **hierarchical statement set** is composed of a specific proposition and a hypothesis or research question. If a conceptual model is included in the framework, the statement set may also contain a general proposition. The proposition is listed first, with the hypothesis or research question immediately following. In some cases, more than one hypothesis may be related to a particular proposition. However, there must be a proposition for each hypothesis stated. This statement set indicates the link between the framework and the methodology.

Constructing a Conceptual Map

Conceptual maps are initiated early in the development of the framework, but refining the map will probably be one of your last steps. Before you can complete the map, the following information must be available:

1. A clear problem and purpose statement.
2. Concepts of interest, including conceptual definitions.
3. Results of an integrative review of the theoretical and empirical literature.
4. Relational statements linking the concepts, expressed literally and diagrammatically.
5. Identification and analysis of existing theories that address the relationships of interest.

6. Identification of existing conceptual models congruent with the developing framework.
7. Linking of proposed relationships with hypotheses, questions, or objectives (hierarchical statement sets).

Some nursing scholars believe that the map should be limited to those concepts included in the study (Fawcett, 1999). However, Artinian (1982) recommended that the map include all the concepts necessary to explain the phenomenon, plainly delineating that portion of the map to be studied. We agree with Artinian. It is important that the map be a full expression of the phenomenon of concern. This strategy is illustrated by Artinian's map of the conceptualization of the effects of role supplementation, presented in Figure 7-3. In this map, the scope of the study is enclosed by a yellow box.

Developing your own concept map entails the following steps. First, arrange the concepts on the page in sequence of occurrence (or causal linkage) from

CONCEPTUALIZATION OF THE EFFECTS OF ROLE SUPPLEMENTATION

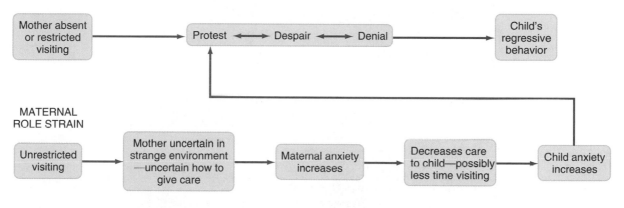

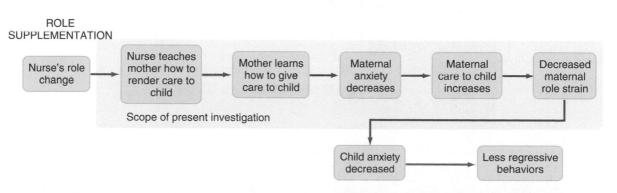

Figure **7-3** Conceptual map outlining scope of present study: conceptualization of the effects of role supplementation.

left to right, with the concepts reflecting the outcomes located on the far right. Concepts that are elements of a more abstract construct can be placed in a frame or box. Sets of closely interrelated concepts can be linked by enclosing them in a frame or circle. Second, using arrows, link the concepts in a way that is consistent with the statement diagrams you previously developed. For some studies, at some point on the map, the path of relationships may diverge, so that there are then two or more paths of concepts. The paths may converge at a later point. Every concept should be linked to at least one other concept. Third, examine the map for completeness by asking yourself the following questions:

- Are all of the concepts in the study also included on the map?
- Are all the concepts on the map defined?
- Does the map clearly portray the phenomenon?
- Does the map accurately reflect all the statements?
- Is there a statement for each of the links portrayed by the map? Is the sequence accurate?

Developing a well-constructed conceptual map requires repeated tries, but persistence pays off. You may need to reexamine the statements identified. Are there some missing links? Are some of the links inaccurately expressed?

As the map takes shape and begins to seem right, show it to trusted colleagues. Can they follow your logic? Do they agree with your links? Can they identify missing elements? Can you explain the map to them? Seek out individuals who have experienced the phenomenon you are mapping. Does the process depicted seem valid to them? Find someone more experienced than you in conceptual mapping to examine your map closely and critically.

Continue to revise your conceptual map until you achieve some degree of consensus with the people you have consulted and you feel a sense of rightness about it. Examine the conceptual map by Kamphuis et al. that is presented in Figure 7-4. Is it consistent with their concepts and statements? Does the process described seem valid to you?

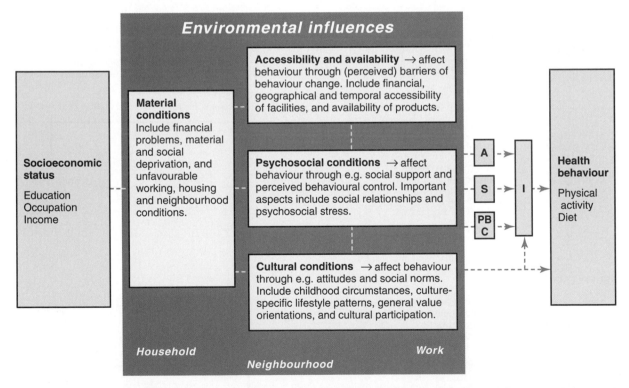

Figure **7-4** Framework of environmental determinants contributing to the explanation of socioeconomic inequalities in health behaviors. The gray panel incorporates four boxes of environmental determinants. The terms *household, neighborhood,* and *work* are examples of the different settings in which these determinants may influence health behaviors. The abbreviations in the right-hand side boxes represent the following constructs: *A* = attitude; *S* = social influences, like social support, subjective norms, and modeling; *PBC* = perceived behavioral control; I = intention. These constructs are derived from the theory of planned behavior (see Ajzen [1991] for more information).

Constructing a Study Framework from Substantive Theory

Developing a framework designed to test statements in a substantive theory requires that all concepts in the framework be obtained from the substantive theory. These concepts must be defined as the theorist defines them. If the theorist has failed to define a concept, develop one that is consistent with the theorist's perspective. Operational definitions must be consistent with the conceptual definitions and should be accepted methods of measurement used for testing the selected theory. Statements (propositions) from the substantive theory must be identified. In a substantive theory, previous studies will have tested at least some of the relational statements. Findings from these studies must be discussed in the literature review or in the presentation of the framework in terms of evidence validating or refuting the relational statements. Hypotheses for the present study must be designed to test one or more statements from the substantive theory.

Hoffman, Given, von Eye, Gift, and Given (2007) developed a study to test the theory of unpleasant symptoms (Lenz, Pugh, Milligan, Gift, & Suppe, 1997). The framework for the theory of unpleasant symptoms is shown in Figure 7-5. The authors described the theory as follows.

The TOUS theorizes that concurrent symptoms (pain, fatigue, and insomnia) may interact and catalyze each other, worsening the overall level of symptom severity experienced by people with lung cancer... The TOUS also highlights four dimensions that characterize the symptom experience: timing (frequency of occurrence and duration), intensity (severity), quality (description of qualifiers), and distress (bother).... Although symptoms comprise a chief component of the TOUS, the theoretical framework has two other components: the antecedent patient factors influencing the symptom experience and the consequences of the symptom experience. Patient factors that influence symptoms include physiologic, psychological, and situational factors... The last component of the TOUS is the consequences of the symptom experience, including performance outcomes such as symptom status.... Finally, the three components of the TOUS are reciprocal, and each component influences every other component (Hoffman et al., 2007, p. 787).

■ *WHAT IS ALREADY KNOWN IN TESTING THIS THEORY*

Studies have examined symptom experiences and reported no differences by gender. (Kurtz et al., 2000; Cooley et al., 2003; Gift et al., 2003; Gift et al., 2004).
• Some studies have found differences by gender (Degner & Sloan, 1995; Hopwood & Stephens, 1995).

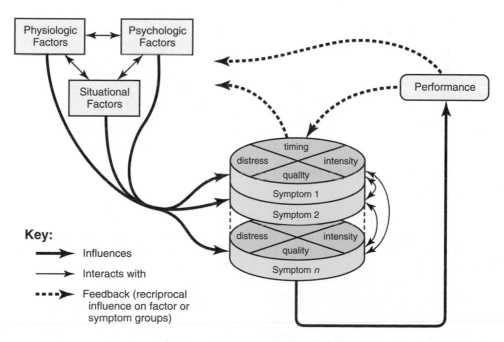

Figure 7-5 Theory of unpleasant symptoms.

- Pain and fatigue were the most common and distressing symptoms among patients with lung cancer (Cooley et al., 2003).
- The presence of pain and fatigue may affect the number of symptoms that people with cancer experience (Given et al., 2001b).
- More than one-third of people diagnosed with lung cancer report insomnia (Cooley et al., 2003).
- Pain, fatigue, and insomnia are the most common and severe symptoms (Fox & Lyon, 2006; Gift et al., 2004; Hoekstra et al., 2006; Miaskowski et al., 2004; Walsh & Rybicki, 2006).
- Four research teams have highlighted the effects of the concurrence of pain, fatigue and insomnia in people with cancer (Beck et al., 2005; Dodd et al., 2001; Given et al., 2001a; Sarna, 1993a; Sarna, 1993b).

■ WHAT THIS STUDY ADDS

The current, gender based study acknowledged the importance of directing research according to a realistic clinical picture of people with lung cancer and focusing on the most common and severe symptoms of pain, fatigue, and insomnia. If pain, fatigue, and insomnia cluster together and are found to interact differently according to gender, then strategies may be developed and implemented to ameliorate the synergistic effects of the symptoms (Hoffman et al., 2007, p. 786).

■ RESEARCH QUESTIONS

For people within 56 days of starting chemotherapy for a new diagnosis of lung cancer:

1. What are the most frequently occurring symptoms in people with lung cancer, and do they differ between men and women?
2. What are the mean severity scores for pain, fatigue, insomnia, and gender?
3. If a relationship exists among pain, fatigue, insomnia, and gender, do the differences remain statistically significant after controlling for age, comorbidities, and stage of cancer?

Constructing a Study Framework on the Basis of a Conceptual Model

Although the testing of extant nursing models is a critical need within nursing, few published studies have been designed for this purpose. One reason is the level of complexity required for such testing. Because conceptual models cannot be tested directly, a middle-range theory based on the conceptual model must be available (or must be developed as a tentative theory). The framework must include both the conceptual model and the middle-range theory. Thus, the conceptual map for the study must illustrate relationships among the constructs of the model, the concepts of the

middle-range theory, and the link between the concepts and relationships in the model and the concepts and relationships in the middle-range theory. Because of this complexity, in our opinion, master's-level students should not attempt the process unless they are collaborating with doctorally prepared nurses. However, master's-level students will be involved in critiquing published studies with such frameworks and applying them in practice situations.

A framework that includes a conceptual model has the following elements:

- Constructs from the conceptual model
- Definitions of constructs from the conceptual model
- Statements linking the constructs
- Concepts that represent portions of the selected constructs
- Conceptual definitions compatible with construct definitions
- Statements linking the concepts that express a tentative or substantive theory
- Selection of variables that represent portions of the concepts
- Operational definitions of the variables compatible with conceptual definitions
- Statement sets
- A conceptual map linking the constructs, concepts, and variables

In some cases, rather than beginning with the choice of a model, the researcher begins developing the framework by identifying concepts relevant to a particular nursing problem. The researcher identifies or develops a theory related to the phenomenon of interest; simultaneously, or perhaps later, the researcher selects all or a portion of a conceptual model compatible with his or her interests. The important issue is not where the development of the framework begins but rather how logically the various elements of the framework are linked and how complete the end product is.

Whittemore and Roy (2002) have developed a middle-range theory of adapting to diabetes mellitus that is derived from the Roy adaptation model, developed through theory and concept synthesis using relevant empirical evidence. The following excerpt contains their description of the process of developing the theoretical model:

The need exists for research in the care of individuals with DM [diabetes mellitus] to be more theoretically grounded. In an extensive review of the topic of DM patient education interventions between 1985 and

1999, only 6% employed a theoretical framework (Fain et al., 1999). In the absence of theory, existing research is fragmented and while voluminous, difficult to interpret. Clearly there is a need for the development of middle-range theories that encompass key elements of living with DM and holistic nursing practice. Promoting health in chronic illness has been suggested to require an understanding of the person's life context, goals, and values. Innovative research and intervention programs require this prerequisite theory development. (Whittemore & Roy, 2002, p. 311)

The researchers conducted an extensive literature review to identify concepts within the nursing literature that are relevant to chronic illness. They selected Pollock's middle-range theory of chronic illness (1986, 1993), based on Roy's adaptation model (Figure 7-6), because it captured key aspects of adapting to DM. The authors analyzed the theory in terms of its origin, meaning, logical adequacy, usefulness, and testability. Several concepts in the DM literature were identified that had the potential to enhance the understanding of the theory—namely, self-management, integration, and health-within-illness. Analyzing the concepts from the Pollock model and from the literature review provided new insights into adapting to DM. A synthesis of Roy's model, Pollock's chronic illness theory, and findings from existing diabetes research were used to develop a new middle-range theory—adapting to DM.

Definitions of adaptation and health from Roy's model and Pollock's theory were expanded, and assumptions of individual creativity and human potential have been added. These additions are consistent with the relationships and propositions from Roy's model and Pollock's middle-range theory.

Adapting to a chronic illness was defined as encompassing internal and external processes that influence responses and behaviors. A person uses conscious awareness and choice to allow for creative personal and environmental integration (Roy, 1997). The goal in living with a chronic illness becomes one of recognizing the realities imposed by the illness and restructuring self and the environment amid this new experience. Psychosocial factors and perception of the impact of illness are as important as physiological factors in adaptation. (Whittemore & Roy, 2002, p. 312)

The goal of nursing in Pollock's theory and the newly developed theory of adapting to diabetes mellitus, consistent with Roy's model, is to facilitate this adaptation. The conceptual map of the newly developed theory of adapting to diabetes mellitus is shown in Figure 7-7. Examine the progression of ideas expressed in the maps illustrating Roy's conceptual map, Pollock's map, and the map of the new theory.

THE CRITICAL ANALYSIS OF FRAMEWORKS: THEORETICAL SUBSTRUCTION

Hinshaw (1979) developed the initial methods for evaluating study frameworks, using theoretical substruction as a strategy. Dulock and Holzemer (1991) have further refined the process. The term substruction is the opposite of *construction* and means "to take apart." With theoretical substruction, a framework of a published study is separated into component parts to evaluate (1) the logical consistency of the theoretical system and (2) the interaction of the framework with the study methodology. It essentially reverses the process for developing a framework described in this chapter. If components of the framework are inferred rather than clearly stated, the evaluator extracts those components and states them as clearly as possible. If a conceptual map is not presented, the evaluator may construct one.

Theoretical substruction must answer two questions: "Is the framework logically adequate?" and "Did the framework guide the methodology of the study?" Gaps and inconsistencies are identified. The conclusions of the study are evaluated in terms of whether

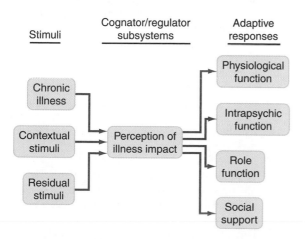

Figure 7-6 Pollock's middle-range theory of chronic illness.

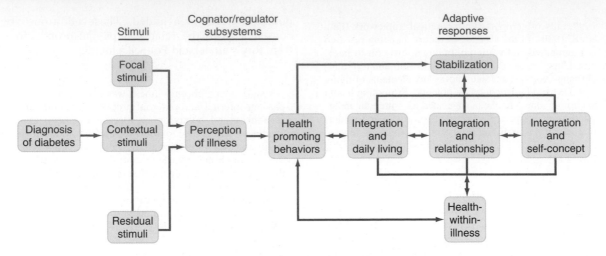

Figure **7-7** Modified theory: adapting to diabetes mellitus.

they are logical, defensible, and congruent with the framework.

To perform theoretical substruction, an evaluator must extract the following elements from the published description of the framework:
- Concepts (and constructs if included)
- Conceptual definitions (and construct definitions if used)
- Operational definitions of concepts
- Conceptual sets linking constructs, concepts, and variables
- General propositions linking the constructs
- Specific propositions linking the concepts
- Hypotheses, research questions, or objectives
- Statement sets linking (a) general propositions, (b) specific propositions, and (c) hypotheses, questions, or objectives
- A conceptual map
- Sampling method and size
- Design
- Data analysis performed in relation to each hypothesis, question, or objective
- Findings related to each hypothesis, question, or objective
- Author's interpretation of findings in relation to the framework

The extracted information is used to analyze the logical structure of the framework and its link with the methodology. The following questions can be used to guide that analysis:

1. Is the framework based on a substantive theory or a tentative theory?
2. Was a conceptual model included in the framework?
3. Are the definitions of constructs consistent with the theorist's definitions?
4. Do the concepts reflect the constructs identified in the framework?
5. Do the variables reflect the concepts identified in the framework?
6. Are the conceptual definitions validated by references to the literature?
7. Do the operational definitions reflect the conceptual definitions?
8. Are the reliability and validity of the operational definitions adequate?
9. Are the propositions logical and defensible?
10. Is evidence from the literature used to validate the propositions?
11. Are the hypotheses, questions, or objectives logically linked to the propositions?
12. Can diagrams of the propositions be linked to the conceptual map?
13. Does the conceptual map adequately explain the phenomenon of concern?
14. Is the design appropriate to test the propositions?
15. Is the sample size adequate to avoid a type II error? (Type II errors are discussed in Chapter 18.)
16. Are the data analyses appropriate for the hypotheses, questions, or objectives?
17. Are the findings for each hypothesis, question, or objective consistent with that proposed by the framework? If not, was the methodology adequate to test the hypothesis, question, or objective?
18. Did the author interpret the findings in terms of the framework?

19. Do the findings validate the framework?
20. Are the findings consistent with those of other studies using the same framework (or testing the same propositions)?

Critical reviews are now being published that examine studies related to selected areas of research. Theoretical substruction is being used to evaluate these studies. One example is Silva's (1986) examination of studies asserting to test nursing models. The use of substruction should strengthen frameworks appearing in published studies. In addition, it will assist the researcher in building a body of knowledge related to a specific theory that can then be applied to clinical practice situations with greater confidence. For further information on critiquing frameworks, see Chapter 26.

SUMMARY

- A framework is the abstract, logical structure of meaning that guides the development of the study and enables the researcher to link the findings to the body of knowledge used in nursing.
- Every study has a framework.
- The framework should be well integrated with the methodology, carefully structured, and clearly presented, whether the study is physiological or psychosocial.
- If a well-established theory is being tested, the framework is derived deductively from the theory.
- A concept is a term that abstractly describes and names an object or a phenomenon, thus providing it with a separate identity or meaning.
- A relational statement declares that a relationship of some kind exists between two or more concepts.
- Relational statements are the core of the framework; it is these statements that are tested through research.
- Developing a framework for a study is one of the most important steps in the research process.
- The steps of the process are (1) selecting and defining concepts, (2) developing statements relating concepts, (3) expressing the statements in hierarchical fashion, and (4) developing a conceptual map.

REFERENCES

Ahrens, S. L. G. (2001). *The development and testing of the Heart Failure Self-Care Inventory: An instrument for measuring heart failure self-care.* Unpublished doctoral dissertation, Wayne State University.

Ailinger, R. L., & Deer, M. R. (1993). Self-care agency in persons with rheumatoid arthritis. *Arthritis Care & Research, 6*(3), 134–140.

Ailinger, R. L., & Deer, M. R. (1997). An examination of the self-care needs of clients with rheumatoid arthritis [including commentary by N. Popovich]. *Rehabilitation Nursing, 22*(3), 135–140.

Ailinger, R. L., Lasus, H., & Braun, M. A. (2003). Revision of the Facts on Osteoporosis Quiz. *Nursing Research, 52*(3), 198–201.

Ailinger, R. L., Moore, J. B., Nguyen, N., & Lasus, H. (2006). Adherence to latent tuberculosis infection therapy among Latino immigrants. *Public Health Nursing, 23*(4): 307–313.

Aish, A. E., & Isenberg, M. (1996). Effects of Orem-based nursing intervention on nutritional self-care of myocardial infarction patients. *International Journal of Nursing Studies, 33*(3), 259–270.

Ajzen, I. (1991). The theory of planned behaviour. *Organizational Behaviour and Human Decision Processes, 50*(2): 179–121.

Ajzen, I., & Fishbein, M. (1980). *Understanding attitudes and predicting social behavior.* Englewood Cliffs, NJ: Prentice-Hall.

Alexander, J. S., Younger, R. E., Cohen, R. M., & Crawford, L. V. (1988). Effectiveness of a nurse-managed program for children with chronic asthma. *Journal of Pediatric Nursing, 3*(5): 312–317.

Amendola, L. R. (1998). *Toward a caring curriculum.* Unpublished doctoral dissertation, University of North Carolina at Greensboro.

Anderberg, P., Lepp, M., Berglund, A. L., & Segesten, K. (2007). Preserving dignity in caring for older adults: A concept analysis. *Journal of Advanced Nursing, 59*(6): 635–643.

Arthur, D., Chong, C., Rujkorakarn, D., Wong, D., & Wongpanarak, N. (2004). A profile of the caring attributes of Hong Kong and Thailand psychiatric nurses. *International Journal of Mental Health Nursing, 13*(2): 100–106.

Arthur, D., Pang, S., & Wong, T. (1998). Caring in context: Caring practices in a sample of Hong Kong nurses. *Contemporary Nurse: A Journal for the Australian Nursing Profession, 7*(4), 198–204.

Arthur, D., Pang, S., Wong, T., Alexander, M. F., Drury, J., Eastwood, et al. (1999). Caring attributes, professional self concept and technological influences in a sample of Registered Nurses in eleven countries. *International Journal of Nursing Studies, 36*(5): 387–396.

Artinian, B. M. (1982). Conceptual mapping: Development of the strategy. *Western Journal of Nursing Research, 4*(4): 379–393.

Artinian, N. T., Magnan, M., Sloan, M., & Lange, M. P. (2002). Self-care behaviors among patients with heart failure. *Heart & Lung, 31*(3): 161–172.

Avant, K. (2000). The Wilson method of concept analysis. In B. L. Rodgers & K. A. Knafl (Eds.), *Concept development in nursing: Foundations, techniques, and applications* (2nd ed., pp. 55–64). Philadelphia: W.B. Saunders.

Baker, L. K. (1991). *Predictors of self-care in adolescents with cystic fibrosis: A test and explication of Orem's theories of self-care and self-care deficit.* Unpublished doctoral dissertation, Wayne State University.

Baker, S. P. (1993). *The relationships of self care agency and self care actions to caregiver strain as perceived by female family caregivers of elderly parents.* Unpublished doctoral dissertation, New York University.

Barnhill, K. O. (2002). *The perception of caring in labor and delivery: A phenomenological study.* Unpublished doctoral dissertation, University of Idaho.

Beatty, E. R. (1991). *Locus-of-control, self-actualization and self-care agency among registered nurses.* Unpublished doctoral dissertation, Columbia University Teachers College.

Beauchesne, M. F. (1989). *An investigation of the relationship between social support and the self care agency of mothers of developmentally disabled children.* Unpublished doctoral dissertation, Boston University.

Beck, S. L., Dudley, W. N., & Barsevick, A. (2005). Pain, sleep disturbance, and fatigue in patients with cancer: Using a mediation model to test a symptom cluster [Online exclusive]. *Oncology Nursing Forum, 32*(3): E48–E55. Retrieved October 20, 2007, from www.ons.org/publications/journals/ONF/Volume32/Issue3/3203542.asp.

Bess, C. J. (1995). *Abilities and limitations of adult type II diabetic patients with integrating of self-care practices into their daily lives.* Unpublished doctoral dissertation, University of Alabama at Birmingham.

Biley, F. C., & Bauer, R. (2005). Bringing the heart back to nursing: human caring practice and education in Germany and the UK. *Theoria Journal of Nursing Theory, 14*(3): 21–25.

Blue, C. L. (1995). The predictive capacity of the theory of reasoned action and the theory of planned behavior in exercise research: An integrated literature review. *Research in Nursing & Health, 18*(2): 105–121.

Bottorff, J. L. (1988). Assessing an instrument in a pilot project: The self-care agency questionnaire. *Canadian Journal of Nursing Research, 20*(1): 7–16.

Brand, J. M. E. (2005). *The lived experiences of six women during adjuvant chemotherapy for stage I or II breast cancer.* Unpublished doctoral dissertation, Ball State University.

Brilowski, G. A., & Wendler, M. C. (2005). An evolutionary concept analysis of caring. *Journal of Advanced Nursing, 50*(6): 641–650.

Broome, M. E. (2000). Integrative literature reviews in the development of concepts. In B. L. Rodgers & K. A. Knafl (Eds.), *Concept development in nursing: Foundations, techniques, and applications* (2nd ed., pp. 231–250). Philadelphia: W.B. Saunders.

Brown, K. L. G. (1996). *Grief as a conditioning factor affecting the self-care agency and self-care of family caregivers of persons with neurotrauma.* Unpublished doctoral dissertation, Wayne State University.

Brunelli, T. (2005). A concept analysis: the grieving process for nurses. *Nursing Forum, 40*(4): 123–128.

Brunton, B., & Beaman, M. (2000). Nurse practitioners' perceptions of their caring behaviors. *Journal of the American Academy of Nurse Practitioners, 12*(11): 451–456.

Buchanan, S., & Ross, E. K. (1995). A concept analysis of caring. *Perspectives: The Journal of the Gerontological Nursing Association, 19*(3): 3–6.

Budo, M. L. D., & Saupe, R. (2005). Ways of care in rural communities: Culture permeating the nursing care [Portuguese]. *Texto & Contexto Enfermagem, 14*(2): 177–185.

Burns, N., & Grove, S. (2007). *Understanding nursing research* (4th ed.). Philadelphia: W.B. Saunders.

Cade, N. V. (2001). Orem's self care deficit theory applied to hypertensive people [Portuguese]. *Revista Latino-Americana de Enfermagem, 9*(3): 43–50.

Callaghan, D. (2005a). Healthy behaviors, self-efficacy, self-care, and basic conditioning factors in older adults. *Journal of Community Health Nursing, 22*(3): 169–178.

Callaghan, D. M. (2005b). The influence of spiritual growth on adolescents' initiative and responsibility for self-care. *Pediatric Nursing, 31*(2): 91–95, 115.

Callaghan, D. (2006a). Basic conditioning factors influences on adolescents' healthy behaviors, self-efficacy, and self-care. *Issues in Comprehensive Pediatric Nursing, 29*(4): 191–204.

Callaghan, D. (2006b). The influence of basic conditioning factors on healthy behaviors, self-efficacy, and self-care in adults. *Journal of Holistic Nursing, 24*(3): 178–185.

Callaghan, D. M. (2003). Health-promoting self-care behaviors, self-care self-efficacy, and self-care agency. *Nursing Science Quarterly, 16*(3): 247–254.

Campbell, J. C., & Soeken, K. L. (1999). Women's responses to battering: A test of the model. *Research in Nursing & Health, 22*(1): 49–58.

Canty, J. L. (1993). *An investigation of life change events, hope and self-care agency in inner city adolescents.* Unpublished doctoral dissertation, University of Miami.

Caron, C. D., & Bowers, B. J. (2000). Methods and application of dimensional analysis: A contribution to concept and knowledge development in nursing. In B. L. Rodgers & K. A. Knafl (Eds.), *Concept development in nursing: Foundations, techniques, and applications* (2nd ed., pp. 285–320). Philadelphia: W.B. Saunders.

Carroll, D. L. (1995). The importance of self-efficacy expectations in elderly patients recovering from coronary artery bypass surgery. *Heart & Lung, 24*(1): 50–59.

Celich, K. L., & Crossetti, Mda. G. (2004). Being with the carer: A dimension of the caring process [Portuguese]. *Revista Gaucha de Enfermagem, 25*(3): 377–385.

Chang, M. C. (2007). Concept analysis of susceptibility [Chinese]. *Chinese Journal of Nursing, 54*(4): 88–93.

Chinn, P. L., & Kramer, M. K. (2007). *Integrated Theory and Knowledge Development in Nursing* (7th ed.). St. Louis: Elsevier.

Choiniere, R., Lafontaine, P., & Edwards, A. C. (2000). Distribution of cardiovascular disease risk factors by socioeconomic status among Canadian adults. *Canadian Medical Association Journal, 162*(9 Suppl): S13–S24.

Christopher, K. A., & Hegedus, K. (2000). Oncology patients' and oncology nurses' perceptions of nurses caring behaviours. *European Journal of Oncology Nursing, 4*(4): 196–206.

Clark, C. S. (2004). *Human caring theory: expansion and explication.* Unpublished doctoral dissertation, California Institute of Integral Studies.

Coates, C. J. (1997). The Caring Efficacy Scale: Nurses' self-reports of caring in practice settings. *Advanced Practice Nursing Quarterly, 3*(1): 53–59.

Coelho, M. J. (2006). Caring gestures in nursing [Portuguese]. *Revista Brasileira de Enfermagem, 59*(6), 745–751.

Coffey, S. (2004). *Development of the concept of covenant between nurse and patient.* Unpublished doctoral dissertation, Catholic University of America.

Coffey, S. (2006). The nurse-patient relationship in cancer care as a shared covenant: A concept analysis. *Advances in Nursing Science, 29*(4): 308–323.

Coffman, M. J. (2004). Cultural caring in nursing practice: A meta-synthesis of qualitative research. *Journal of Cultural Diversity, 11*(3): 100–109.

Cooley, M. E., Short, T. H., & Moriarty, H. J. (2003). Symptom prevalence, distress, and change over time in adults receiving treatment for lung cancer. *Psycho-Oncology, 12*(7): 694–708.

Cortis, J. D., & Kendrick, K. (2003). Nursing ethics, caring and culture. *Nursing Ethics, 10*(1): 77–88.

Cossette, S., Côté, J. K., Pepin, J., Ricard, N., & D'Aoust, L. X. (2006). A dimensional structure of nurse-patient interactions from a caring perspective: Refinement of the Caring Nurse-Patient Interaction Scale (CNPI-Short Scale). *Journal of Advanced Nursing, 55*(2): 198–214.

Cossette, S., Pepin, J., Ricard, N., & Côté, J. (2005). A factorial-dimensional structure of the Caring Nurse-Patient Interaction-Short Scale (CNPI-Short Scale). *International Journal for Human Caring, 9*(2): 31.

Covington, H. (2003). Caring presence: Delineation of a concept for holistic nursing. *Journal of Holistic Nursing, 21*(3): 301–317.

Cowling, W. R., III, & Taliaferro, D. (2004). Emergence of a healing-caring perspective: Contemporary conceptual and theoretical directions. *Journal of Theory Construction & Testing, 8*(2): 54–59.

Cull, V. V. (1995). *Exposure to violence and self-care practices of adolescents.* Unpublished doctoral dissertation, University of Alabama at Birmingham.

Dashiff, C. J. (2003). Self- and dependent-care responsibility of adolescents with IDDM and their parents. *Journal of Family Nursing, 9*(2): 166–183.

Deary, V., Deary, I. J., McKenna, H. P., McCance, T. V., Watson, R., & Hoogbruin, A. L. (2002). Elisions in the field of caring. *Journal of Advanced Nursing, 39*(1): 96–102.

Degner, L. F., & Sloan, J. A. (1995). Symptom distress in newly diagnosed ambulatory cancer patients and as a predictor of survival in lung cancer. *Journal of Pain and Symptom Management, 10*(6): 423–431.

Dellasega, C. (1995). SCOPE: A practical method for assessing the self-care status of elderly persons. *Rehabilitation Nursing Research, 4*(4): 128–135.

Delmar, C. (2006). Caring-ethical phronetic research: epistemological considerations. *International Journal for Human Caring, 10*(1): 22–27.

Denyes, M. J. (1980). *Development of an instrument to measure self-care agency in adolescents.* Unpublished doctoral dissertation, University of Michigan, Ann Arbor.

Denyes, M. J. (1982). Measurement of self-care agency in adolescents [Abstract]. *Nursing Research, 31*(1): 63.

Dodd, M. J. (1984a). Measuring informational intervention for chemotherapy knowledge and self-care behavior. *Research in Nursing & Health, 7*(1): 43–50.

Dodd, M. J. (1984b). Patterns of self-care in cancer patients receiving radiation therapy. *Oncology Nursing Forum, 10*(3): 23–27.

Dodd, M. J. (1987). Efficacy of proactive information on self-care in radiation therapy patients. *Heart & Lung, 16*(5): 538–544.

Dodd, M. J., & Dibble, S. L. (1993). Predictors of self-care: A test of Orem's model. *Oncology Nursing Forum, 20*(6): 895–901.

Dodd, M. J., Larson, P. J., Dibble, S. L., Miaskowski, C., Greenspan, D., MacPhail, L., et al. (1996). Randomized clinical trial of chlorhexidine versus placebo for prevention of oral mucositis in patients receiving chemotherapy. *Oncology Nursing Forum, 23*(6): 921–927.

Dodd, M. J., & Miaskowski, C. (2000). The PRO-SELF program: A self-care intervention program for patients receiving cancer treatment. *Seminars in Oncology Nursing, 16*(4): 300–314.

Dodd, M. J., Miaskowski, C., & Paul, S. M. (2001). Symptom clusters and their effect on the functional status of patients with cancer. *Oncology Nursing Forum, 28*(3): 465–470.

Dowd, T. T. (1994). *Relationship among health state factors, foundational capabilities and urinary incontinence self-care in women.* Unpublished doctoral dissertation, Wayne State University.

Droomers, M., Schrijvers, C. T., van de Mheen, H., & Mackenback, J. P. (1998). Educational differences in leisure-time physical inactivity: a descriptive and explanatory study. *Social Science and Medicine, 47*(11): 1665–1676.

Duffy, J. R. (1990). *An analysis of the relationships among nurse caring behaviors and selected outcomes of care in hospitalized medical and/or surgical patients.* Doctoral Dissertation, Catholic University of America.

Duffy, J. R., & Hoskins, L. M. (2003). The quality-caring model: Blending dual paradigms. *Advances in Nursing Science, 26*(1): 77–88.

Duffy, J. R., Hoskins, L., & Seifert, R. F. (2007). Dimensions of caring: psychometric evaluation of the Caring Assessment Tool. *Advances in Nursing Science, 30*(3), 235–245.

Dulock, H. L., & Holzemer, W. L. (1991). Substruction: Improving the linkage from theory to method. *Nursing Science Quarterly, 4*(2): 83–87.

Easley, R. (2007). Harmony: a concept analysis. *Journal of Advanced Nursing, 59*(5): 551–556.

Eriksson, K. (1992a). Different forms of caring communion. *Nursing Science Quarterly, 5*(2), 93.

Eriksson, K. (1992b). The alleviation of suffering the idea of caring. *Scandinavian Journal of Caring Sciences, 6*(2), 119–123.

Evers, G. C. M., Isenberg, M. A., Philipsen, H., Senten, M., & Brouns, G. (1993). Validity testing of the Dutch translation of the appraisal of the self-care agency A.S.A. scale. *International Journal of Nursing Studies, 30*(4): 331–342.

Fagerström, L., Eriksson, K., & Engberg, I. B. (1998). The patient's perceived caring needs as a message of suffering. *Journal of Advanced Nursing, 28*(5): 978–987.

Fain, J. A., Nettles, A., Funnell, M. M., & Charron, D. (1999). Diabetes patient education research: An integrative literature review. *Diabetes Educator, 25*(6, Suppl.): 7–15.

Fawcett, J. (1999). *The relationship of theory and research.* Norwalk, CT: Appleton-Century-Crofts.

Fealy, G. M. (1995). Professional caring: The moral dimension. *Journal of Advanced Nursing, 22*(6): 1135–1140.

Fialho, A. V. M., Pagliuca, L. M. F., & Soares, E. (2002). The Self-Care Deficit Theory adjustment in home-care in the light of Barnum's model [Portuguese]. *Revista Latino-Americana de Enfermagem, 10*(5): 715–720.

Finfgeld-Connett, D. (2005). Clarification of social support. *Journal of Nursing Scholarship, 37*(1): 4–9.

Finfgeld-Connett, D. (2007). Concept comparison of caring and social support. *International Journal of Nursing Terminologies & Classifications, 18*(2): 58–68.

Fishbein, M. & Ajzen, I. (1975). *Belief, attitude, intention and behavior.* Boston: Addison-Wesley.

Fok, M. S., Alexander, M. F., Wong, T. K., & McFayden, A. K. (2002). Contextualising the Appraisal of Self-Care Agency Scale in Hong Kong. *Contemporary Nurse, 12*(2): 124–134.

Fok, M. S., & Wong, T. K. (2003). Testing Orem's self-care agency and basic conditioning factors in a Chinese community undergoing haemodialysis. *Contemporary Nurse: A Journal for the Australian Nursing Profession, 15*(3): 262–272.

Fok, M. S., & Daly, J. (2003). Clinical Application of Orem's Self-care Model of Nursing in a Chinese Community. In *Advances in Contemporary Transcultural Nursing*: eContent Management Pty Ltd, v.1. 262–272.

Folden, S. L. (1990). *The effect of supportive-educative nursing interventions on poststroke older adults' self-care perceptions*. Unpublished doctoral dissertation, University of Miami.

Folden, S. L. (1993). Effect of a supportive-educative nursing intervention on older adults' perception of self-care after a stroke. *Rehabilitation Nursing, 18*(3): 162–167.

Forbat, L. (2004). The care and abuse of minoritized ethnic groups: the role of statutory services. *Critical Social Policy, 24*(3): 312–331.

Fox, S. W., & Lyon, D. E. (2006). Symptom clusters and quality of life in survivors of lung cancer. *Oncology Nursing Forum, 33*(5): 931–936.

Fredriksson, L. (1999). Modes of relating in a caring conversation: A research synthesis on presence, touch and listening. *Journal of Advanced Nursing, 30*(5): 1167–1176.

Fredriksson, L., & Eriksson, K. (2003). The ethics of the caring conversation. *Nursing Ethics, 10*(2): 138–148.

Freeman, E. M. (1992). *Self-care agency in gay men with HIV infection*. Unpublished doctoral dissertation, University of California, San Francisco.

Frey, M. A., & Denyes, M. J. (1989). Health and illness self-care in adolescents with IDDM: A test of Orem's theory. *Advances in Nursing Science, 12*(1): 67–75.

Frey, M. A., & Fox, M. A. (1990). Assessing and teaching self-care to youths with diabetes mellitus. *Pediatric Nursing, 16*(6): 597–599.

Fridh, I., & Bergbom, I. (2006). To watch: A study of the concept [Norwegian]. *Nordic Journal of Nursing Research & Clinical Studies, 26*(1): 4–8.

Gaffney, K. F., & Moore, J. B. (1996). Testing Orem's theory of self-care deficit: Dependent care agent performance for children. *Nursing Science Quarterly, 9*(4): 160–164.

Gammon, J. (1991). Coping with cancer: The role of self-care. *Nursing Practice, 4*(3): 11–15.

Geden, E., & Taylor, S. (1991). Construct and empirical validity of the Self-as-Carer Inventory. *Nursing Research, 40*(1): 47–50.

Gift, A. G., Jablonski, A., Stommel, M., & Given, C. W. (2004). Symptom clusters in elderly patients with lung cancer. *Oncology Nursing Forum, 31*(2): 202–212.

Gift, A. G., Stommel, M., Jablonski, A., & Given, W. (2003). A cluster of symptoms over time in patients with lung cancer. *Nursing Research, 52*(6): 393–400.

Given, B., Given, C., Azzouz, F., & Stommel, M. (2001a). Physical functioning of elderly cancer patients prior to diagnosis and following initial treatment. *Nursing Research, 50*(4): 222–232.

Given, C. W., Given, B., Azzouz, F., Kozachik, S., & Stommel, M. (2001b). Predictors of pain and fatigue in the year following

diagnosis among elderly cancer patients. *Journal of Pain and Symptom Management, 21*(6): 456–466.

Gomes, M. M. (2007). A concept analysis of relational aggression. *Journal of Psychiatric & Mental Health Nursing, 14*(5): 510–515.

Gramling, K. L. (2004). Ice chips and hope: The coach's story of caring art. *International Journal for Human Caring, 8*(2): 62–64.

Greenfield, P. H. (1989). *A comparison of the self-care ability of employed women who have and have not maintained weight loss*. Unpublished doctoral dissertation, Catholic University of America.

Gregg, M. F., & Magilvy, J. K. (2004). Values in clinical nursing practice and caring. *Japan Journal of Nursing Science, 1*(1): 11–18.

Gulick, E. E. (1987). Parsimony and model confirmation of the ADL self-care scale for multiple sclerosis persons. *Nursing Research, 36*(5): 278–283.

Gulick, E. E. (1988). *The self-administered ADL scale for persons with multiple sclerosis*. In C. Waltz & O. Strickland (Eds.), *The measurement of nursing outcomes* (Vol. 1, pp. 128–159). New York: Springer.

Gulick, E. E. (1989). Model confirmation of the MS-related symptom checklist. *Nursing Research, 38*(3): 147–153.

Haas, D. L. (1990). *The relationship between coping dispositions and power components of dependent-care agency in parents of children with special health care needs*. Unpublished doctoral dissertation, Wayne State University.

Haase, J. E., Leidy, N. K., Coward, T. B., Britt, T., & Penn, P. E. (2000). Simultaneous concept analysis: A strategy for developing multiple interrelated concepts. In B. L. Rodgers & K. A. Knafl (Eds.), *Concept development in nursing: Foundations, techniques, and applications* (2nd ed., pp. 209–230). Philadelphia: W.B. Saunders.

Hagopian, G. A. (1996). The effects of informational audiotapes on knowledge and self-care behaviors of patients undergoing radiation therapy. *Oncology Nursing Forum, 23*(4): 697–700.

Hanson, B. R., & Bickel, L. (1985). Development and testing of the questionnaire on perception of self-care agency. In J. Riehl-Sisca (Ed.), *The science and art of self-care* (pp. 271–278). Norwalk, CT: Appleton-Century-Crofts.

Hanucharurnkul, S. (1989). Predictors of self-care in cancer patients receiving radiotherapy. *Cancer Nursing, 12*(1): 21–27.

Harris, M. A. (2004). *Health-deviation self-care, dependent-care, disclosure, and health of children with perinatal HIV/AIDS*. Unpublished doctoral dissertation, Wayne State University.

Hart, M. A. (1993). *Self-care agency and prenatal care actions: Relationships to pregnancy outcomes*. Unpublished doctoral dissertation, Case Western Reserve University (Health Sciences).

Hart, M. A. (1995). Orem's Self-care Deficit Theory: Research with pregnant women. *Nursing Science Quarterly, 8*(3): 120–126.

Hart, M. A. (1998). Self-care agency before and after childbirth education classes. *International Orem Society Newsletter, 6*(2): 10–11.

Hart, M. A., & Foster, S. N. (1998). Self-care agency in two groups of pregnant women. *Nursing Science Quarterly, 11*(4): 167–171.

Hartley, L. A. (1988). Congruence between teaching and learning self-care: A pilot study. *Nursing Science Quarterly, 1*(4): 161–167.

Hartweg, D. L. (1991). *Health promotion self-care actions of healthy, middle-aged women*. Unpublished doctoral dissertation, Wayne State University.

Hartweg, D. L., & Orem, D. (1991). *Self-care deficit theory*. Newbury Park, CA: Sage.

Helin, K., & Lindström, U. A. (2003). Sacrifice: An ethical dimension of caring that makes suffering meaningful. *Nursing Ethics*, *10*(4): 414–427.

Henderson, A. (2001). Emotional labor and nursing: An underappreciated aspect of caring work. *Nursing Inquiry*, *8*(2): 130–138.

Hinshaw, A. S. (1979). Theoretical substruction: An assessment process. *Western Journal of Nursing Research*, *1*(4): 319–324.

Hoekstra, J., Vernooij-Dassen, M. J., de Vos, R., & Bindels, P. J. (2006). The added value of assessing the "most troublesome" symptom among patients with cancer in the palliative phase. *Patient Education and Counseling*, *65*(2): 223–229.

Hoffman, A. J., Given, B. A., von Eye, A., Gift, A. G., & Given, C. W. (2007). Relationships among pain, fatigue, insomnia, and gender in persons with lung cancer. *Oncology Nursing Forum*, *34*(4): 785–792.

Hopwood, P., & Stephens, R. J. (1995). Symptoms at presentation for treatment in patients with lung cancer: Implications for the evaluation of palliative treatment. The Medical Research Council (MRC) Lung Cancer Working Party. *British Journal of Cancer*, *71*(3): 633–636.

Hsieh, C., Gau, M., Mao, H., & Li, C. (2004). The development and psychometric testing of a self-care scale for dysmenorrhic adolescents. *Journal of Nursing Research*, *12*(2): 119–130.

Hupcey, J. E., & Miller, J. (2006). Community dwelling adults' perception of interpersonal trust vs. trust in health care providers. *Journal of Clinical Nursing*, *15*(9): 1132–1139.

Hurst, C., Montgomery, A. J., Davis, B. L., Killion, C., & Baker, S. (2005). The relationship between social support, self-care agency, and self-care practices of African American women who are HIV-positive. *Journal of Multicultural Nursing & Health*, *11*(3): 11–22.

Hurst, J. D. (1991). *The relationship among self-care agency, risk-taking, and health risks in adolescents*. Unpublished doctoral dissertation, University of Alabama at Birmingham.

Isenberg, M., Evers, G., & Brouns, G. (1987). An international research project to test Orem's self-care deficit theory. In *Proceedings of the International Research Congress*. Edinburgh, Scotland: University of Edinburgh.

James, K. S. (1991). *Factors related to self-care agency and self-care practices of obese adolescents*. Unpublished doctoral dissertation, University of San Diego.

James, W. P., Nelson, M., Ralph, A., & Leather, S. (1997). Socioeconomic determinants of health. The contribution of nutrition to inequalities in health. *British Medical Journal*, *314*(7093): 1545–1549.

Jensen, B. J. (2006). To see with the heart's eye [Danish]. *Sygeplejersken / Danish Journal of Nursing*, *106*(15), 40–43.

Jesek-Hale, S. R. (1994). *Self-care agency and self care in pregnant adolescents: A test of Orem's theory*. Unpublished doctoral dissertation, Rush University, College of Nursing.

Johns, C. (2001). Reflective practice: Revealing the [he]art of caring. *International Journal of Nursing Practice*, *7*(4): 237–245.

Jones, C. B., & Alexander, J. W. (1993). The technology of caring: A synthesis of technology and caring for nursing administration. *Nursing Administration Quarterly*, *17*(2): 11–20.

Joudrey, R., & Gough, J. (1999). Caring and curing revisited: student nurses' perceptions of nurses' and physicians' ethical stances. *Journal of Advanced Nursing*, *29*(5): 1154–1162.

Kamphuis, C. B. M., van Lenthe, F. J., Giskes, K., Brug, J., & Mackenback, J. P. (2007). Perceived environmental determinants of physical activity and fruit and vegetable consumption among high and low socioeconomic groups in the Netherlands. *Health & Place*, *13*(2): 493–503.

Kaplan, G. A., & Lynch, J. W. (1997). Whither studies on the socioeconomic foundations of population health? *American Journal of Public Health*, *87*(9): 1409–1411.

Kearney, B. Y., & Fleischer, B. J. (1979). Development of an instrument to measure exercise of self-care agency. *Research in Nursing & Health*, *2*(1): 25–34.

Kelly, D. (1998). Caring and cancer nursing: Framing the reality using selected social science theory. *Journal of Advanced Nursing*, *28*(4): 728–736.

Kongsaktrakul, C., Suchaxaya, P., Kantawang, S., Schepp, K. G., Visudtibhan, A., & Chinvarun, Y. (2006). A causal model of self-care behavior for adolescents with epilepsy. *Thai Journal of Nursing Research*, *10*(4): 264–275.

Koster, M. K. (1995). *A comparison of the relationship among self-care agency, self-determinism, and absenteeism in two groups of school-age children*. Unpublished doctoral dissertation, University of Texas at Austin.

Kostopoulos, M. R. (1988). The reliability and validity of a nurse performance evaluation tool. In O. L. Strickland & C. F. Waltz (Eds.), *Measurement of nursing outcomes* (Vol. 2, pp. 77–95). New York: Springer.

Kunyk, D., & Olson, J. K. (2001). Clarification of conceptualizations of empathy. *Journal of Advanced Nursing*, *35*(3): 317–325.

Kuo, C. L., Turton, M. A., Lee-Hsieh, J., Tseng, H. F., & Hsu, C. L. (2007). Measuring peer caring behaviors of nursing students: Scale development. *International Journal of Nursing Studies*, *44*(2007): 105–114.

Kurtz, M. E., Kurtz, J. C., Stommel, M., Given, C. W., & Given, B. A. (2000). Symptomatology and loss of physical functioning among geriatric patients with lung cancer. *Journal of Pain and Symptom Management*, *19*(4): 249–256.

Kyle, T. V. (1995). The concept of caring: A review of the literature. *Journal of Advanced Nursing*, *21*(3): 506–514.

Lackey, N. R. (2000). Concept clarification: Using the Norris method in clinical research. In B. L. Rodgers & K. A. Knafl (Eds.), *Concept development in nursing: Foundations, techniques, and applications* (2nd ed., pp. 193–208). Philadelphia: W.B. Saunders.

Lake, P. K. (2004). *Transformation: student nurses' experiences in learning the caring process in nursing*. Unpublished dissertation, University of Texas at Tyler.

Larson, P. J. (1987). Comparison of cancer patients' and professional nurses' perceptions of important caring behaviors. *Heart & Lung*, *16*(2): 187–193.

Lea, A., Watson, R., & Deary, I. J. (1998). Caring in nursing: a multivariate analysis. *Journal of Advanced Nursing*, *28*(3): 662–671.

Lee, M. B. (1999). Power, self-care and health in women living in urban squatter settlements in Karachi, Pakistan: A test of Orem's theory. *Journal of Advanced Nursing, 30*(1): 248–259.

Leh, S. K. (2007). Preconceptions: a concept analysis for nursing. *Nursing Forum, 42*(3): 109–122.

Lenz, E. R., Pugh, L. C., Milligan, R. A., Gift, A., & Suppe, F. (1997). The middle-range theory of unpleasant symptoms: An update. *Advances in Nursing Science, 19*(3): 14–27.

Lewis, S. M. (2003). Practice applications. Caring as being in nursing: Unique or ubiquitous. *Nursing Science Quarterly, 16*(1): 37–43.

Lin, Y., & Chiou, C. (2003). Concept analysis of caring [Chinese]. *Chinese Journal of Nursing, 50*(6): 74–78.

Lindholm, L., Nieminen, A., Mäkelä, C., & Rantanen-Siljamäki, S. (2006). Clinical application research: A Hermeneutical approach to the appropriation of caring science. *Qualitative Health Research, 16*(1): 137–150.

Liu, J. E., Mok, E., & Wong, T. (2006). Caring in nursing: Investigating the meaning of caring from the perspective of cancer patients in Beijing, China. *Journal of Clinical Nursing, 15*(2): 188–196.

Lorensen, M. (1998). Psychometric properties of self-care management and life-quality amongst elderly. *Clinical Effectiveness in Nursing, 2*(2): 78–85.

Lorensen, M., Holter, I., Evers, G., Isenberg, M., & van Achterberg, T. (1993). Cross-cultural testing of the "appraisal of self-care agency": ASA scale in Norway. *International Journal of Nursing Studies, 30*(1): 15–23.

Lorenz, S. G. (2007). Protection: Clarifying the concept for use in nursing practice. *Holistic Nursing Practice, 21*(3): 115–123.

Lucena, Ade. F., & Crossetti, Mda. G. (2004). The meaning of caring in the intensive care unit [Portuguese]. *Revista Gaucha de Enfermagem, 25*(2): 243–256.

Lukkarinen, H., & Hentinen, M. (1997). Self-care agency and factors relating this agency among patients with coronary health disease. *International Journal of Nursing Studies, 34*(4): 295–304.

Maas, M. L., Moorhead, S., Specht, J. P., Schoenfelder, D. P., Swanson, E. A., Johnson, M. L., et al. (2000). Concept development of nursing-sensitive outcomes. In B. L. Rodgers & K. A. Knafl (Eds.), *Concept development in nursing: Foundations, techniques, and applications* (2nd ed., pp. 387–400). Philadelphia: W.B. Saunders.

Mackenbach, J. P., Bos, V., Andersen, O., Cardano, M., Costa, G., Hardin, S., et al. (2003). Widening socioeconomic inequalities in mortality in six Western European countries. *International Journal of Epidemiology, 32*(5): 830–837.

Mapanga, K. G. (1994). *The influence of family and friends' basic conditioning factors, and self-care agency on unmarried teenage primiparas' engagement in a contraceptive practice.* Unpublished doctoral dissertation, Case Western Reserve University (Health Sciences).

Marck, P. (1990). Therapeutic reciprocity: A caring phenomenon. *Advances in Nursing Science, 13*(1): 49–59.

Mattsson-Lidsle, B., & Lindström, U. A. (2001). Consolation: A concept analysis [Swedish]. *Nordic Journal of Nursing Research & Clinical Studies, 21*(3): 47–50.

McBride, S. (1987). Validation of an instrument to measure exercise of self-care agency. *Research in Nursing & Health, 10*(5): 311–316.

McBride, S. H. (1991). Comparative analysis of three instruments designed to measure self-care agency. *Nursing Research, 40*(1): 12–16.

McCaleb, A., & Edgil, A. (1994). Self-concept and self-care practices of healthy adolescents. *Journal of Pediatric Nursing, 9*(4): 233–238.

McCaleb, K. A. (1991). *Self-concept and self-care practices of healthy adolescents.* Unpublished doctoral dissertation, University of Alabama at Birmingham.

McCance, T. V. (2003). Caring in nursing practice: The development of a conceptual framework. *Research & Theory for Nursing Practice, 17*(2): 101–116.

McCance, T. V., McKenna, H. P., & Boore, J. R. (1997). Caring: Dealing with a difficult concept. *International Journal of Nursing Studies, 34*(4): 241–248.

McCance, T. V., McKenna, H. P., & Boore, J. R. (2001). Exploring caring using narrative methodology: An analysis of the approach. *Journal of Advanced Nursing, 33*(3): 350–356.

McDermott, M. A. (1989). *The relationship between learned helplessness and self-care agency in adults as a function of gender and age.* Unpublished doctoral dissertation, New York University.

McIntosh, L. C. (2004). *Nurses' experiences with healing and spirituality.* Unpublished dissertation, University of North Carolina at Greensboro.

Metcalfe, S. A., Metcalfe, S. A. (1996). *Self-care actions as a function of therapeutic self-care demand and self-care agency in individuals with chronic obstructive pulmonary disease.* Unpublished doctoral dissertation, Wayne State University.

Miaskowski, C., Dodd, M., & Lee, K. (2004). Symptom clusters: The new frontier in symptom management research. *Journal of the National Cancer Institute Monographs, 32*: 17–21.

Monsen, R. B. (1988). *Autonomy, coping, and self-care agency in healthy adolescents and in adolescents with spina bifida.* Unpublished doctoral dissertation, University of Alabama at Birmingham.

Monteiro, E. M., da Nobraga, M. M., & de Lima, L. S. (2002). Self-care and the adult with asthma: The systematization of nursing assistance [Portuguese]. *Revista Brasileira de Enfermagem, 55*(2): 134–139.

Moody, L. E. (1989). Building a conceptual map to guide research. *Florida Nursing Review, 4*(1), 1–5.

Moore, J. B. (1993). Predictors of children's self-care performance: Testing the theory of self-care deficit. *Scholarly Inquiry for Nursing Practice: An International Journal, 7*(3): 199–217.

Moore, J. B. (1995). Measuring the self-care practice of children and adolescents: Instrument development. *Maternal-Child Nursing Journal, 23*(3): 101–108.

Moore, J. B., & Gaffney, K. F. (1989). Development of an instrument to measure mother's performance of self-care activities for children. *Advances in Nursing Science, 12*(1): 76–84.

Moore, J. B., & Mosher, R. B. (1997). Adjustment responses of children and their mothers to cancer self-care and anxiety. *Oncology Nursing Forum, 24*(3): 519–525.

Morse, J. (2000). Exploring pragmatic utility: Concept analysis by critically appraising the literature. In B. L. Rodgers & K. A. Knafl (Eds.), *Concept development in nursing: Foundations, techniques, and applications* (2nd ed., pp. 333–352). Philadelphia: W.B. Saunders.

Morse, J. M., Solberg, S. M., Neander, W. L., Bottorff, J. L., & Johnson, J. L. (1990). Concepts of caring and caring as a concept. *Advances in Nursing Science, 13*(1): 1–14.

Mosher, R. B., & Moore, J. B. (1998). The relationship of self-concept and self-care in children with cancer. *Nursing Science Quarterly, 11*(3): 116–122.

Nåden, D., & Saeteren, B. (2006). Cancer patients' perception of being or not being confirmed. *Nursing Ethics, 13*(3): 222–235.

Nahas, V. (1997). Research feature. Muslim patients' perceptions of a caring nurse [Singapore]. *Professional Nurse, 24*(2): 20–23.

Nahcivan, N. O. (2004). A Turkish language equivalence of the exercise of self-care agency scale. *Western Journal of Nursing Research, 26*(7): 813–824.

Ness, A. R., & Powles, J. W. (1997). Fruit and vegetables, and cardiovascular disease: A review. *International Journal of Epidemiology, 26*(1): 1–13.

Newman, M. A. (1979). *Theory development in nursing.* Philadelphia: F.A. Davis.

Newman, M. A. (1999). *Health as expanding consciousness.* Boston: Jones & Bartlett.

Niu, T. (2005). The philosophy of nursing management: A conceptual analysis [Chinese]. *Chinese Journal of Nursing, 52*(5): 5–9.

Noh, C. H., Arthur, D., & Sohng, K. Y. (2002). Relationship between technological influences and caring attributes of Korean nurses. *International Journal of Nursing Practice, 8*(5): 247–256.

Nyberg, J. (1989). *Human care and economics: a nursing study.* Doctoral Dissertation, University of Colorado Health Sciences Center.

O'Berle, K., & Davies, B. (1992). Support and caring: exploring the concepts. *Oncology Nursing Forum, 19*(5): 763–767.

O'Connor, N. A. (1995). *Maieutic dimensions of self-care in aging: Instrument development.* Unpublished doctoral dissertation, Wayne State University.

Orem, D. E. (2001). *Nursing: Concepts of practice* (6th ed.). New York: Mosby.

Page, C., & Ricard, N. (1996). Conceptual and theoretical foundations for an instrument designed to identify self-care requisites in women treated for depression [French]. *Canadian Journal of Nursing Research, 28*(3): 95–112.

Pang, S. M., Wong, T. K., Wang, C. S., Zhang, Z. J., Chan, H. Y., Lam, C. W., et al. (2004). Towards a Chinese definition of nursing. *Journal of Advanced Nursing, 46*(6): 657–670.

Patistea, E. (1999). Nurses' perceptions of caring as documented in theory and research. *Journal of Clinical Nursing, 8*(5): 487.

Pepin, J. I. (1992). Family caring and caring in nursing. *Image: Journal of Nursing Scholarship, 24*(2): 127–131.

Perini, C., Stauffer, Y., Grunder, M., Gandon, M., Datwyler, B., & Hantikainen, V. (2006). The meaning of caring from the viewpoint of patients with wounds due to peripheral vascular disease [German]. *Pflege, 19*(6): 345–355.

Phelan, D. L., Oliveria, S. A., Christos, P. J., Dusza, S. W., & Halpern, A. C. (2003). Skin self-examination in patients at high risk for melanoma: a pilot study. *Oncology Nursing Forum, 30*(6): 1029–1036.

Pipatananond, P., & Hanucharurnkul, S. (2003). Development of the Psychiatric Patient's Caregiver Burden Scale (The PPCBS). *Thai Journal of Nursing Research, 7*(1): 37–48.

Pollock, S. E. (1986). Human response to chronic illness: Physiologic and psychological adaptation. *Nursing Research, 35*(2): 90–95.

Pollock, S. E. (1993). Adaptation to chronic illness: A program of research for testing nursing theory. *Nursing Science Quarterly, 6*(2): 86–92.

Pressly, K. B. (1995). Psychosocial characteristics of CAPD patients and the occurrence of infectious complications. *American Nephrology Nurses' Association Journal, 2*(6): 563–574.

Priest, H. M. (2000). The use of narrative in the study of caring: A critique. *NT Research, 5*(4): 245–252.

Reed, P. (2003). The theory of self-transcendence. In M. Smith & P. Liehr (Eds.), *Middle range theory for nursing.* (pp. 145–165). New York: Springer.

Renker, P. R. (1999). Physical abuse, social support, self-care, and pregnancy outcomes of older adolescents. *JOGNN: Journal of Obstetric, Gynecologic, & Neonatal Nursing, 28*(4): 377–388.

Riesch, S. K., & Hauck, M. R. (1988). The exercise of self-care agency: An analysis of construct and discriminant validity. *Research in Nursing & Health, 11*(4): 245–255.

Riley, C. P. (1988). *Effects of a pulmonary rehabilitation program on dyspnea, self care, and pulmonary function of patients with chronic obstructive pulmonary disease.* Unpublished doctoral dissertation, University of Alabama at Birmingham.

Roberts, K. T., & Fitzgerald, L. (1991). Serenity: caring with perspective. *Scholarly Inquiry for Nursing Practice, 5*(2): 127–146.

Robinson, M. K. (1995). *Determinants of functional status in chronically ill adults.* Unpublished doctoral dissertation, University of Alabama at Birmingham.

Rodgers, B. L. (2000). Concept analysis: An evolutionary view. In B. L. Rodgers & K. A. Knafl (Eds.), *Concept development in nursing: Foundations, techniques, and applications* (2nd ed., pp. 77–102). Philadelphia: W.B. Saunders.

Rodriquez, D. (1999). Medicine or caring science in ancient Greece [Spanish]. *Cultura de los Cuidados, 3*(5), 33–37.

Rogers, B. (2003). Nursing: an ethic of caring. *AAOHN Journal, 51*(4): 155–157.

Rogers, M. (1986). Science of unitary human beings. In V. M. Malinski (Ed.), *Explorations on Martha Rogers' science of unitary human beings* (pp. 3–8). Norwalk, CT: Appleton-Century-Crofts.

Rogers, M. E. (1970). *An introduction to the theoretical basis of nursing.* Philadelphia: F.A. Davis.

Rogers, M. E. (1980). Nursing: A science of unitary man. In J. P. Riehl & C. Roy (Eds.), *Conceptual models for nursing practice* (2nd ed., pp. 329–337). Norwalk, CT: Appleton-Century-Crofts.

Rogers, M. E. (1983). A paradigm for nursing. In I. W. Clements & F. B. Roberts (Eds.), *Family health: A theoretical approach to nursing care* (pp. 219–227). New York: Wiley.

Rogers, M. E. (1988). Nursing science and art: A prospective. *Nursing Science Quarterly, 1*(3): 99–102.

Roper, N. Logan, W., & Tierney, A. (1996). The Roper-Logan-Tierney Model: a model in nursing practice. In P.H. Walker (Ed.), *Blueprint for use of nursing models: education, research, practice, and administration.* National League for Nursing, pp. 289–314.

Roy, C. (1984). *Introduction to nursing: An adaptation model* (2nd ed.). Englewood Cliffs, NJ: Prentice-Hall.

Roy, C. (1988). An explication of the philosophical assumptions of the Roy adaptation model. *Nursing Science Quarterly, 1*(1): 26–34.

Roy, C. (1990). Response to dialogue on a theoretical issue: Strengthening the Roy adaptation model through conceptual clarification. *Nursing Science Quarterly, 3*(2): 64–66.

Roy, C. (1997). Future of the Roy model: Challenge to redefine adaptation. *Nursing Science Quarterly, 10*(1): 42–48.

Roy, C., & Roberts, S. L. (1981). *Theory construction in nursing: An adaptation model.* Englewood Cliffs, NJ: Prentice-Hall.

Sadler, J. (2006). In response to Brilowski, G. A., & Wendler M. (2005). An evolutionary concept analysis of caring. *Journal of Advanced Nursing 50*(6), 641–650.

Sadler, J. J. (2000). A multiphase approach to concept analysis and development. In B. L. Rodgers & K. A. Knafl (Eds.), *Concept development in nursing: Foundations, techniques, and applications* (2nd ed., pp. 251–284). Philadelphia: W.B. Saunders.

Sadler, J. J. (2004). Descriptions of caring uncovered in students' baccalaureate program admission essays. *International Journal for Human Caring, 8*(3): 37–46.

Santos, Z. M., & da Silva, R. M. (2006). Self-care practice lived by hipertensive [sic] woman: Analysis on the health education focus [Portuguese]. *Revista Brasileira de Enfermagem, 59*(2): 206–211.

Sarna, L. (1993a). Correlates of symptom distress in women with lung cancer. *Cancer Practice, 1*(1): 21–28.

Sarna, L. (1993b). Fluctuations in physical function: Adults with non-small cell lung cancer. *Journal of Advanced Nursing, 18*(5): 714–724.

Schantz, M. L. (2007). Compassion: A concept analysis. *Nursing Forum, 42*(2): 48–55.

Schoenhofer, S. O. (2002). Theoretical concerns: Philosophical underpinnings of an emergent methodology for nursing as caring inquiry. *Nursing Science Quarterly, 15*(4): 275–280.

Schott-Baer, D. (1993). Dependent care, caregiver burden, and self-care agency of spouse caregivers. *Cancer Nursing, 16*(3): 230–236.

Schott-Baer, D., Fisher, L., & Gregory, C. (1995). Dependent care, caregiver burden, hardiness and self-care agency of caregivers. *Cancer Nursing, 18*(4): 299–305.

Schumacher, D. L. (2005). *Caring behaviors of preceptors as perceived by new nursing graduate orientees.* Unpublished dissertation, Colorado State University.

Schwartz-Barcott, D., & Kim, H. S. (2000). An expansion and elaboration of the hybrid model of concept development. In B. L. Rodgers & K. A. Knafl (Eds.), *Concept development in nursing: Foundations, techniques, and applications* (2nd ed., pp. 129–160). Philadelphia: W.B. Saunders.

Scott, L. D. (1995). *Correlates of health promotion in elders.* Unpublished doctoral dissertation, Louisiana State University Medical Center in New Orleans School of Nursing.

Scott, P. A. (1995). Care, attention and imaginative identification in nursing practice. *Journal of Advanced Nursing, 21*(6): 1196–1200.

Selye, H. (1976). *The stress of life.* New York: McGraw-Hill.

Sherwood, G. D. (1997). Meta-synthesis of qualitative analyses of caring: Defining a therapeutic model of nursing. *Advanced Practice Nursing Quarterly, 3*(1): 32–42.

da Silva, L. M. (2001). A brief reflection on self-care in hospital discharge planning after a bone marrow transplantation (BMT): A case report [Portuguese]. *Revista Latino-Americana de Enfermagem, 9*(4): 75–82.

Silva, M. C. (1981). Selection of a theoretical framework. In S. D. Krampitz & N. Pavlovich (Eds.), *Readings for nursing research* (pp. 17–28). St. Louis: Mosby.

Silva, M. C. (1986). Research testing nursing theory: State of the art. *Advances in Nursing Science, 9*(1): 1–11.

Simmons, S. J. (1990). *Self-care agency and health-promoting behavior of a military population.* Unpublished doctoral dissertation, Medical College of Georgia.

Slusher, I. L. (1999). Self-care agency and self-care practice of adolescents. *Issues in Comprehensive Pediatric Nursing, 22*(1): 49–58.

Smith, A. (1995). An analysis of altruism: A concept of caring. *Journal of Advanced Nursing, 22*(4): 785–790.

Smith, G. D., & Brunner, E. (1997). Socio-economic differentials in health: The role of nutrition. *Proceedings of the Nutrition Society 56*(1A): 75–90.

Smith, M. C. (1999). Caring and the science of unitary human beings. *Advances in Nursing Science, 21*(4): 14–28.

Smith-Campbell, B. (1999). A case study on expanding the concept of caring from individuals to communities. *Public Health Nursing, 16*(6): 405–411.

Soderhamn, O., & Cliffordson, C. (2001). The internal structure of the Appraisal of Self-care Agency (ASA) scale. *Theoria Journal of Nursing Theory, 10*(4): 5–12.

Söderlund, M. (2003). Qualitative research approaches of relevance for caring sciences [Swedish]. *Nordic Journal of Nursing Research & Clinical Studies, 23*(2): 9–15.

Sourial, S. (1997). An analysis of caring. *Journal of Advanced Nursing, 26*(6): 1189–1192.

Sousa, V. D. (2003). *Testing a conceptual framework for diabetes self-management.* Unpublished doctoral dissertation, Case Western Reserve University (Health Sciences).

Sousa, V. D., & Zauszniewski, J. A. (2005). Toward a theory of diabetes self-care management. *Journal of Theory Construction & Testing, 9*(2): 61–67.

St. Onge, J. L. (1988). *The relationship of self-care agency to health-seeking behaviors in Caucasian and black U.S. veterans.* Unpublished doctoral dissertation, University of South Africa.

Stember, M. L. (1986). Model building as a strategy for theory development. In P. L. Chinn (Ed.), *Nursing research methodology: Issues and implementation* (pp. 103–119). Rockville, MD: Aspen.

Su, Y., Songwathana, P., & Naka, K. (2006). Factor related to self-care among Chinese women with mastectomy in Beijing. *Thai Journal of NursingResearch, 10*(4): 252–263.

Sumner, J. (2006). Concept analysis: the moral construct of caring in nursing as communicative action. *International Journal for Human Caring, 10*(1): 8–16.

Sun, F. K., Long, A., Boore, J., & Tsao, L. I. (2006). Patients and nurses' perceptions of ward environmental factors and support systems in the care of suicidal patients. *Journal of Clinical Nursing, 15*(1), 83–92.

Suppe, F., & Jacox, A. K. (1985). Philosophy of science and the development of nursing theory. In H. H. Werley & J. J. Fitzpatrick (Eds.). *Annual review of nursing research* (Vol. 3, pp. 241–267). New York: Springer.

Swanson, K. M. (1999). Effects of caring, measurement, and time on miscarriage impact and women's well-being. *Nursing Research, 48*(6), 288–298.

Swanson, K. M. (1999). What is known about caring in nursing science: A literary meta-analysis. In A. S. Hinshaw, S. L. Feetham, & J. L. Shaver (Eds.), *Handbook of clinical nursing research,* Thousand Oaks, CA: Sage.

Torres, Gde. V., Davim, R. M., & da Nobrega, M. M. (1999). Application of the nursing process based in Orem's theory: A case study with a pregnant adolescent [Spanish]. *Revista Latino-Americana de Enfermagem, 7*(2): 47–53.

Turkel, M. C., Ray, M. A., & Malinski, V. M. (2001). Research issues. Relational complexity: from grounded theory to instrument development and theoretical testing … synthesis of the research findings from a 5-year program of qualitative and quantitative studies. *Nursing Science Quarterly, 14*(4), 281–287.

U.S. Department of Health and Human Services (US DHHS). (1996). Physical activity and health. A report of the Surgeon General U.S. Department of Health and Human Services, Center for Disease Control and Prevention, National Center for Chronic Disease Prevention and Health Promotion, Atlanta, GA.

van Achterberg, T., Lorensen, M., Isenberg, M. A., Evers, G. C., Levin, E., & Philipsen, H. (1991). The Danish and Dutch version of the Appraisal of Self-care Agency scale, comparing reliability aspects. *Scandinavian Journal of Caring Sciences, 5*(2): 101–108.

Van Duyn, M. A., & Pivonka, E. (2000). Overview of the health benefits of fruit and vegetable consumption for the dietetics professional: Selected literature. *Journal of the American Dietetic Association, 100*(12), 1511–1521.

Van Herten, L. M. (2002). Gezonde levensverwachting naar sociaal-economische status. *TNO Preventie en Gezondheid.*

Van Lenthe, F. M., & Mackenbach, J. P. (2002). Neighbourhood deprivation and overweight: The GLOBE study. *International Journal of Obesity and Related Metabolic Disorders, 26*(2): 234–240.

Vannoy, B. E. (1989). *Relationships among basic conditioning factors, motivational dispositions, and the power element of self-care agency in people beginning a weight loss program.* Unpublished doctoral dissertation, Wayne State University.

Velsor-Friedrich, B., Pigott, T. D., & Louloudes, A. (2004). The effects of a school-based intervention on the self-care and health of African-American inner-city children with asthma. *Journal of Pediatric Nursing, 19*(4): 247–256.

Velsor-Friedrich, B., Pigott, T., & Srof, B. (2005). A practitioner-based asthma intervention program with African American inner-city school children. *Journal of Pediatric Healthcare, 19*(3): 163–171.

Villarruel, A. M. (1995). Mexican-American cultural meanings, expressions, self-care and dependent-care actions associated with experiences of pain. *Research in Nursing & Health, 18*(5): 427–436.

Walker, L. O., & Avant, K. C. (2004). *Strategies for theory construction in nursing* (3rd ed.). Norwalk, CT: Appleton & Lange.

Walsh, D., & Rybicki, L. (2006). Symptom clustering in advanced cancer. *Supportive Care in Cancer, 14*(8): 831–836.

Wang, C. Y. (1997). The cross-cultural applicability of Orem's conceptual framework. *Journal of Cultural Diversity, 4*(2): 44–48.

Wang, C. Y., & Fenske, M. M. (1996). Self-care of adults with non-insulin-dependent diabetes mellitus: Influences of family and friends. *Diabetes Educator, 22*(5): 465–470.

Wang, H. H., & Laffrey, S. C. (2001). A predictive model of well-being and self-care for rural elderly women in Taiwan. *Research in Nursing & Health, 24*(2): 122–132.

Wannamethee, S. G., Shaper, A. G., & Alberti, K. G. (2000). Physical activity, metabolic factors, and the incidence of coronary heart disease and type 2 diabetes. *Archives of Internal Medicine, 160*(14): 2108–2116.

Wannapornsiri, C., Sindhu, S., Phancharoenworakul, K., & Gasemgitvatana, S. (2005). Caring process of Thai women with breast cancer receiving chemotherapy. *Thai Journal of Nursing Research, 9*(2): 121–132.

Watson, R., Deary, I. J., & Hoogbruin, A. L. (2001). A 35-item version of the caring dimensions inventory (CDI-35): Multivariate analysis and application to a longitudinal study involving student nurses. *International Journal of Nursing Studies, 38*(2001): 511–521.

Watson, R., Deary, I. J., & Lea, A. (1999a). A longitudinal study into the perceptions of caring among student nurses using multivariate analysis of the Caring Dimensions Inventory. *Journal of Advanced Nursing, 30*(5): 1080–1089.

Watson, R., Deary, I. J., & Lea, A. (1999b). A longitudinal study into the perceptions of caring and nursing among student nurses. *Journal of Advanced Nursing, 29*(5): 1228–1237.

Watson, R., & Lea, A. (1997). The caring dimensions inventory (CDI): Content validity, reliability and scaling. *Journal of Advanced Nursing, 25*(1): 87–94.

Wattanawech, T., Srimoragot, P., Kasemkitwattana, S., & Kimpee, S. (2003). Influence of selected factors and self-care behavior on abdominal distention in patients with abdominal surgery. *Self-care, Dependent-Care & Nursing, 11*(3): 19–32.

Weaver, M. T. (1987). Perceived self-care agency: A LISREL factor analysis of Bickel and Hanson's questionnaire. *Nursing Research, 36*(6): 381–387.

Weber, N. A. (2000). *Explication of the structure of the secondary concept of women's self-care developed within Orem's self-care deficit theory: Instrumentation, psychometric evaluation and theory-testing.* Unpublished doctoral dissertation, Wayne State University.

Weintraub, F. N., & Hagopian, G. A. (1990). The effect of nursing consultation on anxiety, side effects, and self-care of patients receiving radiation therapy. *Oncology Nursing Forum, 17*(3 Suppl.): 31–36.

White, M. A. M. (2000). *Predictors of self-care agency among community-dwelling older adults.* Unpublished doctoral dissertation, University of Alabama at Birmingham.

Whittemore, R., & Roy, C. (2002). Adapting to diabetes mellitus: A theory synthesis. *Nursing Science Quarterly, 15*(4), 311–317.

Wilde, M. H. (1997). The caring connection in nursing: A concept analysis. *International Journal for Human Caring, 1*(1): 18–24.

Wilde, M. H., & Garvin, S. (2007). A concept analysis of self-monitoring. *Journal of Advanced Nursing, 57*(3): 339–350.

Wilkes, L. M., & Wallis, M. C. (1998). A model of professional nurse caring: Nursing students' experience. *Journal of Advanced Nursing, 27*(3): 582–589.

Wilkinson, J. R. (1998). What it means to care. *Curationis, 21*(2): 2–8.

Willard, G. A. (1990). *Development of an instrument to measure the functional status of hospitalized patients.* Unpublished doctoral dissertation, University of Texas at Austin.

Williams, S. A., & Schreier, A. M. (2004). The effect of education in managing side effects in women receiving chemotherapy for treatment of breast cancer. *Oncology Nursing Forum, 31*(1): E16–E23.

Wilson, F. L., Brown, D. L., & Stephens-Ferris, M. (2006). Can easy-to-read immunization information increase knowledge in urban low-income mothers? *Journal of Pediatric Nursing, 21*(1): 4–12.

Wolf, Z., Giardino, E., Osborne, P., & Ambrose, M. (1994). Dimensions of nurse caring. *Image: Journal of Nursing Scholarship, 26*(2): 107–111.

Wolf, Z. R., Zuzelo, P. R., Costello, R., Cattilico, D., Cooper, K. A., Crothers, R., et al. (2004). Development and testing of the Caring Behaviors Inventory for Elders. *International Journal for Human Caring, 8*(1): 48–54.

Wuest, J. (2000). Concept development situated in the critical paradigm. In B. L. Rodgers & K. A. Knafl (Eds.), *Concept development in nursing: Foundations, techniques, and applications* (2nd ed., pp. 369–387). Philadelphia: W.B. Saunders.

Yonge, O., & Molzahn, A. (2002). Exceptional nontraditional caring practices of nurses. *Scandinavian Journal of Caring Sciences, 16*(4): 399–405.

Zrinyi, M., & Rimar, I. (2005). The effect of nursing intervention on the patient's self-care capability, between hospital admission and release. [Hungarian]. *Nover, 18*(4): 3–11.

Zrinyi, M., & Zekanyne, R. I. (2007). Does self-care agency change between hospital admission and discharge? An Orem-based investigation. *International Nursing Review, 54*(3): 256–262.

CHAPTER **8**

Objectives, Questions, and Hypotheses

Researchers formulate objectives, questions, and hypotheses to bridge the gap between the more abstractly stated research purpose and the detailed plan for data collection and analysis. Objectives, questions, and hypotheses delineate the research variables, the relationships among the variables, and, often, the population to be studied.

Research variables are concepts at various levels of abstraction that are measured, manipulated, or controlled in a study. Concrete concepts, such as temperature, weight, and blood pressure, are referred to as variables in a study; abstract concepts, such as creativity, empathy, and social support, are sometimes referred to as research concepts. Research variables and concepts are conceptually defined, based on the study framework, and are operationally defined to direct their measurement, manipulation, or control in a study.

In this chapter, you will learn how to formulate research objectives, questions, and hypotheses, especially how to test different types of hypotheses through research. The chapter explores ways to select objectives, questions, or hypotheses to direct a study. It concludes with a discussion of variables and suggestions for conceptually and operationally defining variables for a study.

FORMULATING RESEARCH OBJECTIVES

Research objectives are clear, concise, declarative statements that are expressed in the present tense. For clarity, an objective usually focuses on one or two variables (or concepts) and indicates whether the variables are to be identified or described. Objectives can also identify relationships or associations among variables *(relational)*, determine differences between groups or compare groups on selected variables *(differences)*, and predict a dependent variable based on selected independent variables *(prediction)*.

You might use the following formats for developing objectives to guide a study (the type of objective is identified in parentheses):

1. To identify the elements or characteristics of variable *X* in a specified population (Identification)
2. To describe the existence of variable *X* in a specified population (Description)
3. To determine the difference between group 1 and group 2 or to compare groups 1 and 2 on variable *X* in a specified population (Difference)
4. To determine or identify the relationship between variables *X* and *Y* in a specified population (Relational)
5. To determine whether certain independent variables are predictive of a dependent variable (Prediction)

Formulating Objectives in Quantitative Studies

In quantitative research, objectives are developed from the research problem and purpose to clarify the foci of the study, the variables, and population. The following excerpts, from a descriptive study of the education and support needs of younger and older cancer survivors, demonstrate the logical flow from research problem (including the problem significance, background, and statement) and purpose to research objectives (Narsavage & Romeo, 2003).

■ RESEARCH PROBLEM

Cancer rates have continued to rise from the late 1970s to the 1990s, but improved treatments have resulted in increasing rates of survival [problem significance] (Gerlach, Gambosi, & Bowen, 1990).... For decades, regional cancer institutes have designed and implemented programs to educate and provide support to cancer patients and their families. A significant amount of research has focused on the effectiveness of cancer programs in improving knowledge and support but findings are conflicting [problem background] (Narsavage & Romeo, 2003, p. 103).

Cancer has been the second leading cause of death in Northeastern Pennsylvania (NEPA), an area with a large elderly population [problem significance] (Pennsylvania Department of Health, 1998). The Northeast Regional Cancer Institute (NRCI), a nonprofit cooperative network of six hospitals in NEPA, provided educational and support programs designed to help cancer patients and their families survive and manage their illness with improved quality of life [problem background].... As the number of survivors increased and program funding became increasingly limited, there was a need to target programs to the population served. Anecdotal accounts from cancer survivors in NEPA suggested that education and support services were limited [problem statement]. (Narsavage & Romeo, 2003, pp. 104–105)

■ RESEARCH PURPOSE

"To address these concerns, this study examined the use, satisfaction with, and need for cancer education and support services in Northeastern Pennsylvania" by younger and older cancer survivors. (Narsavage & Romeo, 2003, p. 103)

■ RESEARCH OBJECTIVES

"The study was designed to (1) identify what education and support services were being used, (2) measure satisfaction with current programs and services, and (3) identify what future programs and services were desired." (Narsavage & Romeo, 2003, p.105)

In this example, the problem provides a basis for the purpose, and the objectives evolve from the purpose and clearly indicate the foci or goals of the study. The first objective was *identification* of the variables education and support services used by younger and older cancer survivors (population) in Northeastern Pennsylvania (setting). The second objective was *description* of the survivors' satisfaction (variable) with the current programs and services. The third objective was *identification* of the variables future programs and services that are needed in Northeastern Pennsylvania. The findings from this study identified the need for new types of education and support services, such as weekly radio talk shows and online Internet chat rooms for cancer survivors. In addition, future programs can be improved by tailoring them to the age of the cancer survivor. (Narsavage & Romeo, 2003)

Formulating Objectives in Qualitative Studies

The research objectives formulated for quantitative and qualitative studies have many similarities. However, the objectives directing qualitative studies commonly have a broader focus and include variables or concepts that are more complex and abstract than those of quantitative studies (Munhall, 2001). An ethnographic study by Happ, Swigart, Tate, Hoffman, and Arnold (2007) included objectives to direct their investigation of patients' involvement in health-related decisions during prolonged critical illness.

■ RESEARCH PROBLEM

Clinicians increasingly recognize the need to involve patients in decision making before, and, if possible, during prolonged critical illness, but have little guidance as to how and when to do this most effectively [problem significance].... Prior reports of studies containing the number of patients able to communicate treatment preferences or to participate in decisions during an acute or critical illness vary from none to as high as 48%.... Moreover, few reports of studies of treatment decision making indicate the criteria used to make decisional capacity assessments [problem background].... Consequently, empirical knowledge of practice in this important area of patient care is limited [problem statement]. (Happ et al., 2007, pp. 361–362)

■ RESEARCH PURPOSE

The purpose of this study was to "describe patterns of communication of patients involved in health-related decision making during prolonged mechanical ventilation (PMV)." (Happ et al., 2007, p. 362)

■ RESEARCH OBJECTIVES

The objectives of this study were to "describe: (a) characteristics of patients who were involved in health-related decisions; (b) types of health-related decisions made with patient involvement; (c) how patient involvement occurred; and (d) the extent of patient involvement with health-related decisions during PMV." (Happ et al., 2007, p. 361)

In this ethnographic study, the problem statement indicated that inadequate research had been conducted on patient involvement in health-related decisions during critical illness, which provided a basis for the study purpose. All four objectives focused on detailed *descriptions* of the study variables: (1) characteristics of the patients, (2) health-related decision making, and (3) patient involvement in a population of patients on prolonged mechanical ventilation. The findings from this study indicated that families, advanced practice nurses, and physicians were engaging critically ill patients in decision making whenever possible. However, most of the time the patients could not make independent decisions but were able to share decision making with their families and clinicians. These findings emphasize how important it is for families and clinicians to include critically ill patients in health-related decisions at whatever level possible. (Happ et al., 2007)

FORMULATING RESEARCH QUESTIONS

A research question is a concise, interrogative statement that is worded in the present tense and includes one or more variables (or concepts). The research questions focus on (1) the *description* of the variable(s), (2) a determination of *differences* between two or more groups regarding selected variables, (3) an examination of relationships among variables (*relational*), and (4) the use of independent variables to *predict* a dependent variable.

You might use the following formats for research questions developed for a study (the focus for each is shown in parentheses):

1. How is variable X described by a specified population? (Description)
2. Is there a difference between groups 1 and 2 regarding variable X? (Difference)
3. What is the relationship between variables X and Y in a specified population? (Relational)
4. Are independent variables W, X, and Y useful in predicting dependent variable Z? (Prediction)

Formulating Questions in Quantitative Studies

Cox, Teasley, Lacey, Carroll, and Sexton (2007) conducted a comparative descriptive study to examine environment perceptions of professional nurses working in pediatric and nonpediatric settings. The following excerpts from this study demonstrate the flow from research problem and purpose to research questions.

■ *RESEARCH PROBLEM*

The professional practice of nursing within the pediatric environment can be both rewarding and challenging.... Although recruitment and retention may be less of a problem in some pediatric hospitals, ensuring a high-quality work environment of pediatric nurses continues to be a priority for nursing leadership [problem significance]. Efforts by multiple researchers have indicated that job satisfaction can be influenced by group cohesion, nurse-physician collaboration, nursing leadership behavior, job stress, pay, time to do nursing interventions in compliance with best practices, and confidence in one's

ability.... (Ernst et al., 2004) [problem background]... Although these preliminary investigations are important, such findings do not elucidate whether pediatric nurses are more or less satisfied than nurses working within nonpediatric environments.... This study will help fill the gaps in the literature related to the differences in support between nurses who work in pediatric facilities and those who work in general acute care sites [problem statement]. (Cox et al., 2007, pp. 9–10)

■ *RESEARCH PURPOSE*

The purpose of this study was to determine "whether pediatric nurse perceptions of the work environment differed (1) from nurses employed in nonpediatric settings, (2) by the type of pediatric practice setting, or (3) by year of birth." (Cox et al., 2007, p. 9)

■ *RESEARCH QUESTIONS*

The following three research questions were addressed in this study.

1. Are there significant differences in perceptions of support (manager, unit, or peer), intent to stay, workload, and satisfaction between staff nurses who work in pediatric facilities and those who work in general acute care settings?
2. When looking at pediatric nursing alone, do nurses working in one clinical service area have better or worse work environment than nurses working in another?
3. Do pediatric nurses of different ages have different perceptions of the work environment? (Cox et al., 2007, p. 10)

Question 1 focused on examining *differences* in work environment perceptions between nurses in pediatric and nonpediatric settings. Questions 2 and 3 focused on examining *differences* among pediatric nurses based on type of setting and age. All of these questions include variables that were *described* in the study. The results of this comparative descriptive study indicate that "pediatric nurses had more positive perceptions of unit support, workload, and overall nurse satisfaction than their colleagues working in nonpediatric facilities. Specific to pediatrics, younger nurses and those working in critical care settings seemed to be the happiest with their work environment" (Cox et al., 2007, p. 9). The evidence from this study can help nurse managers to retain nurses in pediatric settings.

Formulating Questions in Qualitative Studies

The questions directing qualitative studies are often limited in number, have a broad focus, and include variables or concepts that are more complex and abstract than those included in quantitative studies. Marshall and Rossman (2006) have indicated that questions developed to direct qualitative research might be theoretical ones, which can be studied with different populations or in a variety of sites or the questions could be focused on a particular population or setting. Polzer (2007) conducted a qualitative study to describe African Americans with type 2 diabetes. The goal was to examine the participants' perceptions of the spiritual role of health care providers (HCPs) and its effects on how the participants managed their diabetes. The problem, purpose, and research questions used to direct this study are presented in the following excerpts.

■ *RESEARCH PROBLEM*

The establishment of quality patient/provider relationships is paramount in empowering patients to manage chronic illnesses.... Type 2 diabetes mellitus is a major health problem for African Americans, and is one of the primary causes of morbidity and mortality in this population (Center for Disease Control [CDC], 2005) [problem significance].... For many African Americans, spirituality is a source of support in managing diabetes.... Some, however, may also turn their self-management practices over to God in lieu of following health provider recommendations... In a recent grounded theory study (Polzer & Miles, 2007; parent study),... examined how spirituality affected self-management of diabetes in African Americans. The core construct identified in this study was self-management through a relationship with God. Based on their views, participates fell into one of three typologies: Relationship and Responsibility: God is in the Background; Relationship and Responsibility: God is in the Forefront; and Relationship and Relinquishing of Self-Management: God is Healer.... The three typologies shed light on how African Americans viewed their relationship with God, its impact on self-management, and how these perceptions affected their beliefs about HCPs helping them manage their diabetes [problem background]. Knowledge of these perceptions of spiritual care is important as there is little information related to spiritual interventions for African Americans [problem statement]. (Polzer, 2007, pp. 164–166)

■ *RESEARCH PURPOSE*

Based on the grounded theory study [Polzer & Miles, 2007], a qualitative descriptive study was conducted to examine these perceptions of spiritual care, and further extend the three typologies. (Polzer, 2007, p. 166)

■ *RESEARCH QUESTIONS*

The research questions addressed in this analysis were:
1. What are the perceptions of African Americans with diabetes regarding how, if, and when nurses and other HCPs should address spirituality in their care?
2. How do these perceptions differ by typology of self-management through a relationship with God? (Polzer, 2007, p. 166)

The first study question focused on developing a *description* of African Americans' (population) perceptions of the complex concept of health care providers addressing spirituality in their care. The second question focused on examining *differences* in the African Americans' perceptions based on their relationship with God. Based on her study findings, Polzer (2007) identified the following implications for practice: "The model of the three typologies may help health providers understand the importance of spiritual care for some African Americans, as well as how this care can affect self-management. This information also may assist in developing culturally sensitive interventions to improve self-management of diabetes among African Americans." (p. 173)

FORMULATING HYPOTHESES

A hypothesis is the formal statement of the expected relationship or relationships between two or more variables in a specified population. The hypothesis translates the problem and purpose into a clear explanation or prediction of the expected results or outcomes of the study. This section describes the purpose, sources, and types of hypotheses and the process for developing and testing hypotheses in studies.

Purpose of Hypotheses

The purpose of a hypothesis is similar to that of research objectives and questions. A hypothesis (1) specifies the variables you will manipulate or measure, (2) identifies the population you will examine, (3) indicates the type of research, and (4) directs the conduct of your study. Hypotheses also influence the study design, sampling technique, data collection and analysis methods, and interpretation of findings. Hypotheses differ from objectives and questions by predicting the outcomes of a study, and the research findings indicate support for or rejection of each hypothesis.

Hypothesis testing allows us to generate knowledge by testing theoretical statements or relationships that were identified in previous research, proposed by theorists, or observed in practice. In addition, hypotheses direct the testing of new treatments and are often viewed as tools for uncovering ideas rather than as ends in themselves (Beveridge, 1950).

Sources of Hypotheses

We generate hypotheses by observing phenomena or problems in nursing practice, analyzing theory, and reviewing the literature. Many hypotheses originate from real-life experiences. Clinicians and researchers observe events in the world and identify relationships among these events (theorizing), which are the bases for formulating hypotheses. For example, you may notice that the hospitalized patient who complains the most receives the most pain medicine. The relationship identified is a prediction about events in clinical practice that has potential for empirical testing. You could use a literature review to identify a theory that supports this relationship.

Fagerhaugh and Strauss (1977) developed a theory of pain management and identified the following relationship or proposition: As expressions of pain increase, pain management increases. The researchers developed this proposition through the use of grounded theory research. Additional testing is necessary to determine its usefulness in describing how patients express pain and how that pain is managed

in a variety of practice situations. On the basis of theory and clinical observation, the following hypothesis might be formulated: The more frequently a hospitalized patient complains of pain, the more often doses of analgesic medications are administered.

Some hypotheses are initially generated from relationships expressed in a theory, when the intent of the researcher is to test a theory (Chinn & Kramer, 2008). When a theory is being tested, the propositions (relationships) expressed in the theory are used to generate hypotheses. For example, Jennings-Dozier (1999) tested the theory of planned behavior (TPB) in predicting the intentions of African-American and Latina women to obtain a Pap smear. Figure 8-1 illustrates a model of the TPB developed by Ajzen (1985). This model includes direct and indirect relationships among the concepts, as indicated in the following propositions. These propositions provided the basis for the study hypotheses generated by Jennings-Dozier (1999):

1. External variables (age, education, income, and acculturation) have a direct effect on behavioral beliefs, normative beliefs, and control beliefs.
2. Behavioral beliefs have a direct effect on attitude; normative beliefs have a direct effect on

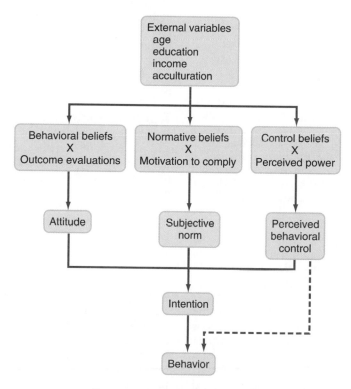

Figure 8-1 The theory of planned behavior.

subjective norm; and control beliefs have a direct effect on perceived behavioral control.

3. Attitude, subjective norm, and perceived behavioral control have a direct effect on intention.
4. Intention has a direct effect on behavior.
5. External variables have an indirect effect on attitude, subjective norm, and perceived control.
6. External variables have an indirect effect on intention.
7. Behavioral beliefs, normative beliefs, and control beliefs have an indirect effect on intention.

Jennings-Dozier's (1999) first hypothesis was as follows:

> Belief-based measures of attitude, subjective norm, and perceived behavioral control would have (a) an indirect effect on intention to obtain a Pap smear and (b) a direct effect on the direct measures of attitude, subjective norm, and perceived behavior control, respectively, which in turn would have (c) direct effects on the intention of African American and Latina women to obtain a Pap smear. (p. 199)

The seven propositions from the TPB, listed previously, can be linked to this study hypothesis in the following way:

Part (a) of the hypothesis tests proposition 7.
Part (b) of the hypothesis tests proposition 2.
Part (c) of the hypothesis tests proposition 3.

Jennings-Dozier's (1999) second hypothesis was as follows.

> External variables (age, level of education, level of income, and level of acculturation for Latinas) would have (a) a direct effect on the belief-based measures of attitude, subjective norm, and perceived behavioral control; (b) an indirect effect on the direct measures of attitude, subjective norms, and perceived behavioral control; and (c) an indirect effect on the intention of African American and Latina women to obtain a Pap smear. (pp. 199–200)

The seven propositions from TPB can be linked to the second study hypothesis in the following way:

Part (a) of the hypothesis tests proposition 1.
Part (b) of the hypothesis tests proposition 5.
Part (c) of the hypothesis tests proposition 6.

These hypotheses were formulated to test the propositions from Ajzen's theory of planned behavior (TPB). The study findings indicated that attitude and perceived behavior control were predictors of a patient's intentions to obtain a Pap smear but that the subjective norms were not. Thus, the study supported some of the relationships in the TPB but not others (Jennings-Dozier, 1999). Further research is needed to determine the effectiveness of the TPB to explain the intentions of women of varying ages, cultures, and socioeconomic level to obtain a Pap smear. The evidence generated from these types of studies could be used to develop and test interventions to encourage and support women in getting Pap smears.

Reviewing the literature and synthesizing findings from different studies can also be used to generate hypotheses. For example, Anderson, Higgins, and Rozmus (1999) synthesized the findings from several studies focused on the outcomes of coronary artery bypass graft (CABG) surgery and formulated the following hypotheses to direct their study:

> 1. CABG patients who stay 1 day in ICU [intensive care unit] begin ambulation in an inpatient cardiac rehabilitation program earlier than patients who stay 2 days in ICU.
> 2. CABG patients who stay 1 day in ICU have a shorter postoperative hospitalization than patients who stay 2 days in ICU. (Anderson et al., 1999, p. 169)

The results of this study supported the first hypothesis because patients who stayed 1 day in the ICU had significantly earlier ambulation than those staying 2 days in the ICU. The researchers rejected the second hypothesis because there was no significant difference in postoperative length of stay between patients who stayed 1 day and those who stayed 2 days in the ICU. These mixed findings indicate the need for this study to be replicated and for further research in this problem area.

Types of Hypotheses

Hypotheses identify different types of relationships and numbers of variables. Studies might have one, three, or more hypotheses, depending on the complexity and scope of the study. The type of hypothesis you develop will be based on the problem and purpose of your study. Hypotheses are described using the terms in the following four categories: (1) associative versus causal, (2) simple versus complex, (3) directional versus nondirectional, and (4) null versus research.

Associative versus Causal Hypotheses

The relationships in hypotheses are identified as associative or causal. An **associative relationship** identifies variables that occur or exist together in practice, and as one variable changes so does the other (Reynolds, 1971). For example, research indicates there is an associative relationship between anxiety and depression, and as a person's depression changes so does the anxiety level. Thus, **associative hypotheses** are developed to examine relationships among variables in a study. The format used for expressing associative hypotheses follows:

1. Variable *X* is related to or associated with variable *Y* in a specified population. (Predicts a relationship between two variables but does not indicate the type of relationship.)
2. An increase in variable *X* is related to an increase in variable *Y* in a specified population. (Predicts a positive relationship.)
3. A decrease in variable *X* is related to a decrease in variable *Y* in a specified population. (Predicts a positive relationship.)
4. An increase in variable *X* is related to a decrease in variable *Y* in a specified population. (Predicts a negative or inverse relationship.)
5. Variables *X* and *Y* can be used to predict variable *Z* in a study. (The independent variables of *X* and *Y* are used to predict the dependent variable *Z* in a predictive correlational study.)

Associative hypotheses identify relationships among variables in a study but do not indicate that one variable causes an effect on another variable.

Reishtein (2005) conducted a predictive correlational study to examine the relationships between symptoms and functional performance in patients with chronic obstructed pulmonary disease (COPD). Reishtein used the following associative hypotheses to guide the study:

1. Positive relationships exist among dyspnea, fatigue, and sleep difficulty in people with COPD;

2. Dyspnea, fatigue, and sleep difficulty are related to functional performance; and

3. Dyspnea, fatigue, and sleep difficulty, taken together, will explain more of the variance in functional performance in people with COPD than any of these symptoms alone. (Reishtein, 2005, p. 40)

Hypothesis 1 predicts positive relationships or associations among the variables of dyspnea, fatigue, and sleep difficulty for patients with COPD. A positive relationship means that the variables change together; thus, they will all increase together in value or all decrease together. These relationships are depicted in the following diagram:

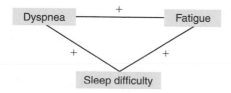

Hypothesis 2 predicts relationships between three variables—dyspnea, fatigue, and sleep difficulty—and the variable functional performance, but it does not identify the type of relationship. These relationships are shown in the following diagram:

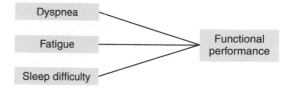

Hypothesis 3 uses the independent variables of dyspnea, fatigue, and sleep difficulty to predict the dependent or outcome variable functional performance in COPD patients. The predictive relationship is shown in the following diagram:

Dyspnea + Fatigue + Sleep difficulty ⟶ Functional performance

The results from Reishtein's (2005) study partially supported hypothesis 1 in that dyspnea had positive, significant relationships with fatigue ($r = 0.43$, $p < 0.001$) and sleep difficulty ($r = 0.39$, $p < 0.001$), but fatigue and sleep difficulty were positively but not significantly related ($r = 0.19$). Hypothesis 2 was also partially supported in that dyspnea ($r = -0.54$, $p < 0.001$) and fatigue ($r = -0.24$, $p < 0.01$) were significantly, negatively related to functional performance, but sleep difficulty ($r = -0.17$) was not. Thus, in hypothesis 3, dyspnea was the most predictive of functional performance with fatigue and sleep difficulty providing limited prediction. Thus, managing dyspnea may be the best way to improve the symptoms and functional performance in patients with COPD. Additional research may distinguish other symptoms that might predict functional performance in COPD patients and thereby help them to manage this disease.

Causal relationships identify a cause-and-effect interaction between two or more variables, which are referred to as independent and dependent variables. The **independent variable** (intervention, treatment, or experimental variable) is manipulated or varied by the researcher to cause an effect on the dependent variable. The **dependent variable** (response or outcome variable) is measured to examine the effect created by the independent variable. A format for stating a causal hypothesis is as follows: The subjects in the experimental group who are exposed to the independent variable *X* demonstrate greater change, dependent variable *Y*, than do the subjects in the control or comparison group who are not exposed to the independent variable.

Artinian, Washington, and Templin (2001, p. 191) studied the "effects of the home telemonitoring and community-based monitoring on blood pressure control in urban African Americans." The following causal hypothesis was used to direct their study:

> Persons who participate in nurse-managed home telemonitoring (HT) plus usual care or who participate in nurse-managed community-based monitoring (CBM) plus usual care will have greater improvement in blood pressure (BP) from baseline to 3 months' follow-up than will persons who receive usual care only. (Artinian et al., 2001, p. 191)

The independent variables are the two types of nurse-managed BP monitoring, HT and CBM, and the dependent variable is BP (systolic and diastolic pressures). The population is clearly identified as African Americans with hypertension, who were recruited from a family community center in Detroit (setting). The findings from this study supported the hypothesis, indicating that the two monitoring interventions, HT and CBM, were significantly more effective than usual care in improving BP (systolic and diastolic pressures) in hypertensive African Americans. A causal arrow (→) is used to show the hypothesized relationships among the independent and dependent variables in the following diagram:

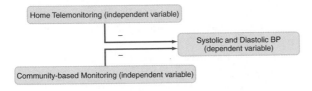

Simple versus Complex Hypotheses

A simple hypothesis predicts the relationship (associative or causal) between two variables. One format for stating a simple associative hypothesis is as follows: Variable X is related to variable Y. A simple causal hypothesis identifies the relationship between one independent variable and one dependent variable, for example, independent variable X causes a change in dependent variable Y. Vasan et al. (2003) studied the relationship of elevated plasma homocysteine levels with the risk for congestive heart failure (CHF) in adults without prior myocardial infarction (MI). A simple, associative hypothesis was developed to direct this study: "We hypothesized that elevated plasma homocysteine levels are associated with an increased risk for CHF" (Vasan et al., 2003, p. 1251). The following diagram demonstrates the positive relationship that was predicted between the two study variables of plasma homocysteine level and risk for CHF:

↑ Plasma Homocysteine Levels —————— $^+$ ↑ Risk for CHF

The results of this 8-year study indicated that elevated plasma homocysteine concentration was related positively and strongly to CHF risk in both men and women who did not have a prior history of an MI. The hypothesis was supported in this study, indicating that nurse practitioners and clinical nurse specialists might examine plasma homocysteine levels in individuals with a family history of CHF and treat those levels as needed.

A complex hypothesis predicts the relationship (associative or causal) among three or more variables. A complex associative hypothesis predicts the relationships among three or more variables, such as the relationships among the variables X, Y, and Z. Complex causal hypotheses also include three or more variables but predict the effects of one independent variable on two (or more) dependent variables or predicting the effects of two or more independent variables on one or more dependent variables. For example, Rawl et al. (2002) studied the effects of a computer-based nursing intervention on the psychological functioning of newly diagnosed cancer patients. The following complex, causal hypothesis was developed to direct their study: "Patients with cancer who received the intervention were hypothesized to have higher psychological functioning scores and lower depression and anxiety scores than those receiving standard care" (Rawl et al., 2002, p. 968).

This causal hypothesis has one independent variable (computer-based nursing intervention) and three dependent variables (psychological functioning, depression, and anxiety scores) and identifies the population of the study (cancer patients). A diagram of this hypothesis follows, with causal arrows (→) indicating the cause-and-effect relationship between the independent variable (IV) and dependent variables (DVs):

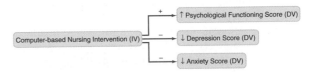

The findings from this study support part of this hypothesis, because the cancer patients exposed to the computer-based nursing intervention had significantly lower depression and anxiety scores but did not have a significant improvement in the psychological functioning score when compared to those subjects receiving standard care. This intervention offers potential benefits for nursing practice, but it requires additional investigation to determine its effectiveness in managing the emotional needs of cancer patients. Often, in practice situations, multiple variables cause an event, or an intervention results in multiple outcomes. Therefore, complex rather than simple causal hypotheses are often more representative of nursing practice.

Nondirectional versus Directional Hypotheses

A nondirectional hypothesis states that a relationship exists but does not predict the nature of the relationship. If the direction of the relationship being studied is not clear in clinical practice or the theoretical or empirical literature, the researcher has no clear indication of the nature of the relationship and states a nondirectional hypothesis. For example, Reishtein's (2005, p. 4) second hypothesis (introduced earlier in this chapter) is nondirectional: "Dyspnea, fatigue, and sleep difficulty are related to functional performance." This hypothesis indicates that dyspnea, fatigue, and sleep difficulty are related to functional performance, but it does not indicate the direction or nature (positive or negative) of the relationship. This hypothesis is nondirectional, complex (four variables), and associative (indicating a relationship exists).

A directional hypothesis states the nature or direction of the relationship between two or more variables. These hypotheses are developed from theoretical statements, findings of previous studies, and clinical experience. As the knowledge on which a study is based increases, the researcher is able to predict the direction of a relationship between the variables being studied. Terms such as *less, more, increase, decrease, greater,* and *smaller* indicate the directions of relationships in hypotheses. Directional hypotheses can be associative or causal and simple or complex.

McDonald, Frakes, Apostolidis, Armstrong, Goldblatt, and Bernardo (2003, p. 226) hypothesized that nurses providing care for patients with a psychiatric diagnosis "(a) estimate a lower probability that the patient was experiencing a myocardial infraction, (b) plan less time for nursing care, (c) delegate more patient care activities to ancillary staff, and (d) do not identify additional ambiguous symptoms as possible evidence of an evolving myocardial infarction." This complex, associative, directional hypothesis was supported by the findings, indicating that nurses provided lower quality of care for acute medical conditions when the patients had a psychiatric diagnosis than when they did not. Evidence from this study indicates that patients with a psychiatric diagnosis are vulnerable when experiencing acute medical problems. It is important for nurses to avoid stereotyping patients

with psychiatric diagnoses and to focus on identifying and managing the patient's medical problem.

A causal hypothesis predicts the effect of an independent variable on a dependent variable, specifying the direction of the relationship. Thus, all causal hypotheses are directional. Efe and Özer (2007) examined the pain-relieving effect of breast-feeding during immunization injections in healthy neonates and used a causal hypothesis to direct their study. "The hypothesis tested was that breast-feeding would decrease the length of crying time, prevent an increase in heart rate, and prevent a decrease in oxygen saturation during vaccination as compared with the control condition (i.e., no breast-feeding)" (Efe & Özer, 2007, p. 11). This causal hypothesis predicted the effect of an intervention or independent variable of breast-feeding during immunization injections on the dependent variables of length of crying time, heart rate, and oxygen saturation. Thus, this is a complex (four variables), directional (decrease crying time and prevent increased heart rate and decreased oxygen saturation), causal hypothesis. The breast-feeding significantly decreased crying time but did not significantly affect the neonates' heart rate or oxygen saturation. Because breast-feeding did decrease neonate crying time during immunizations, nurses might encourage mothers to implement this safe, easy, effective intervention.

Null versus Research Hypotheses

The null hypothesis (H_0), also referred to as a statistical hypothesis, is used for statistical testing and interpretation of statistical outcomes. Even if the null hypothesis is not stated, it is implied, because it is the converse of the research hypothesis (Kerlinger & Lee, 2000). A null hypothesis can be simple or complex and associative or causal. An associative null hypothesis states that there is no relationship between the variables studied. A causal null hypothesis might be stated in one of the following formats:

1. The independent variable has no effect on the dependent variable.
2. The experimental group, who received the independent variable, is no different than the control group for the dependent variable.

Schultz, Drew, and Hewitt (2002) conducted a quasi-experimental study to determine the effectiveness of heparinized and normal saline flushes in maintaining the patency of 24-gauge (G) intermittent peripheral intravenous (IV) catheters in neonates in intensive care. "The hypothesis stated that there would be no significant difference in the duration of patency of a 24 G IV lock in a neonatal patient when flushed with 0.5 mL [millimeters] of heparinized saline (2U/mL), our standard practice, compared with 0.5 mL of 0.9% normal saline" (Schultz et al., 2002, p. 30).

This is a simple, null hypothesis with one independent variable (0.9% normal saline flush) and one dependent variable (patency of 24 G IV catheter). The comparison group received standard care of heparinized saline flush, and the population was neonates in an intensive care setting. The findings of the study did not support the null hypothesis because the catheters flushed with heparinized saline were patent significantly longer than the catheters flushed with normal saline. Thus, the researchers recommended continuing the use of heparinized saline as the standard for flushing 24 G catheters in infants.

A research hypothesis is the alternative hypothesis (H_1 or H_a) to the null. The research hypothesis states that there is a relationship between two or more variables, and it can be simple or complex, nondirectional or directional, and associative or causal. The prediction in a research hypothesis must be based on theoretical statements, previous research findings, or clinical experience. All the previous examples of hypotheses presented in this chapter were research hypotheses except for the one null hypothesis. Researchers have different beliefs about when to state a research hypothesis versus a null hypothesis. Some researchers state the null hypothesis because it is more easily interpreted on the basis of the results of statistical analyses. A researcher will also use the null hypothesis when she or he believes there is no relationship between two or more variables and when there is inadequate theoretical or empirical information to state a research hypothesis. Otherwise it is best to state a research hypothesis that clearly predicts the outcome of a study (Kerlinger & Lee, 2000).

Cheng, Studdiford, Chambers, Diamond, and Paynter (2002) developed both a null hypothesis and a research hypothesis to direct their study of the consistency of patient self-reported blood pressures (BPs) and stored monitor BPs. They developed a simple, associate, null hypothesis: "Patient-reported blood pressures would not consistently match electronically stored pressures" (Cheng et al., 2002, p. 260). They also stated a simple, directional, research hypothesis: "Electronically stored pressures unreported by patients would be higher, on average, than reported pressures" (Cheng et al., 2002, p. 260). The findings from this study encouraged the researchers to reject both the null and research hypotheses and to make the following recommendation for practice: "The reliability of self-reporting of blood pressures for many patients supports the potential usefulness of self-monitoring of blood pressure in hypertension management" (Cheng et al., 2002, p. 259).

Developing Hypotheses

Developing hypotheses requires inductive and deductive thinking. Most people have a predominant way of thinking and will use that thinking pattern in developing hypotheses. *Inductive* thinkers have a tendency to focus on the relationships they observe in clinical practice, and they synthesize these observations to formulate a general statement about the relationships (Chinn & Kramer, 2008). For example, inductive thinkers might note that elderly patients who are not instructed about the reasons for early postoperative ambulation make no effort to get out of bed. *Deductive* thinkers examine more abstract statements from theories or previous research and then formulate a hypothesis for study. Deductive thinkers might translate a statement or proposition, such as "people who receive education about self-care are more capable in caring for themselves," from Orem's (2001) theory into a hypothesis.

The inductive thinker must link the relational statement or hypothesis that was developed from clinical observations with a theoretical framework. Making this connection with the framework requires deductive thinking and improves the usefulness of the study findings. The deductive thinker must use inductive thinking to determine whether the proposition from a theory accurately predicts the relationship of events in clinical practice. Without this real-world experience, the selection of subjects and the identification of ways to measure the variables would be unclear. An example hypothesis is, "Elderly patients who receive an educational program and handout about activity following surgery ambulate earlier and have a shorter hospital stay after surgery than elderly patients who receive standard care."

In formulating a hypothesis, you as a researcher will have several decisions to make. These decisions are directed by the problem studied and by your own expertise and preference. You must decide whether the problem is best investigated with the use of simple or complex hypotheses. Complex hypotheses frequently require complex methodology, and the outcomes may be difficult to interpret. Some beginning researchers prefer the clarity of simple hypotheses.

The research problem and purpose determine whether you will study an associative or a causal relationship. Testing a hypothesis that states a causal relationship requires expertise in implementing a treatment and controlling extraneous variables. Another decision you must make involves the formulation of a research or a null hypothesis. You must make this decision according to what you believe is the most accurate prediction of the relationship between the study variables.

A hypothesis that is clearly and concisely stated gives the greatest direction for conducting a study. For clarity, hypotheses are expressed as declarative statements written in the present tense. Thus, hypotheses must be written without the phrase "There *will be* no relationship...," because the future tense refers to the sample being studied. Hypotheses are statements of relationships about populations, not about study samples. According to mathematical theory regarding generalization, one cannot generalize to the future (Kerlinger & Lee, 2000).

Hypotheses are clearer without the phrase "There is no *significant* difference...," because the level of significance is only a statistical technique applied to sample data (Armstrong, 1981). In addition, hypotheses should not identify methodological points, such as techniques of sampling, measurement, and data analysis (Kerlinger & Lee, 2000). Therefore, statements such as "*measured by*," "in a *random sample* of," or "*using ANOVA* (analysis of variance)" are not appropriate. These phrases limit hypotheses to measurement methods, sampling methods, or data analysis techniques in a single study. Hypotheses must reflect the variables and population outlined in the research problem and should not be limited to a single study. A well-formulated hypothesis clearly identifies the relationship between the variables. There is no set number for how many hypotheses are needed to direct a study, but the number formulated usually reflects the researcher's expertise and the complexity of the problem and purpose. However, most studies contain one to three hypotheses, and the relationships identified in these hypotheses set the limits for a study.

Testing Hypotheses

A hypothesis's value is ultimately derived from whether or not it can be tested in the real world. A testable hypothesis contains variables that can be measured or manipulated in practice. For example, Efe and Özer (2007) manipulated the breast-feeding intervention in their study using set protocol so that the treatment was consistently manipulated for each study situation. They measured crying time in seconds and measured the heart rate and oxygen saturation with a pulse oximeter (Nellcor N180).

Hypotheses are evaluated with statistical analyses. If the hypothesis states an associative relationship, correlational analyses are usually conducted on the data. The Spearman rank order correlation coefficient is often used to analyze ordinal level data, and the Pearson's product-moment correlation coefficient is used for interval and ratio level data (see Chapter 20). These correlational analyses determine the existence, type, and degree of the relationship between the variables studied.

A hypothesis that states a causal relationship is analyzed through the use of statistics that examine differences, such as Mann-Whitney *U*, *t*-test, and analysis of variance (ANOVA) (see Chapter 22). It is the null hypothesis (stated or implied) that is tested. The intent is to determine whether the independent variable had a significant effect on the dependent variable. The level of significance, alpha $(\alpha) = 0.05, 0.01, 0.001$, is set after the generation of causal hypotheses and before the conduct of the study. To learn more about selecting statistical tests and a level of significance for testing hypotheses, see Chapter 18.

The results obtained from testing a hypothesis are described with the use of certain terminology. Research findings do not prove hypotheses true or false; instead, hypotheses are statements of relationships or differences in populations. Even after a series of studies, the word *proven* is not used in scientific language because of the tentative nature of science. Research hypotheses are described as being *supported* or *not supported* in a study. When a null hypothesis is tested, it is either rejected or accepted. Accepting the null hypothesis indicates that no relationship or effect was found among the variables. Rejecting the null hypothesis indicates the possibility that a relationship or difference exists. A study might partially support a complex hypothesis. Efe and Özer's (2007, p. 11) hypothesis stated that "breast-feeding decreases the length of crying time, prevents an increase in heart rate, and prevents a decrease in oxygen saturation during vaccination as compared with the control condition (i.e., no breast feeding)." Their study supported the decreased crying time part of the hypothesis, but it did not support the part of the hypothesis that focused on the prevention of increased heart rate and decreased oxygen saturation. However, the study did provide valuable evidence about the effectiveness of breast-feeding in reducing the pain of immunization injections in infants. In addition, this study provides direction for future research.

SELECTING OBJECTIVES, QUESTIONS, OR HYPOTHESES FOR QUANTITATIVE OR QUALITATIVE RESEARCH

Selecting objectives, questions, or hypotheses for a study is often based on (1) the number and quality of relevant studies conducted on a selected problem (existing knowledge base), (2) the framework of the study, (3) the expertise and preference of the researcher, and (4) the type of study to be conducted (quantitative or qualitative). Commonly, if minimal or no research has been conducted on a problem, investigators state objectives or questions because they do not have the knowledge necessary to formulate hypotheses. The framework for a study indicates whether the intent is to develop or to test theory. Objectives and questions are usually stated to guide theory development, and the focus of a hypothesis is to test theory.

Researcher expertise and preference can also influence the selection of objectives, questions, or hypotheses to direct a study. Moody, Wilson, Smyth, Schwartz, Tittle, and Van Cott (1988) analyzed the focus of nursing practice research from 1977 to 1986 and found that 16% of the studies had research questions and 31% contained hypotheses. The number of nursing studies containing hypotheses continues to grow, and there appears to be a "trend away from descriptive and fact-finding studies toward efforts to establish relationships between variables and to test hypotheses" (Brown, Tanner, & Padrick, 1984, p. 31). The greater use of hypotheses to direct research could indicate the growth of knowledge in selected problem areas and the increasing sophistication of nurse researchers. However, Brown et al. (1984) noted that only 51% of the studies they reviewed contained explicitly stated hypotheses; the other studies had implicit or implied hypotheses. An explicit statement of hypotheses is important to provide clear direction for both the conduct of a study and the use of the findings in practice.

The objectives, questions, or hypotheses designated for study frequently indicate a pattern that the researcher uses in conducting investigations.

Problems can be investigated in a variety of ways. Some researchers start at the core of a problem and work their way outward. Other investigators study a problem from the outside edge and work to the core (Kaplan, 1964). Each study must logically build on the other, as the researcher establishes a pattern for studying a problem area that will affect the quality and quantity of the knowledge generated in that area.

Researchers select objectives, questions, or hypotheses according to the type of study they plan to conduct. Objectives and questions are typically stated when the intent of the study is to identify or describe characteristics of variables, to examine relationships among variables, or both. Thus, objectives or questions are often formulated to direct qualitative and selected quantitative (descriptive and correlational) studies (Table 8-1). However, some experienced researchers can clearly focus and develop a study without using objectives or questions. In these studies, a research purpose directs the research process.

In some qualitative research, the investigator uses only a problem and purpose to direct the study. The specification of objectives or questions might limit the scope of the study and the methods of data collection and analysis (Munhall, 2001). Discovery is important in qualitative research, and sometimes the "research questions may be unclear, the objectives ambiguous, and the final outcome uncertain. Hypotheses and detailed accounts of precise research strategies are neither necessary nor desirable in a well constructed qualitative design" (Aamodt, 1983, p. 399).

Researchers often develop hypotheses when the relationships or results of a study can be anticipated or predicted. Hypotheses are typically used in quantitative research to direct predictive correlational, quasi-experimental, and experimental studies.

IDENTIFYING AND DEFINING STUDY VARIABLES

The research purpose and objectives, questions, and hypotheses identify the variables or concepts to be examined in a study. Variables are qualities, properties,

TABLE 8-1 ▪ Selecting Objectives, Questions, or Hypotheses for Different Types of Research	
Type of Research	**Use of Objectives, Questions, or Hypotheses?**
Qualitative research	Objectives, questions, or none
Quantitative research	
Descriptive studies	Objectives, questions, or none
Correlational studies	Objectives, questions, hypotheses, or none
Quasi-experimental studies	Usually hypotheses
Experimental studies	Hypotheses

or characteristics of persons, things, or situations that change or vary in a study. Variables are characterized by degrees, amounts, and differences within a study. Variables are also concepts of various levels of abstraction that are concisely defined so that they can be measured or manipulated within a study (Kaplan, 1964; Moody, 1990).

The concepts examined in research can be concrete and directly measurable in practice, such as heart rate, hemoglobin value, and tidal volume of the lung. These concrete concepts are usually referred to as *variables* in a study. Other concepts, such as anxiety, coping, and pain, are more abstract and are indirectly observable in the real world (Chinn & Cramer, 2008). Thus, the properties of these concepts are inferred from a combination of measurements. For example, one can infer the properties of anxiety by combining information obtained from (1) observing the signs and symptoms of anxiety (frequent movements, sweating, lack of eye contact, and verbalization of anxiety), (2) examining completed questionnaires or scales (A-state and trait anxiety scales), and (3) measuring physiological responses (galvanic skin response). The concept of anxiety might be represented by the variables "reported anxiety" or "perceived level of anxiety."

In many qualitative studies and in some quantitative studies (descriptive and correlational), the focus is abstract concepts, such as grieving, caring, and promoting health (Marshall & Rossman, 2006; Munhall, 2001). Researchers identify the elements of the study as concepts, not variables. In the ethnographic study previously described, Happ et al. (2007) investigated the concept of health-related decision making by critically ill patients during prolonged mechanical ventilations (PMV). The concept *health-related decision making* was defined as "choices about initiating, continuing, or discontinuing treatment, diagnostics, or therapeutic care activities" (p. 363). In this study, health-related decision making was operationalized to include the following:

> *choices about mechanical ventilation and other therapies, such as invasive diagnostic procedures and placement of central lines and nutritional access devices that may or may not require written informed consent, and about discharge placement. Financial or legal decisions, such as appointment of a power of attorney or signing financial documents to enable insurance payment for health care, were considered health-related in the context of prolonged critical illness. (Happ et al., 2007, p. 363)*

Types of Variables

Variables have been classified into a variety of types to explain their use in research. Some variables are manipulated; others are controlled. Some variables are identified but not measured; others are measured with refined measurement devices. The types of variables presented in this section are independent, dependent, research, extraneous, demographic, moderator, and mediator.

Independent and Dependent Variables

The relationship between independent variables and dependent variables is the basis for formulating hypotheses for correlational, quasi-experimental, and experimental studies. An independent variable is a stimulus or activity that the researcher manipulates or varies to create an effect on the dependent variable. The independent variable is also called an intervention, treatment, or experimental variable.

A dependent variable is the response, behavior, or outcome that the researcher wants to predict or explain. Changes in the dependent variable are presumed to be caused by the independent variable. The dependent variable can also be called an effect or outcome variable or a criterion measure (Kerlinger & Lee, 2000).

The null hypothesis developed by Schultz et al. (2002, p. 30), introduced earlier in the chapter, "stated that there would be no significant difference in the duration of patency of a 24 G IV lock in a neonatal patient when flushed with 0.5 mL [millimeters] of heparinized saline (2U/mL), our standard practice, compared with 0.5 mL of 0.9% normal saline." The independent variable that was manipulated in this study was the 0.5 mL of 0.9% normal saline flush and the dependent variable that was measured was the patency of the 24 G IV. The 0.5 mL of heparinized saline was the standard care for flushing the 24 G IVs of the neonates in the comparison group.

Research Variables or Concepts

Qualitative studies and some quantitative (descriptive and correlational) studies involve the investigation of research variables or concepts. Research variables or concepts are the qualities, properties, or characteristics identified in the research purpose and objectives or questions that are observed or measured in a study. They are used when the intent of the study is to observe or measure variables as they exist in a natural setting without the implementation of a treatment. Thus, no independent variables are manipulated, and no cause-and-effect relationships are examined.

Qualitative studies often focus on abstract concepts. For example, Orne et al. (2000, p. 205) conducted a qualitative phenomenological study of the "experience of being medically uninsured from the perspective of American workers who have lived it." The study was directed by the following research question: "What is the lived experience of being employed but medically uninsured?" (Orne, Fishman, Manka, & Pagnozzi, 2000, p. 205). This study focused on describing the research concept of the experience of medically uninsured in a population of employed adults. We will define this research concept, conceptually and operationally, later in this chapter.

Extraneous Variables

Extraneous variables exist in all studies and can affect the measurement of study variables and the relationships among them. Extraneous variables are of primary concern in quantitative studies, because they can obscure one's understanding of the relational or causal dynamics within the studies. Extraneous variables are classified as (1) recognized or unrecognized and (2) controlled or uncontrolled.

The extraneous variables that are not recognized until the study is in process or are recognized before the study is initiated but cannot be controlled are referred to as **confounding variables**. Sometimes these variables can be measured during the study and controlled statistically during analysis. In other cases, it is not possible to measure a confounding variable, and the variable thus hinders the interpretation of findings. Such extraneous variables must be identified as limitations or areas of study weakness in the discussion section of a research report. As control decreases in quasi-experimental and experimental studies, the potential influence of confounding variables increases.

Researchers attempt to recognize and control as many extraneous variables as possible in quasi-experimental and experimental studies, and specific designs have been developed to control the influence of such variables (see Chapter 11). Schultz et al. (2002) controlled some of the extraneous variables in their study, previously described, by implementing a double-blind experimental design, using specific inclusion and exclusion criteria for sample selection, training the nursing staff participating in the study, and randomizing the subjects to groups. The following excerpt identifies the controls the researchers used in their study to decrease the effect of extraneous variables and bias and to increase the likelihood that the findings are an accurate reflection of reality and not due to error.

Inclusion criteria were all neonates younger than 30 days with a new 24 G IV lock 3/4 inch in length. Exclusion criteria were neonates with central catheters, recent surgery, a diagnosis of disseminated intravascular coagulopathy or idiopathic thrombocytopenia, or current or previous treatment of a patent ductus arteriosis with indomethacin....

■ *EDUCATION OF THE STAFF*

... Competency was established for the flushing procedure by having each nurse pass a quiz on IV lock flush protocol with a score of 90% or higher and show proper IV lock flush technique. All staff nurses completed the requirements to participate in the study....

■ *PROCEDURE*

... Only the first IV lock per infant was included in the study.... Randomization of subjects occurred in the pharmacy on receipt of an order for the study solution and a copy of the informed consent.... Study solutions were prepared, coded, and labeled in the pharmacy and delivered to the NICU [neonatal intensive care unit]. All staff members, including the study investigators, were blinded to the study group. Only the pharmacist knew the results of the randomization. (p. 30)

Environmental variables are a type of extraneous variable that make up the setting in which the study is conducted. Examples are climate, home, health care system, community setting, and governmental organizations. If a researcher is studying humans in an uncontrolled or natural setting, it is impossible and undesirable to control all the environmental variables. In qualitative and some quantitative (descriptive and correlational) studies, researchers make little or no attempt to control environmental variables. Their intent is to study subjects in their natural environment without controlling or altering it. The environmental variables in quasi-experimental and experimental research can be controlled through the use of a study protocol and a laboratory setting or a specially constructed research unit in a hospital.

In intervention effectiveness research, the extraneous variables are referred to as contextual variables. **Contextual variables** are those factors that could influence the implementation of an intervention and thus the outcomes of the study (Sidani & Braden, 1998). These contextual or extraneous factors include social and environmental setting and individual variables that can influence the intervention and study outcomes.

For a study to yield the best understanding of an intervention and its usefulness to practice, the study design must provide for the examination of relevant contextual variables and link them to the study interventions and outcomes. Thus, rather than controlling or preventing the influence of extraneous variables as do quasi-experimental and experimental research, intervention effectiveness research focuses on studying them. Identifying and studying the effects of contextual (extraneous) variables greatly increases the complexity of a study, but it also improves the accuracy of the findings for practice. Intervention effectiveness research is the focus of Chapter 13.

Demographic Variables

Demographic variables are attributes of the subjects that are measured during the study and used to describe the sample. Some common demographic variables examined in nursing research are age, gender, ethnicity, educational level, income, job classification, length of hospital stay, and medical diagnosis. Researchers select demographic variables based on the focus of their study, the demographic variables included in previous studies, and clinical experience. However, age, gender, and ethnicity are essential demographic variables to examine in all types of research. These demographics describe the sample and determine the population for generalization of the findings. More research is needed to improve health care for elderly, women, children, and minorities, and funding agencies often give priority to studies that focus on these individuals.

To obtain data on demographic variables, subjects are asked to complete a demographic or information sheet. When the study is completed, the demographic information is analyzed to provide a picture of the sample, which is called the sample characteristics. Sample characteristics are presented in a table or discussed in the narrative of the research report (or both). As previously discussed, Schultz et al. (2002) studied the effects of heparinized saline versus normal saline in promoting patency of IV catheters in neonates. They summarized their sample characteristics in a table (Table 8-2) and discussed them in the narrative of their article:

Gestational age for the sample ranged from 26 to 42 weeks, with a mean of 33.5 weeks (SD = 3.8). Chronological age ranged from 1 to 30 days, with a mean of 6.8 days (SD = 6.9). Mean birth weight was 2.11 kg (SD = 0.875), with a range from 0.52 to 3.89 kg. There were no statistically significant differences in sex determined by chi-square analysis. There were no statistically significant differences in birth weight, gestational age, or chronological age of subjects between the two groups [experimental and control] based on Student's t-test [see Table 8-2]. (Schultz et al., 2002, p. 31)

The demographic variables in this study were gender, weight, gestational age, and chronological age. The experimental and control groups were compared on these demographic variables to ensure that they were similar before the treatment was implemented. Because the results indicated that the catheters flushed with heparinized saline, which was the standard practice of this agency, were patent significantly longer than the catheters flushed with normal saline, it can be assume that the decreased patency results in the experimental group were due to the effect of the treatment (normal saline flush) rather than demographic or extraneous variables.

TABLE 8-2 Demographic Comparisons				
Variable	Total Sample ($N = 49$)	Experimental Group ($n = 29$)	Control Group ($n = 20$)	p
Gender				
Boys	17	8	9	0.208
Girls	32	21	11	
Weight	M = 2.11	M = 2.17	M = 2.02	0.667
	SD = 0.875	SD = 81	SD = 0.83	
Gestational age	M = 33.47	M = 33.88	M = 33.20	0.685
	SD = 3.81	SD = 3.95	SD = 3.88	
Chronological age	M = 6.80	M = 5.65	M = 8.46	0.210*
	SD = 6.87	SD = 5.01	SD = 8.80	

From Schultz, A. A., Drew, D, & Hewitt, H. (2002). Comparison of normal saline and heparinized saline for patency of IV Locks in neonates. *Applied Nursing Research, 15*(1): 31.

* Significance based on unequal variances.

Moderator and Mediator Variables

Moderator and mediator variables are examined in intervention effectiveness research to improve our understanding of the effect of the intervention on practice-related outcomes. A moderator variable occurs with the intervention (independent variable) and alters the causal relationship between the intervention and the outcomes. Moderator variables include characteristics of the subjects and of the person implementing the intervention. Mediator variables bring about the effects of the intervention after it has occurred and thus influence the outcomes of the study (Sidani & Braden, 1998).

The theoretical model that provides the framework for the study usually identifies the relevant moderator and mediator variables to be examined in the study. The design is developed to examine not only the independent (intervention) and dependent (outcomes) variables but also the moderator, mediator, and contextual variables (see Chapter 13 for a detailed discussion and examples of these types of variables).

OPERATIONALIZING VARIABLES OR CONCEPTS FOR A STUDY

Operationalizing a variable or concept involves developing conceptual and operational definitions. A conceptual definition provides the theoretical meaning of a concept or variable and is derived from a theorist's definition of that concept or is developed through concept analysis. The study framework, which includes concepts and their definitions, provides a basis for conceptually defining the variables. Artinian et al. (2001) studied the effects of two independent variables (home telemonitoring and community-based monitoring) on one dependent variable (blood pressure). The framework for this study was the health belief model, and the proposition studied was that a cue to action is implemented to activate a readiness to change health behaviors. (Strecher & Rosenstock, 1997)

■ *INDEPENDENT VARIABLE—HOME TELEMONITORING*

Conceptual Definition

Home telemonitoring (HT) is a cue to action or a strategy to increase a person's awareness of the need to change behavior. (Strecher & Rosenstock, 1997)

Operational Definition

HT intervention included providing instructions on how to monitor BP in the home three times a week over 12 weeks. In addition, telephone counseling about lifestyle modification was provided once a week for 12 weeks by a specially trained registered nurse. (Artinian et al., 2001)

■ *INDEPENDENT VARIABLE— COMMUNITY-BASED MONITORING*

Conceptual Definition

Community-based monitoring (CBM) is a cue to action or a strategy to increase a person's awareness of the need to change behavior. (Strecher & Rosenstock, 1997)

Operational Definition

CBM intervention required participants to "visit the community center three times a week in the morning to have their BP measured. Participants also received feedback about their BP and weekly education counseling about lifestyle modification and adherence to their medication regimen." (Artinian et al., 2001, p. 193)

■ *DEPENDENT VARIABLE— BLOOD PRESSURE*

Conceptual Definition

BP control requires a change in lifestyle and health behavior that is triggered by educational cues to action. (Strecher & Rosenstock, 1997)

Operational Definition

Both systolic blood pressure (SBP) and diastolic blood pressure (DBP) were measured three times a week. For the HT group, the SBP and DBP "were measured with an electronic home BPLink monitor (model A & D UA 767PC)" and BP monitoring services provided by LifeLink Monitoring, Inc., located in Bearsville, New York. For the CBM, the SBP and DBP were "measured with the BP equipment at the community center" and recorded by a nurse trained by the researcher. (Artinian et al., 2001, p. 194)

Figure 8-2 presents the significant changes in the SBP and DBP for both treatment groups (HT and CBM). The HT and CBM treatment groups had significantly lower SBP and DBP than the usual care group. These monitoring interventions promoted blood pressure control among African Americans, who often have difficulty managing hypertension.

The variables in quasi-experimental and experimental research are narrow and specific in focus and are capable of being quantified (converted to numbers) or manipulated through the use of specified steps. In addition, the variables are objectively defined to reduce researcher bias. The concepts or variables in descriptive and correlational quantitative studies and qualitative studies are usually more abstract and

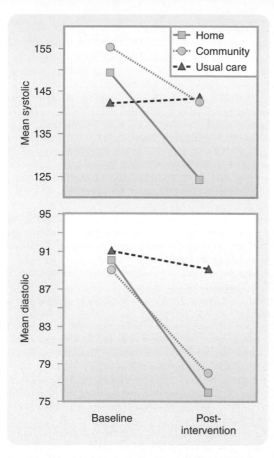

Figure 8-2 Change in SBP and DBP during 3 months for the home telemonitoring, community-based monitoring, and usual care groups. (Home telemonitoring, $n = 6$; community-based monitoring, $n = 6$; usual care only, $n = 9$.)

broadly defined than the variables in quasi-experimental studies.

Some researchers believe that the concepts in qualitative studies do not require operational definitions because sensitizing or experiencing the real situation rather than operationalizing the concepts is most important. **Operational definitions** are thought to limit the investigation so that a phenomenon, such as pain, or a characteristic of a culture, such as health practices, is not completely experienced or understood. In other qualitative studies, the phenomena being examined are not named until the data analysis step (Marshall & Ross, 2006; Munhall, 2001). Thus, some concepts may not be identified or defined until late in the study. For example, Orne et al. (2000, p. 205) conducted their study "with the goal of constructing a vivid depiction of the lived experience of being employed but

medically uninsured." The conceptual definition for the experience of being medically uninsured was identified in the analysis section of the research report in a table format.

■ RESEARCH CONCEPT — EXPERIENCE OF BEING MEDICALLY UNINSURED

Conceptual Definition
Table 8-3 illustrates this definition, including the theme clusters and themes for the experience of being medically uninsured.

Operational Definition
The research concept of the experience of being medically uninsured while working was investigated using audiotaped, face-to-face interviews that were conducted with an unstructured format.

Participants initially were asked to respond to the statement, "Please describe to me as thoroughly as you can, what it is like to be working and without medical insurance." Additional questioning, for clarification, requests for specific examples, and reflective statements were used to encourage the participants to describe their experience in detail. (Orne et al., 2000, p. 206)

Thus, the focus of the study by Orne et al. (2000) was to conceptually define and describe the concept of the experience of being medically uninsured while being employed. The findings from this study could become the basis for additional research to expand our understanding and ability to manage the problems of the medically uninsured population.

TABLE 8-3 Thematic Analysis	
Theme Clusters	**Themes**
A Marginalized Life	Vulnerable on all fronts
	Limits, loss, and hard times
Up against Rocks and Hard Places	The paradox of middle ground
	Entangled in power and politics
Making Choices— Chancing It	Setting priorities—weighing the odds
	Living with compromise
	A game of Russian roulette
Getting By—More or Less	Lucky so far
	Resilience
	Resigned to adversity
	The emotional price tag

From Orne, R. M., Fishman, S. J., Manka, M., & Pagnozzi, M. E. (2000). Living on the edge: A phenomenological study of medically uninsured working Americans. *Research in Nursing & Health, 23*(3): 207.

SUMMARY

- Research objectives, questions, and hypotheses are formulated to bridge the gap between the more abstractly stated research problem and purpose and the detailed design and plan for data collection and analysis.
- Research objectives are clear, concise, declarative statements that are expressed in the present tense.
- A research question is a concise, interrogative statement that is worded in the present tense and consists of one or more variables (or concepts).
- A hypothesis is the formal statement of the expected relationships between two or more variables in a specified population.
- Hypotheses can be described in terms of four categories: (1) associative versus causal, (2) simple versus complex, (3) nondirectional versus directional, and (4) null versus research.
- Selecting objectives, questions, or hypotheses for a study is based on (1) the number and quality of relevant studies conducted on a selected problem (existing knowledge base), (2) the framework of the study, (3) the expertise and preference of the researcher, and (4) the type of study to be conducted (quantitative, qualitative, outcomes, and intervention).
- Variables are qualities, properties, or characteristics of persons, things, or situations that change or vary in a study.
- The types of variables discussed in this chapter are independent, dependent, research, extraneous, demographic, moderator, and mediator.
- An independent variable is a stimulus or intervention that the researcher manipulates or varies to create an effect on the dependent variable.
- A dependent variable is the response, behavior, or outcome that the researcher wants to predict or explain.
- Research variables or concepts are the qualities, properties, or characteristics that are observed or measured in a study.
- Demographic variables are attributes of the subjects that are measured in a study to describe the sample.
- The variables require conceptual and operational definitions, and a conceptual definition provides the theoretical meaning of a concept or variable and is derived from a theorist's definition of the concept or is developed through concept analysis.
- An operational definition is derived from a set of procedures or progressive acts that a researcher performs either to manipulate an independent variable or to measure the existence or degree of existence of the dependent variable.

REFERENCES

Aamodt, A. M. (1983). Problems in doing nursing research: Developing criteria for evaluating qualitative research. *Western Journal of Nursing Research*, 5(4), 398–402.

Ajzen, I. (1985). From intention to action: A theory of planned behavior. In J. Kuhl & J. Beckmann (Eds.), *Action control: From cognition to behavior* (pp. 11–39). New York: Springer.

Anderson, B., Higgins, L., & Rozmus, C. (1999). Critical pathways: Application to selected patient outcomes following coronary artery bypass graft. *Applied Nursing Research*, 12(4), 168–174.

Armstrong, R. L. (1981). Hypothesis formulation. In S. D. Krampitz & N. Pavlovich (Eds.), *Readings for nursing research* (pp. 29–39). St. Louis: Mosby.

Artinian, N. T., Washington, O. G., & Templin, T. N. (2001). Effects of home telemonitoring and community-based monitoring on blood pressure control in urban African Americans: A pilot study. *Heart & Lung*, 30(3), 191–199.

Beveridge, W. B. (1950). *The art of scientific investigation.* New York: Vintage Books.

Brown, J. S., Tanner, C. A., & Padrick, K. P. (1984). Nursing's search for scientific knowledge. *Nursing Research*, 33(1), 26–32.

Center for Disease Control and Prevention. (2005). *Diabetes surveillance report.* Department of Health and Human Services. Retrieved November 26, 2005, from http://www.cdc.gov/diabetes/statistics/prevalence_national.htm.

Cheng, C., Studdiford, J. S., Chambers, C. V., Diamond, J. J., & Paynter, N. (2002). The reliability of patient self-reported blood pressures. *Journal of Clinical Hypertension*, 4(4), 259–264, 273.

Chinn, P. L., & Kramer, M. K. (2008). *Integrated theory and knowledge development in nursing* (7th ed.). St. Louis: Mosby.

Cox, K. S., Teasley, S. L., Lacey, S. R., Carroll, C. A., & Sexton, K. A. (2007). Work environment perceptions of pediatric nurses. *Journal of Pediatric Nursing*, 22(1), 9–14.

Efe, E., & Özer, Z. C. (2007). The use of breast-feeding for pain relief during neonatal immunization injections. *Applied Nursing Research*, 20(1), 10–16.

Ernst, M. E., Messmer, P. R., Franco, M., & Gonzalez, J. L. (2004). Nurses' job satisfaction, stress, and recognition in pediatric setting. *Pediatric Nursing*, 30(3), 219–227.

Fagerhaugh, S. Y., & Strauss, A. (1977). *Politics of pain management.* Menlo Park, CA: Addison-Wesley.

Gerlach, R. W., Gambosi, J. R., & Bowen, R. H. (1990). Cancer survivors' needs reported by survivors and their families. *Journal of Cancer Education*, 5(1), 63–70.

Happ, M. B., Swigart, V. A., Tate, J. A., Hoffman, L. A., & Arnold, R. M. (2007). Patient involvement in health-related decisions during prolonged critical illness. *Research in Nursing & Health*, 30(4), 361–372.

Jennings-Dozier, K. (1999). Predicting intentions to obtain a Pap smear among African American and Latina women: Testing the theory of planned behavior. *Nursing Research*, 48(4), 198–205.

Kaplan, A. (1964). *The conduct of inquiry: Methodology for behavioral science.* New York: Harper & Row.

Kerlinger, F. N., & Lee, H. B. (2000). *Foundations of behavioral research* (4th ed.). Fort Worth, TX: Harcourt College Publishers.

Marshall, C., & Rossman, G. B. (2006). *Designing qualitative research* (4th ed.). Thousand Oaks: CA: Sage.

McDonald, D. D., Frakes, M., Apostolidis, B., Armstrong, B., Goldblatt, S., & Bernardo, D. (2003). Effect of a psychiatric diagnosis on nursing care for nonpsychiatric problems. *Research in Nursing & Health, 26*(3), 225–232.

Moody, L. E. (1990). *Advancing nursing science through research* (Vol. 1). Newbury Park, CA: Sage.

Moody, L. E., Wilson, M. E., Smyth, K., Schwartz, R., Tittle, M., & Van Cott, M. L. (1988). Analysis of a decade of nursing practice research: 1977–1986. *Nursing Research, 37*(6), 374–379.

Munhall, P. L. (2001). *Nursing research: A qualitative perspective* (3rd ed.). Sudbury, MA: Jones & Bartlett and National League for Nursing.

Narsavage, G., & Romeo, E. (2003). Education and support needs of younger and older cancer survivors. *Applied Nursing Research, 16*(2), 103–109.

Orem, D. E. (2001). *Nursing concepts of practice.* St. Louis: Mosby.

Orne, R. M., Fishman, S. J., Manka, M., & Pagnozzi, M. E. (2000). Living on the edge: A phenomenological study of medically uninsured working Americans. *Research in Nursing & Health, 23*(3), 204–212.

Pennsylvania Department of Health. (1998). Number of observed and expected cancer cases by sex and primary site, 1994–1998. *Lackawanna County Health Profile.* Retrieved May 29, 2002, from http://www.health.state.pa.us/pdf/hpa/ststs/profile98/lacka.pdf and http://webserver.health.state.pa.us/health/lib/health/Pennsylvania_cancer.pdf.

Polzer, R. L. (2007). African Americans and diabetes: Spiritual role of the health care provider in self-management. *Research in Nursing & Health, 30*(2), 164–174.

Polzer, R. L., & Miles, M. S. (2007). Spirituality in African Americans with diabetes: Self-management through a relationship with God. *Qualitative Health Research, 17*(2), 176–188.

Rawl, S. M., Given, B. A., Given, C. W., Champion, V. L., Kozachik, S. L., Barton, D., et al. (2002). Intervention to improve psychological functioning for newly diagnosed patients with cancer. *Oncology Nursing Forum, 29*(6), 967–975.

Reishtein, J. L. (2005). Relationship between symptoms and functional performance in COPD. *Research in Nursing & Health, 28*(1), 39–47.

Reynolds, P. D. (1971). *A primer in theory construction.* Indianapolis: Bobbs-Merrill.

Schultz, A. A., Drew, D., & Hewitt, H. (2002). Comparison of normal saline and heparinized saline for patency of IV locks in neonates. *Applied Nursing Research, 15*(1), 28–34.

Sidani, S., & Braden, C. J. (1998). *Evaluating nursing interventions: A theory-driven approach.* Thousand Oaks, CA: Sage.

Strecher, V. J., & Rosenstock, I. M. (1997). The health belief model. In K. Glanz F. M. Lewis & B. K. Rimer (Eds.), *Health behavior and health education: Theory, research and practice* (2nd ed., pp. 41–59). San Francisco: Jossey-Bass.

Vasan, R. S., Beiser, A., D'Agostino, R. B., Levy, D., Selhub, J., Jacques, P. F., et al. (2003). Plasma homocysteine and risk for congestive heart failure in adults without prior myocardial infarction. *Journal of the American Medical Association, 289*(10), 1251–1257.

CHAPTER **9**

Ethics in Research

Nursing research requires not only expertise and diligence but also honesty and integrity. Conducting research ethically starts with the identification of the study topic and continues through the publication of the study. Over the years, ethical codes and regulations have been developed to provide guidelines for (1) the selection of the study purpose, design, and subjects; (2) the collection and analysis of data; (3) the interpretation of results; and (4) the presentation and publication of the study. In 2003, an important regulation titled the Health Insurance Portability and Accountability Act (HIPAA) was enacted to protect the privacy of an individual's health information. HIPAA has had an important impact on researchers and institutional review boards (IRBs), who review health care research for conduct in a variety of settings. This chapter provides an overview of this act and the other U.S. and international regulations that have been developed to promote ethical conduct in research worldwide.

An ethical problem that has received increasing attention since the 1980s is research misconduct. Misconduct has occurred during the performance, reporting, and publication of research, and the Office of Research Integrity (ORI) has investigated a number of research institutions in the United States for fraud (ORI, 2007, June 20). Many disciplines, including nursing, have had episodes of scientific misconduct that have affected the quality of research evidence generated.

Ethical research is essential to generate a sound evidence-based practice for nursing, but what does the ethical conduct of research involve? This is a question that has been debated for many years by researchers,

politicians, philosophers, lawyers, and even research subjects. The debate continues, probably because of the complexity of human rights issues; the focus of research in new, challenging arenas of technology and genetics; the complex ethical codes and regulations governing research; and the various interpretations of these codes and regulations. Even though the phenomenon of the ethical conduct in research defies precise delineation, the historical events, ethical codes, and regulations presented in this chapter provide guidance for nurse researchers. The chapter also discusses the actions essential for conducting research ethically: (1) protecting the rights of human subjects, (2) balancing benefits and risks in a study, (3) obtaining informed consent from subjects, and (4) submitting a research proposal for institutional review. Current ethical issues related to scientific misconduct and the use of animals in research conclude the chapter.

HISTORICAL EVENTS AFFECTING THE DEVELOPMENT OF ETHICAL CODES AND REGULATIONS

The ethical conduct of research has been a focus since the 1940s because of the mistreatment of human subjects in selected studies. Four experimental projects have been highly publicized for their unethical treatment of subjects: (1) Nazi medical experiments, (2) the Tuskegee Syphilis Study, (3) the Willowbrook study, and (4) the Jewish Chronic Disease Hospital study. Although these were biomedical studies and the primary investigators were physicians, there is evidence that nurses were aware of the research, identified potential research subjects, delivered treatments to the subjects, and served as data collectors in these projects. The four projects demonstrate the importance of ethical conduct for anyone reviewing, participating in, and conducting nursing or biomedical research. These four projects and other incidences of unethical treatment of subjects and scientific misconduct in the development, implementation, and reporting of research have influenced the formulation of ethical codes and regulations to direct research today. In addition, the concern for patient privacy with the electronic storage and exchange of health information has resulted in HIPAA privacy regulations (Olsen, 2003).

Nazi Medical Experiments

From 1933 to 1945, the Third Reich in Europe implemented atrocious, unethical activities (Steinfels & Levine, 1976). The programs of the Nazi regime consisted of sterilization, euthanasia, and numerous medical experiments to produce a population of racially pure Germans, or Aryans, who the Nazis maintained were destined to rule the world. The Nazis encouraged population growth among the Aryans ("good Nazis") and sterilized people they regarded as racial enemies, such as the Jews. They also practiced what they called "euthanasia," which involved killing various groups of people whom they considered racially impure, such as the insane, deformed, and senile. In addition, numerous medical experiments were conducted on prisoners of war, as well as racially "valueless" persons who had been confined to concentration camps.

The medical experiments involved exposing subjects to high altitudes, freezing temperatures, malaria, poisons, spotted fever (typhus), and untested drugs and operations, usually without any anesthesia (Steinfels & Levine, 1976). For example, in the hypothermia studies, subjects were immersed in bath temperatures ranging from 2° to 12° C. The researchers noted that "immersion in water 5° C is tolerated by clothed men for 40 to 60 minutes, whereas raising the water temperature to 15° C increases the period of tolerance to four to five hours" (Berger, 1990, p. 1436). These medical experiments were conducted to generate knowledge about human beings but the end result often was to destroy certain groups of people. Extensive examination of the records from some of these studies showed that they were poorly designed and conducted. Thus, they generated little if any useful scientific knowledge.

The Nazi experiments violated numerous rights of human research subjects. The selection of subjects was racially based, demonstrating an unfair selection process. The subjects also had no opportunity to refuse participation; they were prisoners who were coerced or forced to participate. Subjects were frequently killed during the experiments or sustained permanent physical, mental, and social damage as a result (Levine, 1986; Steinfels & Levine, 1976). These studies were not conducted by a few isolated scientists and physicians; they were "the product of coordinated policy-making and planning at high governmental, military, and Nazi Party levels, conducted as an integral part of the total war effort" (Nuremberg Code, 1986, p. 425).

Nuremberg Code

The people involved in the Nazi experiments were brought to trial before the Nuremberg Tribunals, which publicized these unethical activities. The mistreatment of human subjects in these studies led to the development of the Nuremberg Code in 1949. This code contains guidelines for (1) subjects' voluntary consent to participate in research; (2) the right of subjects to withdraw from studies; (3) protection of subjects from physical and mental suffering, injury, disability, and death during studies; and (4) the balance of benefits and risks in a study (Table 9-1). The Nuremberg Code was formulated mainly to direct the conduct of biomedical research; however, the rules it contains are essential to research in other sciences, such as nursing, psychology, and sociology. This code was developed to promote the ethical conduct of research in all countries and can be reviewed online at http://ohsr.od.nih.gov/guidelines/nuremberg.html.

Declaration of Helsinki

The Nuremberg Code provided the basis for the development of the Declaration of Helsinki, which was adopted in 1964 and amended in 1975, 1983, 1989, 1996, 2000, and 2002 by the World Medical Association; it can be viewed online at www.rotrf.org/information/Helsinki_declaration.pdf. The Declaration of Helsinki differentiated therapeutic research from nontherapeutic research. **Therapeutic research** gives the patient an opportunity to receive an experimental treatment that might have beneficial results. **Nontherapeutic research** is conducted to generate knowledge for a discipline, and the results from the study might benefit future patients but will probably not benefit those acting as research subjects.

The Declaration of Helsinki requires that (1) greater care be exercised to protect subjects from harm in nontherapeutic research; (2) there be a strong, independent justification for exposing a healthy volunteer to risk of harm just to gain new scientific information; (3) investigators must protect the life, health, privacy, and dignity of research subjects; and (4) extreme care

TABLE 9-1 ■ The Nuremberg Code

1. The voluntary consent of the human subject is absolutely essential.
2. The experiment should be such as to yield fruitful results for the good of society, unprocurable by other methods or means of study, and not random and unnecessary in nature.
3. The experiment should be so designed and based on the results of animal experimentation and knowledge of the natural history of the disease or other problem under study that the anticipated results will justify the performance of the experiment.
4. The experiment should be so conducted as to avoid all unnecessary physical and mental suffering and injury.
5. No experiment should be conducted where there is a priori reason to believe that death or disabling injury will occur, except, perhaps, in those experiments where the experimental physicians also serve as subjects.
6. The degree of risk to be taken should never exceed that determined by the humanitarian importance of the problem to be solved by the experiment.
7. Proper preparations should be made and adequate facilities provided to protect the experimental subject against even remote possibilities of injury, disability, or death.
8. The experiment should be conducted only by scientifically qualified persons. The highest degree of skill and care should be required through all stages of the experiment of those who conduct or engage in the experiment.
9. During the course of the experiment the human subject should be at liberty to bring the experiment to an end if he has reached the physical or mental state where continuation of the experiment seems to him to be impossible.
10. During the course of the experiment the scientist in charge must be prepared to terminate the experiment at any stage, if he has probable cause to believe, in the exercise of the good faith, superior skill, and careful judgment required of him, that a continuation of the experiment is likely to result in injury, disability, or death to the experimental subject.

From "The Nuremberg Code," in *Ethics and Regulation of Clinical Research* (2nd ed., pp. 425–426), edited by R.J. Levine, 1986, Baltimore–Munich: Urban & Schwarzenberg.

must be taken in making use of placebo-controlled trial and used only in the absence of existing proven therapy (World Medical Association General Assembly, 2002). Thus, this legal document provides an ethical basis for the clinical trials and other research conducted today in the United States and internationally. Clinical trials must focus on improving diagnostic, therapeutic, and prophylactic procedures for patients with selected diseases without exposing subjects to any additional risk of serious or irreversible harm. Most institutions worldwide in which clinical research is conducted have adopted the Declaration

of Helsinki. However, neither this document nor the Nuremberg Code has prevented some investigators from conducting unethical research (Beecher, 1966; Nelson-Marten & Rich, 1999; ORI, 2004).

Tuskegee Syphilis Study

In 1932, the U.S. Public Health Service (U.S. PHS) initiated a study of syphilis in black men in the small, rural town of Tuskegee, Alabama (Brandt, 1978; Rothman, 1982). The study, which continued for 40 years, was conducted to determine the natural course of syphilis in the adult black male. The research subjects were organized into two groups: one group consisted of 400 men who had untreated syphilis and the other consisted of a control group of 200 men without syphilis. Many of the subjects who consented to participate in the study were not informed about the purpose and procedures of the research. Some individuals were unaware that they were subjects in a study.

By 1936, it was apparent that the men with syphilis developed more complications than the control group. Ten years later, the death rate of the group with syphilis was twice as high as that for the control group. The subjects were examined periodically but were not treated for syphilis, even after penicillin was determined to be an effective treatment for the disease in the 1940s (Levine, 1986). Information about an effective treatment for syphilis was withheld from the subjects, and deliberate steps were taken to keep them from receiving treatment (Brandt, 1978).

Published reports of the Tuskegee Syphilis Study first started appearing in 1936, and additional papers were published every 4 to 6 years. No effort was made to stop the study; in fact, in 1969, the U.S. Centers for Disease Control (CDC) decided that it should continue. Numerous individuals were involved in conducting this study, including

> *three generations of doctors serving in the venereal disease division of the U.S. PHS, numerous officials at the Tuskegee Institute and its affiliated hospital, hundreds of doctors in the Macon County and Alabama medical societies, and numerous foundation officials at the Rosenwald Fund and the Milbank Memorial Fund. (Rothman, 1982, p. 5)*

In 1972, an account of the study published in the *Washington Star* sparked public outrage. Only then did the U.S. Department of Health, Education, and Welfare (DHEW) stop the study. The Tuskegee Syphilis Study was investigated and found to be ethically unjustified, but its racial implications were never addressed (Brandt, 1978). There are still many unanswered questions about this study, such as where were the checks and balances in the government and health care systems that should have prevented this unethical study from continuing for 40 years and why was public outrage the only effective means of halting the study?

Willowbrook Study

From the mid-1950s to the early 1970s, Dr. Krugman at Willowbrook, an institution for the mentally retarded, conducted research on hepatitis (Rothman, 1982). The subjects, all children, were "deliberately infected with the hepatitis virus; early subjects were fed extracts of stool from infected individuals and later subjects received injections of more purified virus preparations" (Levine, 1986, p. 70). During the 20-year study, Willowbrook closed its doors to new inmates because of overcrowded conditions. However, the research ward continued to admit new inmates. To gain their child's admission to the institution, the parents were forced to give permission for the child to be a subject in the study.

From the late 1950s to early 1970s, Krugman's research team published several articles describing the study protocol and findings. Beecher (1966) cited the Willowbrook study as an example of unethical research. The investigators defended injecting the children with the virus by citing their own belief that most of the children would have acquired the infection after admission to the institution. The investigators also stressed the benefits the subjects received, which were a cleaner environment, better supervision, and a higher nurse-patient ratio on the research ward (Rothman, 1982). Despite the controversy, this unethical study continued until the early 1970s.

Jewish Chronic Disease Hospital Study

Another highly publicized example of unethical research was a study conducted at the Jewish Chronic Disease Hospital in the 1960s. Its purpose was to determine the patients' rejection responses to live cancer cells. Twenty-two patients were injected with a suspension containing live cancer cells that had been generated from human cancer tissue (Hershey & Miller, 1976; Levine, 1986).

The patients were not informed that they were taking part in research or that the injections they received were live cancer cells. In addition, the Jewish Chronic Disease Hospital Institutional Review Board never reviewed the study; even the physicians caring for the patients were unaware that the study was being conducted. The physician directing the research was

an employee of the Sloan-Kettering Institute for Cancer Research, and there was no indication that this institution had reviewed the research project (Hershey & Miller, 1976). The research project had the potential to cause the human subjects serious or irreversible harm and possibly death.

Other Unethical Studies

In 1966, Henry Beecher published a now classic article describing 22 of the 50 examples of unethical or questionably ethical studies that he had identified in the published literature. The examples, which included the Willowbrook and Jewish Chronic Disease Hospital studies, indicated a variety of ethical problems that were relatively widespread. Consent was mentioned in only 2 of the 50 studies, and many of the investigators had unnecessarily risked the health and lives of their subjects. Beecher (1966, p. 1356) believed that many of the abuses in the research were due to "thoughtlessness and carelessness, not a willful disregard of patients' rights." These studies reinforce the importance of conscientious institutional review and ethical researcher conduct.

U.S. Department of Health, Education, and Welfare Regulations

The continued conduct of harmful, unethical research made additional controls necessary. In 1973, the DHEW published its first set of regulations intended to protect human subjects. By May 1974, clinical researchers were presented with strict regulations for research involving humans, with additional regulations to protect persons having limited capacities to consent, such as the ill, mentally impaired, and dying (Levine, 1986).

In the 1970s, researchers went from a few vague regulations to almost overwhelming guidelines. All research involving human subjects had to undergo full institutional review, even nursing studies that involved minimal or no risks to the human subjects. Institutional review improved the protection of human subjects; however, reviewing all studies, without regard for the degree of risk involved, overwhelmed the review process and greatly prolonged the time required for a study to be approved (Levine, 1986).

National Commission for the Protection of Human Subjects of Biomedical and Behavioral Research

Because the DHEW regulations far from resolved the issue of protecting human subjects in research, the National Commission for the Protection of Human

Subjects of Biomedical and Behavioral Research (1978) was formed. This commission was established by the National Research Act (Public Law 93-348) passed in 1974. The goals of the commission were (1) to identify the basic ethical principles that should underlie the conduct of biomedical and behavioral research involving human subjects and (2) to develop guidelines based on these principles.

The commission developed *The Belmont Report*, which identified three ethical principles as relevant to research involving human subjects: the principles of respect for persons, beneficence, and justice. The principle of respect for persons holds that persons have the right to self-determination and the freedom to participate or not participate in research. The principle of beneficence requires the researcher to do good and "above all, do no harm." The principle of justice holds that human subjects should be treated fairly. The ethical principles in this report continue to influence the conduct of ethical research in the United States and internationally. This commission developed ethical research guidelines based on these three principles, made recommendations to the U.S. Department of Health and Human Services (U.S. DHHS), and was dissolved in 1978 (National Commission for the Protection of Human Subjects of Biomedical and Behavioral Research, 1978).

In response to the commission's recommendations, in 1981 the U.S. DHHS developed a set of federal regulations to protect human research subjects, and these regulations were revised over the years (U.S. DHHS, 1981, 1983, 1991, 2001, 2005). The most current 2005 regulations are part of the Code of Federal Regulations (CFR), Title 45, Part 46, Protection of Human Subjects. These regulations are interpreted by the Office for Human Research Protection (OHRP), an agency within U.S. DHHS, whose functions are described online at www.hhs.gov/ohrp. These regulations provide direction for (1) the protection of human subjects in research, with additional protection for pregnant women, human fetuses, neonates, children, and prisoners; (2) the documentation of informed consent; and (3) the implementation of the institutional review board process (U.S. DHHS, 2005). These regulations apply to all research involving human subjects in the following areas: (1) studies conducted, supported, or otherwise subject to regulations by any federal department or agency; (2) research conducted in educational settings; (3) research involving the use of educational tests, survey procedures, interview procedures, or observation; and (4) research involving the collection or study of existing data, documents, records, pathological specimens, or diagnostic specimens.

Most of the biomedical and behavioral research conducted in the United States is governed by the U.S. DHHS Protection of Human Subjects Regulations (U.S. DHHS, 2005) or the U.S. Food and Drug Administration (FDA) (see www.fda.gov/oc/gcp). The FDA, within the U.S. DHHS, manages the CFR Title 21, Food and Drugs, Part 50, Protection of Human Subjects, and Part 56, Institutional Review Boards. The FDA has additional human subject protection regulations that apply to clinical investigations involving products regulated by the FDA under the Federal Food, Drug, and Cosmetic Act and research that supports applications for research or marketing permits for these products. Thus, these regulations apply to studies of drugs for humans, medical devices for human use, biological products for human use, human dietary supplements, and electronic products and can be viewed online at www.fda.gov/oc/gcp/regulations.html. The physician and nurse researchers conducting clinical trials to generate new drugs and refine existing drug treatments must comply with these FDA regulations. These regulations focus on the protection of human subjects' rights, informed consent (FDA, 2006b), and institutional review boards (FDA, 2006b), with content that is consistent with Title 45, Public Welfare, Part 46, Protection of Human Subjects (U.S. DHHS, 2005).

The U.S. DHHS and FDA regulations provide guidelines to protect subjects in federally and privately funded research by ensuring that their privacy and the confidentiality of the information obtained through research. However, with the advent of electronic access and transfer, the public has become concerned about the potential abuses of the health information of individuals in all circumstances, including research projects. Thus, Public Law 104-191, the Health Insurance Portability and Accountability Act (HIPAA), was enacted in 1996 and implemented in 2003 to protect an individual's health information. The U.S. DHHS developed regulations titled the Standards for Privacy of Individually Identifiable Health Information, and compliance with these regulations is known as the Privacy Rule (U.S. DHHS, 2002, 45 CFR Parts 160 and 164). The HIPAA Privacy Rule established the category of protected health information (PHI), which allows covered entities, such as health plans, health care clearinghouses, and health care providers that transmit health information, to use or disclose PHI to others only in certain situations. These situations are discussed later in this chapter.

The HIPAA Privacy Rule affects not only the health care environment but also the research conducted in this environment. An individual must provide his or her signed permission, or authorization, before his or her PHI can be used or disclosed for research purposes. Researchers must modify their current studies and develop their new research projects to comply with the HIPAA Privacy Rule. The U.S. DHHS developed a website, "HIPAA Privacy Rule: Information for Researchers," to address the impact of this rule on the informed consent and institutional review board processes in research and to answer common questions about the HIPAA (see http://privacyruleandresearch. nih.gov). The full impact of the privacy rule on the protection of individuals' privacy and on the conduct of research is yet to be determined (Conner, Smaldone, Bratts, & Stone, 2003; Olsen, 2003); however, you can view the privacy rule enforcement highlights online at www.hhs.gov/ocr/privacy/enforcement.

In summary, Table 9-2 was developed to clarify the overall objectives and applicability of the HIPAA Privacy Rule, U.S. DHHS Protection of Human Subjects Regulations Title 45 CFR Part 46, and FDA Protection of Human Subjects Regulations Title 21 CFR Parts 50 and 56 (U.S. DHHS, 2007, February 2, b). The specifics of these regulations are discussed later in this chapter in the sections on protecting human rights, obtaining informed consent, and institutional review.

PROTECTION OF HUMAN RIGHTS

Human rights are claims and demands that have been justified in the eyes of an individual or by the consensus of a group of individuals. Having rights is necessary for the self-respect, dignity, and health of an individual (Sasson & Nelson, 1971). Researchers and reviewers of research have an ethical responsibility to recognize and protect the rights of human research subjects. The human rights that require protection in research are (1) the right to self-determination, (2) the right to privacy, (3) the right to anonymity and confidentiality, (4) the right to fair treatment, and (5) the right to protection from discomfort and harm (American Nurses Association [ANA], 2001; American Psychological Association [APA], 2002). Nurses in other countries have developed similar codes of ethics to protect the rights of their patients and to promote ethical conduct in research (Lin et al., 2007).

Right to Self-Determination
The right to self-determination is based on the ethical principle of respect for persons. This principle holds that because humans are capable of self-determination, or controlling their own destiny, they should be treated as autonomous agents who have the freedom to conduct their lives as they choose without

TABLE 9-2 ‖ Clarification of the Focus of Federal Regulations and Impact on Research			
Area of Distinction	**HIPAA Privacy Rule**	**U.S. DHHS Protection of Human Subjects Regulations Title 45 CFR Part 46**	**FDA Protection of Human Subjects Regulations Title 21 CFR Parts 50 and 56**
Overall objective	Establish a federal floor of privacy protections for most individually identifiable health information by establishing conditions for its use and disclosure by certain health care providers, health plans, and health care clearinghouses.	To protect the rights and welfare of human subjects involved in research conducted or supported by U.S. DHHS. Not specifically a privacy regulation.	To protect the rights, safety, and welfare of subjects involved in clinical investigations regulated by the FDA. Not specifically a privacy regulation.
Applicability	Applies to HIPAA-defined covered entities, regardless of the source of funding.	Applies to human subjects' research conducted or supported by U.S. DHHS and research with private funding.	Applies to research involving products regulated by the FDA. Federal support is not necessary for FDA regulations to be applicable. When research subject to FDA jurisdiction is federally funded, both the U.S. DHHS Protection of Human Subjects Regulations and FDA Protection of Human Subjects Regulations apply.

From U.S. Department of Health and Human Services. (2007, February 2, b). How do other privacy protections interact with the privacy rule? *HIPAA Privacy Rule: Information for researchers.* Retrieved October 1, 2007, from http://privacyruleandresearch.nih.gov/pr_05.asp.

external controls. As a researcher, you treat prospective subjects as autonomous agents by informing them about a proposed study and allowing them to voluntarily choose to participate or not. In addition, subjects have the right to withdraw from a study at any time without a penalty (Levine, 1986). Conducting research ethically requires that research subjects' right to self-determination not be violated and that persons with diminished autonomy have additional protection during the conduct of studies.

Preventing Violation of Research Subjects' Right to Self-Determination

A subject's right to self-determination can be violated through the use of (1) coercion, (2) covert data collection, and (3) deception. Coercion occurs when, one person intentionally presents another with an overt threat of harm or the lure of excessive reward to obtain his or her compliance (National Commission for the Protection of Human Subjects of Biomedical and Behavioral Research, 1978). Some subjects are coerced to participate in research because they fear that they will suffer harm or discomfort if they do not participate. For example, some patients believe that their medical or nursing care will be negatively affected if they do not agree to be research subjects. Sometimes students feel forced to participate in research to protect their grades or prevent negative relationships with the faculty conducting the research. Other subjects are coerced to participate in studies because they believe that they cannot refuse the excessive rewards offered, such as large sums of money, specialized health care, special privileges, and jobs. Most nursing studies do not offer excessive rewards to subjects for participating. A few nursing studies have included a small financial reward of $10 to $20 or support for transportation to increase participation, but this usually would not be considered coercive.

An individual's right to self-determination can also be violated if he or she becomes a research subject without realizing it. Some researchers have exposed persons to experimental treatments without their knowledge, a prime example being the Jewish Chronic Disease Hospital study. Most of the patients and their physicians were unaware of the study. The subjects were informed that they were receiving an injection of cells, but the word *cancer* was omitted (Beecher, 1966). With covert data collection, subjects are unaware that research data are being collected because the investigator develops "descriptions of natural phenomena using information that is provided as a matter of normal activity" (Reynolds, 1979, p. 76). This type of data collection has more commonly been used by

psychologists to describe human behavior in a variety of situations, but it has also been used by nursing and other disciplines (APA, 2002). Qualitative researchers have debated this issue, and some believe that certain group and individual behaviors are unobservable within the normal ethical range of research activities, such as the actions of cults or the aggressive or violent behaviors of individuals (Grbich, 1999). However, covert data collection is considered unethical when research deals with sensitive aspects of an individual's behavior, such as illegal conduct, sexual behavior, or drug use (U.S. DHHS, 2005). With the HIPAA Privacy Rule (U.S. DHHS, 2002), the use of any type of covert data collection would be questionable and illegal if PHI data were being used or disclosed.

The use of deception in research can also violate a subject's right to self-determination. Deception is the actual misinforming of subjects for research purposes (Kelman, 1967). A classic example of deception is the Milgram (1963) study, in which the subjects thought they were administering electric shocks to another person. The subjects were unaware that the person was really a professional actor who pretended to feel the shocks. Some subjects experienced severe mental tension, almost to the point of collapse, because of their participation in this study. The use of deception still occurs in some health care, social, and psychological investigations, but it is a controversial research activity (Grbich, 1999). If deception is to be used in a study, you must determine that there is no other way to get the essential research data needed and that the subjects will not be harmed. In addition, the subjects must be informed of the deception once the study is completed, and you must provide them with full disclosure of the study that was conducted (U.S. DHHS, 2005).

Protecting Persons with Diminished Autonomy

Some persons have diminished autonomy or are vulnerable and less advantaged because of legal or mental incompetence, terminal illness, or confinement to an institution (Levine, 1986). These persons require additional protection of their right to self-determination, because they have a decreased ability, or an inability, to give informed consent. In addition, these persons are vulnerable to coercion and deception. The U.S. DHHS (2005) has identified certain vulnerable groups of individuals, including pregnant women, human fetuses, neonates, children, mentally incompetent persons, and prisoners, who require additional protection in the conduct of research. Researchers need to justify their use of subjects with diminished autonomy in a study, and the need for justification increases as the subjects' risk and vulnerability increase. However, in many situations, the knowledge needed to provide evidence-based care to these vulnerable populations can be gained only by studying them.

Legally and Mentally Incompetent Subjects. Neonates and children (minors), the mentally impaired, and unconscious patients are legally or mentally incompetent to give informed consent. These individuals lack the ability to comprehend information about a study and to make decisions regarding participation in or withdrawal from the study. Their vulnerability ranges from minimal to absolute. The use of persons with diminished autonomy as research subjects is more acceptable if (1) the research is therapeutic so that the subjects have the potential to benefit directly from the experimental process, (2) the researcher is willing to use both vulnerable and nonvulnerable individuals as subjects, (3) preclinical and clinical studies have been conducted and provide data for assessing potential risks to subjects, and (4) the risk is minimized and the consent process is strictly followed to secure the rights of the prospective subjects (Levine, 1986; U.S. DHHS, 2005).

Neonates. A neonate is defined as a newborn and is identified as either viable or nonviable on delivery. Viable neonates are able to survive after delivery, if given the benefit of available medical therapy, and can independently maintain a heartbeat and respiration. "A nonviable neonate means that a newborn after delivery, although living, is not viable" (U.S. DHHS, 2005, 45 CFR Section 46.202). Neonates are extremely vulnerable and require extra protection to determine their involvement in research. However, your research may involve viable neonates, neonates of uncertain viability, and nonviable neonates if the following conditions are met: (1) your study is scientifically appropriate and the preclinical and clinical studies have been conducted and provide data for assessing the potential risks to the neonates; (2) your study provides important biomedical knowledge, which cannot be obtained by other means and will not add risk to the neonate; (3) your research has the potential to enhance the probability of survival of the neonate; (4) both parents are fully informed about your research during the consent process; and (5) your research team will have no part in determining the viability of the neonate. In addition, for the "nonviable neonates, the vital functions of the neonate should not be artificially maintained because of the research and the research should not terminate the heartbeat or respiration of the neonate" (U.S. DHHS, 2005, 45 CFR Section 46.205).

Holditch-Davis, Brandon, and Schwartz (2003) conducted a study of preterm infants to increase the understanding of their behaviors related to sleeping and waking and to their infant characteristics and illness severity. The ethical aspects of the study were described as follows: "The study was approved by the institutional committee for protection of human subjects. Infants were enrolled as soon as their medical conditions were no longer critical if an additional hospital stay of at least 1 week was anticipated and informed consent was obtained from the parents" (p. 310). "All other infants, including those with intraventricular hemorrhage, were eligible so that the sample would be representative of preterm infants in intensive care units" (p. 309).

Holditch-Davis et al. (2003) obtained IRB approval for their study and parental consent. They also attempted to ensure that the neonates' conditions were stable to decrease the risks related to the study. They included a variety of neonates with different types of illnesses to increase the representativeness of the sample. All of these activities promoted the ethical conduct of this study according to the U.S. DHHS (2005) regulations.

Children. The unique vulnerability of children makes the decision to include them as research subjects particularly important. To safeguard their interests and protect them from harm, special ethical and regulatory considerations have been put in place for research involving children (Title 45, CFR 46 Subpart D). However, the laws defining the minor status of a child are statutory and vary from state to state. Often a child's competency to consent is governed by age, with incompetence being nonrefutable up to age 7 years (Broome, 1999; Thompson, 1987). Thus, a child younger than 7 years is not believed to be mature enough to assent or consent to research. Developmentally by age 7, a child is capable of concrete operations of thought and can give meaningful assent to participate as a subject in studies (Thompson, 1987). With advancing age and maturity, a child should have a stronger role in the consent process.

To obtain informed consent, federal regulations require both "soliciting the assent of the children (when capable) and the permission of their parents or guardians" (U.S. DHHS, 2005, 45 CFR Section 46.408). "Assent means a child's affirmative agreement to participate in research. Permission to participate in a study means the agreement of parents or guardian to the participation of their child or ward in research" (U.S. DHHS, 2005, 45 CFR Section 46.402). If a child does not assent to participate in the study, he or she should not be included as a subject even if parental permission is obtained.

Using children as research subjects is also influenced by the therapeutic nature of the research and the

TABLE 9-3 ■ Guide to Obtaining Informed Consent Based on the Relationship between a Child's Level of Competence, the Therapeutic Nature of the Research, and Risk versus Benefit

	Nontherapeutic		Therapeutic	
	MMR-LB	MR-LB	MR-HB	MMR-HB
Child, incompetent (general 0–6 yr)				
Parents' consent	Necessary	Necessary	Sufficient*	Sufficient
Child's assent	Optional†	Optional†	Optional	
Child, relatively competent (7 yr and older)				
Parents' consent	Necessary	Necessary	Sufficient‡	Recommended
Child's assent	Necessary	Necessary	Sufficient§	Sufficient

From Thompson, P. J. (1987). Protection of the rights of children as subjects for research. *Journal of Pediatric Nursing, 2*(6): 397.

* A parent's refusal can be superseded by the principle that a parent has no power to forbid the saving of a child's life.

† Children making "deliberate objection" would be precluded from participation by most researchers.

‡ In cases not involving the privacy rights of a "mature minor."

§ In cases involving the privacy rights of a "mature minor."

MMR, More than minimal risk; MR, minimal risk; LB, low benefit; HB, high benefit.

risks versus the benefits. Thompson (1987) developed a guide for obtaining informed consent that is based on the child's level of competence, the therapeutic nature of the research, and the risks versus the benefits (Table 9-3). Children who are experiencing a developmental delay, cognitive deficit, emotional disorder, or physical illness must be considered individually (Broome, 1999; Broome & Stieglitz, 1992).

A child 7 years or older with normal cognitive development can provide assent or dissent to participation in a study, and the process for obtaining the assent should be included in the research proposal. In the assenting process, the child must be given developmentally appropriate information on the study purpose, expectations, and the benefit-risk ratio (discussed later). Videotapes, written materials, demonstrations, diagrams, role-modeling, and peer discussions are methods for communicating study information. The child also needs an opportunity to sign an assent form and to have a copy of this form. An example assent form is presented in Table 9-4. During the study, you must give the child the opportunity to ask questions and to withdraw from the study if he or she desires (Broome, 1999). Assent becomes more complex if the child is bilingual, because the researchers must determine the most appropriate language to use for the consent process for the child and the parents. Holaday, Gonzales, and Mills (2007) included a list of seven questions in their article to assist researchers in determining the language for communication during a study.

In addition to the assent of the child, you must obtain permission from the child's parent or guardian

for the child's participation in a study. In studies of minimal risk, permission from one parent is usually sufficient for the research to be conducted. For research that involves more than minimal risk and has no prospect of direct benefit to the individual subject, "both parents must give their permission unless one parent is deceased, unknown, incompetent, or not reasonably available, or when only one parent has legal responsibility for the care and custody of the child" (U.S. DHHS, 2005, 45 CFR Section 46.408b).

Pregnant Women. Pregnant women require additional protection in research because of the fetus. Federal regulations define *pregnancy* as encompassing the period of time from implantation until delivery. "A woman is assumed to be pregnant if she exhibits any of the pertinent presumptive signs of pregnancy, such as missed menses, until the results of a pregnancy test are negative or until delivery" (U.S. DHHS, 2005, 45 CFR Section 46.202). Research conducted with pregnant women should have the potential to directly benefit the woman or the fetus. If your investigation is thought to provide a direct benefit only to the fetus, you must obtain the consent of the pregnant woman and father. Studies with "pregnant women should include no inducements to terminate the pregnancy and the researcher should have no part in any decision to terminate a pregnancy" (U.S. DHHS, 2005, 45 CFR Section 46.204).

Adults. Because of mental illness, cognitive impairment, or a comatose state, certain adults are incompetent and incapable of giving informed consent. Persons are said to be incompetent if, in the judgment

TABLE 9-4	Sample Assent Form for Children Ages 6 To 12 Years: Pain Interventions for Children with Cancer

Oral Explanation

I am a nurse who would like to know if relaxation, special ways of breathing, and using your mind to think pleasant things help children like you to feel less afraid and feel less hurt when the doctor has to do a bone marrow aspiration or spinal tap. Today, and the next five times you and your parent come to the clinic, I would like for you to answer some questions about the things in the clinic that scare you. I would also like you to tell me about how much pain you felt during the bone marrow or spinal tap. In addition, I would like to videotape (take pictures of) you and your mom and/or dad during the tests. The second time you visit the clinic I would like to meet with you and teach you special ways to relax, breathe, and use your mind to imagine pleasant things. You can use the special imagining and breathing then during your visits to the clinic. I would ask you and your parent to practice the things I teach you at home between your visits to the clinic. At any time you could change your mind and not be in the study anymore.

To Child

1. I want to learn special ways to relax, breathe, and imagine.
2. I want to answer questions about things children may be afraid of when they come to the clinic.
3. I want to tell you how much pain I feel during the tests I have.
4. I will let you videotape me while the doctor does the tests (bone marrow and spinal taps).
If the child says YES, have him/her put an "X" here. _____
If the child says NO, have him/her put an "X" here. _____
Date: _____
Child's signature _____

From Broome, M. E. (1999). Consent (assent) for research with pediatric patients. *Seminars in Oncology Nursing, 15*(2): 101.

of a qualified clinician, they have attributes that ordinarily provide the grounds for designating incompetence (Levine, 1986). Incompetence can be temporary (e.g., inebriation), permanent (e.g., advanced senile dementia), or subjective or transitory (e.g., behavior or symptoms of psychosis).

If an individual is judged incompetent and incapable of consent, you must seek approval from the prospective subject and his or her legally authorized representative. A legally authorized representative means an individual or other body authorized under applicable law to consent on behalf of a prospective subject to the subject's participation in the procedure(s) involved in the research (Levine, 1986). However, individuals can be judged incompetent and can still assent to participate in certain minimal-risk research if they have the ability to understand what they are being asked to do, to make reasonably free choices, and to communicate their choices clearly and unambiguously.

Happ et al. (2007) conducted an ethnographic study to describe family members' and clinicians' interactions with intensive care unit (ICU) patients during their weaning from long-term mechanical ventilation (LTMV). Because some of the ICU patients were incompetent to give informed consent, the researchers obtained their assent if possible and their proxies' or guardians' permission for participation in the study. The following excerpt from this study will guide you in protecting the rights of persons with diminished autonomy by (1) obtaining institutional review board (IRB) approval for your study, (2) ensuring the privacy of patients during data collection, and (3) obtaining informed consent for all study participants based on their physical and mental capabilities.

> The study was approved by the University of Pittsburgh Institutional Review Board.... All patient rooms were private, with the exception of one semiprivate room.... Potential patient participants were identified by ICU clinicians and during rounds with attending physicians and acute care nurse practitioners. Informed consent for participants was obtained from patients, if they were capable of making decisions, or their proxies. Family members ($n = 41$) were enrolled as participants and signed informed consents were usually gathered in conjunction with patient enrollment. Thirty-one enrolled family members (ages 27–74 years) participated in interviews. Clinicians received written and verbal information about the study; 31 clinicians were selected and signed informed consents to participate in interviews on the basis of their involvement in the care of study patients. (Happ et al., 2007, p. 48)

A growing number of people have become permanently incompetent from the advanced stages of senile dementia of the Alzheimer type (SDAT). A minimum of 60% of nursing home residents have this condition (Floyd, 1988). Most long-term care settings have no IRB for research, and the families or guardians of patients in such settings are reluctant to give consent for the patients' participation in research. Nursing research is needed to establish evidence-based interventions for comforting and caring for individuals with SDAT. Thus, there is a need to expand the development of IRBs in long-term care settings and the use of client advocates to assist in the consent process. Levine (1986) identified two approaches that families, guardians, researchers, or institutional review board might use when making decisions on behalf of these incompetent individuals: (1) best interest standard and (2) substituted judgment standard. The best interest standard involves doing what is best for the individual on the basis of balancing risks and benefits. The substituted judgment standard is concerned with determining the course of action that incompetent individuals would take if they were capable of making a choice.

Terminally Ill Subjects. When conducting research on terminally ill subjects, you should determine (1) who will benefit from the research and (2) whether it is ethical to conduct research on individuals who might not benefit from the study (U.S. DHHS, 2005). Participating in research could have greater risks and minimal or no benefits for these subjects. In addition, the dying subject's condition could affect the study results and lead you to misinterpret the results (Watson, 1982). However, Hinds, Burghen, and Pritchard (2007) stressed the importance of conducting end-of-life studies in pediatric oncology to generate evidence that will improve the care for terminally ill children and adolescents and their families.

Some terminally ill individuals are willing subjects because they believe that participating in research is a way to contribute to society before they die. Others want to take part in research because they believe that the experimental process will benefit them. People with acquired immunodeficiency syndrome (AIDS) often want to participate in AIDS research to gain access to experimental drugs and hospitalized care. However, researchers are concerned because some of these individuals do not comply with the research protocol (Arras, 1990). This is a serious dilemma for researchers studying a population with any type of serious or terminal illness, because they must consider the rights of the subjects and be responsible for conducting high-quality research.

Subjects Confined to Institutions. Hospitalized patients have diminished autonomy because they are ill and are confined in settings that are controlled by health care personnel (Levine, 1986). Some hospitalized patients feel obliged to be research subjects because they want to assist a particular practitioner (nurse or physician) with his or her research. Others feel coerced to participate because they fear that their care will be adversely affected if they refuse. Some of these hospitalized patients are survivors of trauma (such as auto accidents, gunshot wounds, or physical and sexual abuse) who are very vulnerable and often have decreased decision-making capacities (McClain, Laughon, Steeves, & Parker, 2007). When conducting research with these types of patients, you must pay careful attention to the informed consent process and make every effort to protect these subjects from feelings of coercion and harm.

In the past, prisoners have experienced diminished autonomy in research projects because of their confinement. They might feel coerced to participate in research because they fear harm if they refuse or because they desire the benefits of early release, special treatment, or monetary gain. Prisoners have been used for drug studies in which there were no health-related benefits and there was possible harm for the prisoners (Levine, 1986). Current regulations regarding research involving prisoners require that "the risks involved in the research are commensurate with risks that would be accepted by nonprisoner volunteers and procedures for the selection of subjects within the prison are fair to all prisoners and immune from arbitrary intervention by prison authorities or prisoners" (U.S. DHHS, 2005, 45 CFR Section 46.305a).

Protecting subjects' rights with diminished autonomy in research is regulated in many other countries as well. In Canada, the ethical conduct of research is governed by the Tri-Council Policy Statement on "Ethical Conduct for Research Involving Human Subjects" (Canadian Institutes of Health Research, Natural Sciences and Engineering Research Council of Canada, and Social Sciences and Humanities Research Council of Canada, 2005). The Council for International Organizations of Medical Sciences (CIOMS) (2002) developed international ethical guidelines for biomedical research involving human subjects, and the guidelines require protection of vulnerable individuals, groups, communities, and populations during research. In summary, researchers must evaluate each prospective subject's capacity for self-determination and protect subjects with diminished autonomy during the research process.

Right to Privacy

Privacy is an individual's right to determine the time, extent, and general circumstances under which personal information will be shared with or withheld from others. This information consists of one's attitudes, beliefs, behaviors, opinions, and records. An individual's privacy was initially protected by the Privacy Act of 1974. As a result of this act, data collection methods were to be scrutinized to protect subjects' privacy, and data cannot be gathered from subjects without their knowledge. Individuals also have the right to access their records and to prevent access by others (U.S. DHHS, 2002, 2005). The intent of this act was to prevent the invasion of privacy that occurs when private information is shared without an individual's knowledge or against his or her will. Invading an individual's privacy might cause loss of dignity, friendships, or employment or create feelings of anxiety, guilt, embarrassment, or shame.

The HIPAA Privacy Rule expanded the protection of an individual's privacy, specifically his or her protected individually identifiable health information, and described the ways in which covered entities can use or disclose this information. Covered entities are the individual's health care provider, health plan, employer, and health care clearinghouse (public or private entity that processes or facilitates the processing of health information). Individually identifiable health information (IIHI)

> is information that is a subset of health information, including demographic information collected from an individual, and: (1) Is created or received by healthcare provider, health plan, or healthcare clearinghouse; and (2) Related to past, present, or future physical or mental health or condition of an individual, the provision of health care to an individual, or the past, present, or future payment for the provision of health care to an individual, and that identifies the individual; or with respect to which there is a reasonable basis to believe that the information can be used to identify the individual. (U.S. DHHS, 2002, 45 CFR, Section 160.103)

According to the HIPAA Privacy Rule, the IIHI is protected health information (PHI) that is transmitted by electronic media, maintained in electronic media, or transmitted or maintained in any other form or medium. Thus, the HIPAA privacy regulations affect nursing research in the following ways: (1) accessing data from a covered entity, such as reviewing a patient's medical record in clinics or hospitals; (2) developing health information, such as the data developed when an intervention is implemented in a study to improve a subject's health; and (3) disclosing data from a study to a colleague in another institution, such as sharing data from a study to facilitate development of an instrument or scale (Olsen, 2003).

The U.S. DHHS developed guidelines to help researchers, health care organizations, and health care providers determine when they can use and disclose IIHI. IIHI can be used or disclosed to a researcher in the following situations:

- The protected health information has been "de-identified" under the HIPAA Privacy Rule. (De-identifying PHI is defined in the following section.)
- The data are part of a limited data set, and a data use agreement with the researcher(s) is in place.
- The individual who is a potential subject for a study authorizes the researcher to use and disclose his or her PHI.
- A waiver or alteration of the authorization requirement is obtained from an IRB or a privacy board (U.S. DHHS, 2007, February 2, a) (see http://privacyruleandresearch.nih.gov/pr_08.asp).

The first two items are discussed in this section of the text. The authorization process is discussed in the section on obtaining informed consent, and the waiver or alteration of authorization requirement is covered in the section on understanding institutional review.

De-identifying Protected Health Information under the Privacy Rule

Covered entities, such as health care providers and agencies, can allow researchers access to health information if the information has been de-identified. De-identifying health data involves removing the 18 elements that could be used to identify an individual or his or her relatives, employer, or household members. The 18 identifying elements are as follows (U.S. DHHS, 2007 February 2, a):

1. Names
2. All geographic subdivisions smaller than a state, including street address, city, county, precinct, zip code, and their equivalent geographical codes, except for the initial three digits of a zip code if, according to the current publicly available data from the Bureau of the Census:
   a. The geographical unit formed by combining all zip codes with the same three initial digits contains more than 20,000 people
   b. The initial three digits of a zip code for all such geographical units containing 20,000 or fewer people are changed to 000
3. All elements of dates (except year) for dates directly related to an individual, including birth date, admission date, discharge date, date of death; and all ages over 89 and all elements of

dates (including year) indicative of such age, except that such ages and elements may be aggregated into a single category of age 90 or older
4. Telephone numbers
5. Facsimile numbers
6. Electronic mail (e-mail) addresses
7. Social security numbers
8. Medical record numbers
9. Health plan beneficiary numbers
10. Account numbers
11. Certificate/license numbers
12. Vehicle identifiers and serial numbers, including license plate numbers
13. Device identifiers and serial numbers
14. Web universal resource locators (URLs)
15. Internet protocol (IP) address numbers
16. Biometric identifiers, including fingerprints and voiceprints
17. Full-face photographic images and any comparable images
18. Any other unique identifying number, characteristic, or code, unless otherwise permitted by the Privacy Rule for re-identification

An individual's health information can also be de-identified using statistical methods. However, the covered entity and you as the researcher must ensure that the individual subject cannot be identified or that there is a very small risk that the subject could be identified from the information used. The statistical method used for de-identification of the health data must be documented, and you must certify that the 18 elements for identification have been removed or revised to ensure that individual is not identified. You must retain this certification information for 6 years.

Limited Data Set and Data Use Agreement
Covered entities (health care provider, health plan, and health care clearinghouse) may use and disclose a limited data set to a researcher for a study without an individual subject's authorization or an IRB waiver. However, a limited data set is considered protected health information, and the covered entity and the researcher must have a data use agreement. The data use agreement limits how the data set may be used and how it will be protected. The HIPAA Privacy Rule requires the data use agreement to do the following (U.S. DHHS, 2002):
1. Specifies the permitted uses and disclosures of the limited data set.
2. Identifies the researcher who is permitted to use or receive the limited data set.

3. Stipulates that the recipient (researcher) will
   a. Not use or disclose the information other than permitted by the agreement.
   b. Use appropriate safeguards to prevent the use or disclosure of the information, except as provided for in the agreement.
   c. Hold any other person (co-researchers, statisticians, or data collectors) to the standards, restrictions, and conditions stated in the data use agreement with respect to the health information.
   d. Not identify the information or contact the individuals whose data are in the limited data set.

Right to Autonomy and Confidentiality
On the basis of the right to privacy, the research subject has the right to anonymity and the right to assume that the data collected will be kept confidential. Anonymity exists if the subject's identity cannot be linked, even by the researcher, with his or her individual responses (ANA, 2001; Sasson & Nelson, 1971). For studies that use de-identified health information or data from a limited data set, the subjects will be anonymous to the researcher. You will be unable to contact these subjects for additional information.

In most studies, researchers desire to know the identity of their subjects and promise that their identity will be kept anonymous from others. However, in these situations, you must receive authorization from the potential subject to use his or her health information, or you must have a waiver or an alteration of the authorization requirement from the IRB (see section on institutional review later in this chapter). Confidentiality is the researcher's management of private information shared by a subject that must not be shared with others without the authorization of the subject. Confidentiality is grounded in the following premises:
- Individuals can share personal information to the extent they wish and are entitled to have secrets.
- One can choose with whom to share personal information.
- People who accept information in confidence have an obligation to maintain confidentiality.
- Professionals, such as researchers, have a "duty to maintain confidentiality that goes beyond ordinary loyalty" (Levine, 1986, p. 164; U.S. DHHS, 2005).

Breach of Confidentiality
A breach of confidentiality can occur when a researcher, by accident or direct action, allows an unauthorized person to gain access to the study raw data. Confidentiality can also be breached in the

reporting or publication of a study when a subject's identity is accidentally revealed, violating the subject's right to anonymity (Ramos, 1989). Breaches of confidentiality can harm subjects psychologically and socially, as well as destroy the trust they had in you. Breaches of confidentiality can be especially harmful to a research subject if they involve (1) religious preferences; (2) sexual practices; (3) employment; (4) racial prejudices; (5) drug use; (6) child abuse; and (7) personal attributes, such as intelligence, honesty, and courage.

Some nurse researchers have encountered health care professionals who believe that they should have access to information about the patients in the hospital and will request to see the data the researchers have collected. Sometimes, family members or close friends would like to see the data collected on specific subjects. Sharing research data in these circumstances is a breach of confidentiality. When requesting permission to conduct a study, you should tell health care professionals, family members, and others in the setting that you will not share the raw data. However, you may elect to share the research report, including a summary of the data and findings from the study, with health care providers, family members, and other interested parties.

Maintaining Confidentiality

Researchers have a responsibility to protect the anonymity of subjects and to maintain the confidentiality of data collected during a study. You can protect anonymity by giving each subject a code number. Keep a master list of the subjects' names and their code numbers in a locked place; for example, subject Mary Jones might be assigned the code number "001." All of the instruments and forms that Mary completes and the data you collect about her during the study will be identified with the "001" code number, not her name. The master list of subjects' names and code numbers is best kept separate from the data collected to protect subjects' anonymity. You should not staple signed consent forms and authorization documents to instruments or other data collection tools, as this would make it easy for unauthorized persons to readily identify the subjects and their responses. Consent forms are often stored with the master list of subjects' names and code numbers. When entering the data collected into the computer, use the code numbers for identification. Then lock the original data collection tools in a secure place.

Another way to protect your subjects' anonymity is to have them generate their own identification codes (Damrosch, 1986). With this approach, each subject generates an individual code from personal information, such as the first letter of a mother's name, the first letter of a father's name, the number of brothers, the number of sisters, and middle initial. Thus, the code would be composed of three letters and two numbers, such as "BD21M." This code would be used on each form that the subject completes. Even you as the researcher would not know the subject's identity, only the subject's code. If the data collected are highly sensitive, you might want to use this type of coding system.

The data collected should undergo group analysis so that an individual cannot be identified by his or her responses. If the subjects are divided into groups for data analysis and there is only one subject in a group, combine that subject's data with that of another group or delete the data. In writing the research report, you should describe the findings in such a way that an individual or a group of individuals cannot be identified by their responses.

Maintaining confidentiality is often more difficult in qualitative research than in quantitative research. The nature of qualitative research requires that the "investigator must be close enough to understand the depth of the question under study, and must present enough direct quotes and detailed description to answer the question" (Ramos, 1989, p. 60). The small number of participants used in a qualitative study and the depth of detail gathered on each participant make it difficult to disguise the participant's identity. Ford and Reutter (1990) have recommended that to maintain confidentiality, the researcher should (1) use pseudonyms instead of the participants' names and (2) distort certain details in the participants' stories while leaving the contents unchanged. You must respect participants' privacy as they decide how much detail and editing of private information are necessary to publish a study (Munhall, 2001a; Orb, Eisenhauer, & Wynaden, 2001).

Researchers should also take precautions during data collection to maintain confidentiality. The interviews conducted with participants are frequently taped and later transcribed, so the participant's name should not be mentioned on the tape. They have the right to know whether anyone other than you will be transcribing information from the interview. In addition, participants should be informed on an ongoing basis that they have the right to withhold information. To critique the rigor and credibility of qualitative research, produce an audit trail so that another researcher could examine the data to confirm the study findings. This process might create a dilemma regarding the confidentiality of participants' data, so you must inform them if other researchers will be examining their data to ensure the credibility of the study findings (Munhall, 2001a; Orb et al., 2001).

Right to Fair Treatment

The right to fair treatment is based on the ethical principle of justice. This principle holds that each person should be treated fairly and should receive what he or she is due or owed. In research, the selection of subjects and their treatment during the course of a study should be fair.

Fair Selection of Subjects

In the past, injustice in subject selection has resulted from social, cultural, racial, and sexual biases in society. For many years, research was conducted on categories of individuals who were thought to be especially suitable as research subjects, such as the poor, charity patients, prisoners, slaves, peasants, dying persons, and others who were considered undesirable (Reynolds, 1979). Researchers often treated these subjects carelessly and had little regard for the harm and discomfort they experienced. The Nazi medical experiments, Tuskegee Syphilis Study, and Willowbrook study all exemplify unfair subject selection and treatment.

The selection of a population and the specific subjects to study should be fair, and the risks and benefits of a study should be fairly distributed on the basis of the subject's efforts, needs, and rights. Subjects should be selected for reasons directly related to the problem being studied and not for "their easy availability, their compromised position, or their manipulability" (National Commission for the Protection of Human Subjects of Biomedical and Behavioral Research, 1978, p. 10).

Another concern with subject selection is that some researchers select certain people as subjects because they like them and want them to receive the specific benefits of a study. Other researchers have been swayed by power or money to make certain individuals subjects so that they can receive potentially beneficial treatments. Random selection of subjects can eliminate some of the researcher bias that might influence subject selection.

A current concern in the conduct of research is finding an adequate number of appropriate subjects to take part in certain studies. As a solution to this problem in the past, some biomedical researchers have offered physicians a finder's fee for identifying research subjects. For example, investigators studying patients with lung cancer would give a physician a fee for every patient with lung cancer the physician referred

to them. However, the HIPAA Privacy Rule requires that individuals give their authorization before PHI can be shared with others. Thus, health care providers cannot recommend individuals for studies without their permission. Researchers can obtain a partial waiver from the IRB or privacy board so that they can obtain PHI necessary to recruit potential subjects (U.S. DHHS, 2002). This makes it more difficult for researchers to find subjects for their studies; however, researchers are encouraged to work closely with their IRBs to facilitate the conduct of quality studies essential for evidence-based practice.

Fair Treatment of Subjects

Researchers and subjects should have a specific agreement about what the subject's participation involves and what the role of the researcher will be (APA, 2002). While conducting a study, you should treat the subjects fairly and respect that agreement. If the data collection requires appointments with the subjects, be on time for each appointment and terminate the data collection process at the agreed-on time. You should not change the activities or procedures that the subject is to perform unless you obtain the subject's consent.

The benefits promised the subjects should be provided. For example, if you promise a subject a copy of the study findings, you should deliver your promise when the study is completed. In addition, subjects who participate in studies should receive equal benefits, regardless of age, race, and socioeconomic level. When possible, the sample should be representative of the study population and should include subjects of various ages, ethnic backgrounds, and socioeconomic status (Williams, 2002). Treating subjects fairly often facilitates the data collection process and decreases subjects' withdrawal from a study (Orb et al., 2001).

Right to Protection from Discomfort and Harm

The right to protection from discomfort and harm is based on the ethical principle of beneficence, which holds that one should do good and, above all, do no harm. According to this principle, members of society should take an active role in preventing discomfort and harm and promoting good in the world around them (Frankena, 1973). Therefore, researchers should conduct their studies to protect subjects from discomfort and harm and try to bring about the greatest possible balance of benefits in comparison with harm.

Discomfort and harm can be physiological, emotional, social, and economic in nature. Reynolds (1979) identified the following five categories of studies, which are based on levels of discomfort and harm: (1) no anticipated effects, (2) temporary discomfort, (3) unusual levels of temporary discomfort, (4) risk of permanent damage, and (5) certainty of permanent damage. Each level is defined in the following discussion.

No Anticipated Effects

In some studies, the subjects expect neither positive nor negative effects. For example, studies that involve reviewing patients' records, students' files, pathology reports, or other documents have no anticipated effects on the subjects. In these types of studies, the researcher does not interact directly with the research subjects. Even in these situations, however, there is a potential risk of invading a subject's privacy. The HIPAA Privacy Rule requires that the agency providing the health information de-identify the 18 essential elements, which could be used to identify an individual, to promote subjects' privacy during a study.

Temporary Discomfort

Studies that cause temporary discomfort are described as minimal-risk studies, in which the discomfort encountered is similar to what the subject would experience in his or her daily life and ceases with the termination of the study. Many nursing studies require the subjects to complete questionnaires or participate in interviews, which usually involve minimal risk. The physical discomforts might be fatigue, headache, or muscle tension. The emotional and social risks might entail the anxiety or embarrassment associated with responding to certain questions. The economic risks might consist of the time spent participating in the study or travel costs to the study site. Participation in many nursing studies is considered a mere inconvenience for the subject, with no foreseeable risks of harm.

Most clinical nursing studies examining the impact of a treatment involve minimal risk. For example, your study might involve examining the effects of exercise on the blood glucose levels of diabetics. During the study, you ask the subjects to test their blood glucose level one extra time per day. There is discomfort when the blood is drawn and a risk of physical changes that might occur with exercise. The subjects might also experience anxiety and fear in association with the additional blood testing, and the testing is an added expense. The diabetic subjects in this study would experience similar discomforts in their daily lives, and the discomforts would cease with the termination of the study.

Unusual Levels of Temporary Discomfort

In studies that involve unusual levels of temporary discomfort, the subjects commonly experience discomfort both during the study and after its termination. For example, subjects might experience a deep vein thrombosis (DVT), prolonged muscle weakness, joint pain, and dizziness after participating in a study that required them to be confined to bed for 10 days to determine the effects of immobility. Studies that require subjects to experience failure, extreme fear, or threats to their identity or to act in unnatural ways involve unusual levels of temporary discomfort. In some qualitative studies, participants are asked questions that reopen old emotional wounds or involve reliving traumatic events (Ford & Reutter, 1990; Munhall, 2001a). For example, asking participants to describe their rape experience could precipitate feelings of extreme fear, anger, and sadness. In these types of studies, you should be vigilant about assessing the participants' discomfort and should refer them for appropriate professional intervention as necessary.

Risk of Permanent Damage

In some studies, subjects have the potential to suffer permanent damage; this potential is more common in biomedical research than in nursing research. For example, medical studies of new drugs and surgical procedures have the potential to cause subjects permanent physical damage. However, nurses have investigated topics that have the potential to damage subjects permanently, both emotionally and socially. Studies examining sensitive information, such as sexual behavior, child abuse, or drug use, can be risky for subjects. These types of studies have the potential to cause permanent damage to a subject's personality or reputation. There are also potential economic risks, such as reduced job performance or loss of employment.

Certainty of Permanent Damage

In some research, such as the Nazi medical experiments and the Tuskegee Syphilis Study, the subjects experience permanent damage. Conducting research that will permanently damage subjects is highly questionable, regardless of the benefits gained. Frequently, the benefits are for other people but not for the subjects. Studies causing permanent damage to subjects violate the fifth principle of the Nuremberg Code (1986, p. 426), which states, "No experiment should be conducted where there is an a priori reason to believe that death or disabling injury will occur except, perhaps, in those experiments where the experimental physicians (or other health professionals) also serve as subjects."

BALANCING BENEFITS AND RISKS FOR A STUDY

Researchers and reviewers of research must examine the balance of benefits and risks in a study. To determine this balance or benefit-risk ratio, you must (1) predict the outcome of your study, (2) assess the actual and potential benefits and risks on the basis of this outcome, and then (3) maximize the benefits and minimize the risks (see Figure 9-1). The outcome of a study is predicted on the basis of previous research, clinical experience, and theory.

Assessment of Benefits

The probability and magnitude of a study's potential benefits must be assessed.

> *A research benefit is defined as something of health-related, psychosocial, or other value to a subject, or something that will contribute to the acquisition of knowledge for evidence-based practice. Money and other compensations for participation in research are not benefits but, rather, are remuneration for research-related inconveniences. (U.S. DHHS, 2005)*

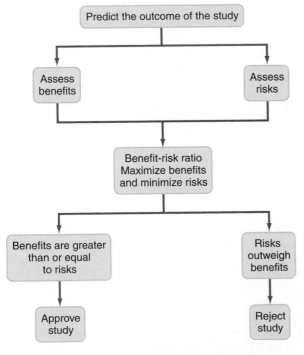

Figure **9-1** Balancing benefits and risks for a study.

In most proposals, the research benefits are described for the individual subjects, subjects' families, and society. Some optimistic researchers overestimate these benefits.

The type of research conducted, whether therapeutic or nontherapeutic, affects the potential benefits for the subjects. In therapeutic nursing research, the individual subject has the potential to benefit from the procedures, such as skin care, range of motion, touch, and other nursing interventions, that are implemented in the study. The benefits might include improvement in the subject's physical condition, which could facilitate emotional and social benefits. In addition, the knowledge generated from the research might expand the subjects' and their families' understanding of health. The conduct of nontherapeutic nursing research does not benefit the subject directly but is important to generate and refine nursing knowledge for practice. By participating in research, subjects have the potential to increase their understanding of the research process and an opportunity to know the findings from a particular study.

Assessment of Risks

You must assess the type, severity, and number of risks that subjects will experience or might experience by participating in your study. The risks involved depend on the purpose of the study and the procedures used to conduct it. Research risks can be physical, emotional, social, and economic in nature and can range from no risk or mere inconvenience to the risk of permanent damage (Levine, 1986; Reynolds, 1979). Studies can have actual (known) risks and potential risks for subjects. In a study of the effects of prolonged bed rest, for example, an actual risk would be muscle weakness and the potential risk would be a DVT. Some studies have actual or potential risks for the subjects' families and society. You must determine the likelihood of the risks and take precautions to protect the rights of subjects when implementing your study.

Benefit-Risk Ratio

The benefit-risk ratio is determined on the basis of the maximized benefits and the minimized risks. The researcher attempts to maximize the benefits and minimize the risks by making changes in the study purpose or procedures or both. If the risks entailed by your study cannot be eliminated or further minimized, you need to justify their existence. If the risks outweigh the benefits, you should revise the study or develop a new study. If the benefits equal or outweigh the risks, you can justify conducting the study, and an institutional review board (IRB) will probably approve it (see Figure 9-1).

Say, for example, that you want to balance the benefits and risks of a study that would examine the effect of an exercise and diet program on the participants' serum lipid values (serum cholesterol, low-density lipoprotein [LDL], and high-density lipoprotein [HDL]) and cardiovascular (CV) risk level. The benefits to the participants are instruction about exercise and diet and information about their serum lipid values and CV risk level at the start of the program and 1 year later. The potential benefits are improved serum lipid values, lowered CV risk level, and better exercise and dietary habits. The risks consist of the discomfort of having blood specimens drawn twice for serum lipid measurements and the time spent participating in the study (Bruce & Grove, 1994). These discomforts are temporary, are no more than what the subject would experience in his or her daily life, and would cease with the termination of the study. The subjects' time participating in the study can be minimized through organization and precise scheduling of research activities. When you examine the ratio of benefits to risks, you find that (1) the benefits are greater in number and importance than the risks and (2) the risks are temporary and can be minimized. Thus, you could justify conducting this study, and it would probably receive approval from the IRB.

The obligation to balance the benefits and risks of studies is the responsibility of the researcher, health professionals, and society. The researcher must balance the benefits and risks of a particular study and protect the subjects from harm during it. Health professionals participate on IRBs to ensure the conduct of ethical research. Society must be concerned with the benefits and risks of the entire enterprise of research and with the protection of all human research subjects from harm.

OBTAINING INFORMED CONSENT

Obtaining informed consent from human subjects is essential for the conduct of ethical research in the United States (FDA, 2006b; U.S. DHHS, 2005) and internationally (CIOMS, 2002; Canadian Institutes of Health Research, Natural Sciences and Engineering Research Council of Canada, Social Sciences and Humanities Research Council of Canada, 2005). Informing is the transmission of essential ideas and content from the investigator to the prospective subject. Consent is the prospective subject's agreement to participate in a study as a subject, which the subject reaches after assimilating essential information. Prospective subjects, to the degree that they are capable, should have the opportunity to choose whether or not to participate in research. The phenomenon of informed consent was formally defined in the first principle of the Nuremberg Code as follows:

> *The voluntary consent of the human subject is absolutely essential.... This means that the person involved should have legal capacity to give consent; should be so situated as to be able to exercise free power of choice, without the intervention of any element of force, fraud, deceit, duress, over-reaching or other ulterior form of constraint or coercion; and should have sufficient knowledge and comprehension of the elements of the subject matter involved as to enable him to make an understanding and enlightened decision. (Nuremberg Code, 1986, p. 425)*

This definition of informed consent provided a basis for the discussion of consent in all subsequent codes and regulations and has general acceptance in the research community. As the definition indicates, informed consent consists of four elements: (1) disclosure of essential information, (2) comprehension, (3) competency, and (4) voluntarism. This section describes the elements of informed consent and the methods of documenting consent.

Information Essential for Consent

Informed consent requires the researcher to disclose specific information to each prospective subject. The following information has been identified as essential content for informed consent in research by CFR 45 Section 46.116 (U.S. DHHS, 2005) and CFR 21 Part 50 (FDA, 2006b).

Introduction of Research Activities

The introduction of the research must indicate that a study is being conducted and provide key information about the study. Each prospective subject is given "a statement that the study involves research, an explanation of the purposes of the research, and the expected duration of the subject's participation" (U.S. DHHS, 2005, CFR 45 Section 46.116). In clinical nursing research, the patient, serving as a subject, must know which nursing activities are research activities and which are routine nursing interventions. If at any point the prospective subjects disagree with your goals or the intent of the study, they can decline participation.

Prospective subjects also need to receive a complete description of the procedures to be followed and identification of any procedures in the study that are experimental (FDA, 2006b; U.S. DHHS, 2005). Thus, you will describe the research variables and the procedures or mechanisms that will be used to observe, examine, manipulate, or measure these variables. In addition, you must inform prospective subjects about when the study procedures will be implemented, how many times, and in what setting.

Description of Risks and Discomforts

Inform prospective subjects about any reasonably foreseeable risks or discomforts (physical, emotional, social, or economic) that might result from the study (FDA, 2006b; U.S. DHHS, 2005). Indicate how the risks of the study have been or will be minimized. If the study involves greater than minimal risk, it is usually a good idea to encourage the prospective subjects to consult another person regarding their participation. A trusted advisor, such as a friend, family member, or another nurse, could serve as a consultant.

Description of Benefits

You should also describe any benefits to the subject or to others that may reasonably be expected from the research (FDA, 2006b; U.S. DHHS, 2005). The study might benefit the current subjects or might generate knowledge that will provide evidence-based care to patients in the future.

Disclosure of Alternatives

You must disclose the "appropriate, alternative procedures or courses of treatment, if any, that might be advantageous to the subject" (U.S. DHHS, 2002, 45 CFR Section 46.116a). For example, the researchers of the Tuskegee Syphilis Study should have informed the subjects with syphilis that penicillin was an effective treatment for their disease.

Assurance of Anonymity and Confidentiality

Prospective subjects must be given a statement describing the extent to which confidentiality of their records will be maintained (FDA, 2006b; U.S. DHHS, 2002, 2005). Thus, your subjects must know that their responses and the information obtained from their records during a study will be kept confidential. You also must assure them that their identity will remain anonymous in presentations, reports, and publications of the study.

Compensation for Participation in Research

For research involving more than minimal risks, the prospective subjects must be given an explanation as to whether any compensation or medical treatments or both are available if injury occurs. If medical treatments are available, describe the type and extent of the treatments. When appropriate, inform the prospective subject as to whether a treatment or procedure may involve potential risks to the subject or her fetus if she is or may become pregnant (FDA, 2006b; U.S. DHHS, 2005).

Offer to Answer Questions

The researcher offers to answer any questions that the prospective subjects may raise. Prospective subjects are provided an "explanation of whom to contact for answers to pertinent questions about the research and research subjects' rights, and whom to contact in the event of a research-related injury" (FDA, 2006b, 21 CFR Section 50.25; U.S. DHHS, 2005, 45 CFR Section 46.116a) as well as a mechanism for contacting that person.

Noncoercive Disclaimer

A noncoercive disclaimer is a statement that participation is voluntary and refusal to participate will involve no penalty or loss of benefits to which the subject is entitled (FDA, 2006b; U.S. DHHS, 2005). This statement can facilitate a relationship between you and your prospective subjects, especially if the relationship has a potential for coercion.

Option to Withdraw

Subjects may discontinue participation or withdraw from a study at any time without penalty or loss of benefits. However, researchers do have the right to ask subjects if they think that they will be able to complete the study, to decrease the number of subjects withdrawing early. There may be circumstances "under which the subject's participation may be terminated by the investigator without regard to the subject's consent" (U.S. DHHS, 2005, 45 CFR Section 46.116b). For example, if a particular treatment becomes potentially dangerous to a subject, you have an obligation to discontinue the subject's participation in the study. Thus, describe for prospective subjects the circumstances under which they might be withdrawn from the study, and make a general statement about the circumstances that could lead to the termination of the entire project.

Consent to Incomplete Disclosure

In some studies, subjects are not completely informed of the study purpose, because that knowledge would alter the subjects' actions. However, prospective subjects must know that certain information is being withheld deliberately. You must ensure that there are no undisclosed risks to the subjects that are more than minimal and truthfully answer the subjects' questions regarding the study. Subjects who are exposed to nondisclosure of information must know when and how they will be debriefed about the study. Debrief the subjects by informing them of the actual purpose of the study and the results that were obtained. If the subjects experience adverse effects related to the study, make every attempt to reconcile the effects (U.S. DHHS, 2005).

Comprehension of Consent Information

Informed consent implies not only the imparting of information by the researcher but also the comprehension of that information by the subject. Studies performed to determine subjects' levels of comprehension after they received the essential information for consent have found the comprehension to be low (Levine, 1986). The amount of information to be taught depends on the subjects' knowledge of research and the specific research project proposed. However, the purpose, benefits, and risks of the study must be presented clearly in the consent form. Subjects need to have a clear understanding of the therapeutic potential of participating in a study. They need to know if the research treatment is going to be nontherapeutic for them but has a potential to benefit future patients.

Federal regulations require that the information given to subjects or their representatives must be in a language they can understand (FDA, 2006b; U.S. DHHS, 2005). Thus, the consent information must be written and verbalized in lay terminology, not professional jargon, and must be presented without the use of loaded or biased terms that might coerce a subject into participating in a study. Meade (1999) identified the following tips for promoting the comprehension of a consent document by potential research subjects:

- Introduce the purpose of the study early in the consent form.
- Outline the study treatment with specificity and conciseness.
- Convey the elements of informed consent in an organized fashion.
- Define technical terms, and be consistent in the use of terminology.
- Use clear terminology, and avoid professional jargon.
- Develop the document using headings, uppercase and lowercase letters, and spacing to make it easy to read.
- Use headings for major elements in the consent form, such as "Purpose," "Benefits," and "Risks."
- Use a readable font, that is, a minimum of 12- to 14-point font for text and a 16- to 18-point font for the headers.
- Address the subject directly, using phrases such as, "You are being asked to take part in this study … "
- Estimate the reading level of the document with the use of a computerized readability formula,

and revise it to achieve no higher than an eighth grade reading level.

Meade (1999) used these tips to simplify a paragraph from an example consent form, as shown in Table 9-5. Once you have developed the consent document, pilot-test it with patients who are comparable to the proposed subjects for the study. These patients can give feedback on the ease of reading, clarity, and understandability of the consent document. You can then revise the document as needed on the basis of the feedback. These guidelines will help you to develop a high-quality consent document that your study subjects can comprehend.

In qualitative research, the participants might comprehend their participation in a study at the beginning, but unexpected events or consequences might occur during the study to obscure that understanding. These events might precipitate a change in the focus of the research and the type of participation by the participants. For example, the topics of an interview might change with an increased need for information from the participants to address these topics. Thus, informed consent is an ongoing, evolving process in qualitative research. The researcher must renegotiate the participants' consent and determine their comprehension of that consent as changes occur in the study. By continually informing and determining the comprehension of participants, you will establish trust with them and promote ethical, high-quality study outcomes (Munhall, 2001a).

Assessment of Subjects' Comprehension

The researcher can take steps to determine the prospective subjects' level of comprehension. Silva (1985) studied the comprehension of information for informed consent by spouses of surgical patients and found that 72 of the 75 spouses adequately comprehended the consent information. Silva assessed the subjects' comprehension of consent information by asking the following questions:

(1) What is the purpose of this study? (2) What risks are involved in the study procedures? (3) What does your participation in this study involve? (4) Approximately how long will your participation in this study take? (5) When can you withdraw from this study? (6) How will your name be associated with the study data? (7) With whom will the study information be shared? and (8) What direct personal benefit will come to you as a result of participating in this study? (Silva, 1985, p. 121)

In complex, high-risk studies, it is more difficult for subjects to comprehend consent information. In some

TABLE 9-5   Simplification of Consent Document

Origin Consent Document

Example A*:

Side effects of the marrow infusion are uncommon and consist primarily of an unusual taste from the preservative, occasional nausea and vomiting, and, rarely, fever and chills. In addition, your chest may feel tight for a while, but that will pass.

Example B†:

The standard approach to treating breast cancer is to give several "cycles" (repeated doses at regularly specified intervals) of a combination of two or more chemotherapy drugs (drugs that kill cancer cells). Recent information suggests that it may be more beneficial to give several cycles of one drug followed by several cycles of another drug. Some researchers think that the second approach may kill more cells that are resistant to chemotherapy. The approach being tested in this study is to administer four cycles of standard chemotherapy (doxorubicin/cyclophosphamide) followed by four cycles of the drug paclitaxel. Researchers hope to show that cancer cells resistant to the doxorubicin/cyclophosphamide chemotherapy may be sensitive to paclitaxel. This may then result in prolonged patient survival and result in a decrease in the number of patients experiencing a recurrence.

Revised Simplified Consent Document

Example A*:

Side effects of getting stem cells:
- An unusual or funny taste in your mouth
- Mild nausea and vomiting
- Fever and chills (rarely)
- Tightness in chest (rarely)

Example B†:

Why is this study being done?
The purpose of this research study is to find out whether adding the drug Taxol (paclitaxel) to a commonly used chemotherapy is better than the commonly used chemotherapy by itself at preventing your cancer from coming back. The study also will see what side effects there are from adding Taxol to the commonly used chemotherapy. Taxol has been found to be effective in treating patients with advanced breast cancer. In this study, we want to see whether Taxol will help to treat patients with early stage breast cancer and whether the side effects seem to be worth the possible benefit.

NCI Model Document Sub-Group: Comprehensive Working Group on Informed Consent, 1998.

* Standard doses versus myeloablative therapy for previously untreated symptomatic multiple myeloma. Phase III. SWOG 9321.

† A randomized trial evaluating the worth of paclitaxel (Taxol) following doxorubicin (Adriamycin)/cyclophosphamide (Cytoxan) in breast cancer.

From "Consent (Assent) for Research with Pediatric Patients," by M.E. Broome, 1999, *Seminars in Oncology Nursing,* 15(2), p. 130.

high-risk studies, the prospective subjects are tested on consent information, and they do not become subjects unless they pass the tests.

Competency to Give Consent

Autonomous individuals, who are capable of understanding and weighing the benefits and risks of a proposed study, are competent to give consent. The competence of the subject is often determined by the researcher (Douglas & Larson, 1986). Persons with diminished autonomy resulting from legal or mental incompetence, terminal illness, or confinement to an institution might not be legally competent to consent to participate in research (see the earlier discussion of the right to self-determination). However, the researcher makes every effort to present the consent information at a level potential subjects can understand, so that they can assent to the research. In addition, the researcher presents the essential information for consent to the legally authorized representative, such as the parents or guardian, of the prospective subject (U.S. DHHS, 2005).

Voluntary Consent

Voluntary consent means that the prospective subject has decided to take part in a study of his or her own volition without coercion or any undue influence. Voluntary consent is obtained after the prospective subject has been given essential information about the study and has shown comprehension of this information (FDA, 2006b; U.S. DHHS, 2005). Some researchers, because of their authority, expertise, or power, have the potential to coerce subjects into participating in research. Researchers must make sure that their persuasion of prospective subjects does not become coercion. Thus, the rewards offered in a study ought to be congruent with the risks taken by the subjects.

Documentation of Informed Consent

The documentation of informed consent depends on (1) the level of risk involved in the study and (2) the discretion of the researcher and those reviewing the study for institutional approval. Most studies require a written consent form, although in some studies, the consent form is waived.

Written Consent Waived

The requirements for written consent may be waived in research that "presents no more than minimal risk of harm to subjects and involves no procedures for which written consent is normally required outside of the research context" (U.S. DHHS, 2005, 45 CFR Section 46.117c). For example, if you were using questionnaires to collect relatively harmless data, you would not need to obtain a signed consent form from the subjects. The subject's completion of the questionnaire may serve as consent. The top of the questionnaire might contain a statement such as "Your completion of this questionnaire indicates your consent to participate in this study."

Written consent is also waived when "the only record linking the subject and the research would be the consent document and the principal risk would be potential harm resulting from a breach of confidentiality. Each subject will be asked whether the subject wants documentation linking the subject with the research, and the subject's wishes will govern" (U.S. DHHS, 2005, 45 CFR Section 46.117c). Thus, in this situation, subjects are given the option to sign or not sign a consent form that links them to the research. The four elements of consent—disclosure, comprehension, competency, and voluntariness—are essential in all studies whether written consent is waived or required.

Written Consent Documents

Short Form Written Consent Document. The short form consent document includes the following statement: "The elements of informed consent required by Section 46.116 [see the section on information essential for consent] have been presented orally to the subject or the subject's legally authorized representative" (U.S. DHHS, 2005, 45 CFR Section 46.117a). The researcher must develop a written summary of what is to be said to the subject in the oral presentation, and the summary must be approved by an IRB. When the oral presentation is made to the subject or to the

subject's representative, a witness is required. The subject or representative must sign the short form consent document. "The witness shall sign both the short form and a copy of the summary, and the person actually obtaining consent shall sign a copy of the summary" (U.S. DHHS, 2005, 45 CFR Section 46.117a). Copies of the summary and short form are given to the subject and the witness; the researcher retains the original documents and must keep these documents for 3 years after the end of the study. The short form written consent documents might be used in studies that present minimal or moderate risk to the subjects.

Formal Written Consent Document. The written consent document or consent form includes the elements of informed consent required by the U.S. DHHS (2005) and FDA (2006b) regulations (see the previous section on information essential for consent). In addition, a consent form might include other information required by the institution where the study is to be conducted or by the agency funding the study. Most universities provide consent form guidelines for researchers to use. A sample consent form is presented in Figure 9-2 with the common essential consent information. The subject can read the consent form, or the researcher can read it to the subject; however, it is wise also to explain the study to the subject. The subject signs the form, and the investigator or research assistant collecting the data witnesses it. This type of consent can be used for minimal to moderate risk studies. All persons signing the consent form must receive a copy of it. The researcher keeps the original consent form for 3 years.

Studies that involve subjects with diminished autonomy require a written consent form. If these prospective subjects have some comprehension of the study and agree to participate as subjects, they must sign the consent form. However, the subject's legally authorized representative also must sign the form. The representative indicates his or her relationship with the subject under the signature (see Figure 9-2).

The written consent form used in a high-risk study often contains the signatures of two witnesses, the researcher and an additional person. The additional person signing as a witness must observe the informed consent process and must not be otherwise connected with the study (Hershey & Miller, 1976). The best witnesses are research subject advocates or patient advocates who are employed in the institution.

Sometimes nurses are asked to sign a consent form as a witness for a biomedical study. They must know the study purpose and procedures and the subject's comprehension of the study before signing the form (Carico & Harrison, 1990). The role of the witness is

Study title: The Needs of Family Members of Critically Ill Adults
Investigator: Linda L. Norris, R.N.

Ms. Norris is a registered nurse studying the emotional and social needs of family members of patients in the Intensive Care Units (**research purpose**). Although the study will not benefit you directly, it will provide information that might enable nurses to identify family members' needs and to assist family members with those needs (**potential benefits**).

The study and its procedures have been approved by the appropriate people and review boards at The University of Texas at Arlington and X hospital (**IRB approval**). The study procedures might cause fatigue for you or your family (**potential risks**). The procedures include: (1) responding to a questionnaire about the needs of family members of critically ill patients and (2) completing a demographic data sheet (**explanation of procedures**). Participation in this study will take approximately 20 minutes (**time commitment**). You are free to ask any questions about the study or about being a subject and you may call Ms. Norris at (999) 999-9999 (work) or (999) 999-9999 (home) if you have further questions (**offer to answer questions**).

Your participation in this study is voluntary; you are under no obligation to participate (**alternative option and voluntary consent**). You have the right to withdraw at any time and the care of your family member and your relationship with the health care team will not be affected (**option to withdraw**).

The study data will be coded so they will not be linked to your name. Your identity will not be revealed while the study is being conducted or when the study is reported or published. All study data will be collected by Ms. Norris, stored in a secure place, and not shared with any other person without your permission (**assurance of anonymity and confidentiality**).

I have read this consent form and voluntarily consent to participate in this study.

(If Appropriate)

_____   _____
Subject's Signature   Date   Legal Representative   Date

I have explained this study to the above subject and to have sought his/her understanding for informed consent

_____
Investigator's Signature   Date

Figure **9-2** Sample consent form.

more important in the consent process if the prospective subject is in awe of the investigator and does not feel free to question the procedures of the study.

Recording of the Consent Process

A researcher might elect to tape-record or obtain a DVD of the consent process. These methods document what was said to the prospective subject and record the subject's questions and the investigator's answers. Tape-recording and DVD are time-consuming and costly, however, and are not appropriate for studies of minimal or moderate risk. If your study is considered high risk, it might be wise to completely document the consent process on tape, because doing so might protect you and your subjects. Both of you would retain a copy of the tape recording or DVD.

Authorization for Research Uses and Disclosure

The HIPAA Privacy Rule provides individuals the right, as research subjects, to authorize covered entities (health care provider, health plan, and health care clearinghouse) to use or disclose their private health information (PHI) for research purposes. This authorization is regulated by the HIPAA and is in addition to the informed consent that is regulated by the U.S. DHHS (2005, CFR 45 Part 46) and the FDA (2006b, CFR 21 Part 50). The authorization focuses on the privacy risks and states how, why, and to whom the PHI will be shared. The authorization form must include the following information:

Authorization Core Elements (see Privacy Rule, 45 CFR Section 164.508[c][1])

- *Description of PHI to be used or disclosed (identifying the information in a specific and meaningful manner).*
- *The name(s) or other specific identification of person(s) or class of persons authorized to make the requested use or disclosure.*
- *The name(s) or other specific identification of the person(s) or class of persons who may use the PHI or to whom the covered entity may make the requested disclosure.*
- *Description of each purpose of the requested use or disclosure. Researchers should note that this element must be study specific, not for future unspecified research.*
- *Authorization expiration date or event that relates to the individual or to the purpose of the use or disclosure (the terms "end of the research study" or "none" may be used for research, including for the creation and maintenance of a research database or repository).*
- *Signature of the individual and date. If the Authorization is signed by an individual's personal representative, a description of the representative's authority to act for the individual. (U.S. DHHS, 2004)*

The authorization information can be included as part of the consent form, but it is probably best to have two separate forms (Olsen, 2003). U.S. DHHS (2004) developed a sample authorization form that is presented in Figure 9-3.

INSTITUTIONAL REVIEW

In institutional review, a committee of the researcher's peers examines his or her study for ethical concerns. The first federal policy statement on protection of human subjects by institutional review was issued by the U.S. PHS in 1966. The statement required that research involving human subjects must be reviewed by a committee of peers or associates to confirm that (1) the rights and welfare of the individuals involved were protected, (2) the appropriate methods were used to secure informed consent, and (3) the potential benefits of the investigation were greater than the risks (Levine, 1986). Internationally, CIOMS (2002) and the Canadian Institutes of Health Research, Natural Sciences and Engineering Research Council of Canada, and Social Sciences and Humanities Research Council of Canada (Canadian Tri-Council) have developed regulations to guide the ethical review of research by peers.

In 1974, DHEW passed the National Research Act, which required that all research involving human subjects undergo institutional review. Currently, both the U.S. DHHS (2005, 45 CFR Sections 46.107–46.115) and the FDA (2006a, 21 CFR Sections 56.101–56.124) have similar regulations for institutional review of research. These regulations describe the membership, functions, and operations of an institutional review board. An institutional review board (IRB) is a committee that reviews research to ensure that the investigator is conducting the research ethically. Universities, hospital corporations, and many managed care centers have IRBs to promote the conduct of ethical research and protect the rights of prospective subjects at their institutions.

Each IRB has at least five members of various backgrounds (cultural, economic, educational, gender, racial) to promote a complete, scholarly, and fair review of research that is commonly conducted in an institution. If an institution regularly reviews studies with vulnerable subjects, such as children, neonates, pregnant women, prisoners, and mentally disabled persons, the IRB should include one or more members with knowledge about and experience in working with these subjects. The members must have sufficient experience and expertise to review a variety of studies, including quantitative, qualitative, outcomes, and intervention research (Munhall, 2001b). The IRB members must not have a conflicting interest related to a study conducted in an institution. Any member having a conflict of interest with a research project being reviewed must excuse himself or herself from the review process, except to provide information requested by the IRB. The IRB also must include other members whose primary concern is nonscientific, such as an ethicist, a lawyer, or a minister. At least one of the IRB members must be someone who is not affiliated with the institution (FDA, 2006b; U.S. DHHS, 2005). The IRBs in hospitals are often composed of physicians, lawyers, scientists, clergy, community laypersons, and, more recently, nurses.

Levels of Reviews Conducted by Institutional Review Boards

The functions and operations of an IRB involve the review of research at three different levels: (1) exempt from review, (2) expedited review, and (3) complete review. The level of the review required for each study is decided by the IRB chairperson or committee, but not by the researcher. Studies are usually exempt from review if they pose no apparent risks for the research subjects. The studies that are usually considered exempt from IRB review by the federal regulations are identified in Table 9-6. For example, studies

AUTHORIZATION TO USE OR DISCLOSE (RELEASE) HEALTH INFORMATION THAT IDENTIFIES YOU FOR A RESEARCH STUDY

REQUIRED ELEMENTS:

If you sign this document, you give permission to [name or other identification of specific health care provider(s) or description of classes of persons, e.g., all doctors, all health care providers] at [name of covered entity or entities] to use or disclose (release) your health information that identifies you for the research study described below:
[Provide a description of the research study, such as the title and purpose of the research.]

The health information that we may use or disclose (release) for this research includes
[complete as appropriate]:
[Provide a description of information to be used or disclosed for the research project. This description may include, for example, all information in a medical record, results of physical examinations, medical history, lab tests, or certain health information indicating or relating to a particular condition.]
The health information listed above may be used by and/or disclosed (released) to:
[Name or class of persons involved in the research; i.e., researchers and their staff**]

[Name of covered entity] is required by law to protect your health information. By signing this document, you authorize [name of covered entity] to use and/or disclose (release) your health information for this research. Those persons who receive your health information may not be required by Federal privacy laws (such as the Privacy Rule) to protect it and may share your information with others without your permission, if permitted by laws governing them.

Please note that [include the appropriate statement]:
- You do not have to sign this Authorization, but if you do not, you may not receive research-related treatment.
  (When the research involves treatment and is conducted by the covered entity or when the covered entity provides health care solely for the purpose of creating protected health information to disclose to a researcher)

- [Name of covered entity] may not condition (withhold or refuse) treating you on whether you sign this Authorization.
  (When the research does not involve research-related treatment by the covered entity or when the covered entity is not providing health care solely for the purpose of creating protected health information to disclose to a researcher)

Please note that [include the appropriate statement]:
- You may change your mind and revoke (take back) this Authorization at any time, except to the extent that [name of covered entity(ies)] has already acted based on this Authorization. To revoke this Authorization, you must write to: [name of the covered entity(ies) and contact information].
  (Where the research study is conducted by an entity other than the covered entity)

- You may change your mind and revoke (take back) this Authorization at any time. Even if you revoke this Authorization, [name or class of persons at the covered entity involved in the research] may still use or disclose health information they already have obtained about you as necessary to maintain the integrity or reliability of the current research. To revoke this Authorization, you must write to: [name of the covered entity(ies) and contact information].
  (Where the research study is conducted by the covered entity)

_____	_____
Signature of participant or participant's personal representative	Date
_____	_____
Printed name of participant or participant's personal representative	If applicable, a description of the personal representative's authority to sign for the participant

** Where a covered entity conducts the research study, the Authorization must list ALL names or other identification, or ALL classes, of persons who will have access through the covered entity to the protected health information (PHI) for the research study (e.g., research collaborators, sponsors, and others who will have access to data that includes PHI). Examples may include, but are not limited to the following:

- Data coordinating centers that will receive and process PHI;
- Sponsors who want access to PHI or who will actualy own the research data; and/or
- Institutional Review Boards or Data Safety and Monitoring Boards.

If the research study is conducted by an entity other than the covered entity, the authorization need only list the name or other identification of the outside researcher (or class of researchers) and any other entity to whom the covered entity is expected to make the disclosure.

Figure **9-3** Sample authorization language for research uses and disclosures of individually identifiable health information by a covered health care provider.

TABLE 9-6 ▪ Research Qualifying for Exemption from Review

Unless otherwise required by department or agency heads, research activities in which the only involvement of human subjects will be in one or more of the following categories are exempt from review:

(1) Research conducted in established or commonly accepted educational settings, involving normal educational practices, such as (i) research on regular and special education instructional strategies, or (ii) research on the effectiveness of or the comparison among instructional techniques, curricula, or classroom management methods.

(2) Research involving the use of educational tests (cognitive, diagnostic, aptitude, achievement), survey procedures, interview procedures or observation of public behavior, unless: (i) information obtained is recorded in such a manner that human subjects can be identified, directly or through identifiers linked to the subjects; and (ii) any disclosure of the human subjects' responses outside the research could reasonably place the subjects at risk of criminal or civil liability or be damaging to the subjects' financial standing, employability, or reputation.

(3) Research involving the use of educational tests (cognitive, diagnostic, aptitude, achievement), survey procedures, interview procedures, or observation of public behavior that is not exempt under paragraph (b)(2) of this section, if: (i) the human subjects are elected or appointed public officials or candidates for public office; or (ii) Federal statute(s) require(s) without exception that the confidentiality of the personally identifiable information will be maintained throughout the research and thereafter.

(4) Research involving the collection or study of existing data, documents, records, pathological specimens, or diagnostic specimens, if these sources are publicly available or if the information is recorded by the investigator in such a manner that subjects cannot be identified, directly or through identifiers linked to the subjects.

(5) Research and demonstration projects which are conducted by or subject to the approval of Department or Agency heads, and which are designed to study, evaluate, or otherwise examine: (i) Public benefit or service programs; (ii) procedures for obtaining benefits or services under those programs; (iii) possible changes in or alternatives to those programs or procedures; or (iv) possible changes in methods or levels of payment for benefits or services under those programs.

(6) Taste and food quality evaluation and consumer acceptance studies, (i) if wholesome foods without additives are consumed or (ii) if a food is consumed that contains a food ingredient at or below the level and for a use found to be safe, or agricultural chemical or environmental contaminant at or below the level found to be safe, by the Food and Drug Administration or approved by the Environmental Protection Agency or the Food Safety and Inspection Service of the U.S. Department of Agriculture.

From U.S. Department of Health and Human Services. (2005, June 23). Protection of human subjects. *Code of Federal Regulations*, Title 45, Part 46. Retrieved October 1, 2007, from www.hhs.gov/ohrp/humansubjects/guidance/45cfr46.htm.

by nurses and other health professionals that have no foreseeable risks or are a mere inconvenience for subjects might be identified as exempt from review by the chairperson of the IRB committee.

Studies that have some risks, which are viewed as minimal, are expedited in the review process. Minimal risk means "that the risks of harm anticipated in the proposed research are not greater, considering probability and magnitude, than those ordinarily encountered in daily life or during the performance of routine physical or psychological examinations or tests" (U.S. DHHS, 2005, 45 CFR Section 46.102). Expedited review procedures can also be used to review minor changes in previously approved research. Under expedited IRB review procedures, the review may be carried out by the IRB chairperson or by one or more experienced reviewers designated by the chairperson from among members of the IRB. In reviewing the research, the reviewers may exercise all of the authorities of the IRB except disapproval of the research. A research activity may be disapproved only after a complete review of the IRB (FDA, 2006b; U.S. DHHS, 2005). Table 9-7 identifies research that usually qualifies for expedited review.

A study that has greater than minimal risks must receive a complete IRB review. To obtain IRB approval, researchers must ensure that

(1) risks to subjects are minimized, (2) risks to subjects are reasonable in relation to anticipated benefits, (3) selection of subjects is equitable, (4) informed consent will be sought from each prospective subject or the subject's legally authorized representative, (5) informed consent will be appropriately documented, (6) the research plan makes adequate provision for monitoring data collection for subjects' safety, and (7) adequate provisions are made to protect the privacy of subjects and to maintain the confidentiality of data. (FDA, 2006b, 21 CFR 56.111; U.S. DHHS, 2005, 45 CFR Section 46.111)

TABLE 9-7 ■ Research Qualifying for Expedited Institutional Review Board Review

Expedited review (by committee chairpersons or designated members) for the following research involving no more than minimal risk is authorized:

1. Collection of hair and nail clippings, in a nondisfiguring manner; deciduous teeth and permanent teeth if patient care indicates a need for extraction.

2. Collection of excreta and external secretions including sweat, uncannulated saliva, placenta removed at delivery, and amniotic fluid at the time of rupture of the membrane before or during labor.

3. Recording of data from subjects 18 years of age or older using noninvasive procedures routinely employed in clinical practice. This includes the use of physical sensors that are applied either to the surface of the body or at a distance and do not involve input of matter or significant amounts of energy into the subject or an invasion of the subject's privacy. It also includes such procedures as weighing, testing sensory acuity, electrocardiography, electroencephalography, thermography, detection of naturally occurring radioactivity, diagnostic echography, and electroretinography. It does not include exposure to electromagnetic radiation outside the visible range (for example, x-rays, microwaves).

4. Collection of blood samples by venipuncture, in amounts not exceeding 450 ml in an 8-week period and no more than two times per week, from subjects 18 years of age or older and who are in good health and not pregnant.

5. Collection of both supragingival and subgingival dental plaque and calculus, provided the procedure is not more invasive than routine prophylactic scaling of the teeth and the process is accomplished in accordance with accepted prophylactic techniques.

6. Voice recordings made for research purposes such as investigations of speech defects.

7. Moderate exercise by healthy volunteers.

8. The study of existing data, documents, records, pathological specimens, or diagnostic specimens.

9. Research on individual or group behavior or characteristics of individuals, such as studies of perception, cognition, game theory, or test development, where the investigator does not manipulate subjects' behavior and research will not involve stress to subjects.

Research on drugs or devices for which an investigational new drug exemption or an investigational device exemption is not required.

From U.S. Department of Health and Human Services. (2005, June 23). Protection of human subjects. *Code of Federal Regulations*, Title 45, Part 46. Retrieved October 1, 2007, from www.hhs.gov/ohrp/humansubjects/guidance/45cfr46.htm.

Amdur (2003) provided a detailed discussion of the role of the IRB in health care research, and this information is a good resource for health care agencies and researchers. The process of seeking approval from a research review committee to conduct a study is described in Chapter 28.

Published studies often indicate that an IRB has approved the research project. For example, Bindler, Massey, Shultz, Mills, and Short (2007) conducted their study to examine metabolic syndrome in a multiethnic sample of schoolchildren. They described the following consent and IRB approval process for their study.

Parents received a flyer about the study (written in English and Spanish languages), which was sent home from school through the children. They could elect to attend an informational program (conducted in both English and Spanish languages) in school one evening. If they signed a consent form, their children were informed about the study and could choose whether to sign an assent form and participate... Participants who spoke English or Spanish were eligible.... The protocol was approved by the Institutional Review Boards of Spokane, Washington, and Washington State University, and the school board of the district where the study was conducted. (Bindler et al., 2007, p. 47)

The subjects in this study were parents and school-age children from different ethnic backgrounds (English and Spanish) who were invited to participate in the study by a flyer sent to all affiliated with the selected school. The parents and children received information about the study in their appropriate language. Then the parents signed consent forms and the children signed assent forms documenting the informed consent process. The two versions of the consent forms (Spanish and English) probably increased the subjects' ability to comprehend the consent form and the purpose of the study. IRB approvals were obtained from both the university and the school district where the study was conducted. Thus, the consent process and IRB approvals were clearly documented in this study

Influence of HIPAA Privacy Rule on Institutional Review Boards

Under the 2003 HIPAA Privacy Rule, IRBs or an institutionally established privacy board can act on requests for a waiver or an alteration of the authorization requirement for a research project. If an IRB and a privacy board both exist in an agency, the approval of only one board is required, and it will probably be the IRB for research projects. Researchers can choose

TABLE 9-8 ▪▪ Comparison of IRB/Privacy Board Responsibilities for HIPAA, U.S. DHHS, and FDA

Area of Distinction	HIPAA Privacy Rule	U.S. DHHS Protection of Human Subjects Regulations Title 45 CFR Part 46	FDA Protection of Human Subjects Regulations Title 21 CFR Parts 50 and 56
Permissions for research	Authorization	Informed consent and authorization	Informed consent and authorization
IRB/privacy board responsibilities	Requires the covered entity to obtain authorization for research use or disclosure of PHI unless a regulatory permission applies. Because of this, the IRB or privacy board would only see requests to waive or alter the authorization requirement. In exercising privacy rule authority, the IRB or privacy board does not review the authorization form.	Requires the covered entity to obtain authorization for research use or disclosure of PHI unless a regulatory permission applies. Because of this, the IRB or privacy board would only see requests to waive or alter the authorization requirement. In exercising privacy rule authority, the IRB or privacy board does not review the authorization form.	The IRB must ensure that informed consent will be sought from, and documented for, each prospective subject or the subject's legally authorized representative, in accordance with, and to the extent required by, FDA regulations. If specified criteria are met, the requirements for either obtaining informed consent or documenting informed consent may be waived. The IRB must review and approve the authorization form if it is combined with the informed consent document. Privacy boards have no authority under the FDA Protection of Human Subjects Regulations.

From U.S. Department of Health and Human Services. (2007, February 2, a). How can covered entities use and disclose protected health information for research and comply with the Privacy Rule? *HIPAA Privacy Rule: Information for researchers.* Retrieved October 1, 2007, from http://privacyruleandresearch.nih.gov/pr_08.asp.

to obtain a signed authorization form from potential subjects or can ask for a waiver or an alteration of the authorization requirement. An altered authorization requirement occurs when an IRB approves a request that some but not all of the required 18 elements be removed from health information that is to be used in research. The researcher can also request a partial or complete waiver of the authorization requirement from the IRB. For a partial waiver, discussed earlier, the researcher obtains PHI to contact and recruit potential subjects for a study. An IRB can give a researcher a complete waiver of authorization in studies where the informed consent requirements might also be waived. Thus, a waiver or alteration of the authorization requirement might occur when the following criteria have been met:

- *The PHI use or disclosure involves no more than minimal risk to the privacy for research subjects based on (1) an adequate plan presented to the IRB to protect the PHI identifiers from improper use of disclosure; (2) an adequate plan exists to destroy the identifiers at the earliest opportunity; and (3) written assurance the PHI will not be reused or disclosed to any other person.*

- *The research could not reasonably be conducted without the waiver or alteration of the Authorization requirement.*
- *The research cannot be done without access to and use of the PHI. (U.S. DHHS, 2003)*

The covered entity (health care provider, health plan, or health care clearinghouse) cannot release the PHI to the researcher until the following documentation has been received: (1) the identity of the approving IRB, (2) the date the waiver or alteration was approved, (3) IRB documentation that the criteria for waiver or alteration have been met, (4) a brief description of the PHI to which the researcher has been granted access or use, (5) a statement as to whether the waiver was approved under normal or expedited review procedures, and (6) the signature of the IRB chair or the chair's designee.

The HIPAA Privacy Rule does not change the IRB membership and functions that are designated under the U.S. DHHS and FDA Regulations. For clarification, the responsibilities of the IRB/privacy board for HIPAA (U.S. DHHS, 2007, February 2, a) and the responsibilities of the IRB under the U.S. DHHS (2005) and FDA (2006a) are outlined in Table 9-8.

RESEARCH MISCONDUCT

The goal of research is to generate sound scientific knowledge, which is possible only through the honest conduct, reporting, and publication of studies. However, since the 1980s, a number of fraudulent studies have been conducted and published in prestigious scientific journals. An example of scientific misconduct was evident in the publications of Dr. Robert Slutsky, a heart specialist at the University of California, San Diego, School of Medicine. He resigned in 1986 when confronted with inconsistencies in his research publications. His publications contained "statistical anomalies that raised the question of data fabrication" (Friedman, 1990, p. 1416). In 6 years, Slutsky published 161 articles, and at one time, he was completing an article every 10 days. Eighteen of the articles were found to be fraudulent and have retraction notations, and 60 articles were judged to be questionable (Friedman, 1990; Henderson, 1990).

Stephen Breuning, a psychologist at the University of Pittsburgh, engaged in deceptive and misleading practices in reporting his research on retarded children. He used his fraudulent research to obtain more than $300,000 in federal grants. In 1988, he was criminally charged with research fraud, pleaded guilty, was fined $20,000, and was sentenced to up to 10 years in prison (Garfield & Welljams-Dorof, 1990).

In response to the increasing incidences of scientific misconduct, the federal government developed the Office of Research Integrity (ORI) in 1989 within the U.S. DHHS. ORI was to supervise the implementation of the rules and regulations related to scientific misconduct and to manage any investigations of scientific misconduct. In 1996, a review and revision of the existing scientific misconduct policy were initiated to (1) develop a uniform research misconduct policy across the agencies of the federal government, (2) establish a policy that addresses behavior that has the potential to affect the integrity of the research record, and (3) develop a procedure to safeguard the handling of allegations of research misconduct. Currently, ORI is responsible for the implementation of CFR 42, Parts 50 and 93, Policies of General Applicability (ORI, 2005).

Role of the Office of Research Integrity in Promoting the Conduct of Ethical Research

Currently, ORI promotes the integrity of biomedical and behavioral research in approximately 4000 institutions worldwide (ORI, 2007, September 10). ORI applies federal policies and regulations to protect the integrity of the U.S. PHS's extramural and intramural research programs. The extramural program provides funding to research institutions, and the intramural program provides funding for research conducted within the federal government. The ORI carries out its responsibilities by doing the following:

- Developing policies, procedures, and regulations related to the detection, investigation, and prevention of research misconduct and the responsible conduct of research
- Reviewing and monitoring research misconduct investigations conducted by applicant and awardee institutions, intramural research programs, and the Office of Inspector General in the Department of Health and Human Services (HHS)
- Recommending research misconduct findings and administrative actions to the assistant secretary for health for decision, subject to appeal
- Assisting the Office of the General Counsel (OGC) to present cases before the HHS departmental appeals board
- Providing technical assistance to institutions that respond to allegations of research misconduct
- Implementing activities and programs to teach responsible conduct of research, promote research integrity, prevent research misconduct, and improve the handling of allegations of research misconduct
- Conducting policy analyses, evaluations, and research to build the knowledge base in research misconduct, research integrity, and prevention and to improve the HHS research integrity policies and procedures
- Administering programs for maintaining institutional assurances, responding to allegations of retaliation against whistleblowers, approving intramural and extramural policies and procedures, and responding to Freedom of Information Act and Privacy Act requests (ORI, 2005)

Since the mid-1990s, ORI has had a major role in the investigation of allegations of misconduct in research within several institutions. "Research misconduct means fabrication, falsification, or plagiarism in processing, performing, or reviewing research, or in reporting research results. It does not include honest error or differences in opinion" (ORI, 2005, 42 CFR Section 93.103). Fabrication in research is the making up of results and recording or reporting them. Falsification of research is manipulating research materials, equipment, or processes, or changing or omitting data or results such that the research is not accurately represented in the research record. Plagiarism is the appropriation of another person's ideas, processes, results, or words without giving appropriate credit, including those obtained through confidential review of others' research proposals and manuscripts.

The ORI classifies research misconduct as (1) an act that involves a significant departure from the acceptable practice of the scientific community for maintaining the integrity of the research record; (2) an act that was committed intentionally; and (3) an allegation that can be proved by a preponderance of evidence. ORI has a section on their website titled "Handling Misconduct" that includes a summary of the allegations and investigations managed by its office from 1992 to 2001 (ORI, 2004). The most common sites for the investigations were medical schools (68%), hospitals (11%), and research institutes (10%). The individuals charged with misconduct were primarily males holding a PhD or medical degree (MD) and were mostly associate professors, professors, and postdoctoral fellows. When research misconduct was documented, the actions taken against the researchers or agencies might have included debarment from receiving federal funding for periods ranging from 18 months to 8 years; prohibition from U.S. PHS advisory service; and other actions requiring supervised research, certification of data, certification of sources, and correction or retraction of articles. The regulations governing ORI and the current investigations and activities of ORI can be viewed online at http://ori.dhhs.gov.

Role of Journal Editors and Researchers in Preventing Scientific Misconduct

Editors of journals also have a major role in monitoring and preventing research misconduct in the published literature. Friedman (1990, p. 1416) identified criteria for classifying a publication as fraudulent, questionable, or valid and indicated research articles were "fraudulent if there was documentation or testimony from coauthors that the publication did not reflect what had actually been done." Articles were considered questionable if no coauthor could produce the original data or if no coauthor had personally observed or performed each phase of the research or participated in the research publication. A research article was considered valid "if some coauthor had personally performed or participated in each aspect of the research and publication" (Friedman, 1990, p. 1416).

Preventing the publication of fraudulent research requires the efforts of authors, coauthors, reviewers, and editors (Hansen & Hansen, 1995; Hawley & Jeffers, 1992; Relman, 1990). Authors who are primary investigators for research projects must be responsible in their conduct, reporting, and publication of research. Coauthors and coworkers should question and, if necessary, challenge the integrity of a researcher's claims. Sometimes, well-known scientists have been added to a research publication as coauthors to give it credibility. Individuals should not be listed as coauthors unless they were actively involved in the conduct and publication of the research.

Peer reviewers have a key role in determining the quality and publishability of a manuscript. They are considered experts in the field, and their role is to examine research for inconsistencies and inaccuracies. Editors must monitor the peer review process and be cautious about publishing manuscripts that are at all questionable. Editors also need procedures for responding to allegations of research misconduct. They must decide what actions to take if the journal contains an article that has proven to be fraudulent. Usually, fraudulent publications require retraction notations and are not to be cited by authors in future publications (ORI, 2005). However, Pfeifer and Snodgrass (1990) studied the continued citation of retracted, invalid scientific literature and found that articles commonly continued to cite retracted articles in U.S. publications and even more so in the literature of other countries.

The publication of fraudulent research is a major concern in medicine and a growing concern in nursing (Rankin & Esteves, 1997). The smaller pool of funds available for research and the greater emphasis on research publications could lead to a higher incidence of fraudulent publications. However, ORI (2007, June 20) has made major advances in addressing scientific misconduct since the regulations were enacted by doing the following:

- Providing a definition of research misconduct
- Designating responsibilities and actions related to research misconduct
- Identifying mechanisms to distribute the policy to scientists
- Designating the membership of investigating committees
- Identifying the administrative actions for acts of research misconduct
- Developing a process for notifying funding agencies and journals of acts of research misconduct
- Providing for public disclosure of the incidents of scientific misconduct

Each researcher is responsible for monitoring the integrity of his or her research protocols, results, and publications. In addition, nursing professionals must foster a spirit of intellectual inquiry, mentor prospective scientists regarding the norms for good science, and stress quality, not quantity, in publications (Wocial, 1995).

ANIMALS AS RESEARCH SUBJECTS

The use of animals as research subjects is a controversial issue of growing concern to nurse researchers. A small but increasing number of nurse scientists are conducting physiological studies that require the use of animals. Many scientists, especially physicians, believe that the current animal rights' movement could threaten the future of health research. Animal rights groups are active in antiresearch campaigns and are backed by massive resources estimated in the millions of dollars (Pardes, West, & Pincus, 1991). Some of the animal rights groups are trying to raise the consciousness of researchers and society to ensure that animals are used wisely in the conduct of research and treated humanely.

Other animal rights groups have tried to frighten the public with sometimes distorted stories about inhumane treatment of animals in research. Some of the activist leaders have made broad comparisons between human life and animal life. For example, a major animal rights group called People for the Ethical Treatment of Animals (PETA) has stated, "There is no rational basis for separating out the human animal. A rat is a pig is a dog is a boy. They're all mammals" (Pardes et al., 1991, p. 1641). Some of these activists have now progressed to violence, using "physical attacks, including real bombs, arson, and vandalism" (Pardes et al., 1991, p. 1642). Even more damage is being done to research through lawsuits that have blocked the conduct of research and the development of new research centers. Medical schools now spend millions of dollars annually for security, public education, and other efforts to defend research.

Two important questions must be addressed: Should animals be used as subjects in research, and if animals are used in research, what mechanisms ensure that they are treated humanely? In regard to the first question, the type of research project developed influences the selection of subjects. Animals are just one of a variety of types of subjects used in research; others are human beings, plants, and computer data sets. If possible, most researchers use nonanimal subjects, because they are generally less expensive. In studies that are low risk, which most nursing studies are, human beings are commonly used as subjects.

Some studies, however, require the use of animals to answer the research question. Approximately 17 to 22 million animals are used in research each year, and 90% of them are rodents, with the combined percentage of dogs and cats being only 1% to 2% (Goodwin & Morrison, 2000). Because animals are deemed valuable subjects for selected research projects, the second question, concerning their humane treatment, must also be answered. At least five separate types of regulations exist to protect research animals from mistreatment. The federal government, state governments, independent accreditation organization, professional societies, and individual institutions work to ensure that research animals are used only when necessary and only under humane conditions. At the federal level, animal research is conducted according to the guidelines of U.S. PHS Policy on Humane Care and Use of Laboratory Animals, which was adopted in 1986 and reprinted essentially unchanged in 1996 and is available on the Office of Laboratory Animal Welfare (OLAW) website at http://grants.nih.gov/grants/olaw/olaw.htm (OLAW, 2007).

The Humane Care and Use of Laboratory Animals Regulations define animal as any live, vertebrate animal used or intended for use in research, research training, experimentation, or biological testing or for related purposes. Any institution proposing research involving animals must have a written Animal Welfare Assurance statement acceptable to the U.S. PHS that documents compliance with the U.S. PHS policy. Every assurance statement is evaluated by the NIH's Office for Protection from Research Risks (OPRR) to determine the adequacy of the institution's proposed program for the care and use of animals in activities conducted or supported by the U.S. PHS (OLAW, 2007).

Institutions' assurance statements about compliance with the U.S. PHS policy have promoted the humane care and treatment of animals in research. In addition, more than 700 institutions conducting health-related research have sought accreditation by the American Association for Accreditation of Laboratory Animal Care (AAALAC), which was developed to ensure the humane treatment of animals in research (Pardes et al., 1991). In conducting research, each investigator must carefully select the type of subject needed; if animals are used as subjects, they require humane treatment.

SUMMARY

- The ethical conduct of research starts with the identification of the study topic and continues through the publication of the study if quality research evidence is going to be developed for practice.
- The debate about ethics and research continues, probably because of (1) the complexity of human rights issues; (2) the focus of research in new, challenging arenas of technology and genetics; (3) the

complex ethical codes and regulations governing research; and (4) the variety of interpretations of these codes and regulations.

- Two historical documents that have had a strong impact on the conduct of research are the Nuremberg Code and the Declaration of Helsinki. More recently, the U.S. Department of Health and Human Services (U.S. DHHS, 2005) and the Food and Drug Administration (FDA, 2006a, 2006b) have promulgated regulations that direct the ethical conduct of research. These regulations include (1) general requirements for informed consent, (2) documentation of informed consent, (3) institutional review board (IRB) review of research, (4) exempt and expedited review procedures for certain kinds of research, and (5) criteria for IRB approval of research.

- The Council for International Organizations of Medical Sciences revises and updates ethical guidelines for biomedical research conducted internationally. The Canadian Institutes of Health Research, Natural Sciences and Engineering Research Council of Canada, and Social Sciences and Humanities Research Council of Canada (Tri-Council) (2005) developed a policy statement to promote the ethical conduct of research in this country.

- A relatively new federal regulation, Public Law 104-191, the Health Insurance Portability and Accountability Act (HIPAA), was enacted in 1996 and implemented in 2003. HIPAA includes privacy rules to protect an individual's protected health information.

- Conducting research ethically requires protection of the human rights of subjects. Human rights are claims and demands that have been justified in the eyes of an individual or by the consensus of a group of individuals. The human rights that require protection in research are (1) self-determination, (2) privacy, (3) anonymity and confidentiality, (4) fair treatment, and (5) protection from discomfort and harm.

- The rights of research subjects can be protected by balancing benefits and risks of a study, securing informed consent, and submitting the research for institutional review.

- To balance the benefits and risks of a study, the type, level, and number of risks are examined, and the potential benefits are identified. If possible, the risks must be minimized and the benefits maximized to achieve the best possible benefit-risk ratio.

- Informed consent involves the transmission of essential information, comprehension of that information, competency to give consent, and voluntary consent of the prospective subject.

- In institutional review, a study is examined for ethical concerns by a committee of peers called an institutional review board (IRB). The IRB conducts three levels of review: exempt, expedited, and complete. The process for accessing protected health information according to the HIPAA Privacy Rule is also detailed.

- Research misconduct includes fabrication, falsification, and plagiarism during the conduct, reporting, or publication of research. The Office of Research Integrity (ORI) was developed to investigate and manage incidents of scientific misconduct so as to protect the integrity of research in all disciplines.

- Another current ethical concern in research is the use of animals as subjects. Two important questions are addressed: Should animals be used as research subjects, and if animals are used in research, what mechanisms ensure that they are treated humanely? The U.S. Public Health Service Policy on Humane Care and Use of Laboratory Animals provides direction for the conduct of research with animals as subjects.

REFERENCES

Amdur, R. (2003). *Institutional review board: Member handbook.* Sudbury, MA: Jones & Bartlett.

American Nurses Association (ANA). (2001). *Code of ethics for nurses with interpretive statements.* Washington, DC: American Nurses Association.

American Psychological Association (APA). (2002). *Ethical principles of psychologists and code of conduct.* Washington, DC: American Psychological Association.

Arras, J. D. (1990). Noncompliance in AIDS research. *Hastings Center Report, 20*(5), 24–32.

Beecher, H. K. (1966). Ethics and clinical research. *New England Journal of Medicine, 274*(24), 1354–1360.

Berger, R. L. (1990). Nazi science: The Dachau hypothermia experiments. *New England Journal of Medicine, 322*(20), 1435–1440.

Bindler, R. C. M., Massey, L. K., Shultz, J. A., Mills, P. E., & Short, R. (2007). Metabolic syndrome in a multiethnic sample of school children: Implications for the pediatric nurse. *Journal of Pediatric Nursing, 22*(1), 43–58.

Brandt, A. M. (1978). Racism and research: The case of the Tuskegee Syphilis Study. *Hastings Center Report, 8*(6), 21–29.

Broome, M. E. (1999). Consent (assent) for research with pediatric patients. *Seminars in Oncology Nursing, 15*(2), 96–103.

Broome, M. E., & Stieglitz, K. A. (1992). The consent process and children. *Research in Nursing & Health, 15*(2), 147–152.

Bruce, S. L., & Grove, S. K. (1994). The effect of a coronary artery risk evaluation program on serum lipid values and cardiovascular risk levels. *Applied Nursing Research, 7*(2), 67–74.

Canadian Institutes of Health Research, Natural Sciences and Engineering Research Council of Canada, and Social Sciences and Humanities Research Council of Canada. (2005). *Tri-Council Policy Statement: Ethical conduct of research involving humans.*

Retrieved October 2, 2002, from http://pre.ethics.gc.ca/english/policystatement/policystatement.cfm.

Carico, J. M., & Harrison, E. R. (1990). Ethical considerations for nurses in biomedical research. *Journal of Neuroscience Nursing*, 22(3), 160–163.

Conner, J. A., Smaldone, A. M., Bratts, T., & Stone, P. W. (2003). HIPAA in 2003 and its meaning for nurse researchers. *Applied Nursing Research*, 16(4), 291–293.

Council for International Organizations of Medical Sciences (CIOMS). (2002). *International ethical guidelines for biomedical research involving human subjects*. Retrieved October 2, 2007, from www.cioms.ch/guidelines_nov_2002_blurb.htm.

Damrosch, S. P. (1986). Ensuring anonymity by use of subject-generated identification codes. *Research in Nursing & Health*, 9(1), 61–63.

Douglas, S., & Larson, E. (1986). There's more to informed consent than information. *Focus on Critical Care*, 13(2), 43–47.

Floyd, J. (1988). Research and informed consent: The dilemma of the cognitively impaired client. *Journal of Psychosocial Nursing and Mental Health Services*, 26(3), 13–21.

Food and Drug Administration (FDA). (2006a, April 1). Institutional review boards. *Code of Federal Regulations,* Title 21, Part 56. Retrieved October 1, 2007, from www.accessdata.fda.gov/scripts/cdrh/cfdocs/cfcfr/CFRsearch.cfm?CFRPart=56.

Food and Drug Administration (FDA). (2006b, April 1). Protection of human subjects (informed consent). *Code of Federal Regulations,* Title 21, Part 50. Retrieved October 1, 2007, from www.accessdata.fda.gov/scripts/cdrh/cfdocs/cfcfr/CFRsearch.cfm?CFRPart=50.

Ford, J. S., & Reutter, L. I. (1990). Ethical dilemmas associated with small samples. *Journal of Advanced Nursing*, 15(2), 187–191.

Frankena, W. K. (1973). *Ethics* (2nd ed.). Englewood Cliffs, NJ: Prentice-Hall.

Friedman, P. J. (1990). Correcting the literature following fraudulent publication. *JAMA*, 263(10), 1416–1419.

Garfield, E., & Welljams-Dorof, A. (1990). The impact of fraudulent research on the scientific literature: The Stephen E. Breuning case. *JAMA*, 263(10), 1424–1426.

Goodwin, F. K., & Morrison, A. R. (2000). Science and self-doubt. *Reason*, 32(5), 22–28.

Grbich, C. (1999). *Qualitative research in health: An introduction*. London: Sage.

Hansen, B. C., & Hansen, K. D. (1995). Academic and scientific misconduct: Issues for nursing educators. *Journal of Professional Nursing*, 11(1), 31–39.

Happ, M. B., Swigart, V. A., Tate, J. A., Arnold, R. M., Sereika, S. M., & Hoffman, L. A. (2007). Family presence and surveillance during weaning from prolonged mechanical ventilation. *Heart & Lung*, 36(1), 47–57.

Hawley, D. J., & Jeffers, J. M. (1992). Scientific misconduct as a dilemma for nursing. *Image: Journal of Nursing Scholarship*, 24(1), 51–55.

Henderson, J. (1990). When scientists fake it. *American Way*, pp. 56–101.

Hershey, N., & Miller, R. D. (1976). *Human experimentation and the law*. Germantown, MD: Aspen.

Hinds, P. S., Burghen, E. A., & Pritchard, M. (2007). Conducting end-of-life studies in pediatric oncology. *Western Journal of Nursing Research*, 29(4), 448–465.

Holaday, B., Gonzales, O., & Mills, D. (2007). Assent of school-age bilingual children. *Western Journal of Nursing Research*, 29(4), 466–485.

Holditch-Davis, D., Brandon, D. H., & Schwartz, T. (2003). Development of behaviors in preterm infants: Relation to sleeping and waking. *Nursing Research*, 52(5), 307–317.

Kelman, H. C. (1967). Human use of human subjects: The problem of deception in social psychological experiments. *Psychological Bulletin*, 67(1), 1–11.

Levine, R. J. (1986). *Ethics and regulation of clinical research* (2nd ed.). Baltimore–Munich: Urban & Schwarzenberg.

Lin, C., Lu, M., Chiang, H, Chung, C., Lin, T., Yin, T. J., & Yang, C. (2007). Using a citizen consensus conference to revise the code of ethics for nurses in Taiwan. *Journal of Nursing Scholarship*, 39(1), 95–101.

McClain, N., Laughon, K., Steeves, R., & Parker, B. (2007). Balancing the needs of scientist and the subject in trauma research. *Western Journal of Nursing Research*, 29(1), 121–128.

Meade, C. D. (1999). Improving understanding of the informed consent process and document. *Seminars in Oncology Nursing*, 15(2), 124–137.

Milgram, S. (1963). Behavioral study of obedience. *Journal of Abnormal and Social Psychology*, 67(4), 371–378.

Munhall, P. L. (2001a). Ethical considerations in qualitative research. In P. L. Munhall (Ed.), *Nursing research: A qualitative perspective* (3rd ed., pp. 537–549). Sudbury, MA: Jones & Bartlett.

Munhall, P. L. (2001b). Institutional review of qualitative research proposals: A task of no small consequence. In P. L. Munhall (Ed.), *Nursing research: A qualitative perspective* (3rd ed., pp. 551–563). Sudbury, MA: Jones & Bartlett.

National Commission for the Protection of Human Subjects of Biomedical and Behavioral Research. (1978). *Belmont report: Ethical principles and guidelines for research involving human subjects* (DHEW Publication No. [05] 78-0012). Washington, DC: U.S. Government Printing Office.

Nelson-Marten, P., & Rich, B. A. (1999). A historical perspective of informed consent in clinical practice and research. *Seminars in Oncology Nursing*, 15(2), 81–88.

Nuremberg Code. (1986). In R. J. Levine (Ed.), *Ethics and regulation of clinical research* (2nd ed., pp. 425–426). Baltimore–Munich: Urban & Schwarzenberg.

Office of Laboratory Animal Welfare (OLAW). (2007). *Public Health Service policy on humane care and use of laboratory animals*. Retrieved October 1, 2007, from http://grants.nih.gov/grants/olaw/olaw.htm.

Office of Research Integrity (ORI). (2004). *Scientific misconduct investigations: 1992–2001*. Retrieved October 1, 2007, from http://ori.dhhs.gov/misconduct/documents/NewInstitutionalResearchMisconductActivity.pdf.

Office of Research Integrity (ORI). (2005, May 17). Public Health Service Policies on Research Misconduct. *Code of Federal Regulations*, Title 42, Part 50 and 93, Policies of General Applicability. Retrieved October 1, 2007, from http://ori.dhhs.gov/documents/FR_Doc_05–9643.shtml.

Office of Research Integrity (ORI). (2007, June 20). Handling misconduct. *Office of Research Integrity*. Retrieved October 1, 2007, from http://ori.dhhs.gov/misconduct.

Office of Research Integrity (ORI). (2007, September 10). About ORI – History. *Office of Research Integrity*. Retrieved October 1, 2007, from http://ori.dhhs.gov/about/history.shtml.

Olsen, D. P. (2003). Methods: HIPAA privacy regulations and nursing research. *Nursing Research, 52*(5), 344–348.

Orb, A., Eisenhauer, L., & Wynaden, D. (2001). Ethics in qualitative research. *Journal of Nursing Scholarship, 33*(1), 93–96.

Pardes, H., West, A., & Pincus, H. A. (1991). Physicians and the animal-rights movement. *New England Journal of Medicine, 324*(23), 1640–1643.

Pfeifer, M. P., & Snodgrass, G. L. (1990). The continued use of retracted, invalid scientific literature. *JAMA, 263*(10), 1420–1423.

Ramos, M. C. (1989). Some ethical implications of qualitative research. *Research in Nursing & Health, 12*(1), 57–63.

Rankin, M., & Esteves, M. D. (1997). Perceptions of scientific misconduct in nursing. *Nursing Research, 46*(5): 270–275.

Relman, A. S. (1990). Publishing biomedical research: Roles and responsibilities. *Hastings Center Report, 20*(5), 23–27.

Reynolds, P. D. (1979). *Ethical dilemmas and social science research.* San Francisco: Jossey-Bass.

Rothman, D. J. (1982). Were Tuskegee and Willowbrook "studies in nature"? *Hastings Center Report, 12*(2), 5–7.

Sasson, R., & Nelson, T. M. (1971). The human experimental subject in context. In J. Jung (Ed.), *The experimenter's dilemma* (pp. 265–296). New York: Harper & Row.

Silva, M. C. (1985). Comprehension of information for informed consent by spouses of surgical patients. *Research in Nursing & Health, 8*(2), 117–124.

Steinfels, P., & Levine, C. (1976). Biomedical ethics and the shadow of Naziism. *Hastings Center Report, 6*(4), 1–20.

Thompson, P. J. (1987). Protection of the rights of children as subjects for research. *Journal of Pediatric Nursing, 2*(6), 392–399.

U.S. Department of Health and Human Services (U.S. DHHS). (1981, January 26). Final regulations amending basic HHS policy for the protection of human research subjects. *Code of Federal Regulations*, Title 45, Part 46.

U.S. Department of Health and Human Services (U.S. DHHS). (1983, March 8). Protection of human subjects. *Code of Federal Regulations*, Title 45, Part 46.

U.S. Department of Health and Human Services (U.S. DHHS). (1991, June 18). Protection of human subjects. *Code of Federal Regulations*, Title 45, Part 46.

U.S. Department of Health and Human Services (U.S. DHHS). (2001, November 23). Protection of human subjects. *Code of Federal Regulations*, Title 45, Part 46.

U.S. Department of Health and Human Services (U.S. DHHS). (2002, August 14). Standards for privacy of individually identifiable health information: Final rule. *Code of Federal Regulations*, Title 45, Public Welfare, Parts 160 and 164. Retrieved October 1, 2007, from www.hhs.gov/ocr/hipaa/privrulepd.pdf.

U.S. Department of Health and Human Services (U.S. DHHS). (2003, September 25). Institutional review boards and the HIPAA Privacy Rule. *HIPAA Privacy Rule: Information for researchers*. Retrieved October 1, 2007, from http://privacyruleandresearch.nih.gov/irbandprivacyrule.asp.

U.S. Department of Health and Human Services (U.S. DHHS). (2004, April). HIPAA authorizations for research. *HIPAA Privacy Rule: Information for researchers*. Retrieved October 1, 2007, from http://privacyruleandresearch.nih.gov/authorization.asp.

U.S. Department of Health and Human Services (U.S. DHHS). (2005, June 23). Protection of human subjects. *Code of Federal Regulations*, Title 45, Part 46. Retrieved October 1, 2007, from www.hhs.gov/ohrp/humansubjects/guidance/45cfr46.htm.

U.S. Department of Health and Human Services (U.S. DHHS). (2007, February 2, a). How can covered entities use and disclose protected health information for research and comply with the Privacy Rule? HIPAA Privacy Rule: Information for researchers. Retrieved October 1, 2007, from http://privacyruleandresearch.nih.gov/pr_08.asp.

U.S. Department of Health and Human Services (U.S. DHHS). (2007, February 2, b). How do other privacy protections interact with the privacy rule? *HIPAA Privacy Rule: Information for researchers*. Retrieved October 1, 2007, from http://privacyruleandresearch.nih.gov/pr_05.asp.

Watson, A. B. (1982). Informed consent of special subjects. *Nursing Research, 31*(1), 43–47.

Williams, A. M. (2002). Issues of consent and data collection in vulnerable populations. *Journal of Neuroscience Nursing, 34*(4), 211–218.

Wocial, L. D. (1995). The role of mentors in promoting integrity and preventing scientific misconduct in nursing research. *Journal of Professional Nursing, 11*(5), 276–280.

World Medical Association (WMA) General Assembly (2002). *World Medical Association Declaration of Helsinki: Ethical principles for medical research involving human subjects*. Washington, DC: WMA General Assembly. Retrieved October 1, 1007, from www.rotrf.org/information/Helsinki_declaration.pdf.

CHAPTER **10**

Understanding Quantitative Research Design

A research design is the blueprint for conducting a study. It maximizes your control over factors that could interfere with the validity of the findings. The research design guides the researcher in planning and implementing the study in a way that is most likely to achieve the intended goal. This control increases the probability that the study results are accurate reflections of reality. Skill in selecting and implementing a research design can improve the quality of the study and thus the usefulness of the findings. A strong design makes it more likely that the study will contribute to the evidence base for practice. Being able to identify the study design and to evaluate design flaws that might threaten the validity of findings is an important part of critically analyzing studies.

The term *research design* is used in two ways. Some consider research design to be the entire strategy for the study, from identification of the problem to final plans for data collection. Others limit design to clearly defined structures within which the study is implemented. In this text, the first definition refers to the research methodology and the second is a definition of the research design.

The design of a study is the end result of a series of decisions you will make concerning how best to implement your study. The design is closely associated with the framework of the study. As a blueprint, the design is not specific to a particular study but rather is a broad pattern or guide that can be applied to many studies. Just as the blueprint for a house must be individualized to the house being built, so the design

must be made specific to a study. Using the problem statement, framework, research questions, and clearly defined variables, you can map out the design to achieve a detailed research plan for collecting and analyzing data. Your research plan specifically directs the execution of your study. Developing a research plan is discussed in Chapter 17.

Elements central to the study design include the presence or absence of a treatment, the number of groups in the sample, the number and timing of measurements, the sampling method, the time frame for data collection, planned comparisons, and the control of extraneous variables. Finding answers to the following questions will help you to develop the design:

1. Is the primary purpose of the study to describe variables and groups within the study situation, to examine relationships, or to examine causality within the study situation?
2. Will a treatment be used?
3. If so, will the researcher control the treatment?
4. Will the sample be pretested before the treatment?
5. Will the sample be randomly selected?
6. Will the sample be studied as a single group or divided into groups?
7. How many groups will there be?
8. What will be the size of each group?
9. Will there be a control group?
10. Will groups be randomly assigned?
11. Will the variables be measured more than once?
12. Will the data be collected cross-sectionally or over time?

13. Have extraneous variables been identified?
14. Are data being collected on extraneous variables?
15. What strategies are being used to control for extraneous variables?
16. What strategies are being used to compare variables or groups?
17. Will data be collected at a single site or at multiple sites?

Developing a study design requires the researcher to consider multiple details such as those listed. The more carefully thought out these details are, the stronger the design. These questions are important because they connect to the logic on which research design is based. To give you the information necessary to understand and answer these questions, this chapter discusses (1) the concepts important to design, (2) design validity, (3) the elements of a good design, and (4) triangulation, a relatively recent approach to research design.

EVIDENCE BASE AND DESIGN

Only the most carefully thought through designs can contribute significantly to the evidence base. By incorporating the elements discussed in this chapter into your design, you will develop a study that is strong enough to be included in the evidence base.

Concepts Important to Design

Many terms used in discussing research design have special meanings within this context. An understanding of these concepts is critical for recognizing the purpose of a specific design. Some of the major concepts used in relation to design are causality, bias, manipulation, control, and validity.

Causality

The first assumption you must make in examining causality is that causes lead to effects. Some of the ideas related to causation emerged from the logical positivist philosophical tradition. Hume, a positivist, proposed that the following three conditions must be met to establish causality: (1) there must be a strong correlation between the proposed cause and the effect, (2) the proposed cause must precede the effect in time, and (3) the cause has to be present whenever the effect occurs. Cause, according to Hume, is not directly observable but must be inferred.

A philosophical group known as essentialists proposed that two concepts must be considered in determining causality: necessary and sufficient. The proposed cause must be necessary for the effect to occur. (The effect cannot occur unless the cause first occurs.) The proposed cause must also be *sufficient* (requiring no other factors) for the effect to occur. This leaves no room for a variable that may sometimes, but not always, serve as the cause of an effect.

John Stuart Mill, another philosopher, added a third idea related to causation. He suggested that, in addition to the preceding criteria for causation, there must be no *alternative explanations* for why a change in one variable seems to lead to a change in a second variable.

Causes are frequently expressed within the propositions of a theory. Testing the accuracy of these theoretical statements indicates the usefulness of the theory. A theoretical understanding of causation is considered important because it improves our ability to predict and, in some cases, to control events in the real world. The purpose of an experimental design is to examine cause and effect. The independent variable in a study is expected to be the cause, and the dependent variable is expected to reflect the effect of the independent variable.

Multicausality

Multicausality, the recognition that a number of interrelating variables can be involved in causing a particular effect, is a more recent idea related to causality. Because of the complexity of causal relationships, a theory is unlikely to identify every variable involved in causing a particular phenomenon. A study is unlikely to include every component influencing a particular change or effect.

Cook and Campbell (1979) have suggested three levels of causal assertions that one must consider in establishing causality. Molar causal laws relate to large and complex objects. Intermediate mediation considers causal factors operating between molar and micro levels. Micromediation examines causal connections at the level of small particles, such as atoms. Cook and Campbell (1979) used the example of turning on a light switch, which causes the light to come on (molar). An electrician would tend to explain the cause of the light coming on in terms of wires and electrical current (intermediate mediation). However, the physicist would explain the cause of the light coming on in terms of ions, atoms, and subparticles (micromediation).

The essentialists' ideas of necessary and sufficient do not hold up well when one views a phenomenon from the perspective of multiple causation. The light switch may not be necessary to turn on the light if the insulation has worn off the electrical wires. Additionally, even though the switch is turned on, the light will not come on if the light bulb is burned out. Although this is a concrete example, it is easy to relate it to common situations in nursing.

Few phenomena in nursing can be clearly reduced to a single cause and a single effect. However, the greater the proportion of causal factors that can be identified and explored, the clearer the understanding of the phenomenon. This greater understanding improves our ability to predict and control. For example, currently nurses have only a limited understanding of patients' preoperative attitudes, knowledge, and behaviors and their effects on postoperative attitudes and behaviors. Nurses assume that high preoperative anxiety leads to less healthy postoperative responses and that providing information before surgery improves healthy responses in the postoperative period. Many nursing studies have examined this particular phenomenon. However, the causal factors involved are complex and have not been clearly delineated. The evidence base in this area is lacking.

Probability

The original criteria for causation required that a variable should cause an identified effect each time the cause occurred. Although this criterion may apply in the basic sciences, such as chemistry or physics, it is unlikely to apply in the health sciences or social sciences. Because of the complexity of the nursing field, nurses deal in probabilities. Probability addresses relative, rather than absolute, causality. From the perspective of probability, a cause will not produce a specific effect each time that particular cause occurs.

Reasoning changes when one thinks in terms of probabilities. The researcher investigates the probability that an effect will occur under specific circumstances. Rather than seeking to prove that A causes B, a researcher would state that if A occurs, there is a 50% probability that B will occur. The reasoning behind probability is more in keeping with the complexity of multicausality. In the example about preoperative attitudes and postoperative outcomes, nurses could seek to predict the probability of unhealthy postoperative patient outcomes when preoperative anxiety levels are high.

Causality and Nursing Philosophy

Traditional theories of prediction and control are built on theories of causality. The first research designs were also based on causality theory. Nursing science must be built within a philosophical framework of multicausality and probability. The strict senses of single causality and of "necessary and sufficient" are not in keeping with the progressively complex, holistic philosophy of nursing. To understand multicausality and increase the probability of being able to predict and control the occurrence of an effect, the researcher must comprehend both wholes and parts.

Practicing nurses must be aware of the molar, intermediate mediational, and micromediational aspects of a particular phenomenon. A variety of differing approaches, reflecting both qualitative and quantitative, descriptive and experimental research, are necessary to develop a knowledge base for nursing. Some see explanation and causality as different and perhaps opposing forms of knowledge. Nevertheless, the nurse must join these forms of knowledge, sometimes within the design of a single study, to acquire the knowledge needed for nursing practice.

Bias

The term bias means to slant away from the true or expected. A biased opinion has failed to include both sides of the question. Cutting fabric on the bias means to cut across the grain of the woven fabric. A biased witness is one who is strongly for or against one side of the situation. A biased scale is one that does not provide a valid measure.

Bias is of great concern in research because of the potential effect on the meaning of the study findings. Any component of the study that deviates or causes a deviation from true measure leads to distorted findings. Many factors related to research can be biased: the researcher, the measurement tools, the individual subjects, the sample, the data, and the statistics. Thus, an important concern in designing a study is to identify possible sources of bias and eliminate or avoid them. If they cannot be avoided, you must design your study to control these sources of bias. Designs, in fact, are developed to reduce the possibilities of bias.

Manipulation

Manipulation tends to have a negative connotation and is associated with one person underhandedly maneuvering a second person so that he or she behaves or thinks in the way the first person desires. Denotatively, to manipulate means to move around or to control the movement of something, such as manipulating a syringe. However, nurses manipulate events or the environment to benefit the patient. Manipulation has a specific meaning when used in experimental or quasi-experimental research; the manipulation is the treatment. For example, in a study on preoperative care, preoperative teaching might be manipulated so that one group receives the treatment and another does not. In a study on oral care, the frequency of care might be manipulated.

In nursing research, when experimental designs are used to explore causal relationships, the nurse must be free to manipulate the variables under study. For example, in a study of pain management, if the freedom to manipulate pain control measures is under the control of someone else, a bias is introduced into the study. In qualitative, descriptive, and correlational studies, the researcher does not attempt to manipulate variables. Instead, the purpose is to describe a situation as it exists.

Control

Control means having the power to direct or manipulate factors to achieve a desired outcome. In a study of pain management, one must be able to control interventions to relieve pain. The idea of control is important in research, particularly in experimental and quasi-experimental studies. The more control the researcher has over the features of the study, the more credible the study findings. The purpose of research designs is to maximize control factors in the study.

Study Validity

Study validity, a measure of the truth or accuracy of a claim, is an important concern throughout the research process. Study validity is central to building an evidence base. Questions of validity refer back to the propositions from which the study was developed and address their approximate truth or falsity. Is the theoretical proposition an accurate reflection of reality? Was the study designed well enough to provide a valid test of the proposition? Validity is a complex idea that is important to the researcher and to those who read the study report and consider using the findings in their practice. Critical analysis of research requires that we think through threats to validity and make judgments about how seriously these threats affect the integrity of the findings. Validity provides a major basis for making decisions about which findings are sufficiently valid to add to the evidence base for patient care.

Cook and Campbell (1979) have described four types of validity: statistical conclusion validity, internal validity, construct validity, and external validity. When conducting a study, you will be confronted with major decisions about the four types of validity. To make these decisions, you must address a variety of questions, such as the following:

1. *Is there a relationship between the two variables? (statistical conclusion validity)*
2. *Given that there is a relationship, is it plausibly causal from one operational variable to the*

other, or would the same relationship have been obtained in the absence of any treatment of any kind? (internal validity)
3. *Given that the relationship is plausibly causal and is reasonably known to be from one variable to another, what are the particular cause-and-effect constructs involved in the relationship? (construct validity)*
4. *Given that there is probably a causal relationship from construct A to construct B, how generalizable is this relationship across persons, settings, and times? (external validity) (Cook & Campbell, 1979, p. 39)*

Statistical Conclusion Validity

The first step in inferring cause is to determine whether the independent and dependent variables are related. You can determine this relationship (covariation) through statistical analysis. Statistical conclusion validity is concerned with whether the conclusions about relationships or differences drawn from statistical analysis are an accurate reflection of the real world.

The second step is to identify differences between groups. There are reasons why false conclusions can be drawn about the presence or absence of a relationship or difference. The reasons for the false conclusions are called *threats to statistical conclusion validity*. These threats are described here.

Low Statistical Power. Low statistical power increases the probability of concluding that there is no significant difference between samples when actually there is a difference (type II error). A type II error is most likely to occur when the sample size is small or when the power of the statistical test to determine differences is low. The concept of statistical power and strategies to improve it are discussed in Chapters 14 and 18.

Violated Assumptions of Statistical Tests. Most statistical tests have assumptions about the data being used, such as that the data are interval data, that the sample was randomly obtained, or that there is a normal distribution of scores to be analyzed. If these assumptions are violated, the statistical analysis may provide inaccurate results. The assumptions of each statistical test are provided in Chapters 20, 21, and 22.

Fishing and the Error Rate Problem. A serious concern in research is incorrectly concluding that a relationship or difference exists when it does not (type I error). The risk of type I error increases when the researcher conducts multiple statistical analyses of relationships or differences; this procedure is referred to as fishing. When fishing is used, a given portion of the analyses shows significant relationships or differences simply by chance. For example, the *t*-test is commonly used to make multiple statistical comparisons of mean differences in a single sample. This procedure increases the risk of a type I error because some of the differences found in the sample occurred by chance and are not actually present in the population. Multivariate statistical techniques have been developed to deal with this error rate problem (Goodwin, 1984). Fishing and error rate problems are discussed in Chapter 18.

Reliability of Measures. The technique of measuring variables must be reliable to reveal true differences. A measure is a reliable measure if it gives the same result each time the same situation or factor is measured. For example, a thermometer would be precise if it showed the same reading when tested repeatedly on the same patient. If a scale is used to measure anxiety, it should give the same score (be reliable) if repeatedly given to the same person in a short time (unless, of course, repeatedly taking the same test causes anxiety to increase or decrease).

Reliability of Treatment Implementation. Treatment standardization ensures that the research treatment is applied consistently each time the treatment is administered. If the method of administering a research treatment varies from one person to another, the chance of detecting a true difference decreases. To control for this lack of standardization, during the planning phase the researcher must ensure that the treatment will be provided in exactly the same way each time it is administered.

Random Irrelevancies in the Experimental Setting. Environmental extraneous variables in complex field settings (e.g., a clinical unit) can influence scores on the dependent variable. These variables increase the difficulty of detecting differences. Consider the activities occurring on a nursing unit. The numbers and variety of staff, patients, crises, and work patterns merge into a complex arena for the implementation of a study. Any of the dynamics of the unit can influence manipulation of the independent variable or measurement of the dependent variable.

Random Heterogeneity of Respondents. Subjects in a treatment group can differ in ways that correlate with the dependent variable. This is referred to as *random heterogeneity*. This difference can influence the outcome of the treatment and prevent detection of a true relationship between the treatment and the dependent variable. For example, subjects may have a variety of responses to preoperative attempts to lower anxiety because of unique characteristics associated with differing levels of anxiety.

Internal Validity

Internal validity is the extent to which the effects detected in the study are a true reflection of reality rather than the result of extraneous variables. Although internal validity should be a concern in all studies, it is addressed more commonly in relation to studies examining causality than in other studies. When examining causality, the researcher must determine whether the independent and dependent variables may have been caused by a third, often unmeasured, variable (an extraneous variable). The possibility of an alternative explanation of cause is sometimes referred to as a rival hypothesis. Any study can contain threats to internal validity, and these validity threats can lead to a false-positive or false-negative conclusion. The researcher must ask, "Is there another reasonable (valid) explanation (rival hypothesis) for the finding other than the one I have proposed?" Threats to internal validity are described here.

History. History is an event that is not related to the planned study but that occurs during the time of the study. History could influence a subject's response to the treatment.

Maturation. In research, maturation is defined as growing older, wiser, stronger, hungrier, more tired, or more experienced during the study. Such unplanned and unrecognized changes can influence the findings of the study.

Testing. Sometimes, the effect being measured (*testing*) can be due to the number of times the subject's responses have been tested. The subject may remember earlier, inaccurate responses and then modify them, thus altering the outcome of the study. The test itself may influence the subject to change attitudes or may increase the subject's knowledge.

Instrumentation. Effects can be due to changes in measurement instruments (instrumentation) between the pretest and the posttest rather than a result of the treatment. For example, a scale that was accurate when the study began (pretest) could now show subjects to weigh 2 lbs less than they actually weigh (posttest). Instrumentation is also involved when people serving as observers or data collectors become more experienced between the pretest and the posttest, thus altering in some way the data they collect.

Statistical Regression. Statistical regression is the movement or regression of extreme scores toward the mean in studies using a pretest-posttest design. The process involved in statistical regression is difficult to understand. When a test or scale is used to measure a variable, some subjects achieve very high or very low scores. In some studies, subjects are selected to be included in a particular group because their scores on a pretest are high or low. A treatment is then performed, and a posttest is administered. However, even with no treatment, subjects who initially achieve very high or very low scores tend to have more moderate scores when retested. Their scores regress toward the mean. Thus, the treatment did not necessarily cause the change. If the pretest scores were low, the posttest may show statistically significant differences (higher scores) from the pretest, leading to the conclusion that the treatment caused the change (type I error). If the pretest scores were high, the posttest scores would tend to be lower (because of a tendency to regress toward the mean) even with no treatment. In this situation, the researcher may mistakenly conclude that the treatment did not cause a change (type II error).

Selection. Selection addresses the process by which subjects are chosen to take part in a study and how subjects are grouped within a study. A selection threat is more likely to occur in studies in which randomization is not possible. In some studies, people selected for the study may differ in some important way from people not selected for the study. In other studies, the threat is due to differences in subjects selected for study groups. For example, people assigned to the control group could be different in some important way from people assigned to the experimental group. This difference in selection could cause the two groups to react differently to the treatment; in this case, the treatment would not have caused the differences in group responses.

Mortality. The mortality threat is due to subjects who drop out of a study before completion. Mortality becomes a threat when (1) those who drop out of a study are a different type of person from those who remain in the study or (2) there is a difference between the kinds of people who drop out of the experimental group and the people who drop out of the control group.

Interactions with Selection. The aforementioned threats can interact with selection to further complicate the validity of the study. The threats most likely to interact with selection are history, maturation, and instrumentation. For example, if the control group you selected for your study has a different history from that of the experimental group, responses to the treatment may be due to this interaction rather than to the treatment.

Ambiguity about the Direction of Causal Influence. Ambiguity about the direction of a causal influence occurs most frequently in correlational studies that address causality. In a study in which variables are measured simultaneously and only once, it may be impossible to determine whether A caused B, B caused A, or the two variables interact in a noncausal way.

Diffusion or Imitation of Treatments. The control group may gain access to the treatment intended for the experimental group (diffusion) or a similar treatment available from another source (imitation). For example, suppose your study examined the effect of teaching specific information to hypertensive patients as a treatment and then measured the effect of the teaching on blood pressure readings and adherence to treatment protocols. Suppose that the control group patients shared the teaching information with the experimental patients (treatment diffusion). This sharing changed the behavior of the control group. The control group patients' responses to the outcome measures may show no differences from those of the experimental group even though the teaching actually did make a difference (type II error).

Compensatory Equalization of Treatments. When the experimental group receives a treatment seen as desirable, such as a new treatment for acquired immunodeficiency syndrome, administrative people and other health professionals may not tolerate the difference and may insist that the control group also receive the treatment. The researcher therefore no longer has a control group and cannot document the effectiveness of the treatment through the study. In health care, both giving and withholding treatments have ethical implications.

Compensatory Rivalry by Respondents Receiving Less Desirable Treatments. For some studies, the design and plan of the study are publicly known. The control group subjects then know the expected difference between their group and the experimental group and may attempt to reduce or reverse the difference. This phenomenon may have occurred in the national hospice study funded by the Health Care Financing Administration (now CMS [Centers for Medicare/Medicaid Studies]) and conducted by Brown University (Greer, Mor, Sherwood, Morris, & Birnbaum, 1983). In this study, 26 hospices were temporarily reimbursed through Medicare while researchers compared the care given at hospices with that given at hospitals. The study made national headlines and was widely discussed in Congress. Health policy decisions related to the reimbursement of hospice care hinged on the findings of the study. The study found no significant differences in care between the two groups, although there were cost differentials. In addition to a selection threat (hospitals providing poor care to dying cancer patients were unlikely to agree to participate in the study), health care professionals in the hospitals selected may have been determined to counter the criticism that the care they provided was poor. This rivalry could have influenced the outcomes of the study and thus threatened its validity.

Resentful Demoralization of Respondents Receiving Less Desirable Treatments. If control group subjects believe that they are receiving less desirable treatment, they may withdraw, give up, or become angry. Changes in behavior resulting from this reaction rather than from the treatment can lead to differences that cannot be attributed to the treatment.

Construct Validity

Construct validity examines the fit between the conceptual definitions and operational definitions of variables. Theoretical constructs or concepts are defined within the framework (conceptual definitions). These conceptual definitions provide the basis for the operational definitions of the variables. Operational definitions (methods of measurement) must validly reflect the theoretical constructs. (Theoretical constructs were discussed in Chapter 7; conceptual and operational definitions of concepts and variables were discussed in Chapter 8.)

Is use of the measure a valid inference about the construct? By examining construct validity, we can determine whether the instrument actually measures the theoretical construct it purports to measure. The process of developing construct validity for an instrument often requires years of scientific work. When selecting methods of measurement, the researcher must determine the previous development of instrument construct validity. (Instrument construct validity is discussed in Chapter 15.) The threats to construct validity are related both to previous instrument development and to the development of measurement techniques as part of the methodology of a particular study. Threats to construct validity are described here.

Inadequate Preoperational Clarification of Constructs. Measurement of a construct stems logically from a concept analysis of the construct, either by the theorist who developed the construct or by the researcher. The conceptual definition should emerge from the concept analysis, and the method of measurement (operational definition) should clearly reflect both. A deficiency in the conceptual or operational definition leads to low construct validity. See Importance of a Conceptual Definition: An Example, in Chapter 7, which discusses the conceptual definition of caring.

Mono-Operation Bias. Mono-operation bias occurs when only one method of measurement is used to assess a construct. When only one method of measurement is used, fewer dimensions of the construct are measured. Construct validity greatly improves if the researcher uses more than one instrument. For example, if anxiety were a dependent variable, more than one measure of anxiety could be used. It is often possible to apply more than one measurement of the dependent variable with little increase in time, effort, or cost.

Monomethod Bias. In monomethod bias, the researcher uses more than one measure of a variable, but all the measures use the same method of recording. Attitude measures, for example, may all be paper and pencil scales. Attitudes that are personal and private, however, may not be detected through the use of paper and pencil tools. Paper and pencil tools may be influenced by feelings of nonaccountability for responses, acquiescence, or social desirability. For example, construct validity would improve if anxiety were measured by a paper and pencil test, verbal messages of anxiety, the galvanic skin response, and the observer's recording of incidence and frequency of behaviors that have been validly linked with anxiety.

Hypothesis Guessing within Experimental Conditions. Hypothesis guessing occurs when subjects within a study guess the hypotheses of the researcher. The validity concern relates to behavioral changes that may occur in the subjects as a consequence of knowing the hypothesis. The extent to which this issue modifies study findings is not currently known.

Evaluation Apprehension. Subjects want researchers to see them in a favorable light. They want to be seen as competent and psychologically healthy. Evaluation apprehension occurs when the subject's responses in the experiment are due to this desire rather than the effects of the independent variable.

Experimenter Expectancies (Rosenthal Effect). The expectancies of the researcher can bias the data. For example, experimenter expectancy occurs if a researcher expects a particular intervention to relieve pain. The data he or she collects may be biased to reflect this expectation. If another researcher who does not believe the intervention would be effective had collected the data, results could have been different. The extent to which this effect actually influences studies is not known. Because of their concern about experimenter expectancy, some researchers are not involved in the data collection process. In other studies, data collectors do not know which subjects are assigned to treatment and control groups.

Another way to control this threat is to design the study so that the various data collectors have different expectations. If the sample size is large enough, the researcher could compare data gathered by the different data collectors. Failing to determine a difference in the data collected by the two groups would give evidence that the construct is valid.

Confounding Constructs and Levels of Constructs. When developing the methodology of a study, you must decide about the intensity of the variable that will be measured or provided as a treatment. This intensity influences the level of the construct that will be reflected in the study. These decisions can affect validity, because the method of measuring the variable influences the outcome of the study and the understanding of the constructs in the study framework.

For example, in reviewing your research, you might find that variable A does not affect variable B when, in fact, it does, but either not at the level of A that was manipulated or not at the level of B that was measured. This issue is a particular problem when A is not linearly related to B or when the effect being studied is weak. To control this threat, you will need to include several levels of A in the design and will have to measure many levels of B. For example, in a study in which A is preoperative teaching and B is anxiety, (1) the instrument being used to measure anxiety measures only high levels of anxiety or (2) the preoperative teaching is provided for 15 minutes but 30 minutes or an hour of teaching is required to cause significant changes in anxiety.

In some cases, there is confounding of variables, which leads to mistaken conclusions. Few measures of a construct are pure measures. Rather, a selected method of measuring a construct can measure a portion of the construct as well as other related constructs. Thus, the measure can lead to confusing results, because the variable measured does not accurately reflect the construct.

Interaction of Different Treatments. The interaction of different treatments is a threat to construct validity if subjects receive more than one treatment in a study. For example, your study might examine the effectiveness of pain relief measures, and subjects might receive medication, massage, distraction, and relaxation strategies. In this case, each one of the treatments interacts with the others, and the effect of any single treatment on pain relief would be impossible to extract. Your study findings could not be generalized to any situation in which patients did not receive all four pain treatments.

Interaction of Testing and Treatment. In some studies, pretesting the subject is thought to modify the effect of the treatment. In this case, the findings can be generalized only to subjects who have been pretested. Although there is some evidence that pretest sensitivity does not have the impact that was once feared, it must be considered in examining the validity of the study. The Solomon Four-Group Design (discussed

in Chapter 11) tests this threat to validity. Repeated posttests can also lead to an interaction of testing and treatment.

Restricted Generalizability Across Constructs. When designing studies, the researcher must consider the impact of the findings on constructs other than those originally conceived in the problem statement. Often, including another measure or two will enable you to generalize the findings to clinical settings, and the translation back to theoretical dimensions will be broader.

External Validity

External validity is concerned with the extent to which study findings can be generalized beyond the sample used in the study. With the most serious threat, the findings would be meaningful only for the group being studied. To some extent, the significance of the study depends on the number of types of people and situations to which the findings can be applied. Sometimes, the factors influencing external validity are subtle and may not be reported in research papers; however, the researcher must be responsible for these factors. Generalization is usually more narrow for a single study than for multiple replications of a study using different samples, perhaps from different populations in different settings. The threats to the ability to generalize the findings (external validity) in terms of study design are described here.

Interaction of Selection and Treatment. Seeking subjects who are willing to participate in a study can be difficult, particularly if the study requires extensive amounts of time or other investments by subjects. If a large number of the persons approached to participate in a study decline to participate, the sample actually selected will be limited in ways that might not be evident at first glance. Only the researcher knows the subjects well. Subjects might be volunteers, "do-gooders," or those with nothing better to do. In this case, generalizing the findings to all members of a population, such as all nurses, all hospitalized patients, or all persons experiencing diabetes, is not easy to justify.

The study must be planned to limit the investment demands on subjects and thereby improve participation. The researcher must report the number of persons who were approached and refused to participate in the study so those who are examining the study can judge any threats to external validity. As the percentage of those who decline to participate increases, external validity decreases. Sufficient data must be collected on the subjects to allow the researcher to be familiar with the characteristics of subjects and, to the extent possible, the characteristics of those who decline to participate. Handwritten notes of verbal remarks made by those who decline and observations of behavior, dress, or other significant factors can be useful in determining selection differences.

Interaction of Setting and Treatment. Bias exists in types of settings and organizations that agree to participate in studies. This bias has been particularly evident in nursing studies. For example, some hospitals welcome nursing studies and encourage employed nurses to conduct studies. Others are resistant to the conduct of nursing research. These two types of hospitals may be different in important ways; thus, there might be an interaction of setting and treatment that limits the generalizability of the findings. As a researcher, you must consider this factor when making statements about the population to which your findings can be generalized.

Interaction of History and Treatment. The circumstances in which a study was conducted (history) influence the treatment and thus the generalizability of the findings. Logically, one can never generalize to the future; however, replicating the study during various periods strengthens the usefulness of findings over time. In critically analyzing studies, you must always consider the period of history during which the study was conducted and the effect of nursing practice and societal events during that period on the reported findings.

Elements of a Good Design

The purpose of design is to set up a situation that maximizes the possibilities of obtaining accurate responses to objectives, questions, or hypotheses. Select a design that is (1) appropriate to the purpose of the study, (2) feasible given realistic constraints, and (3) effective in reducing threats to validity. In most studies, comparisons are the basis of obtaining valid answers. A good design provides the subjects, the setting, and the protocol within which those comparisons can be clearly examined. The comparisons may focus on differences or relationships or both. The study may require that comparisons be made between or among individuals, groups, or variables. A comparison may also be made of measures taken before a treatment (pretest) and measures taken after a treatment (posttest). After these comparisons have been made, you can compare the sample values with statistical tables reflecting population values. In some cases, the study may involve comparing group values with population values.

Designs were developed to reduce threats that might invalidate the comparisons. However, some designs are more effective in reducing threats than others. It may be necessary to modify the design to reduce a particular threat. Before selecting a design, you must identify the threats that are most likely to invalidate your study.

Strategies for reducing threats to validity are sometimes addressed in terms of control. Selecting a design involves decisions related to control of the environment, sample, treatment, and measurement. Increasing control (to reduce threats to validity) will require you to carefully think through every facet of your design. An excellent description of one research team's efforts to develop a good design and control threats to validity is McGuire et al.'s (2000) study, "Maintaining Study Validity in a Changing Clinical Environment." (This paper is available in full text on CINAHL.)

Controlling the Environment

The study environment has a major effect on research outcomes. An uncontrolled environment introduces many extraneous variables into the study situation. Therefore, the study design may include strategies for controlling that environment. In many studies, it is important that the environment be consistent for all subjects. Elements in the environment that may influence the application of a treatment or the measurement of variables must be identified and, when possible, controlled.

Controlling Equivalence of Subjects and Groups

When comparisons are made, it is assumed that the individual units of the comparison are relatively equivalent except for the variables being measured. The researcher does not want to be comparing "apples and oranges." To establish equivalence, the researcher defines sampling criteria. Deviation from this equivalence is a threat to validity. Deviation occurs when sampling criteria have not been adequately defined or when unidentified extraneous variables increase variation in the group.

The most effective strategy for achieving equivalence is random sampling followed by random assignment to groups. However, this strategy does not guarantee equivalence. Even when randomization has been used, the researcher must examine the extent of equivalence by measuring and comparing characteristics for which the groups must be equivalent. This comparison is usually reported in the description of the sample.

Contrary to the aforementioned need for equivalence, groups must be as different as possible in relation to the research variables. Small differences or relationships are more difficult to distinguish than large differences. These differences are often addressed in terms of effect size. Although sample size plays an important role, effect size is maximized by a good design. Effect size is greatest when variance within groups is small.

Control Groups. If the study involves an experimental treatment, the design usually calls for a comparison: Outcome measures for individuals who receive the experimental treatment are compared with outcome measures for those who do not receive the experimental treatment. This comparison requires a control group, subjects who do not receive the experimental treatment.

One threat to validity is the lack of equivalence between the experimental and control groups. This threat is best controlled by random assignment to groups. Another strategy is for the subjects to serve as their own controls. With this design strategy, pretest and posttest measures are taken of the subjects in the absence of a treatment, as well as before and after the treatment. In this case, the timing of measures must be comparable between control and treatment conditions.

Controlling the Treatment

In a well-designed experimental study, the researcher has complete control of any treatment provided. The first step in achieving control is to make a detailed description of the treatment. The next step is to use strategies to ensure consistency in implementing the treatment. Consistency may involve elements of the treatment such as equipment, time, intensity, sequencing, and staff skill.

Variations in the treatment reduce the effect size. It is likely that subjects who receive fewer optimal applications of the treatment will have a smaller response, resulting in more variance in posttest measures for the experimental group. To avoid this problem, the treatment is administered to each subject in exactly the same way. This consideration requires the researcher to think carefully through every element of the treatment to reduce variation wherever possible.

For example, if information is being provided as part of the treatment, some researchers videotape the information, present it to each subject in the same environment, and attempt to decrease variation in the subject's experience before and during the viewing of the videotape. Variations include elements such as time of day, mood, anxiety, experience of pain, interactions with others, and amount of time spent waiting.

In many nursing studies, the researcher does not have complete control of the treatment. It may be costly to control the treatment carefully, it may be difficult to persuade staff to be consistent in the treatment, or the time required to implement a carefully controlled treatment may seem prohibitive. In some cases, the researcher may be studying causal outcomes of an event occurring naturally in the environment.

Regardless of the reason for the researcher's decision, internal validity is reduced when the treatment is inconsistently applied. The risk of a type II error is higher owing to greater variance and a smaller effect size. Thus, studies with uncontrolled treatments need larger samples to reduce the risk of a type II error. External validity may improve if the treatment is studied as it typically occurs clinically. If the study does not reveal a statistically significant difference, then perhaps the typical clinical application of the treatment does not have an important effect on patient outcomes. The question then becomes whether a difference might have been found if the treatment had been consistently applied.

Counterbalancing. In some studies, each subject receives several different treatments sequentially (e.g., relaxation, distraction, and visual imagery) or various levels of the same treatment (e.g., different doses of a drug or varying lengths of relaxation time). Sometimes the application of one treatment can influence the response to later treatments, a phenomenon referred to as a carryover effect. If a carryover effect is known to occur, it is not advisable for a researcher to use this design strategy for the study. However, even when no carryover effect is known, the researcher may take precautions against the possibility that this effect will influence outcomes. In one such precaution, known as counterbalancing, the various treatments are administered in random order rather than being provided consistently in the same sequence.

Controlling Measurement

Measurements play a key role in the validity of a study. Measures must have documented validity and reliability. When measurement is crude or inconsistent, variance within groups is high, and it is more difficult to detect differences or relationships among groups. Thus, the study does not provide a valid test of the hypotheses. However, the consistent implementation of measurements enhances validity. For example, each subject must receive the same instructions about completing scales. Data collectors must be trained and observed for consistency. Designs define the timing of measures (e.g., pretest, posttest). Sometimes, the design calls for multiple measures over time. The researcher must specify the points in time during which measures will be taken. The research report must include a rationale for the timing of measures.

Controlling Extraneous Variables

When designing a study, you must identify variables not included in the design (extraneous variables) that could explain some of the variance that occurs when the study variables are measured. In a good design, the effect of these variables on variance is controlled. The extraneous variables commonly encountered in nursing studies are age, education, gender, social class, severity of illness, level of health, functional status, and attitudes. For a specific study, you must think carefully through the variables that could have an impact on that study.

Design strategies used to control extraneous variables include random sampling, random assignment to groups, selecting subjects that are homogeneous in terms of a particular extraneous variable, selecting a heterogeneous sample, blocking, stratification, matching subjects between groups in relation to a particular variable, and statistical control. Table 10-1 summarizes some nursing studies and the various strategies they have used to control extraneous variables.

Random Sampling. Random sampling increases the probability that subjects with various levels of an extraneous variable are included and are randomly dispersed throughout the groups within the study. This strategy is particularly important for controlling unidentified extraneous variables. Whenever possible, however, extraneous variables must be identified, measured, and reported in the description of the sample.

Random Assignment. Random assignment enhances the probability that subjects with various levels of extraneous variables are equally dispersed in treatment and control groups. Whenever possible, however, this dispersion must be evaluated rather than assumed.

Homogeneity. Homogeneity is a more extreme form of equivalence in which the researcher limits the subjects to only one level of an extraneous variable to reduce its impact on the study findings. To use this strategy, you must have previously identified the extraneous variables. You might choose to include subjects with only one level of an extraneous variable in the study. For example, only subjects between the ages of 20 and 30 years may be included, or only subjects with a particular level of education. The study may include only breast cancer patients who have been diagnosed within 1 month, are at a particular stage of disease and are receiving a specific treatment for cancer. The difficulty with this strategy is that it limits generalization to the types of subjects included in the study. Findings could not justifiably be generalized to types of people excluded from the study.

Heterogeneity. In studies in which random sampling is not used, the researcher may attempt to obtain subjects with a wide variety of characteristics (or who are *heterogeneous*) to reduce the risk of biases. When using the strategy of heterogeneity, you make seek subjects from multiple diverse sources. The strategy is designed to increase generalizability. Characteristics of the sample must be described in the research report.

Blocking. In blocking, the researcher includes subjects with various levels of an extraneous variable in the sample but controls the numbers of subjects at each level of the variable and their random assignment to groups within the study. Designs using blocking are referred to as randomized block designs. The extraneous variable is then used as an independent variable in the data analysis. Therefore, the extraneous variable must be included in the framework and the study hypotheses.

Using this strategy, you might randomly assign equal numbers of subjects in three age categories (younger than 18 years, 18 to 60 years, and older than 60 years) to each group in the study. You could use blocking for several extraneous variables. For example, you could block the study in relation to both age and ethnic background (African American, Hispanic, Caucasian, and Asian). Table 10-2 summarizes an example of this approach.

During data analysis for the randomized block design, each cell in the analysis is treated as a group. Therefore, you must evaluate the cell size for each group and the effect size to ensure adequate power to detect differences. A minimum of 20 subjects per group is recommended. The example described for Table 10-2 would require a minimal sample of 480 subjects.

Stratification. Stratification involves the distribution of subjects throughout the sample, using sampling techniques similar to those used in blocking, but the purpose of the procedure is even distribution throughout the sample. The extraneous variable is not included in the data analysis. Distribution of the extraneous variable is included in the description of the sample.

Matching. To ensure that subjects in the control group are equivalent to subjects in the experimental group, some studies are designed to match subjects in the two groups. Matching is used when a subject in the experimental group is randomly selected and then a subject similar in relation to important extraneous variables is randomly selected for the control group. Clearly, the pool of available subjects would have to be large to accomplish this goal. In quasi-experimental studies, matching may be performed without randomization.

TABLE 10-1	Studies Using Control Strategies for Good Design
Design Strategy	**Example Studies**
Control Group	Hall, W. A., & Hauck, Y. (2007). Getting it right: Australian primiparas' views about breastfeeding: A quasi-experimental study. *International Journal of Nursing Studies, 44*(5), 786–795.
	Kim, H. S. (2007). A randomized controlled trial of a nurse short-message service by cellular phone for people with diabetes. *International Journal of Nursing Studies, 44*(5), 687–692.
	Hee-Sung, K. (2007). Impact of web-based nurse's education on glycosylated haemoglobin in type 2 diabetic patients. *Journal of Clinical Nursing, 16*(7), 1361–1366.
	Hibbard, J. H., Mahoney, E. R., Stock, R., & Tusler, M. (2007). Do increases in patient activation result in improved self-management behaviors? *HSR: Health Services Research, 42*(4), 1443–1463.
	Lett, H. S., Babyak, M. A., Carney, R. M., Burg, M. M., Jaffe, A. S., Catellier, D. J., et al. (2007). Social support and prognosis in patients at increased psychosocial risk recovering from myocardial infarction. *Health Psychology, 26*(4), 418–427.
	Lobchuk, M. M., Degner, L. F., Chateau, D., & Hewitt, D. (2006). Promoting enhanced patient and family caregiver congruence on lung cancer symptom experiences. *Oncology Nursing Forum, 33*(2), 273–282.
Counterbalancing	Cacciola, J. S., Alterman, A. I., McLellan, A. T., Lin, Y., & Lynch, K. G. (2007). Initial evidence for the reliability and validity of a "Lite" version of the Addiction Severity Index. *Drug and Alcohol Dependence, 87*(2–3), 297–302.
	Greer, K. L., Pustay, K. A., Zaun, T. C., & Coppens, P. (2001). A comparison of the effects of toys versus live animals on the communication of patients with dementia of the Alzheimer's type. *Clinical Gerontologist, 24*(3/4), 157–174, 286–293
	Ivarsson, B., Larsson, S., Lührs, C., & Sjöberg, T. (2007). Patients perceptions of information about risks at cardiac surgery. *Patient Education and Counseling, 67*(1–2), 32–38.
	Kotch, J. B., Isbell, P., Weber, D. J., Nguyen, V., Savage, E., Gunn, E., et al. (2007). Hand-washing and diapering equipment reduces disease among children in out-of-home child care centers. *Pediatrics, 120*(1), e29–e36.
Random Sampling	Kim, H. S., & Kim, H. S. (2007). Development of a Family Dynamic Environment Scale for Korean adolescents. *Public Health Nursing, 24*(4), 372–381.
	Martinez-Donate, A. P., Hovell, M. F., Hofstetter, C. R., González-Pérez, G. J., Adams, M. A., & Kotay, A. (2007). Correlates of home smoking bans among Mexican-Americans. *American Journal of Health Promotion, 21*(4), 229–236.
	Tsai, Y. F. (2007). Self-care management and risk factors for depressive symptoms among Taiwanese insntitutionalized older persons. *Nursing Research, 56*(2), 124–131.
	Zaky, H. H., Khattab, H. A., & Galal, D. (2007). Assessing the quality of reproductive health services in Egypt via exit interviews. *Maternal and Child Health Journal, 11*(3), 301–306.
Random Assignment	de Laat, E., Schoonhoven, L., Grypdonck, M., Verbeek, A., de Graaf, R., Pickkers, P., et al. (2007). Early postoperative 30 degrees lateral positioning after coronary artery surgery: Influence on cardiac output. *Journal of Clinical Nursing, 16*(4), 654–661.
	Goyal, D., Gay, C. L., & Lee, K. A. (2007). Patterns of sleep disruption and depressive symptoms in new mothers. *Journal of Perinatal & Neonatal Nursing, 21*(2), 123–129.
	Roman, L. A., Lindsay, J. K., Moore, J. S., Duthie, P. A., Peck, C., Barton, L. R., et al. (2007). Addressing mental health and stress in Medicaid-insured pregnant women using a nurse-community health worker home visiting team. *Public Health Nursing, 24*(3), 239–248.
Homogeneity	Campos de Carvalho, E., Martins, F. T., & dos Santos, C. B. (2007). A pilot study of a relaxation technique for management of nausea and vomiting in patients receiving cancer chemotherapy. *Cancer Nursing, 30*(2), 163–167.
	Courts, N. F., Newton, A. N., & McNeal, L. J. (2005). Husbands and wives living with multiple sclerosis. *Journal of Neuroscience Nursing, 37*(1), 20–27.
	Estok, P. J., Sedlak, C. A., Doheny, M. O., & Hall, R. (2007). Structural model for osteoporosis preventing behavior in postmenopausal women. *Nursing Research, 56*(3), 148–158.
	Ferri Morales, A., Melgar de Correl, G., Avendaño Coy, J., Puchades Belenguer, M. H., & Torres Costoso, A. I. (2003). Qualitative study on the process of searching for health of urinary incontinence in the woman [Spanish]. *Rev Iberoam Fisioter Kinesiol, 6*(2), 74–80.
	Whittemore, R., D'Eramo Melkus, G., & Grey, M. (2005). Metabolic control, self-management and psychosocial adjustment in women with type 2 diabetes. *Journal of Clinical Nursing, 14*(2), 195–203.

Continued

TABLE 10-1 ░░ Studies Using Control Strategies for Good Desigs—*Cont'd*

Design Strategy	Example Studies
Heterogeneity	Benkert, R., Barkauskas, V., Pohl, J., Corser, W., Tanner, C., Wells, M., et al. (2002). Patient satisfaction outcomes in nurse-managed centers. *Outcomes Management, 6*(4), 174–181.
	Martin, L., Farrell, M., Lambrenos, K., & Nayagam, D. (2003). Living with the Ilizarov frame: Adolescent perceptions. *Journal of Advanced Nursing, 43*(5), 478–487.
	Neufeld, A., & Harrison, M. J. (2003). Unfulfilled expectations and negative interactions: Nonsupport in the relationships of women caregivers. *Journal of Advanced Nursing, 41*(4), 323–331.
Blocking	Rousaud, A., Blanch, J., Hautzinger, M., De Lazzari, E., Peri, J. M., Puig, O., et al. (2007). Improvement of psychosocial adjustment to HIV-1 infection through a cognitive-behavioral oriented group psychotherapy program: A pilot study. *AIDS Patient Care and STDs, 21*(3), 212–222.
	Tsay, S. L., Wang, J. C., Lin, K. C., & Chung, U. L. (2005). Effects of acupressure therapy for patients having prolonged mechanical ventilation support. *Journal of Advanced Nursing, 52*(2), 142–150.
Stratification	Beccaro, M., Constantini, M., Giorgi Rossi, P., Miccinesi, G., Grimaldi, M., Bruzzi, P., et al. (2006). Actual and preferred place of death of cancer patients. Results from the Italian survey of the dying of cancer. *Journal of Epidemiology & Community Health, 60*(5), 412–416.
	Carey, T. A. (2006). Estimating treatment duration for psychotherapy in primary care. *Journal of Public Mental Health, 5*(3), 23–28.
	Leslie, E., Coffee, N., Frank, L., Owen, N., Bauman, A., & Hugo, G. (2005). Walkability of local communities: Using geographic information systems to objectively assess relevant environmental attributes. *Health & Place, 13*(1), 111–122.
	Pancorbo-Hidalgo, P. L., Garcia-Fernández, F. P., López-Medina, I. M., & López-Ortega, J. (2005). Protocols and documentation in prevention and treatment of pressure ulcers: The situation in Andalusia (Spain). *Gerokomos, 16*(4), 219–228.
Matching	Arman, M., Backman, M., Carlsson, M., & Hamrin, E. (2006). Women's perceptions and beliefs about the genesis of their breast cancer. *Cancer Nursing, 29*(2), 142–148.
	Gitta, S. N., Wabwire-Mangen, F., Kitimbo, D., Pariyo, G., Centers for Disease Control and Prevention. (2006). Risk factors for neonatal tetanus—Busoga region, Uganda, 2002–2003. *MMWR: Morbidity & Mortality Weekly Report, 55*(Supp 1), 25–30.
	Graham, R. J., Fleegler, E. W., & Robinson, W. M. (2007). Cronic ventilator need in the community: A 2005 pediatric census of Massachusetts. *Pediatrics, 119*(6), e1280–e1287.
	Trevisanuto, D., Micaglio, M., Pitton, M., Magarotto, M., Piva, D., & Zanardo, V. (2006). Laryngeal mask airway: Is the management of neonates requiring positive pressure ventilation at birth changing? *Journal of Neonatal Nursing, 12*(5), 185–192.
Statistical Control (partialing out)	Griffin-Blake, C. S., & DeJoy, D. M. (2006). Evaluation of social-cognitive versus stage-matched, self-help physical activity interventions at the workplace. *American Journal of Health Promotion, 20*(3), 200–209.
	Roberts, J. E., Burchinal, M. R., Jackson, S. C., Hooper, S. R., Roush, J., Mundy, M., et al. (2000). Otitis media in childhood in relation to preschool language and school readiness skills among black children. *Pediatrics, 106*(4), 725–735.
	Roberts, J. E., Burchinal, M. R., & Zeisel, S. A. (2002). Otitis media in early childhood in relation to children's school-age language and academic skills. *Pediatrics, 110*(4), 696–706.
	Wilson, K. M., & Swanson, H. L. (2001). Are mathematics disabilities due to a domain-general or a domain-specific working memory deficit? *Journal of Learning Disabilities, 34*(3), 237–248.

Statistical Control. In some studies, it is not considered feasible to control extraneous variables through the design. However, the researcher recognizes the possible impact of extraneous variables on variance and effect size. Therefore, measures are obtained for the identified extraneous variables. Data analysis strategies that have the capacity to remove (partial out) the variance explained by the extraneous variable are performed before the analysis of differences or relationships between or among the variables of interest in the study. One statistical procedure commonly used

for this purpose is analysis of covariance, described in Chapter 22. Although statistical control seems to be a quick and easy solution to the problem of extraneous variables, its results are not as satisfactory as those of the various methods of design control.

Triangulation

There has been much controversy among researchers about the relative validity of various approaches to research. Designing quantitative experimental studies with rigorous controls may provide strong external

TABLE **10-2** Example of Blocking Using Age and Ethnic Background				
Age	Ethnic Group		Experimental	Control
Younger than 18 years $n = 160$	African American	$n = 40$	$n = 20$	$n = 20$
	Hispanic	$n = 40$	$n = 20$	$n = 20$
	Caucasian	$n = 40$	$n = 20$	$n = 20$
	Asian	$n = 40$	$n = 20$	$n = 20$
19 to 60 years $n = 160$	African American	$n = 40$	$n = 20$	$n = 20$
	Hispanic	$n = 40$	$n = 20$	$n = 20$
	Caucasian	$n = 40$	$n = 20$	$n = 20$
	Asian	$n = 40$	$n = 20$	$n = 20$
Older than 60 years $n = 160$	African American	$n = 40$	$n = 20$	$n = 20$
	Hispanic	$n = 40$	$n = 20$	$n = 20$
	Caucasian	$n = 40$	$n = 20$	$n = 20$
	Asian	$n = 40$	$n = 20$	$n = 20$

validity but questionable or limited internal validity. Qualitative studies may have strong internal validity but questionable external validity. A single approach to measuring a concept may be inadequate to justify a claim that it is a valid measure of a theoretical concept. Testing a single theory may leave the results open to the challenge of rival hypotheses from other theories.

Researchers have been exploring alternative design strategies that might increase the overall validity of studies. The strategy generating the most interest is triangulation. First used by Campbell and Fiske in 1959, triangulation is the combined use of two or more theories, methods, data sources, investigators, or analysis methods in the study of the same phenomenon. Denzin (1989) identified the following four types of triangulation: (1) data triangulation, (2) investigator triangulation, (3) theoretical triangulation, and (4) methodological triangulation. Kimchi, Polivka, and Stevenson (1991) have suggested a fifth type, analysis triangulation. Multiple triangulation is the combination of more than one of these types.

Data Triangulation

Data triangulation involves the collection of data from multiple sources for the same study. For the collection to be considered triangulation, the data must all have the same foci. The intent is to obtain diverse views of the phenomenon under study for purposes of validation (Kimchi et al., 1991). These data sources provide an opportunity for researchers to examine how an event is experienced by different individuals, groups of people, or communities; at different times; or in different settings (Mitchell, 1986).

Longitudinal studies are not a form of triangulation because their purpose is to identify change. When time is triangulated, the purpose is to validate the congruence of the phenomenon over time. For a multisite study to be triangulated, data from the settings must be cross-validated for multisite consistency. When person triangulation is used, data from individuals might be compared for consistency with data obtained from groups. The intent is to use data from one source to validate data from another source (Kimchi et al., 1991).

Investigator Triangulation

In investigator triangulation, two or more investigators with diverse research training backgrounds examine the same phenomenon (Mitchell, 1986). For example, a qualitative researcher and a quantitative researcher might cooperatively design and conduct a study of interest to both. Kimchi et al. (1991, p. 365) have held that investigator triangulation has occurred when "(a) each investigator has a prominent role in the study, (b) the expertise of each investigator is different, and (c) the expertise (disciplinary bias) of each investigator is evident in the study." The use of investigator triangulation removes the potential for bias that may occur in a single-investigator study (Denzin, 1989; Duffy, 1987). Kimchi et al. (1991) suggested that investigator triangulation is difficult to discern from published reports. They advised that, in the future, authors should claim that they have performed investigator triangulation and describe how they achieved it in their study.

Theoretical Triangulation

Theoretical triangulation is the use of all the theoretical interpretations "that could conceivably be applied to a given area" (Denzin, 1989, p. 241) as the framework for a study. Using this strategy, the researcher critically examines various theoretical points of view for utility and power. The researcher then develops competing hypotheses on the basis of the different theoretical perspectives, which are tested using the same data set. We can then place greater confidence in the accepted hypotheses because they have been pitted against rival hypotheses (Denzin, 1989; Mitchell, 1986). This is a tougher test of existing theory in a field of study because alternative theories are examined rather than a single test of a proposition or propositions from one theory. Theoretical triangulation can lead to the development of more powerful substantive theories that have some scientific validation. Denzin (1989) recommended the following steps to achieve theoretical triangulation:

1. *A comprehensive list of all possible interpretations in a given area is constructed. This will involve bringing a variety of theoretical perspectives to bear upon the phenomena at hand (including interactionism, phenomenology, Marxism, feminist theory, semiotics, cultural studies, and so on).*
2. *The actual research is conducted, and empirical materials are collected.*
3. *The multiple theoretical frameworks enumerated in Step 1 are focused on the empirical materials.*
4. *Those interpretations that do not bear on the materials are discarded or set aside.*
5. *Those interpretations that map and make sense of the phenomena are assembled into an interpretive framework that addresses all of the empirical materials.*
6. *A reformulated interpretive system is stated based at all points on the empirical materials just examined and interpreted." (Denzin, 1989, p. 241)*

Currently, few nursing studies meet Denzin's criteria for theoretical triangulation, although some frameworks for nursing studies are developed to compare propositions from more than one theory. For example, Yarcheski, Mahon, and Yarcheski (1999) conducted an empirical test of alternative theories of anger in early adolescents. Kushner and Morrow (2003) proposed triangulating grounded theory, feminist theory, and critical theory.

Methodological Triangulation

Methodological triangulation is the use of two or more research methods in a single study (Mitchell, 1986). The difference can be at the level of design or of data collection. Researchers frequently use methodological triangulation, the most common type of

triangulation, to examine complex concepts. Complex concepts of interest in nursing include caring, sustaining hope during terminal illness, coping with chronic illness, and promoting health.

There are two types of methodological triangulation: within-method triangulation and across-method triangulation (Denzin, 1989). Within-method triangulation, the simpler form, is used when the phenomenon being studied is multidimensional. For example, two or three different quantitative instruments might be used to measure the same phenomenon. Conversely, two or more qualitative methods might be used (Annells, 2006). Examples of different data collection methods are questionnaires, physiological instruments, scales, interviews, and observation techniques. Between-method triangulation involves combining research strategies from two or more research traditions in the same study. For example, methods from qualitative research and quantitative research might be used in the same study (Duffy, 1987; Mitchell, 1986; Morse, 1991; Porter, 1989). From these research traditions, different types of designs, methods of measurement, data collection processes, or data analysis techniques might be used to examine a phenomenon to try to achieve convergent validity.

Mitchell (1986) identified the following four principles that should be applied with methodological triangulation:

(1) The research question must be clearly focused; (2) the strengths and weaknesses of each chosen method must complement each other; (3) the methods must be selected according to their relevance to the phenomenon being studied; and (4) the methodological approach must be monitored throughout the study to make sure the first three principles are followed. (pp. 22–23)

Analysis Triangulation

In analysis triangulation, the same data set is analyzed with the use of two or more differing analyses techniques. The purpose is to evaluate the similarity of findings. The intent is to provide a means of cross-validating the findings (Kimchi et al., 1991).

Pros and Cons of Triangulation

Triangulation may become the research trend of the future. However, before jumping on this bandwagon, we would be prudent to consider the implications of using these strategies. Some are concerned that triangulation will be used in studies for which it is not appropriate. An additional concern is that the popularization of the method will generate a number of triangulated studies that have been poorly conducted. Sohier (1988, p. 740) pointed out that "multiple methods will not compensate for poor design or sloppy research. Ill-conceived measures will compound error rather than reduce it. Unclear questions will not become clearer."

The suggestion that qualitative and quantitative methods be included in the same study has generated considerable controversy in the nursing research community (Clarke & Yaros, 1988; Mitchell, 1986; Morse, 1991; Phillips, 1988a, 1988b; Sims & Sharp, 1998). Myers and Haase (1989) believe that the integration of these two research approaches is inevitable and essential. Clarke and Yaros (1988) have suggested that combining methods is the first step in the development of new methodologies, which are greatly needed to investigate nursing phenomena. Hogan and DeSantis (1991) believe that triangulation of qualitative and quantitative methods will lead to the development of substantive theory. Phillips (1988a, 1988b) has held the position that the two methods are incompatible because they are based on different worldviews. If a single investigator attempted to use both methods in one study, he or she would have to interpret the meaning of the data from two philosophical perspectives. Because researchers tend to acquire their training within a particular research tradition, it may be difficult for them to incorporate another research tradition. As Sandelowski (1995, p. 569) has stated, "a misplaced ecumenicism, definitional drift, and conceptual misappropriation are evident in discussions of triangulation, which has become a technique for everything."

Mitchell (1986) identified a number of problems that investigators may encounter when using this method. These strategies require many observations and result in large volumes of data for analysis. The investigator must have the ability and the desire to deal with complex design, measurement, and analysis issues with limited resources. Mitchell (1986) identified the following issues that the investigator must consider during the data analysis:

- How to combine numerical (quantitative) data and linguistic or textual (qualitative) data
- How to interpret divergent results from numerical data and linguistic data
- What to do with overlapping concepts that emerge from the data and are not clearly differentiated from one another
- Whether and how to weight data sources
- Whether each different method used should be considered equally sensitive and weighted equally

Myers and Haase (1989) provided the following guidelines, which they believe are necessary when one is merging qualitative and quantitative methods. These guidelines are based on the assumption that at least two investigators (one qualitative and one quantitative) are involved in any study combining these two methods.

1. *The world is viewed as a whole, an interactive system with patterns of information exchange between subsystems or levels of reality.*
2. *Both subjective and objective data are recognized as legitimate avenues for gaining understanding.*
3. *Both atomistic and holistic thinking are used in design and analysis.*
4. *The concept of research "participant" includes not only those who are the subjects of the methodology but also those who administer or operate the methodology.*
5. *Maximally conflicting points of view are sought with provision for systematic and controlled confrontation. Respectful, honest, open confrontation on points of view between investigators is essential. Here, conflict is seen as a positive value because it offers potential for expanding questioning and consequent understanding. Confrontation occurs between co-investigators with differing expertise who recognize that both approaches are equally valid and vulnerable. Ability to consider participants' views which may differ from the investigator's perspective is equally important." (Myers & Haase, 1989, p. 300)*

Morse (1991) stated that qualitative and quantitative methods cannot be equally weighted in a research project. The project either (1) is theoretically driven by qualitative methods and incorporates a complementary quantitative component or (2) is theoretically driven by the quantitative method and incorporates a complementary qualitative component. However, each method must be complete in itself and must meet appropriate criteria for rigor. For example, if qualitative interviews are conducted, "the interviews should be continued until saturation is reached, and the content analysis conducted inductively, rather than forcing the data into some preconceived categories to fit the quantitative study or to prove a point" (Morse, 1991, p. 121).

Morse (1991) also noted that the greatest threat to validity of methodological triangulation is not philosophical incompatibility but the use of inadequate or inappropriate samples. The quantitative requirement for large, randomly selected samples is inconsistent with the qualitative requirement that subjects be selected according to how well they represent the phenomena of interest, and sample selection ceases when saturation of data is reached. Morse (1991) did not consider it necessary, however, for the two approaches to use the same samples for the study. In all aspects of a methodologically triangulated study, Morse (1991) observed that strategies must be implemented to maintain the validity for each method. Overall, Morse supported the use of methodological triangulation, believing that it "will strengthen research results and contribute to theory and knowledge development" (Morse, 1991, p. 122).

Duffy (1987, p. 133) held that triangulation, "when used appropriately, combines different methods in a variety of ways to produce richer and more insightful analyses of complex phenomena than can be achieved by either method separately." Coward (1990) opined that the combining of qualitative and quantitative methods will increase support for validity:

> *Construct validity is enhanced when results are stable across multiple measures of a concept. Statistical conclusion validity is enhanced when results are stable across many data sets and methods of analysis. Internal validity is enhanced when results are stable across many potential threats to causal inference. External validity is supported when results are stable across multiple settings, populations, and times." (p. 166)*

Sandelowski (1995) recommended that

> *the concept of triangulation ought to be reserved for designating a technique for conformation employed within paradigms in which convergent and consensual validity are valued and in which it is deemed appropriate to use information from one source to corroborate another. Whether triangulation [is used] or not, the purpose, method of execution, and assumptions in forming any research combinations should be clearly delineated. (p. 573)*

SUMMARY

- Research design is a blueprint for the conduct of a study that maximizes the researcher's control over factors that could interfere with the desired outcomes.

- Before selecting a design, the researcher must understand certain concepts: causality, bias, manipulation, control, and validity.
- The purpose of design is to set up a situation that maximizes the possibilities of obtaining valid answers to research questions or hypotheses.
- A good design provides the subjects, the setting, and the protocol within which these comparisons can be clearly examined.
- Designs were developed to reduce threats to the validity of the comparisons. However, some designs are more effective in reducing threats than others.
- In designing the study, the researcher must identify variables not included in the design (extraneous variables) that could explain some of the variance in measurement of the study variables.
- Triangulation is the combined use of two or more theories, methods, data sources, investigators, or analysis methods to study the same phenomenon.

REFERENCES

Anells, M. (2006). Triangulation of qualitative approaches: Hermeneutic phenomenology and grounded theory. *Journal of Advanced Nursing, 56*(1), 55–61.

Campbell, D. T., & Fiske, D. W. (1959). Convergent and discriminant validation by the multitrait-multimethod matrix. *Psychological Bulletin, 56*(2), 81–105.

Clarke, P. N., & Yaros, P. S. (1988). Research blenders: Commentary and response. *Nursing Science Quarterly, 1*(4), 147–149.

Cook, T. D., & Campbell, D. T. (1979). *Quasi-experimentation: Design and analysis issues for field settings.* Chicago: Rand McNally.

Coward, D. D. (1990). Critical multiplism: A research strategy for nursing science. *Image: Journal of Nursing Scholarship, 22*(3), 163–167.

Denzin, N. K. (1989). *The research act: A theoretical introduction to sociological methods* (3rd ed.). New York: McGraw-Hill.

Duffy, M. E. (1987). Methodological triangulation: A vehicle for merging quantitative and qualitative research methods. *Image: Journal of Nursing Scholarship, 19*(3), 130–133.

Goodwin, L. D. (1984). Increasing efficiency and precision of data analysis: Multivariate vs. univariate statistical techniques. *Nursing Research, 33*(4), 247–249.

Greer, D. S., Mor, V., Sherwood, S., Morris, J. M., & Birnbaum, H. (1983). National hospice study analysis plan. *Journal of Chronic Disease, 36*(11), 737–780.

Hogan, N., & DeSantis, L. (1991). Development of substantive theory in nursing. *Nursing Education Today, 11*(3), 167–171.

Kimchi, J., Polivka, B., & Stevenson, J. S. (1991). Triangulation: Operational definitions. *Nursing Research, 40*(6), 364–366.

Kushner, K. E., & Morrow, R. (2003). Grounded theory, feminist theory, critical theory: Toward theoretical triangulation. *Advances in Nursing Science, 26*(1), 30–43.

McGuire, D. B., DeLoney, V. G., Yeager, K. A., Owen, D. C., Peterson, D. E., Lin, L. S., et al. (2000). Maintaining study validity in a changing clinical environment. *Nursing Research*, *49*(4), 231–235.

Mitchell, E. S. (1986). Multiple triangulation: A methodology for nursing science. *Advances in Nursing Science*, *8*(3), 18–26.

Morse, J. M. (1991). Approaches to qualitative-quantitative methodological triangulation. *Nursing Research*, *40*(1), 120–123.

Myers, S. T., & Haase, J. E. (1989). Guidelines for integration of quantitative and qualitative approaches. *Nursing Research*, *38*(5), 299–301.

Phillips, J. R. (1988b). Research issues: Research blenders. *Nursing Science Quarterly*, *1*(1), 4–5.

Porter, E. J. (1989). The qualitative-quantitative dualism. *Image: Journal of Nursing Scholarship*, *21*(2), 98–102.

Sandelowski, M. (1995). Triangles and crystals: On the geometry of qualitative research. *Research in Nursing & Health*, *18*(6), 569–574.

Sims, J., & Sharp, K. (1998). A critical appraisal of the role of triangulation in nursing research. *International Journal of Nursing Studies*, *35*(1/2), 23–31.

Sohier, R. (1988). Multiple triangulation and contemporary nursing research. *Western Journal of Nursing Research*, *10*(6), 732–742.

Yarcheski, A., Mahon, M. E., & Yarcheski, T. J. (1999). An empirical test of alternate theories of anger in early adolescents. *Nursing Research*, *48*(6), 317–323.

CHAPTER **11**

Selecting a Quantitative Research Design

A design is the blueprint for conducting a study that maximizes control over factors that could interfere with the validity of the findings. A research design gives you greater control and thus improves the validity of your study. To select an appropriate research design, you will need to integrate many elements. Chapter 10 began with questions that will help you select a design or identify by name the design of a study you are appraising. But identifying the design of a published study is not always easy, because many published studies do not identify the design used. Determining the design may require you to put together bits of information from various parts of the research report.

This chapter describes the designs most commonly used in nursing research, using the design categories described in Chapter 3: descriptive, correlational, quasi-experimental, and experimental. Descriptive and correlational designs examine variables in natural environments and do not include researcher-designed treatments or interventions. Quasi-experimental and experimental designs examine the effects of an intervention by comparing differences between groups that have received the intervention and those that have not received the intervention. As you review each design, note the threats to validity controlled by the design, keeping in mind that uncontrolled threats in the design you choose may weaken the validity of your study. Table 11-1 lists the designs discussed in this chapter. After the descriptions of the designs, we provide a series of decision trees that will help you to select the appropriate design or to identify the design used in a published study.

Investigators have always developed designs to meet emerging research needs. In the 1930s, Sir Ronald A. Fisher (1935) developed the first experimental designs, which were published in a book titled *The Design of Experiments*. However, most work on design has been conducted since the 1970s. Since this time, designs have become much more sophisticated and varied. There is no universal standard for categorizing designs. Names of designs change as various authors discuss them. Researchers sometimes merge elements of several designs to meet the research needs of a particular study. From these developments, new designs sometimes emerge.

Originally, only experimental designs were considered of value. In addition, many believed that the only setting in which an experiment can be conducted is a laboratory, where stricter controls can be maintained than in a field or natural setting. This approach is appropriate for the natural sciences but not for the social sciences. From the social sciences have emerged additional quantitative designs (descriptive, correlational, and quasi-experimental), methodological designs, and qualitative designs. The epidemiology, public health, and community health fields have presented time-series designs, health promotion designs, and prevention designs.

At present, nurse researchers are using designs developed in other disciplines, such as psychology, that meet the needs of that discipline. Will these designs be effective in adding to the knowledge base required for nursing? These designs are a useful starting point, but nurse scientists must go beyond these designs to develop designs that will more

TABLE 11-1 ■ Research Designs

Descriptive study designs
  Typical descriptive study designs
  Comparative descriptive study designs
  Time-dimensional designs
    Longitudinal designs
    Cross-sectional designs
    Trend designs
    Event-partitioning designs
  Case study designs
Correlational study designs
  Descriptive correlational designs
  Predictive designs
  Model-testing designs
Quasi-experimental study designs
  Nonequivalent comparison group studies
    One-group posttest-only designs
    Posttest-only designs with comparison group
    One-group pretest-posttest designs
    Pretest and posttest designs with a comparison group
    Pretest and posttest designs with two comparison
      treatments
Pretest and posttest designs with two comparison treatments
  and a standard or routine care group
    Pretest and posttest designs with a removed treatment
    Pretest and posttest designs with a reversed treatment
  Interrupted time-series designs
    Simple interrupted time-series designs
    Interrupted time-series designs with a no-treatment
      comparison group
    Interrupted time-series designs with multiple treatment
      replications
Experimental study designs
  Classic experimental design
  Experimental posttest-only comparison group designs
  Randomized block designs
  Factorial designs
  Nested designs
  Crossover or counterbalanced designs
  Randomized clinical trials

appropriately meet the needs of the nursing community. To go beyond current designs, nurse scientists must have a working knowledge of available designs and of the logic on which they are based. Designs created to meet nursing needs should be congruent with nursing philosophy. They must provide a means for nurses to examine dimensions of nursing within a holistic framework and to review those dimensions over time. Designs must be developed that can seek answers to important nursing questions rather than answering only questions that can be examined by existing designs.

Innovative design strategies are beginning to appear within nursing research. One example is the intervention research design described in Chapter 13. Developing designs to study the outcomes of nursing actions is also important. This emerging field of research in nursing is described in Chapter 12. Nurse researchers must see themselves as credible scientists before they will dare to develop new design strategies that will explore little-understood aspects of nursing. To develop a new design, the researcher must carefully consider possible threats to validity and ways to diminish them. She or he must also be willing to risk the temporary failures that are always inherent in the development of something new.

DESCRIPTIVE STUDY DESIGNS

Descriptive study designs (Table 11-1) are crafted to gain more information about characteristics within a particular field of study. Their purpose is to provide a picture of situations as they naturally happen. In many aspects of nursing, a phenomenon must be clearly delineated before prediction or causality can be examined. A descriptive design may be used to develop theory, identify problems with current practice, justify current practice, make judgments, or determine what others in similar situations are doing. Variables are not manipulated and there is no treatment or intervention. Dependent and independent variables should not be used within a descriptive design, because the design involves no attempt to establish causality.

Descriptive designs vary in levels of complexity. Some contain only two variables, whereas others may have multiple variables. The relationships among variables present an overall picture of the phenomenon being examined, but examination of types and degrees of relationships is not the primary purpose of a descriptive study. Protection against bias (or threat to the validity) in a descriptive design is achieved through (1) links between conceptual and operational definitions of variables, (2) sample selection and size, (3) the use of valid and reliable instruments, and (4) data collection procedures that achieve some environmental control.

Typical Descriptive Study Designs

Figure 11-1 presents the commonly used descriptive study design. The design examines characteristics of a single sample. It identifies a phenomenon of interest and the variables within the phenomenon, develops conceptual and operational definitions of the variables, and describes the variables. The description of

CLARIFICATION ⟶ MEASUREMENT ⟶ DESCRIPTION ⟶ INTERPRETATION

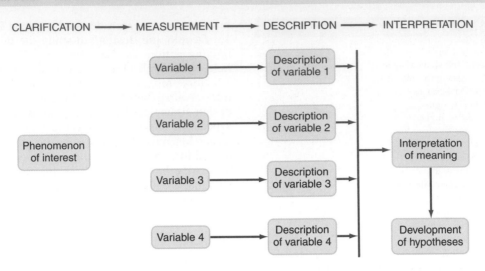

Figure **11-1** Typical descriptive study design.

the variables leads to an interpretation of the theoretical meaning of the findings and provides knowledge of the variables and the study population that can be used for future research in the area.

Most studies contain descriptive components; however, the methodology of some studies is confined to the typical descriptive design. This is a critically important design for acquiring knowledge in an area in which little research has been conducted. An example of a descriptive design is the Rodehorst, Wilhelm, and Stepans (2006) study of asthma in rural elementary school children. The following excerpt describes the design of their study.

Background: Asthma, the leading cause of chronic illness in children, must be managed in both the home and school environments. Identification of children who have risk factors associated with asthma is the first step toward achieving one of the Healthy People 2010 (2000) objectives, which identifies that 25 states will establish a system of surveillance to track asthma mortality, morbidity, access to care, and asthma management. Purpose: The purposes of this research were to: a) identify rural children who are at risk for asthma through written screening; b) assess parameters of respiratory health status of rural school-aged children as indicated by forced expiratory volume at 1 second (FEV[1]), forced vital capacity (FVC), peak expiratory flow (PEF), mean mid-expiratory flow (FEF[25-75]); and c) identify the number of rural school-aged children who sought and obtained follow-up from their primary health care provider and were given a definitive diagnosis of asthma. Framework: The Vulnerable Populations Framework (Flaskerud & Winslow, 1998) was used to organize this study.

Methodology: A prospective descriptive design was utilized for this research. Results: Approximately 12% of the children screened were referred to their primary care provider (PCP) for follow-up care. Of these approximately half of the children were seen by their PCP. Barriers to seeking follow-up care were: a) the child was not symptomatic all the time, b) reluctance to be diagnosed with asthma, and c) others, such as cost and time. Children who were not well controlled identified that they ran out of medicine and their parents did not refill their prescription.

Results from this *descriptive* study indicate that screening for asthma in school may be a way to identify those children who are at risk for asthma, and who are not diagnosed as well as those who are diagnosed with asthma but are not optimally managed. While many parents wanted their children to be screened, follow-up care was not critical to them.

Implications: Nurses working in a school setting are in a prime position to help identify those children with signs and symptoms of asthma. In addition, use of written screenings with or without spirometry may be helpful in identifying children at risk for asthma. Further studies need to be undertaken to determine if written screening is as efficacious as spirometry for school and other ambulatory care settings. (Rodehorst et al., 2006, p. 995; full-text article available in CINAHL)

This is a descriptive study because there is no treatment, the researchers measure the variables of children who are at risk of asthma, (FEV[1]), (FVC), (PEF), (FEF[25-75]); and children who sought and obtained follow-up from their primary health care provider and were given a definitive diagnosis of asthma, and described the results of measuring the variables.

Some descriptive studies use questionnaires (surveys) to describe an identified area of concern. For example, Yoon and Black (2006) distributed a questionnaire to 63 caregivers of children with sickle-cell disease to determine the prevalence and types of complementary therapies used for pain management (full-text article available in CINAHL). Other descriptive studies obtain data from retrospective chart review. For example, Kline and Edwards (2007) conducted a chart review to describe the effectiveness of intrapartum intravenous (I.V.) insulin on antepartum and intrapartum diabetic control of the mother and on the occurrence and severity of hypoglycemia in the neonate (full-text article available in CINAHL).

This is a descriptive design because there is no treatment or intervention, the researchers measured the variables of intrapartum I.V. insulin, antepartum diabetic control, intrapartum diabetic control, and hypoglycemia in the neonate. The results were a description of the measures of these variables.

It is not uncommon for researchers using a descriptive design to combine quantitative descriptive methods and qualitative methods (triangulation of method). To use this strategy, consult with a researcher experienced in using qualitative methods or include this person as a research partner to appropriately collect qualitative data and interpret it. Meghani and Keane (2007) used quantitative and qualitative methods in their study of preference for analgesic treatment for cancer patients among African Americans (the full-text article is available in CINAHL). The authors used demographic data, the Brief Pain Inventory, and in-depth semistructured interviews. Their sample of 35 patients was from three outpatient oncology clinics. Their study identified the major sources of anxiety described by this sample. The goal of their study was to improve our understanding of patient needs and assist in the development of specific interventions that might alleviate the problem.

Comparative Descriptive Designs

The comparative descriptive design (Figure 11-2) examines and describes differences in variables in two or more groups that occur naturally in the setting. Descriptive statistics and inferential statistical analyses may be used to examine differences between or among groups. Commonly, the results obtained from these analyses are not generalized to a population because the description is to a very specific sample and would not necessarily apply to a larger population. An example of this design is the study by Cramer, Chen, Roberts, and Clute (2007) of the social and economic impact of community-based prenatal care. The following extract describes the study.

> Objective: This article describes the evaluation and findings of a community-based prenatal care program, Omaha Healthy Start (OHS), designed to reduce local racial disparities in birth outcomes. Design: This evaluative study used a comparative descriptive design, and Targeting Outcomes of Programs was the conceptual framework for evaluation. Sample: The evaluation followed 3 groups for 2 years: OHS birth mothers ($N = 79$; $N = 157$); non-OHS participant birth mothers ($N = 746$; $N = 774$); and Douglas County birth mothers ($N = 7,962$; $N = 7,987$). Measurement: OHS provided case management, home visits, screening, referral, transportation, and health education to participants. Program outcome measures included low birth weight, infant mortality, adequacy of care, trimester of care, and costs of care. Results: OHS birth outcomes improved during year 2, and there was a 31% cost saving in the average hospital expenditure compared with the nonparticipant groups. Preliminary evaluative analysis indicates that prenatal case management and community outreach can improve birth outcomes for minority women, while producing cost savings. Conclusions: Further prospective study is needed to document trends over a longer period of time regarding the relationship between community-based case management programs for minority populations, birth outcomes, and costs of care. (Cramer et al., 2007; full-text article available in CINAHL)

This is a comparative descriptive design because there is no treatment or intervention; the researchers describe variables of incidence of case management, home visits, screening, referral, transportation, and health education, as well as outcomes of low birth weight, infant mortality, adequacy of care, trimester of care, and costs of care in three groups: OHS birth mothers, non-OHS birth mothers, and Douglas County birth mothers yearly for three years. Results of the study were comparisons across the three years and across the three groups.

Time-Dimensional Designs

Time-dimensional designs were developed within the discipline of epidemiology, a field that studies the occurrence and distribution of disease among populations. These designs examine sequences and patterns of change, growth, or trends over time. The dimension of time, then, becomes an important factor. Within the field of epidemiology, the samples in time-dimensional studies are called cohorts. Originally, cohorts were age categories; however, the concept has been expanded to apply

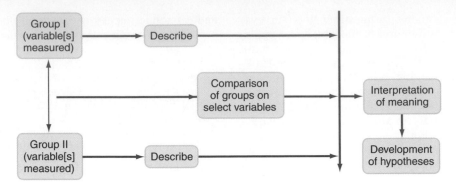

Figure **11-2** Comparative descriptive design.

to groups distinguished by many other variables. Other means of classifying populations that have relevance in relation to time are time of diagnosis, point of entry into a treatment protocol, point of entry into a new lifestyle, and age at which the subject started smoking. An understanding of temporal sequencing is an important prerequisite to examining causality between variables. Thus, the results of these designs lead to description of trends, processes, patterns, and changes over time as well as the development of hypotheses, and are often forerunners of experimental designs.

Epidemiological studies that use time-dimensional designs determine the risk factors or causal factors of illness states. Cause determined in this manner is called inferred causality. These studies also examine trends, patterns, processes, and changes over time. The best-known studies in this area are those on smoking and cancer. Because of the strength of studies that have undergone multiple repetitions, the causal link is strong. The strategy is not as powerful as experimental designs in supporting causality; however, in this situation, as in many nursing contexts, one can never ethically conduct a true experiment. A true experiment requires that there be an experimental group (who would not smoke) and a control group (who smokes). The two groups must be randomly assigned to groups. Therefore, without being provided a choice, some individuals would be required to smoke while others would be required to abstain from smoking over a long period of time.

Epidemiologists use two strategies to examine changes over time: retrospective studies and prospective studies. The norm in epidemiological studies is to use the word *cohorts* to refer to groups of subjects in prospective studies, but the term is generally not used in **retrospective studies**. In retrospective

studies, both the proposed cause and the proposed effect have already occurred. For example, the subjects could have a specific type of cancer, and the researcher could be searching for commonalities among subjects that may have led to the development of that type of cancer. In a **prospective cohort study**, causes may have occurred, but the proposed effect has not.

The Framingham study is the best-known example of a prospective study (U.S. Department of Health and Human Services, 1968). In this study, researchers monitored members of a community for 20 years and examined variables such as dietary patterns, exercise, weight, and blood lipid levels. As the subjects experienced illnesses, such as heart disease, hypertension, or lung disease, their illnesses could be related to previously identified variables.

Prospective studies are considered more powerful than retrospective studies in inferring causality, because the researcher can demonstrate that the risk factors occurred before the illness and are positively related to the illness. Both designs are important for use in nursing studies, because a person's responses to health situations are patterns that developed long before the health situation occurred. These patterns then influence the person's responses to nursing interventions.

Several designs are used to conduct time-dimensional studies: longitudinal, cross-sectional, trend, and event or treatment partitioning.

Longitudinal Designs

Longitudinal designs examine changes in the same subjects over an extended period. They are sometimes called *panel designs* (Figure 11-3). Longitudinal designs are expensive and require a long period of researcher and subject commitment. The area to be

Time 1	Time 2	Time 3	Time 4	Time..n
measure variables	measure variables	measure variables	measure variables	measure variables
Sample 1	Sample 1	Sample 1	Sample 1	Sample 1

Figure **11-3** Longitudinal design.

studied, the variables, and their measurement must be clearly identified before data collection begins. Measurement must be carefully planned and implemented because the measures will be used repeatedly over time. If children are being studied, the measures must be valid for all the ages being studied. To use this design, you must be familiar with how the construct being measured changes, is patterned and trended over time and give a clear rationale for the points of time you have selected for measurement. There is often a bias in selection of subjects because of the requirement for a long-term commitment. In addition, loss of subjects (mortality—not that the subject dies but that the subject quits participating in the study) can be high and can decrease the validity of findings.

Power analysis must be calculated according to the number of subjects expected to complete the study, not the number recruited initially. As a researcher, you must invest considerable energy in developing effective strategies to maintain the sample; Chapter 10 examined some strategies used for this purpose The period during which subjects will be recruited into the study must be carefully planned, and a time line depicting data collection points for each subject must be developed to enable planning for the numbers and availability of data collectors. If this issue is not carefully thought out, data collectors may be confronted with the need to recruit new subjects while they are attempting to collect data scheduled for subjects recruited earlier. You must also decide whether you will use a single data collector to attain all data from a particular subject or whether you will use a different data collector at each point to ensure that data are collected blindly.

Because of the large volumes of data acquired in a longitudinal study, you must give careful attention to strategies for managing the data. The repetition of measures requires that data analysis be carefully thought through. Analyses commonly used are repeated measures analyses of variance, multivariate analyses of variance (MANOVA), regression analysis, cluster analysis, and time-series analysis.

An example of a longitudinal design is the study by Baird and Sands (2006). An abstract of that study follows.

Osteoarthritis (OA) is the most common cause of disability in older adults, which, in turn, leads to poor quality of life (QOL). Disability is caused primarily by the joint degeneration and pain associated with OA.

A randomized pilot study was conducted to test the effectiveness of guided imagery with relaxation (GIR) to improve health-related QOL (HRQOL) in women with OA. A two-group (intervention versus control) *longitudinal design* was used to determine whether GIR leads to better HRQOL in these individuals and whether improvement in HRQOL could be attributed to intervention-associated improvements in pain and mobility. Twenty-eight women were randomized to either the GIR intervention or the control intervention group. Subjects completed a daily journal for a period of 12 weeks.

Using GIR for 12 weeks significantly increased women's HRQOL in comparison to the women who used the control intervention, even after statistically adjusting for changes in pain and mobility. These findings suggest that the effects of GIR on HRQOL are not limited to improvements in pain and mobility. GIR may be an easy-to-use self-management intervention to improve the QOL of older adults. (Baird & Sands, 2006; full-text article available in CINAHL)

Cross-Sectional Designs

Cross-sectional designs examine groups of subjects in various stages of development, trends, patterns, and changes simultaneously with the intent to describe changes in the phenomenon across stages (Figure 11-4). The assumption is that the stages are part of a process that will progress over time. Selecting subjects at various points in the process provides important information about the totality of the process, even though the same subjects are not monitored through the entire process. The processes of development selected for the study might be related to age, position in an educational system, growth pattern, or stages of maturation or personal growth (if they could be clearly enough defined to develop criteria for inclusion within differentiated groups or disease stages). Subjects are then categorized by group, and data on the selected variables are collected at a single point in time.

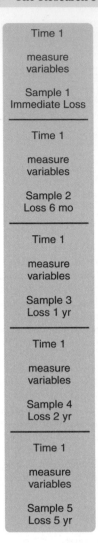

Figure **11-4** Cross-sectional design.

6 months ago, and other groups whose losses occurred 1 year, 2 years, and 5 years ago, respectively. You could study all of these groups during one period of time, but you could describe a pattern of grief reactions over a 5-year period. The design is not as strong as the longitudinal design in which the same participants continue in the study over time and thus eliminate some variance, but it allows some understanding of the phenomenon over time when time allowed for the study is limited.

Sidani et al. (2007) conducted a cross-sectional study titled "Outcomes of Nurse Practitioners in Acute Care: An Exploration." The following excerpts describe the design of their study.

> The purpose of this study was to compare the outcomes achieved by adult patients who did ($n = 78$) and did not ($n = 45$) receive care by acute care nurse practitioners (ACNP), within one week following discharge. A comparative, *cross-sectional design* was used. Consenting patients completed the outcome measures within one week following discharge. The outcomes included satisfaction with care, functional status, symptom resolution, and sense of well-being, which were measured with established instruments.
>
> The two groups of patients were equivalent in terms of their demographic profile and severity of condition. The results indicated that patients who received ACNP care, as compared to those who did not, reported higher levels of satisfaction with care and of physical, psychological, and social functioning. These findings provide preliminary evidence supporting the contribution of ACNPs to high quality care. However, the small sample size limits the generalizability of the study findings. (Sidani et al., 2007; full-text article available in CINAHL)

Trend Designs

Trend designs examine changes in the general population in relation to a particular phenomenon (Figure 11-5). The researcher selects different samples of subjects from the same population at preset intervals of time, and at each selected time, he or she collects data from that particular sample. You must be able to justify generalizing from the samples to the population under study. Analysis involves strategies to predict future

For example, suppose you wish to study grief reactions at various periods after the death of a spouse. With a cross-sectional design, you could study a group of individuals whose spouse had died 1 week ago, another group composed of individuals whose loss occurred

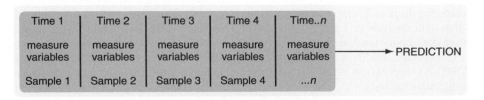

Figure **11-5** Trend design.

trends by examining past trends. An example of this design is the study by Hartley (2003) of "[l]ongitudinal analysis of access to health care, use of preventive health services, and practice of health-related behaviors of Appalachian and non-Appalachian adults in Kentucky." The study is described as follows.

> The purpose of this longitudinal *trend* analysis was to document the extent of disparities in access to health care, use of preventive health services, and practice of health-related behaviors between Appalachian and non-Appalachian adults in Kentucky over a 6-year period. The specific aims were to: (a) examine trends in health insurance coverage, ability to pay for health services, and difficulty with travel to a health facility using the Kentucky Health Interview Survey (KHIS) data; (b) examine preventive health service trends, specifically Pap smears for women and dental visits by adults, using KRIS data; (c) examine physical activity level, body mass index (BMI), and cigarette use using the Behavioral Risk Factor Surveillance System (BRFSS) data; and (d) investigate potential disparities overtime by sex of the participants and area of residence. A longitudinal trend design using secondary data from the KHIS and BRFSS databases was used to examine disparities from 1992 to 1997. Area of residence predicted the probability of difficulty in travel to a health facility, $\chi 2$ (1, N = 3,881) = 151.86, p <= 0.0001. Non-Appalachians had less difficulty traveling to a health facility compared with Appalachians (Odds Ratio = 0.47). Difficulty with travel to a health facility was less likely for those who had at least a high school education compared with those who had not completed high school (Odds Ratio = 0.56), and for those with an income >\$25,000 compared with those who had lower incomes (<\$25,000) (Odds Ratio = 0.52). Multiple regression revealed differences in Body Mass Index (BMI) for years 1996 ($p < 0.0001$) and 1997 ($p < 0.0001$). Appalachians (M = 26.14, SE = 0.08) had a greater BMI than non-Appalachians (M = 25.59, SE = 0.04). The interaction between Region x Year revealed non-Appalachian men had a greater mean BMI in 1997 compared with Appalachian men, a reversing trend in time. Some disparities exist between Appalachians and non-Appalachians in Kentucky and have not changed over time. Compared with non-Appalachians, Appalachians have lower education and income, and greater unemployment creating barriers to access to health care and they use fewer preventive health services and practice fewer health-related behaviors. (Hartley, 2003)

Event-Partitioning Designs

A merger of the cross-sectional or longitudinal and trend designs, the event-partitioning design, is used in some cases to increase sample size and to avoid the effects of history on the validity of findings. Cook and Campbell (1979) referred to these as cohort designs with *treatment partitioning* (Figures 11-6 and 11-7).

The term *treatment* is used loosely here to mean a key event that is thought to lead to change. In a descriptive study, the researcher would not cause or manipulate the key event but rather would clearly define it so that when it occurred naturally, it would be recognized.

For example, you could use the event-partitioning design to study subjects who have completed programs to stop smoking. Smoking behaviors and incidence of smoking-related diseases might be measured at intervals of 1 year for a 5-year period. However, the number of subjects available at one time might be insufficient for you to adequately analyze findings. Therefore, you could use subjects from several programs offered at different times. You would examine the data in terms of the relative time since the subjects' completion of the stop-smoking program, not the absolute length of time. Data would be assumed to be comparable, and a larger sample size would be available for analysis of changes over time.

An example of this design is Barnes-McDowell's (1997) study on home apnea monitoring. The following excerpt describes the study design.

> Sudden Infant Death Syndrome (SIDS) is the leading cause of death in infants between one week and one year of age. The mainstay of therapy to reduce SIDS mortality is evaluation and subsequent home monitoring of infants at risk for SIDS. This study explored the concerns and responses of families of 13 infants to having an infant on a home apnea monitor. These concerns and responses were reported by the mother at three time points in the home apnea monitoring experience. The Neuman Systems Model served as the theoretical basis for the investigation. The study design was longitudinal with event partitioning, and used the following instruments: Hymovich's Parent Perception Inventory, the Feetham Family Functioning Survey, the Monitoring Flowsheet, and the Early Infancy Temperament Questionnaire. Data analysis included repeated measures analyses of variance and correlational coefficients. Maternal concerns and coping response scores were positively correlated with family functioning discrepancy scores at the initiation of monitoring. Parental coping response scores were negatively correlated with infant temperament at the termination of monitoring, as are severity of illness and sibling coping behavior. Patterns were apparent in the frequencies of various concerns and coping strategies at different points in the home monitoring experience. Because nurses are in key positions to coordinate the development of strategies for families to use in coping with the stressor of home apnea monitoring, this study is particularly beneficial to practicing nurses. Information about concerns and coping responses along with determination of the relationship with family functioning and infant temperament provide a basis for nurses to develop interventions to assist families in positively coping with the home apnea monitoring experience. (Barnes-McDowell, 1997)

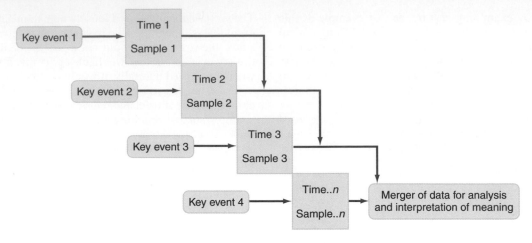

Figure **11-6** Cross-sectional study with treatment partitioning.

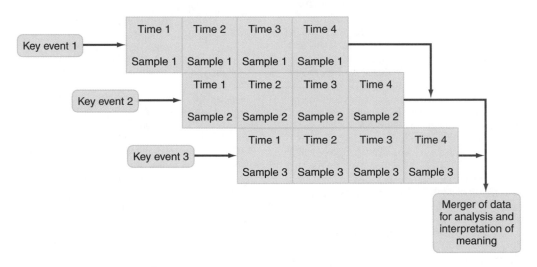

Figure **11-7** Longitudinal design with treatment partitioning.

Case Study Designs

The case study design involves an intensive exploration of a single unit of study, such as a person, family, group, community, or institution, or a small number of subjects who are examined intensively. Although the number of subjects tends to be small, the number of variables involved is usually large. In fact, it is important to examine all variables that might have an impact on the situation being studied.

Case studies were commonly used in nursing research in the 1970s. Their use then declined, but they are beginning to appear in the literature more frequently today. Well-designed case studies are good sources of descriptive information and can be used as evidence for or against theories. Case studies can use a triangulated approach, incorporating both quantitative and qualitative methods in a case study. Sterling and McNally (1992) recommended single-subject case studies for examining process-based nursing practice. The strategy allows the researcher to investigate daily observations and interventions that are a common aspect of nursing practice. Dowd, Withers, Hackwood, and Shuter (2007) used a case study to examine communication impairments.

Communication impairments represent a significant public health issue. Failure to achieve communicative competence has social, emotional, educational and financial costs to the individual and society. A community-based health promotion strategy "Play and Talk" was implemented in a disadvantaged community to enhance communication skills in children prior to school entry. Within the context of the Play and Talk initiative, the parent-child interaction program *You Make the Difference* (YMTD) developed by the Hanen Centre in Ontario, Canada, was piloted and evaluated using a case study design within a collaborative action research framework. An opportunistic sample of eleven mothers participated in the ten-week program. All participants completed pre- and post-program questionnaires and four-week follow-up interviews. Feedback indicated that all mothers who attended the program experienced positive changes in their interactions and communication with their child, and strategies learnt were transferred to and maintained in the home environment. However, longer term follow-up is needed to further validate these results. The overall outcome of the program reinforced the need to provide community-based programs of this type to support the critical role of parents as facilitators of communication development in their children. (Dowd et al., 2007; full-text article available in CINAHL)

Case studies are commonly used in qualitative studies (Sandelowski, 1996). There are even experimental designs for single case studies (Barlow & Hersen, 1984). A variety of sources of information can be collected on each concept of interest through the use of different data collection methods. This approach allows researchers to perform a detailed study of all aspects of a single case. Such a strategy can greatly expand our understanding of the phenomenon under study.

Case studies also can demonstrate the effectiveness of specific therapeutic techniques. In fact, by reporting a case study, the researcher introduces the technique to other practitioners. The case study design also has potential for revealing important findings that can generate new hypotheses for testing. Thus, the case study can lead to the design of large sample studies to examine factors identified through the case study.

How you design a case study depends on the circumstances of the case but usually includes an element of time. History and previous behavior patterns are usually explored in detail. As the case study proceeds, you may become aware of components important to the phenomenon being examined that were not originally built into the study. A case study is likely to have both quantitative

and qualitative elements, and you must incorporate these components into the study design. Methods used to analyze and interpret qualitative data need to be carefully planned. Consultation with a qualitative researcher can strengthen the study. Large volumes of data are generally obtained during a case study. Organizing the findings of a case study into a coherent whole is a difficult but critical component of the study. Generalizing study findings in the statistical sense is not appropriate; however, generalizing the findings to theory is appropriate and important (Barnard, Magyary, Booth, & Eyres, 1987; Crombie & Davies, 1996; Gray, 1998; Yin, 1984).

Not all case studies are research. Many of the articles referring to case studies are clinical practice articles, in which a clinical situation is reported for the purpose of illustrating clinical practice, problems in clinical practice, or changes that need to be made in clinical practice. These articles do not use research methods but rather describe events out of the patient record or the author's personal experience.

SURVEYS

The term survey is used in two ways within scientific thought. It is used in a broad sense to mean any descriptive or correlational study; in this sense, *survey* tends to mean nonexperimental. In a narrower sense, *survey* is used to describe a data collection technique in which the researcher uses questionnaires (collected by mail or in person) or personal interviews to gather data about an identified population.

Surveys, in the narrower definition, are used to gather data that can be acquired through self-report. Because of this limitation in data, some researchers view surveys as rather shallow and as contributing in a limited way to scientific knowledge. This belief has led to a bias in the scientific community against survey research. In this context, the term *survey* is used derisively. However, surveys can be an extremely important source of data. In this text, we use the term *survey* to designate a data collection technique, not a design. Surveys can be used within many designs, including descriptive, correlational, and quasi-experimental studies.

CORRELATIONAL STUDY DESIGNS

Correlational study designs examine relationships among variables. The examination can occur at several levels. The researcher can seek to describe a relationship, predict relationships among variables, or test the relationships proposed by a theoretical proposition.

In any correlational study, a representative sample must be selected for the study. That sample reflects the full range of values possible on the variables being measured. Thus, large samples are required. In correlational designs, a large variance in the variable values is necessary to determine the existence of a relationship. Therefore, correlational designs are unlike experimental designs, in which variance in variable scores is controlled (limited).

In correlational designs, if the range of scores is truncated, the obtained correlational value will be artificially depressed. *Truncated* means that the lowest values and the values either are not measured or are condensed and merged with less extreme values. For example, if an attitude scale were scored from a low score of 1 to a high score of 50, truncated scores might indicate only scores in the range 10 to 40. More extreme scores would be combined with scores within the designated range. If truncation is performed, the researcher may not find a correlation when the variables are actually correlated.

Neophyte researchers tend to make two serious errors with correlational studies. First, they often attempt to establish causality by correlation, reasoning that if two variables are related, one must cause the other. Second, they confuse studies in which differences are examined with studies in which relationships are examined. Although the existence of a difference assumes the existence of a relationship, the design and statistical analysis of studies examining differences are not the same as those examining relationships. If your study examines two or more groups in terms of one or more variables, then you are exploring differences between groups as reflected in scores on the identified variables. If your study examines a single group in terms of two or more variables, then you are exploring relationships between variables. In a correlational study, the relationship examined is that between two or more research variables within an identified situation. Thus, the sample is not separated into groups. Analyses examine variable values in the entire sample. In a correlational design, data from the entire sample are analyzed as a single group.

Descriptive Correlational Designs

A descriptive correlational design examines the relationships that exist in a situation. Using this design facilitates the identification of many interrelationships in a situation in a short time. While the descriptive design discussed earlier may reveal relationships among variables, the descriptive correlational design focuses specifically on relationships among study variables. Descriptive correlational studies may lead to hypotheses for later studies (Figure 11-8).

A descriptive correlational study may examine variables in a situation that has already occurred or is currently occurring. No attempt is made to control or manipulate the situation. As with descriptive studies, variables must be clearly identified and defined. An example of a descriptive correlational design is the study by Kacel, Millar, and Norris (2005) titled "Measurement of Nurse Practitioner Job Satisfaction in a Midwestern State." The following text summarizes the study.

Purpose: To describe the current level of job satisfaction of nurse practitioners (NPs) in one Midwestern state.

Data Sources: This study utilized descriptive correlation design to examine factors that lead to job satisfaction and dissatisfaction among a randomized sample of licensed NPs from a Midwestern state. The sample of 147 NPs (63% return rate) completed self-administered questionnaires about various characteristics of their jobs. Descriptive statistics and correlations were used to analyze the data. The theoretical foundation for the study was Herzberg's Dual Factor Theory of Job Satisfaction.

Conclusions: Overall job satisfaction of NPs was minimally satisfied to satisfied. NPs were most satisfied with intrinsic factors and least satisfied with extrinsic factors of their jobs. Factors NPs were most satisfied with were sense of accomplishment, challenge in work, level of autonomy, patient mix, and ability to deliver quality care. NPs were least satisfied with time off to serve on professional committees, reward distribution, amount of involvement in research, opportunity to receive compensation for services outside normal duties, and monetary bonuses available in addition to salary. NPs with 0-1 year practice experience were the most satisfied with their jobs, but satisfaction scores fell steadily with each additional year of experience, reaching a plateau between the 8th to 11th years of practice. Table 11-2 shows the areas of practice in which NPs were most satisfied and Table 11-3 shows the areas of practice in which NPs were least satisfied.

Implications for Practice: Improving job satisfaction for NPs is critical to recruit and retain advanced practice nurses to enhance access to quality, cost-effective care for all patient populations. Satisfied NPs can potentially reduce healthcare costs associated with employee turnover. Employers must look at extrinsic factors such as compensation and opportunities for professional growth to enhance NP job satisfaction. (Kacel et al., 2005; full-text article available in CINAHL)

This is a correlational study because there is no treatment or intervention, data are obtained from a single group, and correlational statistical analyses are used to examine relationships between variables. Descriptive

MEASUREMENT

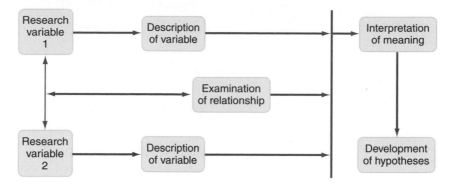

Figure 11-8 Descriptive correlational design.

TABLE 11-2 ■ Items Receiving the Highest Satisfaction		
Scores (Intrinsic Factors)		
Aspect of Job	Mean	SD
Sense of Accomplishment	5.24	0.85
Challenge in Work	5.19	0.84
Level of Autonomy	5.19	0.81
Patient Mix	5.18	0.67
Ability to Deliver Quality Care	5.15	0.78

TABLE 11-3 ■ Items Receiving the Lowest Satisfaction		
Scores (Extrinsic Factors).		
Aspect of Job	Mean	SD
Time Off to Serve on Professional Committees	3.96	1.41
Reward Distribution	3.81	1.34
Amount of Involvement in Research	3.62	1.32
Opportunity to Receive Compensation for Services Outside Normal Duties	3.01	1.52
Monetary Bonuses Available in Addition to Salary	2.69	1.51

statistics are used in this study to a greater extent than correlation analyses. However, correlational analyses were used to examine the relationships of the MNPJSS six subscales with some of the study variables including intrapractice partnership/collegi-ality, challenge/autonomy, professional, social, and community interaction, professional growth, time, and benefits. Statistical values obtained from the correlational analyses are not provided in the published study.

Predictive Designs

Predictive designs are used to predict the value of one variable on the basis of values obtained from another variable or variables. Prediction is one approach you can use to examine causal relationships between variables. Because causal phenomena are being examined, the terms *dependent* and *independent* are used to describe the variables. One variable (the one to be predicted) is classified as the dependent variable, and all other variables (those that are predictors) are classified as independent variables.

The aim of a predictive design is to predict the level of the dependent variable from the independent variables (Figure 11-9). Independent variables most effective in prediction are highly correlated with the dependent variable but not highly correlated with other independent variables used in the study. Predictive designs will require you to develop a theory-based mathematical hypothesis proposing the independent variables that are expected to predict the dependent variable effectively. You can then test the hypothesis using regression analysis. Predictive studies are also used to establish the predictive validity of measurement scales.

Huang et al. (2007) conducted a predictive correlational study called "Stressors, Depressive Symptoms, and Learned Resourcefulness among Taiwanese Adults with Diabetes Mellitus." The following abstract describes this study:

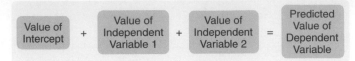

Figure **11-9** Predictive design.

Learned resourcefulness may be an important and necessary resource for people with diabetes to adequately manage their disease. This study used a cross-sectional, descriptive correlation design to examine the relationships of demographic characteristics, stressors, learned resourcefulness, and depressive symptoms among adult Taiwanese with diabetes mellitus. A convenience sample of 131 individuals recruited from outpatient primary care centers from two major hospitals in Taiwan participated in this study. Data were collected with a demographic questionnaire, blood tests, Rosenbaum's self-control schedule, and the Center for Epidemiological Studies depression scale. Data analysis consisted of descriptive statistics and *regression* analysis. Demographic variables (age, gender, education, and income) explained a significant proportion of the variance in depressive symptoms in individuals with diabetes, $R^2 = 0.084$, $F(1, 127) = 2,897$, $p < 0.05$. Among the demographic variables, only age ($R^2 = -0.20, p < 0.05$) was a significant predictor of depressive symptoms. Stressors (duration of diabetes, number of complications, and glycemic control) explained a significant proportion of the variance in depressive symptoms in individuals with diabetes after controlling for the effects of the demographic variables (age, gender, education, and income), adjusted $R^2 = 0.160$, F change $(1, 124) = 3.701$, $p < 0.01$. Among the stressor variables, only HbA_1C ($R^2 = 0.28$, $p < 0.001$) was a significant predictor of depressive symptoms. These results mean that individuals with higher levels of HbA1C also had high scores for depressive symptoms. Findings suggest that individuals with diabetes who had greater learned resourcefulness and better glycemic control also had fewer depressive symptoms. In addition, learned resourcefulness partially mediated the relationship between glycemic control and depressive symptoms. (Huang et al., 2007; full-text article available in CINAHL)

This is a predictive correlational study because both correlational and regression analyses are used. Data are gathered from a single sample of 131 subjects. Correlational analyses were used to examine the relationships among demographic characteristics, stressors, learned resourcefulness, and depressive symptoms. Regression analyses revealed that duration of diabetes, number of complications, and glycemic control predicted depressive symptoms. HbA_1C also predicted depressive symptoms. Learned resourcefulness and better glycemic control resulted in fewer depressive symptoms.

Model-Testing Designs

Some studies are designed specifically to test the accuracy of a hypothesized causal model. The model-testing design requires that all variables relevant to the model be measured. A large, heterogeneous sample is required. All the paths expressing relationships between concepts are identified, and a conceptual map is developed (Figure 11-10). The analysis determines whether or not the data are consistent with the model. For some studies, you might set aside data from some subjects and not include them in the initial path analysis. You might use these data to test the fit of the paths defined by the initial analysis in another data set.

Variables are classified into three categories: exogenous variables, endogenous variables, and residual variables. Exogenous variables are within the theoretical model but are caused by factors outside of this model. Endogenous variables are those whose variation is explained within the theoretical model. Exogenous variables influence the variation of endogenous variables. Residual variables indicate the effect of unmeasured variables not included in the model. These variables explain some of the variance found in the data but not the variance within the model (Mason-Hawkes & Holm, 1989).

In Figure 11-10, the illustration of a model-testing design, paths are drawn to demonstrate directions of cause and effect. The arrows (paths) from the exogenous variables 1, 2, and 3 lead to the endogenous variable 4, indicating that variable 4 is theoretically proposed to be caused by variables 1, 2, and 3. The arrow (path) from endogenous variable 4 to endogenous variable 5 indicates that variable 4 theoretically causes variable 5.

To measure exogenous and endogenous variables, collect data from the subjects and analyze the accuracy of the proposed paths. Initially, these analysis procedures were performed with a series of regression analyses. Statistical procedures have been developed specifically for path analysis using the computer programs LISREL and EQS. Structural equation modeling is a statistical procedure commonly used. Path coefficients are calculated

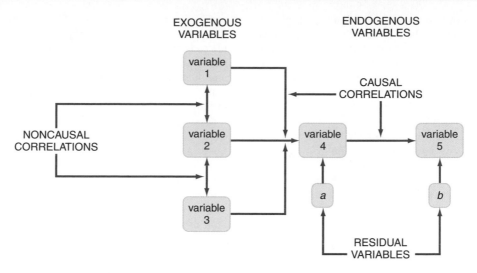

Figure 11-10 Model-testing design.

that indicate the effect that one variable has on another. The amount of variance explained by the model, as well as the fit between the path coefficients and the theoretical model, indicates the accuracy of the theory. Variance that is not accounted for in the statistical analysis is attributed to residual variables (variables *a* and *b*) not included in the analyses (Mason-Hawkes & Holm, 1989).

An example of this design is the Cummings, Estabrooks, Midodzi, Wallin, and Hayduk (2007) test of a model of the influence of organizational characteristics and context on research utilization in nursing.

Background: Despite three decades of empirical investigation into research utilization and a renewed emphasis on evidence-based medicine and evidence-based practice in the past decade, understanding of factors influencing research uptake in nursing remains limited. There is, however, increased awareness that organizational influences are important.

Objectives: To develop and test a theoretical model of organizational influences that predict research utilization by nurses and to assess the influence of varying degrees of context, based on the Promoting Action on Research Implementation in Health Services (PARIHS) framework, on research utilization and other variables.

Methods: The study sample was drawn from a census of registered nurses working in acute care hospitals in Alberta, Canada, accessed through their professional licensing body (*n* = 6,526 nurses; 52.8% response rate). Three variables that measured PARIHS dimensions of context (culture, leadership, and evaluation) were used

to sort cases into one of four mutually exclusive data sets that reflected less positive to more positive context. Then, a theoretical model of hospital-and-unit-level influences on research utilization was developed and tested, using structural equation modeling, and 300 cases were randomly selected from each of the four data sets.

Results: Hospital characteristics that positively influenced research utilization by nurses were staff development, opportunity for nurse-to-nurse collaboration, and staffing and support services. Increased emotional exhaustion led to less reported research utilization and higher rates of patient and nurse adverse events. Nurses working in contexts with more positive culture, leadership, and evaluation also reported significantly more research utilization, staff development, and lower rates of patient and staff adverse events than did nurses working in less positive contexts (i.e., those that lacked positive culture, leadership, or evaluation).

Conclusion: The findings highlight the combined importance of culture, leadership, and evaluation to increase research utilization and improve patient safety. The findings may serve to strengthen the PARIHS framework and to suggest that, although it is not fully developed, the framework is an appropriate guide to implement research into practice. (Cummings et al., 2007; full-text article available in CINAHL)

DEFINING THERAPEUTIC NURSING INTERVENTIONS

In quasi-experimental and experimental studies, an intervention (or protocol) is developed that is expected to result in differences in posttest measures of the treatment and control or comparison groups. This intervention may be physiological, psychosocial, educational, or a combination of these and should be designed to maximize the differences between the groups. Thus, it should be the best intervention possible in the circumstances of the study, an intervention that is expected to improve the outcomes of the experimental group.

The nursing literature has not adequately addressed the methodology for designing interventions for nursing studies. In addition, descriptions of nursing interventions in published studies lack the specificity and clarity given to describing measurement instruments (Egan, Snyder, & Burns, 1992). Thus, nurse researchers provide detailed information about measurement but do not provide sufficient detail to allow a nurse to implement a nursing intervention as it was used in a published nursing study. To some extent, this may reflect the state of knowledge in the nursing field regarding the provision of nursing interventions in clinical practice. Clinical nursing interventions are not well defined; thus, each nurse may use her or his own terminology to describe a particular intervention. In addition, an intervention tends to be applied differently in each case by a single nurse and even less consistently by different nurses.

The Nursing Interventions Classification

The Nursing Interventions Classification (NIC) is a standardized language used to describe treatments performed by nurses. Each intervention consists of a label, a definition, and a set of activities performed by nurses carrying out the intervention. The intervention labels were derived from nursing education and nursing practice. The research methods used to develop the classification included content analysis, surveys, focus groups, similarity analysis, and hierarchical clustering.

Tripp-Reimer Woodworth, McCloskey, and Bulechek (1996), in their analysis of the structure of the NIC interventions, identified three dimensions: focus of care, intensity, and complexity. A high intensity of care is associated with the physiological illness level of the patient and the emergency nature of the illness. The dimension of intensity of care includes indicators of (1) intensity (or acuity) and (2) whether the care is typical or novel. The dimension of focus of care addresses (1) the target of the intervention, ranging from the individual to the system, (2) whether the care action is direct or on behalf of the patient, and (3) the continuum of practice from independent to collaborative actions. The dimension of complexity of care includes continua of degree of knowledge, skill, and urgency of the interventions.

The interventions in the NIC are being subjected to multiple studies examining the effects on different populations and the effects of varying degrees of intensity. Links are being established between the intervention and outcomes at varying points in time after the intervention has been implemented. Studies are also determining the outcomes of each intervention. Outcomes that occur immediately following the intervention are easiest to determine. However, the most important outcomes may be those that occur after a client has been discharged or several weeks or months after the intervention. This information is critical to justifying nursing actions in a cost-conscious market (Stewart & Archbold, 1992, 1993). For a more extensive discussion of the importance of linking interventions with outcomes measures, see Chapter 12. See Table 11-4 for a sample of the work in nursing related to the NIC and the Nursing Outcomes Classification (NOC).

Designing an Intervention for a Nursing Study

The therapeutic nursing intervention provided in a nursing study needs to be carefully designed, clearly described, and well linked to the outcome measures (dependent variables) to be used in the study. Each of these dimensions must be considered to develop consistency in the intervention. The intervention needs to be provided consistently to all subjects. In some studies, you may need to develop a step-by-step protocol in order to control consistency. Educational treatments or educational components of treatments might be audio- or videotaped for consistency.

The first step in designing an intervention should be a thorough review of the clinical and research literature related to the intervention. Because of the sparsity of information in the literature on nursing interventions, you may need to rely on a personal knowledge base emerging from expertise in clinical practice. The nursing actions that are included in the intervention must be spelled out sequentially so that other nurses are able to follow the description and provide the intervention in a consistent manner. The intervention must be consistent in such areas as content, intensity, and length of time. If several caregivers are involved in providing the intervention, take care to protect the integrity of the intervention. You may need to employ a pilot study to refine the intervention so that it can be applied consistently.

QUASI-EXPERIMENTAL STUDY DESIGNS

Quasi-experimental and experimental designs examine causality. The power of the design to accomplish this purpose depends on the extent to which

TABLE 11-4 Work in Nursing Related to the NIC and the Nursing Outcomes Classification (NOC)		
Year	**Author**	**Title**
1995	Davis	AIDS nursing care and standardized nursing language: An application of the Nursing Intervention Classification
1996	Kirby	Classification of advanced practice nursing functions using the Nursing Intervention Classification taxonomy
1996	Micek et al.	Patient outcomes: The link between nursing diagnoses and interventions
1996	Bowles & Naylor	Nursing intervention classification systems
1997	Jones-Baucke	A qualitative study of the implementation of a system to increase nurses' use of standardized nursing languages
1997	Henry & Meade	Nursing classification systems: Necessary but not sufficient for representing "what nurses do" for inclusion in computer-based patient record systems
1997	Redes & Lunney	Validation by school nurses of the Nursing Intervention Classification for computer software
1998	Corbett	Predictors and outcomes of home care for diabetics
1999	Boomsma, Dassen, Dingemans, & van den Heuvel	Nursing interventions in crisis-oriented and long-term psychiatric home care
1999	Coenen, Weis, Schank, & Matheus	Describing parish nurse practice using the Nursing Minimum Data Set
2000	Weis & Schank	Use of a taxonomy to describe parish nurse practice with older adults
2001	Wu & Thompson	Evaluation of the Nursing Intervention Classification for use by flight nurses
2001	O'Connor, Kershaw, & Hameister	Documenting patterns of nursing interventions using cluster analysis
2002	Solari-Twadell	The differentiation of the ministry of parish nursing practice within congregations
2002	Weis, Schank, Coenen, & Matheus	Parish nurse practice with client aggregates
2002	Winters	Primary prevention of agricultural injuries: use of standardized nursing diagnoses, interventions, and outcomes
2003	Blissitt, Roberts, Hinkle, & Kopp	Defining neuroscience nursing practice: The 2001 role delineation study
2003	Mrayyan	Nurse autonomy, nurse job satisfaction and client satisfaction with nursing care: their place in nursing data sets
2003	Jones	Reminiscence therapy for older women with depression: Effects of Nursing Intervention Classification in assisted-living long-term care
2004	Guimarães	Fluid management: a nursing intervention for the patient with fluid volume excess [Portuguese]
2004	Pallarés	Influence of transcultural factors on immigrants populations' needs and nursing diagnosis [Spanish]
2004	Bassoli & Guimaraes	Wound care: Nursing activities in the assistance practice, compared to the activities proposed by the Nursing Intervention Classification (NIC) [Portuguese]
2004	McBride	Postdischarge nursing interventions for stroke survivors and their families
2005	Martins	Nursing interventions for the nursing diagnosis ineffective airway clearance [sic] [Portuguese]
2005	von Krogh, Dale, & Naden	A framework for integrating NANDA, NIC, and NOC terminology in electronic patient records
2006	Figoski & Downey	Perspectives in continuity of care: Facility charging and Nursing Intervention Classification (NIC): the new dynamic duo
2006	Sawada, Porter, Kayama, Setoya, & Miyamato	International nursing. Nursing care delivery in Japanese psychiatric units
2006	Villanueva, Thompson, Macpherson, Meunier, & Hilton	The Neuroscience Nursing 2005 Role Delineation Study: Implications for certification
2007	González-Gancedo & Fernández García	Care plan in a patient with spina bifida. Case report [Spanish]

the actual effects of the experimental treatment (the independent variable) can be detected by measuring the dependent variable. Obtaining an understanding of the true effects of an experimental treatment requires action to control threats to the validity of the findings. Threats to validity are controlled through selection of subjects, control of the environment, manipulation of the treatment, and reliable and valid measurement of the dependent variables. These threats were described in Chapter 10.

Experimental study designs, with their strict control of variance, are the most powerful method of examining causality. For many reasons, both ethical and practical, however, experimental designs cannot always be used in social science research. Quasi-experimental study designs were developed to provide alternative means of examining causality in situations not conducive to experimental controls. Campbell and Stanley first described quasi-experimental designs as a group in 1963, when only experimental designs were considered of any worth. Cook and Campbell expanded this description in 1979. Quasi-experimental designs facilitate the search for knowledge and examination of causality in situations in which complete control is not possible. These designs have been developed to control as many threats to validity as possible in a situation in which at least one of the three components of true experimental design (randomization, comparison groups, and manipulation of the treatment) is lacking.

There are differences of opinion in nursing about the classification of a particular study as quasi-experimental or experimental. The experimental designs emerged from a logical positivist perspective with the purpose of determining cause and effect. The focus is to determine differences between groups using statistical analyses on the basis of decision theory (see Chapter 18 for an explanation of decision theory). The true experimental design (from a logical positivist view) requires the use of random sampling to obtain subjects, random assignment to control and experimental groups, rigorous control of the treatment, and designs that controlled threats to validity. Chapter 14 explains the various sampling methods.

A less rigorous type of experimental design is referred to as the comparative experimental design. Researchers in both nursing and medicine are using it for clinical situations in which the expectation of random sampling is difficult if not impossible to achieve. These studies use convenience samples with random assignment to groups. For example, clinical trials do not use randomly obtained samples but tend to be considered experimental in nature.

These studies are classified as experimental because they have internal validity if the two groups are comparable on variables important to the study, even though there are biases in the original sample. However, these designs do not address threats to statistical conclusion validity and threats to external validity by the nonrandom sample. Threats to external validity have not, in the past, been considered a serious concern because they affect not the claim that the treatment caused a difference but rather the ability to generalize the findings. The importance of external validity, although discounted in the past, is taking on greater importance in the current political and health policy climate. Chapter 12, on outcomes research, explores the concerns some have about the validity of clinical trials.

Random Assignment to Groups

Random assignment to groups is a procedure used to assign subjects to treatment or control groups randomly. Random assignment is most commonly used in nursing and medicine to assign subjects obtained through convenience sampling methods to groups for purposes of comparison. Random assignment used without random sampling is purported to decrease the risk of bias in the selection of groups. However, Ottenbacher (1992) performed a meta-analysis to examine the effect of random assignment versus nonrandom assignment on outcomes. The results failed to reveal significant differences in these two sampling techniques. He suggested that previous assumptions about design strategies should be empirically tested. The term *randomized clinical trial* (RCT) usually means that the study used random assignment of subjects to groups, not that the sample was obtained through random sampling methods.

Traditional approaches to random assignment involve using a random numbers table or flipping an unbiased coin to determine group assignment. However, these procedures can lead to unequal group sizes and thus a decrease in power. Hjelm-Karlsson (1991) suggested using what is referred to as a biased coin design to randomly assign subjects to groups. With this technique, selection of the group to which a particular subject will be assigned is biased in favor of groups that have smaller sample sizes at the point of the assignment of that subject. This strategy is particularly useful when assignment is being made to more than two groups. The researcher can complete calculations for the sequencing of assignment to groups before collecting data, thus freeing the researcher for other activities during this critical period. Hjelm-Karlsson (1991) suggested using cards to make group assignments. The subject numbers and random group assignments are written on cards. As each subject agrees to participate in the study, the next card is drawn from the stack, indicating that subject's number and group assignment.

Stout, Wirtz, Carbonari, and Del Boca (1994) suggested a similar strategy they referred to as *urn randomization*, which they described as follows.

> One would begin the study with two urns, each urn containing a red marble and a blue marble. There is one urn for each level of the stratifying variable; that is, in this example there is an urn for severely ill patients and another urn for the less severe patients. When a subject is ready for randomization, we determine whether or not he/she is severely ill and consult the corresponding urn. From this urn (say, for the severely ill group) we randomly select one marble and note its color. If the marble is red we assign the patient to Treatment A. Then we drop that marble back into the urn *and put a blue marble into the urn as well.* This leaves the "severely ill" urn with one red and two blue marbles. The next time a severely ill patient shows up, the probability that he/she will be assigned to Group B will be 2/3 rather than 2, thus biasing the selection process toward balance. A similar procedure is followed every time a severely ill subject presents for randomization. After each subject is assigned, the marble chosen from the urn is replaced together with a marble of the opposite color. The urn for the less severely ill group is not affected. If a low-severity patient presents for the study, that patient's probability of assignment to either treatment is not affected by the assignment of patients in the other stratum. To some extent, urn randomization can be tailored to maximize balancing or to maximize randomization. (Stout et al., 1994, p. 72)

These authors also provided strategies for balancing several variables simultaneously during random assignment.

Koniak-Griffin et al. (2003) used random assignment in their study of nurse visitation for adolescent mothers. They described their sampling procedure as follows.

> After securing written informed consent in accordance with the University Internal Review Board requirements for pregnant minors, adolescents were randomly assigned, using a computer-based program, into the EIP [early intervention program] or TPHNC [traditional public health nursing care] group, based on specific criteria (maternal age, ethnicity, language, gestation age, geographic region of residence). To avoid contamination of treatment conditions, each PHN provided individualized care on a one-to-one basis to adolescents in only one group. (Koniak-Griffin et al., 2003, p. 129; full-text article available in CINAHL)

Each of the quasi-experimental designs described in this section involves threats to validity owing to constraints in controlling variance. Some achieve greater amounts of control than others. When choosing designs, you must select the design that offers the greatest amount of control possible within your study situation. Even the first designs described in this section, which have low power in terms of establishing causality, can provide useful information on which to design later studies.

Comparison Groups

Control groups, traditionally used in experimental studies, are selected randomly from the same population as the experimental group and receive no treatment. Use of a control group increases the ability of the researcher to detect differences between groups in the real world. Thus, they reduce the risk of error. Control groups are rarely used in nursing or medical studies because of requirements related to consent, ethical issues regarding withholding treatment, and the difficulty of acquiring sufficient potential subjects from which to select a sample.

Comparison groups are not selected using random sampling and do not receive the experimental treatment. There are four types of comparison groups: (1) groups that receive no treatment, (2) groups that receive a placebo treatment, (3) groups that receive the "usual treatment," and (4) groups that receive a second experimental treatment or a different treatment dose for comparison with the first experimental treatment (e.g., clinical trials of drug effectiveness). As a researcher, you should clarify the type of comparison group you are using.

When a study uses a comparison group that receives no treatment, demonstrating statistical significance is easier because there is less variation in the treatments and a greater difference between the two groups. Placebo treatments provide consistency in the comparison group, provide less difference between groups than in no-treatment comparison groups, and would be unethical in some nursing studies. "Usual treatment" is the treatment routinely provided by the health care system. However, usual treatment is uneven and thus is often not standardized across patients. Thus, provision of care may vary from one patient to another depending on the availability of nursing staff and the intensity of care demands being made on nurses at the time the care is provided. Some patients may receive little or no care, whereas others may receive considerably more or better care. There will likely be a greater amount of difference between a patient who received little or no care and patients in the experimental group, and less difference between patients in the "usual care group" who received considerably more care and the experimental group. This wide variation reduces the effect size of the experimental treatment, increases the variance, and decreases the possibility of obtaining a significant difference between groups. The researcher should carefully spell out "usual treatment" and the degree of variation in treatment in the facility in which the study is being conducted.

Nonequivalent Comparison Group Designs

A comparison group is one in which the groups are not selected by random means. Some groups are more nonequivalent than others, and some quasi-experimental designs involve using groups (comparison and treatment) that have evolved naturally rather than being developed randomly. For example, groups might be selected because they are registered for an 8:00 AM class in a university. These groups cannot be considered equivalent because the individuals in the comparison group may be different from individuals in the treatment group. Individuals have selected the group in which they are included rather than being selected by the researcher. Thus, selection becomes a threat to validity.

The approach to statistical analysis is problematic in quasi-experimental designs. Although many researchers use the same approaches to analysis as are used for experimental studies, the selection bias inherent in nonequivalent comparison groups

makes this practice questionable. Reichardt (1979) recommended using multiple statistical analyses to examine the data from various perspectives and to compare levels of significance obtained from each analysis. As a researcher, you must carefully assess the potential threats to validity in interpreting statistical results, because statistical analysis cannot control for threats to validity. The following sections describe examples of nonequivalent comparison group design.

One-Group Posttest-Only Designs

The one-group posttest-only design is referred to as *preexperimental* rather than quasi-experimental because of its weaknesses and the numerous threats to validity. It is inadequate for making causal inferences (Figure 11-11). Usually in this design, no attempt is made to control the selection of subjects who receive the treatment (the experimental group). It is difficult to justify generalizing findings beyond those tested. The group is not pretested; therefore, there is no direct way to measure change. The researcher cannot claim that posttest scores were a consequence (effect) of the treatment if scores before the treatment are unknown. Because there is no comparison group, one does not know whether groups not receiving the treatment would have similar scores on the dependent variable. The one-group posttest-only design is more commonly used in evaluation than in research.

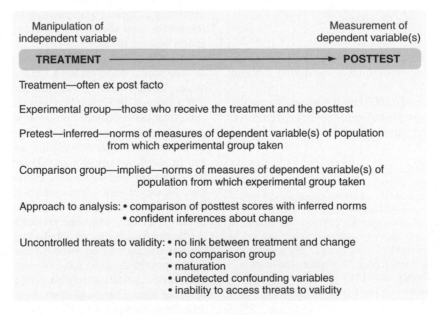

Figure **11-11** One-group posttest-only design.

Cook and Campbell (1979) suggested situations in which the one-group posttest-only design can be appropriate and adequate for inferring causality. For example, the design could be used to determine that a single factory's use of vinyl chloride is causing an increase in the rate of neighborhood and employee cancers. The incidence of cancer in the community at large is known. The fact that vinyl chloride causes cancer and the types of cancer it causes are also known. These norms would then take the place of the pretest and the comparison group. Thus, to use this design intelligently, one must know a great deal about the causal factors interacting within the situation. This is not the usual situation in nursing studies.

Posttest-Only Designs with a Comparison Group

Although the posttest-only design with comparison groups offers an improvement on the previous design, because of the addition of a nonequivalent comparison group, it is still referred to as *preexperimental* (Figure 11-12). The addition of a comparison group can lead to a false confidence in the validity of the findings.

Selection threats are a problem with both groups. The lack of a pretest remains a serious impediment to defining change. Differences in posttest scores between groups may be caused by the treatment or by differential selection processes.

One-Group Pretest-Posttest Designs

Another preexperimental design, the one-group pretest-posttest design, is one of the more commonly used designs. However, it has such serious weaknesses that findings are often uninterpretable (Figure 11-13). Pretest scores cannot adequately serve the same function as a comparison group. Events can occur between the pretest and posttest that alter responses to the posttest. These events then serve as alternative hypotheses to the proposal that the change in posttest scores is due to the treatment. Posttest scores might be altered by (1) maturation processes, (2) administration of the pretest, and (3) changes in instrumentation. Additionally, subjects in many studies using this design are selected on the basis of high or low scores on the pretest. Thus, there is an additional threat that changes in the posttest may be due to regression toward the mean. The addition of a nonequivalent comparison group, as described in the next design, can greatly strengthen the validity of the findings.

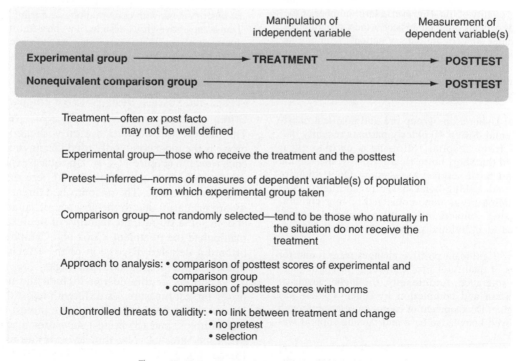

Figure 11-12 Posttest-only design with a comparison group.

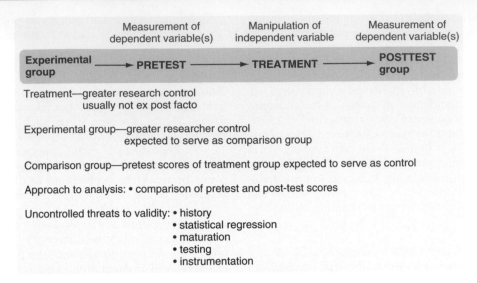

Figure **11-13** One-group pretest-posttest design.

Warrington, Cholowski, and Peters (2003) conducted a one-group pretest-posttest study that they describe as follows.

> *Background:* The benefits of cardiac rehabilitation programmes have been well documented including reductions in mortality, improved physical performance, and improved quality of life. However, a large number of special-needs patients often fail to access these programmes. Of particular concern are elderly patients with chronic illness and disability.
> *Aims:* To evaluate the effectiveness of a home-based cardiac rehabilitation programme in improving health outcomes and rehabilitation access for special-needs patients.
> *Design:* Using a one-group pre and post-test quasi-experimental design 40 elderly patients recently discharged from hospital following a cardiac event completed the Short Form Health Survey, the Angina Quiz, and the Exercise Assessment Questionnaire prior to undertaking home-based rehabilitation. The rehabilitation programme consisted of four community nursing contacts over a 9-week period primarily aimed at individual patient education and carer support.
> *Results:* Significant positive changes were found for measures of quality of life, knowledge of angina, and exercise tolerance. Additionally, the higher levels of participation and completion by older women was encouraging. Development of carer competence through an improved knowledge base and nursing support was also evident.
> While theoretically defensible positive outcomes were found these results need to be replicated in a larger study.

Similarly, the limitations imposed by a single group pretest, post-test design suggest that claims of generalizability need to be limited to the specific variables measured in this study.
> *Conclusion:* The study demonstrated medium term positive health outcomes. These positive findings suggest that home-based rehabilitation using larger samples of older patients with comorbidities, and using randomized comparative group designs, may be a fruitful area in future research. (Warrington et al., 2003; full-text article available in CINAHL)

Pretest and Posttest Designs with a Comparison Group

The **pretest and posttest design** with a comparison group is the most commonly used design in social science research (Figure 11-14). This quasi-experimental design is the first design discussed here that is generally interpretable. The uncontrolled threats to validity are primarily due to the absence of randomization and, in some studies, the inability of the researcher to manipulate the treatment. Cook and Campbell (1979) offered a detailed discussion of the effects of these threats on interpreting study findings.

Variations in this design include the use of (1) proxy pretest measures (a different pretest that correlates with the posttest), (2) separate pretest and posttest samples, and (3) pretest measures at more than one time interval. The first two variations weaken the design, but the last variation greatly strengthens it. In some studies, the comparison group consists of

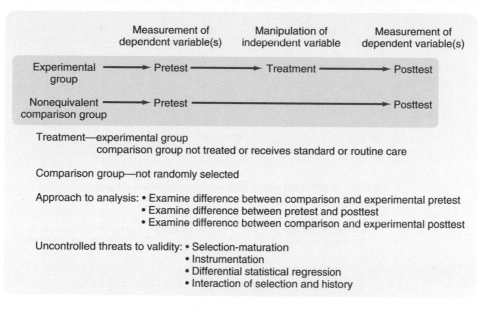

	Measurement of dependent variable(s)	Manipulation of independent variable	Measurement of dependent variable(s)
Experimental group	Pretest	Treatment	Posttest
Nonequivalent comparison group	Pretest		Posttest

Treatment—experimental group
  comparison group not treated or receives standard or routine care

Comparison group—not randomly selected

Approach to analysis: • Examine difference between comparison and experimental pretest
  • Examine difference between pretest and posttest
  • Examine difference between comparison and experimental posttest

Uncontrolled threats to validity: • Selection-maturation
  • Instrumentation
  • Differential statistical regression
  • Interaction of selection and history

Figure 11-14 Pretest and posttest design with a comparison group.

patients cared for before a new treatment was initiated. Data on this comparison group are obtained through chart audit or from electronic databases owned by the facility. Obviously there is no opportunity to control the quality of the data obtained through chart audit. Thus, this strategy weakens the design.

Costanzo, Walker, Yates, McCabe, and Berg (2006) used a pretest-posttest comparison group design in their study of physical activity counseling for older women. They described their design as follows.

Physical inactivity is a major factor in increasing women's risk for chronic disease, disability, and premature mortality. This study compared the effectiveness of five behavioral counseling (BC) sessions with a comparison group receiving one BC session based on the five A's (ask, advise, assist, arrange, and agree) to increase moderate-intensity physical activity, muscle strengthening, and stretching activity. The health promotion model provided the framework for the intervention. A *pretest/posttest comparison group* design was used, with random assignment of 46 women recruited from an urban midwestern community. A significant group interaction was found only for cardiorespiratory fitness (p < 0.001). Significant time effects were found (*p* < 0.001) for both groups in increasing handgrip, leg strength, and flexibility. BC is a promising intervention to achieve physical activity behavior change with older women. (Costanzo et al., 2006; full-text article available in CINAHL)

Pretest and Posttest Designs with Two Comparison Treatments

The two-treatment design is used when two experimental treatments are being compared to determine which is most effective. In most cases, this design is used when one treatment is the currently identified treatment of choice and the researcher has identified a treatment that might lead to even better outcomes (Figure 11-15). This design is strengthened by the addition of one or more of the following: a no-treatment group, a placebo-treatment group, or a usual-treatment group (Figure 11-16).

Côté and Pepler (2002) conducted a study that compared two coping interventions designed for acutely ill HIV-positive men. The following is a description of their study.

Background: People who are HIV-positive now live longer when they have contracted AIDS, and nursing interventions can help improve their quality of life.
Objectives: To test the effects of an intervention based on developing cognitive coping skills as compared to one focused on facilitating the expression of emotions. Both interventions were intended to help regulate emotional response to an exacerbation of HIV-related symptoms.
Method: In a randomized, controlled trial, 90 hospitalized HIV-positive men were randomly assigned to one of three groups: cognitive, expression, or control. The intervention was administered on three consecutive days in 20-30 minute sessions. Preintervention and post-intervention data were gathered on mood, distress, and anxiety.

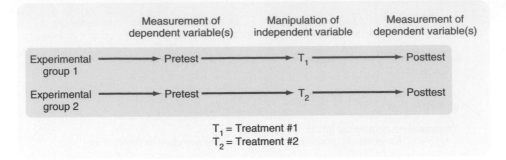

Figure **11-15** Pretest and posttest design with two comparison treatments.

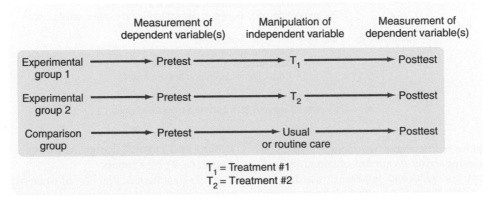

Figure **11-16** Pretest and posttest design with two comparison treatments and a standard or routine care group used as a comparison group.

Results: Both interventions produced a beneficial effect on negative affect (cognitive group $p = 0.002$, expression group $p = 0.011$), and immediately following the first daily session ($p = 0.001$). No change in positive affect was produced by either intervention. Paired t tests indicated a decrease in distress ($p = 0.039$), specifically, of intrusive ideation ($p = 0.03$), for the cognitive group, which also experienced a decrease in anxiety from immediately before to immediately after each session. Conversely, the expressive group experienced an increase in anxiety ($p = 0.018$).

Discussion: The cognitive coping skills nursing intervention was effective in helping to regulate HIV-positive persons' emotional responses to advanced disease. This nursing intervention is feasible for use by skilled practitioners providing daily care. (Côté & Pepler, 2002, p. 237; full-text article available in CINAHL)

Pretest and Posttest Designs with a Removed Treatment

In some cases, gaining access to even a comparison group is not possible. The removed-treatment design with pretest and posttest creates conditions that approximate the conceptual requirements of a control group receiving no treatment. The design is basically a one-group pretest-posttest design. However, after a delay, a third measure of the dependent variable is taken, followed by an interval in which the treatment is removed, followed by a fourth measure of the dependent variable (Figure 11-17). The periods between measures must be equivalent. In nursing situations, the researcher must consider the ethics of removing an effective treatment. Even if doing so is ethically acceptable, the response of subjects to the removal may make interpreting changes difficult.

It is difficult in CINAHL and MEDLINE to locate examples of studies using removed-treatment designs, because the search requires the use of the Boolean terms "removed ADJ treatment" or "removed w treatment." A search in PsychInfo located one study: Schneider (1998) described a study of the effects of virtual reality on symptom distress in children receiving cancer chemotherapy.

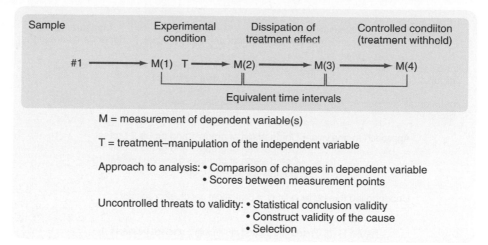

Figure 11-17 Pretest and posttest design with a removed treatment. *M(1)*, pretest; *M(2)*, posttest; *M(3)*, pretest of controlled condition; *M(4)*, posttest of controlled condition.

An interrupted time series design with removed treatment was used to answer the following research questions: (1) Is virtual reality an effective distraction intervention for reducing chemotherapy related symptom distress in children? And (2) Does virtual reality in children have a lasting effect? Hypotheses: (1) There will be differences in measures of symptom distress in a single group of children with cancer who receive a virtual reality distraction intervention during the second chemotherapy treatment and who receive no virtual reality intervention during the first and third chemotherapy treatments. The convenience sample consisted of 11 children receiving outpatient chemotherapy at a clinical cancer center. Measures of symptom distress were obtained at nine time points during three consecutive chemotherapy treatments. Four indicators were used to measure the dependent variable of symptom distress. The Symptom Distress Scale (SDS) (McCorkle & Young, 1978) was considered a general indicator. Specific indicators of symptom distress included the State-Trait Anxiety Inventory for Children (STAIC C-1) (Spielberger et al., 1978) and single item indicators for nausea and vomiting. (Schneider, 1998; full-text article available in PsychInfo)

Pretest and Posttest Designs with a Reversed Treatment

The reversed-treatment nonequivalent control group design with pretest and posttest introduces two independent variables—one expected to produce a positive effect and one expected to produce a negative effect (Figure 11-18). There are two experimental groups, each exposed to one of the treatments. The design tests differences in response to the two treatments. This design is more useful for theory testing than the no-treatment control group design because of its high construct validity of the cause. This means that there are strong theoretical sources that propose that specific treatments cause specific effects. The theoretical causal variable must be rigorously defined to allow differential predictions of directions of effect. To be maximally interpretable, the following two groups must be added: (1) a placebo control group in which the treatment is not expected to affect the dependent variable and (2) a no-treatment control group to provide a baseline.

McConnell (1976) used a reversed-treatment design to test how knowledge of the results affected a subject's attitude toward a motor learning task. The study

tested the hypotheses that a group which has the greatest number of gains in performance in successive trial scores of a motor task will develop a more positive attitude toward the task, and that a group which has the greatest number of gains in performance in successive trial scores will show the greatest change in an already formed attitude. Twelve male and 12 female physical education majors were randomly divided into 2 groups. Each S performed 20 trials of 15 seconds each on a rotary pursuit task, read the directions for the completion of the attitude measuring instrument, and then completed this series of activities was repeated a 2nd time. The difference in the treatment of the 2 groups occurred in the knowledge of results (KR: i.e., time on target). The 1st group received its KR during the 1st 20

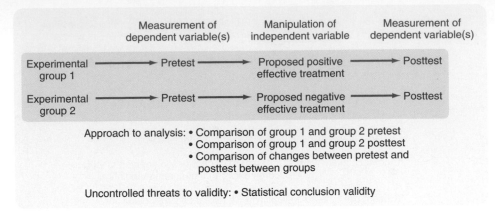

Figure 11-18 Pretest and posttest design with a reversed treatment.

trials to the full second; during the 2nd 20 trials, this group received its KR to .01 second. The other group received the reverse treatment. The difference in treatment caused the Ss in the group being given KR to .01th of a second to achieve more gains in performance than those whose KR was to the full second. Further analyses supported both hypotheses. (McConnell, 1976; abstract available in PsychInfo)

Interrupted Time-Series Designs

The interrupted time-series design is similar to descriptive time designs except that a treatment is applied at some point in the observations. Time-series analyses have some advantages over other quasi-experimental designs. First, repeated pretest observations can assess trends in maturation before the treatment. Second, the repeated pretest observations allow measures of trends in scores before the treatment, decreasing the risk of statistical regression, which would lead to misinterpretation of findings. If you keep records of events that could influence subjects in your study, you can determine whether historical factors that could modify responses to the treatment were in operation between the last pretest and the first posttest.

Some threats, however, are particularly problematic in time-series designs. Record-keeping procedures and definitions of constructs used for data collection tend to change over time. Thus, maintaining consistency can be a problem. The treatment can result in attrition so that the sample before treatment may be different in important ways from the posttreatment group. Seasonal variation or other cyclical influences can be interpreted as treatment effects. Therefore, identifying

cyclical patterns and controlling for them are critical to the analysis of study findings.

McCain and McCleary (1979) have suggested using the autoregressive integrated moving average (ARIMA) statistical model (see Chapter 20) to analyze time-series data. ARIMA is a relatively new statistical model that has some distinct advantages over regression analysis techniques. For adequate statistical analysis, at least 50 measurement points are needed; however, Cook and Campbell (1979) believe that even small numbers of measurement points can provide better information than that obtained in cross-sectional studies. The numbers of measures shown in the designs illustrated in Figures 11-19 through 11-21 are limited by space. They are not meant to suggest limiting measures to the numbers shown.

Simple Interrupted Time-Series Designs

The simple interrupted time-series design is similar to the descriptive time-series study, with the addition of a treatment that occurs or is applied (interrupts the time series) at a given point in time (see Figure 11-19). The treatment, which in some cases is not completely under the control of the researcher, must be clearly defined. There is no control or comparison group in this design. The use of multiple methods to measure the dependent variable greatly strengthens the design. Threats that are well controlled by this design are maturation and statistical regression.

Woods and Dimond (2002) used a simple interrupted time-series design to examine the effect of therapeutic touch on agitated behavior and cortisol in persons with Alzheimer's disease. They described their study as follows.

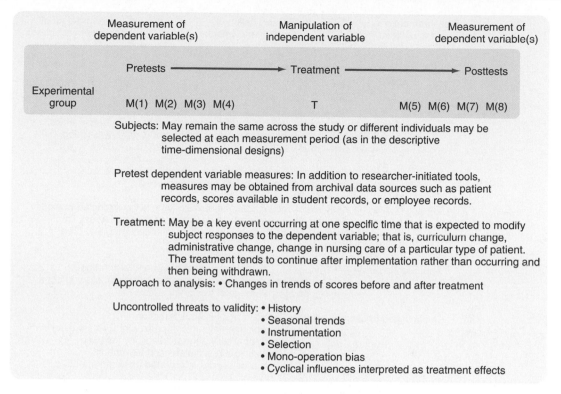

Figure 11-19 Simple interrupted time-series design.

Agitated behavior in persons with Alzheimer's disease (AD) presents a challenge to current interventions. Recent developments in neuroendocrinology suggest that changes in the hypothalamic-pituitary-adrenal (HPA) axis alter the responses of persons with AD to stress. Given the deleterious effects of pharmacological interventions in this vulnerable population, it is essential to explore noninvasive treatments for their potential to decrease a hyper-responsiveness to stress and indirectly decrease detrimental cortisol levels. This within-subject, interrupted time-series study was conducted to test the efficacy of therapeutic touch on decreasing the frequency of agitated behavior and salivary and urine cortisol levels in persons with AD. Ten subjects who were 71 to 84 years old and resided in a special care unit were observed every 20 minutes for 10 hours a day, were monitored 24 hours a day for physical activity, and had samples for salivary and urine cortisol taken daily. The study occurred in 4 phases: 1) baseline (4 days), 2) treatment (therapeutic touch for 5 to 7 minutes 2 times a day for 3 days), 3) post-treatment (11 days), and 4) post-wash-out (3 days). An analysis of variance for repeated measures indicated a significant decrease in overall agitated behavior and in 2 specific behaviors, vocalization and pacing or walking, during treatment and post-treatment.

A decreasing trend over time was noted for salivary and urine cortisol. Although this study does not provide direct clinical evidence to support dysregulation in the HPA axis, it does suggest that environmental and behavioral interventions such as therapeutic touch have the potential to decrease vocalization and pacing, 2 prevalent behaviors, and may mitigate cortisol levels in persons with AD. (Woods & Dimond, 2002; abstract available in CINAHL)

Interrupted Time-Series Designs with a Comparison Group

The addition of a comparison group to the interrupted time-series design greatly strengthens the validity of the findings. The comparison group allows the researcher to examine the differences in trends between groups after the treatment and the persistence of treatment effects over time (Figure 11-20). Although the treatment may continue (e.g., a change in nursing management practices or patient teaching strategies), the initial response to the change may differ from later responses.

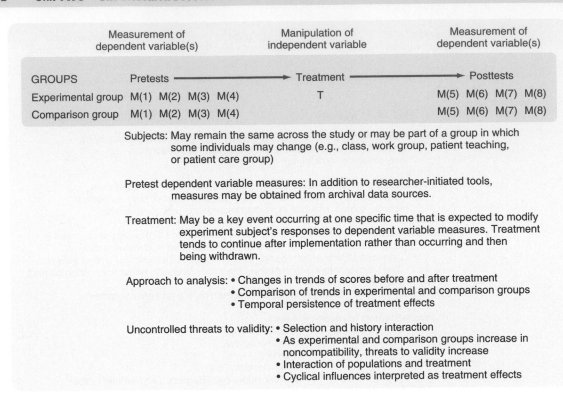

Figure 11-20 Interrupted time-series design with a nonequivalent no-treatment comparison group time series.

Chan, Lu, Tseng, and Chous (2003) used an interrupted time-series design with a comparison group to evaluate an anger control program. The study is described as follows.

The purpose of this study was to evaluate the anger control program in reducing anger expression in patients with schizophrenia. The study had an interrupted time series with nonequivalent comparison group design. Data were collected before the intervention, at the end of the 5th and 10th *group* sessions, and 2 weeks after the 10th (or last) session. A total of 78 patients were assigned to experimental (the anger control program) or *comparison* groups. The Generalized Estimating Equation (GEE) was used to analyze the longitudinal data. The program was found to reduce anger expression in patients with schizophrenia effectively and to increase their anger control ability.

Interrupted Time-Series Designs with Multiple Treatment Replications

The interrupted time-series design with multiple treatment replications is a powerful design for inferring causality (see Figure 11-21). It requires greater researcher control than is usually possible in social science research outside closed institutional settings, such as laboratories or research units. The studies that led researchers to adopt behavior modification techniques used this design. For significant differences to be interpretable, the pretest and posttest scores must be in different directions. Within this design, treatments can be modified by substituting one treatment for another or combining two treatments and examining interaction effects.

EXPERIMENTAL STUDY DESIGNS

Experimental study designs provide the greatest amount of control possible to examine causality more closely. To examine cause, one must eliminate all factors influencing the dependent variable other than the cause (independent variable) being studied. Other factors are eliminated by controlling them. The study is designed to prevent any other element from intruding into observation of the specific cause and effect that the researcher wishes to examine.

The three essential elements of experimental research are (1) randomization, (2) researcher-

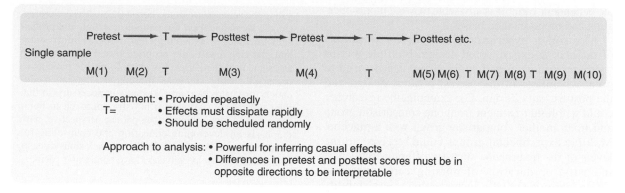

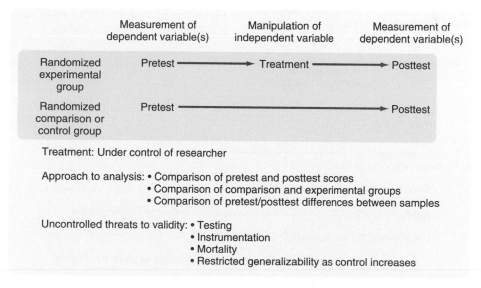

Figure 11-21 Interrupted time-series design with multiple treatment replications.

controlled manipulation of the independent variable, and (3) researcher control of the experimental situation, including a control or comparison group. Experimental designs exert much effort to control variance. Sample criteria are explicit, the independent variable is provided in a precisely defined way, the dependent variables are carefully operationalized, and the situation in which the study is conducted is rigidly controlled to prevent the interference of unstudied factors from modifying the dynamics of the process being studied.

Classic Experimental Design

The original, or classic, experimental design, or pretest-posttest control group design, is still the most commonly used experimental design (Figure 11-22). There are two randomized groups, one receiving the experimental treatment and one receiving no treatment, a placebo treatment, or the usual or standard care. By comparing pretest scores, one can evaluate the effectiveness of randomization in providing equivalent groups. The researcher controls treatment. The dependent variable is measured twice, before and after the manipulation of the independent variable. As with all well-designed studies, the dependent and independent variables are conceptually linked, conceptually defined, and operationalized. Instruments used to measure the dependent variable clearly reflect the conceptual meaning of the variable and have good evidence of reliability and validity. Often, more than one means of measuring

Figure 11-22 The classic experimental design; pretest-posttest control group design.

the dependent variable is advisable to avoid mono-operation and mono-method biases.

Most other experimental designs are variations of the classic experimental design. Multiple groups (both experimental and comparison) can be used to great advantage in the pretest-posttest design and the posttest-only design. For example, the researcher could withhold treatment from one comparison group and treat another comparison group with a placebo. Multiple experimental groups could receive varying levels of the treatments, such as differing frequency, intensity, or duration of nursing care measures. These additions greatly increase the generalizability of the study findings.

Malm, Karlsson, and Fridlund (2007) conducted an experimental study of the effects of a self-care program on health-related quality of life (HRQoL) for pacemaker patients. The study is described as follows.

An experimental, multi-centre, randomized study with a nurse-led intervention was conducted with the aim of evaluating the effects on HRQoL of a 10-month self-care program for pacemaker patients. In the present study, there were no significant differences in HRQoL when comparisons were made between the experimental group and the control group. Results show two main findings for patients in the self-care program ($n = 97$; mean age 71 years): a significantly better HRQoL in terms of experiencing the symptoms that were the reason for pacemaker implantation, as having decreased or disappeared, and a higher level of perceived exertion in a 1 1/2-minute stair test compared with patients who had standard checkups ($n = 115$; mean age 73 years). It is important to actively include pacemaker patients in a self-care program while still in the acute phase in the hospital. Health care professionals should support the patient in a kind and professional manner by providing clear, relevant information, and planning a self-care program based on the nurse's assessment of the patient's needs. To enable patients to manage their life situations, training and continued education for health care professionals is necessary so that their efforts are based on a holistic approach to nursing care and recognition of the patient perspective, with emphasis on developing education and counseling for women, patients with atrial fibrillation/sick sinus disease, and patients whose pacemakers have ventricular pacing.

Experimental Posttest-Only Comparison Group Designs

In some studies, the dependent variable cannot be measured before the treatment. For example, before the beginning of treatment, it is not possible to measure, in a meaningful way, a subject's responses to interventions designed to control nausea from chemotherapy or postoperative pain. Additionally, in some cases, subjects' responses to the posttest can be due, in part, to learning from or having a subjective reaction to the pretest (*pretest sensitization*). If this issue is a concern in your study, you may eliminate the pretest and use an experimental posttest-only design with a comparison group (Figure 11-23). However, you then will not be able to use many powerful statistical analysis techniques within the study. Additionally, the effectiveness of randomization in obtaining equivalent experimental and comparison groups cannot be evaluated in terms of the study variables. Nevertheless, the groups can be evaluated in terms of sample characteristics and other relevant variables.

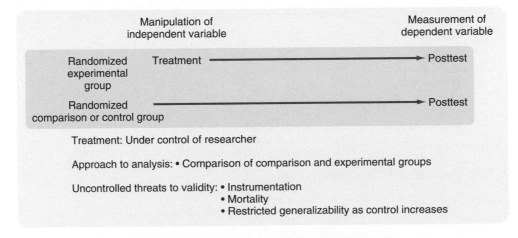

Figure **11-23** Experimental posttest-only comparison group design.

Randomized Blocking Designs

The randomized blocking design uses the two-group pretest-posttest pattern or the two-group posttest pattern with one addition: a blocking variable. The blocking variable, if uncontrolled, is expected to confound the findings of the study. To prevent this confusion, the subjects are rank ordered in relation to the blocking variable.

For example, if effectiveness of a nursing intervention to relieve postchemotherapy nausea were the independent variable in your study, severity of nausea could confound the findings. Subjects would be ranked according to severity of nausea. You would identify and randomly assign the two subjects with the most severe nausea, one to the experimental group and one to the comparison group. You then would identify and randomly assign the two subjects next in rank. You would follow this pattern until the entire sample was randomly assigned as matched pairs. This procedure ensures that the experimental group and the comparison group are equal in relation to the potentially confounding variable.

The effect of blocking can also be accomplished statistically (through the use of analysis of covariance) without categorizing the confounding variable into discrete components. However, for this analysis to be accurate, one must be careful not to violate the assumptions of the statistical procedure (Spector, 1981). An example of this design is the study by Mishel et al. (2003), which was designed to identify moderators of an uncertainty management intervention for men with localized prostate cancer. They described the study as follows.

Background: The effectiveness of psycho-educational interventions for cancer patients is well documented, but less is known about moderating characteristics that determine which subgroups of patients are most likely to benefit.
Objectives: The aim of this study was to determine whether certain individual characteristics of African-American and White men with localized prostate cancer moderated the effects of a psycho-educational Uncertainty Management Intervention on the outcomes of cancer knowledge and patient-provider communication.
Methods: Men were blocked by ethnicity and randomly assigned to one of three conditions: Uncertainty Management Intervention provided to the patient only, Uncertainty Management Intervention supplemented by delivery to the patient and family member, or usual care. The individual characteristics explored were education, sources for information, and intrinsic and extrinsic religiosity. The intervention was implemented for eight weeks and provided by weekly phone calls. Data were collected

at baseline, four months postbaseline, and seven months postbaseline.
Results: Using repeated measures multivariate analysis of variance, findings indicated that there were no significant moderator effects for intrinsic religiosity on any of the outcomes. Lower level of education was a significant moderator for improvement in cancer knowledge. For the outcome of patient-provider communication, fewer sources for cancer information was a significant moderator for the amount told the patient by the nurse and other staff. Less extrinsic religiosity was a significant moderator for three areas of patient provider communication. The three areas are the amount (a) the physician tells the patient; (b) the patient helps with planning treatment; and (c) the patient tells the physician.
Conclusions: Testing for moderator effects provides important information regarding beneficiaries of interventions. In the current study, men's levels of education, amount of sources for information, and extrinsic religiosity influenced the efficacy of the Uncertainty Management Intervention on important outcomes. (Mishel et al., 2003, p. 89; full-text article available in CINAHL)

Factorial Designs

In a factorial design, two or more different characteristics, treatments, or events are independently varied within a single study. This design is a logical approach to examining multiple causality. The simplest arrangement is one in which two treatments or factors are involved and, within each factor, two levels are manipulated (for example, the presence or absence of the treatment); this is referred to as a *2 × 2 factorial design*. This design is illustrated in Figure 11-24, in which the two independent variables are relaxation and distraction as means of relieving pain.

A 2 × 2 factorial design produces a study with four cells (A through D). Each cell must contain an approximately equivalent number of subjects. Cells B and C allow the researcher to examine of each intervention separately. Cell D subjects receive no treatment and serve as a control group. Cell A allows the researcher

Level of Relaxation	Level of Distraction	
	Distraction	No Distraction
Relaxation	A	B
No Relaxation	C	D

Figure 11-24 Example of factorial design.

to examine the interaction between the two independent variables. This design can be used, as in the randomized block design, to control for confounding variables. The confounding variable is included as an independent variable, and interactions between it and the other independent variable are examined (Spector, 1981).

Extensions of the factorial design to more than two levels of variables are referred to as $M \times N$ factorial designs. Within this design, independent variables can have any number of levels within practical limits. Note that a 3×3 design involves 9 cells and requires a much larger sample size. A 4×4 design would require 16 cells. A 4×4 design would allow relaxation to be provided at four levels of intensity, such as no relaxation, relaxation for 10 minutes twice a day, relaxation for 15 minutes three times a day, and relaxation for 20 minutes four times a day. Distraction would be provided at similar levels.

Factorial designs are not limited to two independent variables; however, interpretation of larger numbers becomes more complex and requires greater knowledge of statistical analysis. Factorial designs do allow the examination of theoretically proposed interrelationships between multiple independent variables. However, very large samples are required.

An example of factorial design is the study by Phibbs et al. (2006), which evaluated the impact of a comprehensive geriatric assessment service. An excerpt from that study follows.

Background: The Geriatric Evaluation and Management study was developed to assess the impact of a comprehensive geriatric assessment service on the care of the elderly.

Objectives: We sought to evaluate the cost and clinical impact of inpatient units and outpatient clinics for geriatric evaluation and management.

Research Design: We undertook a prospective, randomized, controlled trial using a 2×2 factorial design, with 1-year follow-up.

Subjects: A total of 1388 participants hospitalized on either a medical or surgical ward at 11 participating Veterans Affairs medical centers were randomized to receive either inpatient geriatric unit (GEMU) or usual inpatient care (UCIP), followed by either outpatient care from a geriatric clinic (GEMC) versus usual outpatient care (UCOP).

Measures: We measured health care utilization and costs.

Results: Patients assigned to the GEMU had a significantly decreased rate of nursing home placement (odds ratio = 0.65; $P = 0.001$). Neither the GEMU nor GEMC had any statistically significant improvement effects on survival and only modest effects on health status. There were statistically insignificant mean cost savings of

$1027 ($P = 0.29$) per inpatient for the GEMU and $1665 ($P = 0.69$) per outpatient for the GEMC.

Conclusions: Inpatient or outpatient geriatric evaluation and management units didn't increase the costs of care. Although there was no effect on survival and only modest effects on SF-36 scores at 1-year follow-up, there was a statistically significant reduction in nursing home admissions for patients treated in the GEMU. (Phibbs et al., 2006)

Nested Designs

In some experimental situations, you may wish to consider the effect of variables that are found only at some levels of the independent variables being studied. Variables found only at certain levels of the independent variable are called nested variables. Possible nested variables are gender, race, socioeconomic status, and education. A nested variable may also be the patients who are cared for on specific nursing units or at different hospitals; the statistical analysis in this case would be conducted as though the unit or hospital were the subject rather than the individual patient. Figure 11-25 illustrates the nested design. In actual practice, nursing units used in this manner would have to be much larger in number than those illustrated, because each unit would be considered a subject and would be randomly assigned to a treatment.

Lewandowski, Good, and Draucker (2005) studied verbal descriptions of pain change. The following excerpt describes their study.

The purpose of this study is to determine how verbal descriptions of pain change with the use of a guided imagery technique. A mixed method, concurrent nested design was used. Participants in the treatment group used the guided imagery technique over a consecutive 4-day period, and those in the control group were monitored. Verbal descriptions of pain were obtained before randomization and at four daily intervals. A total of 210 pain descriptions were obtained across the five time points. Data were analyzed using content analysis. Six categories emerged from the data: pain is never-ending, pain is relative, pain is explainable, pain is torment, pain is restrictive, and pain is changeable. For participants in the treatment group, pain became changeable. The meaning of pain as never-ending was a prominent theme for participants before randomization to treatment and control groups. It remained a strong theme for participants in the control group throughout the 4-day study period; however, pain as never-ending did not resurface for participants in the treatment group.

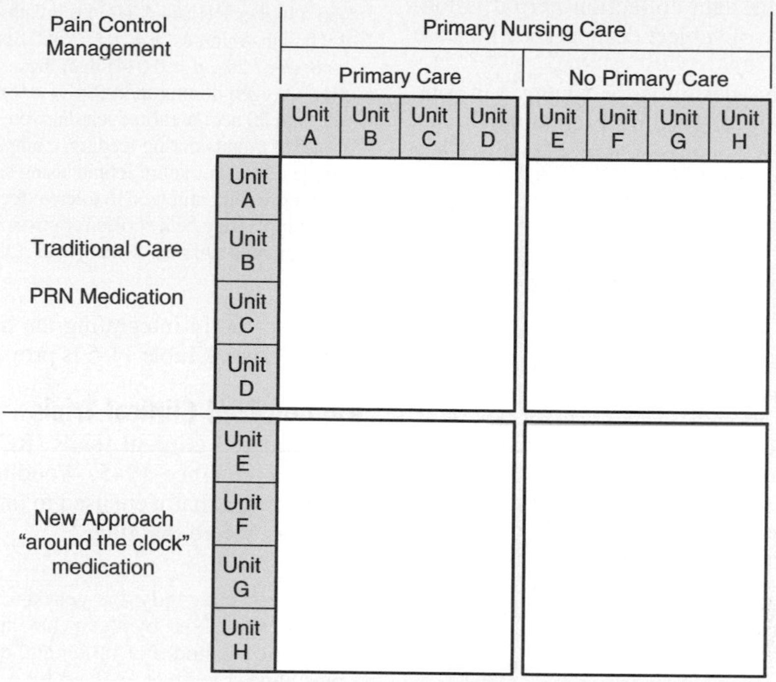

Pain Control Management		Primary Nursing Care							
		Primary Care				No Primary Care			
		Unit A	Unit B	Unit C	Unit D	Unit E	Unit F	Unit G	Unit H
Traditional Care PRN Medication	Unit A								
	Unit B								
	Unit C								
	Unit D								
New Approach "around the clock" medication	Unit E								
	Unit F								
	Unit G								
	Unit H								

Figure 11-25 Nested design.

Crossover or Counterbalanced Designs

In some studies, more than one treatment is administered to each subject. The treatments are provided sequentially rather than concurrently. Comparisons are then made of the effects of the different treatments on the same subject. For example, two different methods known to achieve relaxation might be used as the two treatments. One difficulty with this type of study is that exposure to one treatment may result in effects (called carryover effects) that persist and influence responses of the subject to later treatments. Also, subjects can improve as they become more familiar with the experimental protocol, which is called a practice effect. They may become tired or bored with the study, which is called a fatigue effect. The direct interaction of one treatment with another, such as the use of two drugs, can confound differences in the two treatments.

Crossover, or *counterbalancing*, is a strategy designed to guard against possible erroneous conclusions resulting from carryover effects. With counterbalancing, subjects are randomly assigned to a specific sequencing of treatment conditions. This approach distributes the carryover effects equally throughout all the conditions of the study, thus canceling them out. To prevent an effect related to time, the same amount of time must be allotted to each treatment, and the crossover point must be related to time, not to the condition of the subject.

In addition, the design must allow for an adequate interval between treatments to dissipate the effects of the first treatment; this is referred to as a *washout period*. For example, the design would specify that each treatment would last 6 days and that on the eighth day, each subject would cross over to the alternative treatment after a 2-day washout period.

The researcher also must be alert to the possibility that changes may be due to factors such as disease progression, the healing process, or the effects of treatment of the disease rather than the study treatment. The process of counterbalancing can become complicated when more than two treatments are involved. Counterbalancing is effective only if the carryover effect is essentially the same from treatment A to treatment B as it is from treatment B to treatment A. If one treatment is more fatiguing than the other or more likely to modify response to the other treatment, counterbalancing will not be effective. You can use the crossover design to control variance in your study and thus allow the sample size to be smaller. The sample size required to detect a significant effect is considerably smaller because the subjects serve as their own controls. Because the data collection period is longer, however, the rate of subject dropout may increase (Beck, 1989).

An example of this design is the Chang, Lin, Lin, and Lin (2007) study of feeding premature infants using either single-hole or cross-cut nipple units. They described their study as follows.

The purpose of this study was to compare the amount of total milk intake, feeding time, sucking efficiency, heart rate (HR), respiratory rate (RR), and oxygen saturation (SpO_2) of premature infants when fed with either single-hole or cross-cut nipple units. Twenty stable infants admitted to a level II nursery in a tertiary care center with gestational ages averaging 32.2 +/– 3.2 wks were enrolled. Subjects had an average postmenstrual age of 34.1 +/– 1.6 wks, and average body weight of 1996 +/– 112 gm. A crossover design was used and infants were observed for two consecutive meals separated by a four-hour interval. They were bottle fed with equal feeding amounts using a single-hole and cross-cut nipple administered in random order. Results showed that infants fed with single-hole nipple units took more milk (57.5 +/– 8.3 ml vs. 51.6 +/– 9.5 ml, $p = 0.011$), had a shorter feeding time per meal (11.5 +/– 4.9 min vs. 20.9 +/– 5.0 min, $p < 0.001$), and sucked more efficiently (5.8 +/– 2.5 ml/min vs. 2.7 +/– 1.0 ml/min, $p < 0.001$) compared to those fed through cross-cut nipples. Infants using cross-cut nipple units

had a higher RR (44.4 +/– 4.6 breaths/minutes vs. 40.8 +/– 4.9 breaths/minutes, $p = 0.002$) and SpO_2 (96.1 +/– 1.4% vs. 94.6 +/– 3.2%, $p = 0.044$) than those using single-hole nipples. Oxygen desaturation ($SpO_2 < 90\%$ and lasting for longer than 20 sec) and bradycardia were not recorded in either group of infants during feeding. Compared to using cross-cut nipple units, premature infants using single-hole nipple units take more milk and tend to tolerate feedings better. A single-hole nipple may be a choice for physiologically stable bottle-fed premature infants. (Chang et al., 2007)

To assist you in integrating the information on traditional designs, Table 11-5 is provided.

Randomized Clinical Trials

Randomized clinical trials (RCTs) have been used in medicine since 1945. Wooding (1994) described the strategies that were used to introduce new medical therapies before that time.

Until very recently, the genesis and use of new treatments came about by means having little to do with the scientific method. For millennia, the majority of therapies appear to have evolved by one of three methods: accidental discovery of treatments with unmistakable efficacy; the use of hypotheses alone, without any experimentation; or the utilization of experimentation without

TABLE 11-5 ▪ Comparison of Four Major Types of Design			
Type of Design	**Key Focus**	**Sample Purpose Statement**	**Intervention?**
Descriptive	Describe "what is"	"The purpose of this study was to (a) describe U.S. hospital PR rates and patterns, and (b) explore how U.S. policy and research initiatives might be shaped by the findings." (Minnick et al., 2007, p. 30.)	No
Correlational	Explores relationships among study variables	"The purpose of this study was to determine the relationships between trait anxiety, trait anger, height, weight, patterns of anger expression, and blood pressure in a group of elementary school children" (Howell et al., 2007, p. 18)	No
Quasi-Experimental	Tests causality with suboptimal control	"The purpose of this pilot study was to determine the effects of the addition of coping skills training for obese multiethnic parents whose overweight children were attending a weight management program" (Berry et al., 2007, p. 63)	Yes
Experimental	Tests causality with optimal control	"The purpose of the study was to investigate whether there were time-of-day differences in the effects of morphine on the pain tolerance threshold and circadian plasma BE response to pain" (Rasmussen & Farr, 2003, p. 107)	Yes

controls, randomization, blinding, … or adequate sample sizes. Treatments originating by one of the latter two routes frequently persisted for a very long time despite a lack of unbiased evidence of their efficacy. Bloodletting, purging, and the use of homeopathic dosages of drugs are examples. Failure of a treatment in any particular case was usually attributed by its practitioners to its misuse, to poor diagnosis, or to complicating factors. (Wooding, 1994, p. 26)

The methodology for a clinical trial uses strategies for medical research (Meinert & Tonascia, 1986; Piantadosi, 1997; Pocock, 1996; Whitehead, 1992; Wooding, 1994). The phase I, II, III, and IV clinical trial categories were developed specifically for testing experimental drug therapy. Phase I, the initial testing of a new drug, focuses on determining the best drug dose and identifying safety effects. Phase II trials seek preliminary evidence of efficacy and side effects of the drug dose determined by the phase I trial. Phase I and phase II trials do not include comparison groups or randomization and therefore could not be classified as experimental. They are more similar to pilot studies (Whitehead, 1992).

Phase III trials are comparative definitive studies in which the new drug's effects are compared with those of the drug considered standard therapy. Phase III trials are sometimes referred to as "full-scale definitive clinical trials," suggesting that a decision is made on the basis of the findings as to whether the experimental drug is more effective than standard treatment. In some phase III clinical trials, the sample size is not determined before initiation of data collection. Rather, data are analyzed at intervals to test for significant differences between groups. If a significant difference is found, data collection may be discontinued. Otherwise, the data collection will continue and retesting is initiated after accrual of additional subjects (Meinert & Tonascia, 1986; Whitehead, 1992). Phase IV trials occur after regulatory approval of the drug, are designed to follow patients over time to identify uncommon side effects and test marketing strategies, and do not include a comparison group or randomization (Piantadosi, 1997; Wooding, 1994).

Piantadosi (1997) recommended redefining these stages to be broader and applicable to more types of trials. He suggested using the following terminology: early development, middle development, comparative studies, and late development. In early development trials, researchers would develop and test the treatment mechanism (thus, they could also be called TM trials). Middle development studies would focus on

clinical outcomes and treatment "tolerability." Tolerability would have three components: feasibility, safety, and efficacy; thus, Piantadosi (1997) referred to middle development studies as safety and efficacy trials, or SE trials. In this phase, the researcher would estimate the probability that patients would benefit from the treatment (or experience side effects from it). Performance criteria such as success rate might be used.

Comparative studies, according to Piantadosi (1997), would have defined clinical end points and would address comparative treatment efficacy (so could be called CTE trials). These studies would include a concurrent control group that receives the standard treatment and an experimental group that receives the experimental treatment. Late development studies would be designed to identify uncommon side effects, interactions with other treatments, or unusual complications. They would be developed as expanded safety trials, or ES trials.

Elwood (1998) suggested that clinical trial methodology could be used for prevention intervention studies, as well as testing treatments. Murray (1998) proposed methods of randomizing groups rather than subjects in prevention studies and explores issues related to community-based trials such as sample mortality.

Until recently, the term clinical trial has not been used to describe studies conducted in nursing research. The clinical trial is perceived by many to be the Cadillac of designs. (There are serious criticisms of the clinical trial, however; they are discussed in Chapter 12.)

If the clinical trial is to be used in nursing, the methodology should be redefined to fit the knowledge-building needs of nursing. Sidani and Braden (1998) made a start in this direction by proposing such a methodology, which is described in Chapter 13. Criteria for defining a study as a clinical trial as opposed to referring to it as an experimental study have not been clarified in the nursing literature.

Meinert and Tonascia (1986) defined a clinical trial as a

planned experiment designed to assess the efficacy of a treatment in man by comparing the outcomes in a group of patients treated with the test treatment with those observed in a comparable group of patients receiving a control treatment, where patients in both groups are enrolled, treated, and followed over the same time period. The groups may be established through randomization or some other method of assignment. The outcome measure may be death, a nonfatal clinical event, or a laboratory test. The period of observation may be short or long depending on the outcome measure. (Meinert & Tonascia, 1986, p. 3)

Conceptually, the term *clinical trial*, as it is used in the nursing literature, seems to be associated with a phase III trial and has the following expectations:

1. The study is designed to be a definitive test of the hypothesis that the intervention causes the defined effects.
2. Previous studies have provided evidence that the intervention causes the desired outcome.
3. The intervention is clearly defined, and a protocol has been established for its clinical application.
4. The study is conducted in a clinical setting, not in a laboratory.
5. The design meets the criteria of an experimental study.
6. Subjects are drawn from a reference population through the use of clearly defined criteria. Baseline states are comparable in all groups included in the study. Selected subjects are then randomly assigned to treatment and comparison groups; thus, the term *randomized clinical trial.*
7. Subjects are accrued individually over time as they enter the clinical area, are identified as meeting the study criteria, and agree to participate in the study.
8. The study has high internal validity. The design is rigorous and involves a high level of control of potential sources of bias that will rule out possible alternative causes of the effect. The design may include blinding or double-blinding to accomplish this purpose. **Blinding** means that either the patient or those providing care to the patient are unaware of whether the patient is in the experimental group or the control group. **Double-blinding** means that neither the patient nor the caregivers are aware of the group assignment of the patient.
9. The treatment is equal and consistently applied to all subjects in the experimental group.
10. Dependent variables are measured consistently.
11. The proposed study has been externally reviewed by expert researchers who have approved the design.
12. The study has received external funding sufficient to allow a rigorous design with a sample size adequate to provide a definitive test of the intervention.
13. If the clinical trial results indicate a significant effect of the intervention, the evidence is sufficient to warrant application of the findings in clinical practice.
14. The intervention is defined in sufficient detail so that clinical application can be achieved.

Clinical trials may be carried out simultaneously in multiple geographical locations to increase sample size and resources and to obtain a more representative sample (Meinert & Tonascia, 1986). In this case, the primary researcher must coordinate activities at all the sites. Meinert and Tonascia (1986) indicated that the costs per patient per year of study are less for multi-center studies than for single-center trials. If you plan to use this technique in your research, you must confront several problems. Coordination of a project of this type requires much time and effort. Keeping up with subjects is critical but may be difficult. Communication with and cooperation of staff assisting with the study in the various geographical locations are essential but sometimes difficult. You may encounter attempts to ignore the protocol and provide traditional care (Fetter et al., 1989; Gilliss & Kulkin, 1991; Tyzenhouse, 1981). Meinert and Tonascia (1986) recommended the development of a coordinating center for multisite clinical trials that will be responsible for receiving, editing, processing, analyzing, and storing data generated in the study.

The use of the clinical trial is growing in nursing research. Brooten et al. (1986) conducted a clinical trial of early hospital discharge and home follow-up of very low birth weight infants. Burgess et al. (1987) performed a clinical trial of cardiac rehabilitation. Later studies defined in the literature as clinical trials are those by Clarke (1999); deMoissac & Jensen (1998); Griebel, Wewers, and Baker (1998); Ippoliti and Neumann (1998); Rawl, Easton, Kwiatkowski, Zemen, and Burczyk (1998); and Turner, Clark, Gauthier, and Williams (1998) (all full-text articles available in CINAHL).

An example of a clinical trial in nursing is the study by Krichbaum (2007), which tested the effectiveness of a gerontological advanced practice nurse intervention for elders with hip fracture. The study was funded by a Mentored Research Scientist Award from the National Institutes for Health/National Institute of Nursing Research. The author described the study as follows.

We tested the effectiveness of a nursing intervention model to improve health, function, and return-home outcomes in elders with hip fracture via a 2-year randomized clinical trial. Thirty three elders (age > 65 years) were tracked from hospital discharge to 12 months postfracture. The treatment group had a gerontologic advanced practice nurse as postacute care coordinator for 6 months who intervened with each elder regardless of the postacute care setting, making biweekly visits and/or phone calls. The coordinator assessed health and function, and informed elders, families, long-term care staff, and physicians of the patient's progress. The control group had care based on postacute facility protocols. Nonnormal distribution of data led to nonparametric analysis using Freidman's test with post hoc comparisons (Mann-Whitney U tests, Bonferroni adjustment). The treatment group had better function at 12 months on several activities and instrumental activities of daily living, and no differences in health, depression, or living situation.

STUDIES THAT DO NOT USE TRADITIONAL RESEARCH DESIGNS

In some approaches to research, the research designs described in this chapter cannot be used. These studies tend to be in highly specialized areas that require unique design strategies to accomplish their purposes. Designs for primary prevention and health promotion, secondary analysis, and methodological studies are described here.

Primary Prevention and Health Promotion Studies

To study primary prevention and health promotion as a nurse researcher, you must apply a treatment of primary prevention (the cause) and then attempt to measure the effect (an event that does not occur if the treatment was effective). Primary prevention studies, then, attempt to measure things that do not happen. One cannot select a sample to study, apply a treatment, and then measure an effect. The sample must be the community. The design involves examining changes in the community, and the variables are called indicators. A change in an identified indicator is inferred to be a consequence of the effectiveness of the prevention program (treatment).

Specific indicators would depend on the focus of prevention. For example, nurses in Canada identified oral mucositis as a recurring issue in clinical practice and developed an oral care guide. They used the University Health Network Nursing Research Utilization Model and the Neuman Systems Model as conceptual frameworks.

A flowchart was developed to ensure a coordinated and continuous provision of oral care. Educational presentations were conducted to familiarize nurses and members of the multidisciplinary team of the practice changes. The introduction of the oral care regimen as primary prevention, plus systematic oral assessment and monitoring had the potential to reduce

the occurrence and severity of oral mucositis in patients undergoing autologous stem cell transplantation. (Salvador, 2006)

How might you study the effectiveness of this primary prevention strategy? Because one indicator alone would be insufficient to infer effect, multiple indicators and statistical analyses appropriate for these indicators must be used. For example, you might measure the color of the oral mucosa, moistness in the mouth, severity of oral mucositis, and amount of pain expressed by the patient when eating.

Guinan, McGuckin, and Ali (2002) studied the effect of a comprehensive handwashing program on absenteeism in elementary schools. They described their study as follows.

Handwashing is one of the most important factors in controlling the spread of micro-organisms and in preventing the development of infections. The objective of this study was to determine the effectiveness of a comprehensive handwashing program on absenteeism in elementary grades. Two hundred ninety students from 5 independent schools were enrolled in the study. Each test classroom had a control classroom, and only the test classroom received the intervention (education program and hand sanitizer). Absenteeism data were collected for 3 months. The number of absences was 50.6% lower in the test group ($p < 0.001$). The data strongly suggest that a hand hygiene program that combines education and use of a hand sanitizer in the classroom can lower absenteeism and be cost-effective. (Guinan et al., 2002; full-text article available in CINAHL)

Secondary Analyses

Secondary analysis design involves studying data previously collected in another study. Data are reexamined with the use of different organizations of the data and different statistical analyses from those previously used. The design involves analyzing data to validate the reported findings, examining dimensions previously unexamined, or redirecting the focus of the data to allow comparison with data from other studies (Gleit & Graham, 1989). As data sets accumulate from the research programs of groups of faculty, secondary analyses can be expected to increase. This approach allows the investigators to examine questions related to the data that were not originally posed. These data sets may provide opportunities for junior faculty members or graduate students to become involved in a research program.

Of concern in secondary analyses of data is the tendency of some researchers to write as many papers as possible from the planned analyses of a study to increase the number of their publications—a strategy referred to as "salami slicing." Researchers performing secondary analyses should always identify the original source of data and the previous publications emerging from the analysis of that data set. Aaronson (1994) pointed out the problem with this practice.

> Fundamentally, each paper written from the same study or the same dataset must make a distinct and significant scientific contribution. Presumably this is not only the major overriding criterion used by reviewers, but also the author's intent when writing the paper. When a particular paper is one of several from the same study, project, or dataset, the author's responsibility to identify the source of the data is that much greater. To lead readers to think a report is from a new study or a different dataset than that used in the authors' previous work is dishonest, particularly if the second paper purports to substantiate findings of the first one.... Apart from the overriding concern about "milking the data," the most common objection to multiple articles from a single study is concern about the age of the data.... Concerns in nursing about the number of papers generated from a single study may reflect the emerging status of secondary analysis as a legitimate approach to nursing research....
>
> All of the reasons offered for using secondary analysis—answering new questions with existing data, applying new methods to answer old questions, the real exigencies of cost and feasibility—serve equally to justify the continued use of data collected years ago, by the original investigator of a large project, as well as by others.... The issue remains one of sound science. The question that must be asked is: Does this particular paper make a meaningful and distinct contribution to the scientific literature? (Aaronson, 1994, pp. 61–62)

An example of secondary analysis is Koci and Strickland's (2007) study of the relationship of adolescent physical and sexual abuse with premenstrual syndrome (PMS) in adulthood. Data analyzed from this study were from a longitudinal study of a community sample of 568 women in a database called Nursing Assessment of PMS: Neurometric Indices. A study such as this yields an enormous amount of data that is not examined in the original study. The authors used this large data set to examine another question posed for a secondary analysis. The authors found that "a history of both adolescent physical abuse and sexual abuse was significantly associated with PMS in adulthood. Women with a history of adolescent physical and sexual abuse had significantly more severe PMS patterns with more dysphoria than women without abuse."

Methodological Designs

Methodological designs are used to develop the validity and reliability of instruments to measure constructs used as variables in research. The process is lengthy and complex. The average length of researcher time required to develop a research tool to the point of appropriate use in a study is 5 years. An example of a methodological study is the Reyes, Meininger, Liehr, Chan, and Mueller (2003) study of a scale, funded by the National Institute of Nursing Research (NINR). The study measured anger in adolescents, and the authors explained their study as follows.

> *Background:* The State-Trait Anger Expression Inventory (STAXI), a self-report questionnaire, is designed to measure the experience and expression of anger. Reliability and validity of the STAXI have been well established among African and European Americans aged 13 years and older. However, little is known of the use of this instrument among adolescents younger than 13 years and Hispanic American adolescents.
>
> *Objectives:* Objectives were (a) to test ethnic, sex, and age group differences in STAXI scores in a sample of 11- to 16-year-old African, Hispanic, and European American adolescents; and (b) to assess the psychometric properties of the STAXI among these same adolescents with special emphasis on Hispanic youths, for whom no data are available.
>
> *Methods:* A cross-sectional design was used with stratified quota sampling techniques. Participants ($N = 394$) were African, Hispanic, and European Americans aged 11–16 years and were drawn from one public middle school and two public high schools in Houston, Texas.
>
> *Results:* Internal consistency reliability for the anger scales (STAXI) ranged from 0.61 (anger-in) to 0.91 (state-anger) for the older Hispanic Americans (aged 14–16). No notable differences were seen among the three ethnic groups in regards to internal consistency. Results of factor analyses of the five anger scales were similar to those reported originally by the scale author. Ethnicity and age had statistically significant main effects on the anger scales, and there was only one interaction.
>
> *Discussion:* The use of the STAXI among a tri-ethnic adolescent population is warranted. The anger-in scale may be less reliable, especially among younger adolescents. (Reyes et al., 2003, p. 2; full-text article available in CINAHL)

ALGORITHMS FOR SELECTING RESEARCH DESIGNS

To select a research design, the investigator must follow paths of logical reasoning. You need a calculating mind to explore all the possible consequences of using a particular design in a study. In some ways, selecting a design is like thinking through the moves in a chess game. You must carefully think through the consequences of each option. The research design organizes all the components of the study in a way that is most likely to lead to valid answers to the questions that have been posed.

To help you select the most appropriate design, a series of decision trees is provided here. The first decision tree (Figure 11-26) will help you to identify the type of study you plan to conduct. The next four decision trees (Figures 11-27 through 11-30) will assist you in selecting specific designs for each of the types of studies. Not all of the designs included in these tables have been reviewed in this chapter. Selecting a design is not a rigid, rule-guided task. As a researcher, you have considerable flexibility in choosing a design. The pathways within the decision trees are not absolute and are to be used as guides.

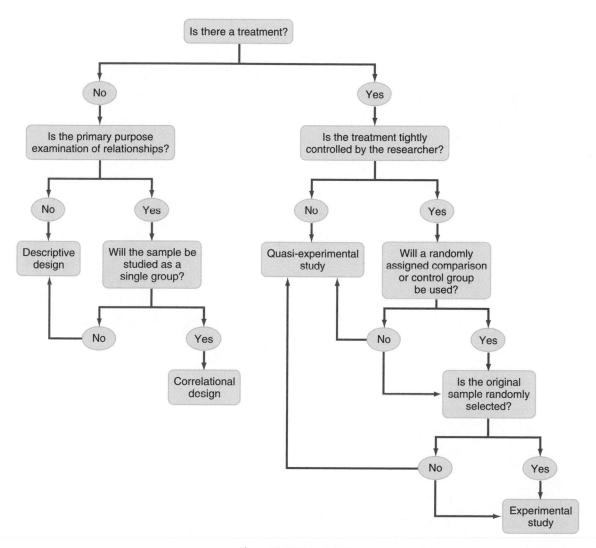

Figure **11-26** Type of study.

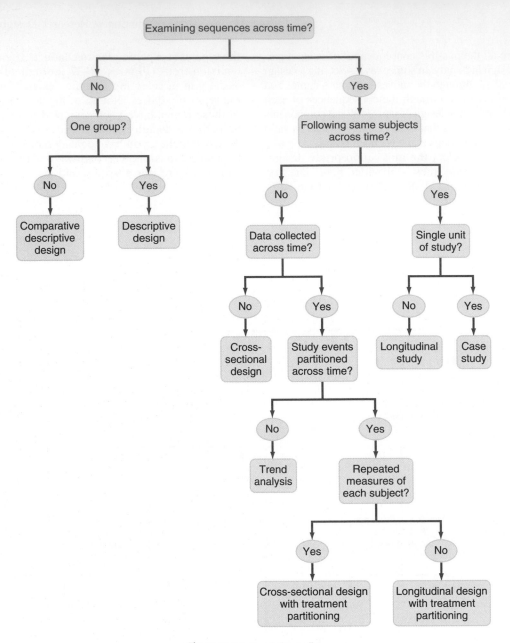

Figure **11-27 Descriptive studies.**

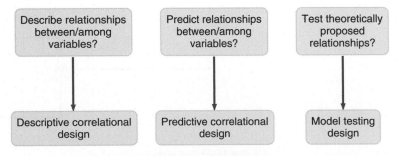

Figure **11-28 Correlational studies.**

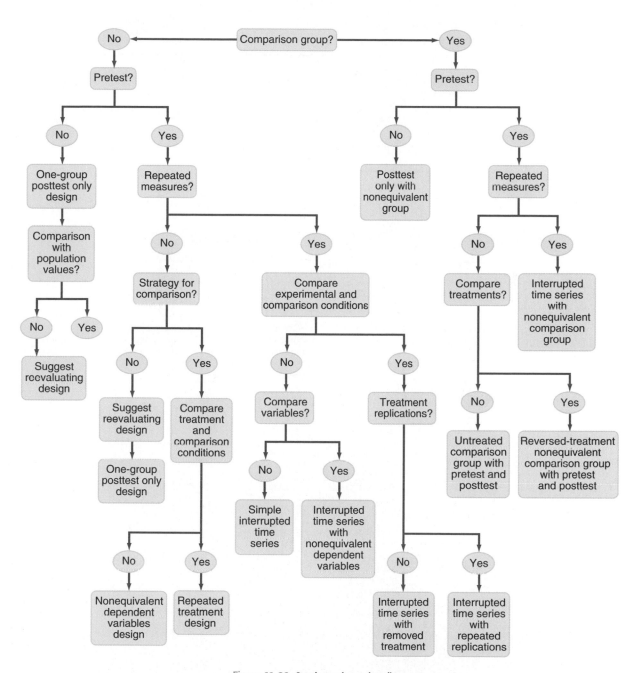

Figure **11-29** Quasi-experimental studies.

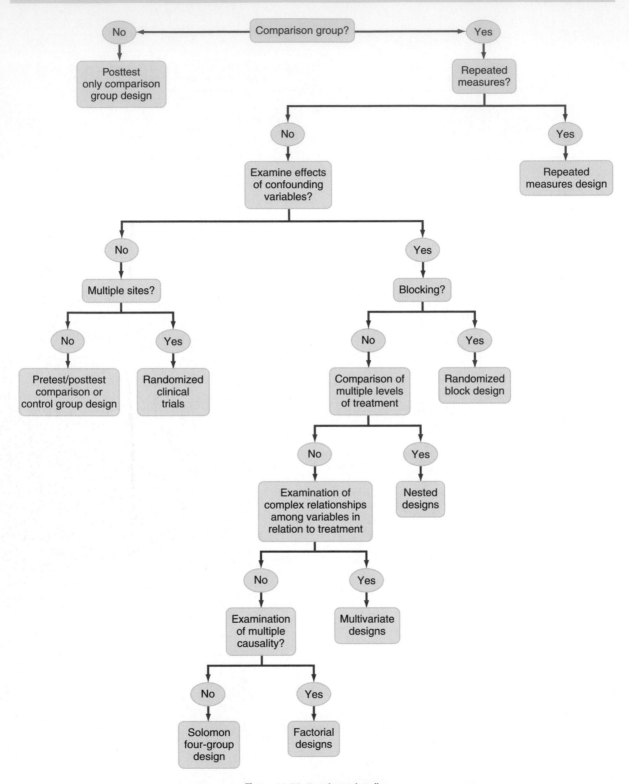

Figure **11-30** Experimental studies.

SUMMARY

- Researchers have developed designs to meet unique research needs as they emerge.
- At present, nursing research is using designs developed by other disciplines, which are a useful starting point, but nurse scientists must go beyond them to develop designs that will more appropriately meet the needs of the knowledge base in nursing.
- Descriptive studies are designed to gain more information about variables within a particular field of study.
- Correlational studies examine relationships between variables.
- Quasi-experimental and experimental designs examine causality. The power of the design to accomplish this purpose depends on the degree to which the actual effects of the experimental treatment (the independent variable) can be detected by measuring the dependent variable.
- Obtaining an understanding of the true effects of an experimental treatment requires action to control threats to the validity of the findings.
- Threats to validity are controlled through selection of subjects, manipulation of the treatment, and reliable measurement of variables.
- Criteria for defining a study as a clinical trial as opposed to referring to it as an experimental study have not been clarified in the nursing literature.
- Studying primary prevention and health promotion involves applying a treatment of primary prevention (the cause) and then attempting to measure the effect (an event that does not occur if the treatment was effective).
- Secondary analysis is the study of data previously collected in another study.
- Methodological studies are designed to develop the validity and reliability of instruments to measure constructs used as variables in research.
- Algorithms for design identification and selection are provided in Figures 11-27 to 11-30.

REFERENCES

Aaronson, L. S. (1994). Milking data or meeting commitments: How many papers from one study? *Nursing Research, 43*(1), 60–62.

Baird, C. L., & Sands, L. P. (2006). Effect of guided imagery with relaxation on health-related quality of life in older women with osteoarthritis. *Research in Nursing & Health, 29*(5), 442–451.

Barlow, D. H., & Hersen, M. (1984). *Single case experimental designs: Strategies for studying behavior change.* New York: Pergamon.

Barnard, K. E., Magyary, D. L., Booth, C. L., & Eyres, S. J. (1987). Longitudinal designs: Considerations and applications to nursing research. *Recent Advances in Nursing, 17*, 37–64.

Barnes-McDowell, B. M. (1997). *Home apnea monitoring: Family functioning, concerns, and coping.* Unpublished doctoral dissertation, University of South Carolina.

Bassoli, S. R. B., & Guimaraes, H. C. Q. (2004). Wound care: Nursing activities in the assistance practice, compared to the activities proposed by the Nursing Intervention Classification (NIC) [Portuguese]. Revista *Paulista De Enfermagem, 23*(2), 108–113.

Beck, S. L. (1989). The crossover design in clinical nursing research. *Nursing Research, 38*(5), 291–293.

Blissitt, P. A., Roberts, S., Hinkle, J. L., & Kopp, E. M. (2003). Defining neuroscience nursing practice: The 2001 role delineation study. *Journal of Neuroscience Nursing, 25*(1), 8–15.

Boomsma, J., Dassen, T., Dingemans, C., & van den Heuvel, W. (1999). Nursing interventions in crisis-oriented and long-term psychiatric home care. *Scandinavian Journal of Caring Science, 13*(1), 41–48.

Bowles, K. H., & Naylor, M. D. (1996). Nursing intervention classification systems. *Journal of Nursing Scholarship, 28*(4), 303–308.

Brooten, D., Kumar, S., Brown, L. P., Butts, P., Finkler, S. A., Bakewell-Sachs, S., et al. (1986). A randomized clinical trial of early hospital discharge and home follow-up of very-low-birth-weight infants. *New England Journal of Medicine, 315*(15), 934–939.

Burgess, A. W., Lerner, D. J., D'Agostino, R. B., Vokonas, P. S., Hartman, C. R., & Gaccione, P. (1987). A randomized control trial of cardiac rehabilitation. *Social Science and Medicine, 24*(4), 359–370.

Campbell, D. T., & Stanley, J. C. (1963). *Experimental and quasi-experimental designs for research.* Chicago: Rand McNally.

Chan, H. Y., Lu, R. B., Tseng, C. L., & Chous, K. R. (2003). Effectiveness of the anger-control program in reducing anger expression in patients with schizophrenia. *Archives of Psychiatric Nursing, 17*(2), 88–95.

Chang, Y. J., Lin, C. P., Lin, Y. J., & Lin, C. H. (2007). Effects of single-hole and cross-cut nipple units on feeding efficiency and physiological parameters in premature infants. *Journal of Nursing Research, 15*(3), 215–223.

Clarke, D. A. (1999). Advancing my health care practice in aromatherapy. *Australian Journal of Holistic Nursing, 6*(1), 32–38.

Coenen, A., Weis, D. M., Schank, M. J., & Matheus, R. (1999). Describing parish nurse practice using the Nursing Minimum Data Set. *Public Health Nursing, 16*(6), 412–416.

Cook, T. D., & Campbell, D. T. (1979). *Quasi-experimentation: Design and analysis issues for field settings.* Chicago: Rand McNally.

Corbett, C. L. F. (1998). *Predictors and outcomes of home care for diabetics.* Unpublished doctoral dissertation, Loyola University of Chicago.

Costanzo, C., Walker, S. M., Yates, B. C., McCabe, B., & Berg, K. (2006). Physical activity counseling for older women. *Western Journal of Nursing Research, 28*(7), 786–810.

Côté, J. K., & Pepler, C. (2002). A randomized trial of a cognitive coping intervention for acutely ill HIV-positive men. *Nursing Research, 51*(4), 237–244.

Cramer, M. E., Chen, L. W., Roberts, S., & Clute, D. (2007). Evaluating the social and economic impact of community-based prentatal care. *Public Health Nursing, 24*(4), 329–336.

Crombie, I. K., & Davies, H. T. O. (1996). *Research in health care: Design, conduct and interpretation of health services research.* New York: Wiley.

Cummings, G. G., Estabrooks, C. A., Midodzi, W. K., Wallin, L., & Hayduk, L. (2007). Influence of organizational characteristics and context on research utilization. *Nursing Research, 56*(4 Suppl), S24–S39.

Davis, K. A. (1995). AIDS nursing care and standardized nursing language: An application of the nursing intervention classification. *Journal of the Association of Nurses in AIDS Care, 6*(6), 37–44.

deMoissac, D., & Jensen, L. (1998). Changing IV administration sets: Is 48 versus 24 hours safe for neutropenic patients with cancer? *Oncology Nursing Forum, 25*(5), 907–913.

Dowd, T., Withers, E., Hackwood, J., & Shuter, P. (2007). An Australian pilot study of a parent-child interaction program: "You make the difference." *Neonatal, Paediatric & Child Health Nursing, 10* (1), 13–19.

Egan, E. C., Snyder, M., & Burns, K. R. (1992). Intervention studies in nursing: Is the effect due to the independent variable? *Nursing Outlook, 40*(4), 187–190.

Elwood, J. M. (1998). *Critical appraisal of epidemiological studies and clinical trials.* New York: Oxford University Press.

Fetter, M. S., Fettham, S. L., D'Apolito, K., Chaze, B. A., Fink, A., Frink, B. B., et al. (1989). Randomized clinical trials: Issues for researchers. *Nursing Research, 38*(2), 117–120.

Figoski, M. R., & Downey, J. (2006). Perspectives in continuity of care. Facility charging and Nursing Intervention Classification (NIC): The new dynamic duo. *Nursing Economics, 24*(2), 102–115.

Fisher, R. A. (1935). *The design of experiments.* New York: Hafner.

Flaskerud, J. H. & Winslow, B. J. (1998). Conceptualizing vulnerable populations health-related research. *Nursing Research, 47*(2), 69-78.

Gilliss, C. L., & Kulkin, I. L. (1991). Monitoring nursing interventions and data collection in a randomized clinical trial. *Western Journal of Nursing Research, 13*(3), 416–422.

Gleit, C., & Graham, B. (1989). Secondary data analysis: A valuable resource. *Nursing Research,* 38(6), 380–381.

González-Gancedo, J., & Fernández García, D. (2007). Care plan in a patient with spina bifida. Case report [Spanish]. *Enfermeria Clinica, 17*(2), 90–95.

Gray, M. (1998). Introducing single case study research design: An overview. *Nurse Researcher, 5*(4), 15–24.

Griebel, B., Wewers, M. E., & Baker, C. A. (1998). The effectiveness of a nurse-managed minimal smoking-cessation intervention among hospitalized patients with cancer. *Oncology Nursing Forum, 25*(5), 897–902.

Guimarães, H. C. Q. (2003). Fluid management: a nursing intervention for the patient with fluid volume excess [Portuguese]. *Barros ALB Revista Latino-Americana de Enfermagem, 11*(6), 734–741.

Guinan, M., McGuckin, M., & Ali, Y. (2002). The effect of a comprehensive handwashing program on absenteeism in elementary schools. *American Journal of Infection Control, 30*(4), 217–220.

Hartley, L. A. (2003). *Longitudinal analysis of access to health care, use of preventive health services, and practice of health-related behaviors of Appalachian and non-Appalachian adults in Kentucky.* Unpublished doctoral dissertation, University of Kentucky.

Henry, S. B., & Meade, C. N. (1997). Nursing classification systems: Necessary but not sufficient for representing "what nurses do" for inclusion in computer-based patient record systems. *Journal of the American Medical Informatics Association, 4*(3), 222–322.

Hjelm-Karlsson, K. (1991). Using the biased coin design for randomization in health care research. *Western Journal of Nursing Research, 13*(2), 284–288.

Huang, C. Y., Sousa, V. D., Chen, H. F., Tu, S. Y., Chang, C. J., & Pan, I. J. (2007). Stressors, depressive symptoms, and learned resourcefulness among Taiwanese adults with diabetes mellitus. *Research & Theory for Nursing Practice, 21*(2), 83–97.

Ippoliti, C., & Neumann, J. (1998). Octreotide in the management of diarrhea induced by graft versus host disease. *Oncology Nursing Forum, 25*(5), 873–878.

Jones, E. D. (2003). Reminiscence therapy for older women with depression: Effects of Nursing Intervention Classification in assisted-living long-term care. *Journal of Gerontological Nursing, 29*(7), 26–33.

Jones-Baucke, D. L. (1997). *A qualitative study of the implementation of a system to increase nurses' use of standardized nursing languages.* Unpublished doctoral dissertation, University of Washington.

Kacel, B., Millar, M., & Norris, D. (2005). Measurement of nurse practitioner job satisfaction in a Midwestern state. *Journal of the American Academy of Nurse Practitioners, 17* (1), 27–32

Kirby, A. E. (1996). *Classification of advanced practice nursing functions using the Nursing Intervention Classification taxonomy.* Unpublished doctoral dissertation, University of Pennsylvania.

Kirchhoff, K. T., & Dille, C. A. (1994). Issues in intervention research: Maintaining integrity. *Applied Nursing Research, 7*(1), 32–46.

Kline, G. A., & Edwards, A. (2007). Antepartum and intrapartum insulin management of type 1 and type 2 diabetic women: Impact on clinically significant neonatal hypoglycemia. *Diabetes Research & Clinical Practice, 7*(22), 223–230.

Koci, A., & Strickland, O. (2007). Relationship of adolescent physical and sexual abuse to perimenstrual symptoms (PMS) in adulthood. *Issues in Mental Health Nursing, 28*(1), 75–87.

Koniak-Griffin, D., Verzemnicks, I. L., Anderson, N. L. R., Brecht, M., Lesser, J., Kim, S., et al. (2003). Nurse visitation for adolescent mothers: Two-year infant health and maternal outcomes. *Nursing Research, 52*(2), 127–136.

Krichbaum, K. (2007). GAPN Postacute care coordination improves hip fracture outcomes. *Western Journal of Nursing Research, 29*(5), 523–544.

Lewandowski, W., Good, M., & Draucker, C. B. (2005). Changes in the meaning of pain with the use of guided imagery. *Pain Management Nursing, 6*(2), 58–67.

Malm, D., Karlsson, J. E., & Fridlund, B. (2007). Effects of a self-care program on the health-related quality of life of pacemaker patients: A nursing intervention study. *Canadian Journal of Cardiovascular Nursing, 17*(1), 15–26.

Martins, I. (2005). Nursing interventions for the nursing diagnosis ineffective airway clearance [sic] [Portuguese]. *Acta Paulista de Enfermagem, 18*(2), 143–149.

Mason-Hawkes, J., & Holm, K. (1989). Causal modeling: a comparison of path analysis and LISREL. *Nursing Research, 38*(5), 312–314.

McBride, K. L., White, C. L., Sourial, R., & Mayo, N. (2004). Postdischarge nursing interventions for stroke survivors and their families. *Journal of Advanced Nursing, 47*(2), 192–200.

McCain, L. J., & McCleary, R. (1979). The statistical analysis of the simple interrupted time-series quasi-experiment. In T. D. Cook & D. T. Campbell (Eds.), *Quasi-experimentation: Design and analysis issues for field settings* (pp. 233–293). Chicago: Rand McNally.

McConnell, A. (1976). Effect of knowledge of results on attitude formed toward a motor learning task. *Research Quarterly, 47*(3), 394–399.

McCorkle, R., & Young, K. (1978). Development of a symptom distress scale. *Cancer Nursing, 1*(5), 373–378.

Meghani, S. H., & Keane, A. (2007). Preference for analgesic treatment for cancer pain among African Americans. *Journal of Pain & Symptom Management, 34*(2), 136–147.

Meinert, C. L., & Tonascia, S. (1986). *Clinical trials: Design, conduct, and analysis.* New York: Oxford University Press.

Micek, W. T., Berry, L., Gilski, D., Kallenbach, A., Link, D., & Scharer, K. (1996). Patient outcomes: The link between nursing diagnoses and interventions. *Journal of Nursing Administration, 26*(11), 29–35.

Mishel, M. H., Germino, B. B., Belyea, M., Stewart, J. L., Bailey, D. E. Jr., Mohler, J, et al. (2003). Moderators of an uncertainty management intervention: for men with localized prostate cancer. *Nursing Research, 52*(2), 89–97.

Mrayyan, M. (2003). Nurse autonomy, nurse job satisfaction and client satisfaction with nursing care: Their place in nursing data sets. *Canadian Journal of Nursing Leadership, 16*(2), 74–82.

Murray, D. M. (1998). *Design and analysis of group-randomized trials.* New York: Oxford University Press.

O'Connor, N. A., Kershaw, T., & Hameister, A. D. (2001). Documenting patterns of nursing interventions using cluster analysis. *Journal of Nursing Measurement, 9*(1), 73–90.

Ottenbacher, K. (1992). Impact of random assignment on study outcome: An empirical examination. *Controlled Clinical Trials, 13*(1), 50–61.

Pallarés, M. A. (2004). Influence of transcultural factors on immigrants populations' needs and nursing diagnosis [Spanish]. *Cultura de los Cuidados, 8*(16), 62–67.

Phibbs, C. S., Holty, J. E., Goldstein, M. K., Garber, A. M., Wang, Y., Feussner, J. R., et al. (2006). The effect of geriatrics evaluation and management on nursing home use and health care costs: Results from a randomized trial. *Medical Care, 44*(1), 91–95.

Piantadosi, S. (1997). *Clinical trials: A methodologic perspective.* New York: Wiley.

Pocock, S. J. (1996). *Clinical trials: A practical approach.* New York: Wiley.

Rawl, S. M., Easton, K. L., Kwiatkowski, S., Zemen, D., & Burczyk, B. (1998). Effectiveness of a nurse-managed follow-up program for rehabilitation patients after discharge. *Rehabilitation Nursing, 23*(4), 204–209.

Redes, S., & Lunney, M. (1997). Validation by school nurses of the Nursing Intervention Classification for computer software. *Computers in Nursing, 15*(6), 333–338.

Reichardt, C. S. (1979). The statistical analysis of data from nonequivalent group designs. In T. D. Cook & D. T. Campbell (Eds.), *Quasi-experimentation: Design and analysis issues for field settings* (pp. 147–206). Chicago: Rand McNally.

Reyes, L. R., Meininger, J. C., Liehr, P., Chan, W., & Mueller, W. H. (2003). Anger in adolescents: Sex, ethnicity, age differences, and psychometric properties. *Nursing Research, 52*(1), 2–11.

Rodehorst, T. K. C., Wilhelm, S. L., & Stepans, M. B. (2006). Screen for asthma: Results from a rural cohort. *Issues in Comprehensive Pediatric Nursing, 29*(4), 205–224.

Salvador, P. T. (2006). Development of an oral care guide for patients undergoing autologous stem cell transplantation. *Canadian Oncology Nursing Journal, 16*(1), 18–20.

Sandelowski, M. (1996). One is the liveliest number: The case orientation of qualitative research. *Research in Nursing & Health, 19*(6), 525–529.

Sawada, A., Porter, S. E., Kayama, M., Setoya, N., & Miyamato, Y. (2006). Nursing care delivery in Japanese psychiatric units. *British Journal of Nursing, 15*(17), 920–925.

Schneider, S. M. (1998). Effects of virtual reality on symptom distress in children receiving cancer chemotherapy. *Dissertation Abstracts International: Section B: The Sciences & Engineering, 59*(5-B), 2126.

Sidani, S., & Braden, C. J. (1998). *Evaluating nursing interventions: A theory-driven approach.* Thousand Oaks, CA: Sage.

Sidani, S., Doran, D., Porter, H., LeFort, S., O'Brien-Pallas, L. L., Zahn, C., et al. (2007). Outcomes of nurse practitioners in acute care: An exploration. *Internet Journal of Advanced Nursing Practice, 8*(1), 15.

Solari-Twadell, P. A. (2004). *The differentiation of the ministry of parish nursing practice within congregations.* Unpublished doctoral dissertation, Loyola University of Chicago.

Spector, P. E. (1981). *Research designs.* Beverly Hills, CA: Sage.

Spielberger, C. D., Edwards, C. D., Lushene, R. E. et al. (1978). *Manual for the State-Trait Anxiety Inventory for Children.* Palo Alto, CA: Consulting Psychologist Press.

Sterling, Y. M., & McNally, J. A. (1992). Single-subject research for nursing practice. *Clinical Nurse Specialist, 6*(1), 21–26.

Stewart, B. J., & Archbold, P. G. (1992). Nursing intervention studies require outcome measures that are sensitive to change, part 1. *Research in Nursing & Health, 15*(6), 477–481.

Stewart, B. J., & Archbold, P. G. (1993). Nursing intervention studies require outcome measures that are sensitive to change, part 2. *Research in Nursing & Health, 16*(1), 77–81.

Stout, R. L., Wirtz, P. W., Carbonari, J. P., & Del Boca, F. K. (1994). Ensuring balanced distribution of prognostic factors in treatment outcome research. *Journal of Studies in Alcoholism, 12*(Suppl.), 70–75.

Tripp-Reimer, T., Woodworth, G., McCloskey, J. C., Bulechek, G. (1996). The dimensional structure of nursing interventions. *Nursing Research, 45*(1), 10–17.

Turner, J. G., Clark, A. J., Gauthier, D. K., & Williams, M. (1998). The effect of therapeutic touch on pain and anxiety in burn patients. *Journal of Advanced Nursing, 28*(1), 10–20.

Tyzenhouse, P. S. (1981). Technical notes: The nursing clinical trial. *Western Journal of Nursing Research, 3*(1), 102–109.

U.S. Department of Health and Human Services . (1968). *The Framingham study: An epidemiological investigation of cardiovascular disease* (USDHHS Publication No. RC667F813). Bethesda, MD: Author.

U.S. Department of Health and Human Services. (2000). *Healthy People 2010: With Understanding and Improving Health and Objectives for Improving Health.* Retrieved May 6, 2008, from www.healthypeople.gov/Publications/.

Villanueva, N. E., Thompson, H. J., Macpherson, B. C., Meunier, K. E., & Hilton, E. (2006). The Neuroscience Nursing 2005 Role Delineation Study: Implications for certification. *Journal of Neuroscience Nursing, 38*(6), 403–408.

von Krogh, G., Dale, C., & Naden, D. (2005). A framework for integrating NANDA, NIC, and NOC terminology in electronic patient records. *Journal of Nursing Scholarship, 37*(3), 275–281.

Warrington, D., Cholowski, K., & Peters, D. (2003). Effectiveness of home-based cardiac rehabilitation for special needs patients. *Journal of Advanced Nursing, 41*(2), 121–129.

Weis, D., & Schank, M. J. (2000). Use of a taxonomy to describe parish nursing practice with older adults. *Geriatric Nursing, 21*(3), 125–131.

Weis, D. M., Schank, M. J., Coenen, A., & Matheus, R. (2002). Parish nurse practice with client aggregates. *Journal of Community Health Nursing, 19*(2), 105–113.

Whitehead, J. (1992). *The design and analysis of sequential clinical trials.* New York: Ellis Horwood.

Winters, J. (2002). Primary prevention of agricultural injuries: Use of standardized nursing diagnosis, interventions, and outcomes. *AAOHN Journal, 50*(6), 271–274.

Wooding, W. M. (1994). *Planning pharmaceutical clinical trials: Basic statistical principles.* New York: Wiley.

Woods, D. Y., & Dimond, M. (2002). The effect of therapeutic touch on agitated behavior and cortisol in persons with Alzheimer's disease. *Biological Research for Nursing, 4*(2), 104–114.

Wu, S. H., & Thompson, C. B. (2001). Evaluation of the Nursing Intervention Classification for use by flight nurses. *Air Medical Journal, 20*(1), 33–37.

Yin, R. (1984). *Applied social research methods series: Vol. 5. Case study research: Design and methods.* Beverly Hills, CA: Sage.

Yoon, S. L., & Black, S. (2006). Comprehensive, integrative management of pain for patients with sickle-cell disease. *Journal of Alternative & Complementary Medicine, 12*(10), 995–1001.

CHAPTER 12
Outcomes Research

A new paradigm for research, outcomes research, has been developing momentum in health care research. Outcomes research focuses on the end results of patient care. To explain the end results, one must also understand the processes used to provide patient care. However, having a focused topic of research outcomes is not sufficient to define outcomes research as a new paradigm. A new paradigm implies new theories, new questions, new approaches to studying the topics of interest, and new methodologies. It suggests a revolution—and in a way, we have a revolution! The strategies used in outcomes research do, to some extent, depart from the accepted scientific methodology for health care research, and they incorporate evaluation methods, epidemiology, and economic theory. Building a scientific base using such methods is controversial. However, the findings of outcome studies are having a powerful impact on the provision of health care and the development of health policy.

The momentum propelling outcomes research comes not from scholars but from policy makers, insurers, and the public. There is a growing demand that providers justify interventions and systems of care in terms of improved patient lives and that costs of care be considered in evaluating treatment outcomes. There has been a major shift in published nursing studies as the number of studies using traditional quantitative or qualitative methods is dwarfed by the number of outcomes studies.

This chapter describes the theoretical basis of outcomes research, provides a brief history of the emerging endeavors to examine outcomes, explains the importance of outcomes research designed to examine nursing practice, and highlights methodologies used in outcomes research. A broad base of literature from a variety of disciplines was used to develop the content for this chapter, in keeping with the multidisciplinary perspective of outcomes research.

THEORETICAL BASIS OF OUTCOMES RESEARCH

The theory on which outcomes research is based emerged from evaluation research (Structure-Process-Outcomes Framework). The theorist Avedis Donabedian (1976, 1978, 1980, 1982, 1987) proposed a theory of quality health care and the process of evaluating it. Quality is the overriding construct of the theory, although Donabedian never defined this concept (Mark, 1995). The cube shown in Figure 12-1 explains the elements of quality health care. The three dimensions of the cube are health, subjects of care, and providers of care. The concept *health* has many aspects; three are shown on the cube: physical-physiological function, psychological function, and social function. Donabedian (1987, p. 4) proposed that "the manner in which we conceive of health and of our responsibility for it, makes a fundamental difference to the concept of quality and, as a result, to the methods that we use to assess and assure the quality of care."

The concept subjects of care has two primary aspects: patient and person. A patient is defined as someone who has already gained access to some care, and a person as someone who may or may not have gained access to care. Each of these concepts is further categorized by the concepts *individual* and *aggregate*. Within patient, the aggregate is a caseload; within person, the aggregate is a target population or a community.

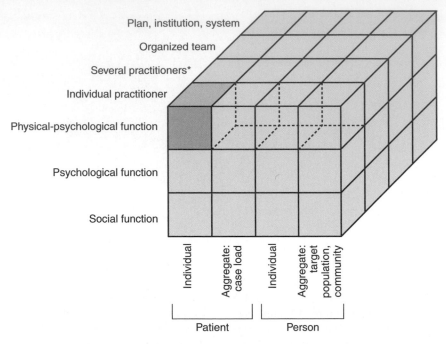

Plan, institution, system
Organized team
Several practitioners*
Individual practitioner

Physical-psychological function

Psychological function

Social function

Individual

Aggregate: case load

Individual

Aggregate: target population, community

Patient   Person

*Of the same profession or of different professions

Figure **12-1** Level and scope of concern as factors in the definition of quality.

The concept **providers of care** shows levels of aggregation and organization of providers. The first level is the individual practitioner. At this level, no consideration is given to anyone else who might be involved in the subject's care, whether individual or aggregate. As the levels progress, providers of care include several practitioners, who might be of the same profession or different professions and "who may be providing care concurrently, as individuals, or jointly, as a team" (Donabedian, 1987, p. 5). At higher levels of aggregation, the provider of care is institutions, programs, or the health care system as a whole.

Donabedian theorized that the dimensions of health are defined by the subjects of care, not by the providers of care, and are based on "what consumers expect, want, or are willing to accept" (Donabedian, 1987, p. 5). Thus, practitioners cannot unilaterally enlarge the definition of *health* to include other aspects; this action requires social consensus that "the scope of professional competence and responsibility embraces these areas of function" (Donabedian, 1987, p. 5). Donabedian indicated, however, that providers of care may make efforts to persuade subjects of care to expand their definition of the dimensions of health.

The **primordial cell** of Donabedian's framework is the physical-physiological function of the individual patient being cared for by the individual practitioner. Examining quality at this level is relatively simple. As one moves outward to include more of the cubical structure, the notions of quality and its assessment become increasingly difficult. When more than one practitioner is involved, both individual and joint contributions to quality must be evaluated. Concepts such as coordination and teamwork must be conceptually and operationally defined. When a person is the subject of care, an important attribute is access. When an aggregate is the subject of care, an important attribute is resource allocation. Access and resource allocation are interrelated, because they each define who gets care, the kind of care received, and how much care is received.

As more elements of the cube are included, conflicts among competing objectives emerge. The chief conflict is between the practitioner's responsibilities to the individual and to the aggregate. The practitioner is expected to have an exclusive commitment to each patient, yet the aggregate demands a commitment to the well-being of the society, leading to ethical dilemmas for the practitioner. Spending more time with an individual patient decreases access for other patients. Society's demand to reduce costs for an overall financing program may require raising costs to the individual. From an examination of the cube, logic would suggest that one could build up quality beginning with the primordial cell and increase by increments with the assumption that each increment would contribute positively to a greater total quality. However, the conflicts among competing objectives may preclude this possibility and lead instead to moral dilemmas.

Donabedian (1987) identified three objects to evaluate when appraising quality: structure, process, and outcome. A complete quality assessment program requires the simultaneous use of all three concepts and an examination of the relationships among the three. However, researchers have had little success in accomplishing this theoretical goal. Studies designed to examine all three concepts would require sufficiently large samples of various structures, each with the various processes being compared and large samples of subjects who have experienced the outcomes of those processes. The funding and the cooperation necessary to accomplish this goal are not yet available.

Evaluating Outcomes

The goal of outcomes research is the evaluation of outcomes as defined by Donabedian. However, this goal is not as simplistic as it might immediately appear. Donabedian's theory requires that identified outcomes be clearly linked with the process that caused the outcome. The researcher must define the process and justify the causal links with the selected outcomes. The identification of desirable outcomes requires dialogue between the subjects of care and the providers of care. Although the providers of care may delineate what is achievable, the subjects of care must clarify what is desirable. The outcomes must also be relevant to the goals of the health professionals, the health care system of which the professionals are a part, and society.

Outcomes are time dependent. Some outcomes may not be apparent for a long period after the process that is purported to cause them, whereas others may be apparent immediately. Some outcomes are temporary, and others are permanent. Thus, an appropriate time frame for determining the selected outcomes must be established.

A final obstacle to outcomes evaluation is attribution. This requires assigning the place and degree of responsibility for the outcomes observed. A particular outcome is often influenced by a multiplicity of factors. Health care represents only one dimension of a complex situation. Patient factors, such as compliance, predisposition to disease, age, propensity to use resources, high-risk behaviors (e.g., smoking), and lifestyle, must also be taken into account. Environmental factors such as air quality, public policies related to smoking, and occupational hazards must also be included. The responsibility for outcomes may be distributed among providers, patients, employers, insurers, and the community.

There is as yet little scientific basis for judging the precise relationship between each of these factors and the selected outcome. Many of the influencing factors may be outside the jurisdiction or influence of the health care system or of the providers within it. One solution to this problem of identifying relevant outcomes is to define a set of proximate outcomes specific to the condition for which care is being provided. Critical pathways and care maps may help the researcher to define at least proximate outcomes. However, proximate outcomes do not provide the degree of evidence of examining the desired outcomes.

Evaluating Process

Clinical management has been, for most health professionals, an art rather than a science. Understanding the process sufficiently to study it must begin with much careful reflection, dialogue, and observation. There are multiple components of clinical management, many of which have not yet been clearly defined or tested. Bergmark and Oscarsson (1991, pp. 139–140) suggested the following questions as important to consider in evaluating process: (1) "What constitutes the therapeutic agent?" (2) "Do practitioners actually do what they say they do?" and (3) "Do practitioners always know what they do?" Current outcomes studies use process variables that are easy to identify. Answers to questions such as those posed by Bergmark and Oscarsson are more difficult to define and will initially require observation, interviews, and the use of qualitative research methodologies. Three components of process that are of particular interest to Donabedian are standards of care, practice styles, and costs of care.

Standards of Care

A standard of care is a norm on which quality of care is judged. Clinical guidelines, critical paths, and care maps define standards of care for particular situations. According to Donabedian (1987), a practitioner has legitimate responsibility to apply available knowledge when managing a dysfunctional state. This management consists of (1) identifying or diagnosing the dysfunction, (2) deciding whether or not to intervene, (3) choosing intervention objectives, (4) selecting methods and techniques to achieve the objectives, and (5) skillfully executing the selected techniques.

Donabedian (1987) recommended the development of criteria to be used as a basis for judging the quality of care. These criteria may take the form of clinical guidelines or care maps based on prior validation that the care contributed to outcomes. The clinical guidelines published by the Agency for Healthcare Research and Quality (AHRQ) establish norms on which the validity of clinical management can be judged. These norms are now established through clinical practice guidelines. However, the core of the problem, from Donabedian's perspective, is clinical judgment. Analysis of the process of making diagnoses and therapeutic decisions is critical to the evaluation of the quality of care. The emergence of decision trees and algorithms is a response to Donabedian's concerns and provides a means of evaluating the adequacy of clinical judgments.

Practice Styles

The style of practice is another dimension of the process of care that influences quality; however, it is problematic to judge what constitutes "goodness" in style and to justify the decisions. Donabedian (1987) identified the following problem-solving styles: (1) routine approaches to care versus flexibility, (2) parsimony versus redundancy, (3) variations in degree of tolerance of uncertainty, (4) propensity to take risks, and (5) preference for type I errors versus type II errors. There are also diverse styles of interpersonal relationships. Westert and Groenewegen (1999, p. 174) suggest that differences in practice styles are a result of differences in opportunities, incentives, and influences. They suggest that "there is an (often implicit) idea of what should be done and how, and this shared (local) standard influences the choices made by individual practitioners. This alternative originates in the borders between economics and sociology and it can be characterized as the social production function approach." Table 12-1 lists studies of practice styles that include nurses.

Costs of Care

A third dimension of the examination of quality of care is cost. There are cost consequences to maintaining a specified level of quality of care. Providing more and better care is likely to increase costs but is also likely to produce savings. Economic benefits (savings) result from preventing illness, preventing complications, maintaining a higher quality of life, or prolonging productive life.

A related issue is who bears the costs of care. Some measures purported to reduce costs have instead simply shifted costs to another party. For example, a hospital might reduce its costs by discharging a particular type of patient early, but total costs could increase if the necessary community-based health care raised costs above those incurred by keeping the patient hospitalized longer. In this case, the third-party provider could experience higher costs. In many cases, the costs are shifted from the health care system to the family as out-of-pocket costs. Studies examining changes in costs of care should consider total costs, which include out-of-pocket costs. Table 12-2 provides examples of studies that examine the costs of care.

Evaluating Structure

Structures of care are the elements of organization and administration that guide the processes of care as well as provider and patient characteristics. The first step in evaluating structure is to identify and describe the elements of the structure. Various administration and management theories could be used to identify the elements of structure. These elements might be leadership, tolerance of innovativeness, organizational hierarchy, decision-making processes, distribution of power, financial management, and administrative decision-making processes.

The second step is to evaluate the impact of various structure elements on the process of care and on outcomes. This evaluation requires comparing different

TABLE 12-1	Studies of Practice Styles of Nurses	
Year	**Authors**	**Title**
1988	Bircumshaw & Chapman	A study to compare the practice style of graduate and non-graduate nurses and midwives: The pilot study
1996	Fullerton, Hollenbach, & Wingard	Practice styles: A comparison of obstetricians and nurse-midwives
1997	Howell-White	Choosing a birth attendant: The influence of a woman's childbirth definition
1999	Byers, Mays, & Mark	Provider satisfaction in Army primary care clinics
2001	Hueston & Lewis-Stevenson	Provider distribution and variations in statewide cesarean section rates
2001	Mark, Byers, & Mays	Primary care outcomes and provider practice styles

structures that provide the same processes of care. In evaluating structures, the unit of measure is the structure. The evaluation requires access to a sufficiently large sample of like structures with similar processes and outcomes, which can then be compared with a sample of another structure providing the same processes and outcomes. For example, in your research you might want to compare various structures providing primary health care, such as the private physician office, the health maintenance organization (HMO), the rural health clinic, the community-oriented primary care clinic, and the nurse-managed center. You might examine surgical care provided within the structures of a private outpatient surgical clinic, a private hospital, a county hospital, and a teaching hospital associated with a health science center. Within each of these examples, the focus of your study would be the impact of structure on processes of care and outcomes

of care. Table 12-3 provides some examples of studies of structures of care.

The federal government mandates nursing homes, home health care agencies, and hospitals to collect and report specifically measured quality variables to the government. This mandate was made because of considerable variation on the quality of care in these structures. Various government agencies analyze the quality of these structures so that they can adequately oversee the quality of care provided to the American public. These data are made available to the general public so that individuals can make their own determination of the quality of care provided by various nursing homes, home health care agencies, or hospitals. Researchers can also access these data for studies of the quality of various structures. To access these data on the Internet, do a search using the phrases *nursing home compare, home health compare,* or *hospital*

TABLE 12-2 Studies Examining Costs of Care

Year	Author	Title
2007	Griffiths, Edwards, Forbes, Harris, & Ritchie	Effectiveness of intermediate care in nursing-led in-patient units
2007	Bradley & Lindsay	Specialist epilepsy nurses for treating epilepsy
2007	Bowles & Baugh	Applying research evidence to optimize telehomecare
2006	Rubin et al.	Replicating the Hospital Elder Life Program in a community hospital and demonstrating effectiveness using quality improvement methodology
2006	Phibbs et al.	The effect of geriatrics evaluation and management on nursing home use and health care costs: Results from a randomized trial
2005	Harris, Richardson, Griffiths, Hallett, Wilson-Barnett	Economic evaluation of a nursing-led inpatient unit: The impact of findings on management decisions of service utility and sustainability
2005	McIsaac	Managing wound care outcomes
2004	Leeper	Nursing outcomes: Percutaneous coronary interventions
2004	Altimier, Eichel, Warner, Tedeschi, & Brown	Developmental care: Changing the NICU physically and behaviorally to promote patient outcomes and contain costs
2004	Challis et al.	The value of specialist clinical assessment of older people prior to entry to care homes
2003	Ahrens, Yancey, & Kollef	Improving family communications at the end of life: Implications for length of stay in the intensive care unit and resource use
2002	Brooten et al.	Lessons learned from testing the quality cost model of advanced practice nursing (APN) transitional care
1999	Kay	Targeting cost containment efforts in Massachusetts nursing homes.
1997	Chisholm, Knapp, Astin, Audini, & Lelliott	The mental health residential care study: The "hidden costs" of provision
1994	Varricchio	Human and indirect costs of home care... for cancer patients
1994	Ward & Brown	Labor and cost in AIDS family caregiving
1992	Harper	Care and cost effectiveness of the clinical care coordinator/patient care associate nursing case management model
1991	Haggerty, Stockdale-Woolley, & Nair	Respi-Care: An innovative home care program for the patient with chronic obstructive pulmonary disease

TABLE 12-3 ▐▐ Studies Examining Various Aspects of Structure

Year	Author	Title
2007	Castle & Engberg	The influence of staffing characteristics on quality of care in nursing homes
2007	Ward, Severs, Dean, & Brooks	Care home versus hospital and own home environments for rehabilitation of older people
2007	Goldman, Vittinghoff, & Dudley	Quality of care in hospitals with a high percent of Medicaid patients
2006	Mor	Defining and measuring quality outcomes in long-term care
2006	Cólon-Emeric et al.	Patterns of medical and nursing staff communication in nursing homes: Implications and insights from complexity science
2005	Wilson et al.	Quality of HIV care provided by nurse practitioners, physician assistants, and physicians
2004	Schnelle et al.	Relationship of nursing home staffing to quality of care
2004	Morgan, Stewart, D'Arcy, & Werezak	Evaluating rural nursing home environments: Dementia special care units versus integrated facilities

compare. In addition to being able to select a specific hospital, nursing home, or home health care agency, you will be able to access considerable general information about quality related to these structures of health care. Do a search for Magnet Hospitals at the American Nurses Credentialing Center at www.nursecredentialing.org/magnet to check for the status of a particular hospital.

FEDERAL GOVERNMENT INVOLVEMENT IN OUTCOMES RESEARCH

Agency for Health Services Research

Nurses participated in the initial federal involvement in studying the quality of health care. In 1959, two National Institutes of Health study sections, the Hospital and Medical Facilities Study Section and the Nursing Study Section, met to discuss concerns about the adequacy and appropriateness of medical care, patient care, and hospital and medical facilities. As a result of their dialogue, a Health Services Research Study Section was initiated. This study section eventually became the Agency for Health Services Research (AHSR). With small amounts of funding from Congress, the AHSR continued to study the effectiveness of health services, primarily supporting the research of economists, epidemiologists, and health policy analysts (White, 1993). Two projects that were to have the greatest impact were small area analyses and the Medical Outcomes Study (MOS).

Small Area Analyses

In the 1970s, an epidemiologist named Wennberg began a series of studies examining small area variations in medical practice across towns and counties.

He found a wide variation in the tonsillectomy rate from one town to another in the New England area that could not be explained by differences such as health status, insurance, and demographics. These findings were replicated for a variety of medical procedures. Investigators began a search for the underlying causes of the variation and their implications for health status (O'Connor, Plume, & Wennberg, 1993; Wennberg, Barry, Fowler, & Mulley, 1993). Studies also revealed that many procedures, such as coronary artery bypass, were being performed on patients who did not have appropriate clinical indications for such surgery (Power, Tunis, & Wagner, 1994).

Medical Outcomes Study

The Medical Outcomes Study (MOS) was the first large-scale study to examine factors influencing patient outcomes. The study was designed to identify elements of physician care associated with favorable patient outcomes. Figure 12-2 shows the conceptual framework for the MOS. MOS failed to control for the effects of nursing interventions, staffing patterns, and nursing practice delivery models on medical outcomes. Coordination of care, counseling, and referral activities more commonly performed by nurses than physicians, were considered in the MOS to be components of medical practice. The abstract of the MOS is provided below:

The Medical Outcomes Study was designed to (1) determine whether variations in patient outcomes are explained by differences in system of care, clinician specialty, and clinicians' technical and interpersonal styles and (2) develop more practical tools for the routine monitoring of patient outcomes in medical practice. Outcomes included clinical end points; physical,

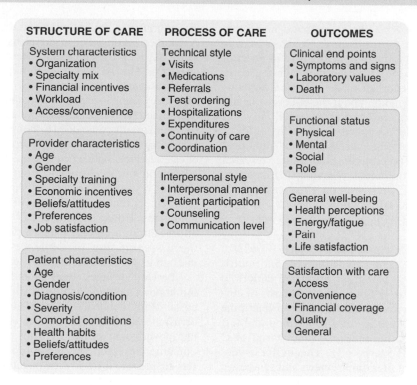

Figure **12-2** The MOS conceptual framework.

social, and role functioning in everyday living; patients' perceptions of their general health and well-being; and satisfaction with treatment. Populations of clinicians (n = 523) were randomly sampled from different health care settings in Boston, MA; Chicago, IL; and Los Angeles, CA. In the cross-sectional study, adult patients (n = 22,462) evaluated their health status and treatment. A sample of these patients (n = 2349) with diabetes, hypertension, coronary heart disease, and/or depression were selected for the longitudinal study. Their hospitalizations and other treatments were monitored and they periodically reported outcomes of care. At the beginning and end of the longitudinal study, Medical Outcomes Study staff performed physical examinations and laboratory tests. Results were reported serially, primarily in The Journal of the American Medical Association. (Tarlov et al., 1989)

Agency for Health Care Policy and Research

In 1989, Congress created the Agency for Health Care Policy and Research (AHCPR) to replace the AHSR. Congress also established the National Advisory Council for Health Care Policy, Research, and Evaluation. The council was required to include (1) health care researchers; (2) health professionals (specifically including nurses); (3) individuals from business, law, ethics, economics, and public policy; and (4) individuals representing the interests of consumers. The budget for AHCPR increased to $1.9 million in 1988, $5.9 million in 1989, and $37.5 million in 1990. Its budget request for 2008 was $329,564,000. This agency has now been renamed the Agency for Healthcare Research and Quality (AHRQ). Their current budget is posted online at www.ahrq.gov.

The AHCPR initiated several major research efforts to examine medical outcomes. Two of the most significant, which are described here, are the Medical Treatment Effectiveness Program (MEDTEP) and a component of MEDTEP referred to as patient outcomes research teams (PORTs) (Greene, Bondy, & Maklan, 1994).

Medical Treatment Effectiveness Program

Congress established MEDTEP in 1989 to be implemented by the AHCPR. The purpose of the program was to improve the effectiveness and appropriateness of medical practice. When the program was mandated, Congress used the term *medical*. However, it was broadly interpreted to include health care in general, particularly—from our perspective—nursing care. The program was charged to develop and disseminate scientific information about the effects of health care services and procedures on patients' survival, health status, functional capacity, and quality of life, a remarkable shift from the narrow focus of traditional medical research. The program funded three research areas: (1) patient outcomes research, (2) database development, and (3) research on effective methods of disseminating the information gathered. For more information on MEDTEP, go to the AHRQ website.

Patient Outcomes Research Team Projects (PORTs)

PORTs were large-scale, multifaceted, and multidisciplinary projects. Congress mandated PORTs to "identify and analyze the outcomes and costs of current alternative practice patterns in order to determine the best treatment strategy and to develop and test methods for reducing inappropriate variations" (U.S. Congress, 1994, p. 67). The PORTs were required to "conduct literature reviews and syntheses; analyze practice variations and associated patient outcomes, using available data augmented by primary data collection where desired; disseminate research findings; and evaluate the effects of dissemination" (U.S. Congress, 1994, p. 67). PORTs might address questions such as "Do patients benefit from the care provided?" "What treatments work best?" "Has the patient's functional status improved?" "According to whose viewpoint?" and "Are health care resources well spent?" (Tanenbaum, 1994; Wood, 1990).

A major task of PORTs was to disseminate their findings and change the practice of health care providers to improve patient outcomes. A framework for dissemination was developed that identified the audiences for disseminated products, the media involved, and the strategies that foster assimilation and adoption of information (Goldberg et al., 1994).

The National Center for Nursing Research, now the National Institute for Nursing Research (NINR), developed a partnership with AHCPR, now the Agency for Health Care Research and Quality (AHRQ), to fund outcomes studies of importance to nursing. Calls for proposals jointly supported by AHRQ and NINR are announced each year. These calls for proposals can be found in NINR's home page at www.nih.gov/ninr.

With a growing budget and strong political support, proponents of the AHCPR were becoming a powerful force. They insisted on a change in health care because of the demand for health care reform that existed throughout the government and among the public. A reauthorization act changed the name of the AHCPR to the Agency for Healthcare Research and Quality (AHRQ). The AHRQ is designated as a scientific research agency. The term policy was removed from the agency name to avoid the perception that the agency determined federal health care policies and regulations. The word quality was added to the agency's name, establishing the AHRQ as the lead federal agency on quality of care research, with a new responsibility to coordinate all federal quality improvement efforts and health services research. The new legislation eliminated the requirement that the AHRQ develop clinical practice guidelines. However, the AHRQ still supports these efforts through evidence-based practice centers and the dissemination of evidence-based guidelines through its National Guideline Clearinghouse.

The United States is not the only country demanding improvements in quality of care and reductions in costs. Many countries are experiencing similar concerns and addressing them in relation to their particular government structures. Thus, the movement into outcomes research and the approaches described in this chapter are a worldwide phenomenon.

Clinical Guideline Panels

Clinical guideline panels incorporate available evidence on health outcomes into sets of recommendations concerning appropriate management strategies for patients with the studied conditions. An important source of guidelines is the National Guideline Clearinghouse (NGC). NGC has clear guidelines for submission of and inclusion of guidelines on their website. Any professional organization may gather a group to develop guidelines on a particular topic. Some groups seek funding for the project; others, such as professional organizations, conduct these efforts as an aspect of their organizational work. Medical schools and nursing schools have submitted guidelines, as have medical and nursing organizations and volunteer agencies such as the American Cancer Society. Guidelines developed across the world are included. Some guidelines are evidence based, whereas others are not. The evidence-based guidelines have considerably more validity. Current guidelines can be obtained from the National Guideline Clearinghouse of AHRQ at www.guideline.gov.

OUTCOMES RESEARCH AND NURSING PRACTICE

Outcome studies provide rich opportunities to build a stronger scientific underpinning for nursing practice.

Nurse researchers have been actively involved in the effort to examine the outcomes of patient care. Ideally, we would like to understand the outcomes of nursing practice within a one-to-one nurse/patient relationship. However, in most cases, more than one nurse cares for a patient. Therefore, the nursing effect is shared. In addition, nurse managers and nurse administrators have control over the nursing staff and the environment of nursing practice, and this affects the autonomy of the nurse to implement practice. Therefore, outcomes research must first focus on how nursing care is organized rather than what nurses do. Then, perhaps, we can begin to determine how what nurses do influences patient outcomes (Lake, 2006). We know that nurses do have an impact on patient outcomes. Kramer, Maguire, and Schmalenberg (2006) indicated that "a growing body of evidence supports a linkage between an empowered shared leadership/governance structure and control over nursing practice." The importance of autonomy in clinical nursing practice is being recognized as critically important to positive patient outcomes. It is important to identify autonomy-enabling structures in the organizational structures of nursing practice. One such structure revealed in a number of nursing studies is Magnet hospitals.

Lake (2006) suggested that we have a black box that holds the causal link between how care is organized and variations in patient outcomes. We cannot see inside the black box, we can only guess right now. Lake (2006) believes the black box contains nursing surveillance, judgment, and action, which are the bases for quality of care. But we cannot yet study it. Do you know how frustrating this is for a nurse researcher? But as we gain more understanding of the organization of nursing care and of the variation in patient outcomes, we will begin to obtain glimpses into the black box and to understand that causal link.

Nursing-Sensitive Patient Outcomes (NSPOs)

A **nursing-sensitive patient outcome** is "sensitive" because it is influenced by nursing. It may not be caused by nursing but is associated with nursing. In various situations, "nursing" might be the individual nurse, nurses as a working group, the approach to nursing practice, the nursing unit, the institution that determines numbers of nurses, salaries, educational levels of nurses, assignments of nurses, workload of nurses, management of nurses, and policies related to nurses and nursing practice. It might even include the architecture of the nursing unit. In whatever form, nursing actions have a role in the outcome, even though acts of other professionals, organizational acts, and patient characteristics and behaviors often

are involved in the outcome. What patient outcomes can you think of that might be nursing-sensitive?

Nursing-sensitive outcomes have become an issue because of national concerns related to the quality of care. "The demand for professional accountability regarding patient outcomes dictates that nurses are able to identify and document outcomes influenced by nursing care" Given and Sherwood (2005, p. 774). Efforts to study nursing-sensitive outcomes were initiated by the American Nurses Association (ANA). In 1994, the ANA, in collaboration with the American Academy of Nursing Expert Panel on Quality Health Care (Mitchell, Ferketich, Jennings, and the American Academy of Nursing Expert Panel on Quality Health Care, 1998), launched a plan to identify indicators of quality nursing practice and to collect and analyze data using these indicators across the United States. The goal was to identify or develop nursing-sensitive quality measures. Donabedian's theory was used as the framework for the project. Together, these indicators were referred to as the ANA **Nursing Care Report Card**. This Nursing Care Report Card could facilitate benchmarking, or setting a desired standard, that would allow comparisons of hospitals in terms of their nursing care quality.

The Acute Care Setting Report Card indicators were as follows:

- Patient satisfaction with pain management, nursing care, overall care, and educational information
- Pressure ulcers
- Patient falls
- Nurse satisfaction
- Nosocomial infection rate
- Direct care staffing mix
- Total nursing care hours per patient per day

No one knew what indicators were sensitive to nursing care provided to patients or what the relationships were between nursing inputs and patient outcomes. Every hospital had a different way of measuring the indicators that the ANA had selected. Persuading them to change to a standardized measure of the indicators for consistency across hospitals was a major endeavor (Jennings, Loan, DePaul, Brosch, & Hildreth, 2001; Rowell, 2001). Multiple pilot studies were conducted as nurse researchers and cooperating hospitals put in place the mechanisms required for data collection. These pilot studies identified multiple problems that had to be resolved before the project could go forward. Researchers learned that not only must the indicators be measured consistently, but data collection must be standardized. As studies continued, indictors were amplified and continue to be tested.

The ANA proposed that all hospitals collect and report on the nursing-sensitive quality indicators. To encourage researchers to collect these indicators, the ANA accredited organizations, and the federal government helped by sharing of the data with key groups. The ANA also encouraged state nurses' associations to lobby state legislatures to include the nursing-sensitive quality indicators in regulations or state law.

In 1998, the ANA provided funding to develop a national database to house data collected using nursing-sensitive quality indicators. The Midwest Research Institute (MRI) and the University of Kansas School of Nursing jointly manage the data. In 2001, data from nursing-sensitive quality indicators were being collected from more than 120 hospitals in 24 states across the United States. Data were analyzed quarterly, and feedback reports were distributed to all participating hospitals. Confidential benchmarking reports were provided to allow hospitals to compare their results with those of other hospitals in the group (Rowell, 2001).

In 1997, the ANA appointed members of the ANA Advisory Committee on Community-based Non-acute Care Indicators to identify a core set of indictors. The committee began by selecting a theoretical base for its work, selecting Evans and Stoddart's (1990) determinants of health model and also Donabedian's model of quality. As its work progressed, the committee chose to synthesize a model to guide the identification and testing of indicators (Figure 12-3). The committee followed the same pattern of work that the previous committee had used to choose the indicators. The following indicators were selected:

- Community based settings
- Pain management
- Staff mix
- Consistency of communication
- Client satisfaction

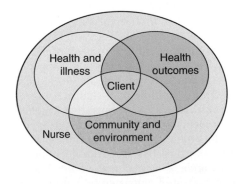

Figure 12-3 Model used by the ANA Advisory Committee to guide identification and testing of community-based nonacute care indicators.

- Prevention of tobacco use
- Cardiovascular risk reduction
- Caregiver activity
- Activities of daily living
- Psychosocial interaction

Other organizations currently involved in efforts to study nursing-sensitive outcomes include The National Quality Forum (NQF), California Nursing Outcomes Coalition, Veterans Affairs Nursing Outcomes Database, the Center for Medicare and Medicaid Services' (CMS) Hospital Quality Initiative, the American Hospital Association, the Federation of American Hospitals, the Joint Commission, and the Agency of Healthcare Research and Quality.

The Joint Commission appointed a group of external experts and stakeholders to provide advice on performance measurement issues. Titled the Advisory Council on Performance Measurement, it is a quasi-independent advisory group with responsibilities that include the initial selection of attributes for core measures and evaluation criteria. In 2007, the Joint Commission had implemented five sets of core performance measures for hospitals (Riehle, Riehle, Hanold, Sprenger, and Loeb, 2007). These sets are in the following areas:

- Heart failure
- Acute myocardial infarction
- Pneumonia
- Pregnancy and related conditions
- Surgical infection prevention

Sets are currently being prepared for the following:

- Intensive care unit (ICU) care
- Surgical care improvement project (SCIP)
- Sepsis
- Inpatient psychiatric care
- Pain management
- Children's asthma care

The National Quality Forum (NQF), with strong financial support from the Robert Wood Johnson Foundation, adopted 15 indicators of health care quality in 2004, which are referred to as the NQF-15. The NQF-15 are as follows:

- Urinary catheter associated urinary tract infection in ICU patients
- Ventilator-associated pneumonia for ICU and high risk nursery patients
- Central line catheter associated blood stream infection (BSI) rate for ICU and HRN
- Death among surgical inpatients (failure to rescue)
- Restraint prevalence (vest and limbs only)
- 30-day mortality risk (risk-adjusted)
- Length of stay for a given condition
- RN education (proportion of total RNs with the credential of bachelor's degree in nursing or higher)

- Smoking cessation counseling for patients with acute myocardial infarction
- Smoking cessation counseling for patients with heart failure
- Smoking cessation counseling for patients with pneumonia
- Recently hospitalized residents with symptoms of delirium (nursing homes)
- Katz Activities of Daily Living Index (home health care and nursing homes)
- Recently hospitalized residents who experience moderate to severe pain (nursing homes)
- Recently hospitalized residents who have pressure ulcers (nursing homes)

These indicators are the first nationally standardized performance measures of nursing sensitive care in acute care hospitals and are designed to assess health care quality, patient safety, and a professional and safe work environment. Although most measures currently used focus on the failure to meet the expected standards, the NQF believes that quality is as much about influencing positive outcomes, as it is about avoiding negative outcomes. Thus, the NQF is interested in developing measures that reflect the positive effects of nursing care. The NQF plans to include newly developed measures as advances in science-linked nursing yields other quality outcome measures. Priority areas for indicators include assessment, patient education, and care coordination (Naylor, 2007). Given and Sherwood (2005) suggested that "patients' outcomes may be measured best in the context of *their* needs, given *their* diagnosis, treatment, and altered life expectations" (p. 774). Given and Sherwood expressed concern that little has been done to examine the relationship between nursing-sensitive patient outcomes and health disparities.

Oncology Nursing Society

The Oncology Nursing Society has taken a leadership role among specialty nursing organizations in developing an evidence-based practice resource area on its website, www.ons.org/outcomes/measures/index.shtml. The site provides nurses with a guide to identify, critically appraise, and use evidence to solve clinical problems. It can also assist nurses—especially advanced practice nurses—who are helping others in developing evidence-based practice protocols. Information on the website indicated that "any healthcare provider, administrator, educator, or student who wants to learn more about the Evidence-Based Practice process or who is involved with implementing such a process may find this resource area informative." The outcomes resource area provides resources

that will help nurses to achieve desired outcomes for people with cancer, including outcome measures, resource cards, and evidence tables. The ONS Outcomes Resource Area (ORA) provides information for both the nurse providing direct patient care and the nurse who is looking for research evidence regarding outcomes. The resource area can be used in conjunction with the Evidence-Based Practice Resource Area (EBPRA), which is focused on the process and resources for evidence-based practice. ONS provides Putting Evidence into Practice (PEP) resources. PEP resource cards can be downloaded or ordered online. Additional information related to interventions for the outcomes including definitions of interventions, evidence tables, meta-analysis and systematic review tables, and references can be found on the ORA website. Another resource is an Outcomes Measures section that provides detailed information on measuring outcomes specific to oncology patients (e.g., pain, nausea and vomiting, peripheral neuropathies, and mucositis). Within each outcome, you will find definitions, an overview of measuring the outcome, and tables of instruments recommended for measurement. Additional resources related to measurement of the outcome are also available. All resources on the ORA can be easily printed from PDF files. Articles related to PEPs are published regularly in the *Oncology Nursing Forum.* A list of Oncology Nursing-Sensitive Outcomes is provided on the ORA website, and those available in 2007 are listed in Table 12-4. Because this incredible site is accessible to the public, all nurses can use this information to improve patient outcomes. A separate web page is provided for each nursing-sensitive outcome.

Advanced Practice Nursing Outcomes Research

Studies of outcomes of advanced practice nurses (APNs) are now appearing in the literature. APNs are RNs educationally prepared at the master's or doctoral level. These practitioners have expertise in a particular area of clinical specialization and provide direct patient care. The ANA recognizes four types of APNs: certified registered nurse anesthetists (CRNA), certified nurse midwives (CNMs), clinical nurse specialists (CNSs), and nurse practitioners (NPs). Of interest in studying APNs is the number of years they have practiced, which researchers are finding to be related to quality of care. There are two aspects of years of practice that may influence the quality of care they provide: the number of years of clinical practice before becoming an APN and the number of years of practice as an APN.

TABLE 12-4	Oncology Nursing-Sensitive Outcomes: A Classification with Exemplars

Symptom Experience

Pain
Fatigue
Insomnia
Nausea
Constipation
Anorexia
Breathlessness
Diarrhea
Altered skin/mucous membranes
Neutropenia

Functional Status

ADL (activities of daily living)
IADL (instrumental activities of daily living)
Role functioning
Activity tolerance
Ability to carry out usual activities
Nutritional status

Safety (preventable adverse events)

Infections
Falls
Skin ulcers
Extravasation incidents
Hypersensitive reactions

Psychological Distress

Anxiety
Depression
Spiritual distress

Economic (incorporate this category into all categories)

Length of stay
Unexpected re-admissions
Emergency visits
Out-of-pocket costs (family)
Cost per patient day
Cost per episode of care

From Given, B., Beck, S., Etland, C., Gobel, B. H., Lamkin, L., & Marsee, V. D. (2004). *Nursing-sensitive patient outcomes.* Oncology Nursing Society. Retrieved November 16, 2007, from www.ons.org/outcomes/measures/outcomes.shtml.

Another interest in terms of outcome research is what happens during the process of APN care. This care involves a set of activities within, among, and between practitioners and patients and includes both technical and interpersonal elements. This process of care is complex and somewhat mysterious. However, clearly describing what occurs during this process of care is essential to developing a comprehensive understanding of how APNs affect outcomes. Although researchers have provided descriptions of APN care, considerable detailed work must still be done to more thoroughly describe the activities and interactions that occur between APNs and patients during the process of care (Cunningham, 2004).

The next step is to establish the relationship between APN interventions and outcomes. The outcomes must be clearly defined and measurable or observable. One critical outcome is cost. Outcomes may require risk adjustments for factors that may confound the results, such as comorbidity, stage of illness, severity of illness, and demographic characteristics.

Failure to use rigor in measurement will limit your ability to interpret study findings meaningfully. It is important for variables to be measured using the same measurement methods across studies so that results are more readily compared. Understanding which outcomes are sensitive to APN interventions is critical to building knowledge in this area. We need a classification of outcomes of APN practice. Ingersoll, McIntosh, and Williams (2000) generated a beginning list of 27 relevant outcome indicators of APN practice. The nine highest outcomes were the following:

- Satisfaction with care delivered
- Symptom resolution or reduction
- Perception of being well cared for
- Compliance or adherence with treatment plan
- Knowledge of patients and families
- Trust of care provider
- Collaboration among care providers
- Frequency and type of procedures ordered
- Quality of life

These outcomes will require empirical validation. This means that the outcome measures will need to be tested repeatedly in nursing studies. No studies have, as yet, specified which APN interventions were responsible for what outcomes or how the outcomes were affected by the interventions. Cunningham (2004) posed the following critical questions in relation to APN outcomes:

1. What are the mechanisms by which APNs are able to consistently improve outcomes?
2. Is it just that they provided the interventions described by the researchers?
3. Was something key about those interventions within the populations studied?
4. What about the interpersonal components of care? (p. 228)

Linking APN nursing interventions to outcomes requires that we be able to quantify (reduce to numbers) an episode of nursing care using a measurement method that adequately captures what nurses actually do (Hughes et al., 2002). Information must be provided on type and frequency, range, emphasis, and dose intensity of the intervention. Outcomes are context dependent and should be evaluated within specific populations and settings. It has not been clear at this point in APN research which conditions or settings are most likely to benefit from APN interventions (Cunningham, 2004; Sox, 2000). Cunningham (2004) cautioned:

[A]ll outcome measurement must be considered within the context of time. The effects of healthcare interventions may not be discernable immediately or be sustained over time. Longitudinal measures provide information about the patterns and trajectories of outcomes. Understanding the duration of an intervention's effect allows for the planning and delivery of effective health care. (p. 227)

If you are interested in becoming involved in APN-led multidisciplinary outcomes measurements projects, Kleinpell and Gawlinski (2005) recommended the following process:

- Find/identify outcomes variables that the APN can impact.
- Organize a team.
- Clarify current knowledge of the practice issue to be improved.
- Understand sources of variation.
- Select practices and strategies for improvement.
- Plan.
- Do the interventions according to your plan.
- Check/analyze/review data and results.
- Put improvement into effect, hold the gains you have achieved, and apply the lessons you have learned.

Practice-Based Research Networks (PBRNs)

PBRNs are a group of practices focused on patient care, and they are affiliated in order to analyze their clinical practices in communities. A Web-based search and a survey of PBRNs yielded 111 PBRNs (Tierney et al., 2007). The 86 who met the criteria for primary care PBRNs contained 1871 practices, 12,957 physicians, and 14.7 million patients. Minority and underinsured patients were overrepresented. The average PBRN was young; half had published three or fewer studies. Three-quarters were affiliated with universities. There were four primary care specialties represented in PBRN practices: family medicine, pediatrics, general internal medicine, and family nurse practitioners.

The primary research foci were prevention, diabetes, cardiovascular risk, and mental health. There are two networks of advanced practice registered nurses: APRNet and MNCCRN.

APRNet (Advanced Practice Registered Nurses' Research Network) was funded in 2000 by a grant to Yale University School of Nursing in collaboration with Boston College, the University of Connecticut, the Universities of Massachusetts at Amherst and Worcester, and the University of Rhode Island. The focus of APRNet is to provide primary care. The purpose of the network is to "conduct and facilitate practice-based research relevant to APRN primary care practice; develop culturally competent, evidence-based practice models for APRNs; and translate research findings into primary care practice" (McCloskey, Grey, Deshefy-Longhi, & Grey, 2003).

Midwest Nursing Centers Consortium Research Network (MNCCRN), a practice-based research network (PBRN) funded by the AHRQ, is the only PBRN in the United States comprising exclusively clinical nurse specialists. Its focus is to deliver primary health care with a particular emphasis on reducing health disparities. The network conducts community-based participatory research that will ultimately inform practice, education, and health policy (Anderko, Lundeen, S., & Bartz, 2006).

METHODOLOGIES FOR OUTCOMES STUDIES

A research tradition for the outcomes paradigm is still emerging. A research tradition defines acceptable research methodologies. The lack of an established set of methodologies should encourage greater creativity in seeking new strategies for studying the phenomena of concern. Small single studies using untried methodologies may be useful. Research teams must develop research programs with a planned sequence of studies focused on a particular outcome concern. The PORTs defined a research process for conducting programs of funded outcomes studies. These programs are complex and may consist of multiple studies using a variety of research strategies whose findings must be merged to formulate conclusions.

Although implementing a research program as extensive as a PORT would be unrealistic without funding, ideas for developing the methodology of outcomes research programs on a smaller scale may be generated through an examination of these plans. For example, measurement methods used in PORTs are available for smaller studies. The following steps were constructed combining PORT plans proposed by

Freund, Dittus, Fitzgerald, and Heck (1990), Sledge (1993), and Turk and Rudy (1994):

1. Perform a critical review of the published literature or a meta-analysis.
2. Conduct large database analyses on the basis of the results of the critical literature review.
3. Identify outcomes measures for use in the study, and evaluate their sensitivity to change.
4. Identify variables that might affect the outcomes.
5. Achieve consensus on definitions for all variables to be used in the research program.
6. Develop assessment instruments or techniques.
7. Conduct patient surveys or focus groups to gain information on outcomes, such as level of functional status and perceived pain, and on how these outcomes may improve or regress over time.
8. Determine patterns of care. (Who provides care at what points of time for what purposes?)
9. Perform a cohort analysis: Monitor a cohort of patients—some of whom will receive one treatment and others of whom will not receive the treatment—to assess changes in outcomes over time. Use a telephone survey at selected intervals to gather information. Evaluate the proportion of patients who improve, as well as the group mean differences.
10. Determine, through follow-up studies, differences in patient selection or interventions that are associated with different outcomes. Evaluate the durability of change by conducting sufficiently long follow-up. Determine the percentage of patients dropping out of groups receiving different treatments, and, when possible, determine their reasons for dropping out.
11. Determine the clinical significance of improvement, as well as the statistical significance.
12. Determine the cost-benefit and cost-effectiveness of the treatments under evaluation.
13. Use decision analyses to synthesize information about patients' outcomes and preferences for various types of outcomes.
14. Disseminate information to both patients and health care providers about which individuals would and which would not benefit from the procedure.
15. Conduct a clinical trial to evaluate the effects of the intervention.
16. Incorporate findings into treatment guidelines.
17. Modify provider and patient behavior so that proven, effective treatment is given to those who are most likely to benefit.

The PORTs recognized the need to allow diversity in research strategies, measures, and analyses to facilitate methodological advances (Fowler, Cleary, Magaziner, Patrick, & Benjamin, 1994). Creative flexibility is often necessary to develop ways to answer new questions. Finding ways to determine the impact of a condition on a person's life is difficult. Interpreting results can also be problematic, because clinical significance is considered as important as statistical significance. This issue requires a judgment by the research team as to what constitutes clinical significance in their particular area of study.

The following section describes some of the sampling issues, research strategies, measurements, and statistical approaches that researchers use when conducting outcomes studies. These descriptions are not sufficient to guide you in using the approaches described; rather they provide a broad overview of a variety of methodologies being used. For additional information, refer to the citations in each section. Outcomes studies cross a variety of disciplines; thus, the emerging methodologies are being enriched by a cross-pollination of ideas, some of which are new to nursing research.

Samples and Sampling

The preferred methods of obtaining samples are different in outcomes studies; random sampling is not considered desirable and is seldom used. Heterogeneous, rather than homogeneous, samples are obtained. Rather than using sampling criteria that restrict subjects included in the study to decrease possible biases and that reduce the variance and increase the possibility of identifying a statistically significant difference, outcomes researchers seek large heterogeneous samples that reflect, as much as possible, all patients who would be receiving care in the real world. Samples, then, must include, for example, patients with various comorbidities and patients with varying levels of health status. In addition, persons should be identified who do not receive treatment for their condition. Devising ways to evaluate the representativeness of such samples is problematic. Developing strategies to locate untreated individuals and include them in follow-up studies is a challenge.

Traditional researchers and statisticians argue that when patients are not selected randomly, biases and confounding variables are more likely to occur and that this issue is a particular problem when the sample size is small. In nonexperimental studies, variation is likely to be greater, resulting in a higher risk of a type II error. Traditional analysts consider nonrandomized studies to be based on observational data and therefore do not view them as credible (Orchard, 1994). Using this argument, traditionalists claim that the findings of most outcomes studies are not valid and should not be used to establish guidelines for clinical practice or to build a body of knowledge.

Slade, Kuipers, and Priebe (2002) suggested the following:

> Research questions are designed so that they can be answered by Randomized Controlled Trials (RCTs). Specifically, the use of RCTs involves the identification of an intervention which is given to patients in the experimental group, but not the control group. This encourages the asking of particular types of research questions, typically of the form "Does intervention X work for disorder Y?" It will be argued that the RCT methodology limits the questions that can be asked, and hence can restrict the potential findings from research. Furthermore, if different questions were being asked, the RCTs would not always be the best methodology to employ.... The question "Which patients with condition Y does intervention X work for?" may prove to have more clinical relevance, and answering this question may involve asking the question "How does intervention X work"?, a question which cannot be answered just by using RCTs. (Slade et al., 2002, pp. 12–13)

Large Databases as Sample Sources

One source of samples for outcomes studies is large databases. Two broad categories of databases emerge from patient care encounters: clinical databases and administrative databases, as illustrated by Figure 12-4. **Clinical databases** were created by providers such as hospitals, HMOs, and health care professionals. The clinical data are generated either as a result of routine documentation of care or in relation to a research protocol. Some databases are data registries that have been developed to gather data related to a particular disease, such as cancer (Lee & Goldman, 1989). With a clinical database, you can link observations made by many practitioners over long periods. Links can be made between the process of care and outcomes (Mitchell et al., 1994; Moses, 1995).

Administrative databases are created by insurance companies, government agencies, and others not directly involved in providing patient care. Administrative databases have standardized sets of data for enormous numbers of patients and providers (Deyo et al., 1994; McDonald & Hui, 1991). An example is the Medicare database managed by the Centers for Medicare & Medicaid Services (CMS). These large databases can be used to determine the incidence or prevalence of disease, geographical variations in medical care utilization, characteristics of medical care, outcomes of care, and complementarity with clinical trials. Wray et al. (1995) cautioned, however, that analyses should be restricted to outcomes specific to a particular subgroup of patients, rather than one adverse outcome of all disease states.

There are problems with the quality of data in the large databases. Hundreds of individuals in a variety of settings have gathered and entered these data. There have been few quality checks on the data, and within the same data sets, records may have different lengths and structures. Missing data are common. Sampling and measurement errors are inherent in all large databases. Sampling error results from the way in which cases are selected for inclusion in the database; measurement error emerges from problems related to the operational definition of concepts. Thus, the reliability and validity of the data are a concern (Davis, 1990; Lange & Jacox, 1993).

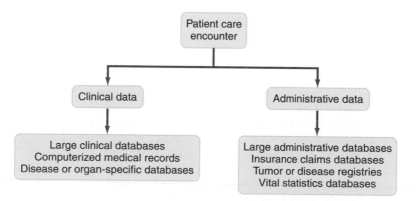

Figure 12-4 Types of databases emanating from patient care encounters.

Large databases are used in outcomes studies to examine patient care outcomes. The outcomes that can be examined are limited to those recorded in the database and thus tend to be general. Existing databases can be used for analyses such as (1) assessing nursing care delivery models; (2) varying nursing practices; or (3) evaluating patients' risk of hospital-acquired infection, hospital-acquired pressure ulcer, or falls. Lange and Jacox (1993) identified the following important health policy questions related to nursing that should be examined through the use of large databases:

1. *What is standard nursing practice in various settings?*
2. *What is the relationship between variations in nursing practice and patient outcomes?*
3. *What are the effects of different nursing staff mixes on patient outcomes and costs?*
4. *What are the total costs for episodes of treatment of specific conditions, and what part of those are attributable to nursing care?*
5. *Who is being reimbursed for nursing care delivery? (Lange & Jacox, 1993, p. 207)*

To examine these questions, nurses must develop the statistical and methodological skills needed for working with large databases. Large databases contain patient and institutional information from huge numbers of patients. They exist in computer-readable form, require special statistical methods and computer techniques, and can be used by researchers who were not involved in the creation of the database.

Regrettably, nursing data are noticeably missing from these large databases and thus from the funded health policy studies using them. A nursing minimum data set has been repeatedly recommended for inclusion in these databases (Werley, Devine, Zorn, Ryan, & Westra, 1991; Werley & Lang, 1988; Zielstorff, Hudgings, Grobe, and the National Commission on Nursing Implementation Project Task Force on Nursing Information Systems, 1993). This minimum data set would comprise a set of variables necessary and sufficient to describe an episode of illness or the care given by a provider. The ANA has mandated the formation of a steering committee on databases to support clinical nursing practice. The following nursing classification schemes are being used in national databases:

- The North American Nursing Diagnosis Association (NANDA) classification
- The Omaha System: Applications for Community Health Nursing classification
- The Home Health Care Classification

- The Nursing Interventions Classification (NIC)
- The Nursing Outcomes Classification (NOC)

Temple (1990, p. 211) expressed the following concerns regarding the use of large data sets rather than controlled trials to assess the effectiveness of treatments: "We have traveled this route before with uncontrolled observations. It has always been hoped, and has often been asserted, that uncontrolled databases can be adjusted in some way that will allow valid comparisons of treatments. I know of no systematic attempt to document this." Outcomes researchers counter these criticisms by pointing out that experimental studies lack external validity and are not useful for application in clinical settings. They claim that clinicians are not using the findings from clinical trials because they are not representative of the patients seeking care.

Research Strategies for Outcomes Studies

Outcomes research programs usually consist of studies with a mix of strategies carried out sequentially. Although these strategies could be referred to as designs, for some the term *design* as used in Chapters 10 and 11 is inconsistent with the use of the term here. Research strategies for outcomes studies have emerged from a variety of disciplines, and innovative new strategies continue to appear in the literature. Strategies for outcomes studies tend to have less control than traditional research designs and cannot be as easily categorized. The research strategies for outcomes studies described in this section are only a sampling from the literature; they are consensus knowledge building, practice pattern profiling, prospective cohort studies, retrospective cohort studies, population-based studies, clinical decision analysis, study of the effectiveness of interdisciplinary teams, geographical analyses, economic studies, ethical studies, and defining and testing of interventions.

Consensus Knowledge Building

Consensus knowledge building is usually performed by a multidisciplinary group representing a variety of constituencies. Initially, the group conducts an extensive international search of the literature on the topic of concern, including unpublished studies, studies in progress, dissertations, and theses. Several separate reviews may be performed, focusing on specific questions about the outcomes of care, diagnosis, prevention, or prognosis. Because meta-analytic methods often cannot be applied to the literature pertinent to PORTs, systematic approaches to critique and synthesis have been developed to identify relevant studies and gather and analyze data abstracted from the studies (Powe, Turner, Maklan, & Ersek, 1994).

The results are dispersed to researchers and clinical experts in the field, who are asked to carefully examine the material and then participate in a consensus conference. The consensus conference yields clinical guidelines, which are published and widely distributed to clinicians. The clinical guidelines are also used as practice norms to study process and outcomes in that field. Gaps in the knowledge base are identified and research priorities determined by the consensus group.

Preliminary steps in this process might include conducting extensive integrative reviews and seeking consensus from a multidisciplinary research team and locally available clinicians. A review could be accomplished by establishing a website and conducting dialogue with experts via the Internet. The review could be published in Sigma Theta Tau's online journal, *Knowledge Synthesis in Nursing*, and then dialogue related to the review could be conducted over the Internet. The Delphi method has also been used to seek consensus (Tork, Dassen, & Lohrmann, 2008).

Practice Pattern Profiling

Practice pattern profiling is an epidemiological technique that focuses on patterns of care rather than individual occurrences of care. Researchers use large database analysis to identify a provider's pattern of practice and compare it with that of similar providers or with an accepted standard of practice. The technique has been used to determine overutilization and underutilization of services, to determine costs associated with a particular provider's care, to uncover problems related to efficiency and quality of care, and to assess provider performance. The provider being profiled could be an individual practitioner, a group of practitioners, or a health care organization, such as a hospital or an HMO.

The provider's pattern is expressed as a rate aggregated over time for a defined population of patients under the provider's care. For example, the analysis might examine the number of sigmoidoscopy claims filed per 100 Medicare patients seen by the provider in a given year. Analyses might examine (1) whether diabetic patients have had at least one annual serum glucose test and have received an ophthalmology examination or (2) the frequency of flu shots, Papanicolaou smears, and mammograms for various target populations (Lasker, Shapiro, & Tucker, 1992; McNeil, Pedersen, & Gatsonis, 1992).

Profiling can be used when the data contain hierarchical groupings: Patients could be grouped by nurse, nurses by unit, and units by larger organizations. The analysis uses regression equations to examine the relationship of an outcome to the characteristics of the various groupings. To be effective, the analysis must include data on the different sources of variability that might contribute to a given outcome.

The structure of the analysis reflects the structure of the data. For example, patient characteristics could be data on disease severity, comorbidity, emergent status, behavioral characteristics, socioeconomic status, and demographics. Nurse characteristics might consist of level of education, specialty status, years of practice, age, gender, and certifications. Unit characteristics could comprise number of beds, nursing management style used on the unit, ratio of patients to nurses, and the proportion of staff who are RNs (McNeil et al., 1992).

Profiles are designed to generate some type of action, such as to inform the provider that his or her rates are too high or too low compared with the norm. By examining aggregate patterns of practice, profiling can be used to compare the care provided by different organizations or received by different populations of patients. Critical pathways or care maps can then be used to determine the proportion of patients who diverged from the pathway for a particular nurse, group of nurses, or group of nursing units. Profiling can be used to improve quality, assess provider performance, and review utilization.

Profiling does not address methods of improving outcomes, although this process can identify problem areas. It can be used to determine how performance should be changed to improve outcomes and who should make those changes. Profiling can also identify outliers, allowing more detailed examination of these individuals.

The databases currently being used for profiling are not ideal, because they were developed for other purposes. Only broad outcomes can be examined, such as morbidity and mortality, complications, readmissions, and frequency of utilization of various services (Lasker et al., 1992; McNeil et al., 1992). Table 12-5 lists examples of the large database measures that might be used in profiling.

Prospective Cohort Studies

A prospective cohort study is an epidemiological study in which the researcher identifies a group of people who are at risk for experiencing a particular event. Sample sizes for these studies often must be very large, particularly if only a small portion of the at-risk group will experience the event. The entire group is followed over time to determine the point at which the event occurs, variables associated with the event, and outcomes for those who experienced the event compared with those who did not.

TABLE 12-5 ■ Examples of Large Database Measures Used in Profiling

Quality of Care Issue	Measures	Example	Criteria
Access	Proportion of population receiving care during the year, classified by age and sex	Percentage of children under age 2 seen for at least one well-care visit	National
		Percentage of children seen in emergency rooms for any reason, for trauma, and for medical problems	Trends
Preventive	Portion of population in specific age and sex groups receiving recommended tests or procedures	Percentage of children by group having recommended immunizations in previous year	National recommendation
		Percentage of women age 50 and over having mammography in past year	National recommendation
		Percentage of deliveries with prenatal care beginning in first trimester	National recommendation
Diagnosis	Percentage of population diagnosed (and under care) for specific chronic conditions by age and sex	Percentage of adults diagnosed at one or more visits as having essential hypertension by age and sex	Epidemiological data on prevalence of hypertension
Treatment	Medications Average number of new prescriptions or antibiotics per person per year	Average number of new prescriptions per person per year	Trends and comparison data
	Surgery Rate of surgical procedures per year; total, inpatient, and ambulatory (if applicable)	Cesarean section rate for all deliveries	Trends and comparison data
Outcomes	Hospital readmissions within 3 months of discharge	Percentage of readmissions for some condition Percentage of readmission identifying a complication	Comparison data and trends

Reproduced in part from Steinwachs, D. M., Weiner, J. P., & Shapiro, S. (1989). Management information systems and quality. In N. Goldfield & D. B. Nash (Eds.), *Providing quality care: The challenge to clinicians* (pp. 160–180). Philadelphia: American College of Physicians.

The Harvard Nurses Health Study, which is still being conducted, is an example of a prospective cohort study. This study recruited 100,000 nurses to determine the long-term consequences of the use of birth control pills. Every 2 years, nurses complete a questionnaire about their health and health behaviors. The study has now been in progress for more than 20 years. Multiple studies reported in the literature have used the large data set yielded by the Harvard study. Prospective cohort nursing studies could be conducted on a smaller scale on other populations, such as patients identified as being at high risk for the development of pressure ulcers.

Retrospective Cohort Studies

A retrospective cohort study is an epidemiological study in which the researcher identifies a group of people who have experienced a particular event. This is a common research technique used in the epidemiology field to study occupational exposure to chemicals. Events of interest to nursing that could be studied in this manner include a procedure, an episode of care, a nursing intervention, and a diagnosis. Nurses might use a retrospective cohort study to follow a cohort of women who had received a mastectomy for breast cancer or of patients in whom a urinary bladder catheter was placed during and after surgery. The cohort is evaluated after the event to determine the occurrence of changes in health status, usually the development of a particular disease or death. Nurses might be interested in the pattern of recovery after an event or, in the case of catheterization, the incidence of bladder infections in the months after surgery.

On the basis of the study findings, epidemiologists calculate relative risk of the identified change in health for the group. For example, if death were the occurrence of interest, the expected number of deaths would be determined. The observed number of deaths divided by the expected number of deaths and multiplied by 100 yields a *standardized mortality ratio* (SMR), which is regarded as a measure of the relative risk of the studied group to die of a particular condition. In nursing studies, patients might be followed over time after discharge from a health care facility (Swaen & Meijers, 1988).

In retrospective studies, researchers commonly ask patients to recall information relevant to their previous health status. This information is often used to determine the amount of change occurring before and after an intervention. Recall can easily be distorted, however, misleading researchers, and thus it should be used with caution. Herrmann (1995) identified three sources of distortion in recall: (1) the question posed to the subject may be conceived or expressed incorrectly, (2) the recall process may be in error, and (3) the research design used to measure recall can result in the recall's appearing to be different from what actually occurred. Herrmann (1995, p. AS90) also identified four bases of recall:

Direct recall: The subject "accesses the memory without having to think or search memory," resulting in correct information.
Indirect recall: The subject "accesses the memory after thinking or searching memory," resulting in correct information.
Limited recall: "Access to the memory does not occur but information that suggests the contents of the memory is accessed," resulting in an educated guess.
No recall: "Neither the memory nor information relevant to the memory may be accessed," resulting in a wild guess.

The following abstract is from a retrospective cohort study of the impact of an anemia clinic on emergency room visits and hospitalizations in patients with anemia of CKD pre-dialysis by Perkins et al. (2007).

■ *ABSTRACT*

Aim: There is limited data regarding the impact on hospital resource use of a dedicated, nurse-managed anemia clinic in patients with pre-end stage chronic kidney disease.

Methods: A retrospective cohort study was conducted comparing patients with pre-end stage anemia of chronic kidney disease enrolled in an algorithmic anemia clinic ($N = 27$, treatment group) with un-enrolled patients with chronic kidney disease ($N = 22$, control group). The treatment group received algorithmic treatment with recombinant human erythropoietin and intravenous iron sucrose, while controls received usual care.

The primary outcomes investigated were emergency room visits and hospitalizations during a 1-year period.

Results: The two groups were similar at baseline. During the first year of clinic enrollment, the mean hemoglobin values improved in the treatment group from baseline and compared with controls (11.6 +/− 1.2 g/dL vs. 10.3 +/− 1.0 g/dL, $p < 0.05$). The relative risk of an emergency room visit (RR 0.18, 95% CI 0.05–0.67, $p < 0.05$) and hospitalization (RR [relative risk] 0.20, 95% CI 0.06–0.67, $p < 0.05$) were reduced in the treatment group versus the control group. The average length of hospital stay was also reduced (6.8 days vs. 9.5 days, $p = 0.05$).

Conclusion: Enrollment in a dedicated nurse-managed anemia clinic is significantly associated with reduced emergency room visits and hospitalizations in patients with pre-end stage CKD. These associative findings justify future prospective analyses to establish causality. (Perkins et al., 2007, pp. 167–74)

Population-Based Studies

Population-based studies are also important in outcomes research. Conditions must be studied in the context of the community rather than of the medical system. With this method, all cases of a condition occurring in the defined population are included, rather than only patients treated at a particular health care facility, because the latter could introduce a selection bias. The researcher might make efforts to include individuals with the condition who had not received treatment.

Community-based norms of tests and survey instruments obtained in this manner provide a clearer picture of the range of values than the limited spectrum of patients seen in specialty clinics. Estimates of instrument sensitivity and specificity are more accurate. This method enables researchers to understand the natural history of a condition or of the long-term risks and benefits of a particular intervention (Guess et al., 1995).

Geller et al. (2007) conducted "A study of health outcomes in school children: Key challenges and lessons learned from the Framingham Schools' Natural History of Nevi Study." The following is an abstract of their study.

■ *ABSTRACT*

Background: We describe the planning, recruitment, key challenges, and lessons learned in the development of a study of the evolution of nevi (moles) among children in a school setting.

Methods: This population-based study of digital photography and dermoscopy of the child's back (overview, close-up, and dermoscopic images) and genetic specimens took place among fifth graders in the Framingham, Massachusetts School System. Schoolchildren and their parents completed baseline surveys on sun protection practices, sunburns, and past ultraviolet exposures, including summer and vacation experiences.

Results: Prestudy outreach was conducted with children, parents, nurses, administrators, and pediatricians. Of the 691 Framingham families with a fifth grader (aged 10–11), 443 consented to complete surveys and undergo digital photography and dermoscopy during the school's routine scoliosis testing. Of the 443 families providing consent, 369 agreed to genetic testing. We identified key factors to consider when implementing school-based studies: (a) pilot studies to demonstrate feasibility, (b) inclusion of school administration and parents, (c) grassroots approach with multiple contacts, and (d) embedding research studies within preexisting school health services.

Conclusions: Launching an observational study within the school environment required an academic/school collaboration across numerous disciplines including dermatology, epidemiology, genetics, medical photography, school health, community health education, and most notably, the need for the presence of a full-time study nurse in the school. A large school system proved to be an excellent resource to conduct this first prospective study on the evolution of moles in US schoolchildren. The key challenges and lessons learned may be applicable to other investigators launching school-based initiatives. (Geller et al., 2007, pp. 312-318)

Clinical Decision Analysis

Clinical decision analysis is a systematic method of describing clinical problems, identifying possible diagnostic and management courses of action, assessing the probability and value of various outcomes, and then calculating the optimal course of action. Decision analysis is based on the following four assumptions: (1) decisions can be quantified; (2) all possible courses of action can be identified and evaluated; (3) the different values of outcomes, viewed from the perspective of the nurse, patient, payer, and administrator, can be examined; and (4) the analysis allows selection of an optimal course of therapy.

To perform the analysis, the researchers must define the boundaries of what is being defined as the clinical in terms of a logical sequence of events over time. All the possible courses of action are then determined. These courses of action are usually represented in a decision tree consisting of a starting point, available alternatives, probable events, and outcomes. Next, researchers define the goals and objectives for resolving the problem. They then calculate the probability that each path of the decision tree will occur. For each potential path, there is an outcome. Each outcome is assigned a value. These values may be expressed in terms of money, morbidity incidents, quality-of-life measures, or length of stay. Figure 12-5 presents a simplified decision tree for breech delivery in obstetrics. An optimal course of action is identified according to which decision maximizes the chances of the most desirable outcomes (Crane, 1988; Keeler, 1994; Sonnenberg et al., 1994).

Studies analyzing clinical decisions have primarily used questionnaires and interviews. However, determining the clinical decisions of practitioners is not an easy task. Much of patient care involves the clinician and the patient alone. The underlying theories of care and the processes of care are hidden from view. Thus, it is difficult for clinicians to compare their approaches to care. Among physicians, care delivered by other physicians is rarely observed (O'Connor et al., 1993). Studies have found that physicians have difficulty recalling their decisions and providing rationales for them (Chaput de Saintonge & Hattersley, 1985; Kirwan, Chaput de Saintonge, Joyce, Holmes, & Currey, 1986). Simulation would be an effective strategy for analyzing clinical decisions.

Unsworth (2001) described the following strategies for studying clinical decision making:

1. The clinician conducts semistructured interviews.
2. The clinician listens to an audiotape of the clinician-client dialogue and uses this to recall her or his reasoning processes (audio-assisted recall).
3. The clinician uses video footage to prompt recall of reasoning processes (video-assisted recall).
4. The clinician writes notes as he or she solves a problem.
5. The clinician provides verbal commentary during interaction with the client (the think-aloud method).
6. The clinician presents his or her reasoning about a clinician-client session afterward from memory.
7. The clinician uses a head-mounted video camera with video-assisted recall.

Chaput de Saintonge, Kirway, Evans, and Crane (1988) proposed a strategy for analyzing clinical decisions using "paper patients." The techniques seem to parallel the decisions clinicians have made in the clinical setting. In their study, 10 common clinical variables used to evaluate the status of patients with rheumatoid arthritis were collected at two points on 30 patients participating in a clinical trial, at the time

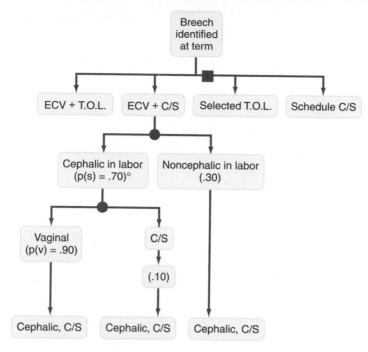

Figure **12-5** Simplified decision tree for breech delivery. (Numbers in parentheses refer to estimated probability of event.)

of entry and 1 year later. Twenty of the patients were duplicated throughout the table to check the consistency of responses, making 50 responses in all. The variables were presented to rheumatologists on a single sheet of paper labeled "before" and "after a year." Physicians were asked to indicate the extent of change in each patient's condition using a visual analogue scale (VAS) with the ends labeled "greatest possible deterioration" and "greatest possible improvement." They were also asked whether they considered the change clinically important. Then they were asked to indicate the relative importance of each variable, rating the variables on a scale of 1 to 100.

Regression analyses were performed in which the VAS values were used as the dependent variable. With increasing VAS values, judgments of clinical importance changed from "not important" to "important." This change occurred over a 5 mm length of the scale or less. (VAS scales are traditionally 100 mm in length.) The researchers designated the midpoint of this transition zone as the "threshold value of clinical importance." To test the consistency of responses, the researchers used the Spearman rank correlation to compare responses to the duplicate cases. They then developed a consensus model by weighing each physician's responses on the basis of the Spearman coefficient.

The VAS scores were multiplied by the Spearman coefficient. These VAS scores were then used as the dependent variable in another regression analysis. This method is useful in identifying the variables important in the making of clinical decisions and the consistency with which practitioners make their decisions.

Standing (2007) conducted a study of clinical decision-making of nursing students as they progressed to practicing RNs. The following is an abstract of the study.

■ *ABSTRACT*

Aim: This paper is a report of a study to explore, from the perspective of nursing students, how they acquire clinical decision-making skills and how well-prepared they feel in this respect regarding their responsibilities as Registered Nurses.

Background: Previous research has focused mainly on exploring experienced nurses' judgment and decision-making. Some studies have elicited senior nursing students' understanding of the process, but none has explored the development of clinical decision-making skills throughout the educational program and in the first year as a Registered Nurse.

Method: A volunteer sample of 20 respondents, broadly representative of the student cohort regarding qualifications, age, gender and nursing specialty, was recruited. A longitudinal hermeneutic phenomenological study was carried out from 2000 to 2004, using interviews, reflective journals, care studies, critical incident analyses and document analysis.

Findings: Ten conceptions of nursing and 10 perceptions of clinical decision-making were identified and a growing pattern of inter-relationships between them became apparent. A 'matrix model' was developed by cross-referencing the two thematic categories within the timeline of respondents' developmental journey through significant milestones and changing contexts. As Registered Nurses they found having to 'think on your feet' without the 'comfort blanket' of student status both a stressful and formative learning experience.

Conclusion: Further collaboration between education and health service partners is recommended to integrate clinical decision-making throughout the nursing curriculum, enhance the development of such vital skills, and facilitate the transition from student to Registered Nurse. (Standing, 2007, pp. 257–269)

Study of the Effectiveness of Interdisciplinary Teams

According to Schmitt, Farrell, and Heinemann (1988), interdisciplinary teams have the following characteristics:

(1) Multiple health disciplines are involved in the care of the same patients, (2) the disciplines encompass a diversity of dissimilar knowledge and skills required by the patients, (3) the plan of care reflects an integrated set of goals shared by the providers of care, and (4) the team members share information and coordinate their services through a systematic communication process. (p. 753)

Part of the communication process consists of regularly scheduled face-to-face meetings. The assumption is that collaborative team approaches provide more effective care than nonteam approaches or than noncollaborative multidisciplinary approaches (parallel care).

Interdisciplinary teams are becoming more common as health care changes. Examples are hospice care teams, home health teams, and psychiatric care teams. Studying the effectiveness of interdisciplinary teams is difficult, however. The characteristics that make team care more effective have not been identified. Researchers usually focus on evaluating a single team rather than conducting comparison studies. The outcomes of team care are also multidimensional, requiring the use of multiple dependent variables.

Evaluation studies examining team care often examine only posttreatment data without baseline data. If groups are compared, there is no evidence that the groups were similar in terms of important variables before the intervention. Involvement of family members with the team has not been examined. Clearly, this is an important focus of research requiring more rigorous designs than have previously been used.

Lujan, Ostwald, and Ortiz (2007) conducted a study of the effectiveness of an interdisciplinary team using a diabetes intervention. The following abstract describes the study.

■ *ABSTRACT*

Purpose: The purpose of this randomized controlled trial is to determine the effectiveness of an intervention led by promotoras (community lay workers) on the glycemic control, diabetes knowledge, and diabetes health beliefs of Mexican Americans with type 2 diabetes living in a major city on the Texas-Mexico border.

Methods: One hundred fifty Mexican American participants were recruited at a Catholic faith-based clinic and randomized into 2 groups. Personal characteristics, acculturation, baseline hemoglobin A1C level, diabetes knowledge, and diabetes health beliefs were measured. The intervention was culturally specific and consisted of participative group education, telephone contact, and follow-up using inspirational faith-based health behavior change postcards. The A1C levels, diabetes knowledge, and diabetes health beliefs were measured 3 and 6 months postbaseline, and the mean change between the groups was analyzed.

Results: The 80% female sample, with a mean age of 58 years, demonstrated low acculturation, income, education, health insurance coverage, and strong Catholicism. No significant changes were noted at the 3-month assessment, but the mean change of the A1C levels, $F(1, 148) = 10.28, p < 0.001$, and the diabetes knowledge scores, $F(1, 148) = 9.0, p < 0.002$, of the intervention group improved significantly at 6 months, adjusting for health insurance coverage. The health belief scores decreased in both groups.

Conclusions: The intervention resulted in decreased A1C levels and increased diabetes knowledge, suggesting that using promotoras as part of an interdisciplinary team can result in positive outcomes for Mexican Americans who have type 2 diabetes. Clinical implications and recommendations for future research are suggested. (Lujan et al., 2007, pp. 660–670)

Geographical Analyses

Geographical analyses examine variations in health status, health services, patterns of care, or patterns of use by geographical area and are sometimes referred to as small area analyses. Variations may be associated with sociodemographic, economic, medical, cultural, or behavioral characteristics. Locality-specific factors of a health care system, such as capacity, access, and convenience, may play a role in explaining variations. The social setting, environment, living conditions, and community may also be important factors.

The interactions between the characteristics of a locality and of its inhabitants are complex. The characteristics of the total community may transcend the characteristics of individuals within the community and may influence subgroup behavior. High educational levels in the community are commonly associated with greater access to information and receptiveness to ideas from outside the community.

Regression analyses are commonly used to develop models using all the risk factors and the characteristics of the community. Results are often displayed through the use of maps (Kieffer, Alexander, & Mor, 1992). After the analysis, the researcher must determine whether differences in rates are due to chance alone and whether high rates are too high. From a more theoretical perspective, the researcher must then explain the geographical variation uncovered by the analysis (Volinn, Diehr, Ciol, & Loeser, 1994).

Geographical information systems (GISs) can provide an important tool for performing geographical analyses. A GIS uses relational databases to facilitate processing of spatial information. The software tools in a GIS can be used for mapping, data summaries, and analysis of spatial relationships. GISs have the capability of modeling data flows so that the effect of proposed changes in interventions applied to individuals or communities on outcomes can be modeled (Auffrey, 1998).

Metzel and Giordano (2007) conducted a geographical analysis of the locations of employment services and people with disabilities. The following abstract describes the study.

■ *ABSTRACT*

Vocational Rehabilitation (VR) services and One-Stop Career Centers (One-Stops) are the 2 principal public services intended to increase the employment rates of people with disabilities through employment and training services. As a first step in assessing accessibility of the locations of employment services, this study compared the location of VRs and One-Stops with areas of high numbers of nonemployment among people with disabilities and high numbers of unemployment in the general population. Using geographic information science and the spatial technique of the Local Indicators of Spatial Association (LISA), we analyzed the locations of the 2 programs and the concentrations of nonemployed people with disabilities at national and intrastate scales. We found that areas with high numbers of nonemployed people with disabilities are geographically underserved by both VRs and One-Stops, which raises questions about site selection and geographic accessibility. (Metzel & Giordano, 2007, pp. 88–97)

Economic Studies

Many of the problems studied in health services research address concerns related to the efficient use of scarce resources and, thus, to economics. Health economists are concerned with the costs and benefits of alternative treatments or ways of identifying the most efficient means of care. The economist's definition of *efficiency* is the least expensive method of achieving a desired end while obtaining the maximum benefit from available resources. If available resources must be shared with other programs or other types of patients, an economic study can determine whether changing the distribution of resources will increase total benefit or welfare.

To determine the efficiency of a treatment, the economist conducts a cost-effectiveness analysis. This technique uses a single measure of outcomes, and all other factors are expressed in monetary terms as net cost per unit of output (Ludbrook, 1990). Cost-effectiveness analyses compare different ways of accomplishing a clinical goal, such as diagnosing a condition, treating an illness, or providing a service. The alternative approaches are compared in terms of costs and benefits. The purpose is to identify the strategy that provides the most value for the money. There are always trade-offs between costs and benefits (Oster, 1988). Stone (1998) described the methodology for performing a cost-effectiveness analysis.

It is time for nurses to take a more active role in conducting cost-effectiveness research. Nurses are well positioned to evaluate health care practices and have the incentive to conduct the studies. Nursing practice is seldom a subject of cost-effectiveness analyses. The knowledge gained from this effort could enable nurses to refine their practice by substituting interventions that maximize nurses' time to the best advantage, in terms of the patient's health, for interventions that offer less gain (Siegel, 1998).

As Lieu and Newman (1998) have pointed out:

"Cost-effective" does not necessarily mean "cost-saving" (Doubilet, Weinstein, & McNeil, 1986). Many health interventions, even preventive ones, do not save money (Tengs et al., 1995). Rather, a service should be called cost-effective if its benefits are judged worth the costs. Recently, a consensus panel supported by the National Institutes of Health published recommendations that define standards for conducting cost-effectiveness analysis (Gold, Siegel, Russell, & Weinstein, 1996). Cost-effectiveness analysis is only one of several methods that can be used for the economic evaluation of health services (Drummond, Stoddart, & Torrance, 1987). Although these methods are useful, an intervention cannot be cost-effective without being effective. (Lieu & Newman, 1998, p. 1043)

To examine overall benefits, researchers perform a cost-benefit analysis. With this method, the costs and benefits of alternative ways of using resources are assessed in monetary terms, and the use that produces the greatest net benefit is chosen. The costs included in an economic study are defined in exact ways. The actual costs associated with an activity, not prices, must be used. Cost is not the same as price. In most cases, price is greater than cost. Costs are a measure of the actual use of resources rather than the price charged. Charges are a poor reflection of actual costs. Costs that might be included in a cost-benefit analysis are costs to the provider, costs to third-party payers (e.g., insurance), out-of-pocket costs, and opportunity costs.

Out-of-pocket *costs* are expenses incurred by the patient or family or both that are not reimbursable by the insurance company; they include costs of buying supplies, dressings, medications, and special food, transportation expenses, and unreimbursable care expenses.

Opportunity costs are lost opportunities that the patient, family member, or others experience. For example, a family member might have been able to earn more money if he or she had not had to stay home to care for the patient. The child might have been able to advance her education if she had not had to drop out of school for a semester to care for a parent. A husband might have been able to take a better job if the family could have moved to another town rather than stay in place to enable a member to receive specific medical care.

Opportunity costs are often not included in overall costs. This omission results in an underestimation of costs and an overestimation of benefit. For example, one can demonstrate that caring for an acutely ill patient at home is cost-effective if one does not consider out-of-pocket costs and opportunity costs. However, the total costs of providing the care, regardless of who pays or who receives the money, must be included. In performing such a study, it is important to state whose costs are being considered and who is to weigh the benefits against the consequences.

Allred, Arford, Mauldin, and Goodwin (1998) critiqued the seven nursing studies between 1992 and 1996 in which cost-effectiveness analyses were performed. They found these studies to be equivalent in quality to those from other disciplines. They concluded that more emphasis must be placed on cost-effectiveness analyses in nursing research, and they provided guidelines for conducting these studies.

Stone (1998) has described the recommended guidelines for journal reports of cost-effectiveness analyses. Cost-effectiveness studies should be used as aids in decision making rather than as the end decision. If a cost-effectiveness study is conducted to inform those who make resource allocation decisions, a standard reference case should be presented to allow the decision makers to compare a proposed new health intervention with existing practice.

Mason, Freemantle, Gibson, and New (2005) conducted an economic analysis of the SPLINT clinical trial. The following is an abstract of that study.

■ ABSTRACT

Objective: To determine the cost-effectiveness of specialist nurse-led clinics provided to improve lipid and blood pressure control in diabetic patients receiving hospital-based care.

Research Design and Methods: A policy of targeting improved care through specialist nurse-led clinics is evaluated using a novel method, linking the cost-effectiveness of antihypertensive and lipid-lowering treatments with the cost and level of behavioral change achieved by the specialist nurse-led clinics. Treatment cost-effectiveness is modeled from the U.K. Prospective Diabetes Study and Heart Protection Study treatment trials, whereas specialist nurse-led clinics are evaluated using the Specialist Nurse-Led Clinics to Improve Control of Hypertension and Hyperlipidemia in Diabetes (SPLINT) trial.

Results: Good lipid and blood pressure control are cost-effective treatment goals for patients with diabetes. Modeling findings from treatment trials, blood pressure lowering is estimated to be cost saving and life prolonging (−1,400 dollars/quality-adjusted life-year [QALY]), whereas lipid-lowering is estimated to be highly cost-effective (8,230 dollars/QALY). Investing in nurse-led clinics to help achieve these benefits imposes an addition on treatment cost-effectiveness leading to higher estimates: 4,020 dollars/QALY and 19,950 dollars/QALY, respectively. For both clinics combined, the estimated cost-effectiveness is 9,070 dollars/QALY. Using an acceptability threshold of 50,000 dollars/QALY, the likelihood that blood pressure-lowering clinics are cost-effective is 77%, lipid clinics 99%, and combined clinics 83%.

Conclusions: A method is described for evaluating the cost-effectiveness of policies to change patient uptake of health care. Such policies are less attractive than treatment cost-effectiveness (which implies cost-less self-implementation). However, specialist nurse-led clinics, as an adjunct to hospital-based diabetic care, combining both lipid and blood pressure control, appear effective and likely to provide excellent value for money. (Mason et al., 2005, pp. 40–46)

Ethical Studies

Outcomes studies often lead to policies for allocating scarce resources. Ethicists take the position that moral principles, such as justice, constrain the use of costs and benefits to choose treatments that might maximize the benefit per unit cost. Value commitments are inherent in choices about research methods and about the selection and interpretation of outcome variables, and researchers should acknowledge these commitments. "The choices researchers make should be documented and the reasons for those choices should be given explicitly in publications and presentations so that readers and other users of the information are enabled and expected to bear more responsibility for interpreting and applying the findings appropriately" (Lynn & Virnig, 1995, p. AS292). Veatch (1993) proposed that by analyzing the implications of rationing decisions in terms of the principles of justice and autonomy, we would establish more acceptable criteria than we would by using outcomes predictors alone. As an example, Veatch performed an ethical analysis of the use of outcome predictors in decisions related to the early withdrawal of life support. Ethical studies should play an important role in outcomes programs of research.

Schwartz (2004) performed an ethical analysis of postmortem sperm retrieval. The following is an abstract of that analysis.

■ *ABSTRACT*

Reproductive technologists are developing new and more powerful means to assist reproduction, including postmortem sperm retrieval. This rapid technological development could lead to ethical concerns for nurses and nurse practitioners. In this article, I will present an overview of relevant literature and discussion of postmortem sperm retrieval. Topics discussed include the postmortem sperm retrieval process, public awareness of this process, ethical theories and principles related to this process, and case law related to this process. With the availability of increasingly complex and advanced reproductive technologies, including postmortem sperm retrieval, nurses and nurse practitioners need knowledge about the legal and ethical principles and the ramifications involved in this issue. (Schwartz, 2004, pp. 183–188)

Measurement Methods

The selection of appropriate outcome variables is critical to the success of a study (Bernstein & Hilborne, 1993). As in any study, the researcher must evaluate the evidence of validity and the reliability of the measurement methods. Outcomes selected for nursing studies should be those most consistent with nursing practice and theory (Harris & Warren, 1995). In some studies, rather than selecting the final outcome of care, which may not occur for months or years, researchers use measures of intermediate end points. *Intermediate end points* are events or markers that act as precursors to the final outcome. It is important, however, to document the validity of the intermediate end point in predicting the outcome (Freedman & Schatzkin, 1992). In early outcomes studies, researchers selected outcome measures that they could easily obtain rather than those most desirable for outcomes studies.

Table 12-6 identifies characteristics important to evaluate in selecting methods of measuring outcomes. In evaluating a particular outcome measure, the researcher should consult the literature for previous studies that have used that particular method of measurement, including the publication describing development of the method of measurement. Information related to the measurement can be organized into a table such as Table 12-7, which allows others to easily compare several methods of measuring a particular outcome.

Outcomes researchers are moving away from classic measurement theory as a means of evaluating the reliability of measurement methods. They are interested in identifying change in measures over time in a subject, and instruments developed through the use of classical measurement theory are often not sensitive to these changes. It is also important to determine the magnitude of change that can be detected. In addition, measures may detect change within a particular range of values but may not be sensitive to changes outside that range. The sensitivity to change of many commonly used outcome measures has not been examined (Deyo & Carter, 1992; Felson, Anderson, & Meenan, 1990). Studies must be conducted specifically to determine the sensitivity of measures before they are used in outcomes studies. As the sensitivity of a measure increases, statistical power increases, allowing smaller sample sizes to detect significant differences.

Creative methods of collecting data on instruments for large outcomes studies must be explored. In a busy office or clinic setting, the typical strategy of having clerks or other staff administer questionnaires or scales to patients is time intensive and costly and may result in lost data. Greist et al. (1997) recommended using

TABLE 12-6 ▪ ▪ Characteristics of Outcomes Assessment Instruments

Characteristic	Considerations in Patient Outcomes Evaluation	References

Applicability	Consider purpose of instruments
	Discriminate between subjects at a point in time Predict future outcomes
	Evaluate changes within subjects over time
	Screen for problems
	Provide case-mix adjustment
	Assess quality of care
	Consider whether
	Norms are established for clinical population of interest
	Instrument format is compatible with assessment approach (e.g., observer rated versus self-administered)
	Setting in which instrument was developed
		Deyo & Carter, 1992
		Stewart et al., 1989
		Guyatt, Walter, &
		  Norman, 1987
		Feinstein, Josephy, &
		  Wells, 1986
		Deyo, 1984

Practicality
(clinical utility)
	The instrument:
	Includes outcomes important to the patient
	Is short and easy to administer (low respondent burden)
	Questions are easy to understand and acceptable to patients and interviewers
	Scores reflect condition severity, condition-specific features, and discriminate those with conditions from those without
	Is easily scored and scores are readily understandable
	Level of measurement allows a change score to be determined
	Provides information that is clinically useful
	Performance or capacity based
	Includes patient rating of magnitude of effort and support needed for performance of physical tasks
		Leidy, 1991
		Nelson, Landgraf, Hays,
		  Wasson, & Kirk, 1990
		Stewart et al., 1989
		Lohr, 1988
		Bombardier &
		  Tugwell, 1987
		Feinstein et al., 1986
		Kirshner & Guyatt, 1985
		Deyo, 1984

Comprehensive- ness	Generic measures are designed to summarize a spectrum of concepts applied to different impairments, illnesses, patients, and populations Disease-specific measures are designed to assess specific patients with specific conditions or diagnoses Dimensions of the instrument; a core set of physical, mental, and role function desirable	Nelson et al., 1990 Patrick & Deyo, 1989 Deyo, 1984
Reliability	Can be influenced by day-to-day variations in patients, differences between observers, items in the scale, mode of administration This is the critical determinant of usefulness of an instrument Designed for discriminative purpose	Nelson et al., 1990 Spitzer, 1987 Guyatt , Walter, & Norman, 1987 Deyo, 1984
Validity	No consensus of what are scientifically admissible criteria for many indices No "gold standard" exists for establishing criterion validity for many indices	Spitzer, 1987 Deyo, 1984

Responsiveness	Not yet indexed for virtually any evaluative measures
	Coarse scale rating may not detect changes
	Aggregated scores may obscure changes in subscales
	Useful for determining sample size and statistical power
	Reliable instruments are likely to be responsive but reliability not adequate as sole index of consistent results over time
	Consider detail in scaling
	As baseline variability of score changes within stable subjects, may need larger treatment effects to demonstrate efficacy
	Consider temporal relationship between intervention and outcome
		Stewart & Archbold, 1992
		Leidy, 1991
		Jaeschke, Singer, &
		  Guyatt, 1989
		Bombardier &
		  Tugwell, 1987
		Guyatt, Walter, &
		  Norman, 1987
		Deyo & Centor, 1986
		Deyo, 1984

From Harris M. R., & Warren, J. J. (1995). Patient outcomes: Assessment issues for the CNS. *Clinical Nurse Specialist, 9*(2), 82.

the computer and the telephone to collect such data. Computers containing the instrument can be placed in locations convenient to patients, so the instrument can be completed with a minimum of staff involvement.

Another option is telephone interviews using the computer. The traditional telephone method of using interviewers to ask questions is costly. However, the same interactive voice response (IVR) technology used in voicemail can be used in telephone interviewing by computer. Interactive voice response allows the patient to respond to yes-no and multiple-choice questions by pressing numbers on the keypad or by saying "yes" or "no" or a number from 0 to 9. Patients can record answers in their own voices.

TABLE **12-7** Characteristics of the Katz Activities of Daily Living (ADL) Scale: A Proposed Outcome Instrument	
Characteristic	**References**
Applicability	
Purpose is to objectively evaluate results of treatment in chronically ill and aging populations	Katz, Downs, Cash, & Grotz, 1970
Used in case-mix adjustments	Fries, 1990
Scale discriminates well on disability in elderly population, norms easily referenced	Spector, 1990
Ratings judgment based on direct observation and caregiver reports, known differences in observed vs. reported ratings	Spector, 1990
Practicality	Katz et al., 1970
Brief, 6 items with 3 levels of dependency	
Can be used by clinicians and non-clinicians	Spector, 1990
Measures performance (not ability)	Katz et al., 1970
Aggregate score represents increasing level of dependency	Spector, 1990
Comprehensiveness	Katz et al., 1970
Includes bathing, dressing, toileting, transfer, continence, and eating	
Does not explain etiology of level of performance	Kane & Bayer, 1991
Generic measure (not disease-specific)	
Reliability	Kane & Bayer, 1991
Performance may be influenced by motivational, social, and environmental factors	
High internal consistency reported	Spector, 1990
Validity	Spector, 1990
Content and construct validity assessments are acceptable	
Responsiveness	
No published reports that quantify relationship of scale change to minimal clinically important change	

From Harris M. R., & Warren, J. J. (1995). Patient outcomes: Assessment issues for the CNS. *Clinical Nurse Specialist, 9*(2), 85.

Measuring the frequency and nature of care activities of various staff has been problematic in studies where the goal is to evaluate the process of care. Strategies commonly used are chart review, time and motion studies, work sampling, and retrospective recall. None of these is a satisfactory indicator of the actual care (Hale, Thomas, Bond, & Todd, 1997). Holmes, Teresi, Lindeman, and Glandon (1997) recommended the use of barcode methodology to measure service inputs. The barcodes capture what care is provided, for whom, by whom, and at what time. Barcoded service sheets and a portable barcode reader are used with an accompanying database management system.

Analysis of Measurement Reliability

Estimating the reliability of outcome measures through the use of classic measurement theory may be problematic. The traditional concept of measurement reliability was developed to evaluate quantities that were not expected to change over time in an individual. This assessment of reliability is irrelevant, or only partially relevant, to assessing the suitability or precision of measures selected because of their sensitivity to change within the individual over time.

Traditional evaluations of measurement methods assume that any change in group values is a result of variation among individuals. Patient change, however, results in changes within one individual. With classical measurement theory analysis, a measure that did not vary among individuals would have zero (or poor) reliability. This measure, however, may be an excellent measure of change over time if individuals change on that measure (even if group averages do not change much). Thus, it is inappropriate to assess the reliability of difference scores according to the internal consistency of measures (Collins & Johnston, 1995).

In some outcomes studies, measures obtained from individuals are used as indicators of characteristics of a group. The data from the measures are aggregated to reflect the group. In this case, the researcher must assess the extent to which the responses represent the group. Although the group mean is usually expected to serve this purpose, it may not adequately represent the group. Verran, Mark, and Lamb (1992) described techniques that can be employed to examine the psychometric properties of instruments used to describe group-level phenomena. Items of the instrument should be assessed for content validity to determine how well they measure group-level concepts. Reliability and validity must be assessed at the aggregated level rather than the individual level.

Commonly, multiple outcomes measures are used in outcomes studies. Researchers wish to evaluate all relevant effects of care. However, quantity of measures is not necessarily evidence of the quality of the measures. The measures most relevant to the treatment should be selected. Measures selected should not be closely correlated. Interpreting the results of studies in which multiple outcomes have been used can be problematic. For example, Felson et al. (1990, p. 141) asked, "Which is the better therapy, the one that shows a change in 6 outcome measures out of 12 tested or the one that shows a change in 4 of the 12 measures? What if the 4 that demonstrate change with one therapy are not the same as the 6 that show a change in another therapy?" If multiple comparisons are made, it is important to make statistical adjustments for them; the risk of a type I error is greater when multiple comparisons are made.

Some researchers recommend combining various measures into a single summary score (DesHarnais, McMahon, & Wroblewski, 1991; Felson et al., 1990). However, such global composite measures have not been widely used. The various measures used in such an index may not be equally weighted and may be difficult to combine. Also, clinicians may not readily interpret the composite index value.

The focus of most measures developed for outcomes studies has been the individual patient. However, a number of organizations are now developing measures of the quality of performance of systems of care. In 1990, the Consortium Research on Indicators of System Performance (CRISP) project began to develop indicators of the quality of performance of integrated delivery systems. From the perspective of CRISP, the success of a health system is associated with its ability to decrease the number of episodes of diseases in the population. Therefore, the impact of the delivery system on the community is considered an important measure of performance. CRISP has developed a number of indicators now in use by consortium members, who pay to participate in the studies (Bergman, 1994).

The Joint Commission is also applying outcomes data to quality management efforts in hospitals using the Indicator Measurement System (IMSystem) (McCormick, 1990; Nadzim, Turpin, Hanold, & White, 1993). The National Committee for Quality Assurance, the organization that accredits managed care plans, has developed a tool (HEDIS) for comparing managed care plans. Comparisons involve more than 60 measures, including patient satisfaction, quality of care, and financial stability (Guadagnoli & McNeil, 1994). Researchers

at the Henry Ford Health Systems' Center for Health System Studies in Detroit have evolved 80 performance indicators to evaluate health systems (Anderson, 1991).

Statistical Methods for Outcomes Studies

Although outcomes researchers test for statistical significance of their findings, this is not considered sufficient to judge the findings as important. Their focus is the clinical significance of study findings (see Chapter 18 for more information on clinical significance). In analyzing data, outcomes researchers have moved away from statistical analyses that use the mean to test for group differences. They place greater importance on analyzing change scores and use exploratory methods for examining the data to identify outliers.

Analysis of Change

With the focus on outcomes studies has come a renewed interest in methods of analyzing change. Gottman and Rushe (1993) reported that the first book addressing change in research, *Problems in Measuring Change* edited by Harris (1967), is the basis for most current approaches to analyzing change. Since then, a number of new ideas have emerged regarding the analysis of change (e.g., in studies by Collins & Horn, 1991; Rovine & Von Eye, 1991; Von Eye, 1990a, 1990b). However, many researchers are unfamiliar with these new ideas and continue to base their reasoning on Harris's 1967 book. Gottman and Rushe (1993) suggested that many beliefs related to the analysis of change are based on little more than the following fallacies:

Fallacy 1: In change, regression toward the mean is an unavoidable law of nature.
Fallacy 2: The difference score between premeasurement and postmeasurement is unreliable.
Fallacy 3: Analysis of covariance (ANCOVA, or related methods such as path analysis) is the way to analyze change.
Fallacy 4: Two points (pretest and posttest) are adequate for the study of change.
Fallacy 5: The correlation between change and initial level is always negative.

Outcomes researchers are also questioning the method of analyzing change. Collins and Johnston (1995) have suggested that the recommended analysis method of regressing pretest scores on outcome scores and basing the analysis of change on residual change scores is overly conservative and tends to understate the extent of real change. There are serious questions about the conceptual meaning of these residual change scores.

For some outcomes, the changes may be nonlinear or may go up and down rather than always increasing. Thus, it is as important to uncover patterns of change as it is to test for statistically significant differences at various time points. Some changes may occur in relation to stages of recovery or improvement. These changes may occur over weeks, months, or even years. A more complete picture of the process of recovery can be obtained by examining the process in greater detail and over a broader range. With this approach, the examiner can develop a recovery curve, which provides a model of the recovery process and can then be tested (Collins & Johnston, 1995; Ottenbacher, Johnson, & Hojem, 1995).

Analysis of Improvement
In addition to reporting the mean improvement score for all patients treated, it is important to report what percentage of patients improve. Do all patients improve slightly, or is there a divergence among patients, with some improving greatly and others not improving at all? This divergence may best be illustrated by plotting the data. Researchers studying a particular treatment or approach to care might develop a standard or index of varying degrees of improvement that might occur. The index would allow better comparisons of the effectiveness of various treatments. Characteristics of patients who experience varying degrees of improvement should be described, and outliers should be carefully examined. This step requires that the study design include baseline measures of patient status, such as demographic characteristics, functional status, and disease severity measures. An analysis of improvement will allow better judgments of the appropriate use of various treatments (Felson et al., 1990).

Variance Analysis
Variance analysis is used to track individual and group variance from a specific critical pathway. The goal is to decrease preventable variance in process, thus helping patients and their families achieve optimal outcomes. Some of the variance is due to comorbidities. You may find that keeping a patient with comorbidities on the desired pathway may require you to utilize more resources early in the patient's care. Thus, it is important to track both variance and comorbidities. Studies examining variations from pathways may make it easier for health care providers to tailor existing critical pathways for specific comorbidities.

Variance analysis can also be used to identify at-risk patients who might benefit from the services of a case manager. Variance analysis tracking is expressed through the use of graphics, and the expected pathway is plotted on the graph. The care providers plot deviations (negative variance) on the graph, allowing

immediate comparison with the expected pathway. Deviations may be related to the patient, the system, or the provider (Tidwell, 1993).

Longitudinal Guttman Simplex Model
The longitudinal Guttman simplex (LGS) model is an extension of the Guttman scale that involves times, as well as items and persons. For example, an LGS model of mobility might involve the following items:
   M1: moving unassisted from bed to chair
   M2: moving unassisted from bed to another room
   M3: moving unassisted up stairs
Table 12-8 shows hypothetical data collected with this measure on three patients at three periods, showing a pattern of improving ability over time (Collins & Johnston, 1995).

Latent Transition Analysis
Latent transition analysis (LTA) is used in situations in which stages or categories of recovery have been defined and transitions between stages can be identified. To use the analysis method, the researchers assign each member of the population in a single category or stage for a given point of time. However, stage membership changes over time. The analysis tests stage membership to provide a realistic picture of development. Collins and Johnston (1995) described an example of this type of analysis with a hypothetical model of recovery from functional neglect after stroke.

TABLE 12-8	Sample Data Using Longitudinal Guttman Scale		
	Functional Items		
	M1	**M2**	**M3**
Patient A			
Time 1	Fail	Fail	Fail
Time 2	Pass	Fail	Fail
Time 3	Pass	Pass	Fail
Patient B			
Time 1	Fail	Fail	Fail
Time 2	Pass	Pass	Fail
Time 3	Pass	Pass	Fail
Patient C			
Time 1	Pass	Fail	Fail
Time 2	Pass	Pass	Fail
Time 3	Pass	Pass	Pass

From Collins, L. M., & Johnston, M. V. (1995). Analysis of stage-sequential change in rehabilitation research. *American Journal of Physical Medicine and Rehabilitation, 74*(2), 167.
M1, Moving unassisted from bed to chair; *M2,* moving unassisted from bed to another room; *M3,* moving unassisted up stairs.

Let's assume that we can define a study subpopulation displaying four latent stages or types of functional neglect: sensory limitations (S), cognitive limitations (C), both (S and C) or patients may recover and adapt to the point that they are functional (F). ... Membership in each category is inferred from several clinical symptoms or test items, which supposedly go together but in fact may not for some patients. The items have some error and are imperfect indicators of true (latent) stage membership. Our objective is to estimate in which category a patient probably falls at any point in time and the probability of movement between stages over time, conditional on previous stage membership....Suppose we use a large number of times periodically to monitor progress, testing the same group of patients at multiple points in time. We record which items the patient passes and which the patient does not. (p. 47)

After the use of a computerized program designed to perform latent transition analysis, the researchers obtained the results (Table 12-9). Only two points of time are shown here, although the program can handle up to five points in time.

The first line of the table contains the estimate of the proportion of patients in each of the four stages at Time 1. In this example, 30% of the sample had both S and C limitations, 30% had S limitations, and 40%

TABLE **12-9** ▪▪ A Hypothetical Latent Transition Model of Recovery from Neglect Following Stroke				
	Latent Status			
	F	C	S	S and C
Total Marginal Proportions				
Time 1 proportions	0.0	0.40	0.30	0.30
Time 2 proportions	0.27	0.25	0.30	0.18
	Time 2 Latent Status			
Time 1 Latent Status	**F***	**C**	**S**	**S and C**
Time 1 to Time 2 Transition *Proportions with Rows*				
Functional (F)	0	0	0	0
Cognitive limitation (C)	0.46	0.54	0.0	0.0
Sensory limitation (S)	0.30	0.0	0.70	0.0
S and C	0.0	0.10	0.30	0.60

From Collins, L. M., & Johnston, M. V. (1995). Analysis of stage-sequential change in rehabilitation research. *American Journal of Physical Medicine and Rehabilitation, 74*(2), 168.
* No patients were functional at time 1.

had C limitations, and none was functional. At Time 2, the proportion in each functional limitation appears to have declined, except sensory limitations, which is unchanged, and 27% are now in the functional stage. The bottom half of the table is a matrix of transition probabilities that reveals patterns of change. Of patients who started with S, 30% improved; however, the overall percentage at S remained the same because 30% of the patients who started at S and C moved to the S category. Of patients who initially had C problems alone, 46% moved to the functional category.

A third set of quantities estimated by the full latent transition analysis model but not shown in the table are the relationships between items and stage memberships. This relationship indicates the probability that when a subject moves from one category to another, each item will also change to reflect the new stage membership. Thus, this relationship determines the effectiveness of the test items or clinical symptoms as indicators of stage membership.

Multilevel Analysis

Multilevel analysis is used in epidemiology to study how environmental factors (aggregate-level characteristics) and individual attributes and behaviors (individual-level characteristics) interact to influence individual-level health behaviors and disease risks. For example, the risk that an adolescent will start smoking is associated with the following variables: (1) attributes of the child (e.g., self-esteem, academic achievement, refusal skills), (2) attributes of the child's family (e.g., parental attitudes toward smoking, smoking behavior of parents), (3) general characteristics of the community (e.g., ease of minors' access to cigarettes, school policies regarding smoking, city smoking ordinances, social norms of students toward smoking), and (4) general social factors (e.g., geographical region, economic policies that influence the price of cigarettes). The researchers might ask, "Does smoking status covary with the level of restriction of smoking in public places after we have controlled for the individual-level variables that influence smoking risks?" (Von Korff, Koepsell, Curry, & Diehr, 1992).

DISSEMINATING OUTCOMES RESEARCH FINDINGS

Including plans for the dissemination of findings as a component of a program of research is a new idea within nursing, if one considers the process of dissemination to be more than publishing the results in professional journals. As we discuss in Unit Three of this text, strategies for the dissemination of research findings tend to be performed by groups other than the original researchers. The transfer of knowledge from nurse researchers to nurse clinicians has been, for the most part, ineffective.

Nursing, as a discipline, has not yet addressed the various constituencies for nursing research knowledge. A research team conducting a program of outcomes research must identify its constituencies. These should include (1) the clinicians, who will apply the knowledge to practice; (2) the public, who may make health care decisions on the basis of the information; (3) health care institutions, which must evaluate care in their facilities on the basis of the information; (4) health policy makers, who may set standards on the basis of the information; and (5) researchers, who may use the information in designing new studies. Disseminating information to these various constituencies through presentations at meetings and publications in a wide diversity of journals and magazines, as well as releasing the information to the news media, requires careful planning. Mattson and Donovan (1994) suggested that dissemination involves strategies for debunking myths, addressing issues related to feasibility, communicating effectively, and identifying opinion leaders.

SUMMARY

- Outcomes research examines the end results of patient care.
- The scientific approaches used in outcomes studies differ in some important ways from those used in traditional research.
- Donabedian (1987) developed the theory on which outcomes research is based.
- Quality is the overriding construct of the theory, although Donabedian never defined this concept.
- The three major concepts of the theory are health, subjects of care, and providers of care.
- Donabedian identified three objects of evaluation in appraising quality: structure, process, and outcome.
- The goal of outcomes research is to evaluate outcomes as defined by Donabedian, whose theory requires that identified outcomes be clearly linked with the process that caused the outcome.
- Clinical guideline panels are developed to incorporate available evidence on health outcomes.
- Outcome studies provide rich opportunities to build a stronger scientific underpinning for nursing practice.

- A nursing-sensitive patient outcome is "sensitive" because it is influenced by nursing.
- Organizations currently involved in efforts to study nursing-sensitive outcomes include the American Nurses Association, the National Quality Forum (NQF), the California Nursing Outcomes Coalition, the Veterans Affairs Nursing Outcomes Database, the Center for Medicare and Medicaid Services' (CMS) Hospital Quality Initiative, the American Hospital Association, the Federation of American Hospitals, the Joint Commission on Accreditation of Healthcare Organizations, and the Agency of Healthcare Research and Quality.
- Another interest in terms of outcome research is what happens during the process of advanced practice nurses care.
- Practice-based research networks (PBRNs) are a group of practices that focus on patient care and are affiliated in order to analyze their clinical practices in communities.
- Outcome designs tend to have less control than traditional research designs and, except for the clinical trial, seldom use random samples; rather, they use large representative samples.
- Statistical approaches used in outcomes studies include new approaches to examining measurement reliability, strategies to analyze change, and the analysis of improvement.

REFERENCES

Ahrens, T., Yancey, V., & Kollef, M. (2003). Improving family communications at the end of life: Implications for length of stay in the intensive care unit and resource use. *American Journal of Critical Care, 12*(4), 317–323.

Allred, C. A., Arford, P. H., Mauldin, P. D., & Goodwin, L. K. (1998). Cost-effectiveness analysis in the nursing literature, 1992–1996. *Image: Journal of Nursing Scholarship, 30*(3), 235–242.

Altimier, L. B., Eichel, M., Warner, B., Tedeschi, L., & Brown, B. (2004). Developmental care: Changing the NICU physically and behaviorally to promote patient outcomes and contain costs. *Neonatal Intensive Care, 17*(2), 35–39.

Anderko, L., Lundeen, S., & Bartz, C. (2006). The Midwest Nursing Centers Consortium Research Network: Translating research into practice. *Policy, Politics & Nursing Practice, 7*(2), 101–109.

Anderson, H. J. (1991). Sizing up systems: Researchers to test performance measures. *Hospitals, 65*(20), 33–34.

Auffrey, C. (1998). Geographic information systems as a tool for community health research and practice. *Nursing Research Methods*. Retrieved March 24, 2003, from www.nursing.uc.edu/nrm/AUFFREY51598.htm.

Bergman, R. (1994). Are my outcomes better than yours? *Hospital Health Network, 68*(15), 113–116.

Bergmark, A., & Oscarsson, L. (1991). Does anybody really know what they are doing? Some comments related to methodology of treatment service research. *British Journal of Addiction, 86*(2), 139–142.

Bernstein, S. J., & Hilborne, L. H. (1993). Clinical indicators: The road to quality care? *Joint Commission Journal on Quality Improvement, 19*(11), 501–509.

Bircumshaw, D., & Chapman, C. M. (1988). A study to compare the practice style of graduate and non-graduate nurses and midwives: The pilot study. *Journal of Advanced Nursing, 13*(5), 605–614.

Bombardier, C., & Tugwell, P. (1987). Methodological considerations in functional assessment. *Journal of Rheumatology, 14*(Suppl. 15), 7–10.

Bowles, K. H., & Baugh, A. C. (2007). Applying research evidence to optimize telehomecare. *Journal of Cardiovascular Nursing, 22*(1), 5–15.

Bradley, P., & Lindsay, B. (2007). Specialist epilepsy nurses for treating epilepsy. *Cochrane Database of Systematic Reviews,* (4), CD001907.

Brooten, D., Naylor, M. D., York, R., Brown, L. P., Munro, P. H., Hollingsworth, A. O., et al. (2002). Lessons learned from testing the quality cost model of advanced practice nursing (APN) transitional care. *Journal of Nursing Scholarship, 34*(4), 369–375.

Byers, V. L., Mays, M. Z., & Mark, D. D. (1999). Provider satisfaction in Army primary care clinics. *Military Medicine, 164*(2), 132–135.

Castle, N. G., & Engberg, J. (2007). The influence of staffing characteristics on quality of care in nursing homes. *Health Services Research, 42*(5), 1822–1847.

Challis, D., Clarkson, P., Williamson, J., Hughes, J., Venables, D., Burns, A., et al. (2004). The value of specialist clinical assessment of older people prior to entry to care homes. *Age & Ageing, 33*(1), 25–34.

Chaput de Saintonge, D. M., & Hattersley, L. A. (1985). Antibiotics for otitis media: Can we help doctors agree? *Family Practice, 2*(4), 205–212.

Chaput de Saintonge, D. M., Kirway, J. R., Evans, S. J., & Crane, G. J. (1988). How can we design trials to detect clinically important changes in disease severity? *British Journal of Clinical Pharmacology, 26*(4), 355–362.

Chisholm, D., Knapp, M., Astin, J., Audini, B., & Lelliott, B. (1997). The mental health residential care study: The "hidden costs" of provision. *Health & Social Care in the Community, 5*(3), 162–172.

Collins, L. M., & Horn, J. L. (1991). *Best methods for the analysis of change: Recent advances, unanswered questions, future directions.* Washington, DC: American Psychological Association.

Collins, L. M., & Johnston, M. V. (1995). Analysis of stage-sequential change in rehabilitation research. *American Journal of Physical Medicine and Rehabilitation, 74*(2),163–170.

Cólon-Emeric, C. S., Ammarell, N., Bailey, D., Corazzini, K., Lekan-Rutledge, D., Piven, M. L., et al. (2006). Patterns of medical and nursing staff communication in nursing homes: Implications and insights from complexity science. *Qualitative Health Research, 16*(2), 173–188.

Crane, V. S. (1988). Economic aspects of clinical decision making: Applications of clinical decision analysis. *American Journal of Hospital Pharmacy, 45*(3), 548–553.

Cunningham, R. S. (2004). Advanced practice nursing outcomes: A review of selected empirical literature. *Oncology Nursing Forum, 31*(2), 219–230.

Davis, K. (1990). Use of data registries to evaluate medical procedures: Coronary artery surgery study and the balloon valvuloplasty registry. *International Journal of Technology Assessment in Health Care, 6*(2), 203–210.

DesHarnais, S., McMahon, L. F., Jr., & Wroblewski, R. (1991). Measuring outcomes of hospital care using multiple risk-adjusted indexes. *HSR: Health Services Research, 26*(4), 425–445.

Deyo, R. A. (1984). Measuring functional outcomes in therapeutic trials for chronic disease. *Controlled Clinical Trials, 5*(3), 223–240.

Deyo, R. A., & Carter, W. B. (1992). Strategies for improving and expanding the application of health status measures in clinical settings. *Medical Care, 30*(5 Suppl.), MS176–M186.

Deyo, R. A., & Centor, R. M. (1986). Assessing the responsiveness of functional scales to clinical change: An analogy to diagnostic test performance. *Journal of Chronic Disease, 39*(11), 897–906.

Deyo, R. A., Taylor, V. M., Diehr, P., Conrad, D., Cherkin, D. C., Ciol, M., et al. (1994). Analysis of automated administrative and survey databases to study patterns and outcomes of care. *Spine, 19*(18 Suppl.), 2083S–2091S.

Donabedian, A. (1976). *Benefits in medical care programs.* Cambridge, MA: Harvard University Press.

Donabedian, A. (1978). *Needed research in quality assessment and monitoring.* Hyattsville, MD: U.S. Department of Health, Education, and Welfare, Public Health Service, National Center for Health Services Research.

Donabedian, A. (1980). *Explorations in quality assessment and monitoring.* Ann Arbor, MI: Health Administration Press.

Donabedian, A. (1982). *The criteria and standards of quality.* Ann Arbor, MI: Health Administration Press.

Donabedian, A. (1987). Some basic issues in evaluating the quality of health care. In L. T. Rinke (Ed.), *Outcome measures in home care* (Vol. I, pp. 3–28). New York: National League for Nursing. (Original work published 1976.)

Doubilet, P., Weinstein, M. C., & McNeil, B. H. (1986). Use and misuse of the term "cost effective" in medicine. *New England Journal of Medicine, 314*(4), 253–255.

Drummond, M. F., Stoddart, G. L., & Torrance, G. W. (1987). *Method for the economic evaluation of health care programs.* New York: Oxford University Press.

Evans, R. G., & Stoddart, G. L. (1990). Producing health, consuming health care. *Social Science and Medicine, 31*(12), 1347–1363.

Feinstein, A. R., Josephy, B. R., & Wells, C. K. (1986). Scientific and clinical problems in indexes of functional disability. *Annals of Internal Medicine, 105*(3), 413–420.

Felson, D. T., Anderson, J. J., & Meenan, R. F. (1990). Time for changes in the design, analysis, and reporting of rheumatoid arthritis clinical trials. *Arthritis and Rheumatism, 33*(1), 140–149.

Fowler, F. J., Jr., Cleary, P. D., Magaziner, J., Patrick, D. L., & Benjamin, K. L. (1994). Methodological issues in measuring patient-reported outcomes: The agenda of the work group on outcomes assessment. *Medical Care, 32*(7 Suppl.), JS65–JS76.

Freedman, L. S., & Schatzkin, A. (1992). Sample size for studying intermediate endpoints within intervention trials or observational studies. *American Journal of Epidemiology, 136*(9), 1148–1159.

Freund, D. A., Dittus, R. S., Fitzgerald, J., & Heck, D. (1990). Assessing and improving outcomes: Total knee replacement. *HSR: Health Services Research, 25*(5), 723–726.

Fries, B. E. (1990). Comparing case-mix systems for nursing home payment. *Health Care Financing Review, 11*(4), 103–119.

Fullerton, J. T., Hollenbach, K. A., & Wingard, D. L. (1996). Research exchange. Practice styles: A comparison of obstetricians and nurse-midwives. *Journal of Nurse-Midwifery, 41*(3), 243–250.

Geller, A. C., Oliveria, S. A., Bishop, M., Buckminster, M., Brooks, K. R., & Halpern, A. C. (2007). Study of health outcomes in school children: Key challenges and lessons learned from the Framingham Schools' Natural History of Nevi Study. *Journal of School Health, 77*(6), 312–318.

Given, B., & Sherwood, P. R. (2005). Nursing-sensitive patient outcomes: A white paper. *Oncology Nursing Forum, 32*(4), 773–784.

Gold, M. R., Siegel, J. E., Russell, L. B., & Weinstein, M. C. (Eds.). (1996). *Cost-effectiveness in health and medicine.* New York: Oxford University Press.

Goldberg, H. I., Cummings, M. A., Steinberg, E. P., Ricci, E. M., Shannon, T., Soumerai, S. B., et al. (1994). Deliberations on the dissemination of PORT products: Translating research findings into improved patient outcomes. *Medical Care, 32*(7 Suppl.), JS90–JS110.

Goldman, L. E., Vittinghoff, E., & Dudley, R. A. (2007). Quality of care in hospitals with a high percent of Medicaid patients. *Medical Care, 45*(6), 579–583.

Gottman, J. M., & Rushe, R. H. (1993). The analysis of change: Issues, fallacies, and new ideas. *Journal of Consulting and Clinical Psychology, 61*(6), 907–910.

Greene, R., Bondy, P. K., & Maklan, C. W. (1994). The national medical effectiveness research initiative. *Diabetes Care, 17*(Suppl. 1), 45–49.

Greist, J. H., Jefferson, J. W., Wenzel, K. W., Kobak, K. A., Bailey, T. M., Katzelnich, D. J., et al. (1997). The telephone assessment program: Efficient patient monitoring and clinician feedback. *M.D. Computing, 14*(5), 382–387.

Griffiths, P. D., Edwards, M. H., Forbes, A., Harris, R. L., & Ritchie, G. (2007). Effectiveness of intermediate care in nursing-led in-patient units. *Cochrane Database of Systematic Reviews,* (2), CD002214.

Guadagnoli, E., & McNeil, B. J. (1994). Outcomes research: Hope for the future or the latest rage? *Inquiry, 31*(1), 14–24.

Guess, H. A., Jacobsen, S. J., Girman, C. J., Oesterling, J. E., Chute, C. G., Panser, L. A., et al. (1995). The role of community-based longitudinal studies in evaluating treatment effects. Example: Benign prostatic hyperplasia. *Medical Care, 33*(4 Suppl.), AS26–AS35.

Guyatt, G., Walter, S., & Norman, G. (1987). Measuring change over time: Assessing the usefulness of evaluative instruments. *Journal of Chronic Disease, 40*(2), 171–178.

Hale, C. A., Thomas, L. H., Bond, S., & Todd, C. (1997). The nursing record as a research tool to identify nursing interventions. *Journal of Clinical Nursing, 6*(3), 207–214.

Haggerty, M. C., Stockdale-Woolley, R., & Nair, S. (1991). Respi-Care: An innovative home care program for the patient with chronic obstructive pulmonary disease. *Chest, 100*(3), 607–612.

Harper, R. W. (1992). *Care and cost effectiveness of the clinical care coordinator/patient care associate nursing case management model.* Unpublished doctoral dissertation, University of California, San Francisco.

Harris, C. W. (Ed.). (1967). *Problems in measuring change.* Madison: University of Wisconsin Press.

Harris, M. R., & Warren, J. J. (1995). Patient outcomes: Assessment issues for the CNS. *Clinical Nurse Specialist, 9*(2), 82–86.

Harris, R., Richardson, G., Griffiths, P., Hallett, N., Wilson-Barnett, J. (2005). Economic evaluation of a nursing-led inpatient unit: The impact of findings on management decisions of service utility and sustainability. *Journal of Nursing Management, 13*(5), 428–438.

Herrmann, D. (1995). Reporting current, past, and changed health status: What we know about distortion. *Medical Care, 33*(4 Suppl.), AS89–AS94.

Holmes, D., Teresi, J., Lindeman, D. A., & Glandon, G. L. (1997). Measurement of personal care inputs in chronic care settings. *Journal of Mental Health and Aging, 3*(1), 119–127.

Howell-White, S. (1997). Choosing a birth attendant: The influence of a woman's childbirth definition. *Social Science & Medicine, 45*(6), 925–936.

Hueston, W. J., & Lewis-Stevenson, S. (2001). Provider distribution and variations in statewide cesarean section rates. *Journal of Community Health, 26*(1), 1–10.

Hughes, L. C., Robinson, L. A., Cooley, M. E., Nuamah, I., Grobe, S. J., & McCorkle, R. (2002). Describing an episode of home nursing care for elderly postsurgical cancer patients. *Nursing Research, 51*(2), 110–118.

Ingersoll, G. L., McIntosh, E., & Williams, M. (2000). Nurse-sensitive outcomes of advanced practice. *Journal of Advanced Nursing, 32*(5), 1272–1282.

Jaeschke, R., Singer, J., & Guyatt, G. H. (1989). Measurement of health status: Ascertaining the minimal clinically important difference. *Controlled Clinical Trials, 10*(4), 407–415.

Jennings, B. M., Loan, L. A., DePaul, D., Brosch, L. R., & Hildreth, P. (2001). Lessons learned while collecting ANA indicator data. *Journal of Nursing Administration, 31*(3), 121–129.

Kane, R. A., & Bayer, A. J. (1991). Assessment of functional status. In M. S. J. Pathy (Ed.), *Principles and practices of geriatric medicine* (2nd ed., pp. 265–277). New York: Wiley.

Katz, S., Downs, T. D., Cash, H. R., & Grotz, R. C. (1970). Progress in the development of the Index of ADL. *Gerontologist, 10*(1), 20–30.

Kay, C. M. (1999). *Targeting cost containment efforts in Massachusetts nursing homes.* Unpublished doctoral dissertation, Brandeis University, The Florence Heller Graduate School for Advanced Studies in Social Welfare.

Keeler, E. B. (1994). Decision analysis and cost-effectiveness analysis in women's health care. *Clinical Obstetrics and Gynecology, 37*(1), 207–215.

Kieffer, E., Alexander, G. R., & Mor, J. (1992). Area-level predictors of use of prenatal care in diverse populations. *Public Health Reports, 107*(6), 653–658.

Kirshner, B., & Guyatt, G. (1985). A methodological framework for assessing health indices. *Journal of Chronic Diseases, 38*(1), 27–36.

Kirwan, J. R., Chaput de Saintonge, D. M., Joyce, C. R. B., Holmes, J., & Currey, H. L. F. (1986). Inability of rheumatologists to describe their true policies for assessing rheumatoid arthritis. *Annals of Rheumatic Diseases, 45*(2), 156–161.

Kleinpell, R., & Gawlinski, A. (2005). Assessing outcomes in advanced practice nursing practice: The use of quality indicators and evidence-based practice. *AACN Clinical Issues, 16*(1), 43–57.

Kramer, M., Maguire, P., & Schmalenberg, C. (2006). Excellence through evidence: The what, when, and where of clinical autonomy. *Journal of Nursing Administration, 36*(10), 479–491.

Lake, E. T. (2006). Multilevel models in health outcomes research Part I: Theory, design, and measurement. *Applied Nursing Research, 19*(1), 51–53.

Lange, L. L., & Jacox, A. (1993). Using large data bases in nursing and health policy research. *Journal of Professional Nursing, 9*(4), 204–211.

Lasker, R. D., Shapiro, D. W., & Tucker, A. M. (1992). Realizing the potential of practice pattern profiling. *Inquiry, 29*(3), 287–297.

Lee, T. H., & Goldman, L. (1989). Development and analysis of observational data bases. *Journal of the American College of Cardiology, 14*(3, Suppl. A), 44A–47A.

Leeper, B. (2004). Nursing outcomes: Percutaneous coronary interventions. *Journal of Cardiovascular Nursing, 19*(5), 346–353.

Leidy, N. K. (1991). Survey measures of functional ability and disability of pulmonary patients. In B. L. Metzger (Ed.), *Synthesis conference on altered functioning: Impairment and disability* (pp. 52–79). Indianapolis: Nursing Center Press of Sigma Theta Tau International.

Lewis, B. E. (1995). HMO outcomes research: Lessons from the field. *Journal of Ambulatory Care Management, 18*(1), 47–55.

Lieu, T. A., & Newman, T. B. (1998). Issues in studying the effectiveness of health services for children: Improving the quality of healthcare for children: An agenda for research. *HSR: Health Services Research, 4*(33), 1041–1058.

Lohr, K. N. (1988). Outcome measurement: Concepts and questions. *Inquiry, 25*(1), 37–50.

Ludbrook, A.(1990). Using economic appraisal in health services research. *Health Bulletin, 48*(2), 81–90.

Lujan, J., Ostwald, S. K., & Ortiz, M. (2007). Promotora diabetes intervention for Mexican Americans. *The Diabetes Educator, 33*(4), 660–670.

Lynn, J., & Virnig, B. A. (1995). Assessing the significance of treatment effects: Comments from the perspective of ethics. *Medical Care, 33*(4), AS292–AS298.

Mark, B. A. (1995). The black box of patient outcomes research. *Image: Journal of Nursing Scholarship, 27*(1), 42.

Mark, D. D., Byers, V. L., & Mays, M. Z. (2001). Primary care outcomes and provider practice styles. *Military Medicine, 166*(10), 875–880.

Mason, J. M., Freemantle, N., Gibson, J. M., & New, J. P. (2005). Specialist nurse-led clinics to improve control of hypertension and hyperlipidemia in diabetes: Economic analysis of the SPLINT trial. *Diabetes Care, 28*(1), 40–46.

Mattson, M. E., & Donovan, D. M. (1994). Clinical applications: The transition from research to practice. *Journal of Studies on Alcohol, 12*(Suppl.), 163–166.

McCloskey, B., Grey, M., Deshefy-Longhi, T., & Grey, L. (2003). APRN practice patterns in primary care. *Nurse Practitioner: American Journal of Primary Health Care, 28*(4), 39–44.

McCormick, B. (1990). Outcomes in action: The JCAHO's clinical indicators. *Hospitals, 64*(19), 34–38.

McDonald, C. J., & Hui, S. L. (1991). The analysis of humongous databases: Problems and promises. *Statistics in Medicine, 10*(4), 511–518.

McIsaac, C. (2005). Managing wound care outcomes. *Ostomy Wound Management, 51*(4), 54–56, 58, 60 passim.

McNeil, B. J., Pedersen, S. H., & Gatsonis, C. (1992). Current issues in profiling quality of care. *Inquiry, 29*(3), 298–307.

Metzel, D. S., & Giordano, A. (2007). Locations of employment services and people with disabilities: A geographical analysis of accessibility. *Journal of Disability Policy Studies, 18*(2), 88–97.

Mitchell, J. B., Bubolz, T., Pail, J. E., Pashos, C. L., Escarce, J. J., Muhlbaier, L. H., et al. (1994). Using Medicare claims for outcomes research. *Medical Care, 32*(7 Suppl.), JS38–JS51.

Mitchell, P. H., Ferketich, S., Jennings, B. M., & American Academy of Nursing Expert Panel on Quality Health Care. (1998). Quality health outcomes model, *Image: Journal of Nursing Scholarship, 30*(1), 43–46.

Mor, V. (2006). Defining and measuring quality outcomes in long term care. *Journal of the American Medical Directors Association, 7*(8), 532–538; discussion 532–540.

Morgan, D. G., Stewart, N. J., D'Arcy, K. C., & Werezak, L. J. (2004). Evaluating rural nursing home environments: Dementia special care units versus integrated facilities. *Aging & Mental Health, 8*(3), 25–265.

Moses, L. E. (1995). Measuring effects without randomized trials? Options, problems, challenges. *Medical Care, 33*(4), AS8–AS14.

Nadzim, D. M., Turpin, R., Hanold, L. S., & White, R. E. (1993). Data-driven performance improvement in health care: The Joint Commission's Indicator Measurement System (IMSystem). *Joint Commission Journal on Quality Improvement, 19*(11), 492–500.

Naylor, M. D. (2007). Advancing the science in the measurement of health care quality influenced by nurses. *Medical Care Research & Review, 64*(2 Suppl.), 144S–169S.

Nelson, E. C., Landgraf, J. M., Hays, R. D., Wasson, J. H., & Kirk, J. W. (1990). The functional status of patients: How can it be measured in physicians' offices? *Medical Care, 28*(12), 1111–1126.

O'Connor, G. T., Plume, S. K., & Wennberg, J. E. (1993). Regional organization for outcomes research. *Annals of the New York Academy of Sciences, 703*, 44–51.

Orchard, C. (1994). Comparing healthcare outcomes. *British Medical Journal, 308*(6942), 1493–1496.

Oster, G. (1988). Economic aspects of clinical decision making: Applications in patient care. *American Journal of Hospital Pharmacy, 45*(3), 543–547.

Ottenbacher, K. J., Johnson, M. B., & Hojem, M. (1995). The significance of clinical change and clinical change of significance: Issues and methods. *American Journal of Occupational Therapy, 42*(3), 156–163.

Patrick, D. L., & Deyo, R. A. (1989). Generic and disease-specific measures in assessing health status and quality of life. *Medical Care, 27*(3 Suppl.), S217–S232.

Perkins, R., Olson, S., Hanson, J., Lee, J., Stiles, K., & Lebrun, C. (2007). Impact of an anemia clinic on emergency room visits and hospitalizations in patients with anemia of CKD pre-dialysis. *Nephrology Nursing Journal, 34*(2), 167–174, 182.

Phibbs, C. S., Holty, J. C., Goldstein, M. K., Garber, A. M., Wang, Y., Feussner, J. R., et al. (2006). The effect of geriatrics evaluation and management on nursing home use and health care costs: Results from a randomized trial. *Medical Care, 44*(1), 91–95.

Powe, N. R., Turner, J. A., Maklan, C. W., & Ersek, M. (1994). Alternative methods for formal literature review and meta-analysis in AHCPR patient outcomes research teams. *Medical Care, 32*(7), JS22–JS37.

Power, E. J., Tunis, S. R., & Wagner, J. L. (1994). Technology assessment and public health. *Annual Review of Public Health, 15*, 561–579.

Riehle, A. I., Hanold, L. S., Sprenger, S. L., & Loeb, J. M. (2007). Specifying and standardizing performance measures for use at a national level: Implications for nursing-sensitive care performance measures. *Medical Care Research & Review, 64*(2 Suppl.), 64S–81S.

Rovine, M. J. & Von Eye, A. (1991). *Applied computational statistics in longitudinal research.* San Diego, CA: Academic Press.

Rowell, P. (2001). Lessons learned while collecting ANA indicator data: The American Nurses Association responds, *Journal of Nursing Administration, 31*(3), 130–131.

Rubin, F. H., Williams, J. T., Lescisin, D. A., Mook, W. J., Hassan, S., & Innouye, S. K. (2006). Replicating the Hospital Elder Life Program in a community hospital and demonstrating effectiveness using quality improvement methodology. *Journal of the American Geriatrics Society, 54*(6), 969–974.

Schmitt, M. H., Farrell, M. P., & Heinemann, G. D. (1988). Conceptual and methodological problems in studying the effects of interdisciplinary geriatric teams. *Gerontologist, 28*(6), 753–764.

Schnelle, J. F., Simmons, S. F., Harrington, C., Cadogan, M., Garcia, E., & Bates-Jensen, B. M. (2004). Relationship of nursing home staffing to quality of care. *Health Services Research, 39*(2), 225–250.

Schwartz, D. A. (2004). Postmortem sperm retrieval: An ethical analysis. *Clinical Excellence for Nurse Practitioners, 8*(4), 183–188.

Siegel, J. E. (1998). Cost-effectiveness analysis and nursing research: Is there a fit? *Image: Journal of Nursing Scholarship, 30*(3), 221–222.

Slade, M., Kuipers, E., & Priebe, S. (2002). Mental health services research methodology. *International Review of Psychiatry, 14*(1), 12–18.

Sledge, C. B. (1993). Why do outcomes research? *Orthopedics, 16*(10), 1093–1096.

Sonnenberg, F. A., Roberts, M. S., Tsevat, J., Wong, J. B., Barry, M., & Kent, D. L. (1994). Toward a peer review process for medical decision analysis models. *Medical Care, 32*(7), JS52–JS64.

Sox, H. C. (2000). Independent primary care practice by nurse practitioners. *JAMA, 283*(1), 106–108.

Spector, W. D. (1990). Functional disability scales. In B. Spilker (Ed.), *Quality of life assessments in clinical trials* (pp. 115–129). New York: Raven Press.

Spitzer, W. O. (1987). State of science 1986: Quality of life and functional status as target variables for research. *Journal of Chronic Disease, 40*(6), 465–471.

Standing, M. (2007). Clinical decision-making skills on the developmental journal from student to registered nurse: A longitudinal inquiry. *Journal of Advanced Nursing, 60*(3), 257–269.

Stewart, A. L., Greenfield, S., Hays, R. D., Wells, K., Rogers, W. H., Berry, S. D., et al. (1989). Functional status and well-being of patients with chronic conditions. *JAMA, 262*(7), 907–913.

Stewart, B. J., & Archbold, P. G. (1992). Nursing intervention studies require outcome measures that are sensitive to change: Part 2. *Research in Nursing & Health, 16*(1), 77–81.

Stone, D. W. (1998). Methods for conducting and reporting cost-effectiveness analysis in nursing. *Image: Journal of Nursing Scholarship, 30*(3), 229–234.

Swaen, G. M. H., & Meijers, J. M. M. (1988). Influence of design characteristics on the outcomes of retrospective cohort studies. *British Journal of Industrial Medicine, 45*(9), 624–629.

Tanenbaum, S. J. (1994). Knowing and acting in medical practice: The epistemological politics of outcomes research. *Journal of Health Politics, Policy and Law, 19*(1), 27–44.

Tarlov, A. R., Ware, J. E. Jr., Greenfield, S., Nelson, E. C., Perrin, E., & Zubkoff, M. (1989). The medical outcomes study: An application of methods for monitoring the results of medical care. *JAMA, 262*(7), 925–930.

Temple, R. (1990). Problems in the use of large data sets to assess effectiveness. *International Journal of Technology Assessment in Health Care, 6*(2), 211–219.

Tengs, T. O., Adams, M. E., Pliskin, J. S., Safran, D. G., Siegel, J. E., Weinstein, M. C., et al. (1995). Five hundred life-saving interventions and their cost-effectiveness. *Risk Analysis, 15*(3), 369–390.

Tidwell, S. L. (1993). A graphic tool for tracking variance and comorbidities in cardiac surgery case management. *Progress in Cardiovascular Nursing, 8*(2), 6–19.

Tierney, W. M., Caitlin, C., Oppenheimer, M. P. H., Hudson, B. L., Benz, J., Finn, A., et al. (2007). A national survey of primary care practice-based research networks. *Annals of Family Medicine, 5*(3), 242–250.

Tork, H. K., Dassen, T., & Lohrmann, C. (2008). Care dependency of children in Egypt. *Journal of Clinical Nursing, 17*(3), 287–295.

Turk, D. C., & Rudy, T. E. (1994). Methods for evaluating treatment outcomes: Ways to overcome potential obstacles. *Spine, 19*(15), 1759–1763.

Unsworth, C. A. (2001). Using a head-mounted video camera to study clinical reasoning. *American Journal of Occupational Therapy, 55*(5), 582–588.

U.S. Congress, Office of Technology Assessment. (1994). *Identifying health technologies that work: Searching for evidence* (Publication No. OTA-H-608). Washington, DC: U.S. Government Printing Office.

Varricchio, C. (1994). Human and indirect costs of home care... for cancer patients. *Nursing Outlook, 42*(4), 151–157.

Veatch, R., M. (1993). Justice and outcomes research: The ethical limits. *Journal of Clinical Ethics, 4*(3), 258–261.

Verran, J. A., Mark, B. A., & Lamb, G. (1992). Psychometric examination of instruments using aggregated data. *Research in Nursing & Health, 15*(3), 237–240.

Volinn, E., Diehr, P., Ciol, M. A., & Loeser, J. D. (1994). Why does geographic variation in health care practices matter (and seven questions to ask in evaluating studies on geographic variation)? *Spine, 19*(18S), 2092S–2100S.

Von Eye, A. (Ed.). (1990a). *Statistical methods in longitudinal research: Vol. 1. Principles and structuring change.* Boston: Academic Press.

Von Eye, A. (Ed.). (1990b). *Statistical methods in longitudinal research: Vol. 2. Time series and categorical longitudinal data.* Boston: Academic Press.

Von Korff, M., Koepsell, T., Curry, S., & Diehr, P. (1992). Multi-level analysis in epidemiologic research on health behaviors and outcomes. *American Journal of Epidemiology, 135*(10), 1077–1082.

Ward, D., & Brown, M. A. (1994). Labor and cost in AIDS family caregiving. *Western Journal of Nursing Research, 16*(1), 1–25.

Ward, D., Severs, M., Dean, T., & Brooks, N. (2007). Care home versus hospital and own home environments for rehabilitation of older people. *Cochrane Database of Systematic Reviews,* (2), CD003164.

Wennberg, J. E., Barry, M. J., Fowler, F. J., & Mulley, A. (1993). Outcomes Research, PORTs, and health care reform. *Annals of the New York Academy of Sciences, 703*, 52–62.

Werley, H., Devine, E., Zorn, C., Ryan, P., & Westra, B. (1991). The nursing minimum data set: Abstraction tool for standardized, comparable, essential data. *American Journal of Public Health, 81*(4), 421–426.

Werley, H., & Lang, N. (1988). *Identification of the nursing minimum data set.* New York: Springer.

Westert, G. P., & Groenewegen, P. P. (1999). Medical practice variations: Changing the theoretical approach. *Scandinavian Journal of Public Health, 27*(3), 173–180.

White, K. L. (1993). Health care research: Old wine in new bottles. *Pharos of Alpha Omega Alpha Honor Medical Society, 56*(3), 12–16.

Wilson, I. B., Landon, B. E., Hirschhorn, L. R., McInnes, K., Ding, L., Marsden, P. V., et al. (2005). Quality of HIV care provided by nurse practitioners, physician assistants, and physicians. *Annals of Internal Medicine, 143*(10), 729–736.

Wood, L. W. (1990). Medical treatment effectiveness research. *Journal of Occupational Medicine, 32*(12), 1173–1174.

Wray, N. P., Ashton, C. M., Kuykendall, D. H., Petersen, N. J., Souchek, J., & Hollingsworth, J. C. (1995). Selecting disease-outcome pairs for monitoring the quality of hospital care. *Medical Care, 33*(1), 75–89.

Zielstorff, R., Hudgings, C., Grobe, S., & National Commission on Nursing Implementation Project Task Force on Nursing Information Systems. (1993). *Next generation nursing information systems: Essential characteristics for professional practice.* Washington, DC: American Nurses Association.

CHAPTER 13
Intervention Research

This chapter describes a revolutionary new approach to intervention research that holds great promise for designing and testing nursing interventions. The approach is very new, and you are unlikely to find many published studies using the techniques. A growing number of scholars are beginning to seriously question the current approach to testing interventions, the "true experiment," because modifications in the original design have decreased its validity (Adelman, 1986; Bergmark & Oscarsson, 1991; Chen, 1990; Egan, Snyder, & Burns, 1992; Fawcett et al., 1994; Lipsey, 1993; Nolan & Grant, 1993; Rothman & Thomas, 1994; Scott & Sechrest, 1989; Sechrest, Ametrano, & Ametrano, 1983; Sidani & Braden, 1998; Sidani, Epstein, & Moritz, 2003; Yeaton & Sechrest, 1981). The presentation of the new methodology for designing and testing interventions in this chapter is heavily based on two decisive books that reflect this new approach, Sidani and Braden's (1998) *Evaluating Nursing Interventions: A Theory-Driven Approach* and Rothman and Thomas's (1994) *Intervention Research: Design and Development for Human Service*, and on the works of scholars on which these books are based.

This chapter defines the term *nursing intervention*, discusses problems with the "true experiment," provides an overview of intervention research, and describes the process of conducting intervention research. The intervention research process consists of planning the project, gathering information, developing an intervention theory, designing the intervention, establishing an observation system, testing the intervention, collecting and analyzing data, and disseminating results. Examples of the steps of intervention research are provided from published studies.

WHAT ARE NURSING INTERVENTIONS?

Nursing interventions are defined as "deliberative cognitive, physical, or verbal activities performed with, or on behalf of, individuals and their families [that] are directed toward accomplishing particular therapeutic objectives relative to individuals' health and well-being" (Grobe, 1996, p. 50). We would expand this definition to include nursing interventions that are performed with, or on behalf of, communities. Sidani and Braden (1998, p. 8) defined interventions as "treatments, therapies, procedures, or actions implemented by health professionals to and with clients, in a particular situation, to move the clients' condition toward desired health outcomes that are beneficial to the clients."

A nursing intervention can be defined in terms of (1) a single act (e.g., changing the position of a patient), (2) a series of actions at a given point in time (e.g., management by an intensive care nurse of an abrupt increase in the intracranial pressure of a patient with brain injury, responding to the grief of a family whose loved one has died), (3) a series of actions over time (e.g., implementing a protocol for the management of a newly diagnosed diabetic patient by a primary care nurse practitioner, management of a chronically depressed patient), or (4) a series of acts performed collaboratively with other professionals (e.g., implementing a clinical pathway, conducting a program to reduce smoking in a community). Rather than targeting patients, some interventions target health care providers (e.g., a continuing education program), the setting (e.g., a change in staffing pattern), or the care delivery (e.g., a change in the structure of care).

317

Historically, nursing interventions have tended to be viewed as discrete actions, for example, "Position the limb with sandbags," "Raise the head of the bed 30 degrees," or "Explore the need for attention with the patient." There is little conceptualization of how these discrete actions fit together (McCloskey & Bulechek, 2008). Interventions must be described more broadly as all of the actions required to address a particular problem (Abraham, Chalifoux, & Evers, 1992).

Some of the purposes of interventions are risk reduction, treatment or resolution of a health-related problem or symptom, management of a problem or symptom, and prevention of complications associated with a problem. Some interventions have multiple purposes or multiple outcomes or both. Desired outcomes vary with the purpose and might include continued absence of a problem, resolution of a problem, successful management of a problem, or absence of complications (Sidani & Braden, 1998).

The terminology and operationalization of a nursing intervention varies with the clinical setting and among individual nurses. Each nurse may describe a particular intervention differently. Nursing intervention vocabulary varies in different settings, such as intensive care, home care, extended care, and primary care. There is little consistency in how interventions are performed. An intervention is often applied differently each time by a single nurse and is even less consistently applied by different nurses. Even in published nursing studies, descriptions of interventions tested lack the specificity and clarity given to describing the methods of measurement used in a study (Egan et al., 1992).

The problem with definition and operationalization of nursing interventions is illustrated by the work of Schmelzer and Wright (1993a, 1993b), gastroenterology nurses who, in 1993, began a series of studies that examined the procedure for administering an enema. They found no research in nursing or medical literature that tested the effectiveness of various enema procedures. There is no scientific evidence to justify the use of various procedures for administering enemas. The amount of solution, temperature of solution, speed of administration, content of the solution (soap suds, normal saline, water), positioning of the patient, measurement of expected outcomes, or possible complications are based on tradition and have no scientific basis.

For their first study, Schmelzer and Wright (1996) conducted telephone interviews with nurses across the country in an effort to identify patterns in the methods used to administer enemas. They found none. They developed a protocol for administering enemas

and pilot-tested it on hospitalized patients awaiting liver transplantation. In their subsequent study, using a sample of liver transplant patients, these researchers tested for differences in the effects of different enema solutions (Schmelzer et al., 2000). Schmelzer (1999–2001) then conducted a study funded by the National Institute for Nursing Research to compare the effects of three enema solutions on the bowel mucosa. Well subjects were paid $100 for each of three enemas, after which a small biopsy specimen was collected.

The strategy that these researchers adopted must be used to test the effectiveness of many current nursing interventions. What methods should be used for this testing, however? The "true experiment," quasi-experimental studies, or the new intervention research methods? The "gold standard" has been the "true experiment."

PROBLEMS WITH THE TRUE EXPERIMENT

Clark (1998) pointed out that the true experiment is based on a logical-positivist approach to research, an atheoretical strategy that focuses on discovering laws through the accumulation of facts. Few nurse researchers hold to the logical-positivist perspective. The logical-positivist approach is not consistent with nursing philosophy or with the theory-based approach through which nursing is building its body of knowledge.

Traditionally, adherence to rigid rules was required to define a study as a true experiment (Fisher, 1935). These rules were (1) random sampling from individuals representative of the population, (2) equivalence of groups, (3) complete control of the treatment by the researcher, (4) a control group that receives no treatment or a placebo treatment, (5) control of the environment in which the study is conducted, and (6) precise measurement of hypothesized outcomes. True experiments powerfully demonstrate the validity of the cause. However, the method is easier to apply when studying corn (as Fisher did) than when studying humans (as we do).

Studying humans requires modifications in the true experiment that have weakened the power of the design and threatened its validity. Because of requirements related to the use of human subjects and problems related to accessing sufficient numbers of subjects, most health care researchers have abandoned random sampling. This change has decreased the representativeness of the sample. Subjects in "true experiments" (e.g., clinical trials) are increasingly unlike the target population. Compared with the patients in a typical clinical practice, subjects selected for experimental studies are less likely to include, for example, individuals who have comorbidities; who are being cared for by a primary care provider; who are not receiving treatment; who are in a managed care program or health maintenance organization (HMO); who receive Medicare benefits; who are uninsured, undereducated, or poor; or who are members of minority groups. Treatments affect various groups differently and for some groups have no effect. Knowing how various groups are affected has become increasingly important with the advent of managed care (Orchid, 1994). Equivalence of groups, a critical element of the experimental design, continues to be addressed through random assignment. In analyzing data from clinical trials, however, Ottenbacher (1992) found random assignment ineffective in making groups more equivalent.

Complete control of the intervention is a problem in many experimental studies. Often clinicians, unskilled staff, or family members—rather than the researchers—apply the intervention. It is sometimes difficult to determine the extent to which (or even whether) a subject received the defined experimental treatment. Sometimes the intervention must be modified to meet the needs of particular subjects, a practice problematic to the assumptions of the experimental design. Comparison groups are often given the usual treatment, but the "usual treatment" or "standard care" is seldom defined. In most cases, there is wide variation in usual treatment that makes valid comparisons with the treatment group problematic and increases the risk of a type II error.

Dependent variables selected to test the intervention sometimes do not reflect actual outcomes. In many clinical situations, the desired outcomes occur a considerable time after the intervention, making them difficult, if not impossible, to measure during a reasonable period (in a funded study). Intermediate outcomes may be substituted, with the assumption that end outcomes can be inferred from intermediate outcomes, a questionable assumption in many cases (Orchid, 1994).

"True experiments," as they were originally designed, are the most effective way to determine the validity of the cause; modifications make them less valid. Using quasi-experimental designs creates more threats to internal validity. A number of problems related to the newly defined "true experiment" threaten the validity of statistical conclusion, the most important of which is the absence of a random sample. External validity is threatened by problems with representativeness.

As a nurse researcher, to what extent can you deviate from the original definition of a true experiment and be justified in using the term to refer to your study? To what extent can quasi-experimental studies justifiably replace the true experiment as a means to validate the effectiveness of an intervention? Does an atheoretical, modified true experiment provide sufficient evidence to justify implementing an intervention in clinical practice?

With the growing demand for evidence-based practice, it is essential that nursing interventions be clearly defined and tested for effectiveness, including those that have become part of nursing through history, tradition, or trial and error, and that new interventions be designed and tested to address unresolved nursing problems (Abraham et al., 1992). What strategies, however, do we use to accomplish this goal?

INTERVENTION RESEARCH

Intervention research is a revolutionary new methodology that holds great promise as a more effective way of testing interventions. It shifts the focus from causal connection to causal explanation. In causal connection, the focus of a study is to provide evidence that the intervention causes the outcome. In causal explanation, in addition to demonstrating that the intervention causes the outcome, the researcher must provide scientific evidence to explain why the intervention causes changes in outcomes, how it does so, or both. Causal explanation is theory based. Thus, research focused on causal explanation is guided by theory, and the findings are expressed theoretically. Researchers employ a broad base of methodologies, including qualitative ones, to examine the effectiveness of the intervention (Rothman & Thomas, 1994; Sidani & Braden, 1998).

It is becoming increasingly clear that the design and testing of a nursing intervention require an extensive program of research rather than a single well-designed study (Rothman & Thomas, 1994; Sidani & Braden, 1998). It is also clear that a larger portion of nursing studies must focus on designing and testing interventions.

PROCESS OF INTERVENTION RESEARCH

The process of intervention research described here was derived from strategies currently being used in a variety of disciplines, including evaluation research and the design and development approach used in engineering. To begin the process, the researcher launches an extensive search for relevant information that can be applied to the development of an intervention theory. The intervention theory guides the design and development of an intervention, which is then extensively tested, refined, and retested. When the intervention is sufficiently refined and evidence of effectiveness has been obtained, field testing is used to ensure that the intervention can be effectively implemented in clinical settings. The researcher uses the results of these field tests to further refine the intervention and improve its clinical application. An observation system is developed for use throughout the design and development process, allowing the researcher to observe events related to the intervention naturalistically and to analyze these observations. Efforts to disseminate the newly refined intervention are extensive and are planned as an integral part of the research program.

Project Planning

Because an intervention research project comprises multiple studies conducted over a period of years, nurse researchers are advised to engage in careful planning before initiating the project. You will need to determine issues such as (1) who will be included on your project team, (2) how the team will function, and (3) whether or not to use participatory research methods, which stipulate the inclusion of stakeholders and key informants as members of the project team.

Forming a Project Team

Because of the nature of intervention research, you may need to gather a multidisciplinary project team to facilitate distribution of the work and a broader generation of ideas. Because both quantitative data and qualitative data will be gathered during the research program, your team should include members experienced in various qualitative and quantitative data collection and analysis approaches. Including a team member with marketing expertise will be beneficial, because the final step of the project will be to market the intervention. Teams are enhanced by the inclusion of undergraduate, master's, and doctoral nursing students.

Recruiting colleagues located in other areas of the country or the world for the research team can add an important dimension, permitting multisite evaluation studies. To achieve this goal, (1) contact researchers with similar interests; (2) attend specialty conferences related to the research area, during which you can dialogue with researchers and possibly extend an invitation to participate in the project; (3) invite colleagues to join the project after presentations at a professional meeting; (4) develop a project website that invites other researchers to participate; and (5) develop or participate in an Internet mailing list (Listserv) or a blog

related to the topic. The process of developing a team is dynamic rather than static, with changes occurring as development of the research program continues.

Work of the Project Team

There is almost always a core group in a project team that carries on most of the work, maintains group activities, and encourages the achievement of tasks. However, other people can contribute in lesser ways to benefit the project. For example, you may want to establish liaison groups from the clinical facilities in which the intervention will be studied. In some cases, the addition of other advisory groups can be helpful.

The initial focus of the team is to clarify the problem. In analyzing identified problems, the team should answer the questions listed in Table 13-1. Considering these questions may provide new insights that redefine of the problem and may lead to a more effective intervention. Sidani and Braden (1998) have cautioned the project team to be alert to the risk of making a type III

TABLE 13-1 ▪ Problem Analysis Questions

1. For whom is the situation a problem?
2. What are the negative consequences of the problem for the affected individuals?
3. What are the negative consequences of the problem for the community (health care providers, system, or agency)?
4. Who (if anyone) benefits from conditions as they are now?
5. How do they benefit?
6. Who should share the responsibility for "solving" the problem?
7. What (or whose) behaviors must change for patients to consider the problem solved?
8. What conditions must change to establish or support needed change?
9. What is an acceptable level of change?
10. At what level should the problem be addressed?
11. Is this a multilevel problem requiring action at various levels of change?
12. Is it feasible (technically, financially, politically) to make changes at each identified level?
13. What (or whose) behaviors must change for providers to consider the problem solved?
14. Who are stakeholders?
15. What does each stakeholder have invested in the status quo?
16. Who might support change?
17. Who might function as champion?

Questions 1 through 12 adapted from Fawcett, S. B., Suarez-Belcazar, Y., Belcazar, F. E., White, G. W., Paine, A. L., Blanchard, K. A., et al. (1994). Conducting intervention research: The design and development process. In J. Rothman & E. J. Thomas (Eds.), *Intervention Research: Design and Development for Human Service* (pp. 25–54). New York: Haworth Press.

error. A type III error is the risk of asking the wrong question—a question that does not address the problem of concern. This error is most likely to occur when the researchers do not thoroughly analyze the problem and, as a result, have a fuzzy or inaccurate understanding of the issue of concern. The solution, then, does not fit the problem. A study conducted on the basis of a type III error provides the right answer to the wrong question, leading to the incorrect conclusion that the newly designed intervention will resolve the problem.

Once the problem to be examined is clarified, you must establish your goals and objectives. Project team tasks include gathering information, developing an intervention theory, designing the intervention, establishing an observation system, testing the intervention, collecting and analyzing data, and disseminating the intervention. Seeking funding for the various studies of the project will be an ongoing effort.

Using Participatory Research Methods

Some supporters of intervention research recommend establishing a participatory research strategy, which involves including representatives from all groups that will be affected by the change (stakeholders) as collaborators. (For more details on participatory research methods, see Chapter 23.) This strategy facilitates broad-based support for the new intervention from the target population, the professional community, and the general public. Disadvantaged groups are recommended as stakeholders in interventions that would or should affect members of that group (Fawcett et al., 1994). Table 13-2 lists examples of stakeholder groups.

TABLE 13-2   Examples of Stakeholder Groups
Clinical nurses
Physicians
Pharmacists
Administrators
Other allied health professionals
Third-party payers
Chaplains
Representatives of the target population
Families living in poverty
Residents of low-income groups
Ethnic groups
Groups for whom English is a second language
People with poor access to care
People not currently receiving care
Institutionalized psychiatric patients
Recipients of public health services
Representatives of rural communities
Youths
People with physical disabilities

The selection of key informants is also recommended, unless the researchers are currently practicing in the setting or settings in which the intervention will be implemented (Fawcett et al., 1994). Key informants can help researchers become familiar with settings. Whether the setting is a clinical agency or an element of the community, key informants can help researchers to understand local ways and gain access to the settings. Interactions with key informants can also help you to identify what you and your research team can offer to the setting and how to articulate the benefits of the project to groups or organizations. Key informants in stakeholder groups—such as "natural leaders," advocates, community leaders, and service providers—can furnish information useful for determining and addressing the concerns or needs of these groups as the intervention project is being planned (Fawcett et al., 1994).

If you choose a participatory research approach, your project team will consist of the researchers, stakeholders, and key informants. At the initial meeting, members of the team familiar with the process of intervention research can explain the process to the team. Next, the team can discuss the problem and possible solutions. One rule of team meetings should be that team members will avoid imposing their views of the problem or its solution on the group but, rather, will attempt to understand issues of importance to others on the project team. Use consensus to arrive at decisions. Involve all members of the team in activities such as reviewing and integrating literature and other information gathered, developing the intervention theory, designing studies, interpreting results, and disseminating findings (Fawcett et al., 1994).

Gathering Information

Conduct an extensive search for information related to the project. This gathering of information is considerably more extensive than the traditional literature review. Various methods are used to gather information. These include the methods listed in Table 13-3, which uncover in-depth information on the topics listed in Table 13-4. It is particularly important to gather sources of information about the intervention. In designing your study, you and your team do not need to reinvent the wheel. Therefore, researchers must know what others have done to address the problem.

Potential sources of information about interventions for the problem of concern are listed in Table 13-5 and discussed here. As you explore each source of information, be sure to address the queries listed in Table 13-6. Information gathered from all sources

TABLE 13-3 Information Gathering Sources
Integrative reviews of the literature
News media
Consumer publications
Position papers
Standards or guidelines
Meta-analyses
Introspection related to personal experience
Observation
Case studies
Qualitative studies
Focus groups
Consensus conferences
Concept analyses
Foundational studies
Health policy analyses
Ethical analyses
Health services research
Retrospective chart reviews
Outcomes studies
Descriptive and correlational studies, including regression analyses and path analyses
Q-sorts
Delphi studies
Methodological studies to develop or validate methods of measurement

TABLE 13-4 Topic for Information Gathering
Problem
Nature of the problem (actual or potential)
Manifestations
Causative factors
Level of severity
Variation in different patient populations
Variation in different conditions
Intervention
How people who have actually experienced the problem have addressed it
Previous interventions designed to address the problem
Unsuccessful interventions
Value to target population
Sensitivity to cultural diversity
Biases or prejudices
Processes underlying the intervention effects
Intervention actions
Components
Mode of delivery
Strength of dosage
Amount
Frequency
Duration
Mediating Processes
Patient characteristics
Setting characteristics
Intervener characteristics
Expected Outcomes
Contextual factors
Environmental factors
Patient characteristics
Provider factors
Health care system factors

requires careful analysis and synthesis. Undergraduate, master's, and doctoral nursing students, as well as clinicians, working with the project team, could play a major role in gathering and synthesizing information.

Taxonomies

An intervention taxonomy is an organized categorization of all interventions performed by nurses. A number of classifications of nursing interventions have been developed: the Nursing Diagnosis Taxonomy (Warren & Hoskins, 1995), Home Health Care Classifications (Saba, 1995), the Omaha System (Martin & Scheet, 1995), the Nursing Interventions Classification (NIC) (Bulechek & McCloskey, 1999; Bulechek, McCloskey, & Donahue, 1995; and the Nursing Intervention Lexicon and Taxonomy (NILT) (Grobe, 1996). Grobe (1996, p. 50) suggested that "theoretically, a validated taxonomy that describes and categorizes nursing interventions can represent the essence of nursing knowledge about care phenomena and their relationship to one another and to the overall concept of care." Although taxonomies may contain brief definitions of interventions, they do not provide sufficient detail to allow one to implement the intervention. Also, the actions identified in taxonomies may be too discrete for testing and may not be linked to the resolution of a particular patient problem (Sidani & Braden, 1998).

Databases

Many health care agencies have databases that store information about patient care activities. Researchers can use these databases for secondary analyses examining many of the topics listed in Table 13-3. For example, a group of 17 home health care agencies in Tarrant County, Texas, arranged to establish a joint patient care database. All the home care nurses were provided with laptops linked to the database. They entered data related to their patient care visits into the database and were able to access information about a patient while in the patient's home. The central database site employed nurses with master's degrees and a statistician, as well as computer technicians. Reports

TABLE 13-5   Sources of Information about Interventions
Nursing intervention taxonomies
Computerized databases containing data on nursing interventions
Nursing textbooks
State-of-the-art journal articles on nursing interventions
Previous intervention studies (theses, dissertations, publications)
Clinical guidelines: www.guidelines.gov
Critical pathways
Intervention protocols
Interviews with patients who have experienced the problem and related interventions
Interviews with providers who have addressed the problem
Interviews with researchers who have tested previous interventions
Probing of personal experiences
Observations of care provided to patients with the problem
Consumer groups who are stakeholders (e.g., Gilda Clubs, Reach for Recovery)

TABLE 13-6   Queries Relevant to All Sources
1. Are there existing interventions or practices that have been successful?
2. What made a particular practice effective?
3. Are there existing interventions or practices that were unsuccessful?
4. What caused them to fail?
5. Which events appeared to be critical to success (or failure)?
6. What conditions (e.g., organizational features, patient characteristics, broader environmental factors) may have been critical to success (or failure)?
7. What specific procedures were used in the practice?
8. Was information provided to patients or change agents about how and under what conditions to act?
9. Were modeling, role-playing, practice, feedback, or other training procedures used?
10. What positive consequences, such as rewards or incentives, and negative consequences, such as penalties or disincentives, helped establish and maintain desired changes?
11. What environmental barriers, policies, or regulations were removed to make it easier for the changes to occur?
12. What proportion of people experiencing a specific cluster of symptoms were diagnosed (correctly or not) as having a particular diagnosis, and of this group, who received what treatment?
13. Should a treatment or procedure have been performed?
14. Did persons with a particular diagnosis receive appropriate treatment?
15. What proportion of people with the cluster of symptoms did not receive treatment?

from the database were generated and sent to the individual nursing homes. Data could be pooled for analysis purposes. It was possible to query the database for information on patients receiving a particular intervention. Researchers could search the database to obtain information related to patient characteristics, the timing of the intervention in relation to the emergence of the problem, costs, outcomes, and characteristics of the intervener.

Textbooks

Textbooks often provide little or no instruction on how the interventions listed should be implemented. If they provide any information, it is usually in the form of a long list of actions that nurses should take in a particular patient situation. The lists given for the same patient situation vary with the textbook (McCloskey & Bulechek, 1992). One exception is a textbook by Bulechek and McCloskey (1999) titled *Nursing Interventions: Effective Nursing Treatments*, which is organized by the NIC taxonomy and provides detailed descriptions of nursing interventions with a known research base. Two more recent publications describing nursing interventions for clinical practice are Gulanick and Myers's (2007) *Nursing Care Plans: Nursing Diagnosis and Intervention* and Elkin, Perry, and Potter's (2007) *Nursing Interventions and Clinical Skills*. Available also are Eslinger's (2002) *Neuropsychological Interventions: Clinical Research and Practice* and Steckler and Linnan's (2002) *Process Evaluation for Public Health Interventions and Research.*

Adapted from Fawcett, S. B., Suarez-Belcazar, Y., Belcazar, F. E., White, G. W., Paine, A. L., Blanchard, K. A., et al. (1994). Conducting intervention research: The design and development process. In J. Rothman & E. J. Thomas (Eds.), *Intervention research: Design and development for human service,* (pp. 25–54). New York: Haworth Press.

State-of-the-Art Journal Articles

Articles delineating state-of-the-art care in relation to particular patient care situations are appearing in nursing journals. These articles generally result from an extensive review of the literature and may be a good source of information when available. They often contain a discussion of the problem and elements of an intervention theory and propose strategies for future research. References cited in such articles can often add valuable information to that obtained by computer search. Letters to the editor sections of practice journals are also good sources of information about the strategies clinicians use.

Previous Studies

Previous studies are also an important source of information about the intervention. A previous study usually discusses the problem, describes the intervention procedure, presents measurement methods for variables, offers approaches to design and analysis, gives information that can be used to determine effect size, and discusses problems related to the intervention or the research methodology. Your examination of previous studies should include theses and dissertations that may not be published. A search for other unpublished studies may yield valuable information. Use of nursing listservs can be an effective way to seek unpublished studies. As with state-of-the-art journals, references from previous studies often yield sources not identified through computer searches.

Clinical Guidelines

The Agency for Healthcare Research and Quality (AHRQ) and other organizations have developed clinical guidelines for patient care situations. These guidelines are available at the National Guideline Clearinghouse website at www.guidelines.gov and at the AHRQ website at www.ahcpr.gov; they are discussed in Chapters 2 and 27. Clinical guidelines define the standard of care for particular patient situations, are interdisciplinary, and are based on an extensive review of the literature focused on findings from previous studies. Although these guidelines are not specific to nursing, elements of the guidelines specify nursing actions.

Critical or Clinical Pathways

Health care agencies often develop critical or clinical pathways that define the expected care activities and the expected outcomes of the care in specific patient care situations. Critical pathways may be developed through the use of findings from previous research, analyses of agency databases, and clinical experiences of the practitioners in the agency. Some agencies consider their critical pathways to be proprietary information, limiting the possibilities of testing them and publishing the results. However, written documentation related to the pathway or interaction with committee members involved in developing the pathway can help you and other researchers to specify the problem, define the intervention, and obtain information related to moderator or mediator variables (see later discussion) and outcomes.

Evidence-Based Practice

When designing an intervention for a study, it is critical that you be aware of and current in your knowledge of evidence-based practice in the area of the intervention. Check the date that current guidelines were reviewed. Search the literature for recent interventions that may have been developed since the latest review. Broaden your search beyond the particular intervention of interest to you to include interventions in the relevant area of practice.

Provider Interviews

Clinicians are an important source of information about the intervention. They have firsthand experience in implementing interventions for the patient problem. They are more familiar than most with the nuances and variations of the situation. Their knowledge often is not sought and seldom is available in journal articles. Information from these sources about unsuccessful practices is particularly valuable (Fawcett et al., 1994).

Researcher Interviews

Interviews with researchers who have developed or tested previous interventions for the problem of concern can provide excellent information to guide the development and testing of a new intervention. Obtaining information from such interviews can often help the project team avoid repeating mistakes in designing the intervention or in developing the methodology for testing it. You can contact these researchers by phone, e-mail, webcasting, or letter. In some cases, it may be important for you to visit a site for an interview (Fawcett et al., 1994).

Patient Interviews

Patients who have experienced the problem under study can provide valuable information often not available from other sources. They offer a completely different perspective from that of providers. Patients, their family members, or both may have used interventions not documented in the literature and may have insights about what is lacking in the intervention that may not have been considered (Fawcett et al., 1994).

Probing of Personal Experience

Because of the sparseness of information in the literature on nursing interventions, you may have to rely heavily on a personal knowledge base emerging from expertise in clinical practice. You can elicit this knowledge through introspection and dialogue with colleagues.

Observations of Patient Care

Observations of patient care are essential in determining the dynamics of the process of patient care, because in many cases, the care activities are so familiar to clinicians that, in describing it, they leave out components important to the overall process. These observations will be components of the observation system described later in the chapter.

Developing an Intervention Theory

Use the knowledge obtained through a synthesis of collected information to develop a middle-range intervention theory. An intervention theory is explanatory and combines characteristics of descriptive, middle-range theories and prescriptive, practice theories. A descriptive theory describes the causal processes occurring. A prescriptive theory specifies what must be done to achieve the desired effects, including (1) the components, intensity, and duration required; (2) the human and material resources needed; and (3) the procedures to be followed to produce the desired outcomes.

An intervention theory is also action oriented, guiding the team on how to design, test, and implement the intervention. The intervention theory should contain conceptual definitions, propositions, hypotheses, and any empirical generalizations available from previous studies (Chen, 1990; Chen & Rossi, 1989; Finney & Moos, 1989; Rothman & Thomas, 1994; Sidani & Braden, 1998). The theory will be further refined during the design and development process. Master's and doctoral nursing students, working in collaboration with faculty researchers or with the project team, can provide valuable input for the development of the intervention theory by (1) conducting literature reviews and synthesis; (2) developing class papers related to the intervention theory; (3) conducting class discussions about the intervention theory, which are then communicated to the project team; or (4) meeting with the project team to participate in discussions during development of the intervention theory.

An intervention theory must include a careful description of the problem the intervention will address, the intervening actions that must be implemented to address the problem, moderator variables that might change the impact of the intervention, mediator variables that might alter the effect of the intervention, and expected outcomes of the intervention. Table 13-7 lists the components of an intervention theory. Further detail about developing each intervention theory element is provided in the following discussion.

Problem

The problem that the intervention theory addresses might be one of alterations in function or of inadequacies

TABLE 13-7   Elements of Intervention Theory

Problem

Nature of the problem
Manifestations
Causative factors
Level of severity
Variation in different patient populations
Variation in different conditions

Critical Inputs

Activities to be performed
Procedures to be followed
Amounts of the intervention elements (intensity)
Frequency of the intervention
Duration of the intervention

Mediating Processes

Stages of change that occur after the intervention
Mediating variables that bring about treatment effects
Hypothesized relations among mediating variables

Expected Outcomes

Aspects of health status affected
Physical
Mental v Social
Spiritual v Timing and pattern of changes
Hypothesized interrelationships among outcomes
Extraneous Factors
Contextual factors
Environmental factors
Patient characteristics

Treatment Delivery System Resources

Setting
Equipment
Intervener characteristics

in functioning that have the potential of resulting in dysfunction. The problem might also be expressed as a nursing diagnosis. Your theoretical description of the problem must include a discussion of its causal dynamics and how the problem is manifested. You must address the causal processes through which the intervention is expected to affect the problem. You must also clarify variations of the problem in different populations and in different conditions. The following excerpt, from a study by Colling and Buettner (2002), is an example description of a problem that an intervention theory might address.

Physical aggression, wandering, problematic vocalizations, and passivity are well-documented behaviors which often accompany dementing illnesses especially during the middle to late stages of cognitive and physical impairment (Kolanowski, 1999). (Colling & Buettner, 2002, p. 16)

Buettner (1999) acknowledged nursing home residents with dementia often sit for hours with little stimulation or activity within their reach. In addition, the more advanced the course of the dementia, the fewer visits the individual had from family and friends. Supporting literature shows nursing home residents have nothing to do during 60% to 80% of their waking hours. It was during this time of boredom and inactivity that most disturbing behaviors occurred (Cohen-Mansfield & Werner, 1998). It appeared certain disturbing behaviors were an attempt by residents to create their own activity because nursing facilities often do not have funds to continually supply residents with social recreational items. (Colling & Buettner, 2002, p. 17)

Intervention

The theoretical presentation of the intervention must specify what actions, procedures, and intervention strength are required to produce the desired effects. Causal interactions among various elements of the intervention must be explored.

Strong interventions contain large amounts of the elements constituting the intervention. Strength of intervention is defined in terms of amount, frequency, and duration. Intensity of an intervention defines the amount of each activity that must be given and the frequency with which each activity is implemented. Duration of an intervention is the total length of time the intervention is to be implemented (Scott & Sechrest, 1989; Sechrest et al., 1983; Sidani & Braden, 1998; Yeaton & Sechrest, 1981). For example, if the intervention were mouth care for stomatitis (controlling for severity, white blood count, and day in the treatment cycle), strength would be (1) the amount or concentration of mouth solution used, (2) the frequency with which the mouth care was given, and (3) the number of days (duration) that the mouth care was provided.

Some interventions are relatively simple, and others may be complex. The complexity of the intervention is determined by the type and number of activities to be performed. Complex, multicomponent interventions may require multiple, highly skilled interveners. The research team must explore the effect of moderator variables (see later discussion) on the effectiveness of the intervention. The theoretical presentation given here guides the operational development of an intervention design by Colling and Buettner (2002).

The authors hypothesized isolation, inactivity, and disturbing behaviors would be reduced by enriching the environment with readily accessible, attractive recreational items. They also expected that unmet needs for socialization, comforting activities, and freedom to take and use things from the environment would reduce inactivity, isolation, and need-driven behaviors.

The purpose of this project was first to design and test easy-to-make, recreational items for nursing home residents. The items were to be fabricated by community volunteers, who were trained to make, deliver, and use the items during visits. (Colling & Buettner, 2002, p. 17)

The Simple Pleasures project consisted of the design and production of sensorimotor recreational items by staff, volunteers, and families. There was also an educational component to this part of the intervention. Everyone was trained to make specific items based on talents and interests, and were taught about making a visit with the items. Twenty-three items were selected from the original 30 items tested. Families, staff, and residents used the items freely, as needed. "How to use" instruction sheets were included in the training manual. (Colling & Buettner, 2002, p. 17)

Two models were used for the model of delivery. Residents were able to select items freely that were displayed on the "Simple Pleasures cart." Visitors and staff were also invited to select items from the Simple Pleasures activity area to use during their visits. (Colling & Buettner, 2002, p. 19)

At the end of the project, a training manual was published which included instructions for making and using each item. (Colling & Buettner, 2002, p. 18).

Table 13-8 lists examples of items developed and what behaviors the items were used for.

Moderator Variables

A moderator variable is, in effect, a separate independent variable affecting outcomes. A moderator variable alters the causal relationship between the intervention and the outcomes. The moderator effect occurs simultaneously with the intervention effect. A moderator variable also may interact with elements of the intervention to alter the direction or strength of changes caused by the intervention. Thus, a moderator variable could cause the intervention to have a negative rather than a positive effect or to have a less powerful effect on outcomes. Moderator variables could also increase the maximum effectiveness of the treatment. An understanding of the causal links between moderator variables and the intervention is critical to implementing an effective intervention in various patient care situations. Moderator variables may be characteristics of patients or of interveners, or

TABLE 13-8 ▪ Simple Pleasures Activities

Name of Item	Behavior Item Used For
Activity apron	Repetitive motor patterns
Stuffed butterfly or fish	Verbal repetitiveness
Cart for wandering	Wandering and taking med cart
Electronic busy box	Passivity
Fishing box	Hand restlessness
Fleece covered hot water bottle	Screaming
Flower arranging	Hand restlessness
Electronic busy box	Passivity
Hang the laundry	Wandering and restlessness
Home decorator books	Sad, weepy, upset
Latch box-doors	Verbal agitation
Look inside purse	Wandering, upset, hand restlessness
Message magnets	Difficulty making needs known
Muffs	General agitation and anxiety
Rings on hooks game	Motor restlessness
Sewing cards	Passivity and hand restlessness
Squeezies	Anxiety and hand restlessness
Table ball game	Wandering and trying to leave
Tablecloth with activities	Boredom, isolation, hand restlessness
Tetherball game	Verbal or motor repetitiveness
Vests/sensory	Verbal or motor repetitiveness
Wave machines	Repetitive hand movements

From Fitzsimmons, S., & Buettner, L. L. (2002). Therapeutic recreation interventions for need-driven dementia-compromised behaviors in community-dwelling elders. *American Journal of Alzheimer's Disease & Other Dementias, 17*(6), 367–381.

they may be situational (Baron & Kenny, 1986; Lindley & Walker, 1993).

One of the most familiar moderators is the effect of stress on learning from the intervention of patient education. The causal relationship in this case can be modeled as follows:

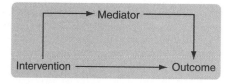

The level of stress occurring during patient education can change the effect of the education. In very low stress, the patient may not experience a need to know what he or she is being taught; thus, learning is reduced. High stress during patient education interferes with the patient's ability to incorporate and apply the information provided and thus reduces learning. Moderate stress during patient education maximizes the effect of the intervention.

The level of stress also has a direct effect (as an independent variable) on learning. The relationship of stress in this case could be modeled as follows:

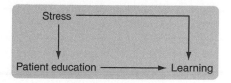

Colling and Buettner (2002), in developing their intervention, used the middle-range theory of the Needs-Driven Dementia-Compromised Behavior Model (Algase et al., 1996).

Needs Driven Behaviors include wandering, vocalizing and physical aggression. These behaviors may be perceived as disruptive or dysfunctional, however, they represent the most integrated response the person can give. The person is limited by the dementing condition; they have strengths from their basic abilities and personality; and they have constraints, challenges, and supports from the immediate environment. The needs driven behaviors are an effort by the person with dementia to pursue a goal or to express a need. The behaviors are the result of an interaction of Background Factors (neurological, cognitive, general health, and psychosocial) and Proximal Factors (personal, physical environment, and social environment). A moderator variable in this situation could be interaction with another person such as a staff person, family member or friend.

Mediator Variables and Processes

A **mediator variable** brings about treatment effects after the treatment has occurred. The effectiveness of the treatment process relies on mediator variables. The intervention may have a direct effect on the outcomes, a direct effect on the mediator or mediators, and an indirect effect on outcomes through the mediator variables. The relationship could be modeled as follows:

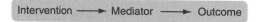

In other cases, the effect of the intervention occurs only through its effect on the mediator, as follows:

Intervention ⟶ Mediator ⟶ Outcome

The expected outcomes of an intervention are the result of a transformational process that occurs as a series of changes in participants and mediator variables after the intervention has been initiated. The series of changes are referred to as mediating processes. For any intervention, a number of mediating processes may ensue before the implementation leads to the outcomes. Although broadly the intervention causes the outcomes, defining the mediating processes explains exactly how the intervention causes the outcomes.

To understand each mediating process, the researcher must dissect the causal processes to identify hypothesized relations among the mediator variables that result in the outcomes. Because the same variable can function as a mediator in some situations and as a moderator in other situations, it is important for the intervention theory to specify the mediator-moderator role of the different variables important to the understanding of the phenomenon of interest. The stages of change through which a participant progresses in the transition to the desired state can be expressed in the map of the intervention theory (Baron & Kenny, 1986; Lindley & Walker, 1993; Sidani & Braden, 1998).

Colling and Buettner (2002) provided the following discussion of mediating processes in their intervention theory:

> Two models were used for the mode of delivery. Residents were able to select items freely that were displayed on the "Simple Pleasures cart." Visitors and staff were also invited to select items from the Simple Pleasures activity area to use during their visits. These modes manipulated model factors relating to the person and the physical and social environment. The amount of stimulation and the frequency of the stimulation were studied during the research project. The use of videotaped observation of residents allowed the research staff to determine the average duration each item was used. For example, the tetherball was used by 47 residents with an average MMSE score of 6.8, for an average time of 21 minutes. (Colling & Buettner, 2002, p. 19)
>
> Part of the transformational process centered on the education of the staff, volunteers, and family members. As a result, there were a series of changes that occurred. These included more visits, more socializing, less boredom, less self-stimulating behavior (e.g., entering another resident's room and rummaging, passively sitting at the nursing station). The results showed fewer disturbing behaviors occurred. (Colling & Buettner, 2002, p. 19)

Expected Outcomes

Outcomes are determined by the problem and purpose of the intervention and are the various effects of the intervention. They reflect the changes that occur as a consequence of the intervention. Outcomes may be physical, mental, social, spiritual, or any combination of these types. The timing and pattern of changes must also be specified. Timing is the point in time after the intervention that a change is expected to occur. Some changes occur immediately after an intervention, whereas others may not appear for some time. Mediators are referred to in some studies as intermediate outcomes. Hypothesized interrelationships among the outcomes must be indicated in the theory.

Extraneous Factors

Extraneous variables are elements of the environment or characteristics of the patient that significantly affect the problem, the treatment process, or the outcomes. Unlike mediator variables, extraneous factors tend not to be well understood and often are unidentifiable until a study has been initiated. They are seldom included in explanations of the causal links between intervention and outcomes. Thus, they are extraneous to existing theoretical explanations of cause. They are sometimes referred to as confounding variables. If the researcher recognizes their potential effect, extraneous factors may be held constant (not allowed to vary) or measured so that they can be statistically controlled during analysis. Careful analyses may indicate that some variables defined as extraneous are actually moderator or mediator variables (Sidani & Braden, 1998).

Patient Characteristics

Researchers are increasingly attending to the influence of individual characteristics on the patients' response to illness or to treatment. Sidani and Braden (1998, p. 64) pointed out that "client characteristics may affect the clients' general susceptibility to illness; the nature and extent of the presenting problem; the design and selection of interventions; the clients' beliefs, values, and preferences for treatments; and the clients' response to illness and to treatment." Patient characteristics also affect the extent to which the patient becomes involved in health-promoting lifestyles.

Patient characteristics of importance to a particular intervention can be identified (1) during the information-gathering period, (2) through pilot studies designed to test the intervention, and (3) through the established observation system. The intervention theory must identify and categorize patient characteristics that have the potential of influencing response to the treatment (Frank-Stromborg, Pender, Walker, & Sechrist, 1990; Johnson, Ratner, Bottroff, & Hayduk, 1993). As the nurse researcher, you must identify or develop methods to measure patient characteristics relevant to the intervention using the observation system. Table 13-9 lists patient characteristics that researchers have identified as influencing the response to illness or treatment.

TABLE 13-9 ▪ Patient Characteristics

Personal Characteristics

Demographic characteristics (age, gender, education, ethnicity)
Personality traits
Emotional status
Cognitive processes
Beliefs and attitudes
Values
Resourcefulness
Sense of mastery
Perceived self-competence
Lifestyle
Learning style preference
Behavior
Cognitive processes
Cultural norms
Affect
Anxiety
Depression

Illness or Health-Related Characteristics

Physiological and physical functioning
Biological characteristics
Psychosocial functioning
Individual's definition of health
Value for health
Beliefs about health and illness
Severity of illness
Stage of illness
Perceived symptom burden
Functional status
Ability to perform activities of daily living
Number of symptoms experienced
Available Resources
Social support
Employment
Health care cost coverage
Income
Coping strategies

TABLE 13-10 ▪ Intervener Characteristics

Personal Characteristics

Age
Gender
Ethnicity
Communication skills
Demeanor
Friendliness
Courtesy
Sensitivity
Being gentle and understanding
Tone of voice
Body language
Appearance
Attractiveness
Neatness
Method of presentation
Maturity
Emotional well-being
Perceptual and cognitive style
Expectancies
Economic incentives

Professional Competencies

Skills needed to implement intervention
Educational background
Discipline
Specialty training
Level of competence or expertise
Beliefs and attitudes toward health and health care
Preferences for treatment modalities
Manual dexterity
Job satisfaction

Environmental Factors

An intervention "occurs in a sociocultural, economic, political, and organizational context, any part of which may affect both the processes and the outcomes, usually in ways we little understand" (Hegyvary, 1992, p. 21). Two environmental factors of particular importance to the problem, the intervention, and the outcomes in many intervention theories are intervener characteristics and setting characteristics.

Intervener Characteristics. Interveners are individuals who help to deliver the study intervention. They are usually health care professionals functioning in the role of clinicians or researchers. In some cases, however, the intervener may be a family member, a neighbor, the patient, or an unskilled staff person employed within the treatment delivery system. The personal and professional characteristics of interveners affect interpersonal and technical aspects related to implementing the intervention. Thus, it is essential for researchers to identify important intervener characteristics in the intervention theory. Develop measurement methods that you can use to gather data on the interveners for the observation system. Table 13-10 lists some of the personal and professional intervener characteristics identified by Sidani and Braden (1998) that might modify the implementation of an intervention.

Setting Characteristics. The setting in which the intervention will be delivered has a potential influence on the expected intervention outcomes. For example, variation in the clinical activities performed by the staff nurses in different settings can affect outcomes. The setting can serve as a moderator variable either by facilitating or impeding implementation of the intervention or by muting or intensifying intervention effects (Conrad & Conrad, 1994). In addition, the setting may modify the way the intervention is implemented. Such influences can threaten the external validity of conclusions and cannot be ignored.

Other aspects of the setting that the intervention theory must address are the resources needed to carry out the activities of the intervention. Resources include (1) equipment, (2) space for the intervention, (3) the availability of adequately educated professional interveners with the experience needed to provide the intervention, (4) adequate support staff, (5) a political-social environment that facilitates implementation of the intervention, and (6) access to telephones and computers (Sidani & Braden, 1998). Table 13-11 lists some of the setting characteristics identified by Sidani and Braden (1998).

Health Care System. In today's health care arena, factors related to the system of care within which the intervention is provided may play an important role in the effectiveness of the intervention. The system of care may be a managed care system, a health maintenance organization (HMO), a home health care

system, a nursing home corporation, the community, a primary care provider's office, a public health clinic in the community, or the patient's home. In some cases, the patient may be the community, and a group of committed citizens may be the health care system of interest.

Developing a Conceptual Map of the Intervention Theory

The researcher should develop a map illustrating the elements of the intervention and the causal links among them. Elements must be clearly defined, and causal links explained. Your map should show all causal pathways described in the intervention theory, including moderator and mediator variables. List all of the testable propositions that the theory has generated.

Designing the Intervention

During the design period, and guided by the intervention theory, the project team specifies the procedural elements of the intervention and develops an observation system (Fawcett et al., 1994). The intervention may be (1) a strategy, (2) a technique, (3) a program, (4) informational or training materials, (5) environmental design variables, (6) a motivational system, or (7) a new or modified policy. The intervention must be specified in sufficient detail to allow interveners to implement it consistently.

During the design process, the intervention will emerge in stages, as it is repeatedly tested, redesigned, and retested. Training materials and programs for interveners also must be developed and repeatedly tested and revised. Design criteria are established to evaluate the implementation of the intervention and outcomes.

In addition to a detailed development of the intervention, an operational development of the design guided by the theory should include the following activities:

- Define the target population.
- List acceptable strategies for selecting a sample.
- Identify subgroups that might show differential effects of the intervention.
- Specify essential characteristics of interventionists.
- Determine study variables.
- Indicate appropriate measures of variables.
- Specify the appropriate time or times to measure outcomes.
- Indicate what analyses to perform and what relationships to test on the basis of the relationships among the treatment and the moderator, mediator, and outcome variables specified by the intervention theory.

Intervention Fidelity

Intervention fidelity occurs when the interventionist reliably and competently delivers the experimen-

TABLE 13-11 ■ Setting Characteristics
Personal Features
Access to participants
Convenience to participants
Availability of equipment
Physical layout and attractiveness
Noise level
Ambient temperature
Light
Comfort of furniture
Provision for privacy
Room interior design or decoration
Familiarity to participants
General ambience
Psychosocial Features
Organizational culture
Norms and policies
Standards and protocols of care
Composition of interdisciplinary health care team
Differences in skill mix of providers
Number of providers
Type of institution
Geographical context
Staff satisfaction
Stress levels of staff
Leadership style
Professional practice model

tal treatment (Stein et al., 2007). An interventionist is a person who has been formally prepared to provide a particular intervention and is accountable for the fidelity of the intervention. Methods to adhere to the intervention protocol are critical to the success of an intervention study. The internal validity of a study requires the independent variable (the intervention) to be administered systematically and consistently. The interventionists must conform to the intervention protocol and have sufficient competence to administer the intervention. The behaviors proscribed by the intervention protocol are delivered in sessions or classes designed to prepare the interventionists. Strategies to improve intervention fidelity may include intervention manuals, formal training, and clinical supervision. To evaluate intervention fidelity, before and during the study, coders may be used to evaluate audio or audiovisual tapes, to observe of the interventionist during practice, and to apply other means using rating scales. These coders are part of the observation system described later. The coders' observation activities may occur during pilot studies and periodically during the study. They are implemented during the study to test for drift. Drift is a gradual change in the consistency in treatment delivery over the course of the study.

Interventionists

Interventionist behaviors in relation to the administration of the intervention are usually evaluated in pilot tests before a study has been initiated and during the period of the study. Three behaviors of interventionists concern us here: (1) those prescribed by the intervention, (2) those that are universal in therapeutic interactions, and (3) those proscribed by the intervention. These three constitute the distinctiveness and purity of the intervention. Prescribed behaviors are those that are elements of the interventions. Universal behaviors are those that any practitioner in the situation would commonly do, such as establishing rapport with the patient, explaining the goals of the interventionist, or explaining the intervention process to the patient. Proscribed behaviors are those that the interventionist must not do or discuss. For example it is essential that the interventionist not use strategies from competing interventions, as this will weaken the capacity to test for differences in the experimental intervention and comparison interventions (Stein et al., 2007).

Establishing an Observation System

The use of an observation system is a novel idea in nursing research. They are not used frequently. However, the observation system is one of the important strengths of intervention research. It is designed and

implemented before any changes are made in the patient care situation. An observation system allows you and other researchers to (1) observe events related to the phenomenon naturalistically, (2) discover the extent of the problem, (3) observe the intervention being implemented, and (4) detect effects of the intervention. Patients affected by the problem under study can help identify behaviors and environmental conditions that must be observed. Observations should be made also of patient characteristics, intervener characteristics, setting characteristics, dynamics of the health care system, and use of resources (Fawcett et al., 1994; Sidani & Braden, 1998). Possible elements of the observation system are listed in Table 13-12.

Observations lead to insights about what must be changed by the intervention or in the system so that the intervention can be effective. The observation system also serves as a means of feedback for refining early prototypes of the intervention and, thus, is closely tied to designing and pilot-testing the intervention. Behavioral events that are elements of the intervention or that are components of the environment that could influence the effectiveness of the intervention must be defined and observed. The observation activities provide information that is important for specifying the procedural elements of the intervention. These elements include (1) the use of information, (2) the use of skills, (3) training, (4) environmental change strategies, (5) the policy changes or enforcement strategies used, and (6) reinforcement and punishment procedures (Fawcett et al., 1994; Sidani & Braden, 1998).

Nursing students at all levels of education could participate in the observation system. The system could give undergraduate students the chance to participate clinically in nursing research activities. Students involved in research projects, theses, or dissertations might gather or analyze data for the observational system.

The observational methods used and the extent of observations vary with the financial and personnel resources available. The observation system should be developed based on knowledge acquired through the information-gathering process. The observation system must include measures of variables in the setting that might affect the problem, the intervention, or the outcomes. Possible elements of the observation system are listed in Table 13-12.

Researchers must design the observation system carefully and include methods for measuring the elements of interest. Your procedures should be specified in enough detail that they can be replicated. Observers must be carefully trained. Observations must be made before initiation of the intervention, during the intervention,

TABLE 13-12 ■ Elements of Observation System

Before the Intervention

Characteristics of the problem
Patient characteristics
Characteristics of patients with the problem who receive the
  intervention
Characteristics of patients with the problem who do not receive
  the intervention
Intervention characteristics
Elements of intervention
Intensity of intervention
Duration of intervention
Use of the intervention
Intervener characteristics
Professional and personal characteristics
Setting characteristics
Resources used (e.g., equipment and supplies)
Physical layout
Staff
Organizational support
Events occurring during the study that affected the intervention

During the Intervention

Problem characteristics
Patient characteristics
Who were the target population?
How many participants were recruited?
How many who were approached refused to participate?
What reasons did they give for refusal?
What were the characteristics of the participants?
What were the characteristics of those who refused to
  participate?
How do those who accepted and those who refused compare
  with the target population?
Intervention characteristics
Elements of intervention
Intensity of intervention
Duration of intervention
Intervener characteristics
Professional and personal characteristics
Were training sessions provided?
Content of training sessions
What interveners attended training sessions?
How did interveners relate to participants?
Did more than one intervener care for a participant?
Setting characteristics
Administrative arrangements made
Events occurring during intervention that might affect
  implementation
Type of equipment used
Was the same type of equipment used for all participants?

After the Intervention

Process of outcomes

and after the intervention. Your observation system must allow monitoring of the extent to which the intervention was implemented as planned during the period in which it was provided.

The types of measurement you will use depend on a number of factors, such as (1) the number of individuals and behaviors being observed, (2) the length of observations, (3) the size of observation intervals during an observation session, and (4) the availability of observers. You might include measures such as tape-recorded interviews, field notes of observers, coding forms, checklists, knowledge tests, scales to measure aspects such as attitudes or beliefs, measures of physiological dimensions of the patient state, videotapes of the intervention being provided, and event logs. In addition to measures for direct observation, you may need to establish measures for patients or interveners to self-monitor or self-report about events that are difficult for you or your team to observe directly (Barlow, Hayes, & Nelson, 1989).

The validity and reliability of measurement methods used must be evaluated. You must develop criteria for the observer to apply when determining whether or not the event being studied has occurred. Use these criteria to determine the start of an observation period (Fawcett et al., 1994). Steps of the observation process are listed in Table 13-13.

Testing the Intervention

The intervention is tested in stages, revised, and retested until a satisfactorily designed intervention emerges.

TABLE 13-13 ■ Steps of the Observation Process

1. Determine elements that must be observed on the basis of the intervention theory.
2. Develop methods of measuring essential elements.
3. Develop criteria for determining whether or not the event to be observed has occurred.
4. Select observers.
5. Train observers.
6. Develop scoring instructions to guide recording of desired behaviors or products.
7. Develop a schedule of observations to include the following:
   a. What is happening before the intervention is implemented
   b. What is happening during the intervention
   c. What changes occur after the intervention
8. Perform preliminary analysis of preintervention data.
9. Apply preliminary analysis results to further develop the intervention.
10. Analyze changes in environment and behaviors before, during, and after the intervention.
11. Refine intervention theory.

The stages of testing are (1) development of a prototype, (2) analogue testing, (3) pilot testing, (4) formal testing, (5) advanced testing, and (6) field testing.

Developing a Prototype

A prototype is a primitive design that has evolved to the point that it can be tested clinically. The prototype is defined by the intervention theory. Developing a prototype involves establishing and selecting a mode of delivering the intervention. Considerable refinement would be required before a prototype could be used in an intervention study (Fawcett et al., 1994).

Analogue Testing

For some interventions, before the pilot test, it is useful to test prototypes in analogue situations, using actors to play roles in the intervention. Members of the project team, staff from the settings to be used for the project, or nursing students might perform these roles. The actor interveners follow the intervention steps prescribed by the prototype. Videotapes of the proceedings will allow you to carefully analyze the adequacy of the prototype. Observers also make notes during the prototype test of missing elements, insights gained, or questions that the project team must explore (Fawcett et al., 1994).

Pilot Testing

Multiple pilot tests are needed for intervention research. These pilot studies are used for the following purposes:

1. To determine whether the prototype will work.
2. To guide refinement of the prototype. The intervention is first evaluated according to standards established in that particular care situation. The established design criteria are then used to evaluate the effectiveness of the prototype. This evaluation enables the researchers to optimize the intervention before further testing.
3. To test and refine instructions, manuals, or training programs.
4. To determine whether the intervention has been described in sufficient detail to allow clinicians and other researchers to replicate the work. Clinicians should also be queried about their reasoning and decisions during the implementation of the intervention.
5. To examine reliability, validity, and usability of measurement methods in the target population.
6. To test the design.
7. To determine unanticipated effects.

Pilot tests should be conducted in settings similar to those in which the intervention will be used and with subjects similar to those who will typically be receiving the intervention. Use observation techniques to gather the information you will need to revise the prototype. Pilot tests are ideal for graduate nursing student research projects, theses, or dissertations conducted in collaboration with the project team. Colling and Buettner (2002) described the development of their observational system and intervention as follows.

> The Simple Pleasures project began in a pilot test site, which was used to evaluate the safety and appeal of the 30 original recreation items. During this pilot testing period, the research team eliminated seven of the Simple Pleasures recreational items. The team also determined color and texture preference, and decided how to best make the items accessible. (Colling & Buettner, 2002, p. 17)
>
> The research component then began using a clinical crossover design at two nursing homes with a 1-month 'wash-out' period between sites. The research was carried out on two 40-bed special care units for 6 months each. Data were collected through random videotaping, family interviews, direct observations, and questionnaires. (Colling & Buettner, 2002, p. 18)
>
> In addition to the videotaped information, primary professional caregivers provided information on disturbing behaviors at four time points by filling out the Cohen-Mansfield Agitation Inventory (CMAI) (Cohen-Mansfield, 1996), Mini-Mental State Examination (MMSE) (Folstein, Folstein, & McHugh, 1975), Geriatric Depression Scale (GDS) (Sheikh & Yesavage, 1986), and Minimum Data Set (MDS) medication listing (Rantz & Popejoy, 1998). The actual number of visits was reported on a unit log-in system. The research team also maintained a volunteer count during the project. During the research component of the project, the following questions were examined:
>
> - Will age-related and stage-appropriate recreational items, constructed by families and volunteers, positively affect frequency and quality of visits?
> - Will an increased supply of the Simple Pleasure items increase time spent in purposeful activity, and decrease disturbing behaviors?
> - Which items are most appropriate for residents at different functional levels and behavioral needs?

Three different Simple Pleasures items were introduced each week at a short staff in-service and family education session. Staff, family, and visitors were asked to try the various items and provide feedback to the research team.

> *Results:* Families at both sites reported significantly more visits during the intervention phase of the project ($p < 0.006, p < 0.000$). Families at both sites also reported using recreational items during visits significantly more often ($p < 0.000, p < 0.001$), and said they were more satisfied with their visits ($p < 0.001, p < 0.000$).

During the intervention phase, residents at both facilities who were inactive dramatically declined, and residents were more involved with the recreational items and other residents. During the intervention phase at research Site 1, there was a significant drop in agitation ($p < 0.001$). There was a slight drop in agitation at Site 2, but the change was not statistically significant. (Colling & Buettner, 2002, p. 18)

Formal Testing

The most desirable formal test of the intervention is a conventional experimental design to determine whether the intervention causes the intended effects. The design should be as rigorous as possible. Use power analyses to determine a sample size sufficient to avoid a type II error. Perform analyses to ensure that the treatment and control groups are comparable on important variables. Use measurement instruments whose reliability and validity has been documented. Report the effect size for each outcome examined. The observation system established before the initiation of testing is continued, and patient characteristics, intervener characteristics, and setting characteristics are measured (Sidani & Braden, 1998). Two-way analysis of variance (ANOVA) or multivariate analysis of covariance (ANCOVA) is commonly used to test for effects of the intervention.

Identifying the Required Resources. The formal test of an intervention must occur in a setting that can provide the required resources to implement the intervention optimally. The nature of the intervention and its level of complexity define the resources needed. The resources required include (1) institutional support for testing the intervention, (2) the availability of equipment and materials needed to administer the intervention, (3) the availability of target participants who would benefit most from the intervention, and (4) interveners with the full range of skills needed to implement the intervention. If any of these resources is at a level less than required, delivery of the intervention may vary, affecting the intervention outcomes (Chen, 1990; Lipsey, 1993; Rosen & Proctor, 1978; Sidani & Braden, 1998).

Maintaining the Integrity of the Intervention. In a formal test of an intervention, it is critical that the integrity of the intervention be maintained. Integrity of an intervention is the extent to which the intervention is implemented as it was designed. The design defines what activities are to be done and when, where, how, and by whom they are to be carried out.

Lack of intervention integrity is a discrepancy between what was planned and what was actually delivered. It may occur if the intervention is not clearly described or if the interveners do not have a clear understanding of what activities to perform, when, or with whom. Lack of integrity can occur because interveners were not sufficiently trained or lacked guidance during the period of formal testing. In some cases, interveners may not interpret instructions as the researchers expected. This is most likely to occur when elements of the intervention are not well defined and clearly circumscribed, leading to different interpretations by the interveners (Kirchhoff & Dille, 1994; Rezmovic, 1984; Sechrest et al., 1983; Sidani & Braden, 1998; Yeaton & Sechrest, 1981).

Loss of integrity can also occur because participants are exposed to different elements of the intervention or given different levels of strengths of the intervention. Loss of integrity may occur because the intervention is not provided in a consistent manner, interveners tailor the intervention to the needs of individual patients, or the intervention requires the participants to implement the intervention in settings away from the intervener's immediate supervision. These differences lead to disparities in levels of outcomes and can result in an inability to detect significant treatment effects; thus, they may lead to incorrect conclusions about the effectiveness of the intervention (Rezmovic, 1984; Rossi & Freemen, 1993; Sidani & Braden, 1998; Yeaton & Sechrest, 1981). Level of response and motivation of subjects is another factor that causes outcomes to vary. Factors affecting intervention integrity are listed in Table 13-14.

TABLE 13-14 ▪ Factors Affecting Integrity of Intervention

Inadequate training of interveners
Poorly defined intervention
Variation in strength of intervention provided
Variation in elements of intervention provided
Ease in implementing intervention activities
Intervention's level of complexity
Inadequate planning
Inadequate guidance during study
Level of interveners' skill
Level of staff commitment to the intervention
Level of organizational commitment to the intervention
Number of interveners
Number of sites involved in implementing the intervention
Level of compliance of staff with treatment protocol
Interactional style of interveners
Changes in organization policies after initiation of study
Changes in brand of equipment used
Changes in composition of interveners

Kirchhoff and Dille (1994) described problems they experienced in maintaining the integrity of their study intervention:

In 1983 a study was conducted on the Rehabilitation Nursing Unit at University of Utah Hospital to test the effectiveness of a decontamination procedure on vinyl urinary leg and bed bags. Rehabilitation patients with bladder dysfunction use two urine bags, a daytime leg bag (for concealment under clothing) and a nighttime larger-volume bed bag. Because the usually closed urinary drainage system is disrupted at least twice daily, a procedure for decontamination was necessary if the bags were to be reused safely rather than discarded daily....

The solution instilled into bags daily was a 1:3 solution of bleach to water with a contact time of at least 30 minutes (Hashisaki et al., 1984). Based on that study's results of effective decontamination, the bag replacement schedule was changed from daily to weekly at a considerable savings....

Four years later cost-conscious nurses proposed a 4-week in-hospital reuse for the bags. Because the bags are marketed as single-use disposable items, this time frame needed to be carefully tested....

In the decontamination study, the frequency, regularity, and daily nature of the intervention called for several individuals participating solely from a scheduling perspective. Because of the long-term nature of this study (3-year funding period), vacation time and other leave time had to be considered....

In this study, communication occurred with the obvious: the Rehabilitation Unit nursing staff, the attending physicians, nursing and hospital administration, and the epidemiology nurses. Inadvertently, the not so obvious did not receive or recall study information: the per diem nurses who floated to the unit, the rehabilitation residents who rotated in and out of the unit every 3 months, and the housekeepers. These three groups of people had the potential to influence results, affect subject accrual, and contribute to missing or altered data if they were not informed about the study requirements. Per diem staff either had not been taught about the protocol or performed the former standard for the procedure. Residents who were not informed believed that the study would limit a patient's progression in bladder management and were reluctant to have their patients entered into the study. At times the housekeepers inadvertently discarded the drainage equipment as it was air drying, which resulted in the loss of data and affected costs of the grant.

Using the procedure as a performance checklist, observations of the staff's performance of the procedure were completed before and during the study at least every 6 months. At the same time, the study progress was reviewed and the staff was questioned about activities they were required to perform for the study. These included how to label and use the bags, what to do when problems arise, the criteria for inclusion in the study, and the differences between the experimental and control groups. On subsequent observations, this time period also was used to discuss reported or discovered concerns about the individual's performance....

Despite the intensive planning and compliance checks, problems arose. Housekeeping personnel discarded bags that were air-drying. Per diem staff discarded the bags, performed the procedure incorrectly, or neglected to do it at all. Discoveries were made by the nursing staff or study staff that bags had been mislabeled, applied to the wrong patient, or had incomplete information on the bag label. When a few staff devised a method of hanging the leg bag to dry by knotting its tubing, the effect of air-drying was reduced. In all these instances, individual staff members were contacted and the situation was corrected....

Although it appears that a number of problems were uncovered, close monitoring showed these problems before there was major impact on the integrity of the study. When close monitoring does not occur, a lack of problems may really be a lack of discovery. A false sense of security can result. (Kirchhoff & Dille, 1994, pp. 32–36)

On the basis of these experiences, which they were good enough to share with us, Kirchhoff and colleagues modified their intervention protocol for future studies (Dille & Kirchhoff, 1993; Dille, Kirchhoff, Sullivan, & Larson, 1993).

Advanced Testing

Advanced testing of the intervention occurs after sufficient evidence is available that the intervention is effective in achieving desired outcomes. This stage of testing might begin after a single, well-designed study indicates a satisfactory effect size but is more likely to be initiated after a series of studies in which the intervention is modified or the findings are replicated. Advanced testing focuses on identifying variations in effectiveness based on patient characteristics, intervener characteristics, and setting characteristics.

Testing Variations in Effectiveness Based on Variations in Patient Characteristics. Intervention effects that have been determined through the use of a sample of white, middle-class Americans may not have the same effect with other groups. The intervention should be tested in various ethnic groups. Pilot tests may reveal a need to refine the intervention to make it culturally appropriate. The poor and undereducated may respond differently to interventions, because (1) they have a different view of health and of preventive behaviors and (2) they may not understand educational components of interventions that were designed for people with a higher level of education. For the same reasons, scales designed for the white middle class may not be effective measures in different ethnic groups or in the undereducated. Thus, modifications in the intervention and in the design may be necessary.

Studies also must be conducted to examine the effect of the intervention on groups with comorbidities or differing levels of severity of illness. Other variations in patient characteristics, such as age, gender, and diagnosis, may be important to examine. Characteristics specific to the intervention may be identified as important for determining differential effects. If sufficiently large samples were obtained in the initial study, these patient characteristics may be available from the observation system and may involve secondary analyses of available data.

Testing Variations in Effectiveness Based on Setting. If your setting is held constant, so that all interventions are provided in the same place, under the same conditions, and among all subjects, the effects of your setting will be potentially confounded with the treatment effects. Therefore, one component of testing the intervention is to set up multisite projects, in which the settings are varied and the effects of the settings on outcomes are examined (Sidani & Braden, 1998).

Testing Variations in Effectiveness Based on Variations in Intervener Characteristics. The initial study examining the effectiveness of an intervention is usually conducted under ideal conditions. Ideal conditions involve the selection of highly educated interveners judged to be experts in the field of practice related to the intervention. However, after the intervention is found to be effective, questions arise regarding the use of less well-prepared interveners to provide the intervention. Studies should be conducted to determine variations in the effectiveness of the intervention based on the competencies of interveners.

Testing Variations in Effectiveness Based on Strength of an Intervention. The strategy of testing the variations of an intervention's strength is used to determine the amount of treatment that provides optimal strength in achieving the desired outcome. To test this issue, the researcher must be able to provide varying doses of the intervention. You might vary the intensity of the intervention, the length of time of a single treatment, the frequency of an intervention, or the span of time over which the intervention is continued or repeated.

Path Analyses. Path analyses examine the causal processes through which each component of an intervention has its effect, including moderator and mediator variables. The design tests the validity of the intervention theory. Reliable measures of each of the processes and each of the outcome variables are included in the design. Structural equation analysis examines the contribution of each component to the outcome (Sidani & Braden, 1998).

Preference Clinical Trials. In the typical clinical trial, subjects are randomized into groups. However, in some cases, patient preference is an important variable. The effect of active choice on outcomes is important to understand. Wennberg, Barry, Fowler, and Mulley (1993, p. 56) indicated that "when symptom reduction and improvement in the quality of life are the main effects of treatment and the proper decision involves the evaluation of risk aversion and degree of botheredness, then these topics cannot be ignored; they must be made the object of investigation." Thus, in preference clinical trials, rather than being randomized to subject groups, patients choose among all treatments available.

Treatment Matching. Treatment matching compares the relative effectiveness of various treatments. Treatment matching designs are used when the following conditions are met: (1) there is no clearly superior treatment for all individuals with a given problem; (2) a number of treatments with some proven efficacy have comparable effectiveness for undifferentiated groups of subjects; and (3) there is evidence of differential outcomes, either within or among treatments, for defined subtypes of patients (Donovan et al., 1994). No control group is used. The researcher selects sampling criteria to promote heterogeneity rather than homogeneity. Randomization is used, but stratification, matching, and other strategies can be used to obtain balanced distribution. Creative sampling methods may be required to fulfill sampling requirements (Carroll, Kadden, Donovan, Zweben, & Rounsaville, 1994; Connors et al., 1994; DiClemente et al., 1990; Miller & Cooney, 1994; Zweben et al., 1994).

Testing the Effectiveness of Individual Components of Complex Interventions. In complex interventions, whether all elements of the intervention or only some of them are causing the expected outcomes is not always clear. It is important in such cases to conduct studies to examine the differential effects of intervention elements.

West, Aiken, and Todd (1993) have described a series of designs that can be used to test the effectiveness of various components of such a treatment; these strategies are summarized on the following pages. Used as components of an intervention effectiveness research program, these strategies must be conducted with the guidance of the intervention theory and implementation of the observation system.

Dismantling Strategy (Subtraction Design). In dismantling strategy, the full version of the program is compared with a reduced version in which one or more components have been removed. Criteria for selecting components to delete vary but are often based on theory or on information from the literature. Components that are expensive or difficult to provide may also be selected for deletion. Components are removed one at a time, and the reduced set is tested against the full version until a single base component remains. When programs are complex and include many components, various mixes of components may be tested.

Constructive Strategy. In constructive strategy, a base intervention is identified. A component that is expected to increase the effectiveness of the base intervention is added, and the two interventions are tested. There must be a theoretical rationale for the selection of components to add to the base intervention. The components are added one at a time, and each set of components is tested for effectiveness until the full set of possible combinations has been studied. With the use of the dismantling strategy in large programs, various mixes of components may be tested.

Factorial ANOVA Designs. Commonly used in psychology, factorial ANOVA designs are potentially the most powerful way to examine all possible combinations of an intervention. Factorial designs used in intervention trials are usually limited to a 2×2 design, examining the presence or absence of two intervention components. Factorial ANOVA designs usually involve a multisite project with a large sample size to achieve adequate statistical power. The complexity of the design increases with the number of components in the intervention.

Fractional Factorial Designs. Fractional factorial designs are simplifications of the factorial designs. The researcher systematically selects a portion of all possible intervention component combinations to implement. Such a design requires the researcher to be willing to assume that the effects of higher-order interactions (multiple combination effects) are negligible.

Response Surface Methodology. With response surface methodology, the dose response can be applied to more than one dimension of a treatment. If several interventions are constructed that represent a number of combinations of differing levels of strength for each component and the outcome is plotted for each combination, the plotted figure is referred to as a response surface. Researchers can use this methodology to determine which combination of components produces the optimum outcome.

Results of previous response surface analyses have shown that increasing the strength of a component does not always increase its effectiveness. When two individually effective components are combined, the resulting program may be more or less effective than each component alone or may not change the effect. A researcher can improve a program sequentially by refining each component and then studying the combined effects. Developing an optimal program is often an evolutionary process.

Field Tests

Field tests are conducted in clinical settings in which the intervention will typically be implemented. Field tests are ideal for graduate nursing student projects. These studies evaluate the effectiveness of the intervention when implemented in uncontrolled situations. Rather than being controlled, patient characteristics are allowed to vary and are measured. Sampling criteria are limited to the selection of only those patients experiencing the problem. No other constraints are imposed.

The observation system is in operation, and patient characteristics, intervener characteristics, and setting characteristics are measured. Outcome variables are measured at least once before the treatment and once afterward. Repeated measures of outcome variables are often performed during the posttest period (Fawcett et al., 1994; Sidani & Braden, 1998). Design criteria against which the intervention is judged are listed in Table 13-15.

Collecting and Analyzing Data

Data from the observation system, pilot tests, the formal study, and field tests are collected and analyzed continuously. Data analysis goes beyond testing for statistical significance. Two-way analysis of variance, regression

---

TABLE 13-15 ■ Criteria for Intervention Design

1. The intervention is effective.
2. The intervention is replicable by typical interveners.
3. The intervention is simple to use.
4. The intervention is practical.
5. The intervention is adaptable to various contexts.
6. The intervention is compatible with local customs and values.

Adapted from Fawcett, S. B., Suarez-Belcazar, Y., Belcazar, F. E., White, G. W., Paine, A .L., Blanchard, K. A., et al. (1994). Conducting intervention research: The design and development process. In J. Rothman & E. J. Thomas (Eds.), *Intervention research: Design and development for human service,* (pp. 25–54). New York: Haworth Press.

analyses, path analyses, and residual analyses are commonly used.

Exploratory analysis techniques provide important information for determining, for instance, when initial interventions should be implemented and whether supplemental procedures are necessary. Residual analyses may identify subjects who respond differently to the intervention. Qualitative analyses are used when appropriate. Ongoing graphing of phases of the intervention and outcomes over time provide critical information. Data from the project constitute an excellent source for secondary analyses by nursing students.

Dissemination

Once field testing and evaluation are completed, your intervention is ready for dissemination. In nursing, dissemination has traditionally involved presenting the findings at professional meetings, describing the intervention in professional journals, and reporting studies documenting its effect on outcomes. Researchers may report their results by traditional means throughout the process of developing and evaluating the intervention. These contributions are vital to the development of science in nursing.

You should also consider a higher level of dissemination. Nurse researchers might think about viewing the intervention as a product and its dissemination in terms of marketing and selling a product (Fawcett et al., 1994). This would be an important consideration if the user's initial implementation required a considerable investment of time, perhaps to consult with or request assistance from members of the project team. In this case, the process of dissemination would involve choosing a brand name, establishing a price, and setting standards for the intervention's use.

Choosing a Brand Name

Give your intervention a name that is intuitively appealing. It may address the purpose, patients, or setting of the intervention. The name may link the intervention to an established concept in a theory. Establishing a brand name allows adopters to recognize the intervention and differentiate it from similar, but perhaps less effective, interventions. The name of the intervention will come to be associated with its effectiveness, dependability, or efficiency (Fawcett et al., 1994). Do you think "Simple Pleasures" was a good brand name for Colling and Buettner's intervention?

Setting a Price

In setting a price for the intervention, determine or define the market for your product and the discre-

tionary budget of potential adopters. In this period of managed care, when health care corporations are competing for patients by hospitals seeking Magnet status and demonstrating more effective outcomes than their competitors, the motivation to purchase well-designed interventions with demonstrated positive outcomes is high. In 1994, the American Nurses Credentialing Center developed the Magnet Recognition Program to recognize facilities that provide excellent nursing care. To achieve Magnet status, the facility must meet 14 standards with 63 criteria.

Other factors that you and your research team must consider in setting the price are (1) the cost of providing materials related to the intervention; (2) the costs of staff time for phone calls, mailing material, maintaining files, and so on; (3) organizational requirements; (4) the cost of training; and (5) the cost of technical support that may be required after the intervention is implemented. If your goal is the widespread adoption of the intervention with a simple training procedure and little need for ongoing technical support, you might set the price very low, only sufficient to recover costs. However, you are offering a comprehensive or complex treatment program that will require considerable involvement of the researchers or other technical personnel, a higher price might be appropriate (Fawcett et al., 1994).

Setting Standards for Use

The project team must establish guidelines for using the intervention correctly that adopters must agree to before they receive it. Develop specifications regarding conditions under which the intervention can be used. The project should be protected by a patent or copyright until your costs are recovered. This arrangement helps ensure the integrity of the process and the quality of the product (Fawcett et al., 1994).

Identifying Potential Markets

To identify all of the potential markets for your intervention, you and your product team should answer the following questions:

- Which people can benefit personally from our intervention?
- Who (with the use of the intervention) could contribute most to solving the problem?
- Is broad-based adoption our goal (i.e., saturation of the market), or do we seek more restricted use by selected adopters?
- Which market segments—types of health or human service organizations—would most likely adopt and benefit from our intervention if they were aware of it?

- Which media approach—public service announcements, direct mail, or other strategies—would be most appropriate and feasible for informing our targeted market segment?

Identifying potential early adopters may encourage others in the identified market to adopt the intervention. Early adopters tend to have relatively greater resources, sophistication, education, and willingness to try innovative practices. These characteristics may put them in more frequent contact with their colleagues, increasing the chances that other adopters will become aware of the benefits of using your intervention (Fawcett et al., 1994). See Chapter 27 for a discussion of early adopters.

Creating a Demand for the Intervention

Anyone marketing the intervention must persuade potential purchasers that it will actually benefit them. Strategies designed to market innovations include modeling the innovation, arranging sampling of the innovation and its benefits, and advertising. Modeling involves showing experts, celebrities, or others easily identifiable by the market segment using the intervention and benefiting from its use.

In sampling, allow potential purchasers to try out portions of the product. This process might consist of demonstrations of the intervention and opportunities to review materials at regional and national professional conferences.

Advertising campaigns can highlight desired features of the intervention, such as its relative effectiveness, low cost, and decreased time and effort for users. Incentives to encourage adoption, such as describing support services available, can positively influence purchasers. Ultimately, however, these strategies will work only if your product is more effective, is lower in cost, or requires less user time than similar interventions on the market (Fawcett et al., 1994).

Encouraging Appropriate Adaptation

Adaptation involves changing the intervention to fit local conditions and is sometimes referred to as reinvention. Elements of the intervention may be modified or deleted, or new elements may be added. There is a tension between maintaining the quality of an intervention and allowing others to adapt it. Allowing adaptation may increase the speed with which an intervention is adopted, but it may also diminish the intervention's effectiveness. The project team should permit (or even encourage) necessary adaptation, but only under the condition defined by the team. Your team should be allowed to collect and analyze data related to the adaptation or see reports of ongoing analysis by the adapting facility. It is important for the team to determine whether the changed intervention continues to meet the established standards for the intervention (Fawcett et al., 1994).

Providing Technical Support for Adopters

The researchers and their staff are the primary experts on the intervention. Adopters may require technical support with troubleshooting or adapting the intervention to their specific needs (Fawcett et al., 1994).

JUST YOU AND ME: IMPLEMENTING AN INTERVENTION THEORY STUDY ON A SMALL SCALE

Reading this chapter can be overwhelming. It may seem that unless you have a couple of million dollar grants and a huge research team, you might as well forget doing an intervention theory study. And then you think about the Simple Pleasures project. How feasible is it to consider using intervention theory strategies to implement an idea that has been running around the corners of your mind as you read this chapter?

We suggest considering it. You do need some partners who are as committed as you are. You must realize that such a project requires a long-term effort. It is a series of studies and time invested in theoretical thinking and theory development. It may require that you invest some time building your knowledge in areas in which you are not yet well informed. You can start small and build as you begin your first steps. Contact researchers who have been involved in intervention theory work. They can help you to avoid some of the mistakes they made. They may also be willing to guide you across time. The nursing discipline needs more intervention theory projects. The potential contribution to the body of knowledge for nursing is great.

SUMMARY

- This chapter describes a revolutionary new approach to intervention research that holds great promise for designing and testing nursing.
- Nursing interventions are defined as "deliberative cognitive, physical, or verbal activities performed with, or on behalf of, individuals and their families [that] are directed toward accomplishing particular therapeutic objectives relative to individuals' health and well-being" (Grobe, 1996, p. 50).

- An intervention research project consists of multiple studies conducted over a period of years by a project team that may include nursing students.
- Some teams use a participatory research method that involves community groups.
- An intervention theory must include (1) a careful description of the problem to be addressed, (2) the intervening actions that must be implemented to address the problem, (3) moderator variables that might change the impact of the intervention, (4) mediator variables that might alter the effect of the intervention, and (5) expected outcomes of the intervention.
- The intervention theory guides the design and development of an intervention, which is then extensively tested, refined, and retested.
- Advanced testing of the intervention occurs after sufficient evidence is available to determine that the intervention is effective in achieving desired outcomes.
- When the intervention is sufficiently refined and evidence of effectiveness has been obtained, the intervention is field-tested to ensure that it can be effectively implemented in clinical settings.
- An observation system is developed for use throughout the design and development process. This system allows the researchers to observe events related to the intervention naturalistically and to analyze these observations.
- Dissemination efforts are more extensive than in traditional experimental studies and involve choosing a brand name, establishing a price, and setting standards for the intervention's use.

REFERENCES

Abraham, I. L., Chalifoux, Z. L., & Evers, G. C. M. (1992). Conditions, interventions, and outcomes: A qualitative analysis of nursing research (1981–1990). In U.S. Department of Health and Human Services, Public Health Service, *Patient outcomes research: Examining the effectiveness of nursing practice. Proceedings of the State of the Science Conference sponsored by the National Center for Nursing Research, September 11–13, 1991* (DHHS Publication #93–3411, pp. 70–87). Rockville, MD: U.S. Government Printing Office.

Adelman, H. S. (1986). Intervention theory and evaluating efficacy. *Evaluation Review, 10*(1), 65–83.

Algase, D., Beck, C., Kolanowski, A., Whall, A., Berent, S., Richards, K., & Beattie, E. (1996). Need-driven dementia-compromised behavior: An alternative view of disruptive behavior. *American Journal of Alzheimer's Disease, 11*(6), 10–19.

Barlow, D. H., Hayes, S. C., & Nelson, R. O. (1989). *The scientist practitioner: Research and accountability in clinical and educational settings.* New York: Pergamon Press.

Baron, R. M., & Kenny, D. A. (1986). The moderator mediator variable distinction in social psychological research: Conceptual, strategic, and statistical considerations. *Journal of Personality and Social Psychology, 51*(6), 1173–1183.

Bergmark, A., & Oscarsson, L. (1991). Does anybody really know what they are doing? Some comments related to methodology of treatment service research. *British Journal of Addiction, 86*(2), 139–142.

Buettner, L. (1999). Simple pleasures: A multilevel sensorimotor intervention for nursing home residents with dementia. *American Journal of Alzheimer's Disease, 14*(1), 41–52.

Bulechek, G. M., McCloskey, J. C. (2008). *Nursing interventions: Effective nursing treatments.* Philadelphia: W. B. Saunders.

Bulechek, G. M., McCloskey, J. C., & Donahue, W. J. (1995). Nursing interventions classifications (NIC): A language to describe nursing treatments. In N.M. Lang (Ed.), *Nursing data systems: An emerging framework: Data system advances for clinical nursing practice.* Washington, DC: American Nurses Publishing.

Carroll, K. M., Kadden, R. M., Donovan, D. M., Zweben, A., Rounsaville, B. J. (1994). Implementing treatment and protecting the validity of the independent variable in treatment matching studies. *Journal on Studies of Alcohol, 12*(Suppl.), 149–155.

Chen, H. T. (1990). *Theory-driven evaluations.* Newbury Park, CA: Sage.

Chen, H. T., Rossi, P. H. (1989). Issues in the theory-driven perspective. *Evaluation and Program Planning, 12*(4), 199–306.

Clark, A. M. (1998). The qualitative-quantitative debate: Moving from positivism and confrontation to post-positivism and reconciliation. *Journal of Advanced Nursing, 27*(6), 1242–1249.

Cohen-Mansfield, J. (1996). Conceptualization of agitation: Results based on the Cohen-Mansfield Agitation Inventory and the Agitation Behavior Mapping Instrument. *International Psychogeriatrics, 8*(Suppl 3), 309–315.

Colling, K. B., & Buettner, L. L. (2002). Simple Pleasures: Interventions from the Need-Driven Dementia-Compromised behavior model. *Journal of Gerontological Nursing, 28*(10), 16–20.

Connors, G. J., Allen, J. P., Cooney, N. L., DiClemente, C. C., Tonigan, J. S., & Anton, R. F. (1994). Assessment issues and strategies in alcoholism treatment matching research. *Journal of Studies on Alcohol, 12*(Suppl.), 92–100.

Conrad, K. J., & Conrad, K. M. (1994). Reassessing validity threats in experiments: Focus on construct validity. *New Directions for Program Evaluation, 63,* 5–26.

Diclemente, C.C., & Hughes, S.O. (1990). Stages of change profiles in outpatient alcoholism treatment. *Journal of Substance Abuse 2*(2), 217–235.

Dille, C. A., & Kirchhoff, K. T. (1993). Decontamination of vinyl urinary drainage bags with bleach. *Rehabilitation Nursing, 18*(5), 292–295, 355–356.

Dille, C. A., Kirchhoff, K. T., Sullivan, J. J., & Larson, E. (1993). Increasing the wearing time of vinyl urinary drainage bags by decontamination with bleach. *Archives of Physical Medicine & Rehabilitation, 74*(4), 431–437.

Donovan, D. M., Kadden, R. M., DiClemente, C. C., Carroll, K. M., Longabaugh, R., Zweben, A., et al. (1994). Issues in the selection and development of therapies in alcoholism treatment matching research. *Journal of Studies on Alcohol, 12*(Suppl.), 138–148.

Egan, E. C., Snyder, M., & Burns, K. R. (1992). Intervention studies in nursing: Is the effect due to the independent variable? *Nursing Outlook, 40*(4), 187–190.

Elkin, M. K., Perry, A. G., & Potter, P. A. (2007). *Nursing interventions and clinical skills.* (4th ed.) St. Louis, MO: Mosby.

Eslinger, P. J. (2002). *Neuropsychological interventions: Clinical research and practice.* New York: Guilford Press.

Fawcett, S. B., Suarez-Belcazar, Y., Balcazar, F. E., White, G. W., Paine, A. L., Blanchard, K. A., et al. (1994). Conducting intervention research: The design and development process. In J. Rothman & E. J. Thomas (Eds.), *Intervention research: Design and development for human service* (pp. 25–54). New York: Haworth Press.

Finney, J. W., & Moos, R. H. (1989). Theory and method in treatment evaluation. *Evaluation and Program Planning, 12*(4), 307–316.

Fisher, R. A. (1935). *The design of experiments.* New York: Hafner.

Folstein, M.F., Folstein, P.R. & McHugh, P.R. (1975). "Mini-Mental State": A practical method for grading the cognitive state of patients for the clinician. *Journal of Psychiatric Research, 12,* 189–198.

Frank-Stromborg, M., Pender, N. J., Walker, S. N., & Sechrist, K. R. (1990). Determinants of health-promoting lifestyle in ambulatory cancer patients. *Social Science and Medicine, 31*(10), 1159–1168.

Grobe, S. J. (1996). The nursing intervention lexicon and taxonomy: Implications for representing nursing care data in automated patient records. *Holistic Nursing Practice, 11*(1), 48–63.

Gulanick, M., & Myers, J. L. (2007). *Nursing care plans: Nursing diagnosis and intervention.* (6th ed.) St. Louis, MO: Mosby.

Hashisaki, P., Swenson, J., Mooney, B., Epstein, B., & Bowcutt, C. (1984). Decontamination of urinary bags for rehabilitation patients. *Archives of Physical Medicine & Rehabilitation, 65*(8), 474–476.

Hegyvary, S. T. (1992). Outcomes research: Integrating nursing practice into the world view. In U.S. Department of Health and Human Services, Public Health Service, *Patient outcomes research: Examining the effectiveness of nursing practice. Proceedings of the State of the Science Conference sponsored by the National Center for Nursing Research, September 11–13, 1991* (DHHS Publication #93–3411). Rockville, MD: U.S. Government Printing Office.

Johnson, J. L., Ratner, P. A., Bottroff, J. L., & Hayduk, L. A. (1993). An exploration of Pender's health promotion model using LISREL. *Nursing Research, 42*(3), 132–138.

Kirchhoff, K. T., & Dille, C. A. (1994). Issues in intervention research: Maintaining integrity. *Applied Nursing Research, 7*(1), 32–46.

Kolanowski, A. M. (1999). An overview of the need-driven dementia compromised behavior model. *Journal of Gerontological Nursing, 25*(9), 7–16.

Lindley, P., & Walker, S. N. (1993). Theoretical and methodological differentiation of moderation and mediation. *Nursing Research, 42*(5), 276–279.

Lipsey, M. W. (1993). Theory as method: Small theories of treatments. *New Directions for Program Evaluation, 57,* 5–38.

Martin, K. S., & Scheet, N. J. (1995). The Omaha system: Nursing diagnoses, interventions, and client outcomes. In N. M. Lang (Ed.), *Nursing data systems: An emerging framework: Data systems advances for clinical nursing practice.* Washington, DC: American Nurses Publishing.

McCloskey, J. C., & Bulechek, G. M. (Eds.). (2008). *Nursing interventions classification (NIC)* 5th ed. St. Louis, MO: Mosby-Year Book.

Miller, W. R., & Cooney, N. L. (1994). Designing studies to investigate client-treatment matching. *Journal of Studies on Alcohol, 12*(Suppl.), 38–45.

Nolan, M., & Grant, G. (1993). Service evaluation: Time to open both eyes. *Journal of Advanced Nursing, 18*(9), 1434–1496.

Orchid, C. (1994). Comparing healthcare outcomes. *British Medical Journal, 308*(6942), 1493–1496.

Ottenbacher, K. (1992). Impact of random assignment on study outcome: An empirical examination. *Controlled Clinical Trials, 13*(1), 50–61.

Rantz, M.R., & Popejoy, L.L. (1998). *Using MDS Quality Indicators to Improve Outcomes.* Gaithersburg, MD: Aspen.

Rezmovic, E. L. (1984). Assessing treatment implementation amid the slings and arrows of reality. *Evaluation Review, 8*(2), 187–204.

Rosen, A., & Proctor, E. K. (1978). Specifying the treatment process: The basis for effectiveness research. *Journal of Social Service Research, 2*(1), 25–43.

Rossi, P. H., & Freeman, H. E. (1993). *Evaluation: A systematic approach* (5th ed.). Newbury Park, CA: Sage.

Rothman, J., & Thomas, E. J. (Eds.). (1994). *Intervention research: Design and development for human service.* New York: Haworth Press.

Saba, V. K. (1995). Home Health Care Classifications (HHCCs): Nursing diagnoses and nursing interventions. In N. M. Lang (Ed.), *Nursing data systems: An emerging framework: Data system advances for clinical nursing practice.* Washington, DC: American Nurses Publishing.

Schmelzer, M. (1999–2001). Safety and effectiveness of large volume enema solutions. *National Institutes of Health Research Enhancement Award (AREA).* NIH grant number R15NR04867-01. Unpublished paper.

Schmelzer, M., Case, P., Chappell, S., & Wright, K. (2000). Colonic cleansing, fluid absorption, and discomfort following tap water and soapsuds enemas. *Applied Nursing Research, 13*(2), 83–91.

Schmelzer, M., & Wright, K. (1993a). Risky enemas: What's the ideal solution? *American Journal of Nursing, 93*(2), 21.

Schmelzer, M., & Wright, K. (1993b). Say nope to soap. *American Journal of Nursing, 93*(3), 21.

Schmelzer, M., & Wright, K. (1996). Enema administration techniques used by experienced registered nurses. *Gastroenterology Nursing, 19*(5), 171–175.

Scott, A. G., & Sechrest, L. (1989). Strength of theory and theory of strength. *Evaluation and Program Planning, 12*(4), 329–336.

Sechrest, L., Ametrano, D., & Ametrano, I. M. (1983). Evaluations of social programs. In C. E. Walker (Ed.), *The handbook of clinical psychology* (pp. 129–166). Homewood, IL: Dow Jones-Irwin.

Sheikh, J.I., & Yesavage, J.A. (1986). Geriatric Depression Scale (GDS): Recent evidence and development of a shorter version. *Clinical Gerontologist, 5,* 265.

Sidani, S. & Braden, C.J. (1998). *Evaluating nursing interventions: A theory-driven approach*. Thousand Oaks, CA: Sage.

Sidani, S., Epstein, D. R., & Moritz, P. (2003). Focus on research methods. An alternative paradigm for clinical nursing research: An exemplar. *Research in Nursing & Health*, 26(3), 244–255.

Steckler, A., & Linnan, L. (Eds.). (2002). *Process evaluation for public health interventions and research*. San Francisco: Jossey-Bass.

Stein, K. F., Sargent, J. T., & Rafaels, N. (2007). Intervention research: establishing fidelity of the independent variable in nursing clinical trials. *Nursing Research*, 56(1), 54–62.

Warren, J. J., & Hoskins, L. M. (1995). NANDAs nursing diagnosis taxonomy: A nursing database. In N. M. Lang (Ed.), *Nursing data systems: An emerging framework: Data system advances for clinical nursing practice*. Washington, DC: American Nurses Publishing.

Wennberg, J. E., Barry, M. J., Fowler, F. J., & Mulley, K. A. (1993). Outcomes research, PORTs, and health care reform. *Annals of the New York Academy of Sciences*, 703, 52–62.

West, S. G., Aiken, L. S., & Todd, M. (1993). Probing the effects of individual components in multiple component prevention programs. *American Journal of Community Psychology*, 21(5), 571–605.

Yeaton, W. H., & Sechrest, L. (1981). Critical dimensions in the choice and maintenance of successful treatments: Strength, integrity, and effectiveness. *Journal of Consulting and Clinical Psychology*, 49(2), 156–167.

Zweben, A., Donovan, D. M., Randall, C. L., Barrett, D., Dermen, K., Kabela, E., et al. (1994). Issues in the development of subject recruitment strategies and eligibility criteria in multisite trials of matching. *Journal of Studies on Alcohol*, 12(Suppl.), 62–69.

CHAPTER 14
Sampling

Many of us have preconceived notions about samples and sampling, which we acquired from television commercials, polls of public opinion, market researchers, and newspaper reports of research findings. The advertiser boasts that four of five doctors recommend its product; the newscaster announces that John Jones is predicted to win the senate election by a margin of 3 to 1; the newspaper reports that scientists' studies have found that taking a statin drug, such as atorvastatin (Lipitor), significantly reduces the risk of coronary artery disease.

All of these examples use sampling techniques. Some of the outcomes, however, are more valid than others, partly because of the sampling techniques used. In most instances, television, newspapers, and advertisements do not explain their sampling techniques. You may hold opinions about the adequacy of these techniques, but there is not enough information to make a judgment.

The sampling component is an important part of the research process that needs to be carefully thought out and clearly described. To achieve these goals, you and other researchers must understand the techniques of sampling and the reasoning behind them. With this knowledge, you can make intelligent judgments about sampling when you are critically appraising studies or developing a sampling plan for your own study. This chapter examines sampling theory and concepts, sampling plans, probability and nonprobability sampling methods for quantitative research, nonprobability sampling methods for qualitative research, sample size, and settings for conducting studies. The chapter concludes with a discussion of the process for acquiring and retaining subjects for a sample in a variety of settings.

SAMPLING THEORY

Sampling involves selecting a group of people, events, behaviors, or other elements with which to conduct a study. A sampling plan defines the process of making the sample selections; sample denotes the selected group of people or elements included in a study. Sampling decisions have a major impact on the meaning and generalizability of the findings.

Sampling theory was developed to determine mathematically the most effective way to acquire a sample that would accurately reflect the population under study. The theoretical, mathematical rationale for decisions related to sampling emerged from survey research, although the techniques were first applied to experimental research by agricultural scientists. One of the most important surveys that stimulated improvements in sampling techniques was the United States census. Researchers have adopted the assumptions of sampling theory identified for the census surveys and incorporated them within the research process.

Key concepts of sampling theory are (1) populations, (2) elements, (3) sampling criteria, (4) representativeness, (5) sampling errors, (6) randomization, (7) sampling frames, and (8) sampling plans. The following sections explain these concepts; and later in the chapter, these concepts are used to explain a variety of sampling methods.

Populations and Elements

The population is a particular type of individual or element, such as people with type 2 diabetes, who are the focus of the research. The target population is the entire set of individuals or elements who meet the

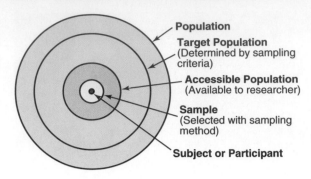

Figure **14-1** Population, sample, and subject selected for a study.

sampling criteria, such as women who are 18 years and older with a new diagnosis of type 2 diabetes. Figure 14-1 demonstrates the relationships among the population, target population, and accessible populations. An accessible population is the portion of the target population to which the researcher has reasonable access. The accessible population might be elements within a country, state, city, hospital, or nursing unit, such as the diabetics in primary care clinics in Fort Worth, Texas. The sample is obtained from the accessible population by a particular sampling method, such as simple random sampling. The individual units of the population and sample are called elements. An element can be a person, event, behavior, or any other single unit of study. When elements are persons, they are usually referred to as subjects in quantitative, outcomes, and interventions research and participants in qualitative research (see Figure 14-1). The findings from a study are generalized first to the accessible population and then, more abstractly, to the target population.

Generalizing means that the findings can be applied to more than just the sample under study. Because of the importance of generalizing, there are risks to defining the accessible population too narrowly. For example, a narrow definition of the accessible population reduces the ability to generalize from the study sample to the target population and, thus, diminishes the meaningfulness of the findings. Biases may be introduced that make generalization to the broader target population difficult to defend. If the accessible population is defined as individuals in a white, upper-middle-class setting, one cannot generalize to nonwhite or lower-income populations. These biases are similar to those that may be encountered in a nonrandom sample.

In some studies, the entire population is the target of the study. These studies are referred to as population

studies (Barhyte, Redman, & Neill, 1990). Many of these studies use data available in large databases, such as the census data or other government-maintained databases. Epidemiologists often use entire populations for their large database studies. In other studies, the entire population of interest in the study is small and well defined. For example, one could conduct a study in which the defined population was all living recipients of heart and lung transplants.

In some cases, a hypothetical population is defined. A hypothetical population assumes the presence of a population that cannot be defined according to sampling theory rules, which require a list of all members of the population. For example, individuals who successfully lose weight would be a hypothetical population. The number of individuals in the population, who they are, how much weight they have lost, how long they have kept it off, or how they achieved the weight loss is unknown. Some populations are elusive and constantly changing. For example, listing all women in active labor in the United States, all people grieving the loss of a loved one, or all people coming into an emergency department would be impossible.

Sampling or Eligibility Criteria

Sampling criteria, also referred to as eligibility criteria, include a list of characteristics essential for membership or eligibility in the target population. The criteria are developed from the research problem, the purpose, a review of literature, the conceptual and operational definitions of the study variables, and the design. The sampling criteria determine the target population, and the sample is selected from the accessible population within the target population (see Figure 14-1). When the study is complete, the findings are generalized from the sample to the accessible population and then to the target population.

You might identify broad sampling criteria for a study, such as all adults over 18 years of age able to read and write English. These criteria ensure a large target population of heterogeneous or diverse potential subjects. A heterogeneous sample increases your ability to generalize the findings to a larger target population. In descriptive or correlational studies, the sampling criteria may be defined to ensure a heterogeneous population with a broad range of values for the variables being studied. The sampling criteria may be specific and designed to make the population as homogeneous or similar as possible or to control for extraneous variables. In quasi-experimental or experimental studies, the primary purpose of sampling criteria is to limit the effect of extraneous variables on the particular interaction between the independent and dependent variables. Subjects are selected to maximize the effects of the independent variable and minimize the effects of variation in other extraneous variables so they have a limited impact on the dependent variable scores.

Sampling criteria may include characteristics such as the ability to read, to write responses on the data collection instruments or forms, and to comprehend and communicate using the English language. Age limitations are often specified, such as adults 18 years and older. Subjects may be limited to those who are not participating in any other study. Persons who are able to participate fully in the procedure for obtaining informed consent are often selected as subjects. If potential subjects have diminished autonomy or are unable to give informed consent, consent must be obtained from their legal representative. Thus, persons who are legally or mentally incompetent, terminally ill, or confined to an institution are more difficult to access as subjects. However, sampling criteria should not become so restrictive that the researcher cannot find an adequate number of subjects.

A study might have inclusion or exclusion sampling criteria (or both). Inclusion sampling criteria are those characteristics that a subject or element must possess to be part of the target population. Exclusion sampling criteria are those characteristics that can cause a person or element to be excluded from the target population. For example, Andrews, Felton, Wewers, Waller, and Tingen (2007) clearly identified their inclusion and exclusion sampling criteria for their quasi-experimental study of the effect of a smoking cessation intervention on smoking abstinence in African American women residing in public housing.

> Inclusion criteria for this study were: (a) nonpregnant or nonbreastfeeding African American female; (b) over 18 years of age; (c) current daily smoker; (d) planning to quit smoking within the next 6 months; and (e) resident of intervention community or comparison community, and/or female relative or close friend of resident of these communities. Exclusion criteria were: (a) diagnosis of mental health disorder; (b) unstable angina or recent myocardial infarction within the past month; (c) plans to move within the next 6 months; and (d) in precontemplation stage of quitting. (Andrews et al., 2007, p. 47)

Andrews et al.'s (2007) inclusion and exclusion sampling criteria precisely designated the attributes of the subjects who made up the target population.

The researchers narrowly defined these sampling criteria, probably to promote the selection of a homogeneous sample of female African Americans with a documented smoking problem. Because this was a quasi-experiment study, the specific sampling criteria decreased the effects of extraneous variables so the effect of the smoking cessation intervention (independent variable) could be determined on the women's smoking abstinence (dependent variable).

Researchers must provide logical reasons for their inclusion and exclusion sampling criteria. Larson (1994) suggested that some groups, such as women, ethnic minorities, the elderly, and the poor, are unnecessarily excluded from many studies. A review of approved research protocols in one tertiary care center (1989–1990) revealed that 75% of studies listed exclusion criteria, many of which were not justified by the researchers. The most common exclusions for which no justification was provided were age, socioeconomic status, and race. Exclusion criteria limit the generalization of the study findings and should be carefully considered before being used in a study. Andrews et al.'s (2007) study focused on a minority, adult, female population, and there was no exclusion based on age (age greater than 18 years). The exclusion criteria—mental illness, unstable angina, plans to move, and the precontemplation stage of quitting—seem appropriate for the study to decrease the effects of extraneous variables.

Representativeness

For a sample to be representative, it must be like the target population in as many ways as possible. It is especially important that the sample be representative in relation to the variables you are studying and to other factors that may influence the study variables. For example, if your study examines attitudes toward acquired immunodeficiency syndrome (AIDS), the sample should represent the distribution of attitudes toward AIDS that exists in the specified population. In addition, a sample must represent the demographic characteristics, such as age, gender, ethnicity, income, and education, which often influence study variables.

The accessible population must be representative of the target population. If the accessible population is limited to a particular setting or type of setting, the individuals seeking care at that setting may be different from those who would seek care for the same problem in other settings or from those who self-manage their problems. Studies conducted in private hospitals usually exclude the poor, and other settings could exclude the elderly or the undereducated. People who do not have access to care are usually excluded from health-focused studies. Subjects in research centers and the care they receive are different from patients and the care they receive in community clinics, public hospitals, veterans' hospitals, and rural health clinics. Obese individuals who chose to enter a program to lose weight may differ from those who did not enter a program. All of these factors limit representativeness and, in turn, limit our understanding of the phenomena important in practice.

Representativeness is usually evaluated by comparing the numerical values of the sample (a statistic such as the mean) with the same values from the target population. A numerical value of a population is called a parameter. We can estimate the population parameter by identifying the values obtained in previous studies examining the same variables. The accuracy with which the population parameters have been estimated within a study is referred to as precision. Precision in estimating parameters requires well-developed methods of measurement that are used repeatedly among several studies. You can define parameters by conducting a series of descriptive and correlational studies, each of which examines a different segment of the target population. Then perform a meta-analysis to estimate the population parameter.

Sampling Error

The difference between a sample statistic and a population parameter is called the sampling error (Figure 14-2). A large sampling error means that the sample is not providing a precise picture of the population; it is not representative. Sampling error is usually larger with small samples and decreases as the sample size increases. Sampling error reduces the power of a study, or the ability of the statistical analyses conducted to detect differences between groups or to describe the relationships between variables. Sampling error occurs as a result of random variation and systematic variation.

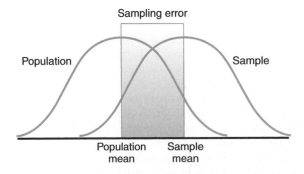

Figure **14-2** Sampling error.

Random Variation

Random variation is the expected difference in values that occurs when one examines different subjects from the same sample. If the mean is used to describe the sample, the values of individuals in that sample will not all be exactly the same as the sample mean. Individual subjects' values vary from the value of the sample mean. The difference is random because the value of each subject is likely to vary in a different direction. Some values are higher and others are lower than the sample mean. Thus, the values are randomly scattered around the mean. As the sample size becomes larger, overall variation in sample values decreases, with more values being close to the sample mean. As the sample size increases, the sample mean is also more likely to have a value similar to that of the population mean.

Systematic Variation

Systematic variation, or systematic bias, is a consequence of selecting subjects whose measurement values are different, or vary, in some specific way from the population. Because the subjects have something in common, their values tend to be similar to those of others in the sample but different in some way from those of the population as a whole. These values do not vary randomly around the population mean. Most of the variation from the mean is in the same direction; it is systematic. All the values in the sample may tend to be higher or lower than the population mean.

For example, if all the subjects in a study examining some type of health care knowledge have an intelligence quotient (IQ) higher than 120, many of their scores will likely be higher than the mean of a population that includes individuals with a wide variation in IQ, such as IQs that range from 90 to 130. The IQs of the subjects have introduced a systematic bias. This situation could occur, for example, if all the subjects were college students, which has been the case in the development of many measurement methods in psychology.

Because of systematic variance, the sample mean is different from the population mean. The extent of the difference is the sampling error. Exclusion criteria tend to increase the systematic bias in the sample and thus increase the sampling error. An extreme example of this problem is the highly restrictive sampling criteria used in some clinical trials that result in a large sampling error and greatly diminished representativeness.

If the method of selecting subjects produces a sample with a systematic bias, increasing the sample size will not decrease the sampling error. When a systematic bias occurs in an experimental study, it can lead the researcher to believe that a treatment has made a difference when, in actuality, the values would be different even without the treatment. This situation usually occurs because of an interaction of the systematic bias with the treatment.

Systematic variation or bias is most likely to occur when the sampling process is not random. However, even in a random sample, systematic variation can occur if potential subjects decline participation. Thus, systematic bias increases as the subjects' refusal rate increases. A refusal rate is the number or percentage of subjects who declined to participate in the study. High refusal rates to participate in a study have been linked to individuals with serious physical and emotional illnesses, low socioeconomic status, and weak social networks (Neumark, Stommel, Given, & Given, 2001). The higher the refusal rate, the less the sample is representative of the target population. The refusal rate is calculated by dividing the number of potential subjects refusing to participate by the number of potential subjects meeting sampling criteria and multiplying the results by 100%. For example if 200 potential subjects met the sampling criteria and 40 refused to participate in the study, the refusal rate is 20%.

> Refusal rate = 40 (number refusing) ÷ 200 (number meeting sampling criteria) = 0.2 × 100% = 20%

Sometimes researchers provide an acceptance rate, or the number or percentage of the subjects who agree to participate in a study, rather than a refusal rate. The acceptance rate is calculated by dividing the number of potential subjects who agree to participate in a study by the number of potential subjects who meet sampling criteria and multiplying the result by 100%. If you know the refusal rate, you can subtract the refusal rate from 100% to obtain the acceptance rate. In the example mentioned earlier, 200 potential subjects met the sampling criteria; 160 agreed to participate in the study and 40 refused.

> Acceptance rate = 160 (number accepting) ÷ 200 (number meeting sampling criteria) = 0.8 × 100% = 80%

> Acceptance rate = 100% − Refusal rate 100% − 20% = 80%

Andrews et al. (2007) described the screening of their potential subjects, identified those who did not meet sample criteria, and indicated the acceptance rate for their study, introduced earlier in this chapter.

A total of 157 women from both communities were screened during the recruitment period. Of those screened, 16 were ineligible for the following reasons: 8 were in the precontemplation state of change; 3 did not live in the defined housing developments or had no family or friends who lived in the housing developments; 2 had not smoked in the previous 24 hours and had baseline carbon monoxide (CO) rates <8; and 3 were <18 years of age. Of the 141 remaining women eligible to participate, 103 (73%) volunteered to participate. (Andrews et al., 2007, pp. 47–48)

Andrews et al. (2007) had a 73% acceptance rate, which is somewhat low and could indicate a systematic bias in the subjects who chose to participate in this study. In addition, the researchers did not provide a rationale for the potential subjects' refusal to participate (27% refusal rate), nor did they discuss if there were any differences between those who did participate and those who refused to participate. The 73% acceptance rate and the lack of rationale for subjects' refusals are study limitations that could affect the sample's representativeness of the target population. These sampling limitations decrease the researchers' ability to generalize their findings (Peat, Mellis, Williams, & Xuan, 2002). The calculations for the acceptance and refusal rates for this study are presented here:

> Acceptance rate = 103 (number accepting) ÷ 141 (number meeting sampling criteria) = 0.730 × 100% = 73%

> Refusal rate = 38 (number refusing) ÷ 141 (number meeting sampling criteria) = 0.2695 × 100% = 26.95% = 27%

Systematic variation can also occur in studies with high sample mortality. Sample mortality or attrition is the withdrawal or loss of subjects from a study. Systematic variation is greatest when a high number of subjects withdraw from the study before the data have been collected or when a large number of subjects withdraw from one group but not the other in the study (Kerlinger & Lee, 2000). In studies involving a treatment, subjects in the control group who do not receive the treatment may be more likely to withdraw from the study. Sample mortality or attrition should be reported in the published study to determine if the final sample represents the target population. Sample attrition is calculated by dividing the number of subjects withdrawing from a study by the sample size and multiplying the results by 100%. The opposite of the attrition rate is the retention rate. For example, if a study had a sample size of 160 and 40 people withdrew from the study, the attrition rate would be 25%. In that same example, if 40 subjects withdrew from the study, then 120 subjects were retained. The calculations of the attrition and retention rates are presented here:

Attrition rate = 40 (number withdrawing) ÷ 160 (sample size) = 0.25 × 100% = 25%

Retention rate = 120 (number retained) ÷ 160 (sample size) = 0.75 × 100% = 75%

Andrews et al. (2007) described their study attrition as follows:

Of the 103 women who completed the baseline data collection, 13 were lost to attrition, yielding a retention rate of 87.4% during the 6-month study period. Seven participants (13%) dropped out of the comparison community [group] and six participants (12%) dropped out of the intervention community [group]. There were no differences in age [t (101) = 0.38, p = 0.71], income [t (92) = 0.55, p = 0.58], education [χ^2 (8, N = 103) = 6.24, p = 0.62], and employment status [χ^2 (2, N = 103) = 0.66, p = 0.72] between the participants who remained in the study and those who were lost to attrition. (Andrews et al., 2007, p. 51)

The calculations for the attrition and retention rates for the Andrews et al. (2007) study are presented here:

Attrition rate = 13 (number withdrawing) ÷ 103 (sample size) = 0.126 × 100% = 12.6%

Retention rate = 90 (number retained) ÷ 103 (sample size) = 0.874 × 100% = 87.4%

Andrews et al. (2007) had a strong retention rate of 87.4%, when you consider this was a 6-month long intervention study focused on smoking cessation. The attrition from the treatment group (6 subjects) was essentially the same as that for the comparison group (7 subjects), indicating the groups were comparable for retention. In addition, the researchers found no differences in the demographic variables (age, income, education levels, and employment status) between those who remained in the study and those lost to attrition. These are study strengths that increased the sample's representativeness of the target population; however, indicating the reasons for the loss of the 13 subjects would have added to the quality of the study report.

Randomization

From a sampling theory point of view, randomization means that each individual in the population should have a greater than zero opportunity to be selected for the sample. The method of achieving this opportunity is referred to as random sampling. In experimental studies that use a control group, subjects are randomly selected and then randomly assigned to either the control group or the experimental group. The use of the term control group is limited to those studies using random sampling and random assignment to the treatment and control groups. If nonrandom sampling methods are used for sample selection, the group not receiving a treatment is referred to as a comparison group, because there is a greater possibility of preexisting differences between that group and the group receiving the treatment.

Random sampling increases the extent to which the sample is representative of the target population. However, random sampling must take place in an accessible population that is representative of the target population. Exclusion criteria limit true randomness. Thus, a study that uses random sampling techniques may have such restrictive sampling criteria that the sample is not truly random. In any case, it is rarely possible to obtain a purely random sample for nursing studies because of informed consent requirements. Even if the original sample is random, persons who volunteer or consent to participate in a study may differ in important ways from those who are not willing to participate. Methods of achieving random sampling are described later in the chapter.

Sampling Frames

For each person in the target or accessible population to have an opportunity to be selected for the sample, each person in the population must be identified. To accomplish this goal, the researcher must acquire a list of every member of the population through the use of the sampling criteria to define membership. This listing of members of the population is referred to as the sampling frame. The researcher then selects subjects from the sampling frame using a sampling plan. Rivers et al. (2003) studied predictors of nurses' acceptance of an intravenous catheter safety device and described their sampling frame as follows: "The sampling frame consisted of full-time direct patient care registered nurses (N = 742), who had used the Protective® Plus IV [intravenous] catheter device to initiate intravenous procedures at this hospital. Temporary (contract), supplemental, and part-time nurses and licensed practical nurses were excluded" (p. 250).

Sampling Plans

A **sampling plan** describes the strategies that will be used to obtain a sample for a study. The plan is developed to enhance representativeness, reduce systematic bias, and decrease the sampling error (Brent, Scott, & Spencer, 1988; Peat et al., 2002). Thus, sampling strategies have been devised to accomplish these three tasks and to optimize sample selection. The sampling plan may use probability (random) sampling methods or nonprobability (nonrandom) sampling methods.

A **sampling method** is the process of selecting a group of people, events, behaviors, or other elements that represent the population being studied. A sampling method is similar to a design; it is not specific to a study. The sampling plan provides detail about the use of a sampling method in a specific study. The sampling plan must be described in detail for purposes of critique, replication, and future meta-analyses. The following sections describe different types of probability and nonprobability sampling methods.

PROBABILITY (RANDOM) SAMPLING METHODS

Probability sampling methods have been developed to ensure some degree of precision in estimations of the population parameters. Thus, probability samples reduce sampling error. The term **probability sampling method** refers to the fact that every member (element) of the population has a probability higher than zero of being selected for the sample. Inferential statistical analyses are based on the assumption that the sample from which data were derived has been obtained randomly. Thus, probability sampling methods are often referred to as **random sampling methods**. These samples are more likely to represent the population than are samples obtained with nonprobability sampling methods. All subsets of the population, which may differ from one another but contribute to the parameters of the population, have a chance to be represented in the sample. Probability sampling methods are most commonly used in quantitative and outcomes research.

There is less opportunity for systematic bias if subjects are selected randomly, although it is possible for a systematic bias to occur by chance. Using random sampling, the researcher cannot decide that person X will be a better subject for the study than person Y.

In addition, a researcher cannot exclude a subset of people from selection as subjects because he or she does not agree with them, does not like them, or finds them hard to deal with. Potential subjects cannot be excluded because they are too sick, not sick enough, coping too well, or not coping adequately. The researcher, who has a vested interest in the study, could (consciously or unconsciously) select subjects whose conditions or behaviors are consistent with the study hypothesis. It is tempting to exclude uncooperative or assertive individuals. Random sampling leaves the selection to chance and, thus, increases the validity of the study.

Theoretically, to obtain a probability sample, the researcher must develop a sampling frame that includes every element in the population. The sample must be randomly selected from the sampling frame. Thus, according to sampling theory, it is not possible to select a sample randomly from a population that cannot be clearly defined. Four sampling designs have been developed to achieve probability sampling: simple random sampling, stratified random sampling, cluster sampling, and systematic sampling.

Simple Random Sampling

Simple random sampling is the most basic of the probability sampling methods. To achieve simple random sampling, elements are selected at random from the sampling frame. This goal can be accomplished in a variety of ways, limited only by the imagination of the researcher. If the sampling frame is small, the researcher can write names on slips of paper, place the names in a container, mix well, and then draw out one at a time until the desired sample size has been reached. Another technique is to assign a number to each name in the sampling frame. In large population sets, elements may already have assigned numbers. For example, numbers are assigned to medical records, organizational memberships, and licenses. The researcher can then select these numbers randomly to obtain a sample.

There can be some differences in the probability for the selection of each element, depending on whether the selected element's name or number is replaced before the next name or number is selected. Selection with replacement, the most conservative random sampling approach, provides exactly equal opportunities for each element to be selected (Kerlinger & Lee, 2000). For example, if the researcher draws names out of a hat to obtain a sample, each name must be replaced before the next name is drawn to ensure equal opportunity for each subject.

Selection without replacement gives each element different levels of probability for selection. For example, if the researcher is selecting 10 subjects from a population of 50, the first name has a 1 in 5 chance, or a 0.2 probability, of being selected. If the first name is not replaced, the second name has a 9 in 49 chance, or a 0.18 probability, of being selected. As further names are drawn, the probability of being selected decreases.

There are many ways to achieve random selection, such as with the use of a computer, a random numbers table, or a roulette wheel. The most common method of random selection is the computer, which can be programmed to randomly select a sample from the sampling frame with replacement. However, some researchers still use a table of random numbers to select a random sample. Table 14-1 shows a section from a random numbers table. To use a table of random numbers, the researcher places a pencil or a finger on the table with the eyes closed. The number touched is the starting place. Moving the pencil or finger up, down, right, or left, the researcher uses the numbers in order until the desired sample size is obtained. For example, the researcher places a pencil on 58 in Table 14-1, which is in the fourth column from the left and fourth row down. If five subjects are to be selected from a population of 100 and the researcher decides to go across the column to the right, the subject numbers chosen are 58, 25, 15, 55, and 38. Table 14-1 is useful only if the population number is less than 100. However, tables are available for larger populations, such as the random numbers table provided in Appendix A.

Flynn (2007, p. 200) used simple random sampling in her study that "explored associations between organizational support for nursing practice in home health care agencies and (a) the frequency of nurse-reported adverse events, (b) nurse-assessed quality of care, (c) nurse job satisfaction, and (d) nurses' intentions to leave their employing agency." The following excerpt from her study describes the process used to obtain the random sample.

To obtain a sample of registered nurses (RNs) currently employed in home health staff nurse positions, 645 names were randomly selected to receive a mailed research packet from a list of subscribers to a prominent journal for home health care nurses [sampling frame]. All 645 of the randomly selected subscribers [sampling method] resided in the United States. A total of 25 surveys were returned by the post office as undeliverable. Of the 620 delivered surveys, a response rate of 52.4% produced surveys from 325 nurse respondents. Among these respondents, 68 indicated that they no longer practice in home health care and an additional 120 indicated that although they worked in home health care, they were not employed in staff RN positions. Thus, the sample for the current study consisted of 137 RNs [sample size], employed as home health staff nurses, from 38 states. (Flynn, 2007, p. 204)

Flynn (2007) used simple random sampling to obtain her sample from 38 different states. However, the sampling frame was a list of subscribers to a journal, and home health nurses who did not subscribe to this journal were excluded and might differ in some way from the subscribers. In addition, the researcher had a 52.4% response rate, which is strong for a mailed survey. However, the final sample size was small because only 137 of the RNs who responded met the study sample criteria. Simple random sampling increased the sample's representativeness of the target population, but the sampling frame and sample size problems decreased the sample's representativeness.

Stratified Random Sampling

Stratified random sampling is used when the researcher knows some of the variables in the population that are critical to achieving representativeness. Variables commonly used for stratification are age, gender, ethnicity, socioeconomic status, diagnosis, geographical region, type of institution, type of care, care provider, and site of care. The variable or variables chosen for stratification must be correlated with the dependent variables being examined in the study. Subjects within each stratum are expected to be more alike (homogeneous) in

TABLE **14-1**	Section from a Random Numbers Table								
06	84	10	22	56	72	25	70	69	43
07	63	10	34	66	39	54	02	33	85
03	19	63	93	72	52	13	30	44	40
77	32	69	58	25	15	55	38	19	62
20	01	94	54	66	88	43	91	34	28

relation to the study variables than they are to be like subjects in other strata or the total sample. In stratified random sampling, the subjects are randomly selected on the basis of their classification into the selected strata.

For example, if in conducting your research you selected a stratified random sample of 100 adult subjects using age as the variable for stratification, the sample might include 25 subjects in the age range 18 to 39 years, 25 subjects in the age range 40 to 59 years, 25 subjects in the age range 60 to 79 years, and 25 subjects 80 years or older. Stratification ensures that all levels of the identified variable, in this example age, are adequately represented in the sample. With a stratified random sample, you could use a smaller sample size to achieve the same degree of representativeness as a large sample acquired through simple random sampling. Sampling error decreases, power increases, data collection time is reduced, and the cost of the study is lower if stratification is used.

One question that arises in relation to stratification is whether each stratum should have equivalent numbers of subjects in the sample (termed **disproportionate sampling**) or whether the numbers of subjects should be selected in proportion to their occurrence in the population (termed **proportionate sampling**). For example, if stratification is being achieved by ethnicity and the population is 60% Caucasian, 20% African American, 15% Mexican American, and 5% Asian, your research team would have to decide whether to select equal numbers of each ethnic group or to calculate a proportion of the sample. Good arguments exist for both approaches. Stratification is not as useful if one stratum contains only a small number of subjects. In the aforementioned situation, if proportions are used and the sample size is 100, the study would include only five Asians, hardly enough to be representative. If equal numbers of each group are used, each group would contain at least 25 subjects; however, the Caucasian group would be underrepresented. In this case, mathematically weighting the findings from each stratum can equalize the representation to ensure proportional contributions of each stratum to the total score of the sample. Most textbooks on sampling describe this procedure (Cochran, 1977; Levy & Lemsbow, 1980; Yates, 1981).

Ulrich et al. (2006) used a stratified random sampling method to obtain their sample of nurse practitioners (NPs) and physician assistants (PAs) for the purpose of studying their ethical conflict associated with managed care. The following excerpt from this study describes the sampling method used to obtain the final sample of 1536 providers (833 NPs and 689 PAs).

A self-administered questionnaire was mailed to an initial stratified random sample [sampling method] of 3,900 NPs and PAs practicing in the United States. The sample was selected from the national lists provided by Medical Marketing Services, and independently owned organization that manages medical industry lists (www. mmslists.com/main.asp). The list for PAs was derived from the American Academy of Physicians Assistants (AAPA), and a comprehensive list of NPs was derived from the medical and nursing boards of the 50 states and the District of Columbia [sampling frames for NPs and PAs].... After undeliverable (1.9%) and other disqualified (13.2% i.e., no longer practicing, non-primary-care practitioner) were removed, the overall adjusted response rate was 50.6%. (Ulrich et al., 2006, p. 393)

The study sampling frames for the NPs and PAs are representative of all 50 states and the District of Columbia, and the lists for the sampling frames were from quality sources. The study has a strong response rate of 50.6% for the mailed questionnaires, and the researchers identified why certain respondents were disqualified. The final sample was large (1536 subjects) with strong representation for both NPs (833 subjects) and PAs (689 subjects). The study sample might have been stronger with a more equal number of NP and PA subjects. However, the sample was a great strength of this study and appeared to represent the target population of NPs and PAs currently practicing in primary care.

Cluster Sampling

Cluster sampling is used in two situations. The first situation is when a simple random sample would be prohibitive in terms of travel time and cost. Imagine trying to arrange personal meetings with 100 people, each in a different part of the United States. The second situation is in cases in which the individual elements making up the population are not known, thus preventing the development of a sampling frame. For example, there is no list of all the open-heart surgery patients in the United States. In these cases, it is often possible to obtain lists of institutions or organizations with which the elements of interest are associated.

In **cluster sampling**, the researcher develops a sampling frame that includes a list of all the states, cities, institutions, or organizations with which elements of the identified population would be linked. States, cities, institutions, or organizations are selected randomly as units from which to obtain elements for the sample. In some cases, this random selection continues through several stages and is then referred to as **multistage cluster sampling**. For example, the researcher might first randomly select states, then randomly select cities within the sampled states. Hospitals within the randomly selected cities might then be randomly selected. Within the hospitals, nursing units might be randomly selected. At this level, either all the patients on the nursing unit who fit the criteria for the study might be included or patients could be randomly selected.

Cluster sampling provides a means for obtaining a larger sample at a lower cost. However, it has some disadvantages. Data from subjects associated with the same institution are likely to be correlated and thus not completely independent. This correlation can cause a decrease in precision and an increase in sampling error. However, such disadvantages can be offset to some extent by the use of a larger sample.

Mitchell, Woods, & Lentz (1994) used multistage cluster sampling in their study differentiating women with three perimenstrual symptom patterns. They described their sampling procedure as follows.

> The community sample of healthy women participating in this study was obtained through a multistage sampling procedure commonly used in epidemiological studies. First, census block groups were selected using age, income, and ethnicity to facilitate the selection of a sample of menstruating women between the ages of 18 and 45 with a wide range of incomes. The ethnic mix was representative of the northwestern metropolitan area that was sampled. Second, street segments were identified and randomly ordered by computer from the selected census block groups. Third, residential telephone numbers for every household within the computer-generated street segments were obtained from a city directory. Finally, telephone contact was made with 5,755 households, and 1,135 women between the ages of 18 and 45 were identified.
>
> Criteria for inclusion were as follows: age between 18 and 45, not currently pregnant, not being treated for a gynecological problem, having menstrual periods, and the ability to write and understand English. Women taking birth control pills (BCPs) were included in the original data collection but were excluded from the analysis for this study to avoid confounding the sample selection and results with effects of exogenous hormones.
>
> Six hundred fifty-six eligible women who satisfied all the inclusion criteria completed an in-home interview and received instructions about keeping the Washington Women's Health Diary (WWHD). Three hundred forty-three women returned at least one complete cycle of daily data. Of these 343 women, 47 were taking BCPs [birth control pills], leaving 296 women who were not on any ovarian hormones. A total of 142 of these women fell into one of the three subgroups of interest for this study. The remaining 154 women fell into one of 25 other possible symptom severity subgroups that were not part of this study. (Mitchell et al., 1994, pp. 26–27)

Mitchell et al. (1994) clearly described the different clusters (census block groups, street segments, and residential telephone numbers) of subjects that were used to randomly select the sample. In addition, the sample size of 142 subjects is a strength but is somewhat limited because 656 women met the inclusion criteria. Overall, this sampling method strengthens this study and produces a sample that probably represents the target population.

Systematic Sampling

Systematic sampling can be conducted when an ordered list of all members of the population is available. The process involves selecting every kth individual on the list, using a starting point selected randomly. If the initial starting point is not random, the sample is not a probability sample. To use this design in your research, you must know the number of elements in the population and the size of the sample desired. Divide the population size by the desired sample size, giving k, the size of the gap between elements selected from the list. For example, if the population size is $N = 1200$ and the desired sample size is $n = 100$, then you could calculate the value of k:

$$k = \text{Population size} \div \text{Sample size}$$
$$\text{Example: } k = 1200 \div 100 = 12$$

Thus, $k = 12$, which means that every twelfth person on the list would be included in the sample. Some argue that this procedure does not truly give each element an opportunity to be included in the sample; it provides a random but not equal chance for inclusion.

Researchers must be careful to determine that the original list has not been set up with any ordering that could be meaningful in relation to the study. The process is based on the assumption that the order of the list is random in relation to the variables being studied. If the order of the list is related to the study, systematic bias is introduced. In addition to this risk, it is difficult to compute sampling error with the use of this design. For additional information about systematic sampling, see Floyd (1993).

Tolle, Tilden, Rosenfeld, and Hickman (2000) used systematic sampling to study family reports of the barriers to optimal care of the dying. They described their sampling plan as follows.

> After approval of Institutional Review Boards at both the University and the Oregon Health Division, death certificates for all Oregon deaths occurring in the 14 months between November 1996 and December 1997 were systematically randomly sampled, excluding

decedents under the age of 18 years and deaths attributable to suicide, homicide, accident or those undergoing medical examiner review. Out of a sampling frame of $N = 24,074$, the systematic random sample yielded 1,458 death certificates. Although the name of a family contact is listed on each death certificate, Oregon death certificates do not list an address or telephone number for family contacts. As a result, case finding for family contacts was unsuccessful for 44% of the sample. Using newspaper obituaries and published telephone directories, a total of 816 family contacts were located, of whom 59% ($n = 475$) agreed to participate.... Of those who refused, the most frequent reason mentioned for not participating was that talking about the death would be too painful. (Tolle et al., 2000, p. 311)

The systematic sampling plan used by Tolle et al. (2000) has both strengths and weaknesses. Because their sampling frame was 24,074 death certificates and their desired sample size was 1458, they systematically selected every 16th death certificate to identify families for inclusion in their study. Two potential areas of bias are that 44% of the families identified on the originally selected 1458 death certificates could not be contacted. Of the 816 families contacted, 41% refused to participate. The families who could not be contacted or refused to participate might differ in some way from those who did participate, which decreases the sample's representativeness of the target population. However, the representativeness of the sample is strengthened by the sample size, $N = 475$, and the use of a probability sampling method.

NONPROBABILITY (NONRANDOM) SAMPLING METHODS IN QUANTITATIVE RESEARCH

In nonprobability sampling, not every element of the population has an opportunity to be included in the sample. Thus, nonprobability sampling methods increase the likelihood of obtaining samples that are not representative of their target populations. However, the majority of nursing studies use nonprobability sampling, especially convenience sampling, to select study samples. An analysis of nursing studies published in six nursing journals from 1977 to 1986 revealed that 91% of the studies used nonrandom sampling methods and only 9% used random sampling, which is a trend that appears to continue today (Moody et al., 1988).

There are several types of nonprobability (nonrandom) sampling designs. Each addresses a different research need. The five nonprobability sampling designs described in this textbook are (1) convenience sampling, (2) quota sampling, (3) purposive sampling, (4) network sampling, and (5) theoretical sampling. These sampling methods are used in both quantitative and qualitative research. However, convenience sampling and quota sampling are used more often in quantitative than in qualitative studies and are discussed in this section. Purposive sampling, network sampling, and theoretical sampling are used more frequently in qualitative studies than in quantitative studies and are discussed later in this chapter.

Convenience (Accidental) Sampling

In convenience sampling, subjects are included in the study because they happened to be in the right place at the right time. Researchers simply enter available subjects into the study until they have reached the desired sample size. Convenience sampling, also called accidental sampling, is considered a weak approach to sampling because it provides little opportunity to control for biases. Multiple biases may exist in convenience sampling; these biases range from minimal to serious.

Researchers must identify and describe known biases in their samples. You can identify biases by carefully thinking through the sample criteria used to determine the target population and then taking steps to improve the representativeness of the sample. For example, in a study of home care management of patients with complex health care needs, educational level would be an important extraneous variable. One solution for controlling this extraneous variable would be to redefine the sampling criteria to include only those with a high school education. Doing so would limit the extent of generalization but decrease the bias created by educational level. Another option would be to select a population known to include individuals with a wide variety of educational levels. Data could be collected on educational level so that the description of the sample would include information on educational level. With this information, one could judge the extent to which the sample was representative with respect to educational level.

Decisions related to sample selection must be carefully described to enable others to evaluate the possibility of biases. In addition, data must be gathered to allow a thorough description of the sample that can also be used to evaluate for possible biases. Data on the sample can be used to compare the sample with other samples and for estimating the parameters of populations through meta-analyses.

Many strategies are available for selecting a convenience sample. A classroom of students might be used.

Patients who attend a clinic on a specific day, subjects who attend a support group, patients currently admitted to a hospital with a specific diagnosis, and every fifth person who enters the emergency department are examples of types of commonly selected convenience samples.

Convenience samples are inexpensive and accessible, and they usually require less time to acquire than other types of samples. Convenience samples provide means to conduct studies on topics that could not be examined through the use of probability sampling. Thus, convenience sampling enables researchers to acquire information in unexplored areas. According to Kerlinger and Lee (2000), a convenience sample is probably not that bad when it is used with reasonable knowledge and care in implementing a study. Health care studies are usually conducted with particular types of patients experiencing varying numbers of health problems; these patients often have limited desires to participate in research. Thus, researchers often find it very difficult to recruit subjects for their studies and frequently must use a sample of convenience versus random sampling to obtain their sample.

Bay, Hagerty, and Williams (2007) used convenience sampling to describe the depressive symptoms of individuals following mild-to-moderate traumatic brain injury (TBI). The following excerpt describes their sampling method.

A convenience sample was recruited from five outpatient TBI programs that offered outpatient therapies for those with neurological disorders. Human investigation procedures with the injured person and their relative/significant other (R/SO) were obtained for each clinical site and written consent was obtained from the injured person and their R/SO. All centers were affiliated with large trauma hospitals in the Midwest and recruitment procedures were similar across settings.... All persons completed the survey information in the same order, during the same testing session (unless too fatigued), and in the presence of a data collector.... An incentive payment was offered to compensate participants for their time.... Seventy-five persons with mild or moderate TBI participated in the study. (Bay et al., 2007, p. 4)

Bay et al.'s (2007) convenience sample has several strengths and a few weaknesses. The consistent recruitment of the participants and the inclusion of five traumatic brain injury programs across the Midwest as settings are strengths of the sample. It would have been helpful if the acceptance or refusal rate for the study had been addressed to determine possible sample bias. The individuals with traumatic brain injury have decreased ability to consent to research so consent was obtained from these individuals and their relative/significant others, indicating ethical treatment of the subjects during the sampling process. The data were collected at one session, so no attrition was noted during the study. The subjects were compensated for their time during the study, which usually increases the acceptance and retention rates for a study. The sample size of 75 might have been larger but was strong considering the type of patient studied. Most of the actions of the researchers during the sampling process decreased the potential for bias and improved this convenience sample's representativeness of the target population.

Quota Sampling

Quota sampling uses a convenience sampling technique with an added feature, a strategy to ensure the inclusion of subject types that are likely to be underrepresented in the convenience sample, such as women, minority groups, the elderly, the poor, the rich, and the undereducated. This method may also be used to mimic the known characteristics of the target population or to ensure adequate numbers of subjects in each stratum for the planned statistical analyses. The technique is similar to that used in stratified random sampling. If necessary, mathematical weighting can be used to adjust sample values so that they are consistent with the proportion of subgroups found in the population. Quota sampling offers an improvement over convenience sampling and tends to decrease potential biases. In most studies in which convenience samples are used, quota sampling could be used and should be considered.

McCain et al. (2003) used quota sampling to study the effects of stress management on the psychoneuroimmunology outcomes in persons with HIV infection. They described their sample selection as follows.

Quota sampling was used to achieve appropriate sample representation by gender, at a ratio of 4 males:1 female (20%). Gender subgroups were next stratified by pre-baseline CD4$^+$ cell counts to equilibrate study groups by initial CD4$^+$ counts and, indirectly, by stage of illness....

Enrolled in the study were 148 individuals, 29 females (20%) and 119 males.... Study attrition was within the expected range, with 112 participants completing the intervention groups or initial waiting period (76% retention) and 102 individuals completing the 6-month follow-up visit (69% retention). The attrition rate did not differ among study groups. (McCain et al., 2003, pp. 105–106)

McCain et al. (2003) used quota sampling to ensure a gender distribution of 80% males and 20% females in the study and to achieve study groups that were equal based on patients' CD4+ counts and stage of illness. The stratification by gender and CD4+ count decreased the potential for bias in the sampling method, promoted equality in the study groups, and improved the sample's representativeness of the target population. The researchers also addressed the attrition rate in terms of the total sample and the groups and indicated that this probably did not affect the study findings. The strengths of this study's sampling process decreased the likelihood of sampling error, which is often associated with nonprobability sampling.

NONPROBABILITY SAMPLING METHODS USED IN QUALITATIVE RESEARCH

Qualitative research is conducted to gain insights and discover meaning about a particular experience, situation, cultural element, or historical event. The intent is an in-depth understanding of a purposefully selected sample and not the generalization of the findings from a randomly selected sample to a target population, as in quantitative research. Thus, in qualitative research, experiences, events, and incidents are more the focus of sampling than people (Patton, 2002; Sandelowski, 1995, 2000). The researcher attempts to select participants who can provide extensive information about the experience or event being studied. For example, if the goal of your study was to describe the phenomenon of living with chronic pain, you would purposefully select participants who were articulate and reflective, had a history of chronic pain, and were willing to share their chronic pain experience (Coyne, 1997).

Three common sampling methods used in qualitative research are purposive sampling, snowball sampling, and theoretical sampling. These sampling methods enable the researcher to select the specific participants who will provide the most extensive information about the phenomenon, event, or situation being studied (Marshall & Rossman, 2006). The sample selection process can have a profound effect on the quality of the research and should be described in enough depth to promote the interpretation of the findings and the replication of the study (Munhall, 2001; Patton, 2002).

Purposive Sampling

In purposive sampling, sometimes referred to as *judgmental* or *selective sampling*, the researcher consciously selects certain participants, elements, events, or incidents to include in the study. In purposive sampling, qualitative researchers select information-rich cases, or those cases that can teach them a great deal about the central focus or purpose of the study (Green & Thorogood, 2004; Patton, 2002). Efforts might be made to include typical and atypical participants or situations. Researchers also seek critical cases, or those cases that make a point clearly or are extremely important in understanding the purpose of the study (Munhall, 2001). The researcher might select participants of various ages, those with differing diagnoses or illness severity, or those who received an ineffective treatment versus an effective treatment for their illness.

This sampling plan has been criticized because it is difficult to evaluate the precision of the researcher's judgment. How does one determine that the patient or element was typical or atypical, good or bad, effective or ineffective? Thus, researchers need to indicate the characteristics that they desire in participants and provide a rationale for selecting these types of participants to obtain essential data for their study. Purposive sampling method is used in qualitative research to gain insight into a new area of study or to obtain in-depth understanding of a complex experience or event.

Bakitas (2007) used purposive sampling in conducting her qualitative study to describe the symptom experiences and the impact of chemotherapy-induced peripheral neuropathy (CIPN) on function and everyday life for 28 cancer patients. She described her sample as follows.

> After approval by university and cancer center institutional review boards, purposive sampling (Lincoln & Guba, 1985) was used to identify participants from a rural, National Center Institute-designated, comprehensive cancer center on a maximally diverse set of personal, disease, and CIPN characteristics. Patients were eligible if identified by a clinician or self as having tingling, burning, numbness, "pins-and-needles," shock-like, or painful sensations bilaterally in the feet or hands that were not present prior to receiving chemotherapy but that were related temporally to the initiation of chemotherapy. Patients were excluded if they had preexisting neuropathy not related to chemotherapy. (Bakitas, 2007, p. 324)

In this example, Bakitas (2007) used purposive sampling to select participants who were information rich for her sample. Thus, the study participants were recruited from a large, national cancer center so they would have maximal diverse personal, disease, and CIPN characteristics. The sample inclusion and exclusion criteria are clearly identified to ensure that the participants are experiencing CIPN and not neuropathy resulting from another condition. Bakitas (2007) provided a strong rationale for the number (28) and types of patients selected for her study. These sampling strengths promote the conduct of a sound qualitative study.

Network Sampling

Network sampling, sometimes referred to as "snowballing," holds promise for locating samples difficult or impossible to obtain in other ways or who had not been previously identified for study. Network sampling takes advantage of social networks and the fact that friends tend to have characteristics in common. When you have found a few participants with the necessary criteria, you can ask for their assistance in getting in touch with others with similar characteristics. The first few participants are often obtained through a convenience sampling method, and the sample size is expanded using network sampling. This sampling method is occasionally used in quantitative studies, but it is more commonly used in qualitative studies (Marshall & Rossman, 2006; Munhall, 2001). In qualitative research, network sampling is an effective strategy for identifying participants who know other potential participants who can provide the greatest insight and essential information about an experience or event that is identified for study (Patton, 2002). This strategy is also particularly useful for finding participants in socially devalued populations such as alcoholics, child abusers, sex offenders, drug addicts, and criminals. These individuals are seldom willing to make themselves known. Other groups, such as widows, grieving siblings, or those successful at lifestyle changes, can be located using this strategy. These individuals are outside the existing health care system and are difficult to find. Obviously, biases are built into the sampling process, because the participants are not independent of one another. However, the participants selected have the expertise to provide the essential information needed to address the study purpose.

Coté-Arsenault and Morrison-Beedy (2001) conducted a phenomenological study titled "Women's Voices Reflecting Changed Expectations for Pregnancy after Perinatal Loss." They used network or snowball sampling and described the sampling plan for their study as follows.

Following IRB [institutional review board] approval, a snowball [network] sampling approach was used to recruit women who had experienced at least one perinatal loss and a minimum of one subsequent pregnancy. Recruitment was accomplished using various sources: personal contacts, the local perinatal loss support group, and flyers placed within the university community and local community health settings.... The sample consisted of 21 women with diverse pregnancy and loss histories....

The diversity of childbearing experiences was extensive, encompassing one woman who was currently pregnant, a woman who had given birth 14 weeks before, and women whose last birth was more than two decades prior to this study. The women had experienced from 1 to 7 losses which occurred throughout the three trimesters of pregnancy and at birth. All currently had living children. (Coté-Arsenault & Morrison-Beedy, 2001, p. 241)

The researchers clearly identified the networks (personal contacts, loss support group, and flyers) that were used to recruit study participants. This sampling plan successfully identified women with diverse childbearing experiences, who provided detailed, information-rich data on the expectations for pregnancy after perinatal loss. The sample size of 21 is strong for a qualitative study.

Theoretical Sampling

Theoretical sampling is usually used in grounded theory research to advance the development of a selected theory throughout the research process (Munhall, 2001). The researcher gathers data from any individual or group that can provide relevant data for theory generation. The data are considered relevant if they include information that generates, delimits, and saturates the theoretical codes in the study needed for theory generation. A code is saturated if it is complete and the researcher can see how it fits in the theory. Thus, the researcher continues to seek sources and gather data until the codes are saturated and the theory evolves from the codes and the data. Diversity in the sample is encouraged so the theory developed covers a wide range of behavior in varied situations (Patton, 2002).

Rew (2003) conducted a grounded theory study to develop a theory of taking care of oneself that was grounded in the experiences of homeless youth. The study incorporated theoretical sampling, and the sampling method was described as follows.

Theoretical sampling of homeless youths living temporarily in an urban area was used to insure a wide range of self-care experiences. Potential participants were recruited from youths seeking health and social services from a street outreach program (i.e., a clinic set up in a church basement) in central Texas. Criteria for inclusion were: (a) 16–20 years of age, (b) ability to understand and speak English, and (c) willingness to volunteer for an interview. This age group represented the majority of youths seeking services from this program. Fifteen youths (7 males, 6 females, and 2 transgendered) who were an average of 18.8 years of age volunteered to participate. Saturation (sufficient or adequate data had been collected to meet the goal of the study) was reached at the end of 12 interviews; three additional participants were recruited to verify the findings (Morse, 1998). These participants had been homeless for an average of 4.0 years. In the past year, the majority ($n = 13$) had lived in 'squats,' which are temporary campsites claimed by youths and other homeless persons. (Rew, 2003, p. 235)

Rew (2003) clearly identified the sampling method and the type of participants who were recruited for the study. The number of participants interviewed to reach data saturation was addressed, and three additional interviews were conducted to verify the findings. Adequate data were collected, and codes were saturated to ensure the development of a grounded theory of "Taking Care of Oneself in a High Risk Environment." This descriptive theory of self-care for homeless/street youth included three categories: becoming aware of oneself, staying alive with limited resources, and handling one's own health.

SAMPLE SIZE IN QUANTITATIVE RESEARCH

One of the questions beginning researchers commonly ask is, "What size sample should I use?" Historically, the response to this question has been that a sample should contain at least 30 subjects. There is no logical reason for the selection of this number, and in most cases, 30 subjects is an inadequate sample size.

Currently, the deciding factor in determining an adequate sample size for correlational, quasi-experimental, and experimental studies is power. Power is the capacity of the study to detect differences or relationships that actually exist in the population. Expressed another way, power is the capacity to correctly reject a null hypothesis. The minimum acceptable power for a study is 0.80 (80%). If you do not have sufficient power to detect differences or relationships that exist in the population, you might question the advisability

of conducting the study. You determine the sample size needed to obtain sufficient power by performing a power analysis. The statistical procedures used to perform power analyses are described in Chapter 18.

An increasing number of nurse researchers are using power analysis to determine sample size, but it is essential that the results of the power analyses be included in the published studies. Not conducting a power analysis for a study or omitting the power analysis results in a published study are significant problems if the study failed to detect significant differences or relationships, which might be due to an inadequate sample size. Beck (1994) reviewed the reporting of power analysis in three nursing research journals from 1988 through 1992. Power analysis was reported in only eight studies published in *Nursing Research*, nine studies in *Research in Nursing & Health*, and three studies in *Western Journal of Nursing Research*. Currently, many published studies still do not include a discussion of power analysis, and a number of studies lack the power to detect significant relationships or differences.

The adequacy of sample sizes must be more carefully evaluated in future nursing studies before data collection. Studies with inadequate sample sizes should not be approved for data collection unless they are preliminary pilot studies conducted before a planned larger study. If it is not possible for you to obtain a larger sample because of time or numbers of available subjects, you should redesign your study so that the available sample is adequate for the planned analyses. If you cannot obtain a sufficient sample size, you should not conduct the study.

Large sample sizes are difficult to obtain in nursing studies, require long data collection periods, and are costly. Therefore, in developing the methodology for a study, you must evaluate the elements of the methodology that affect the required sample size. Kraemer and Thiemann (1987) identified the following factors that must be taken into consideration in determining sample size:

1. The more stringent the significance level (e.g., 0.001 versus 0.05), the greater the necessary sample size.
2. Two-tailed statistical tests require larger sample sizes than one-tailed tests. (Tailedness of statistical tests is explained in Chapter 18.)
3. The smaller the effect size, the larger the necessary sample size.
4. The larger the power required, the larger the necessary sample size.
5. The smaller the sample size, the smaller the power of the study.

The factors that must be considered in decisions about sample size (because they affect power) are the effect size, the type of study, the number of variables, the sensitivity of the measurement methods, and the data analysis techniques. These factors are discussed in the following sections.

Effect Size

Effect is the presence of a phenomenon. If a phenomenon exists, it is not absent, and thus, the null hypothesis is in error. However, effect is best understood when not considered in a dichotomous way—that is, as either present or absent. If a phenomenon exists, it exists to some degree. Effect size (ES) is the extent of the presence of a phenomenon in a population. *Effect,* in this case, is used in a broader sense than that of "cause and effect." For example, you might examine the impact of distraction on the experience of pain during an injection. To examine this question, you might obtain a sample of subjects receiving injections and measure differences in the experience of pain in a group of subjects who were distracted during injection and a group of subjects who were not distracted. The null hypothesis would be that there is no difference in the amount of pain experienced by the group receiving distraction versus the one receiving no distraction. If this were so, you would say that the effect of distraction on the experience of pain was zero. In another study, you might be interested in using the Pearson product moment correlation *r* to examine the relationship between coping and anxiety. Your null hypothesis is that the population *r* would be zero or coping is not related to anxiety (Cohen, 1988).

In a study, it is easier to detect large differences between groups than to detect small differences. Thus, smaller samples can detect large *ES*s; smaller effect sizes require larger samples. Broadly speaking, a small *ES* would be <0.3, a medium *ES* would be about 0.3 to 0.5, and a large *ES* would be >0.5. Extremely small *ES*s, such as <0.2, may not be clinically important because the relationships between the variables are small and the differences between the treatment and comparison groups are limited. Knowing the effect size that would be regarded as clinically important allows us to limit the sample to the size needed to detect that level of *ES* (Kraemer & Thiemann, 1987). A result is clinically significant if the effect is large enough to alter clinical decisions. For example, in a comparison of glass thermometers with electronic thermometers, an effect size of 0.1 °F in oral temperature is probably not important enough to influence selection of a particular type of thermometer.

*ES*s vary according to the population being studied. Thus, we must determine the ES for the particular relationship or effect being studied in a selected population. The most desirable source of this information is evidence from previous studies (Melnyk & Fineout-Overholt, 2005). The correlation value (*r*) is equal to the *ES* for the relationship between two variables. For example, if depression is correlated with anxiety at $r = 0.45$, then the $ES = 0.45$. In published studies with treatments, the means and standard deviations can be used to calculate the *ES*. For example, if the mean weight loss for the treatment or intervention group is 5 pounds per month with a standard deviation *(SD)* of 4.5 and the mean weight loss of the control or comparison group is 1 pound per month with a $SD = 6.5$, you can calculate the *ES*.

ES = Mean of the treatment group – Mean of the control group ÷ Standard deviation of control or comparison group

$$ES = 5 - 1 \div 6.5 = 4 \div 6.5 = 0.615 = 0.62$$

This calculation, however, can be used only as an estimate of *ES* for the study. If the researcher changes the measurement method used, the design of the study, or the population being studied, the *ES* will be altered. The best estimate of a population parameter of *ES* is obtained from a meta-analysis in which an estimated population effect size is calculated through the use of statistical values from all studies included in the analysis (Cohen, 1988).

If few relevant studies have been conducted in the area of interest, small pilot studies can be performed, and data analysis results used to calculate the *ES*. If pilot studies are not feasible, dummy power table analysis can be used to calculate the smallest *ES* with clinical or theoretical value. Yarandi (1991) described the process of calculating a dummy power table. If all else fails, *ES* can be estimated as small, medium, or large. Numerical values would be assigned to these estimates, and the power analysis performed. Cohen (1988) has indicated the numerical values for small, medium, and large effects on the basis of specific statistical procedures. In new areas of research, *ES*s are usually small (< 0.3) (Borenstein & Cohen, 1989).

Im et al. (2007, p. 296) conducted a power analysis to identify the sample size they needed to "determine ethnic differences in reported cancer pain experiences among four of the most common ethic groups in the United States, Hispanic, non-Hispanic [N-H] White, N-H African American, and N-H Asian." They included the following discussion of power analysis in their published study.

Four hundred eighty [480] cancer patients (105 Hispanic, 148 N-H Whites, 109 N-H African Americans, and 118 Asians) were recruited through both Internet ($n = 204$) and community ($n = 276$) settings. To test the differences in cancer pain, symptoms accompanying pain, and functional status according to the four ethnic groups (Hypothesis 1), a conventional effect size of 0.20 (Cohen, 1988) was assumed. With alpha = 0.05, 68 participants per ethnic group would be needed to detect a statistically significant difference with power greater than 0.80 (Cohen, 1988). The Internet settings for recruitment were Internet cancer support groups identified through Google, MSN, and Yahoo searchers. The community settings were cancer clinics and cancer support groups across the United States that were identified also by Internet searchers. (Im et al., 2007, p. 297)

Im et al. (2007) identified the small *ES* of 0.2 for their study because this is a relatively new area of research for the four ethnic groups. The researchers indicated that a minimum of 68 subjects would be needed for each ethnic group to achieve a power of 0.8 to detect significant differences in this study. Thus, the minimum sample size needed was 272, and the researchers greatly exceeded that minimum sample size by obtaining a sample of 480. Another important strength of this study was that each ethnic group had more than 100 subjects, when a minimum of 68 subjects was required. The total sample size (480 subjects) and the number of subjects in each ethnic group enabled the researchers to detect significant differences among the four ethnic groups. The study findings indicated that there were ethnic differences in types of pain, symptoms, and functional status for cancer patients, which needs to be considered in caring for these patients.

Type of Study

Descriptive case studies tend to use small samples. Groups are not compared, and problems related to sampling error and generalization have little relevance for such studies. A small sample size may better serve the researcher who is interested in examining a situation in depth from various perspectives. Other descriptive studies, particularly those using survey questionnaires, and correlational studies often require large samples. In these studies, multiple variables may be examined, and extraneous variables are likely to affect subject responses to the variables under study. Statistical comparisons are often made among multiple subgroups in the sample, requiring that an adequate sample be available for each subgroup being analyzed. In addition, subjects are likely to be heterogeneous in terms of demographic variables, and

measurement tools are sometimes not adequately refined. Although target populations may have been identified, sampling frames may not be available, and parameters have not usually been well defined by previous studies. All of these factors lower the power of the study and require increases in sample size (Kraemer & Thiemann, 1987).

In the past, quasi-experimental and experimental studies often used smaller samples than descriptive and correlational studies. As control in the study increases, the sample size can decrease and still approximate the population. Instruments in these studies tend to be refined, thus improving precision. However, sample size must be sufficient to achieve an acceptable level of power (0.8) and thereby reduce the risk of a type II error (indicating the study findings are nonsignificant, when they are really significant) (Kraemer & Thiemann, 1987).

The study design influences power, but the design with the greatest power may not always be the most valid design to use. The experimental design with the greatest power is the pretest-posttest design with a historical control or comparison group. However, this design may have questionable validity because of the historical control group. Can the researcher demonstrate that the historical control group is comparable to the experimental group? The repeated measures design will increase power if the trait being assessed is relatively stable over time. Designs that use blocking or stratification usually require an increase in the total sample size. The sample size increases in proportion to the number of cells included in the data analysis. Designs that use matched pairs of subjects have greater power and thus require a smaller sample. The higher the degree of correlation between subjects on the variable on which the subjects are matched, the greater the power (Kraemer & Thiemann, 1987).

Kraemer and Thiemann (1987) classified studies as *exploratory* or *confirmatory*. According to their approach, confirmatory studies should be conducted only after a large body of knowledge has been gathered through exploratory studies. Confirmatory studies are expected to have large samples and to use random sampling techniques. These expectations are lessened for exploratory studies. Exploratory studies are not intended for generalization to large populations. They are designed to increase the knowledge of the field of study. For example, pilot or preliminary studies to test a methodology or provide estimates of an *ES* are often conducted before a larger study. In other studies, the variables, not the subjects, are the primary area of concern. Several studies may examine the same variables using different populations. In these types of studies, the specific population used may be somewhat incidental. Data from these studies may be used to define population parameters. This information can then be used to conduct confirmatory studies using large, randomly selected samples.

Confirmatory studies, such as those testing the effects of nursing interventions on patient outcomes or those testing the fit of a theoretical model, require large sample sizes. Clinical trials are being conducted in nursing for these purposes. The power of these large, complex studies must be carefully analyzed (Leidy & Weissfeld, 1991). For the large sample sizes to be obtained, subjects are acquired in a number of clinical settings, sometimes in various parts of the country. Kraemer and Thiemann (1987) believe that these studies should not be performed until extensive information is available from exploratory studies. This information should include meta-analysis and the definition of a population *ES*.

Number of Variables

As the number of variables under study grows, the needed sample size may also increase. Adding variables such as age, gender, ethnicity, and education to the analysis plan (just to be on the safe side) can increase the sample size by a factor of 5 to 10 if the selected variables are uncorrelated with the dependent variable. In this case, instead of a sample of 50, you may need a sample of 250 to 500 if you plan to use the variables in the statistical analyses. (Using them only to describe the sample does not cause a problem in terms of power.) If the variables are highly correlated with the dependent variable, however, the effect size will increase, and the sample size can be reduced.

Therefore, variables included in the data analysis must be carefully selected. They should be essential to the research purpose or should have a documented strong relationship with the dependent variable (Kraemer & Thiemann, 1987). Sometimes researchers have obtained sufficient sample size for the primary analyses but failed to plan for analyses involving subgroups, such as analyzing the data by age categories or by ethnic groups, which require a larger sample size. The inclusion of multiple dependent variables also increases the sample size needed.

Measurement Sensitivity

Well-developed instruments measure phenomena with precision. A thermometer, for example, measures body temperature precisely. Tools measuring psychosocial variables tend to be less precise. However, a tool with strong reliability and validity tends to measure more precisely than a tool that is less well developed.

Variance tends to be higher in a less well-developed tool than in one that is well developed. An instrument with a smaller variance is preferred because the power of a test always decreases when within-group variance increases (Kraemer & Thiemann, 1987). For example, if you were measuring anxiety and the actual anxiety score for several subjects was 80, the subjects' scores on a less well-developed tool might range from 70 to 90, whereas a well-developed tool would tend to show a score closer to the actual score of 80 for each subject. As variance in instrument scores increases, the sample size needed to gain an accurate understanding of the phenomenon under study increases.

The range of measured values influences power. For example, a variable might be measured in 10 equally spaced values, ranging from 0 to 9. *ES*s vary according to how near the value is to the population mean. If the mean value is 5, *ES*s are much larger in the extreme values and lower for values near the mean. If you decided to use only subjects with values of 0 and 9, the *ES* would be large, and the sample could be small. The credibility of the study might be questionable, however, because the values of most individuals would not be 0 or 9 but rather would tend to be in the middle range of values. If you decided to include subjects who have values in the range of 3 to 6, excluding the extreme scores, the *ES* would be small, and you would require a much larger sample. The wider the range of values sampled, the larger the *ES* (Kraemer & Thiemann, 1987). A strong measurement method has validity and reliability and measures variables at the interval or ratio level. The stronger the measurement methods used in a study, the smaller the sample that is needed to identify significant relationships among variables and differences between groups.

Data Analysis Techniques

Data analysis techniques vary in their ability to detect differences in the data. Statisticians refer to this as the power of the statistical analysis. For your data analysis, choose the most powerful statistical test appropriate to the data. Overall, parametric statistical analyses are more powerful than nonparametric techniques in detecting differences and should be used if the data meet criteria for parametric analysis. In many cases, however, nonparametric techniques are more powerful if your data do not meet the assumptions of parametric techniques. Parametric techniques vary widely in their capacity to distinguish fine differences and relationships in the data. Parametric and nonparametric analyses are discussed in Chapter 18.

There is also an interaction between the measurement sensitivity and the power of the data analysis technique. The power of the analysis technique increases as precision in measurement increases. Larger samples must be used when the power of the planned statistical analysis is low.

For some statistical procedures, such as the *t*-test and analysis of variance (ANOVA), having equal group sizes increases power, because the effect size is maximized. The more unequal the group sizes are, the smaller the effect size. Therefore, in unequal groups, the total sample size must be larger (Kraemer & Thiemann, 1987).

The chi-square (χ^2) test is the weakest of the statistical tests and requires very large sample sizes to achieve acceptable levels of power. As the number of categories in your study grows, the sample size needed increases. Also, if there are small numbers in some of the categories, you must increase the sample size. Kraemer and Thiemann (1987) have recommended that the chi-square test be used only when no other options are available. In addition, the number of categories should be limited to those essential to the study.

SAMPLE SIZE IN QUALITATIVE RESEARCH

In quantitative research, the sample size must be large enough to identify relationships among variables or to determine differences between groups. However, in qualitative research, the focus is on the quality of information obtained from the person, situation, event, or documents sampled versus the size of the sample (Patton, 2002; Sandelowski, 1995). The sample size and sampling plan are determined by the purpose of the study. Thus, the sample size required is determined by the depth of information that is needed to gain insight into a phenomenon, describe a cultural element, develop a theory, or describe a historical event. The sample size can be too small when the data collected lacks adequate depth or richness. Thus, an inadequate sample size can reduce the quality and credibility of the research findings. Many qualitative researchers use purposive sampling methods to select the specific participants, events, or situations that they believe will provide them the rich data needed to gain insights and discover new meaning in an area of study (Sandelowski, 2000).

The number of participants in a qualitative study is adequate when saturation of information is achieved in the study area. Saturation of data occurs when additional sampling provides no new information, only redundancy of previously collected data. Important factors that must be considered in determining sample size to achieve saturation of data are (1) scope of the study, (2) nature of the topic, (3) quality of the data,

and (4) study design (Marshall & Rossman, 2006; Morse, 2000; Munhall, 2001; Patton, 2002).

Scope of the Study

If the scope of your study is broad, you will need extensive data to address the study purpose, and it will take longer to reach data saturation. Thus, a study with a purpose that has a broad scope will require more sampling of participants, events, or documents than would a study with a narrow scope (Morse, 2000). A study that has a clear focus and provides focused data collection usually has richer, more credible findings. Thus, the depth of your study's scope and its clarity of the focus will influence the number of participants you will need for the sample. For example, fewer participants would be needed to describe the phenomenon of chronic pain in adults with rheumatoid arthritis than would be needed to describe the phenomenon of chronic pain in the elderly. A study of chronic pain in the elderly has a much broader focus, with less clarity, than a study of chronic pain experienced by adults with a specific medical diagnosis of rheumatoid arthritis.

Nature of the Topic

If the topic of your study is clear and the participants can easily discuss it, fewer individuals are needed to obtain the essential data. If the topic is difficult to define and awkward for people to discuss, however, you will probably need a larger number of participants to saturate the data (Morse, 2000; Patton, 2002). For example, a phenomenological study of the experience of an adult living with a history of child sexual abuse is a sensitive, complex topic to investigate. This type of topic would probably require a greater number of participants and increased interview time to collect the essential data.

Quality of the Data

The quality of information obtained from an interview, observation, or document review influences the sample size. The higher the quality and richness of the data, the fewer participants you will need to saturate data in the area of study. Quality data are best obtained from articulate, well-informed, and communicative participants (Sandelowski, 1995). These participants are able to share more rich data in a clear and concise manner. In addition, participants who have more time to be interviewed usually provide data with greater depth and breadth. Qualitative studies require that you critically appraise the quality of the participants, events, or documents studied; the richness of the data collected; and the adequacy of the sample size based on the findings.

Study Design

Some studies are designed to increase the number of interviews with participants. The more interviews conducted with a participant, the greater the quality of the data collected. For example, a study design that includes an interview both before an event and after the event would produce more data than a single interview. Designs that involve interviewing a family or a group of individuals produce more data than an interview with a single study participant. In critically appraising a qualitative study, determine if the sample size is adequate for the design of the study.

Bakitas (2007) conducted a qualitative study to explore and describe the symptom experience and the resulting impact of chemotherapy-induced peripheral neuropathy (CIPN) on function and everyday life for patients with cancer. We introduced this study earlier in this chapter as an example of a study with purposive sampling, where the sampling method, sample criteria, and setting were described. The following excerpt describes Bakitas's rationale for the sample size used to collect data in her study.

> After approval by university and cancer center institutional review boards, purposive sampling (Lincoln & Guba, 1985) was used to identify participants…. The total number of participants was determined during the course of the study by the number needed to obtain saturation (theoretical completeness) of the concept being explored. Theoretical saturation was defined as the point at which no additional information that could form a new category of data was collected (Glaser & Strauss, 1967; Sandelowski, 2000…).
>
> After recruitment of 20 participants, theoretical sampling was used to more fully explicate the emerging themes and issues; only extreme (e.g., severe or prolonged) or deviant (e.g., unique CIPN experience from Phase II investigational drug) cases of CIPN were sought. Data redundancy or saturation seemed apparent after 27 interviews. To strengthen this conclusion, an additional interview was conducted and analyzed. Because no new codes or themes were revealed in Participant 28, enrollment was closed. (Bakitas, 2007, p. 324)

Bakitas's (2007) study has many strengths in the area of sampling, including quality sampling methods (purpose and theoretical), strong sample size ($N = 28$), and conscientious participants. She provided extensive detail of her sampling process that included both purposive and theoretical sampling methods to ensure an adequate number of data-rich participants were interviewed to achieve depth and breadth in the data. The sample size of 20 from purposive sampling seemed strong, because rich, detailed data were collected from these participants. By using theoretical sampling to select seven more participants, Bakitas was able to more fully identify themes and issues and to saturate the data. Bakitas conducted a final interview to strengthen the study conclusions, resulting in a sample size of 28 for the study. The scope of the study, nature of the topic, and quality of the data were addressed and seemed to support the sample size. The report would have been strengthened by a discussion of refusal and attrition rates for the study, but the sample and data collected were extremely strong, increasing the validity of the study findings. The study results indicated "diverse symptom patterns and degrees of physical symptoms and distress from mild to severe, emotional distress, alterations in functional ability, and social role impairment. Comprehensive clinical and research measures are needed to assess the full spectrum of CIPN effects on everyday life" (Bakitas, 2007, p. 323).

RESEARCH SETTINGS

The setting is the location where a study is conducted. There are three common settings for conducting nursing research: natural, partially controlled, and highly controlled. A natural setting, or *field setting*, is an uncontrolled, real-life situation or environment (Peat et al., 2002). Conducting a study in a natural setting means that the researcher does not manipulate or change the environment for the study. Descriptive and correlational quantitative studies and qualitative studies are often conducted in natural settings. For example, Bakitas (2007), discussed previously, made no attempt to manipulate the setting when she conducted the interviews for her qualitative study; she even allowed participants to select the setting most convenient to and comfortable for them. All data were conducted in natural settings, with 21 participants interviewed in a private cancer center office, 6 in their homes, and 1 by telephone. The intent of the study was to describe the cancer patients' symptoms and function as they exist in a natural environment.

A partially controlled setting is an environment that the researcher manipulates or modifies in some way. An increasing number of nursing studies, usually correlational, quasi-experimental, and experimental studies, are being conducted in partially controlled settings. Rivers et al. (2003), in a study that was introduced earlier in the discussion of sampling frame, conducted a predictive correlational study to determine predictors of nurses' acceptance of an intravenous catheter safety device. These researchers described their setting as follows:

A 900-bed urban teaching hospital in Texas implemented a new intravenous Protectiv® Plus IV catheter safety needle device in September 1999. Data collection was implemented in December 2000 to ensure that all training had been accomplished and that the device was implemented in all areas. All the nurses on the various 36 nursing units/areas where RNs initiate IV therapy were surveyed by a 34-item, self-administered questionnaire. The units included medical surgical units, intensive care, cardiovascular transplant units, surgical preoperative and postoperative, day surgery, maternal and neonatal units, emergency and urgent care areas, oncology clinic and others. (Rivers et al., 2003, p. 250)

Rivers et al. (2003) selected a teaching hospital, which provides a partially controlled setting in terms of the units that have IVs, nurses' training within the hospital and in particular for the IV safety device, and the safety climate or requirements of the workplace. However, the researchers did not control other aspects of the environment, such as the nurses' previous work experience; interactions of the nurses regarding their training and use of the IV safety device on different units; and the data collection process, which was a self-administered questionnaire.

A highly controlled setting is an artificially constructed environment developed for the sole purpose of conducting research. Laboratories, research or experimental centers, and test units in hospitals or other health care agencies are highly controlled settings where experimental studies are often conducted. This type of setting reduces the influence of extraneous variables, which enables the researcher to examine accurately the effect of one variable on another. Highly controlled settings are commonly used to conduct experimental research. Rasmussen and Farr (2003) conducted an experimental study of the effects of morphine and time of day on pain and beta-endorphin in a sample of Dilute Brown Agouti (DBA) mice. This study was conducted in a laboratory using a selected type of mouse, and the setting is described as follows:

The mice were housed individually in clear styrene cages in a private, controlled-access room in the laboratory animal facilities of the Comparative Medicine Department. Individual housing was used to reduce social conflict and stress, which have been shown to bring about stress-induced analgesia. … The presence of other mice in the room prevented isolation stress. Food and water were allowed ad libitum. A 12:12 light/dark cycle, with lights on at 0600, and a room temperature of 22 ± 1 °C were maintained throughout the study. Experiments timed for the dark phase were performed under dim red lights. (Rasmussen & Farr, 2003, p. 107)

The study included the use of a highly controlled laboratory setting in terms of the housing of the mice, the light and temperature of the environment, implementation of the treatments, and the measurements of the dependent variables. Only with animals could this type of setting control be achieved in the conduct of a study. This type of highly controlled setting removes the impact of numerous extraneous variables, so the effects of the independent variables on the dependent variables can be clearly determined. However, because this research was conducted on animals, the findings cannot be generalized to humans, and additional research is needed to determine the effects of the independent variables of morphine and time of day on the dependent variables of pain and beta-endorphins in humans.

RECRUITING AND RETAINING SUBJECTS

Once you and your research team have made a decision about the size of the sample, your next step is to develop a plan for recruiting subjects. Recruitment strategies differ, depending on the type of study and the setting. Special attention must focus on recruiting subjects who tend to be underrepresented in studies, such as minorities, women, children, and the elderly (Corbie-Smith, Thomas, Williams, & Moody-Ayers, 1999; Fulmer, 2001; Hendrickson, 2007; Rice, Bunker, Kang, Howell, & Weaver, 2007). The sampling plan, initiated at the beginning of data collection, is almost always more difficult than expected. In addition to subject recruitment, retaining acquired subjects is critical to achieve an acceptable sample size and requires you to consider the effects of the data collection strategies on subject attrition. Problems with retaining subjects increase as the data collection period lengthens. Some researchers never obtain their planned sample size because of problems they encounter as they try to recruit and retain subjects. These researchers often are forced to complete their study with a smaller sample size, which could decrease the power of the study and produce nonsignificant results. With the additional studies being conducted in health care, recruiting and retaining subjects have become more complex issues for researchers to manage.

Recruiting Subjects

The effective recruitment of subjects is crucial to the success of a study. Few studies have examined the effectiveness of various strategies of subject recruitment. Most information available to guide researchers comes from the personal experiences of skilled researchers. Some of the factors that influence a subject's decision to participate in a study are the attitudes and ethics of the researchers, the subject's need for a treatment, the subject's interest in the study topic, fear of the unknown, time and travel constraints, financial compensation, and the nature of the informed consent (Madsen et al., 2002; Papadopoulos & Lees, 2002; Sullivan-Bolyai et al., 2007).

The researcher's initial approach to a potential subject usually strongly affects his or her decision about participating in the study. Therefore, your approach must be pleasant, positive, informative, and nonaggressive. Explain the importance of the study, and clarify exactly what the subject will be asked to do, how much of the subject's time will be involved, and what the duration of the study will be. Subjects are valuable resources, and the researcher must communicate this value to the potential subject. High-pressure techniques, such as insisting that the subject make an instant decision to participate in a study, usually lead to resistance and a higher rate of refusals. If the study involves minorities, the researcher must be culturally competent or knowledgeable and skilled in relating to the particular ethnic group being studied (Papadopoulos & Lees, 2002). Hendrickson (2007) used a video for recruiting Hispanic women for her study, and she provided all the details related to the study in the subjects' own language in the video. This greatly improved the subjects' understanding of the study and the consent process.

If a potential subject refuses to participate in a study, you must accept the refusal gracefully—in terms of body language, as well as words. Your actions can influence the decision of other potential subjects who observe or hear about the encounter. Studies in which a high proportion of individuals refuse to participate have a serious validity problem. The sample is likely to be biased, because often only a certain type of individual has agreed to participate. Therefore, keep records of the numbers of persons who refuse and, if possible, their reasons for refusal. With this information, you can include the refusal rate in the published research report with the reasons for refusal. It would also be helpful if you could determine if the potential subjects who refused to participate differ from those who agreed to participate in the study. This information will help you to determine the representativeness of your sample.

Recruiting minority subjects for a study can be particularly problematic. Minority individuals may be difficult to locate and are often reluctant to participate in studies because of feelings of being "used" while receiving no personal benefit from their involvement or because of their distrust of the medical community (Corbie-Smith et al., 1999). Pletsch, Howe, and Tenney (1995, p. 211) recommended using "feasibility analysis, developing partnerships with target groups and community members, using active face-to-face recruitment, and using process evaluation techniques to recruit members of minority groups as subjects of a study."

If you are using data collectors in your study, verify that they are following the sampling plan, especially in random samples. When the data collectors encounter difficult subjects or are unable to make contact easily, they may simply shift to the next person without informing the principal investigator. This behavior could violate the rules of random sampling and bias the sample. If data collectors do not understand, or do not believe in, the importance of randomization, their decisions and actions can undermine the intent of the sampling plan. Thus, data collectors must be carefully selected and thoroughly trained. Develop a plan for the supervision and follow-up of data collectors to increase their accountability.

If you conduct a survey study, you may never have personal contact with the subjects. To recruit such subjects, you must rely on the use of attention-getting techniques, persuasively written material, and strategies for following up on individuals who do not respond to the initial written or e-mail communication. Because of the serious problems of low response rates in survey studies, using strategies to raise the response rate is critical. For instance, we have received a teabag or packet of instant coffee with a questionnaire, accompanied by a recommendation in the letter to have a cup of tea or coffee "on" the researcher while we take a break from work to complete the questionnaire. Creativity is required in the use of such strategies, because they tend to lose their effect on groups who receive questionnaires frequently (such as faculty). In some cases, small amounts of money (fifty cents to a dollar) are enclosed with the letter, which may suggest that the recipient buy a soft drink or that the money is a small offering for completing the questionnaire. This strategy imposes some sense of obligation on the recipient to complete the questionnaire, but it is not thought to be coercive (Baker, 1985). Also, you should plan mailings to avoid holidays or times of the year when workloads are high for potential subjects, possibly reducing the return rate.

Researchers frequently use the Internet to recruit subjects and to collect survey data. This method makes it easier for you to contact potential subjects and for the subjects to provide the requested data. However, an increased number of surveys are being sent by the Internet, which can decrease the response rate of potential subjects who are frequently surveyed.

In studies with surveys, the letter (in hard copy or e-mail) to potential subjects must be carefully composed. It may be your only chance to persuade the subject to invest the time needed to complete the questionnaire. You must sell the reader on the importance of both your study and his or her response. The tone of your letter will be the potential subject's only image of you as a person; yet, for many subjects, their response to the perception of you as a person most influences their decision about completing the questionnaire. Seek examples of letters sent by researchers who have had high response rates, and save letters you receive that you responded positively to. You also might pilot-test your letter on individuals who can give you feedback about their reactions to the letter's tone.

The use of follow-up e-mails, letters, or cards has been repeatedly shown to raise response rates to surveys. The timing is important. If too long a period has lapsed, the potential subject may have deleted the questionnaire from his or her e-mail box or discard the mailed copy. Sending the follow-up too soon, however, could be offensive. Baker (1985) described her strategies for following up on questionnaires:

Before the questionnaires are emailed or mailed, precise plans need to be made for monitoring the return of each questionnaire as a means of follow-up procedure. A bar graph could be developed to record the return of each questionnaire as a means of suggesting when the follow-up mailing or email should occur. The cumulative number and percentage of responses would then be logged on the graph to reflect the overall data collection process. When the daily responses decline, a follow-up, first-class mailing or email could be sent, containing another questionnaire and a modified cover letter. Study participants and questionnaires are assigned the same code numbers, and nonrespondents are identified by checking the list of code numbers of unreturned questionnaires. A third follow-up questionnaire with a further modified cover letter could be emailed or mailed to increase the return rate for the questionnaires.

The factors involved in the decision of whether to respond to a questionnaire are not well understood. One obvious factor is the time required to respond; this includes the time needed to orient to the directions and the emotional energy necessary to deal with the threats and anxieties generated by the questions. There is also a cognitive demand for thinking. Subjects seem to make a judgment about the relevance of the research topic and the potential for personal application of findings. Previous experience with questionnaires is also a deciding factor.

Traditionally, subjects for nursing studies have been sought in the hospital setting. However, access to these subjects is becoming more difficult—in part because of the larger numbers of nurses and other health care professionals now conducting research. The largest involvement of research subjects within a health care agency usually occurs with medical research and mainly with clinical trials that include large samples (Hellard, Sinclair, Forbes, & Fairley, 2001; Sullivan-Bolyai et al., 2007). Nurse researchers and other clinicians are now recruiting subjects from a variety of settings. An initial phase of recruitment may involve obtaining community and institutional support for the study. Support from other health care professionals, such as nurses and physicians, may be critical to the successful recruitment of subjects.

Recruitment of subjects for clinical trials requires a different set of strategies because the recruitment may be occurring simultaneously in several sites (perhaps in different cities). Many of these studies never achieve their planned sample size. The number of subjects meeting the sampling criteria who are available in the selected clinical sites may not be as large as anticipated. Researchers must often screen twice as many patients as are required for the study to obtain a sufficient sample size. Screening logs must be kept during the recruiting period to record data on patients who met the criteria but were not entered into the study. Researchers commonly underestimate the amount of time required to recruit subjects for a clinical study. In addition to defining the number of subjects and the time set aside for recruitment, it may be helpful to develop short-term or interim recruitment goals designed to maintain a constant rate of patient entry. Hellard et al. (2001) studied methods to improve the recruitment and retention of subjects in clinical trials and found that the four most important strategies were to (1) use nonaggressive recruitment methods, (2) maintain regular contact with the participants, (3) ensure that the participants are kept well informed of the study's progress, and (4) constantly encourage subjects to continue participation. Another source is Sullivan-Bolyai et al. (2007), who identified the barriers and strategies to improve the recruitment of study participants from clinical settings (Table 14-2).

Studies may also benefit from the endorsement of community leaders, such as city officials; key civic leaders; and leaders of social, educational, religious, or labor groups. In some cases, these groups may be involved in planning the study, leading to a sense of community ownership of the project. Community groups may also help researchers to recruit subjects for the study. Sometimes, subjects who meet the sampling criteria are found in the groups assisting with

TABLE 14-2 ⬛⬛ Barriers to Recruitment with Actions and Strategies for Engaging Health Care Providers in the Referral Process

Barriers and/or Action	Strategies
HIPAA Create alternative recruitment methods	Clinicians distribute letters to potential study participants Obtain institutional review board waiver of authorization requirement for the use or disclosure of personal health information Work with clinics to secure a consent that meets HIPAA regulations and allows the staff to provide names and contact information of patients with specific conditions that may be of interest to researchers Recognize and acknowledge the burden that recruitment places on health care providers
Work burden Create compensations	Salary support Provide educational incentives (e.g., purchase laptop, journals, books, pay for conference attendance in the field under study) for health care providers who do not normally have access to such opportunities as part of their job Assess administrative and/or managerial perceptions of health care providers' recruitment-related responsibilities and if salary support is given, how that money will be used Discuss the designated recruitment tasks and responsibilities with the assigned staff to determine their perceptions and expectations
Financial disincentives Recognize that patient numbers and/or productivity may be linked to the clinic's livelihood	Assess the clinic's financial situation and determine if it is realistic, pragmatic, or feasible to use that site, especially if its funding depends on patient numbers Help keep participants linked to the clinical site while they are participating in the study
Provider competition Create a partnership with health care providers involved in recruitment so that they are rewarded and acknowledged for their participation in the research process	Develop a research proposal that reflects the clinical site's philosophical and policy perspectives Include health care providers in the development of a study Hire and pay a clinical staff member to be responsible for introducing the study to potential participants Link recruitment activities to nursing clinical ladder or organization values Maintain open communication between the clinical and research teams regarding the workings of the study
Provider concerns Demystify research process Develop a team atmosphere and a spirit of "we're all in this together"	Assess health care providers' perceptions of research Encourage health care providers to participate in developing the research proposal Include health care providers in developing study-related manuscripts Include providers in research team meetings at a mutually convenient time Express appreciation on an ongoing basis for health care providers' involvement in recruitment process Share recruitment status information on a monthly basis with health care providers Share pilot or feasibility data with health care providers to support the study rationale and choice of specific methods
Desire to protect patients Work with health care providers to acknowledge and respect patient decision-making abilities Encourage healthy partnerships between patients and health care providers	Acknowledge responsibility of health care providers to protect patients from harm Address concerns of health care providers by emphasizing the pilot data that supports the protocol Model respectful partnerships with study participants

From Sullivan-Bolyai, S., Bova, C., Deatrick, J. A., Knafl, K., Grey, M., Leung, K., et al. (2007). Barriers and strategies for recruiting study participants in clinical settings. *Western Journal of Nursing Research, 29*(4), 498–499.

the study. Endorsement may involve letters of support and, in some cases, funding. These activities can add legitimacy to your study and make involvement in the study more attractive to potential subjects (Alvarez, Vasquez, Mayorga, Feaster, & Mitrani, 2006).

Media support can be helpful in recruiting subjects. Researchers can place advertisements in local newspapers and church and neighborhood bulletins. Radio stations can make public service announcements. Members of the research team can speak to groups relevant to the study population. Your team can place posters in public places, such as supermarkets, drugstores, and public laundries. With permission, you can set up tables in shopping malls with a member of the research team present to recruit subjects.

Dombeck (2003) used multiple recruitment strategies to obtain a sample of 36 nurses for a qualitative ethnographic study to explore how nurses construe and understand their professional culture, including gender and race, and their professional personhood. The following excerpt from her study describes the different recruitment strategies used and the numbers of subjects obtained with each strategy.

> The purposeful sampling procedures used were aimed at obtaining a diverse group of nurse participants who were also articulate and willing to give time to this research. Recruiting a diverse sample for a profession in which most of the dominant voices are White middle-class women was a challenge. The first approach to recruitment was to place notices on bulletin boards of local hospitals and in the newsletter of the local nursing organization. This initial effort yielded 9 White women (non-Hispanic Caucasian) and 1 man. During the initial interactions the male participant reported that the other nurses who are men that he knew would welcome the opportunity to participate in a group with other men to tell stories of nursing. The plans for such a group were announced through flyers and by word of mouth. Within a short time 13 men were recruited. During early group meetings key informants among the men and one of the women suggested that the African American nurses they knew would prefer to be in a group with other such nurses. Shortly after the decision was announced to place recruits in racially homogenous groups, several African American nurses from diverse settings volunteered to be in the study. (Dombeck, 2003, p. 354)

Retaining Subjects

One of the serious problems in many studies is subject retention. Often, subject attrition cannot be avoided. Subjects move, die, or withdraw from a treatment. If you must collect data at several points over time, subject mortality can become a problem. Subjects who move frequently and those without phones pose a particular problem. A number of strategies have been found to be effective in maintaining the sample. For instance, it is a good idea to obtain the names, addresses, and phone numbers (cell and home numbers if possible) of at least two family members or friends when you enroll the subject in the study. Ask if the subject would agree to give you access to unlisted phone numbers in the event that the subject changes his or her number.

In some studies, the subject is reimbursed for participation. A bonus payment may be included for completing a certain phase of the study. Gifts can be used in place of money. Sending greeting cards for birthdays and holidays helps maintain contact. Rudy, Estok, Kerr, and Menzel (1994) compared the effect on recruitment and retention of money versus gifts. They found no differential effect on recruitment but found that money was more effective than gifts in retaining subjects in longitudinal studies. However, the researchers pointed out the moral issues related to providing monetary payment to subjects. This strategy can compromise the voluntariness of participation in a study and particularly has the potential of exploiting low-income persons.

Collecting data takes time. Always keep in mind that the subject's time is valuable and should be used frugally. During data collection, it is easy to begin taking the subject for granted. Taking time for social amenities with subjects may pay off. However, take care that these interactions do not influence the data being collected. Beyond that, nurturing subjects participating in the study is critical. In some situations, providing refreshments and pleasant surroundings helps. Often, during the data collection phase, you also must nurture others who interact with the subjects; these may be volunteers, family, staff, students, or other professionals. It is important to maintain a pleasant climate for the data collection process, which will pay off in the quality of data collected and the retention of subjects.

Qualitative studies and longitudinal studies require extensive time commitment from the subjects. They are asked to participate in detailed interviews or to complete numerous forms at various intervals during a study (Marshall & Rossman, 2006; Patton, 2002). Sometimes data are collected with diaries that require daily entries over a set period of time. These studies face the greatest risk of participant mortality. Barnard, Magyary, Booth, and Eyres (1987) described the extensive sample maintenance procedures required for their longitudinal study in the following excerpt.

> Sometimes the researcher needs to invest a great deal of time and money in sample maintenance. For example, for the 13-month assessment point in our current study of high-social-risk mothers and children, a research assistant picks up the mother and child at home (a 45-minute drive), brings them to the clinic for testing, and then drives them home again. In addition, the mother is given up to $10 to cover babysitting costs for her other children and is sent a free copy of the videotape we make of her and her child. Without these elaborate arrangements, we feel that our attrition rate would be very high. (Barnard et al., 1987, p. 47)

In summary, subjects who have a personal investment in the study are more likely to continue participating. This investment occurs through interactions with and nurturing by the researcher. A combination of the subject's personal belief in the significance of the study, perceived altruistic motives of the researcher in conducting the study, the ethical actions of the researcher, and nurturing support provided by the researcher during data collection can greatly diminish subject attrition (Madsen et al., 2002). The recruitment and retention of subjects will continue to be significant challenges for researchers, and creative strategies are needed to manage these challenges.

SUMMARY

- Sampling involves selecting a group of people, events, behaviors, or other elements with which to conduct a study. Sampling denotes the process of making the selections; sample denotes the selected group of elements.
- A sampling plan is developed to increase representativeness, decrease systematic bias, and decrease the sampling error; there are two main types: probability and nonprobability sampling plans.
- Four sampling designs have been developed to achieve probability sampling: simple random sampling, stratified random sampling, cluster sampling, and systematic sampling.
- In nonprobability (nonrandom) sampling, not every element of the population has an opportunity for selection in the sample. The five nonprobability sampling designs described in this textbook are (1) convenience sampling, (2) quota sampling, (3) purposive sampling, (4) network sampling, and (5) theoretical sampling.
- In quantitative studies, sample size is best determined by a power analysis, which is calculated using the level of significance ($\alpha = 0.05$, 0.01, or 0.001), standard power of 0.8, and effect size.

- The number of participants in a qualitative study is adequate when saturation of information is achieved in the study area, which occurs when additional sampling provides no new information, only redundancy of previously collected data. Important factors that must be considered in determining sample size to achieve saturation of data are (1) scope of the study, (2) nature of the topic, (3) quality of the data, and (4) study design.
- The three common settings for conducting nursing research are natural, partially controlled, and highly controlled. A natural setting, or field setting, is an uncontrolled, real-life situation or environment. A partially controlled setting is an environment that the researcher has manipulated or modified in some way. A highly controlled setting is an artificially constructed environment developed for the sole purpose of conducting research.
- Recruiting and retaining subjects have become significant challenges in research, and this chapter includes some strategies to assist researchers with these challenges so their samples might be more representative of their target population.

REFERENCES

Alvarez, R. A., Vasquez, E., Mayorga, C. C., Feaster, D. J., & Mitrani, V. B. (2006). Increasing minority research participation through community organization outreach. *Western Journal of Nursing Research*, 28(5), 541–560.

Andrews, J. O., Felton, G., Wewers, M. E., Waller, J., & Tingen, M. (2007). The effect of a multi-component smoking cessation intervention in African American women residing in public housing. *Research in Nursing & Health*, 30(1), 45–60.

Baker, C. M. (1985). Maximizing mailed questionnaire responses. *Image: Journal of Nursing Scholarship*, 17(4), 118–121.

Bakitas, M. A. (2007). Background noise: The experience of chemotherapy-induced peripheral neuropathy. *Nursing Research*, 56(5), 323–331.

Barhyte, D. Y., Redman, B. K., & Neill, K. M. (1990). Population or sample: Design decision. *Nursing Research*, 39(5), 309–310.

Barnard, K. E., Magyary, D. L., Booth, C. L., & Eyres, S. J. (1987). Longitudinal designs: Considerations and applications to nursing research. *Recent Advances in Nursing*, 17, 37–64.

Bay, E., Hagerty, B. M., & Williams, R. A. (2007). Depressive symptomatology after mild-to-moderate traumatic brain injury: A comparison of three measures. *Archives of Psychiatric Nursing*, 21(1), 2–11.

Beck, C. T. (1994). Statistical power analysis in pediatric nursing research. *Issues in Comprehensive Pediatric Nursing*, 17(2), 73–80.

Borenstein, M., & Cohen, J. (1989). *Statistical power analysis* (Release: 1.00). Hillsdale, NJ: Erlbaum.

Brent, E. E., Jr., Scott, J. K., & Spencer, J. C. (1988). Ex-Sample™: An expert system to assist in designing sampling plans. *User's guide and reference manual* (Version 2.0). Columbia, MO: The Idea Works.

Cochran, W. G. (1977). *Sampling techniques* (3rd ed.). New York: Wiley.

Cohen, J. (1988). *Statistical power analysis for the behavioral sciences* (2nd ed.). New York: Academic Press.

Corbie-Smith, G., Thomas, S. B., Williams, M. V., & Moody-Ayers, S. (1999). Attitudes and beliefs of African Americans toward participation in medical research. *Journal of General Internal Medicine, 14*(9), 537–546.

Coté-Arsenault, D., & Morrison-Beedy, D. (2001). Women's voices reflecting changed expectations for pregnancy after perinatal loss. *Journal of Nursing Scholarship, 33*(3), 239–244.

Coyne, I. T. (1997). Sampling in qualitative research. Purposeful and theoretical sampling; merging or clear boundaries. *Journal of Advanced Nursing, 26*(3), 623–630.

Dombeck, M. T. (2003). Work narratives: Gender and race in professional personhood. *Research in Nursing & Health, 26*(5), 351–365.

Floyd, J. A. (1993). Systematic sampling: Theory and clinical methods. *Nursing Research, 42*(5), 290–293.

Flynn, L. (2007). Extending work environment research into home health settings. *Western Journal of nursing Research 29*(2), 200–212.

Fulmer, T. (2001). Recruiting older adults in our studies [Editorial]. *Applied Nursing Research, 14*(2), 63.

Glaser, B. G., & Strauss, A. L. (1967). *The discovery of grounded theory: Strategies for qualitative research.* Chicago: Aldine.

Green, J., & Thorogood, N. (2004). *Qualitative methods for health research.* Thousand Oaks, CA: Sage.

Hellard, M. E., Sinclair, M. I., Forbes, A. B., & Fairley, C. K. (2001). Methods used to maintain a high level of participant involvement in a clinical trial. *Journal of Epidemiology and Community Health, 55*(5), 348–351.

Hendrickson, S. G. (2007). Video recruitment of non-English-speaking participants. *Western Journal of Nursing Research, 29*(2), 232–242.

Im, E., Chee, W., Guevara, E., Liu, Y., Lim, H., Tsai, H., et al. (2007). Gender and ethnic differences in cancer pain experience: A multiethnic survey in the United States. *Nursing Research, 56*(5), 296–306.

Kerlinger, F. N. & Lee, H. B. (2000). *Foundations of behavioral research* (4th ed.). Fort Worth, TX: Harcourt College Publishers.

Kraemer, H. C., & Thiemann, S. (1987). *How many subjects? Statistical power analysis in research.* Newbury Park, CA: Sage.

Larson, E. (1994). Exclusion of certain groups from clinical research. *Image: Journal of Nursing Scholarship, 26*(3), 185–190.

Leidy, N. K., & Weissfeld, L. A. (1991). Sample sizes and power computation for clinical intervention trials. *Western Journal of Nursing Research, 13*(1), 138–144.

Levy, P. S., & Lemsbow, S. (1980). *Sampling for health professionals.* Belmont, CA: Lifetime Learning.

Lincoln, Y. S., & Guba, E. G. (1985). *Naturalistic inquiry.* Beverly Hills, CA: Sage.

Madsen, S. M., Mirza, M. R., Holm, S., Hilsted, K. L., Kampmann, K., & Riis, P. (2002). Attitudes towards clinical research amongst participants and nonparticipants. *Journal of Internal Medicine, 251*(2), 156–168.

Marshall, C., & Rossman, G. B. (2006). *Designing qualitative research* (4th ed.). Thousand Oaks, CA: Sage.

McCain, N. L., Munjas, B. A., Munro, C. L., Elswick, R. K., Jr., Robins, J. L. W., Ferreira-Gonzalez, A., et al. (2003). Effects of stress management on PNI-based outcomes in persons with HIV disease. *Research in Nursing & Health, 26*(2), 102–117.

Melnyk, B. M., & Fineout-Overholt, E. (2005). *Evidence-based practice in nursing & healthcare: A guide to best practice.* Philadelphia: Lippincott Williams & Wilkins.

Mitchell, E. S., Woods, N. F., & Lentz, M. J. (1994). Differentiation of women with three perimenstrual symptom patterns. *Nursing Research, 43*(1), 25–30.

Moody, L. E., Wilson, M. E., Smyth, K., Schwartz, R., Tittle, M., & Van Cott, M. L. (1988). Analysis of a decade of nursing practice research: 1977–1986. *Nursing Research, 37*(6), 374–379.

Morse, J. M. (1998). Designing funded qualitative research. In N. K. Denzin & Y. S. Lincoln (Eds.), *Strategies of qualitative inquiry* (pp. 56–85). Thousand Oaks, CA: Sage.

Morse, J. M. (2000). Determining sample size. *Qualitative Health Research, 10*(1), 3–5.

Munhall, P. L. (2001). *Nursing research: A qualitative perspective* (3rd ed.). Sudbury, MA: Jones & Bartlett.

Neumark, D. E., Stommel, M., Given, C. W., & Given, B. A. (2001). Brief report: Research design and subject characteristics predicting nonparticipation in panel survey of older families with cancer. *Nursing Research, 50*(6), 363–368.

Papadopoulos, I., & Lees, S. (2002). Developing culturally competent researchers. *Journal of Advanced Nursing, 37*(3), 258–264.

Patton, M. Q. (2002). *Qualitative evaluation and research methods* (3rd ed.). Thousand Oaks, CA: Sage.

Peat, J. K., Mellis, C., Williams, K., & Xuan, W. (2002). *Health science research: A handbook of quantitative methods.* Thousand Oaks, CA: Sage.

Pletsch, P. K., Howe, C., & Tenney, M. (1995). Recruitment of minority subjects for intervention research. *Image: Journal of Nursing Scholarship, 27*(3), 211–215.

Rasmussen, N. A., & Farr, L. A. (2003). Effects of morphine and time of day on pain and beta-endorphin. *Biological Research for Nursing, 5*(2), 105–116.

Rew, L. (2003). A theory of taking care of oneself grounded in experiences of homeless youth. *Nursing Research, 52*(4), 234–241.

Rice, M., Bunker, K. D., Kang, D., Howell, C. C., & Weaver, M. (2007). Accessing and recruiting children for research in schools. *Western Journal of Nursing Research, 29*(4), 501–514.

Rivers, D. L., Aday, L. A., Frankowski, R. F., Felknor, S., White, D., & Nichols, B. (2003). Predictors of nurses' acceptance of an intravenous catheter safety device. *Nursing Research, 52*(4), 249–255.

Rudy, E. B., Estok, P. J., Kerr, M. E., & Menzel, L. (1994). Research incentives: Money versus gifts. *Nursing Research, 43*(4), 253–255.

Sandelowski, M. (1995). Sample size in qualitative research. *Research in Nursing & Health, 18*(2), 179–183.

Sandelowski, M. (2000). Combining qualitative and quantitative sampling, data collection, and analysis techniques in mixed-method studies. *Research in Nursing & Health, 23*(3), 246–255.

Sullivan-Bolyai, S., Bova, C., Deatrick, J. A., Knafl, K., Grey, M., Leung, K., et al. (2007). Barriers and strategies for recruiting study participants in clinical settings. *Western Journal of Nursing Research, 29*(4), 486–500.

Tolle, S. W., Tilden, V. P., Rosenfeld, A. G., & Hickman, S. E. (2000). Family reports of barriers to optimal care of the dying. *Nursing Research*, *49*(6), 310–317.

Ulrich, C. M., Danis, M., Ratcliffe, S. J., Garrett-Mayer, E., Koziol, D., Soeken, K. L., et al. (2006). Ethical conflict in nurse practitioners and physician assistants in managed care. *Nursing Research*, *55*(6), 391–401.

Yarandi, H. N. (1991). Planning sample sizes: Comparison of factor level means. *Nursing Research*, *40*(1), 57–58.

Yates, F. (1981). *Sampling methods for censuses and surveys*. New York: Macmillan.

CHAPTER **15**

Measurement Concepts

Measurement is the process of assigning "numbers to objects (or events or situations) in accord with some rule" (Kaplan, 1963, p. 177). The numbers assigned can indicate numerical values or categories. Instrumentation, a component of measurement, is the application of specific rules to develop a measurement device (instrument). Instrumentation produces trustworthy evidence that we can use to evaluate the outcomes of research.

The rules of measurement ensure that values or categories are assigned consistently from one subject (or event) to another and, eventually, if the measurement strategy is found to be meaningful, from one study to another. The rules of measurement established for research are similar to those used in nursing practice. For example, when nurses measure the urine output from patients, they use an accurate measurement container, observe the amount of urine in the container in a consistent way, and precisely record the urine output on the chart. This practice ensures accuracy and precision and reduces the amount of error. When one is measuring the abdominal girth to detect changes in ascites, the skin on the abdomen is marked to ensure that the measurement is always taken the same distance below the waist. With this method, any change in measurement can be attributed to a change in ascites rather than an inadvertent change in the measurement site. Developing accurate and precise measures of concepts important to nursing practice is a major focus of nursing research.

It is important for researchers to understand the logic within measurement theory so they can select, use, and develop quality measurement methods for their studies. As with most theories, measurement theory uses terms with meanings that can be best understood within the context of the theory. The following explanation of the logic of measurement theory includes definitions of directness of measurement, measurement error, levels of measurement, reference of measurement, reliability, validity, accuracy, precision, sensitivity, specificity, and likelihood ratio. The chapter concludes with a discussion of the process for appraising validity in qualitative research.

DIRECTNESS OF MEASUREMENT

Measurement begins by clarifying the object, characteristic, or element to be measured. Only then can one identify or develop strategies or methods to measure it. In some cases, identification of the measurement object and measurement strategies can be simple and straightforward, as when we are measuring concrete factors, such as a person's height or wrist circumference; this is referred to as direct measurement. Health care technology has made direct measures of concrete elements—such as height, weight, temperature, time, space, movement, heart rate, and respiration—familiar to us. Technology is also available to measure many bodily functions and biological and chemical characteristics. The focus of measurement theory in these instances is in the accuracy and precision of the measurement method. Nurses are also experienced in gathering direct measures of attribute or demographic variables, such as age, gender, ethnic origin, diagnosis, marital status, income, and education.

Often in nursing, however, the characteristic we want to measure is an abstract idea, such as pain, stress, depression, anxiety, caring, or coping. If the element to be measured is abstract, it is best clarified through a conceptual definition. We can then use the conceptual definition to select or develop appropriate means of measuring the concept. The instrument or measurement strategy used in the study must match the conceptual definition. An abstract concept is not measured directly; instead, indicators or attributes of the concept are used to represent the abstraction. This is referred to as indirect measurement. For example, indicators of coping skills might be the frequency or accuracy of identifying the problem, the creativity in selecting solutions, and the speed or effectiveness in resolving the problem. Rarely, if ever, can a single measurement strategy completely examine or measure all the aspects of an abstract concept.

MEASUREMENT ERROR

There is no perfect measure. Error is inherent in any measurement strategy. Measurement error is the difference between what exists in reality and what a research instrument measures. Measurement error exists in both direct and indirect measures and can be random or systematic. Direct measures, which are considered to be highly accurate, are subject to error. For example, the scale may not be accurate, laboratory equipment may be precisely calibrated but may change with use, or the tape measure may not be placed in the same location or held at the same tension for each measurement.

There is also error in indirect measures. Efforts to measure concepts usually result in measuring only part of the concept or measures that identify an aspect of the concept but also contain other elements that are not part of the concept. Figure 15-1 shows a Venn diagram of the concept A measured by instrument A-1. As the figure shows, A-1 does not measure all of A. In addition, some of what A-1 measures is outside the concept of A. Both of these situations are examples of errors in measurement.

Types of Measurement Errors

Two types of errors are of concern in measurement: random error and systematic error. To understand these types of errors, we must first understand the elements of a score on an instrument or an observation. According to measurement theory, there are three components to a measurement score: the true score (T), the observed score (O), and the error score (E). The true score is what we would obtain if there was no error in measurement. Because there is always some measurement error, the true score is never known. The observed score is the measure obtained. The error

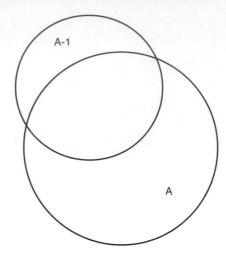

Figure **15-1** Measurement error when measuring a concept.

score is the amount of random error in the measurement process. The theoretical equation of these three measures is as follows:

$$\text{Observed score} = \text{True score} + \text{Random error}$$

This equation is a means of conceptualizing random error and not a basis for calculating it. Because the true score is never known, the random error is never known, only estimated. Theoretically, the smaller the error score, the more closely the observed score reflects the true score. Therefore, using measurement strategies that reduce the error score improves the accuracy of the measurement.

A number of factors can occur during the measurement process that increase random error. They are (1) transient personal factors, such as fatigue, hunger, attention span, health, mood, mental set, and motivation; (2) situational factors, such as a hot stuffy room, distractions, the presence of significant others, rapport with the researcher, and the playfulness or seriousness of the situation; (3) variations in the administration of the measurement procedure, such as interviews in which wording or sequence of questions is varied, questions are added or deleted, or researchers code responses differently; and (4) processing of data, such as errors in coding, accidentally marking the wrong column, punching the wrong key when entering data into the computer, or incorrectly totaling instrument scores.

Random error causes individuals' observed scores to vary haphazardly around their true score. For example, with random error, one subject's observed score may be higher than his or her true score, whereas another subject's observed score may be lower than

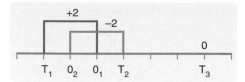

Figure **15-2** Conceptualization of random error.

his or her true score. According to measurement theory, the sum of random errors is expected to be zero, and the random error score (E) is not expected to correlate with the true score (T). Thus, random error does not influence the direction of the mean but, rather, increases the amount of unexplained variance around the mean. When this occurs, estimation of the true score is less precise.

If you were to measure a variable for three subjects and diagram the random error, it might appear as shown in Figure 15-2. The difference between the true score of subject 1 (T_1) and the observed score (O_1) is two positive measurement intervals. The difference between the true score (T_2) and observed score (O_2) for subject 2 is two negative measurement intervals. The difference between the true score (T_3) and observed score (O_3) for subject 3 is zero. The random error for these three subjects is zero ($+2 - 2 + 0 = 0$). In viewing this example, one must remember that this is only a means of conceptualizing random error.

Measurement error that is not random is referred to as **systematic error**. A scale that weighed subjects 2 pounds more than their true weights demonstrates systematic error. All of the body weights would be higher, and, as a result, the mean would be higher than it should be. Systematic error occurs because something else is being measured in addition to the concept. A conceptualization of systematic error is presented in Figure 15-3. Systematic error (represented by shaded area in the figure) is due to the part of A-1 that is outside of A. This part of A-1 measures factors other than A and will bias scores in a particular direction.

Systematic error is considered part of T (true score) and reflects the true measure of A-1, not A. Adding the true score (with systematic error) to the random error (which is 0) yields the observed score, as shown by the following equations:

T (true score with systematic error) + E (random error of 0) = O (observed score)

or

T + E = O

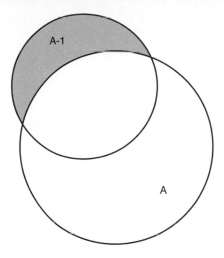

Figure **15-3** Conceptualization of systematic error.

You will incur some systematic error in almost any measure; however, a close link between the abstract theoretical concept and the development of the instrument can greatly decrease systematic error. Because of the importance of this factor in a study, researchers spend considerable time and effort refining their measurement instruments to decrease systematic error.

Another effective means of diminishing systematic error is to use more than one measure of an attribute or a concept and to compare the measures. To make this comparison, researchers use a variety of data collection methods, such as interview and observation. Campbell and Fiske (1959) developed a technique of using more than one method to measure a concept, referred to as the **multimethod-multitrait technique**. More recently, the technique has been described as a version of methodological triangulation, as discussed in Chapter 10. These techniques allow researchers to measure more dimensions of the abstract concept, and the effect of the systematic error on the composite observed score decreases. Figure 15-4 illustrates how more dimensions of concept A are measured through the use of four instruments, designated A-1, A-2, A-3, and A-4.

For example, a researcher could decrease systematic error in measures of anxiety by (1) administering Taylor's Manifest Anxiety Scale, (2) recording blood pressure readings, (3) asking the subject about anxious feelings, and (4) observing the subject's behavior. Multimethod techniques decrease systematic error by combining the values in some way to give a single observed score of anxiety for each subject. Sometimes, however, it may be difficult logically to justify

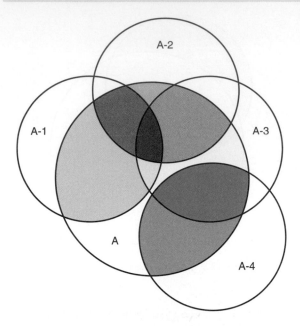

Figure **15-4** Multiple measures of an abstract concept.

combining scores from various measures, and triangulation may be the most appropriate approach. Using triangulation, the researcher decreases systematic error by performing a series of bivariate (two variable) correlations on the matrix of values.

In some studies, researchers use instruments to examine relationships. Consider a hypothesis that tests the relationship between concept A and concept B. In Figure 15-5, the shaded area enclosed in the dark lines represents the true relationship between concepts A and B. If two instruments (A-1 and B-1) are used to

examine the relationship between concepts A and B, the part of the true relationship actually reflected by these measures is represented by light colored areas in Figure 15-6. Because two instruments provide a more accurate measure of concepts A and B, more of the true relationship between concepts A and B can be measured.

If additional instruments (A-2 and B-2) are used to measure concepts A and B, more of the true relationship might be reflected. Figure 15-7 demonstrates the parts of the true relationship with four colors that might be reflected if two instruments are used to measure concept A (A-1 and A-2) and two instruments to measure concept B (B-1 and B-2).

LEVELS OF MEASUREMENT

The traditional levels of measurement have been used for so long that the categorization system has been considered absolute and inviolate. In 1946, Stevens organized the rules for assigning numbers to objects so that a hierarchy in measurement was established. The levels of measurement, from lower to higher, are nominal, ordinal, interval, and ratio.

Nominal-Scale Measurement

Nominal-scale measurement is the lowest of the four measurement categories. It is used when data can be organized into categories of a defined property but the categories cannot be ordered. For example, ethnicity is nominal data with categories such as African American,

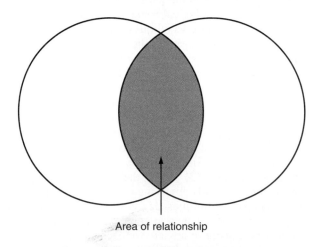

Figure **15-5** True relationship of concepts A and B.

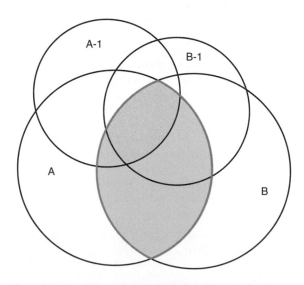

Figure **15-6** Examining a relationship using one measure of each concept.

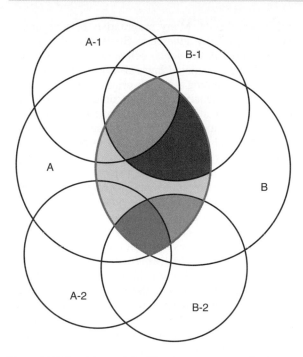

Figure **15-7** Examining a relationship using two measures of each concept.

Caucasian, or Hispanic. One cannot say that one category is higher than another or that category A (African American) is closer to category B (Caucasian) than to category C (Hispanic). The categories differ in quality but not quantity. Therefore, one cannot say that subject A possesses more of the property being categorized than does subject B. (*Rule:* **The categories must be unorderable.**) Categories must be established so that each datum will fit into only one of the categories. (*Rule:* **The categories must be exclusive.**) All the data must fit into the established categories. (*Rule:* **The categories must be exhaustive.**) Data such as gender, marital status, and diagnoses are examples of nominal data. When data are coded for entry into the computer, the categories are assigned numbers. For example, gender may be classified as 1 = male, 2 = female. The numbers assigned to categories in nominal measurement are used only as labels and cannot be used for mathematical calculations.

Ordinal-Scale Measurement

Data that can be measured at the ordinal-scale level can be assigned to categories of an attribute that can be ranked. There are rules for how one ranks data. As with nominal-scale data, the categories must be exclusive and exhaustive. With ordinal-scale data, the quantity of the attribute possessed can be identified.

However, it cannot be demonstrated that the intervals between the ranked categories are equal. Therefore, ordinal data are considered to have unequal intervals. Scales with unequal intervals are sometimes referred to as ordered metric scales.

Many scales used in nursing research are ordinal levels of measure. For example, one could rank intensity of pain, degrees of coping, levels of mobility, ability to provide self-care, or daily amount of exercise on an ordinal scale. For daily exercise, the scale could be 0 = no exercise; 1 = moderate exercise, no sweating; 2 = exercise to the point of sweating; 3 = strenuous exercise with sweating for at least 30 minutes per day; 4 = strenuous exercise with sweating for at least 1 hour per day. This type of scale may be referred to as a metric ordinal scale.

Interval-Scale Measurement

In interval-scale measurement, distances between intervals of the scale are numerically equal. Such measurements also follow the previously mentioned rules: mutually exclusive categories, exhaustive categories, and rank ordering. Interval scales are assumed to be a continuum of values. Thus, the researcher can identify the magnitude of the attribute much more precisely. However, it is not possible to provide the absolute amount of the attribute because of the absence of a zero point on the interval scale.

Fahrenheit and centigrade temperatures are commonly used as examples of interval scales. A difference between a temperature of 70 °F and one of 80 °F is the same as the difference between a temperature of 30 °F and one of 40 °F. We can measure changes in temperature precisely. However, it is not possible to say that a temperature of 0 °C means the absence of temperature.

Ratio-Level Measurement

Ratio-level measurements are the highest form of measure and meet all the rules of the lower forms of measures: mutually exclusive categories, exhaustive categories, rank ordering, equal spacing between intervals, and a continuum of values. In addition, ratio-level measures have absolute zero points. Weight, length, and volume are common examples of ratio scales. Each has an absolute zero point, at which a value of zero indicates the absence of the property being measured: Zero weight means the absence of weight. In addition, because of the absolute zero point, one can justifiably say that object A weighs twice as much as object B, or that container A holds three times as much as container B. Laboratory values are also an example of ratio level of measurement where the individual with a fasting blood sugar (FBS) of 180 has an FBS twice that of an individual with a normal FBS of 90. To help expand your understanding of levels of measurement (nominal, ordinal, interval, and ratio) and to apply this knowledge, Grove (2007) developed a statistical workbook focused on examining the levels of measurement, sampling methods, and statistical results in published studies.

The Importance of Level of Measurement for Statistical Analyses

An important rule of measurement is that one should use the highest level of measurement possible. For example, you can collect data on age (measured) in a variety of ways: (1) you can obtain the actual age of each subject (ratio level of measurement); (2) you can ask subjects to indicate their age by selecting from a group of categories, such as 20 to 29, 30 to 39, and so on (ordinal level of measurement); or (3) you can use a bivariate measure such as under 65 and over 65 (nominal level of measurement). The highest level of measurement in this case is the actual age of each subject. If you need age categories for specific analyses in your research, the computer can be instructed to establish them from the initial age data.

The level of measurement is associated with the types of statistical analyses that can be performed on the data. Mathematical operations are limited in the lower levels of measurement. With nominal levels of measurement, only summary statistics, such as frequencies, percentages, and contingency correlation procedures, can be used. In the age example, however, you can perform more sophisticated analyses if you have obtained the actual age of each subject. The age variable is measured at the ratio level (actual age of the subject) so the data can be entered into the computer and analyzed with stronger statistical techniques. Variables measured at the interval or ratio level can be analyzed with the strongest statistical techniques available.

Controversy over Measurement Levels

In recent years, controversy has erupted over justification for the system used to categorize measurement levels, dividing researchers into two factions: the fundamentalists and the pragmatists. *Pragmatists* regard measurement as occurring on a continuum rather than by discrete categories, whereas *fundamentalists* adhere rigidly to the original system of categorization.

The primary focus of the controversy relates to the practice of classifying data into the categories ordinal and interval. The controversy developed because, according to the fundamentalists, many of the current statistical analysis techniques can be used only

with interval data. Many pragmatists believe that if researchers rigidly adhered to Stevens's rules, few if any measures in the social sciences would meet the criteria to be considered interval-level data. They also believe that violating Stevens's criteria does not lead to serious consequences for the outcomes of data analysis. Thus, pragmatists often treat ordinal data as interval data, using statistical methods to analyze them such as the *t*-test and analysis of variance (ANOVA), which are traditionally reserved for interval or ratio level data. Fundamentalists insist that the analysis of ordinal data be limited to statistical procedures designed for ordinal data, such as nonparametric procedures.

There is also a controversy about the statistical operations that can justifiably be performed with scores from the various levels of measure (Armstrong, 1981, 1984; Knapp, 1984, 1990). For example, can one calculate a mean using ordinal data? Fundamentalists believe that appropriate statistical analysis is contingent on the level of measurement. They disagree with the contention that the scaling procedures used for most psychosocial instruments provide interval-level data. This is related to scale definition, which we discuss in Chapter 16.

For example, the Likert scale uses the scale points "strongly disagree," "disagree," "uncertain," "agree," and "strongly agree." Numerical values (e.g., 1, 2, 3, 4, and 5, respectively) are assigned to these categories. Fundamentalists claim that equal intervals do not exist between these categories. It is not possible to prove that there is the same magnitude of feeling between "uncertain" and "agree" as there is between "agree" and "strongly agree." Therefore, they hold, parametric analyses cannot be used. Pragmatists believe that with many measures taken at the ordinal level, such as scaling procedures, an underlying interval continuum is present that justifies the use of parametric statistics.

Our position is more like that of the pragmatists than of the fundamentalists. Many nurse researchers analyze data from Likert scales as though the data were interval level. However, some of the data in nursing research are obtained through the use of crude measurement methods that can be classified only into the lower levels of measurement. Therefore, we have included the nonparametric statistical procedures needed for their analysis in the statistical chapters.

REFERENCE TESTING OF MEASUREMENT

Referencing involves comparing a subject's score against a standard. Two types of testing involve referencing: norm-referenced testing and criterion-referenced testing. Norm-referenced testing addresses the question "How does the average person score on this test?" It involves the use of standardization that has been developed over several years, with extensive reliability and validity data available. Standardization involves collecting data from thousands of subjects expected to have a broad range of scores on the instrument. From these scores, population parameters such as the mean and standard deviation (described in Chapter 19) can be developed. Evidence of the reliability and validity of the instrument can also be evaluated through the use of the methods described later in this chapter. The best-known norm-referenced test is the Minnesota Multiphasic Personality Inventory (MMPI), which is used commonly in psychology and occasionally in nursing research.

Criterion-referenced testing asks the question "What is desirable in the perfect subject?" It involves comparing a subject's score with a criterion of achievement that includes the definition of target behaviors. When the subject has mastered these behaviors, he or she is considered proficient in the behavior. The criterion might be a level of knowledge or desirable patient outcome measures. Criterion measures are not as useful in research as they might be in evaluation studies or evaluation of clinical expertise. Faculty use criterion measures to evaluate student performance in clinical agencies. For example, a clinical evaluation form would include the critical behaviors the student is expected to master in a pediatric course to be clinically competent to care for pediatric patients at the end of the course.

RELIABILITY

The reliability of a measure denotes the consistency of measures obtained in the use of a particular instrument and indicates the extent of random error in the measurement method. For example, if the same measurement scale is administered to the same individuals at two different times, the measurement is reliable if the individuals' responses to the items remain the same (assuming that nothing has occurred to change their responses). For example, if you measure oral temperatures of 10 individuals every 5 minutes 10 times using the same thermometer for all measures of all individuals, and at each measurement the individuals' temperatures change, being sometimes higher than before and sometimes lower, you begin to question the reliability of the thermometer. If two data collectors observe the same event and record their observations on a carefully designed data collection instrument, the measurement would be reliable if the recordings from the two data collectors are comparable. The equivalence

of their results would indicate the reliability of the measurement technique. If responses vary each time a measure is performed, there is a chance that the instrument is not reliable—that is, that it yields data with a large random error.

Reliability plays an important role in the selection of scales for use in a study. Researchers need instruments that are reliable and provide values with only a small amount of random error. Reliable instruments enhance the power of a study to detect significant differences or relationships actually occurring in the population under study. Therefore, it is important to test the reliability of an instrument before using it in a study. Estimates of reliability are specific to the sample being tested. Thus, high reported reliability values on an established instrument do not guarantee that its reliability will be satisfactory in another sample or with a different population. Therefore, you must perform reliability testing on each instrument used in your study before you perform other statistical analyses. The reliability values must be included in published reports of the study.

Reliability testing examines the amount of random error in the measurement technique. It is concerned with characteristics such as dependability, consistency, precision, and comparability. Because all measurement techniques contain some random error, reliability exists in degrees and is usually expressed as a form of correlation coefficient, with 1.00 indicating perfect reliability and 0.00 indicating no reliability. A reliability coefficient of 0.80 is considered the lowest acceptable value for a well-developed psychosocial measurement instrument. The coefficient of 0.80 (or 80%) indicates the instrument is 80% reliable with 20% random error (Grove, 2007). For a newly developed psychosocial instrument, a reliability coefficient of 0.70 is considered acceptable as the researcher refines the instrument to achieve a reliability of ≥ 0.80. Higher levels of reliability (0.90 to 0.99) are essential for physiological measures that are used to determine "critical" physiological functions such as cardiac output. Reliability testing focuses on the following three aspects of reliability: stability, equivalence, and homogeneity.

Stability

Stability is concerned with the consistency of repeated measures of the same attribute with the use of the same scale or instrument over time. It is usually referred to as test-retest reliability. This measure of reliability is generally used with physical measures, technological measures, and paper-and-pencil scales. The technique requires an assumption that the factor to be measured remains the same at the two testing times and that any change in the value or score is a consequence of random error.

Physical measures and equipment can be tested and then immediately retested, or the equipment can be used for a time and then retested to determine the necessary frequency of recalibration. For example, the diagnosis of osteoporosis is made by bone mineral density (BMD) study of the hip, spine, and wrist. The BMD score is determined with the dual-energy x-ray absorptiometry (DEXA or DXA) scan. Because the BMD does not change rapidly in people even with treatment, the test-retest over a week time period should demonstrate reliable or consistent DXA scan scores for patients.

With paper-and-pencil measures, a period of 2 weeks to 1 month is recommended between the two testing times. After retesting, the investigator performs a correlational analysis on the scores from the two measures. A high correlation coefficient indicates high stability of measurement by the instrument. Test-retest reliability has not proved to be as effective with paper-and-pencil measures as originally anticipated. The procedure presents a number of problems. Subjects may remember their responses at the first testing time, leading to overestimation of the reliability. Subjects may actually be changed by the first testing and therefore may respond to the second test differently, leading to underestimation of the reliability.

Test-retest reliability requires the assumption that the factor being measured has not changed between the measurement points. Many of the phenomena studied in nursing, such as hope, coping, and anxiety, do change over short intervals. Thus, the assumption that if the instrument is reliable, values will not change between the two measurement periods may not be justifiable. If the factor being measured does change, the test is not a measure of reliability. In fact, if the measures stay the same even though the factor being measured actually has changed, the instrument may lack reliability.

Equivalence

Equivalence compares two versions of the same paper-and-pencil instrument or two observers measuring the same event. Comparison of two observers is referred to as interrater reliability. Comparison of two paper-and-pencil instruments is referred to as alternate-forms reliability or parallel-forms reliability. Alternative forms of instruments are of more concern in the development of normative knowledge testing. When repeated measures are part of the design, however, alternative forms of measurement, although

not commonly used, would improve the design. Demonstrating that one is actually testing the same content in both tests is extremely complex, and thus, the procedure is rarely used in clinical research.

Determining interrater reliability is a more immediate concern in research and is used in many observational studies. Interrater reliability values must be reported in any study in which observational data are collected or judgments are made by two or more data gatherers. Two techniques determine interrater reliability. Both techniques require that two or more raters independently observe and record the same event using the protocol developed for the study or that the same rater observes and records an event on two occasions. To adequately judge interrater reliability, the raters must observe at least 10 subjects or events (Washington & Moss, 1988). A DVD can be used to record the same event on two occasions. Every data collector used in the study must be tested for interrater reliability.

The first procedure for calculating interrater reliability requires a simple computation involving a comparison of the agreements obtained between raters on the coding form with the number of possible agreements. This calculation is performed through the use of the following equation:

$$\frac{\text{Number of agreements}}{\text{Number of possible agreements}} = \text{Interrater reliability}$$

This formula tends to overestimate reliability, a particularly serious problem if the rating requires only a dichotomous judgment. In this case, there is a 50% probability that the raters will agree on a particular item through chance alone. Appropriate correlational techniques can be used to provide a more accurate estimate of interrater reliability. If more than two raters are involved, a statistical procedure to calculate coefficient alpha (discussed later in this chapter) may be used. ANOVA may also be used to test for differences among raters. There is no absolute value below which interrater reliability is unacceptable. However, any value below 0.80 should generate serious concern about the reliability of the data or of the data gatherer (or both). The interrater reliability value is best to be ≥ 0.90, which means 90% reliability and 10% random error. The process for determining interrater reliability and the value achieved must be included in research reports.

When raters know they are being watched, their accuracy and consistency are considerably better than when they believe they are not being watched. Thus, interrater reliability declines (sometimes dramatically) when the raters are assessed covertly (Topf, 1988). You can develop strategies to monitor and reduce the decline in interrater reliability, but they may entail considerable time and expense.

The coding of data into categories, which is a frequent step done in qualitative research, has received little attention in regard to reliability. Two types of reliability are related to categorizing data: unitizing reliability and interpretive reliability. Unitizing reliability assesses the extent to which each judge (data collector, coder, researcher) consistently identifies the same units within the data as appropriate for coding. This is of concern in observational studies and studies using text transcribed from interviews. In observational studies, the data collector must select particular units of what is being observed as appropriate to record and code. Of concern is the extent to which two data collectors observing the same event would select the same units to record. In studies using transcribed text from interviews, the researcher must select particular units of the transcribed text to code into preselected categories. To what extent would two individuals reading the same text select the same passages to code into categories (Garvin, Kennedy, & Cissna, 1988)?

In some studies, the selection of units for coding is simple and straightforward. For example, a unit may begin when a person starts talking. In other studies, however, the identification of an appropriate unit for coding may require some level of inference or judgment on the part of the rater. For example, if the unit began when the baby awakened, the rater would have to determine at what point the baby was indeed awake. Studies in which every event in the unit is coded require less inference than studies in which only select acts in the unit are to be coded. In all cases, reliability improves when the researcher clearly identifies the units to be coded rather than relying on the judgment of the coder (Marshall & Rossman, 2006; Washington & Moss, 1988). Guetzkow's (1950) index (U) can be used to calculate unitizing reliability (Garvin et al., 1988).

Interpretive reliability assesses the extent to which each judge assigns the same category to a given unit of data. Most studies using categories report only a global level of reliability in which the overall rate of reliability is examined. The most commonly used measure of global reliability is Guetzkow's (1950) P, which reports the extent to which the judges agree in the selection of categories. A more desirable method of calculating the extent of agreement between judges is Cohen's (1960) Kappa statistic. However, global measures of interpretive reliability provide no information on the degree of consistency in assigning data to a particular category. Category-by-category measures of reliability include the assumption that some categories are more difficult to use than others and thus have a

lower reliability. To use this method of evaluating reliability, you must (1) statistically analyze the reliability category by category, (2) determine the equality of the frequency distribution among categories, and (3) examine the possibility that coders may be systematically confusing some categories (Garvin et al., 1988).

Homogeneity

Tests of instrument homogeneity, used primarily with paper-and-pencil tests, address the correlation of various items within the instrument. The original approach to determining homogeneity was split-half reliability. This strategy was a way of obtaining test-retest reliability without administering the test twice. Rather, the instrument items were split in odd-even or first-last halves, and a correlational procedure was performed between the two halves. Researchers have generally used the Spearman-Brown correlation formula for this procedure. One of the problems with the procedure was that although items were usually split into odd-even items, it was possible to split them in a variety of ways. Each approach to splitting the items would yield a different reliability coefficient. Therefore, the researcher could continue to split the items in various ways until a satisfactorily high coefficient was obtained.

More recently, testing the homogeneity of all the items in the instrument has been seen as a better approach to determining reliability. Although the mathematics of the procedure are complex, the logic is simple. One way to view it is as though one conducted split-half reliabilities in all the ways possible and then averaged the scores to obtain one reliability score. Homogeneity testing examines the extent to which all the items in the instrument consistently measure the construct. It is a test of internal consistency. The statistical procedures used for this process are Cronbach's alpha coefficient for interval and ratio level data and, when the data are dichotomous, the Kuder-Richardson formula (K-R 20).

If the Cronbach's alpha coefficient value were 1.00, each item in the instrument would be measuring exactly the same thing. When this occurs, one might question the need for more than one item. A slightly lower coefficient (0.8 to 0.9) indicates an instrument that will reflect more richly the fine discriminations in levels of the construct. Magnitude of the instrument reliability can then be discerned more clearly. Bakas, Champion, Perkins, Farran, and Williams (2006) conducted a psychometric study to test the revised 15-item Bakas Caregiving Outcomes Scale (BCOS) and provided the following internal consistency and test-retest reliability data to support the 15-item BCOS reliability.

The original 10-item BCOS was improved by adding five items addressing financial well-being, level of energy, role functioning, physical functioning, and general health [resulting in the 15-item BCOS]. (p. 346)

■ *INTERNAL CONSISTENCY RELIABILITY AND TEST-RETEST RELIABILITY*

Internal consistency reliability for the 15-item BCOS was supported by a Cronbach's alpha of 0.90 ($n = 147$); the 10-item BCOS had an alpha = 0.85. A small subsample ($n = 36$) also completed the BCOS 2 weeks later, with Cronbach's alpha of 0.81 for the 15-item BCOS and 0.75 for the 10-item BCOS. The ICC [intraclass correlation coefficient] assessing 2-week test-retest reliability were 0.66 for the 15-item BCOS and 0.68 for the 10-item BCOS. (Bakas et al., 2006, p. 350; full-text article available in CINAHL)

Other approaches to testing internal consistency are (1) Cohen's Kappa statistic, which determines the percentage of agreement with the probability of chance being taken out; (2) correlating each item with the total score for the instrument; and (3) correlating each item with each other item in the instrument. This procedure, often used in instrument development, allows researchers to identify items that are not highly correlated and delete them from the instrument. Factor analysis may also be used to develop instrument reliability. The number of factors being measured influences the instrument's reliability and total scores may be more reliable than subscores in determining reliability. After performing the factor analysis, the researcher can delete instrument items with low factor weights. After these items have been deleted, reliability scores on the instrument will be higher. For instruments with more than one factor, correlations can be performed between items and factor scores. Estok, Sedlak, Doheny, and Hall (2007) conducted a study to develop a structural model for osteoporosis preventing behaviors in postmenopausal women and one of the scales they used was the Osteoporosis Self-Efficacy Scale (OSES). The researchers documented the reliability of this scale by providing internal consistency reliability (Cronbach alpha) for the total scale and subscales (identified through factor analysis) for previous studies and the current study.

The OSES "was used to avoid subject fatigue. There are two subscales: Osteoporosis Self-Efficacy Exercise Scale (items 1-6) and Osteoporosis Self-Efficacy Calcium Scale (items 7-12). Scoring is done by multiplying item response by 10 and summing them; the possible score ranged for each subscale is 0 to 600. The reliability coefficient for the total tool and the two subscales was $\alpha = 0.90$. For the present study, they were $\alpha = 0.95$ to 0.96 and 0.96 to 0.98 respectively." (Estok et al., 2007, p. 150; full-text article available in CINAHL)

It is essential that an instrument be both reliable and valid for measuring a study variable in a population. If the instrument has low reliability values, then it cannot be valid because its measurement is inconsistent. An instrument that is reliable cannot be assumed to be valid for a particular study or population. Thus, you will need to determine the validity of the instrument you are using for your study, which you can accomplish in a variety of ways.

VALIDITY

The validity of an instrument determines the extent to which it actually reflects the abstract construct being examined. Validity has been discussed in the literature in terms of three primary types: content validity, predictive validity, and construct validity. Within each of these types, subtypes have been identified. These multiple types of validity were very confusing, especially because the types were not discrete but interrelated.

Currently, validity is considered a single broad method of measurement evaluation that is referred to as construct validity and includes content and predictive validity (Berk, 1990; Rew, Stuppy, & Becker, 1988). All of the previously identified types of validity are now considered evidence of construct validity. In 1985, in its *Standards for Educational and Psychological Testing,* the American Psychological Association (APA) published standards used to judge the evidence of validity. This important work greatly extends our understanding of what validity is and how to achieve it. According to the APA, validity addresses the appropriateness, meaningfulness, and usefulness of the specific inferences made from instrument scores. It is important to note that it is the inferences made from the scores, not the scores themselves, that are important to validate (Goodwin & Goodwin, 1991).

Validity, like reliability, is not an all-or-nothing phenomenon but, rather, a matter of degree. No instrument is completely valid. Thus, one determines a measure's degree of validity rather than whether or not it has validity. Defining the validity of an instrument requires years of work. Many equate the validity of the instrument with the rigorousness of the researcher. The assumption is that because the researcher develops the instrument, the researcher also develops the validity. However, this is to some extent an erroneous assumption, as Brinberg and McGrath (1985) have pointed out.

> Validity is not a commodity that can be purchased with techniques. Validity, as we will treat it, is a concept designating an ideal state—to be pursued, but not to be attained. As the roots of the word imply, validity has to do with truth, strength, and value. The discourse of our field has often been in tones that seem to imply that validity is a tangible "resource," and that if one can acquire a sufficient amount of it, by applying appropriate techniques, one has somehow "won" at the game called research. We reject this view. In our views, validity is not like money—to gain and lose, to count and display. Rather, validity is like integrity, character, or quality, to be assessed relative to purposes and circumstances. (Brinberg & McGrath, 1985, p. 13)

Figure 15-8 illustrates validity (the shaded area) by the extent to which the instrument A-1 reflects concept A. As measurement of the concept improves, validity improves. The extent to which the instrument A-1 measures items other than the concept is referred to as systematic error (also identified as the unshaded area of A-1 in Figure 15-8). As **systematic error** decreases, validity increases.

Validity varies from one sample to another and from one situation to another; therefore, validity testing actually validates the use of an instrument for a specific group or purpose rather than the instrument itself. An instrument may be valid in one situation but not valid in another. Therefore, validity should be reexamined in each study situation, but this often does not happen.

Because many instruments used in nursing studies were developed for use in other disciplines, it is important that any measure chosen for a nursing study be valid in terms of nursing knowledge. Nagley and Byers (1987) provided an example of a study in which a measure of cognitive function was used to gauge confusion. However, the instrument did not capture the nursing meaning of *confusion*. Nurses consider persons confused who do not know their age or location. The aforementioned measure of cognitive function does not categorize such persons as confused.

Content-Related Validity Evidence

Content-related validity evidence examines the extent to which the method of measurement includes all the major elements relevant to the construct being measured. This evidence is obtained from the following three sources: the literature, representatives of the relevant populations, and content experts.

In the 1970s, the only type of validity that most studies addressed was referred to as **face validity**, which verified basically that the instrument looked like it was valid or gave the appearance of measuring the content it was suppose to measure. This approach is no longer considered acceptable evidence for validity. However, it is still an important aspect of the usefulness of the instrument, because the willingness of subjects to complete the instrument relates to their perception that the instrument measures the content they agreed to provide (Lynn, 1986; Thomas, Hathaway, & Arheart, 1992).

Documentation of content-related validity evidence begins with development of the instrument. The first step of instrument development is to identify *what* is to be measured; this is referred to as the *universe* or *domain* of the construct. You can determine your domain through a concept analysis or an extensive literature search. Qualitative methods can also be used for this purpose. Johnson and Rogers (2006) developed the Medication-Taking Questionnaire based on purposeful action dimensions to determine individuals' decision-making process for adherence to medication treatment for hypertension. They described their initial instrument development process as follows.

> A total of 20 items (need, $n = 8$; effectiveness, $n = 6$; and safe, $n = 6$) were initially developed to tap the three underlying dimensions of purposeful action based on the statements given by participants in a qualitative study (Johnson, 2002; Johnson et al., 1999). The method for

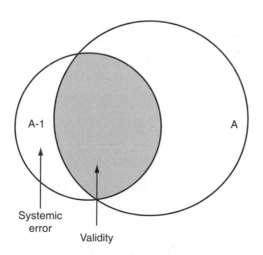

Figure **15-8** Representation of instrument validity.

item construction was guided by the principles outlined in DeVellis (1991) and Streiner and Norman (1995)... The MTQ: Purposeful Action items were arranged in a 7-point, Likert-type format describing responses base on agreement (7 = *always agree*, 6 = *very frequently agree*, 5 = *usually agree*, and 4 = *occasionally agree*, 3 = *rarely agree*, 2 = *almost never agree*, 1 = *never agree*). The 7-reponse option was used in an attempt to obtain optimal variance while discouraging a ceiling effect (Steiner & Norman, 1995). Higher scores for the MTQ: Purposeful Action indicated greater intent to take medications based on perceived need, effectiveness, and safety. (Johnson & Rogers, 2006, p. 339; full-text article available in CINAHL)

You must describe the procedures used to develop or select items for the instrument that represent the domain of the construct. One helpful strategy commonly used is to develop a blueprint or matrix, such as is used in developing test items for an examination. However, before developing such items, the blueprint specifications must be submitted to an expert panel to validate that they are appropriate, accurate, and representative. At least five experts are recommended, although a minimum of three experts is acceptable if you cannot locate additional individuals with expertise in the area (Lynn, 1986). You might seek out individuals with expertise in various fields, for example, one with knowledge of instrument development, a second with clinical expertise in an appropriate field of practice, and a third with expertise in another discipline relevant to the content area.

Give the experts specific guidelines for judging the appropriateness, accuracy, and representativeness of the specifications. Berk (1990) recommended that the experts first make independent assessments and then meet for a group discussion of the specifications. You can then revise the specifications and resubmit them to the experts for a final independent assessment. Davis (1992) recommended that the researcher provide expert reviewers with theoretical definitions of concepts and a list of which instrument items are expected to measure each of the concepts. Ask the reviewers to judge how well each of the concepts has been represented in the instrument.

You then need to determine how to measure the domain. The item format, item content, and procedures for generating items must be carefully described. Items are then constructed for each cell in the matrix, or observational methods are designated to gather data related to a specific cell. You will be expected to describe the specifications used in constructing items or selecting observations. Sources of content for items must be documented. Then you can assemble, refine, and arrange the items in a suitable order before submitting them to the content experts for evaluation. Specific instructions for evaluating each item and the total instrument must be given to the experts.

Use the content validity index (CVI) developed by Waltz and Bausell (1981) to obtain a numerical value that reflects the level of content-related validity evidence. With this instrument, experts rate the content relevance of each item using a 4-point rating scale. Lynn (1986, p. 384) recommended standardizing the options on this scale to read as follows: "1 = not relevant; 2 = unable to assess relevance without item revision or item is in need of such revision that it would no longer be relevant; 3 = relevant but needs minor alteration; 4 = very relevant and succinct." In addition to evaluating existing items, ask the experts to identify important areas not included in the instrument. As presented earlier, Johnson and Rogers (2006) developed the Medication-Taking Questionnaire (MTQ): Purposeful Action and described their content validity testing process and outcomes as follows.

Content validity testing was undertaken to determine clarity and relevance of content. Participants and experts were given verbal instructions and a packet consisting of a consent form, written instructions, clarity instrument, content validity instrument, and demographic questionnaire. The clarity instrument asked participants to rate items as clear or unclear (Imle & Atwood, 1988). Participants were given a definition of each subscale and asked to rate each item's relevancy using a 4-point scale from 1 (irrelevant) to 4 (extremely relevant; Lynn, 1986). Space was provided to make comments after each rating procedure. (p. 339)

Items met clarity criterion if 70% of participants rated the item as clear and the content validity criterion if 80% of participants rated the item as 3 or 4 (Imle & Atwood, 1988; Lynn, 1986). The comments from the clarity and content validity criterion were used to revise the MTQ: Purposeful Action items and subscales...

Of the 20 MTQ: Purpose Action items, 19 achieved clarity and content validity agreement. The 1 item that had an unacceptable clarity agreement was eventually eliminated from the questionnaire. Professionals expressed a concern about the lack of specificity in the questions, but that was not an issue for the hypertensive participants. For example, one professional indicated that the item, "Blood pressure pills keep me from having problems," lacked specificity. Because the purpose of this questionnaire was to establish a general screening tool for individuals who potentially may choose not to take their medications rather than to create a diagnostic tool, the participants' scores were given priority. Of the 20 items [see Table 15-1 for the 20 items in the original questionnaire], 12 underwent minor grammatical revisions guided by the comments of both the participants and professionals. For example, items were made specific to blood pressure and the term medication was changed to pills. Several items were reworded, or the tense of the verb was changed. (Johnson & Rogers, 2006, pp. 341–342)

Before sending the instrument to experts for evaluation, decide how many experts must agree on each item and on the total instrument in order for the content to be considered valid. Items that do not achieve minimum agreement by the expert panel must be either eliminated from the instrument or revised. Johnson and Rogers (2006) described their panel of reviewers, who were health professionals and patients prescribed antihypertensive medications, for their MTQ: Purposeful Action MTQ in the following except.

Content validity testing was conducted in a sample of five hypertensive patients and five health care professionals who examined the MTQ: Purposeful Action for clarity and content relevance (Imle & Atwood, 1988; Lynn, 1986). Professionals were invited to participate in the study based on their known experience with antihypertensive treatment and included two family physicians, a cardiology nurse practitioner, a nurse working with a statewide cardiovascular disease program, and a nurse

TABLE **15-1** Medication-Taking Questionnaire: Purposeful Action Initial 20 Items Statistics				
	M	SD	Item-Total Correlation	Mann-Whitney Adherence p Values[a]
Perceived need				
My blood pressure pills keep me from having a stroke.	5.8	1.5	0.58	0.08
I need to take my blood pressure pills.	6.4	1.4	0.77	0.01
I take my blood pressure pills for my health.	6.5	1.3	0.75	0.01
Blood pressure pills keep me from having health-related problems.	5.7	1.5	0.63	0.17
I could have health problems if I do not take my blood pressure pills.	6.1	1.3	0.74	0.13
It's not a problem if I miss my blood pressure pills.[b]	5.1	2.0	0.30	0.02
I would rather treat my blood pressure without pills.[b]	4.1	2.3	0.37	0.26
I am OK if I do not take my blood pressure pills.[b]	5.6	1.8	0.64	0.012
Perceived effectiveness				
My blood pressure will come down enough without pills.[b]	5.4	1.8	0.40	0.10
I will have problems if I don't take my blood pressure pills.	6.1	1.4	0.63	0.001
My blood pressure pills control my blood pressure.	6.0	1.4	0.66	0.46
Blood pressure pills benefit my health.	6.1	1.4	0.74	0.01
I feel better when I take my blood pressure pills.	5.4	1.8	0.56	0.01
I have problems finding pills that will control my blood pressure.[b]	5.7	1.8	0.09	0.059
Perceived as safe				
The side effects from my blood pressure pills are a problem.[b]	5.2	1.9	0.40	0.10
The side effects from my blood pressure pills are harmful.[b]	5.6	1.8	0.63	0.27
My blood pressure pills are safe.	5.8	1.4	0.66	0.47
Taking my blood pressure pills is not a problem because they benefit my health.	6.0	1.4	0.74	0.02
My blood pressure pills cause other health problems.[b]	5.4	1.8	0.56	0.35
I will become dependent on my blood pressure pills.[b]	3.9	2.3	−0.5	0.20

From Johnson, M. J., & Rogers, S. (2006). Development of the Purposeful Action Medication-Taking Questionnaire. *Western Journal of Nursing Research, 28*(3), 344.

a. Difference between low (scored 1–3) versus high (scored 7–10) adherence.

b. Reverse coded.

researcher who had published articles on adherence. All professionals were Anglo American and were nearly equally divided with regard to gender.

Participants for the content validity phase who had been prescribed antihypertensive medications and lived in a situation in which they managed their own medications were recruited through healthy aging clinics, worksite wellness programs, hospital outpatient clinics, and hospital emergency departments in the intermountain west. The five hypertensive participants were Anglo American, had at least a high school education and ranged in age from 48 to 90 years ($M = 62.0 \pm 16.4$). (Johnson & Rogers, 2006, p. 338)

Johnson and Rogers (2006) provided excellent detail about the development of their questionnaire and the process for determining content validity. They also provided extensive information about the expert review panel for conducting the content validity testing. The strength of the review panel is that it included both health professionals and patients taking medications for hypertension. The MTQ: Purposeful Action was a Likert scale with 7-point response options (described earlier), so it would be clearer if the researchers had called the MTQ a scale versus a questionnaire.

With some modifications, this procedure can also be used with existing instruments, many of which have never been evaluated for content-related validity. With the permission of the author or researcher who developed the instrument, you could revise the instrument to improve its content-related validity (Lynn, 1986). In addition, Berk (1990) has suggested that the panel of experts or judges asked to evaluate the instrument items for content validity also examine it in terms of readability and the possibility that its language might offend subjects or data gatherers.

Readability of an Instrument

Readability is an essential element of the validity and reliability of an instrument. Assessing an instrument's level of readability is relatively simple and takes about 20 minutes. There are more than 30 readability formulas. These formulas count language elements in the document. They then use this information to estimate the degree of difficulty a reader may have in comprehending the text. Readability formulas are now a standard part of word-processing software. Table 15-2 provides instructions for using the Fog formula to determine the readability of a measurement method.

Although readability has never been formally identified as a component of content validity, it should be. How valid is content that is incomprehensible? Miller and Bodie (1994) suggested that the researcher should

TABLE 15-2   How to Find the Fog Index (Fog Formula)

1. Pick a sample of writing 100 to 125 words long. Count the average number of words per sentence. In counting, treat independent clauses as separate sentences. "In school we studied; we learned; we improved" is three sentences.
2. Count the words of three syllables or more. Do not count: (a) capitalized words, (b) combinations of short words such as butterfly or manpower, or (c) verbs made into three syllables by adding "–es" or "–ed" such as trespasses or created. Divide the count of long words by the number of words in the passage to get the percentage.
3. Add the results from no. 1 (average sentence length) and no. 2 (percentage of long words). Multiply the sum by 0.4. Ignore the numbers after the decimal point.
4. The result is the years of schooling needed to easily understand the passage tested. Few readers have more than 17 years of schooling, so give any passage higher than 17 a Fog Index of 17-plus.

Adapted from Gunning, R., & Kallan, R. A. (1994). *How to take the fog out of business writing*. Chicago: Dartnell. The Fog Index[SM] is a service mark licensed exclusively to RK Communication Consultants by D. and M. Mueller.

directly assess the reading comprehension level of the study population before using a formula to calculate an instrument's readability. They indicated that it is a mistake to assume that someone's literacy is equivalent to the last grade level the individual completed. They recommended that researchers use the Classroom Reading Inventory (CRI), which is based on the Flesch, Space, Dale, and Fry reading comprehension scales (Silvaroli, 1986). This instrument determines the level at which an individual can comprehend written material without assistance. Johnson and Rogers (2006) described the readability of their MTQ: Purposeful Action as follows.

Items were worded at approximately a sixth-grade reading level, evaluated by using the Flesch-Kincaid grade-level assessment program in Microsoft Word (2000) (Rasin, 1997). Items ranged from a 1.0 to 6.2 grade level, with a 3.5 grade level readability score for the overall questionnaire. (Johnson & Rogers, 2006, p. 339)

Evidence of Validity from Factor Analysis

Exploratory factor analysis can be performed to examine relationships among the various items of the instrument. Items that are closely related are clustered into a factor. The analysis may reveal the presence of several factors, which may indicate that the instrument reflects several constructs rather than a single construct. The researcher can validate the number of constructs in the instrument and measurement equivalence among comparison groups through the use of confirmatory factor analysis (Goodwin & Goodwin, 1991; Stommel, Wang, Given, & Given, 1992; Teel & Verran, 1991). Items that do not fall into a factor (and thus do not correlate with other items) may be deleted. We further describe validity from factor analysis in Chapter 20.

Johnson and Rogers (2006) conducted an exploratory factor analysis (EFA) to determine the factor structure for their MTQ: Purposeful Action. The EFA identifies the specific factors or subscales for the scale and the items that fit each of these subscales. The original scale had 20 items sorted into three subscales (labeled perceived need, perceived effectiveness, and perceived as safe) that were identified in Table 15-1. The EFA and the results are described as follows:

Factor analysis is a grouping technique that allows for evaluation of the dimensionality of scales (Munro, 2001; Nunnally & Bernstein, 1994). A principle axis factoring solution with an oblimen rotation, considered the best analysis for achieving a theoretical solution uncontaminated by unique and random error variability was undertaken....

The EFA yielded two interpretable factors [see Table 15-3], which eliminated six additional items because of factor loadings < 0.40. The first factor merged the need and effectiveness items along with one item from the Safe subscale. This factor was renamed treatment benefits (benefits). The second factor, renamed medication safety (safety), was reduced to three of the original safe subscales items.

The Benefits subscale retained nine items that focused on the actual perceived benefits of treatment, such as preventing a stroke, controlling blood pressure, preventing further health problems, and feeling better when taking medications, which indicated a desire to control blood pressure to maintain and promote health and well-being. The subscale had an eigenvalue of 5.5 and a total item variance explained by the factor of 46%....

The Safety subscale (three items) focused on side effects of medications. This subscale had an eigenvalue of 1.9 and a total item variance explained by the factor of 16%...Together, the two factor solution had a coefficient alpha [Cronbach alpha] of 0.87 and an explained variance of 62%. (Johnson & Rogers, 2006, pp. 343–346)

Johnson and Rogers (2006) initially developed a 20-item scale with three subscales (see Table 15-1). Based on the content validity testing and the EFA, the scale was reduced from 20 to 12 items that were organized into two subscales (treatment benefit and medication safety) (see Table 15-3). These researchers provide an excellent rationale for the revisions that they made

in their MTQ: Purposeful Action. In this study, the revised scale demonstrated homogeneity reliability (Cronbach alpha = 0.87) and construct validity through content validity testing and EFA. Johnson and Rogers (2006, p. 348) also conducted confirmatory factor analysis that "supported the hypothesis that benefits and safety underlie the cognitive component of medication taking in hypertensive medications."

Evidence of Validity from Structural Analysis

Structural analysis is now being used to examine the structure of relationships among the various items of an instrument. This approach provides insights beyond that provided by factor analysis. Factor analysis determines what items group together. Structural analysis determines how each item is related to other items. Thus, structural analysis goes a step beyond factor analysis. The exact relationship of each item in a factor is examined through correlational analyses.

Evidence of Validity from Contrasting (or Known) Groups

To test the instrument's validity, identify groups that are expected (or known) to have contrasting scores on the instrument. Generate hypotheses about the expected response of each of these known groups to the construct. Next, select samples from at least two groups that are expected to have opposing responses to the items in the instrument. Hagerty and Patusky (1995) developed a measure called the Sense of Belonging Instrument (SOBI). They tested the instrument on the following three groups: community college students, clients diagnosed with major depression, and retired Roman Catholic nuns, as described in the following excerpt.

The community college sample was chosen for its heterogeneous mix of students and ease of access. Depressed clients were included based on the literature and the researcher's clinical experience that interpersonal relationships and feeling "connected" are difficult when one is depressed. It was hypothesized that the depressed group would score significantly lower on the SOBI than the student group. The nuns were selected to examine the performance of the SOBI with a group that, in accordance with the theoretical basis of the instrument, should score significantly higher than the depressed and student groups. (Hagerty & Patusky, 1995, p. 10)

The nuns had the highest sense of belonging, the student groups followed, and the depressed group had the lowest sense of belonging. This test increased the validity of the instrument in that the scores of groups were as anticipated.

TABLE 15-3 Principal Axis Factor Analysis with Oblimen Rotation Pattern (and Structure in Parentheses) Coefficients for the MTQ: Purposeful Action Two-Factor Solution

	Factor Loadings					% Variance	
	1		2	h^2	Eigen-value	Explained	Coefficient α
Treatment benefits					5.5	45.9	0.90
I need to take my blood pressure pills.	0.84	(0.85) (0.34)		0.73			
Taking my blood pressure pills is not a problem because they benefit my health.	0.82	(0.84) (0.35)		0.72			
I could have problems if I do not take my blood pressure pills.	0.81	(0.84) (0.21)		0.70			
Blood pressure pills keep me from having health-related problems.	0.81	(0.79) (0.16)		0.63			
My blood pressure pills keep me from having a stroke.	0.75	(0.75) (0.23)		0.55			
I feel better when I take my blood pressure pills.	0.74	(0.74) (0.21)		0.55			
My blood pressure pills control my blood pressure.	0.74	(0.74) (0.26)		0.55			
I am OK if I do not take my blood pressure pills.[a]	0.72	(0.71)		0.52			
My blood pressure will come down enough without pills.[a]	0.54	(0.48)		0.30			
Medication safety					1.9	15.6	0.80
The side effects from my blood pressure pills are harmful.[a]	(0.19)		0.87 (0.86)	0.74			
The side effects from my blood pressure pills are a problem.[a]	(0.27)		0.84 (0.86)	0.74			
My blood pressure pills cause other health problems.[a]	(0.29)		0.82 (0.83)	0.70			
Total					7.4	61.5	0.88

From Johnson, M. J., & Rogers, S. (2006). Development of the Purposeful Action Medication-Taking Questionnaire. *Western Journal of Nursing Research, 28*(3), 345.

Note: n = 229.

[a] Item required reverse coding. Factor loadings in parenthesis represent structure coefficients. If patterned or structure coefficient is not listed, the value was < 0.15.

Evidence of Validity from Examining Convergence

In many cases, several instruments are available to measure a construct, for example, depression. But, for a number of possible reasons, the existing instruments may not be satisfactory for a particular purpose or a particular population. Therefore, the researcher may choose to develop a new instrument for a study. In examining the validity of the new instrument, it is important to determine how closely the existing instruments measure the same construct as the newly developed instrument (convergent validity). Administer all of the instruments (the new one and the existing ones) to a sample concurrently, and then evaluate the results using correlational analyses. If the measures are highly positively correlated, the validity of each instrument is strengthened. Johnson and Rogers (2006) strengthened the validity of their 12-item MTQ: Purposeful Action and its subscales (benefit and safety) by correlating them with a variety of other instruments (Hamilton Health Belief Model Hypertension [HBM] Scale with the HBM subscales of Susceptibility, Severity, Benefits, and Barriers; Lifestyle Busyness Questionnaire with Busyness and Routine subscales; and Blood Pressure

TABLE 15-4	Validity Correlation Coefficients for the MTQ: Purposeful Action and Subscales		
	MTQ: Purposeful Action	MTQ Benefit Subscale	MTQ Safe Subscale
Hamilton HBM Scale[a]	0.30**	0.43**	−0.12
HBM: Susceptibility subscale	0.36**	0.41**	0.01
HBM: Severity subscale	0.00	0.12	−0.27**
HBM: Benefits subscale	0.58**	0.63**	0.19
HBM: Barriers subscale	−0.49**	−0.42**	−0.41**
Lifestyle Busyness Questionnaire[b]	0.08	0.11	−0.02
Busyness subscale	0.10	0.13	0.01
Routine subscale	−0.07	−0.06	−0.06
Blood Pressure Feedback Log[c]			
Adherent	0.53**	0.54**	0.25*
Nonadherent	−0.60**	−0.50**	−0.53**

From Johnson, M. J., & Rogers, S. (2006). Development of the Purposeful Action Medication-Taking Questionnaire. *Western Journal of Nursing Research, 28*(3), 346.
Note: HBM is the Health Belief Model Hypertension Scale.
[a] $n = 107$.
[b] $n = 104$.
[c] $n = 102$.
* $p < 0.05$, two-tailed.
** $p < 0.01$, two-tailed.

Feedback Log). The results of these correlations are presented in Table 15-4. The significant positive correlations of 0.3 to 0.63 between the existing scales (Hamilton HBM Scale with Susceptibility and Benefits subscales and the Blood Pressure Feedback Log for adherent group) and the MTQ and the benefits subscale add to the construct validity of these instruments. This is an example of evidence of validity from examining convergence, which was strong for the MTQ and the benefit subscale but not the safety subscale.

Evidence of Validity from Examining Divergence

Sometimes, instruments can be located that measure a construct opposite to the construct measured by the newly developed instrument (divergent validity). For example, if the newly developed instrument measures hope, you and your research team could search for an instrument that measures despair. If possible, you could administer this instrument and the instruments used to test convergent validity at the same time. You will perform correlational procedures with all the measures of the construct. If the divergent measure negatively correlates with other measures, validity for each of the instruments is strengthened. Johnson and Rogers (2006) also obtained evidence of validity from examining divergence for their MTQ: Purposeful Action. In Table 15-4, you will note that the MTQ and the subscales benefits and safety were significantly, negatively correlated with HBM Barriers subscale and the Blood Pressure Feedback Log for nonadherent hypertensive patients. These scales measure the opposite construct from the MTQ and its subscales, so these significant negative correlations indicated that the construct validity was strengthened for these instruments.

Evidence of Validity from Discriminant Analysis

Sometimes, instruments have been developed to measure constructs closely related to the construct measured by the newly developed instrument. If such instruments can be located, you can strengthen the validity of the two instruments by testing the extent to which the two instruments can finely discriminate between these related concepts. Testing of this discrimination involves administering the two instruments simultaneously to a sample and then performing a discriminant analysis. Chapter 21 discusses discriminant analysis.

Evidence of Validity from Prediction of Future Events

The ability to predict future performance or attitudes on the basis of instrument scores adds to an instrument's validity. For example, nurse researchers might want to determine the ability of a scale that measures health-related behaviors to predict the future health status of individuals. One approach might be to examine reported stress levels of these individuals for the past 3 years. The validity of the Holmes and Rahe Life Events Scale, for example, could be tested in this manner. Miller (1981) discussed the validity and reliability of the Holmes and Rahe Life Events Scale in measuring stress levels in a variety of populations. The accuracy of predictive validity is determined through regression analysis.

Evidence of Validity from Prediction of Concurrent Events

Validity can be tested by examining the ability to predict the current value of one measure on the basis of the value obtained on the measure of another concept. For example, you might be able to predict the self-esteem score of an individual who had a high score on an instrument to measure coping. For example, a person who received a high score on coping might be expected to also have a high self-esteem score. If these results held true in a study in which both measures were obtained concurrently, the two instruments would have evidence of concurrent validity.

Successive Verification of Validity

After the initial development of an instrument, other researchers begin using the instrument in unrelated studies. Each of these studies adds to the validity information on the instrument. Thus, there is a successive verification of the validity of the instrument over time. For example, when additional researchers use the MTQ: Purposeful Action in their studies, this will add or subtract from the validity of this questionnaire.

ACCURACY AND PRECISION OF PHYSIOLOGICAL MEASURES

Accuracy and precision of physiological and biochemical measures tend not to be reported in published studies. These routine physiological measures are assumed to be accurate and precise, an assumption that is not always correct. The most common physiological measures used in nursing studies are blood pressure, heart rate, weight, and temperature. These measures are often obtained from the patient's record with no consideration given to their accuracy. It is important to consider the possibility of differences between the obtained value and the true value of physiological measures. Thus, researchers using physiological measures must provide evidence of the accuracy of their measures (Gift & Soeken, 1988).

The evaluation of physiological measures may require a slightly different perspective from that applied to behavioral measures, in that standards for physiological measures are defined by the National Bureau of Standards rather than the APA. The construct by which physiological accuracy is judged consists of human physiology and the mechanics of physiological equipment. However, the process is similar to that used for behavioral measures and must be addressed. Gift and Soeken (1988) identified the following five terms as critical to the evaluation of physiological measures: accuracy, selectivity, precision, sensitivity, and error.

Accuracy

Accuracy is comparable to validity, in which evidence of content-related validity addresses the extent to which the instrument measured the domain defined in the study. For example, measures of pulse oximetry could be compared with arterial blood gas measures,

and pulse oximetry should produce comparable values to blood gases to be considered an accurate measure. The researcher must be able to document the extent to which the measure is an effective predictive clinical instrument. For example, peak expiratory flow rate can predict asthma episodes.

Selectivity

Selectivity, an element of accuracy, is "the ability to identify correctly the signal under study and to distinguish it from other signals" (Gift & Soeken, 1988, p. 129). Because body systems interact, the researcher must choose instruments that have selectivity for the dimension being studied. For example, electrocardiographic readings allow one to differentiate electrical signals coming from the myocardium from similar signals coming from skeletal muscles.

To determine the content validity of biochemical measures, contact experts in the laboratory procedure and ask them to evaluate the procedure used for collection, analysis, and scoring. You might also ask them to judge the appropriateness of the measure for the construct being measured. Use contrasted groups' techniques by selecting a group of subjects known to have high values on the biochemical measures and comparing them with a group of subjects known to have low values on the same measure. In addition, to obtain concurrent validity, compare the results of the test with results from the use of a known, valid method (DeKeyser & Pugh, 1990).

Precision

Precision is the degree of consistency or reproducibility of measurements made with physiological instruments. Precision is comparable to reliability. The precision of most physiological instruments is determined by the manufacturer and is part of quality control testing. Because of fluctuations in most physiological measures, test-retest reliability is inappropriate. Engstrom (1988, p. 389) stated that assessment of precision for physiological variables that yield continuous data must include "mean, minimal, and maximal differences; standard deviation of the net differences; technical error of measurement; and indices of agreement." She suggested displaying these differences graphically and recommended exploratory data analysis (EDA) techniques for summarizing differences. Correlation coefficients are not adequate tests of the precision of physiological measures.

Two procedures are commonly used to determine the precision of biochemical measures. One is the Levy-Jennings chart. For each analysis method, a control sample is analyzed daily for 20 to 30 days. The control sample contains a known amount of the substance being tested. The mean, the standard deviation, and the known value of the sample are used to prepare a graph of the daily test results. Only 1 value of 22 is expected to be greater than or less than 2 standard deviations from the mean. If two or more values are more than 2 standard deviations from the mean, the method is unreliable in that laboratory. Another method of determining the precision of biochemical measures is the duplicate measurement method. The same technician performs duplicate measures on randomly selected specimens for a specific number of days. Results will be the same each day if there is perfect precision. Results are plotted on a graph, and the standard deviation is calculated on the basis of difference scores. The use of correlation coefficients is not recommended (DeKeyser & Pugh, 1990).

Sensitivity

Sensitivity of physiological measures relates to "the amount of change of a parameter that can be measured precisely" (Gift & Soeken, 1988, p. 130). If changes are expected to be small, the instrument must be very sensitive to detect the changes. Thus, sensitivity is associated with effect size (see Chapter 14). With some instruments, sensitivity may vary at the ends of the spectrum. This is referred to as the *frequency response*. The stability of the instrument is also related to sensitivity. This feature may be judged in terms of the ability of the system to resume a steady state after a disturbance in input. For electrical systems, this feature is referred to as *freedom from drift* (Gift & Soeken, 1988).

Error

Sources of error in physiological measures can be grouped into the following five categories: environment, user, subject, machine, and interpretation. The environment affects both the machine and the subject. Environmental factors include temperature, barometric pressure, and static electricity. User errors are caused by the person using the instrument and may be associated with variations by the same user, different users, changes in supplies, or procedures used to operate the equipment. Subject errors occur when the subject alters the machine or the machine alters the subject. In some cases, the machine may not be used to its full capacity. Machine error may be related to calibration or to the stability of the machine. Signals transmitted from the machine are also a source of error and can cause misinterpretation (Gift & Soeken, 1988).

Sources of error in biochemical measures are biological, preanalytical, analytical, and postanalytical. Biological variability in biochemical measures is due

to factors such as age, gender, and body size. Variability in the same individual is due to factors such as diurnal rhythms, seasonal cycles, and aging. Preanalytical variability is due to errors in collecting and handling of specimens. These errors include sampling the wrong patients; using an incorrect container, preservative, or label; lysis of cells; and evaporation. Preanalytical variability may also be due to patient intake of food or drugs, exercise, or emotional stress. Analytical variability is associated with the method used for analysis and may be due to materials, equipment, procedures, and personnel used. The major source of postanalytical variability is transcription error. You can greatly reduce this source of error by entering data into the computer directly (DeKeyser & Pugh, 1990).

In Estok et al.'s (2007) study, introduced earlier in this chapter, the researchers used a dual-energy x-ray absorptiometry (DXA) scan to measure the bone mineral density (BMD) of their subjects. They provided a strong description of this physiological measurement device by discussing the accuracy, precision, and potential for error of the DXA. In addition, they described the scoring for the DXA scan, with the results being standardized using World Health Organization evidence-based guidelines for determining normal, osteopenia, and osteroporosis diagnoses. The DXA scan measurement method, the process for obtaining the BMD scores, and the meaning of the scores are described in the following excerpt:

There is low precision error and low radiation exposure in the DXA, and it can be used to measure multiple skeletal sites (Wahner & Fogelman, 1994). Measurements of bone mineral density of the AP [anterior posterior] lumbar spine (L1-L4, anterior posterior) and femur were made using the Lunar model DPX-IQ or DPX-A dual-energy X-ray obsorptiometer. The DXA takes only a few minutes and can be used to predict future risk of factures in asymptomatic patients (NOF [National Osteoporosis Foundation], 2003). The results are expressed as a *T*-score and/or age-matched *Z* scores. The *T*-score is independent of age … and is used to compare the DXA result with the mean peak bone mass of a young adult in terms of a standard deviation (*SD*). At any skeletal site, a decrease in bone mass of 1 *SD* approximately doubles the relative risk of subsequent fracture. Scores were coded using the World Health organization [WHO] Study Group (1994) prescribed categories: 0 = normal (*T*-score above −1 *SD* in both sites); 1 = osteopenia (*T*-score between −1 and −2.5 *SD* in one or both sites); 2 = osteoporosis (*T*-score below −2.5 *SD* in one or both sites). (Estok et al., 2007, pp. 150–151)

USE OF SENSITIVITY, SPECIFICITY, AND LIKELIHOOD RATIOS TO DETERMINE THE QUALITY OF DIAGNOSTIC TESTS

An important part of evidence-based practice is the use of quality diagnostic tests to determine the presence or absence of disease. Clinicians want to know what laboratory or imaging study to order to help screen for or diagnose a disease. When you order a test, how can you be sure that the results are valid or accurate? The accuracy of a screening test or a test used to confirm a diagnosis is evaluated in terms of its ability to correctly assess the presence or absence of a disease or condition as compared to a gold standard. The gold standard is the most accurate means of currently diagnosing a particular disease and serves as a basis for comparison with newly developed diagnostic or screening tests. If the test is positive, what is the probability that the disease is present? If the test is negative, what is the probability that the disease is not present? When you talk to the patient about the results of their tests, how sure are you that they do or do not have the disease? *Sensitivity* and *specificity* are the terms used to describe the accuracy of a screening or diagnostic test (Table 15-5). There are four possible outcomes of a screening test for a disease: (1) true positive, which accurately identifies the presence of a disease; (2) false positive, which indicates a disease is present when it is not; (3) true negative, which indicates accurately that a disease is not present; or (4) false negative, which indicates that a disease is not present when it is (Grove, 2007). The 2×2 contingency table shown in Table 15-5 will help you to visualize sensitivity and specificity and these four outcomes (Melnyk & Fineout-Overholt, 2005).

Sensitivity and specificity can be calculated based on research findings and clinical practice outcomes to determine the most accurate diagnostic or screening tool to use in identifying the presence or absence of a disease for a population of patients. The calculations for sensitivity and specificity are provided as follows:

> Sensitivity calculation = Probability of disease
> = a/(a + c) = True positive rate

> Specificity calculation = Probability of no disease
> = d/(b+d) = True negative rate

Sensitivity is the proportion of patients with the disease who have a positive test result or true positive. The ways the researcher or clinician might refer to the test sensitivity include the following:

- *Highly sensitive test* is very good at identifying the diseased patient.
- If a test is highly sensitive, it has a low percentage of false negatives.
- *Low sensitivity test* is limited in identifying the patient with a disease.
- If a test has low sensitivity, it has a high percentage of false negatives.
- Therefore, if a sensitive test has negative results, the patient is less likely to have the disease.
- Use the acronym SnNout, which is read: High sensitivity (Sn), test is negative (N), rules the disease out (out).

Specificity of a screening or diagnostic test is the proportion of patients without the disease who have a negative test result or true negative. The ways the researcher or clinician might refer to the test specificity include the following:

- *Highly specific test* is very good at identifying the patients without a disease.
- If a test is very specific, it has a low percentage of false positives.
- *Low specificity test* is limited in identifying patients without disease.
- If a test has low specificity, it has a high percentage of false positives.
- Therefore, if a specific test has positive results the patient is more likely to have the disease.
- Use the acronym SpPin, which is read: High specificity (Sp), test is positive (P), rules the disease in (in).

TABLE 15-5	Results of Sensitivity and Specificity of Screening Tests		
Diagnostic Test Result	Disease Present	Disease Not Present or Absent	Total
Positive test	a (true positive)	b (false positive)	a + b
Negative test	c (false negative)	d (true negative)	c + d
Total	a + c	b + d	a + b + c + d

Grove, S. K. (2007). *Statistics for health care research: A practical workbook*. Philadelphia: Saunders, p. 335.

a = The number of people who have the disease and the test is positive (true positive).

b = The number of people who do not have the disease and the test is positive (false positive).

c = The number of people who have the disease and the test is negative (false negative).

d = The number of people who do not have the disease and the test is negative (true negative).

Porter, Fleisher, Kohane, and Mandl (2003) conducted a prospective observational study to assess predictive value of parents reporting the medical history and physical signs of dehydration in their children. Their study included 132 parent-child dyads. The primary outcome was percentage of dehydration and secondary outcomes were clinically important acidosis and hospital admission. They also compared the reports of physical signs of dehydration made by the parents and the nurse. Their study results indicated that parent reports of physical symptoms and history had a higher sensitivity (range 73% to 100%) than specificity (range 0% to 49%) for predicting dehydration of

5% or greater in their child (Table 15-6). The nurse reports of physical signs for clinically important dehydration were always more specific (33% to 93%) than the parents (17% to 82%) and usually more sensitive (10% to 100%) than the parents (0% to 91%) (Table 15-7) (Porter et al., 2003). In this study, the nurses' diagnostic ability to determine clinically important dehydration is the gold standard used as a basis for comparison of the parents' diagnostic ability. As expected, the nurses' were more sensitive and specific in diagnosing clinically important dehydration in children than were parents, but the parents were very sensitive in reporting the child's history that predicated

TABLE 15-6 ■ Value of Parent Reported History for Prediction of Clinically Important Dehydration

Historical Element (Total No. of Parents = 132)	% Sensitivity (95% CI)	% Specificity (95% CI)
Decreased oral intake	100 (75–100)	18 (8–28)
Decreased urine output	100 (75–100)	26 (15–37)
History of any vomiting during illness	100 (75–100)	3 (0–7)
History of vomiting in past 12 hours	73 (37–92)	6 (0–12)
History of any diarrhea during illness	91 (63–99)	28 (17–39)
History of diarrhea in past 12 hours	82 (50–97)	38 (26–50)
Contact with PCP by telephone ($n - 131$)	91 (63–99)	23 (12–34)
Contact with PCP in office ($n = 131$)	100 (75–100)	49 (36–62)
Previous trial of clear liquids ($n = 131$)	100 (75–100)	22 (12–32)

From Porter, S. C., Fleisher, G. R., Kohane, I. S., & Mandl, K. D. (2003). The value of parental report for diagnosis and management of dehydration in the emergency department. *Annals of Emergency Medicine, 41*(2), 201.
PCP, primary care provider.
CI, Confidence interval

TABLE 15-7 ■ Diagnostic Value of Parents' and Nurses' Report of Physical Signs for Clinical Important Dehydration

Physical Sign (No. of Parents/No. of Nurses)	% Sensitivity		% Specificity	
	Parent (95% CI)	Nurse (95% CI)	Parent (95% CI)	Nurse (95% CI)
Ill appearance (71/68)*	91 (63–99)	90 (60–99)	17 (7–26)	33 (21–45)
Sunken fontanelle[†] (13/11)	0 (0–84)	100 (2–100)	82 (48–98)	90 (56–100)
Sunken eyes (71/68)	64 (33–86)	70 (38–91)	37 (15–58)	59 (47–72)
Decreased tears[‡] (67/42)	91 (63–99)	100 (33–100)	25 (14–36)	33 (21–45)
Dry mouth (71/68)	64 (33–86)	100 (73–100)	42 (35–48)	49 (36–62)
Weak cry[§] (71/41)	54 (25–80)	25 (1–75)	27 (16–38)	78 (65–92)
Cool extremities (71/68)	27 (8–63)	10 (1–40)	73 (62–84)	93 (87–100)

From Porter, S. C., Fleisher, G.R., Kohane, I. S., & Mandl, K. D. (2003). The value of parental report for diagnosis and management of dehydration in the emergency department. *Annals of Emergency Medicine, 41*(2), 202.
[*] The total number of patients for this outcome equals 71. Three patients from the subset of 71 did not have nursing assessments for physical signs completed.
[†] Subset of 32 infants <9 months of age with only 2 cases of significant dehydration.
[‡] Parents and nurses could answer "no opportunity to observe," resulting in missing data for parents (4 patients) and nurses (26 patients).
[§] Nurses could answer "no opportunity to observe," resulting in missing data (27 patients).

dehydration. In developing a diagnostic or screening test, researchers must achieve the highest sensitivity and specificity possible, and clinicians must select the most sensitive and specific screening test to diagnose diseases in their patients (Craig & Smyth, 2007; Grove, 2007). However, the screening test selected for detecting a disease is affected by cost as well as sensitivity and specificity.

Likelihood ratios (LRs) are additional calculations that can help researchers to determine the accuracy of diagnostic or screening tests, which are based on the sensitivity and specificity results. The LRs are calculated to determine the likelihood that a positive test result is a true positive and a negative test result is a true negative. The ratio of the true positive results to false positive results is known as the positive LR (Craig & Smyth, 2007). The positive LR is calculated as follows:

Positive LR = Sensitivity ÷ 100% − Specificity

Positive LR for sunken fontanelle diagnosed by nurse = 100% ÷ 100% − 90% = 100% ÷ 10% = 10

The **negative LR** is the ratio of true negative results to false negative results, and it is calculated as follows:

Negative LR = 100% − Sensitivity ÷ Specificity

Negative LR for sunken fontanelle diagnosed by nurse = 100% − 100% ÷ 90% = 0 ÷ 90% = 0

The very high LRs (or those that are above 10) rule in the disease or indicate that the patient has the disease. The very low LRs (or those that are < 0.1) virtually rule out the chance that the patient has the disease (Melnyk & Fineout-Overholt, 2005). Understanding sensitivity, specificity, and LR increases your ability to read clinical studies and to determine the most accurate diagnostic test to use in clinical practice.

VALIDITY IN QUALITATIVE RESEARCH

One of the most serious concerns related to qualitative research has been the lack of strategies to determine the validity of the measurements that led to the development of theory. Qualitative researchers tend to work alone. Biases in their work, which threaten validity, can easily go undetected. Miles and Huberman (1994) have cautioned the qualitative researcher to be alert to the occurrence of the *holistic fallacy*. This fallacy occurs as the researcher becomes more and more sure that his or her conclusions are correct and that the model does, in fact, explain the situation. This feeling should arouse suspicion and alert the researcher

to validate his or her findings. Miles and Huberman (1994) have described 12 strategies for examining the validity of qualitative measures:

Checking for representativeness. Qualitative measurement can be biased by either the attention of the researcher or a bias in the people from whom they obtain their measures. To ensure that measures are representative of the entire population, the researcher looks for sources of data not easily accessible. The researcher assumes that observed actions are representative of actions that occur when the researcher is not present. However, efforts must be made to determine whether this is so.

Checking for researcher effects. In many cases, the researcher's presence can alter behavior, leading to invalid measures. To avoid this effect, the researcher must (1) remain on the site long enough to become familiar, (2) use unobtrusive measures, and (3) seek input from informants or study participants.

Triangulating. The qualitative researcher must compare all the measures from different sources to determine the validity of the findings.

Weighing the evidence. Qualitative research involves reducing large amounts of data during the process of coming to conclusions. In this process, some evidence is captured from this mass of data and is used in reaching conclusions. The researcher needs to review the strength of the captured data to validate the conclusions. The researcher determines the strength of the evidence from the source, the circumstances of data collection, and the researcher's efforts to validate the evidence. The researcher must search actively for reasons why the evidence should not be trusted.

Making contrasts and comparisons. Contrasts between subjects or events in relation to the study conclusions must be examined. An example would be an action that nursing supervisors consider to be very important but that staff nurses regard as simply another administrative activity. The two extreme positions must be examined. A decision must then be made about whether the difference is a significant one.

Checking the meaning of outliers. Exceptions to findings must be identified and examined. These exceptions are referred to as **outliers**. The outliers provide a way to test the generality of the findings. Therefore, in the selection of subjects, it may be important to seek individuals who seem to be outliers.

Using extreme cases. Certain types of outliers, referred to as *extreme cases,* can be useful in confirming conclusions. The researcher can compare the extreme case with the theoretical model that was developed and determine the key factor that causes the model not to fit the case. Purposive sampling is often used to ensure that extreme cases are included.

Ruling out spurious relations. The strategy of ruling out spurious relations requires the examination of relationships identified in the model to consider the possibility of a third variable influencing the situation.

Replicating a finding. Documenting the findings from several independent sources increases the dependability of the findings and diminishes the risk of the holistic fallacy. The findings can be tested either with new data collected later in the study or with data from another site or data set. The second option is more rigorous.

Checking out rival explanations. The qualitative researcher is taught to keep several hypotheses in mind and constantly to compare the plausibility of each with the possibility that one of the others is more accurate. Near the end of data analysis, however, when the researcher is more emotionally "wedded to" one idea, it is useful to have someone not involved in the research act as a devil's advocate. Questions such as "What could disprove the hypothesis?" or, conversely, "What does the present hypothesis disprove?" should be asked. Evidence that does not fit the hypothesis must be carefully examined.

Looking for negative evidence. A search for negative evidence naturally flows from the searches for outliers and rival explanations. In this step, there is an active search for disconfirmation of what is believed to be true. The researcher goes back through the data, seeking evidence to disconfirm the conclusions. However, the inability to find disconfirming evidence never decisively confirms the conclusions reached by the researcher. In some cases, independent verification, through examination of the data by a second qualitative researcher, is sought.

Obtaining feedback from informants or study participants. Conclusions should be given to the participants, and feedback is sought from them about the accuracy of the causal network developed. Although researchers have been getting feedback from participants throughout the analysis period, feedback after completion of the model provides a different type of verification of the information.

SUMMARY

- Measurement is the process of assigning numbers to objects, events, or situations in accord with some rule.
- Instrumentation is the application of specific rules to develop a measurement device or instrument.
- Measurement theory and the rules within this theory have been developed to direct the measurement of abstract and concrete concepts.
- There is direct measurement and indirect measurement.
- Health care technology has made researchers familiar with direct measures of concrete elements, such as height, weight, heart rate, temperature, and blood pressure, very familiar.
- Indirect measurement is used with abstract concepts, when the concepts are not measured directly, but when the indicators or attributes of the concepts are used to represent the abstraction.

- Measurement error is the difference between what exists in reality and what is measured by a research instrument.
- The levels of measurement, from lower to higher, are nominal, ordinal, interval, and ratio.
- Reliability refers to how consistently the measurement technique measures the concept of interest.
- The validity of an instrument is determined by the extent to which the instrument actually reflects the abstract construct being examined.
- Evaluation of physiological measures requires a different perspective from that of behavioral measures and requires evaluation for accuracy, precision, selectivity, and sensitivity.
- The accuracy of screening or diagnostic tests is determined by calculating the sensitivity, specificity, and likelihood ratios for the test.
- One of the most serious concerns related to qualitative research has been the lack of strategies to determine the validity of the measurements that led to the development of theory. However, strategies are being identified to examine the validity of qualitative measures.

REFERENCES

American Psychological Association's Committee to Develop Standards. (1985). *Standards for educational and psychological testing.* Washington, DC: American Psychological Association.

Armstrong, G. D. (1981). Parametric statistics and ordinal data: A pervasive misconception. *Nursing Research, 30*(1), 60–62.

Armstrong, G. D. (1984). Parametric statistics [Letter]. *Nursing Research, 33*(1), 54.

Bakas, T., Champion, V., Perkins, S. M., Farran, C. J., & Williams, L. S. (2006). Psychometric testing of the revised 15-item Bakas Caregiving Outcomes Scale. *Nursing Research, 55*(5), 346–355.

Berk, R. A. (1990). Importance of expert judgment in content-related validity evidence. *Western Journal of Nursing Research, 12*(5), 659–671.

Brinberg, D., & McGrath, J. E. (1985). *Validity and the research process.* Beverly Hills, CA: Sage.

Campbell, D. T., & Fiske, D. W. (1959). Convergent and discriminant validation by the multitrait-multimethod matrix. *Psychological Bulletin, 56*(2), 81–105.

Cohen, J. A. (1960). A coefficient of agreement for nominal scales. *Education and Psychological Measurement, 20*(1), 37–46.

Craig, J. V., & Smyth, R. L. (2007). *The evidence-base practice manual for nurses* (2nd ed.). Edinburgh, Scotland: Churchill Livingstone.

Davis, L. L. (1992). Instrument review: Getting the most from a panel of experts. *Applied Nursing Research, 5*(4), 194–197.

DeKeyser, F. G., & Pugh, L. C. (1990). Assessment of the reliability and validity of biochemical measures. *Nursing Research, 39*(5), 314–317.

DeVellis, R. F. (1991). *Scale development: Theory and applications.* Newbury Park, CA: Sage.

Engstrom, J. L. (1988). Assessment of the reliability of physical measures. *Research in Nursing & Health, 11*(6), 383–389.

Estok, P. J., Sedlak, C. A., Doheny, M. O., & Hall, R. (2007). Structural model for osteoporosis preventing behavior in postmenopausal women. *Nursing Research, 56*(3), 149–158.

Garvin, B. J., Kennedy, C. W., & Cissna, K. N. (1988). Reliability in category coding systems. *Nursing Research, 37*(1), 52–55.

Gift, A. G., & Soeken, K. L. (1988). Assessment of physiologic instruments. *Heart & Lung, 17*(2), 128–133.

Goodwin, L. D., & Goodwin, W. L. (1991). Estimating construct validity. *Research in Nursing & Health, 14*(3), 235–243.

Grove, S. K. (2007). *Statistics for health care research: A practical workbook.* Philadelphia: Saunders.

Guetzkow, H. (1950). Unitizing and categorizing problems in coding qualitative data. *Journal of Clinical Psychology, 6*(1), 47–58.

Gunning, R., & Kallan, R. A. (1994). *How to take the fog out of business writing.* Chicago: Dartnell.

Hagerty, B. M. K., & Patusky, K. (1995). Developing a measure of sense of belonging. *Nursing Research, 44*(1), 9–13.

Imle, M. A., & Atwood, J. R. (1988). Retaining qualitative validity while gaining reliability and validity: Development of the Transition to Parenthood Concerns Scale. *Advanced Nursing Science, 11*(1), 61–75.

Johnson, M. J. (2002). *The development and testing of three medication-taking questionnaires for the medication adherence model constructs for hypertensive patients. Unpublished doctoral dissertation.* University of Utah, Salt Lake City, UT.

Johnson, M. J., & Rogers, S. (2006). Development of the Purposeful Action Medication-Taking Questionnaire. *Western Journal of Nursing Research, 28*(3), 335–351.

Johnson, M. J., Williams, M., & Marshall, E. S. (1999). Adherent and nonadherent medication-taking elderly hypertensive patients. *Clinical Nursing Research, 8*(4), 318–335.

Kaplan, A. (1963). *The conduct of inquiry: Methodology for behavioral science.* New York: Harper & Row.

Knapp, T. R. (1984). Parametric statistics [Letter]. *Nursing Research, 33*(1), 54.

Knapp, T. R. (1990). Treating ordinal scales as interval scales: An attempt to resolve the controversy. *Nursing Research, 39*(2), 121–123.

Lynn, M. R. (1986). Determination and quantification of content validity. *Nursing Research, 35*(6), 382–385.

Marshall, C., & Rossman, G. B. (2006). *Designing qualitative research* (4th ed.). Thousand Oaks, CA: Sage.

Melnyk, B. M., & Fineout-Overholt, E. (2005). *Evidence-based practice in nursing & healthcare: A guide to best practice.* Philadelphia: Lippincott Williams & Wilkins.

Miles, M. B., & Huberman, A. M. (1994). *Qualitative data analysis: A sourcebook of new methods* (2nd ed.). Beverly Hills, CA: Sage.

Miller, B., & Bodie, M. (1994). Determination of reading comprehension level for effective patient health-education materials. *Nursing Research, 43*(2), 118–119.

Miller, T. W. (1981). Life events scaling: Clinical methodological issues. *Nursing Research, 30*(5), 316–320A.

Munro, B. H. (2001). *Statistical methods for health care research* (3rd ed.). Philadelphia: Lippincott.

Nagley, S. J., & Byers, P. H. (1987). Clinical construct validity. *Journal of Advanced Nursing, 12*(5), 617–619.

National Osteoporosis Foundation (NOF). (2003). *Stand up to osteoporosis* [Brochure]. Washington, DC: Author.

Nunnally, J. C., & Bernstein, I. H. (1994). *Psychometric theory* (3rd ed.). New York: McGraw-Hill.

Porter, S. C., Fleisher, G. R., Kohane, I. S., & Mandl, K. D. (2003). The value of parental report for diagnosis and management of dehydration in the emergency department. *Annals of Emergency Medicine, 41*(2), 196–205.

Rasin, J. H. (1997). Measurement issues with the elderly. In M. Frank-Stromberg & S. J. Olsen (Eds.), *Instruments for clinical health-care research* (2nd ed.), pp. 44–53. Boston: Jones & Bartlett.

Rew, L., Stuppy, D., & Becker, H. (1988). Construct validity in instrument development: A vital link between nursing practice, research, and theory. *Advances in Nursing Science, 10*(4), 10–22.

Silvaroli, N. J. (1986). *Classroom reading inventory* (5th ed.). Dubuque, IA: William C. Brown.

Stevens, S. S. (1946). On the theory of scales of measurement. *Science, 103*(2684), 677–680.

Stommel, M., Wang, S., Given, C. W., & Given, B. (1992). Confirmatory factor analysis (CFA) as a method to assess measurement equivalence. *Research in Nursing & Health, 15*(5), 399–405.

Streiner, D. L., & Norman, G. R. (1995). *Health measurement scales: A practical guide to their development and use* (2nd ed.). Oxford, England: Oxford University Press.

Teel, C., & Verran, J. A. (1991). Factor comparison across studies. *Research in Nursing & Health, 14*(1), 67–72.

Thomas, S. D., Hathaway, D. K., & Arheart, K. L. (1992). Face validity. *Western Journal of Nursing Research, 14*(1), 109–112.

Topf, M. (1988). Interrater reliability decline under covert assessment. *Nursing Research, 37*(1), 47–49.

Wahner, H. W., & Fogelman, I. (1994). The evaluation of osteoporosis: Dual energy x-ray absorptiometry in clinical practice. In H. W. Wahner & I. Fogelman (Eds.), *Mayo clinic proceedings* (pp. 178–195). London: Mayo Clinic.

Waltz, C. W., & Bausell, R. B. (1981). *Nursing Research: Design, statistics and computer analysis.* Philadelphia: F.A. Davis.

Washington, C. C., & Moss, M. (1988). Pragmatic aspects of establishing interrater reliability in research. *Nursing Research, 37*(3), 190–191.

World Health Organization Study Group. (1994). *Assessment of fracture risk and its application to screening for postmenopausal osteoporosis.* Geneva, Switzerland: World Health Organization.

CHAPTER 16

Measurement Methods Used in Developing Evidence for Practice

Nursing studies examine a wide variety of phenomena and thus require an extensive array of measurement methods. However, nurse researchers have sometimes found limited instruments available to measure phenomena central to the studies needed to development evidence for practice. Measurement methods used in older nursing studies were often developed for a specific study, and there was little documented proof of their validity and reliability. Since the early 1980s, nurse researchers have made it a priority to develop valid and reliable instruments to measure phenomena of concern to nursing. As a result, the number and quality of measurement methods have greatly increased.

Knowledge of measurement methods is important at all levels of nursing. To critically appraise a study, not only must the nurse researcher have some knowledge of measurement theory, but she or he must also understand the state of the art for developing measures to examine the phenomena under study. When evaluating someone else's research, you might, for example, want to know whether the researcher was using an older tool that had been surpassed by a number of more recently developed instruments. It might help you to know that measuring a particular phenomenon has been a problem with which nurse researchers have struggled for a number of years. Your understanding of the successes and struggles in measuring nursing phenomena may stimulate your creative thinking and lead you to contribute your own research to the development of measurement approaches. Some nursing phenomena have not been adequately examined because reliable and valid instruments are not available to measure them, which makes it difficult for

nurse researchers to generate the essential evidence needed for practice (Craig & Smyth, 2007; Malloch & Porter-O'Grady, 2006).

This chapter describes the common measurement approaches used in nursing research, including physiological measures, observations, interviews, questionnaires, and scales. Other methods of measurement discussed include Q methodology, the Delphi technique, projective techniques, and diaries. This chapter also describes the process for locating existing instruments, determining their reliability and validity, and assessing their readability. Directions are provided for describing an instrument in a written report. The chapter concludes with a description of the process of scale construction and issues related to translating an instrument into another language.

PHYSIOLOGICAL MEASUREMENT

Much of nursing practice is oriented toward physiological dimensions of health. Therefore, many of our questions require us to be able to measure these dimensions. Of particular importance are studies linking physiological and psychosocial variables. In 1993, the National Institute of Nursing Research (NINR) expressed a need for increased numbers of physiologically based nursing studies inasmuch as 85% of NINR-funded studies involved nonphysiological variables. According to NINR staff, a review of physiological studies funded by the NINR found that "the biological measurements used in the funded grants often were not state-of-the-science, and the biological theory underlying the measurements often was underutilized" (Cowan, Heinrich, Lucas, Sigmon, & Hinshaw,

1993, p. 4). This report suggested an increase not only in the number of biologically based studies but also in the quality of measurements used in these studies. The NINR's (2006) number one strategy for building the science of nursing for 2006 to 2010 is the "integrating of biological and behavior science for better health" (see NINR Web site at www.nih.gov/ninr). Due in part to these funding priorities and in part to the demands for outcome studies with physiological measures, the number of studies including physiological measures has dramatically increased. For example, physiological instruments exist to precisely measure nutritional status, wound healing, and sleep patterns.

Physiological measures can be acquired in a variety of ways. The following sections describe how to obtain physiological measures by self-report, observation, direct or indirect measurement, laboratory tests, electronic monitoring, and the creative development of new instruments. The measurement of physiological variables across time is also addressed. The section concludes with a discussion of how to select physiological variables for a particular study.

Obtaining Physiological Measures by Self-Report

Self-report has been used effectively to obtain physiological information and may be particularly useful when the subjects are not in closely monitored settings such as hospitals, clinics, or research facilities. Phenomena that have been or could be measured by self-report include hours of sleep, patterns of daily activities, eating patterns, dieting patterns, stool frequency and consistency, patterns of joint stiffness, variations in degree of mobility, fear of falling, health status, and exercise patterns. For some variables, self-reporting may be the only means of obtaining the information. Such may be the case when the subject experiences a physiological phenomenon, but it cannot be observed or measured by others. Nonobservable physiological phenomena include pain (Adachi, Shimada, & Usui, 2003; Chung, Ng, & Wong, 2002; Im et al., 2007), angina (DeVon & Zerwic, 2003), nausea, dizziness, indigestion, patterns of hunger or thirst, hot flashes, variations in cognition, visual phenomena, tinnitus, pruritus (Ro, Ha, Kim, & Yeom, 2002), fatigue, and dyspnea (Kapella, Larson, Patel, Covey, & Berry, 2006). Pope (1995) pointed out that sound is an essential and constant component of the human condition, but its importance to health has been little recognized. Although one can measure sounds, one cannot measure sound perception and sensitivity. Pope has recommended the development of instruments to measure these responses and

specifically pointed out the potential impact of these variables in settings such as critical care units.

Kapella et al. (2006) examined relationships among the physiological variables of fatigue, dyspnea, and functional status in chronic obstructive pulmonary disease (COPD) patients. These variables were measured with self-report instruments, and the measurement of dyspnea is described in the following excerpt.

> Dyspnea was measured with the Chronic Respiratory Disease Questionnaire (CRQ).... The CRQ is a disease-specific measure that was developed for use in people with COPD (Guyatt, Berman, Townsend, Pugsley, & Chambers, 1987). With the CRQ Dyspnea Scale, participants rate the dyspnea they experience during selected activities that they perform on a regular basis. It is a five-item scale with a potential range from 1 = *extremely short of breath* to 7 = *not at all short of breath*. A self-report form of the CRQ (Williams, Singh, Sewell, Guyatt, & Morgan, 2001) was used here. Cronbach's alpha for the CRQ in this study was 0.84. (Kapella et al., 2006. p. 12)

The self-report CRQ Dyspnea Scale seemed to be a valid and reliable method for measuring the dyspnea experienced by patients with COPD. Kapella et al. (2006) indicated the scale was developed just for people with COPD, which adds to the validity of the scale. Sources that documented the development of the scale's validity and reliability were identified. In addition, the CRQ Dyspnea Scale was reliable in this study, as indicated by the Cronbach alpha = 0.84. Using self-report measures may enable nurses to ask research questions that were not previously considered, which could be an important means to build knowledge in areas not yet explored. The insight gained could alter the way nurses manage patient situations that are now considered problematic and thereby improve patient outcomes.

Obtaining Physiological Measures by Observation

Researchers sometimes obtain data on physiological parameters by using observational data collection measures. These measures provide criteria for quantifying various levels or states of physiological functioning. In addition to collecting clinical data, this method provides a means to gather data from the observations of caregivers. This source of data has been particularly useful in studies involving persons with Alzheimer's disease, advanced cancer, and severe mental illness. Observation is also an effective way to gather data on the frail elderly, infants, and young children. Studies involving home health agencies and hospices often use observation tools to record physiological dimensions of patient status. These data are sometimes stored electronically and are available to researchers for large database analysis.

Small and Melnyk (2006) studied the early predictors of post-hospital adjustment problems in critically ill toddlers and preschool children. The researchers measured the mother's participation in the child's care during hospitalization using an observational checklist that was completed by the primary nurse. The following excerpt describes the measurement method used and its validity and reliability.

Maternal participation was assessed using the Index of Parent Participation (IPP; Melnyk, Alpert-Gillis, Hensel, Cable-Beiling, & Rubenstein, 1997). The primary nurses used the 36-item dichotomous scale to identify which care behaviors the participant mothers were involved in with their ill or injured children during the prior 4 hours (e.g., set up child's food tray, talked with child about the need for a test). The instrument is scored by summing the total number of parental care behaviors indicated, then dividing by the total number of possible care behaviors to yield a percentage score. Prior researchers have demonstrated acceptable content and face validity (Melnyk et al., 1997). An interrater reliability of 0.80 or higher was maintained throughout the primary study period as determined by having a nurse researcher independently complete the IPP questionnaire on a random sample of parents that the primary nurses also were rating. Prior Cronbach's alphas for this index ranged between 0.77 and 0.87 (Melnyk, 1994; Melnyk et al., 1997). The Cronbach's alpha for this sample was 0.93. (Small & Melnyk, 2006, p. 626)

Obtaining Physiological Measures Directly or Indirectly

Physiological variables can be measured either directly or indirectly. Direct measures are more accurate because there is an objective measurement of the study variable. For example, patients might be asked to report any irregular heartbeats over 24 hours, which is an indirect measurement of heart rhythm, and each patient's heart could be monitored with a holter monitor over the same 24-hour timeframe (direct measure of heart rhythm). Whenever possible, researchers usually select direct measures of their study variables due to the accuracy and precision of these measurement methods. However, if a direct measurement method does not exist, an indirect measurement method could be used in the initial investigation of a physiological variable. Sometimes researchers use both direct and indirect measurement methods to expand

the understanding of a physiological variable. For example, Dubbert, White, Grothe, O'Jile, and Kirchner (2006) studied the physical activity of patients who are severely mentally ill. These researchers measured the variable physical activity with indirect and direct measurement methods that are described in the following excerpt.

■ SELF-REPORTED PHYSICAL ACTIVITY [INDIRECT MEASURE]

The 42-item Community Health Activities Model Program for Seniors (CHAMPS) ... was used to assess frequency and duration of a variety of physical activities for the previous 4 weeks. The CHAMPS yields estimates of kilocalorie (kcal) energy expenditure per unit time and physical activity frequency. In nonclinical samples, CHAMPS scores have test-retest reliability intraclass correlations (ICCS) $R = 0.76$ for moderate and $R = 0.66$ for total estimated kcal expenditure over 6 months and validity correlations in the $R = 0.20$ to 0.30 range with performance on a 6-minute walk test....

■ OBJECTIVELY MEASURED PHYSICAL ACTIVITY [DIRECT MEASUREMENT]

Participants wore RT3 (Stayhealthy, Inc., Monrovia, CA) accelerometers to obtain objective estimates of daily physical activity. The RT3 instrument, about the size of a pager, measures acceleration of movement along three axes, which was averaged into a composite score (i.e., vector movement [VM], representing the overall magnitude of activity for each minute. RT3 software transformed VM into an estimate of energy expenditure (i.e., kcal per day and per hour), using participant's height, weight, age, and gender. (Dubbert et al., 2006, p. 206)

Obtaining Physiological Measures from Laboratory Tests

Laboratory tests are usually very precise and accurate and provide direct measures of many physiological variables. Biochemical measures such as the activated partial thromboplastin time must be obtained through invasive procedures. Sometimes these invasive procedures are part of routine patient care, and the researcher can obtain the results from the patient's record. Although nurses are now performing some biochemical measures in the nursing unit, these measures often require laboratory analysis. When invasive procedures are not part of routine care but are instead performed specifically for a study, great care must be taken to protect the subjects and to follow guidelines for informed consent and institutional approval. The patient (or his or her insurer) cannot be billed for invasive procedures that are not part of routine care;

thus, the researcher must seek external funding or the institution in which the patient is receiving care must agree to forego billing for the procedure.

The researcher must also carefully consider the accuracy and precision of laboratory measures and the method of collecting specimens. Kreman et al. (2006) examined the effects of motivational interviewing on selected physiological outcomes in hyperlipidemic persons. One of the physiological outcomes was a lipid profile laboratory test that was collected before and after the motivational treatment. The following excerpt describes the measurement of the subjects' lipid levels.

■ *LIPID PROFILE*

A fasting lipid profile included total cholesterol, LDL-C [low-density-lipoprotein cholesterol], and HDL-C [high-density-lipoprotein cholesterol], which were drawn at baseline and at 3 months to examine changes over time. Participants were instructed to fast for 12 hours and avoid alcohol consumption for 24 hours prior to having their blood drawn. Samples were drawn in the participants' homes, spun down on-site, and transported to a certified clinical laboratory within 4 hours. (Kreman et al., 2006, p. 168)

These researchers picked an accurate and precise way to assess the lipid status of their subjects by measuring their total cholesterol, LDL-C, and HDL-C. By educating the subjects about fasting, controlling the collection of the blood samples, and ensuring the blood was analyzed in a certified lab, the researchers strengthened the precision and accuracy of their laboratory tests that directly measured patients' lipid statuses.

Obtaining Physiological Measures through Electronic Monitoring

The availability of electronic monitoring equipment has greatly increased the possibilities of physiological measurement in nursing studies, particularly in critical care environments. Understanding the processes of electronic monitoring can make the procedure less formidable to those critically appraising published studies and those considering using the method for measurement.

To use electronic monitoring, usually you will place sensors on or within your subject. The sensors measure changes in body functions such as electrical energy. Many sensors need an external stimulus to trigger the measurement process. Transducers convert the electrical signal to numerical data. Electrical signals often include interference signals as well as the desired signal, so you may choose to use an amplifier to decrease interference and amplify the desired signal. The electrical signal is then digitized (converted to numerical digits or values) and stored on magnetic tape. In addition, it is immediately displayed on a monitor. The display equipment may be visual or auditory, or both. A writing recorder provides a printed version of the data. One type of display equipment is an oscilloscope that displays the data as a waveform, and it may provide information such as time, phase, voltage, or frequency of the data. Some electronic equipment simultaneously records multiple physiological measures that are displayed on a monitor. The equipment is often linked to a computer, which allows the researcher to review the data, and the computer often contains complex software for detailed analysis of the data and will provide a printed report of the analysis (DeKeyser & Pugh, 1991; Pugh & DeKeyser, 1995). Figure 16-1 illustrates the process of electronic measurement.

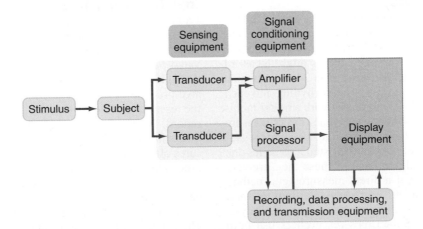

Figure **16-1** Process of electronic measurement.

The advantages of using electronic monitoring equipment are the collection of accurate and precise data, recording of data accurately within a computerized system, potential for collection of large amounts of data frequently over time, and the transmission of data electronically for analysis. One disadvantage of using sensors to measure physiological variables is that the presence of a transducer within the body can alter the reading. For example, the presence of a flow transducer in a blood vessel can partially block the vessel and thus alter blood flow. The reading, then, is not an accurate reflection of the flow.

Paratz and Lipman (2006) examined the effects of manual hyperinflation (MHI) on the hemodynamics and plasma catecholamines of ventilated patients. Electronic sensors were used to measure many of the variables in this study, and the measurement of the diastolic pressure, mean arterial pressure (MAP), pulmonary artery occlusion pressure (PAOP), and cardiac output (CO) are described in the following excerpt.

> Diastolic and MAP were recorded (Merlin pressure module M1006reA; Hewlett Packard) 1 minute before, during disconnection from the ventilator, at 1, 2, and 3 minutes during MHI, and at 1 and 5 minutes after MHI. The information was down-loaded to a computerized information system. PAOP was taken immediately before and after MHI at end of expiration. CO was measured by the Vigilance Cardiac Output System (Baxter Edwards Critical Care, Irwin, CA). This system employs a heated filament wrapped around a balloon flotation pulmonary artery catheter, which is positioned in the right atrium and ventricle. (Paratz & Lipman, 2006, p. 263)

Paratz and Lipman (2006) provided a detailed description of the electronic monitoring equipment they used to measure their study variables. They also detailed when the measurements of variables were obtained, the recording of data, and the preparation of the data for analysis, which were done electronically to reduce the potential for error and increase the accuracy of the data.

Creative Development of Physiological Measures

Some studies require imaginative approaches to measuring phenomena that are traditionally observed in clinical practice but are not measured. The first step in this process is to recognize that the phenomenon being observed by the nurse can be measured. Once that idea has emerged, one can begin envisioning various means of measuring the phenomenon.

Ro et al. (2002) selected a creative treatment and a creative physiological approach to measuring its effect. They describe their study as follows.

> This study was designed to investigate the effects of aromatherapy on pruritus in patients with chronic renal failure undergoing hemodialysis. The participants were 29 adult patients living in Seoul, Korea. Thirteen patients were assigned to the experimental group and received the aromatherapy massage on the arm 3 times a week for 4 weeks. Pruritus score, skin pH, stratum corneum hydration, and pruritus-related biochemical markers were measured before and after the treatment. The results showed that pruritus score was significantly decreased after aromatherapy. Skin pH showed no significant changes in either group while stratum corneum hydration increased significantly in the experimental group after aromatherapy. The results support the use of aromatherapy as a useful and effective method of managing pruritus in patients undergoing hemodialysis. (Ro et al., 2002; full-text article available in CINAHL)

As new physiological measurements are developed, they must be compared with previous methods to determine the best strategy for measuring each physiological outcome based on the patient's condition. Schallom, Sona, McSweeney, and Mazuski (2007) conducted a study to compare forehead and digit oximetry in surgical/trauma patients who were at risk for decreased peripheral perfusion. Previous research had shown that the measurement of pulse oximetry was often impaired in critically ill patients and that the forehead reflectance oximetry may be less susceptible to poor tissue perfusion and might improve the accuracy of oxygen saturation measurement. The following excerpt describes the measurement of oxygen saturation using both the forehead and digit oximetry devices. Figure 16-2 shows the Nellcor N-595 oximeter and Max-Fast forehead sensor.

> Pulse oximetry forehead reflectance (Max-Fast) sensors [Figure 16-2] were placed above the supraorbital ridge of consenting patients and secured in place with latex-free adjustable head band with a Velcro (Velcro USA, Manchester, NH) attachment. The existing pulse oximeter digit was not manipulated (Max A; digit 2). Patients were fitted with digit (Max A; digit 1); both digit 1 and forehead (Max-Fast) sensors were attached to a Nellcor N-595 (v 3.3.0) oximeter. The exiting digit sensor (Max A; digit 2), placed by the bedside nurse before study enrollment, was connected to a multiparameter monitor (Phillips CMS).... Digit sensors were placed on opposing hands to reduce the risk of optical/light interference during data collection. (Schallom et al., 2007, pp. 189–190)

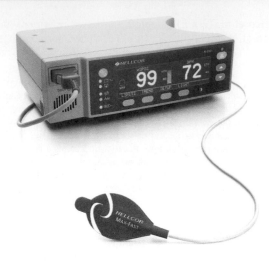

Figure **16-2** Nellcor N-595 oximeter and Max-Fast forehead sensor.

These researchers detailed the devices they used to obtain the oxygen saturation values and the placement of these devices to prevent error in the measurement process. They provided a picture of the devices and how to apply them to a patient and described the precision and accuracy of the devices in the narrative of the research article. Schallom et al. (2007, p. 188) found that "there were fewer unsuccessful measurements with the forehead oximetry technique." Thus, they concluded that the "forehead sensors improve measurement of oxygen saturation in critically ill surgical/trauma patients."

Obtaining Physiological Measures across Time

Many nursing studies using physiological measurement methods focus on a single point in time. Thus, there is insufficient information on normal variations in physiological measures across time, and much less information on changes in physiological measures across time in individuals with abnormal physiological states. In some cases, physiological states demonstrate cyclic activity and are associated with circadian rhythms and day-night patterns. When a clinician observes variation in a physiological value, it is important to know whether the variation is within the normal range or signals a change in the patient's condition. Thus, additional studies need to be conducted to describe patterns of physiological function over time.

Faulkner, Hathaway, and Tolley (2003, p. 10) studied the effects of age, sex, race, body mass index, and Tanner's stage on short-term evoked cardiovascular

autonomic tests (i.e., Valsalva ratio and change in heart rate with deep breathing) and 24-hour heart rate variability (HRV) in a sample of healthy adolescents. The researchers also identified normative indices of both short-term evoked and 24-hour HRV in this age group. The following excerpt identifies the measurement of the cardiovascular autonomic function and HRV over 24 hours.

Cardiovascular autonomic function typically is measured by a battery of short-term evoked cardiovascular reflex tests originally developed by Clarke and Ewing. These reflex tests evaluate heart rate and blood pressure changes to postural and respiratory maneuvers and include beat-to-beat (R-R) variation with the expiration-to-inspiration ratio, change in heart rate with deep breathing and with the Valsalva maneuver, and alteration in blood pressure response to postural change. The process of evaluating an individual's responses to the reflex tests allows for the detection of the "beat-to-beat" balance of sympathetic and parasympathetic modulation of the cardiac cycle, which can be altered by physical or psychologic stress.

The reflex tests were conducted in a temperature-controlled laboratory, maintained at 25 °C to 27 °C, and minimized environmental noise. Data collection of ECG [electrocardiogram] recordings was completed with a Power Macintosh 9500 computer with the AcqKnowledge III BIOPAC data acquisition and analysis system (Biopac Systems, Goleta, CA)....

In addition to evoked cardiovascular autonomic measures, 24-hour ambulatory heart rate monitoring with power spectral analysis was obtained on subjects. Power spectral analysis of HRV quantifies and discriminates between sympathetic and parasympathetic autonomic modulation of heart rate during a 24-hour period by recording the frequency oscillations of R-R variation. (Faulkner et al., 2003, p. 16)

Faulkner et al. (2003) clearly described their measurement of selective physiological variables over time to identify normal patterns of HRV in healthy adolescents. Their measurement methods seemed to be accurate and precisely implemented to obtained quality data.

Selecting a Physiological Measure

Researchers designing a physiological study have less assistance in selecting methods of measurement than do those conducting studies using psychosocial variables. Multiple books and electronic sources are available that discuss various methods for measuring psychosocial variables. In addition, numerous articles in nursing journals describe the development of psychosocial variables or discuss various means of measuring a particular psychosocial variable. However, literature guiding the selection of physiological variables is less available. You might consider the following factors when selecting a physiological measure for a study:

1. What physiological variables are relevant to the study?
2. Do the variables need to be measured continuously or at a particular point in time?
3. Are repeated measures needed?
4. Do certain characteristics of the population under study place limits on the measurement approaches that can be used?
5. How has the variable been measured in previous research?
6. Is more than one measurement method available to measure the physiological variable being studied?
7. Which measurement method is the most accurate and precise for the population you are studying?
8. Could the study be designed to include more than one measurement method for the variable being studied?
9. Where can the measurement device(s) be obtained to measure the physiological variable being studied?
10. Can the measurement device be obtained from the manufacturer for use in the study, or must it be purchased?

It is more difficult to identify previous research on physiological measures than it is to find research on psychosocial measures. The sources most commonly used to identify physiological measurement methods are previous studies that have measured a particular physiological variable. Literature reviews or meta-analyses can provide reference lists of relevant studies. Because the measure might have been used in studies unrelated to the current research topic, it is usually important to examine the research literature broadly.

Physiological measures must be linked conceptually with the framework of the study. The logic of operationalizing the concept in a particular way must be well thought out and expressed clearly. It is often a good idea to use diverse physiological measures of a single concept, which reduces the impact of extraneous variables that might affect measurement. The operationalization of a physiological variable in a study should clearly indicate the physiological measure to be used. The link of the physiological variable to the concept in the framework must be made explicit in the published report of your study.

You also must evaluate the accuracy and precision of physiological measures. Until recently, researchers commonly used information from the equipment manufacturer to describe the accuracy of measurement. This information is useful but not sufficient to evaluate accuracy and precision. The accuracy and precision of physiological measures are discussed in Chapter 15.

One field of research in which considerable effort has been put forth to develop and evaluate measures is wound healing. Identifying valid and reliable measurement methods is important for comparing the effectiveness of various methods of treating a wound. Measurement strategies that have been applied include tracing the outline of the wound, inspecting the wound with a hand-held scanner, using electronic cameras, employing a structured light-scanning device, and applying a computer vision method based on image processing. Other strategies involve measuring wound volume by filling it with various substances such as normal saline, plaster of Paris, or a high-viscosity vinyl polysiloxane (Gentzkow, 1995; Harding, 1995). Thomas (1997) developed a model for the perfect wound-healing instrument and evaluated existing tools in terms of the model. A number of studies have been conducted to compare the accuracy and precision of these measures (Etris, Pribble, & LaBrecque, 1994; Hansen, Sparrow, Kokate, Leland, & Iaizzo, 1997; Liskay, Mion, & Davis, 1993; Melhuish, Plassman, & Harding, 1994). Researchers have not yet reached a consensus on the most desirable method of measurement, and methodological studies in this area continue.

You will need to consider problems you might encounter when using various approaches to physiological measurement. One factor of concern is the sensitivity of the measure. Will the measure detect differences finely enough to avoid a type II error? Physiological measures are usually norm referenced. Thus, data obtained from a subject will be compared with a norm, as well as with other subjects. You will need to determine whether the norm used for comparison is relevant for the population you are studying. For example, Schallom et al. (2007) compared the effectiveness of the digit versus the forehead oximetry in accurately measuring oxygen saturation in surgical/trauma patients. These patients had decreased peripheral perfusion; thus, their oxygen saturation was best measured by the forehead versus the digit oximetry. How labile is the measure? Some measures vary within the individual from time to time, even when conditions are similar. Circadian rhythms, activities, emotions, dietary intake, or posture can also affect physiological measures, as indicated by Faulkner et al. (2003). To what extent will these factors affect the ability to interpret measurement outcomes?

Many measurement strategies require the use of specialized equipment. In many cases, the equipment is available in the patient care area and is part of routine patient care in that unit. Otherwise, the researcher may need to purchase, rent, or borrow the equipment specifically for the study. You will need to be skilled in operating the equipment or obtain the assistance of someone who has these skills. Make sure that the equipment is operated in an optimal fashion and is used in a consistent manner. Sometimes equipment must be recalibrated, or reset, regularly to ensure consistent readings. For example, weight scales are recalibrated periodically to ensure that the weight indicated is accurate and precise. According to federal guidelines, recalibration must be performed as follows:

- In accordance with the manufacturers' instructions
- In accordance with criteria set up by the laboratory
- At least every 6 months
- After major preventive maintenance or replacement of a critical part
- When quality control indicates a need for recalibration

When publishing the results of a physiological study, you must describe the measurement technique in considerable detail to allow an adequate critical appraisal of your study, enable others to replicate your study, and promote clinical application of the results. At present, few replications of physiological studies have been reported in the nursing literature. A detailed description of physiological measures in a research report includes (1) a description of the equipment or device used in performing the measurement, (2) the name of the equipment manufacturer, (3) an account of the accuracy and precision of the equipment or device based on previous research and the manufacturer, (4) an explanation of the exact procedure followed to measure the physiological variable, and (5) an overview of the process the device used to record, retrieve, and store data. The examples discussed in this section can be used as models for describing the methods for obtaining and precisely implementing physiological measures in research to obtain accurate measures of physiological variables.

OBSERVATIONAL MEASUREMENT

Observational measurement is the use of unstructured and structured inspection to gauge a study variable. This section focuses on structured observational measurement, and unstructured measurement is described in Chapter 23. Although measurement by observation is most common in qualitative research, it is used to some extent in all types of studies (Marshall & Rossman, 2006). First you must decide what you want to observe, and then determine how to ensure that every variable is observed in a similar manner in each instance. Therefore, much attention must be given to training data collectors, especially when the observations are complex and examined over time. You must create opportunities for the observational technique to be pilot-tested and to generate data on interrater reliability. Observational measurement tends to be more subjective than other types of measurement and is thus often seen as less credible. However, in many cases, observation is the only possible way to obtain important evidence for practice.

Structured Observations

The first step in a structured observation is to define carefully what is to be inspected or observed in a study. From that point, you will direct your concern toward how the observations are to be made, recorded, and coded. In most cases, you and your research team will develop a category system for organizing and sorting the behaviors or events being observed. The extent to which these categories are exhaustive varies with the study.

Category Systems

The observational categories should be mutually exclusive. If the categories overlap, the observer will be faced with making judgments regarding what category should contain each observed behavior, and data collection may not be consistent. In some category systems, only the behavior that is of interest is recorded. Most category systems require the observer to make some inference from the observed event to the category. The greater the degree of inference required, the more difficult the category system is to use. Some systems are applicable in a wide variety of studies, whereas others are specific to the study for which they were designed. The number of categories used varies considerably with the study. An optimal number for ease of use and therefore effectiveness of observation is 15 to 20 categories.

Checklists

Checklists are techniques used to establish whether a behavior occurred. The observer places a tally mark on a data collection form each time he or she witnesses the behavior. Behavior other than that on the checklist is ignored. In some studies, the observer may place multiple tally marks in various categories while witnessing a particular event. However, in other studies, the observer is required to select a single category in which to place the tally mark. Minnick, Mion, Johnson, Catrambone, and Leipzig (2007) used a checklist to structure their observations of the prevalence and variation of physical restraint use in acute care settings. They provided a detailed description of their measurement process that included extensive training of data collectors and checks for interrater reliability, which was extremely high (>98%) in this study.

Data collection included direct observation and nurse report. The data collector (DC) informed the unit's charge nurse of his or her presence and then determined the overall census and number of patients by gender, ventilatory status, and age category (less than 65, 65 and older). The DC inquired about the PR [physical restraint] use and recorded the nurse's stated reasons for use, age, ventilatory status, and gender of each restrained individual. The DC also made a unit tour to verify the reports of use. DCs were not authorized to review charts.

Site contacts conducted two to three unannounced reliability checks per data collector during the 18-day period. A research team member, the site contact, and a data collector participated in additional reliability checks usually 7 days after the first reliability check to decrease technique variability within and between institutions.... High levels of interrater reliability (>98%) were maintained. (Minnick et al., 2007, p. 32)

Rating Scales

Rating scales, which we will discuss later in this chapter, can be used for observation as well as for self-reporting. A rating scale allows the observer to rate the behavior or event on a scale. This method provides more information for analysis than does the use of dichotomous data, which indicate only that the behavior either occurred or did not occur.

Drankiewicz and Dundes (2003) used observational methods in their study of handwashing among female college students, which is described in the following section.

Our study used observation methods similar to those used by Guinan et al. (1997) in that we observed handwashing behavior among students after bathroom use. Whereas the observers in the study by Guinan et al. were out in the open but unknown as observers by the participants, in our study, the principal investigator conducted observations of handwashing behavior from inside a bathroom stall. This vantage point was selected to minimize

the Hawthorne effect that can result from the presence of a suspected observer. The principal investigator conducted observations over a 3-month period, February to April 2002, in 2 bathrooms at the college. The identity of those observed was not recorded. One of the bathrooms was in a building housing classrooms and the other was in a campus recreational area. The layout of both bathrooms consisted of a row of 5 toilets, with a row of 5 sinks situated in front of the stalls. The bathrooms had ample supplies of handwashing soap in dispensers located next to each sink and paper-towel dispensers were stocked with easy-to-access towels. Observations made from inside a bathroom stall took place at various times during the day including lunchtime, dinnertime, and during the transitional period between day classes. Although the door to the principal investigator's stall was closed, there was sufficient space next to the door's hinges to allow her to observe handwashing behavior. We did not seek the consent of those under observation because, as delineated in institutional review board guidelines, we fell under research exempt from obtaining consent because we conducted observational research in a public area and did not record the data in such a manner that human participants could be identified, either directly or through identifiers linked to the participants. Nor could any disclosure of the human participants' responses reasonably place them at risk of criminal or civil liability or damage their employability or reputation. Duration of the wash was recorded using a digital stopwatch. Data collected included time, location, whether the hands were washed, if soap was used among those who washed their hands, the duration of the handwashing, and the number of other persons present in the sink area at the time a student exited the toilet stall. (Drankiewicz & Dundes, 2003; full-text article available in CINAHL)

INTERVIEWS

Interviews involve verbal communication during which the subject provides information to the researcher. Although this measurement strategy is most common in qualitative and descriptive studies, it can be used in other types of studies as well. There are various approaches to conducting an interview. They range from the totally unstructured interview in which the subject completely controls content (see Chapter 23) to interviews in which the subject responds to a questionnaire that the researcher has carefully designed. Although most interviews are conducted face to face, telephone interviews are becoming more common (Burnard, 1994). Chapple (1997) pointed out that most interviews in nursing studies have concerned those in relatively powerless positions in society. To successfully interview persons in positions of power, you may have to vary the approach.

Using the interview method for measurement requires careful, detailed work, and it has almost become a science in itself. Excellent books are available on the techniques of developing interview questions (Briggs, 1986; Converse & Presser, 1986; Dillman, 1978; Dillon, 1990; Fowler, 1990; Gorden, 1987; McCracken, 1988; McLaughlin, 1990; Mishler, 1986; Schuman, 1981). If you plan to use this strategy, consult a text on interview methodology before designing your instrument. Because nurses frequently use interview techniques in nursing assessment, the dynamics of interviewing are familiar; however, using this technique for measurement in research requires greater sophistication.

Structured Interviews

Structured interviews are verbal interactions with subjects that allow the researcher to exercise increasing amounts of control over the content of the interview to obtain essential data for a study. The researcher designs the questions before data collection begins, and the order of the questions is specified. In some cases, the interviewer is allowed to further explain the meaning of the question or modify the way in which the question is asked so that the subject can better understand it. In more structured interviews, the interviewer is required to ask the question precisely as it has been designed. If the subject does not understand the question, the interviewer can only repeat it. The subject may be limited to a range of responses previously developed by the researcher, similar to those in a questionnaire. If the possible responses are lengthy or complex, they may be printed on a card so that the subject can review them before selecting a response.

Designing Interview Questions

The process for developing and sequencing interview questions is similar to the process used to design questionnaires and will be explained in the section on questionnaires. Briefly, questions progress from broad and general to narrow and specific. Questions are grouped by topic, with fairly "safe" topics being addressed first and sensitive topics reserved until late in the interview process. Less interesting data such as age, educational level, income, and other demographic information are usually collected last. These data should not be collected during an interview if they can be obtained from another source such as a patient record. The wording of questions in an interview will depend on the educational level of the subjects. Different subjects may interpret the wording of certain questions in a variety of ways, and the researcher must anticipate this possibility. After the interview protocol has been developed, seek feedback from an expert on interview technique and also from a content expert.

Pretesting the Interview Protocol

Once you and your research team have satisfactorily developed the protocol, you will need to pretest or pilot-test it on subjects similar to those who will be included in your study. This pretest will allow you to identify problems in the design of questions, sequencing of questions, or procedure for recording responses. It also will give you a chance to assess the reliability and validity of the interview instrument.

Training Interviewers

Skilled interviewing requires practice, and interviewers must be familiar with the content of the interview. They must anticipate situations that might occur during the interview and develop strategies for dealing with them. One of the most effective methods of developing a polished approach is role-playing. Playing the role of the subject can give the interviewer insight into the experience and thus facilitate an effective response to unscripted situations.

The interviewer must establish a permissive atmosphere in which the subject is encouraged to respond to sensitive topics. He or she must also develop an unbiased verbal and nonverbal manner. The wording of a question, the tone of voice, a raised eyebrow, or a shifting body position can all communicate a positive or negative reaction to the subject's responses—either of which can alter the data.

Preparing for an Interview

If you are serving as the interviewer and expect the meeting to be lengthy, you will need to make an appointment. Make sure that you are nicely dressed but not overdressed, and be prompt. Choose a site for the interview that is quiet, private, and provides a pleasant environment. Before the appointment, carefully plan the instructions you will give to the subject. For example, you might say, "I am going to ask you a series of questions about ... Before you answer each question you need to ... Select your answer from the following ..., and then you may elaborate on your response. I will record your answer and then, if it is not clear, I may ask you to explain some aspect further."

Probing

Interviewers use **probing** to obtain more information in a specific area of the interview. In some cases, you may have to repeat a question. If your subject answers, "I don't know," you may have to press for a response. In other situations, you may have to explain the question further or ask the subject to explain statements that she or he has made. At a deeper level, you may pick up on a comment the subject made and begin asking questions to better understand what the subject meant. Probes should be neutral to avoid biasing the subject's responses. Probing needs to be done within reasonable guidelines so that the subject does not feel that he or she is being cross-examined.

Recording Interview Data

Data obtained from interviews are recorded, either during the interview or immediately afterward. The recording may be in the form of handwritten notes, DVD recordings, or audiotape recordings. If you hand-record your notes, you must have the skill to identify key ideas (or capture essential data) in an interview and concisely record this information. Data must be recorded without distracting the interviewee. Some interviewees have difficulty responding if it is obvious that the interviewer is taking notes or taping the conversation. In such a case, the interviewer may need to record data *after* completing the interview. If you would prefer to tape-record the interview, you must first obtain the subject's permission, and plan to prepare verbatim transcriptions of the tapes before data analysis. In some studies, researchers use content analysis to capture the meaning within the data (see Chapter 23).

Advantages and Disadvantages of Interviews

Interviewing is a flexible technique that can allow the researcher to explore greater depth of meaning than she or he can obtain with other techniques. Use your interpersonal skills to encourage your subject's cooperation and elicit more information. The response rate to interviews is higher than that to questionnaires, and thus interviews can offer a more representative sample. Interviews allow researchers to collect data from subjects who are unable or unlikely to complete questionnaires, such as the very ill or those whose reading, writing, and ability to express themselves are marginal.

Interviews are a form of self-report, and the researcher must assume that the information provided is accurate. Interviewing requires much more time than needed for questionnaires and scales and is thus more costly. Because of time and cost, sample size is usually limited. Subject bias is always a threat to the validity of the findings, as is inconsistency in data collection from one subject to another.

Dzurec and Coleman (1995) used hermeneutics to study the experience of interviewing from the perspective of the interviewer. They found that an unspoken power gradient was present during an interview that made the process difficult for the interviewer. The insight gained from the interview process and from relating to the interviewee as a person made the process seem worthwhile. As respondents indicated, "You find out stuff you never even thought to ask" (Dzurec & Coleman, 1995, p. 245). Recommendations emerging from the study included the following:

(a) Identifying one's agenda for conducting an interview and sharing it with interviewees in a way comfortable for the interviewer; (b) staying in touch with personal discomforts of the interviewer-interviewee relationship, for example, their disparate roles, knowledge levels, and health and social status; (c) allowing the interview to follow its own course, even if structured by an interview format; and (d) conducting retrospective analyses of interview data to guide subsequent interviews. (Dzurec & Coleman, 1995, p. 245)

Interviewing children requires a special understanding of the art of asking children questions. The interviewer must use words that children tend to use to define situations and events. He or she also must be familiar with the language skills that exist at varying stages of development. Children view topics differently than adults do. Their perception of time, past and present, is also different. Holaday and Turner-Henson (1989) provided detailed suggestions for developing an interview guide or questionnaire appropriate for children.

Some researchers use a combination of open-ended or unstructured interview questions and structured interview questions to gather the data needed for a study. For example, Harralson (2007, p. 96) used quantitative and qualitative methods to examine the "factors associated with delay in seeking emergency medical attention for acute ischemic symptoms in a sample of predominantly African American women." Harralson interviewed female patients who presented with symptoms of acute myocardial infarction (AMI) in a large, urban teaching hospital in the United States. The following excerpt describes the interview process used in this study.

■ *STRUCTURED INTERVIEW*

The study used a structured interview to explore the variables of interest. The 45-minute interview included questions pertaining to sociodemographics, social support, general physical health, medical comorbidities, perceived and practical barriers to seeking health care, and CHD [coronary heart disease] symptoms and severity. Open-ended questions addressed the patients' experiences from symptom onset until a decision was made to seek medical attention. Open-ended questions included questions about patients' physical and emotional feelings during the experience, decision-making processes (i.e., who they told and who they sought advice from), and beliefs about what was happening to them at the onset of the symptoms of AMI.

The structured interview was developed specifically for this study on the basis of a systematic review of the literature that examined concepts and factors associated with delay in seeking medical treatment. In addition, several nurses, cardiologists, and social scientists reviewed the interview.

To reduce recall bias in this study, interviews were conducted within 5 days of the acute ischemic event. This recall time frame is similar to time periods used in other studies reviewed in the background section. (Harralson, 2007, p. 98)

QUESTIONNAIRES

A questionnaire is a printed self-report form designed to elicit information that can be obtained from a subject's written responses. The information derived through questionnaires is similar to that obtained by interview, but the questions tend to have less depth. The subject is unable to elaborate on responses or ask for questions to be clarified, and the data collector cannot use probe strategies. However, questions are presented in a consistent manner, and there is less opportunity for bias than in an interview.

Questionnaires can be designed to determine facts about the subject or persons known by the subject; facts about events or situations known by the subject; or beliefs, attitudes, opinions, levels of knowledge, or intentions of the subject. Questionnaires can be distributed to large samples directly or indirectly through e-mail or mail. The design, development, and administration of questionnaires have been the topics of many excellent books that focus on survey techniques (Berdie, Anderson, & Niebuhr, 1986; Converse & Presser, 1986; Fox & Tracy, 1986; Sudman & Bradburn, 1982). Two nursing methodology texts (Shelley, 1984; Waltz, Strickland, & Lenz, 1991) provide detailed explanations of the questionnaire development procedure.

Although questions on a questionnaire appear easy to design, a well-designed item requires considerable effort. Like interviews, questionnaires can have varying degrees of structure. Some questionnaires ask open-ended questions that require written responses. Others ask closed-ended questions with options that the researcher has selected.

Data from open-ended questions are often difficult to interpret, and content analysis may be used to extract meaning. Open-ended questionnaire items are not advised if your data are being obtained from large samples. Researchers are now using computers to gather questionnaire data (Saris, 1991). Computers are set up at the data collection site, the questionnaire is presented on screen, and subjects respond by using the keyboard or mouse. Data are stored in a computer file and are immediately available for analysis. Data entry errors are greatly reduced. Questionnaires can also be e-mailed to subjects, or subjects can be directed to a website where they can complete the questionnaire online, allowing the data to be stored and analyzed immediately. Thus, researchers can keep track of the number of subjects completing their questionnaire and the evolving results.

Development of Questionnaires

The first step in either selecting or developing a questionnaire is to identify the information desired. For this purpose, you and your research team would develop a blueprint or table of specifications. The blueprint identifies the essential content to be covered by the questionnaire, and the content must be at the educational level of the potential subjects. It is difficult to stick to the blueprint when designing the questionnaire because it is tempting to add "just one more question" that seems a "neat idea" or a question that someone insists "really should be included." As a questionnaire lengthens, however, fewer subjects are willing to respond and more questions are left blank.

The second step is to search the literature for questionnaires or items in questionnaires that match the blueprint criteria. Sometimes published studies include questionnaires, but frequently you must contact the authors of a study to receive a copy of their questionnaire. Unlike scaling instruments, questionnaires are seldom copyrighted. Researchers are encouraged to use questions in exactly the same form as those in previous studies to enhance the accuracy when results of the two studies are compared. However, questions that are poorly written need to be modified, even if rewriting makes it more difficult to directly compare results.

In some cases, you may find a questionnaire in the literature that matches the questionnaire blueprint that you have developed for your study. However, you may have to add items to or delete items from an existing questionnaire to accommodate your blueprint. In some situations, items from several questionnaires are combined to develop an appropriate questionnaire.

An item on a questionnaire has two parts: a lead-in question (or stem) and a response set. Each lead-in question must be carefully designed and clearly expressed. Problems include ambiguous or vague language, leading questions that influence the response, questions that assume a preexisting state of affairs, and double questions.

In some cases, respondents will interpret terms used in the lead-in question in one way when the researcher intended a different meaning. For example, the researcher might ask how heavy the traffic is in the neighborhood in which the family lives. The researcher might be asking about automobile traffic, but the respondent interprets the question in relation to drug traffic. The researcher might define *neighborhood* as a region composed of a three-block area, whereas the respondent considers a neighborhood to be a much larger area. *Family* could be defined as those living in one house or as all close blood relations (Converse & Presser, 1986). If a question includes a term that is unfamiliar to the respondent or for which several meanings are possible, the term must be defined.

Leading questions suggest the answer the researcher desires. These types of questions often include value-laden words and indicate the researcher's bias. For example, a researcher might ask, "Do you believe physicians should be coddled on the nursing unit?" or "All hospitals are bad places to work, aren't they?" These examples are extreme, and leading questions are usually constructed more subtly. The degree of formality with which the question is expressed and the permissive tone of the questions are, in many cases, important for obtaining a true measure. A permissive tone suggests that any of the possible responses will be acceptable.

Questions implying a preexisting state of affairs lead the respondent to admit to a previous behavior regardless of how she or he answers. Examples are "How long has it been since you used drugs?" or, to an adolescent, "Do you use a condom when you have sex?"

Double questions ask for more than one bit of information, for example, "Do you like critical care nursing and working closely with physicians?" It would be possible for the respondent to like working in critical care settings but dislike working closely with physicians. In this case, the question would be impossible to answer accurately. A similar question is, "Was the in-service program educational and interesting?"

Questions with double negatives are also difficult to answer. For example, one might ask, "Do you believe nurses should not question doctors' orders? Yes or No." In this case, it is difficult to determine the meaning of a yes or no. Thus, the subjects' responses are uninterpretable.

Each item in a questionnaire has a **response set** that provides the parameters within which the respondent can answer. This response set can be open and flexible, as it is with open-ended questions, or it can be narrow and directive, as it is with closed-ended questions. For example, an open-ended question might have a response set of three blank lines. With closed-ended questions, the response set includes a specific list of alternatives from which to select.

Response sets can be constructed in a variety of ways. The cardinal rule is that every possible answer must have a response category. If the sample includes respondents who might not have an answer, then include a response category of "don't know" or "uncertain." If the information sought is factual, include "other" as one of the possible responses. However, recognize that the item "other" is essentially lost data. Even if the response is followed by a statement such as "Please explain," it is rarely possible to analyze the data meaningfully. If a large number of subjects (greater than 10%) select the alternative "other," the alternatives included in the response set might not be appropriate for the population studied.

The simplest response set is the dichotomous yes/no option. Arranging responses vertically preceded by a blank will reduce errors. For example,

_____Yes
_____No
is better than
_____Yes_____ No

because in the latter example, the respondent might not be sure whether to indicate *yes* by placing a response before or after the Yes.

Response sets must be mutually exclusive, which might not be the case in the following response set:

_____ Working full-time
_____ Full-time graduate student
_____ Working part-time
_____ Part-time graduate student

Burns (1986) used a questionnaire to examine smoking patterns of nurses in Texas. Items from that questionnaire, which demonstrates a variety of response

Select the response that most accurately describes you and mark it on the attached Scantron sheet.

1. Do you currently smoke cigarettes?

   a. no
   b. yes

2. How old were you when you started smoking?

   a. under 15
   b. 15 years   e. 18 years   h. 21 years
   c. 16 years   f. 19 years   i. 22 years
   d. 17 years   g. 20 years   j. older than 22 years

3. Before entering your basic (GENERIC) nursing education program,
   on the average, about how many cigarettes a day did you smoke?

   a. didn't smoke at all   d. 15–24 cigarettes/day
   b. didn't smoke every day   e. 25–39 cigarettes/day
   c. less than 15 cigarettes/day   f. 40 or more cigarettes/day

4. During your basic (GENERIC) nursing education program,
   on the average, about how many cigarettes a day did you smoke?

   a. didn't smoke at all   d. 15–24 cigarettes/day
   b. didn't smoke every day   e. 25–39 cigarettes/day
   c. less than 15 cigarettes/day   f. 40 or more cigarettes/day

5. How many organized programs have you attended to help you quit smoking?

   a. none   d. three   g. six
   b. one   e. four   h. seven
   c. two   f. five   i. eight

6. What is the longest single period you have stopped smoking?

   a. have never stopped   e. more than 1 month but less than 1 year
   b. less than a day   f. more than 1 year but less than 3 years
   c. less than a week   g. 3 years or more
   d. less than a month

7. Aside from what you think you actually could do, which would you most like to do?

   a. quit smoking   d. not sure at this time
   b. cut down   e. smoke as much as now
   c. cut down just a little

Figure **16-3** Example of items from a smoking questionnaire.

sets, are presented in Figure 16-3. Each question should clearly instruct the subject how to respond (i.e., choose one, mark all that apply), or instructions should be included at the beginning of the questionnaire. The subject must know whether to circle, underline, or fill in a circle as he or she responds to items. Clear instructions are difficult to construct and usually require several attempts, and each pilot should be tested on naive subjects who are willing and able to express their reactions to the instructions.

After the questionnaire items have been developed, you will need to carefully plan how they will be ordered. Questions related to a specific topic must be grouped together. General items are included first, with progression to more specific items. More important items might be included first, with subsequent progression to items of lesser importance. Questions of a sensitive nature or those that might be threatening should appear last on the questionnaire. In some cases, the response to one item may influence the response to another. If so, their order must be carefully considered. Any open-ended questions should be presented last because their responses will require more time than needed for closed-ended questions.

The general trend is to ask for demographic data about the subject at the end of the questionnaire.

Optical scanning sheets or teleforms may be used to speed up data entry on computer and decrease errors (see Chapter 17 about teleform development). As society becomes more digital, teleforms are becoming common. However, subjects who are not familiar with these sheets may make errors when entering their responses (thus decreasing measurement validity).

A cover letter explaining the purpose of the study, the name of the researcher, the approximate amount of time required to complete the form, and organizations or institutions supporting the study must accompany your questionnaire. Instructions include an address to which the questionnaire can be returned. This address must be at the end of the questionnaire, as well as on the cover letter and envelope. Respondents often discard both the envelope and the cover letter and, after completing the questionnaire, do not know where to send it. It is also wise to provide a stamped, addressed envelope for the subject to return the questionnaire. If possible, the best way to provide questionnaires to potential subjects is by e-mailing a web address for them to access the questionnaire. Subjects can easily complete the questionnaire in their own time, and their responses are automatically submitted at the end of the questionnaire. Sending questionnaires by e-mail have many advantages but one disadvantage is being able to access only individuals with e-mail. Thus, researchers need to determine if the population they are studying has e-mail access.

Your questionnaire must be pilot-tested to determine the clarity of questions, effectiveness of instructions, completeness of response sets, time required to complete the questionnaire, and success of data collection techniques. As with any pilot test, the subjects and techniques must be as similar as possible to those planned for the main study. In some cases, the open-ended questions are included in a pilot test to obtain information for the development of closed-ended response sets for the main study.

Questionnaire Validity

One of the greatest risks in developing response sets is leaving out an important alternative or response. For example, if the questionnaire item addressed the job position of nurses working in a hospital and the sample included nursing students, a category must be added to represent the student role. When seeking opinions, there is a risk of obtaining a response from an individual who actually has no opinion on the research topic. When an item requests knowledge that the respondent does not possess, the subject's guessing interferes with obtaining a true measure of the study variables.

The response rate to questionnaires is generally lower than that with other forms of self-reporting, particularly if the questionnaires are mailed out. If the response rate is lower than 50%, the representativeness of the sample is seriously in question. The response rate for mailed questionnaires is usually small (25% to 30%), so researchers are frequently unable to obtain a representative sample, even with randomization. There does seem to be a stronger response rate for questionnaires that are sent by e-mail. Strategies that can increase the response rate for a mailed questionnaire are covered in Chapter 17.

Commonly, respondents fail to respond to all the questions. This problem, especially with long questionnaires, can threaten the validity of the instrument. In some cases, the respondent will write in an answer if she or he does not agree with the available choices, or the respondent may write comments in the margin. Generally, these responses cannot be included in the analysis; however, you should keep a record of such responses. Before distributing the questionnaires, determine which questions are critical to the research topic. If any of these questions is omitted in a questionnaire, do not include the results of that question in the analysis.

Consistency in the way the questionnaire is administered is important to validity. For example, administering some questionnaires in a group setting, mailing others, and e-mailing others is not wise. There should not be a mix of mailing or e-mailing to business addresses and to home addresses. If questionnaires are administered in person, the administration must be consistent. Several problems in consistency can occur: (1) Some subjects may ask to take the form home to complete it and return it later, whereas others will complete it in the presence of the data collector; (2) some subjects may complete the form themselves, whereas others may ask a family member to write the responses that the respondent dictates; and (3) in some cases, a secretary or colleague may complete the form, rather than the individual whose response you are seeking. These situations lead to biases in responses that are unknown to the researcher, and they alter the true measure of the variables.

Analysis of Questionnaire Data

Data from questionnaires are usually ordinal in nature, which limits analysis for the most part to summary statistics and nonparametric statistics. However, in some cases, ordinal data from questionnaires are treated as interval data, and t-tests or analyses of variance (ANOVA) are used to test for differences between responses of various subsets of the sample. Discriminant analysis may be used to determine the ability to predict membership in various groups from responses to particular questions.

SCALES

Scales, a form of self-report, are a more precise means of measuring phenomena than are questionnaires. The majority of scales have been developed to measure psychosocial variables. However, self-reports can be obtained on physiological variables such as pain, nausea, or functional capacity by using scaling techniques. Scaling is based on mathematical theory, and there is a branch of science whose primary concern is the development of measurement scales. From the point of view of scaling theory, considerable measurement error (random error) and systematic error are expected in a single item. Therefore, in most scales, the various items on the scale are summed to obtain a single score, and these scales are referred to as **summated scales**. Less random error and systematic error exist when using the total score of a scale. Using several items in a scale to measure a concept is comparable to using several instruments to measure a concept (see Figure 15-7 in Chapter 15). The various items in a scale increase the dimensions of the concept that are reflected in the instrument. The types of scales described include rating scales, the Likert scale, semantic differentials, and visual analogue scales.

Rating Scales

A rating scale, the crudest form of scaling technique, lists an ordered series of categories of a variable that are assumed to be based on an underlying continuum. A numerical value is assigned to each category, and the fineness of the distinctions between categories varies with the scale. The general public commonly uses rating scales. In conversations one can hear statements such as "On a scale of 1 to 10, I would rank that …" Rating scales are easy to develop; however, one must be careful to avoid end statements that are so extreme that no subject will select them. A rating scale could be used to rate the degree of cooperativeness of the patient or the value placed by the subject on nurse-patient interactions. This type of scale is often used in observational measurement to guide data collection. The Faces Pain Scale is a commonly used rating scale to assess the pain of children in clinical practice, and it has proven to be valid and reliable over the years (Figure 16-4). Pain in adults is often assessed with a numeric rating scale (NRS) like the one presented in Figure 16-5.

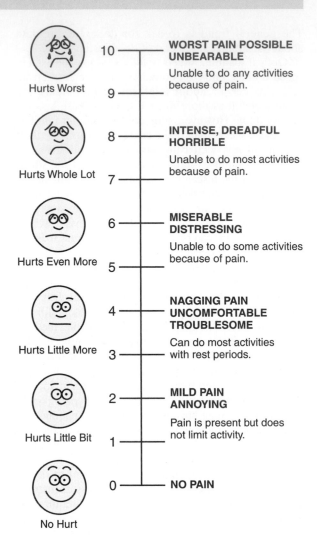

Figure **16-4** FACES Pain Scale.

Likert Scale

The Likert scale determines the opinion or attitude of a subject and contains a number of declarative statements with a scale after each statement. The Likert scale is the most commonly used of the scaling techniques. The original version of the scale included five response categories. Each response category was assigned a value, with a value of 1 given to the most negative response and a value of 5 to the most positive response (Nunnally & Bernstein, 1994).

Response choices in a Likert scale most commonly address agreement, evaluation, or frequency. Agreement options may include statements such as *strongly agree, agree, uncertain, disagree*, and *strongly disagree*. Evaluation responses ask the

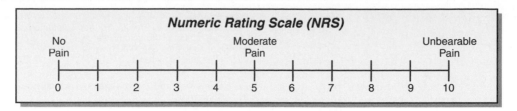

Figure **16-5** Numerical Rating Scale (NRS).

respondent for an evaluative rating along a good/bad dimension, such as positive to negative or excellent to terrible. Frequency responses may include statements such as *never, rarely, sometimes, frequently,* and *all the time.* The terms used are versatile and must be selected for their appropriateness to the stem (Spector, 1992). Sometimes seven options are given, sometimes only four.

Use of the uncertain or neutral category is controversial because it allows the subject to avoid making a clear choice of positive or negative statements. Thus, sometimes only four or six options are offered, with the uncertain category omitted. This type of scale is referred to as a **forced choice** version. Sometimes respondents will become annoyed at forced choice items and refuse to complete them. Researchers who use the forced choice version consider an item that is left blank as a response of "uncertain." However, responses of "uncertain" are difficult to interpret, and if a large number of respondents select that option or leave the question blank, the data may be of little value.

How the researcher phrases item stems depends on the type of judgment that the respondent is being asked to make. Agreement items are declarative statements such as "Nurses should be held accountable for managing a patient's pain." Frequency items can be behaviors, events, or circumstances to which the respondent can indicate how often they occur. A frequency stem might be "You read research articles in nursing journals." An evaluation stem could be "The effectiveness of 'X' drug for relief of nausea after chemotherapy." Items must be clear, concise, and concrete (Spector, 1992).

An instrument using a Likert scale usually consists of 10 to 20 items, each addressing an element of the concept being measured. Half the statements should be expressed positively and half negatively to avoid inserting bias into the responses. Scale values of negatively expressed items must be reversed before analysis. Usually, the values obtained from each item in the instrument are summed to obtain a single score

for each subject. Although the values of each item are technically ordinal-level data, the summed score is often treated as interval-level data, thus allowing more sophisticated statistical analyses. Some researchers now treat each item as interval-level data. The Zung Depression Scale is a Likert scale used to assess the level of depression in patients in clinical practice (Figure 16-6). This scale has four response options, which include *none or a little of the time* = 1, *some of the time* = 2, *good part of the time* = 3, and *most of the time* = 4. The scores on the scale can range from 20 to 80 with the interpretation of the scores being: below 50, within normal range, no psychopathology; 50–59, presence of minimal to mild depression; 60–69, presence of moderate to marked depression; and 70 and over, presence of severe to extreme depression. This scale was developed in the 1960s and has extensive testing through research; it is frequently used in clinical practice as a screening tool for depression (Zung, 1965).

Flaskerud (1988) reported difficulty using the Likert scale with some cultural groups. Hispanic and Vietnamese subjects had difficulty understanding the request to select one of four or five possible responses and insisted on responding to each item with a simple yes or no. Additional explanation did not sway them from this position. The reason for this difficulty is not understood.

Semantic Differentials

The **semantic differential scale** was developed by Osgood, Suci, and Tannenbaum (1957) to measure attitudes or beliefs. It is now used more broadly to measure variations in views of a concept. A semantic differential scale consists of two opposite adjectives with a seven-point scale between them. The subject is to select one point on the scale that best describes his or her view of the concept being examined. The scale is designed to measure the connotative meaning of the concept to the subject. Although the adjectives may not seem to be particularly related to the concept being examined, the technique can be used to distinguish varying degrees

Instructions
Read each sentence carefully. For each statement, check the bubble in the column that best corresponds to how often you have felt that way during the past two weeks.

For statements 5 and 7, if you are on a diet, answer as if you were not.

Please check a response for each of the 20 items.	None or a little of the time	Some of the time	Good part of the time	Most or all of the time
1 I feel downhearted, blue, and sad	O	O	O	O
2 Morning is when I feel the best	O	O	O	O
3 I have crying spells or feel like it	O	O	O	O
4 I have trouble sleeping through the night	O	O	O	O
5 I eat as much as I used to	O	O	O	O
6 I enjoy looking at, talking to, and being with attractive women/men	O	O	O	O
7 I notice that I am losing weight	O	O	O	O
8 I have trouble with constipation	O	O	O	O
9 My heart beats faster than usual	O	O	O	O
10 I get tired for no reason	O	O	O	O
11 My mind is as clear as it used to be	O	O	O	O
12 I find it easy to do the things I used to do	O	O	O	O
13 I am restless and can't keep still	O	O	O	O
14 I feel hopeful about the future	O	O	O	O
15 I am more irritable than usual	O	O	O	O
16 I find it easy to make decisions	O	O	O	O
17 I feel that I am useful and needed	O	O	O	O
18 My life is pretty full	O	O	O	O
19 I feel that others would be better off if I were dead	O	O	O	O
20 I still enjoy the things I used to do	O	O	O	O

Figure **16-6** Zung Self-Rating Depression Scale (SDS).

of positive and negative attitudes toward a concept. Figure 16-7 illustrates the form used for this type of scale.

In a semantic differential scale, values from 1 to 7 are assigned to each of the spaces, with 1 being the most negative response and 7 the most positive. Placement of negative responses to the left or right of the scale should be randomly varied to avoid global responses (in which the subject places checks in the same column of each scale). Each line is considered one scale. The values for the scales are summed to obtain one score for each subject. Factor analysis is used to determine the factor structure, which is expected to reflect three factors or dimensions: evaluation, potency, and activity. The researcher must explain theoretically why

particular items on the scale cluster together in the factor analysis. Thus, development of the instrument contributes to theory development. Factor analysis is also used to evaluate the validity of the instrument. With some of these instruments, three factor scores, each representing one of the dimensions, are used to describe the subject's responses and are a basis for further analysis (Nunnally & Bernstein, 1994).

Visual Analogue Scales
One of the problems with scaling procedures is the difficulty of obtaining a fine discrimination of values. An effort to resolve this problem is the **visual analogue scale**, sometimes referred to as *magnitude scaling* (Gift, 1989). This technique seems to provide

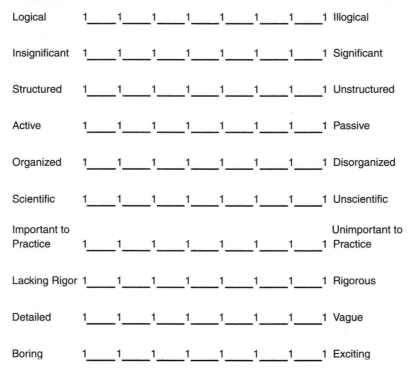

Nursing Research

Logical	1____1____1____1____1____1____1____1	Illogical
Insignificant	1____1____1____1____1____1____1____1	Significant
Structured	1____1____1____1____1____1____1____1	Unstructured
Active	1____1____1____1____1____1____1____1	Passive
Organized	1____1____1____1____1____1____1____1	Disorganized
Scientific	1____1____1____1____1____1____1____1	Unscientific
Important to Practice	1____1____1____1____1____1____1____1	Unimportant to Practice
Lacking Rigor	1____1____1____1____1____1____1____1	Rigorous
Detailed	1____1____1____1____1____1____1____1	Vague
Boring	1____1____1____1____1____1____1____1	Exciting

Figure **16-7** Example items from a semantic differential scale to measure nursing research.

interval-level data, and some researchers argue that it provides ratio-level data (Sennott-Miller, Murdaugh, & Hinshaw, 1988). It is particularly useful in scaling stimuli (Lodge, 1981). This scaling technique has been used to measure pain, mood, anxiety, alertness, craving for cigarettes, quality of sleep, attitudes toward environmental conditions, functional abilities, and severity of clinical symptoms (Wewers & Lowe, 1990).

The stimuli must be defined in a way that the subject clearly understands. Only one major cue should appear for each scale. The scale is a line 100 mm in length with right-angle stops at each end. The line may be horizontal or vertical. Bipolar anchors are placed beyond each end of the line. The anchors should *not* be placed underneath or above the line before the stop. These end anchors should include the entire range of sensations possible in the phenomenon being measured. Examples include "all" and "none," "best" and "worst," and "no pain" and "pain as bad as it could possibly be." These scales can be developed for children by using pictorial anchors at each end of the line rather than words (Lee & Kieckhefer, 1989).

The subject is asked to place a mark through the line to indicate the intensity of the stimulus. A ruler is then used to measure the distance between the left end of the line and the mark placed by the subject. This measure is the value of the stimulus. The scale is designed to be used while the subject is seated. Whether use of the scale from the supine position influences the results by altering perception of the length of the line has yet to be determined (Gift, 1989).

Wewers and Lowe (1990) have published an extensive evaluation of the reliability and validity of visual analogue scales, although reliability is difficult to determine. Because most of the variables measured with the tool are labile, test-retest consistency is not applicable, and because a single measure is obtained, internal consistency cannot be examined. The visual analogue scale is more sensitive to small changes than numerical and rating scales are and can discriminate between two dimensions of pain. Comparisons of the scale with other instruments measuring the same construct have had varying results and are difficult to interpret. An example of a visual analogue scale is shown in Figure 16-8.

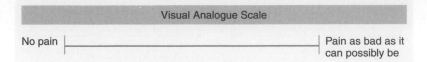

Figure **16-8** Example of a visual analogue scale to measure pain.

Q-SORT METHODOLOGY

Q-sort methodology is a technique of comparative rating that preserves the subjective point of view of the individual (McKeown & Thomas, 1988). Cards are used to categorize the importance placed on various words or phrases in relation to the other words or phrases in the list. Each phrase is placed on a separate card. The number of cards should range from 40 to 100 (Tetting, 1988). The subject is instructed to sort the cards into a designated number of piles, usually 7 to 10 piles ranging from the most to the least important. However, the subject is limited in the number of cards that may be placed in each pile. If the subject must sort 59 cards, category 1 (of greatest importance) may allow only 2 cards; category 2, 5 cards; category 3, 10 cards; category 4, 25 cards; category 5, 10 cards; category 6, 5 cards; and category 7 (the least important), 2 cards. Thus, placement of the cards fits the pattern of a normal curve. The subject is usually advised to select first the cards that he or she wishes to place in the two extreme categories and then work toward the middle category (which contains the largest number of cards), rearranging cards until he or she is satisfied with the results.

The Q-sort method can also be used to determine the priority of items or the most important items to include in the development of a scale. In the previously mentioned example, the behaviors sorted into categories 1, 2, and 3 might be organized into a 17-item scale. Correlational or factor analysis is used to analyze the data (Dennis, 1986; Tetting, 1988). Simpson (1989) suggested using the Q-sort method for cross-cultural research, with pictures rather than words used for nonliterate groups.

The Q-sort technique is used in the Control Preferences Scale, a general measure of a unidimensional construct involving consumer preferences about participating in decisions regarding their treatment. The Control Preferences Scale is administered by having each subject sort a series of cards through successive paired comparisons (Degner, 1998). Luniewski, Riegle, and White (1999) used a Q-sort technique in their study of effective education for patients with heart failure. Patients were asked to sort 12 cards with questions related to the content of discharge teaching for patients with heart failure.

DELPHI TECHNIQUE

The **Delphi technique** measures the judgments of a group of experts for the purpose of making decisions, assessing priorities, or making forecasts. Using this technique allows a wide variety of experts to express opinions and provide feedback, nationally and internationally, without meeting together. When the Delphi technique is used, the opinions of individuals cannot be altered by the persuasive behavior of a few people at a meeting. Three types of Delphi techniques have been identified: classic Delphi, policy Delphi, and decision Delphi. In classic Delphi, the focus is on reaching consensus. In policy Delphi, the aim is not consensus but rather to identify and understand a variety of viewpoints. In decision Delphi, the panel consists of individuals in decision-making positions. The purpose is to come to a decision (Beretta, 1996; Crisp, Pelletier, Duffield, Adams, & Nagy, 1997). Some nursing specialty organizations have established their research priorities by using Delphi techniques (Rudy, 1996). Mitchell (1998) assessed the validity of the Delphi technique in nursing education planning and found that 98.1% of the predicted events had either occurred or were still expected to occur.

To implement the technique, the researcher identifies a panel of experts, but the criteria used to determine that a member of the panel is an expert are unclear. Members of the panel remain anonymous, even to each other. A questionnaire is developed that addresses the topics of concern. Although most questions call for closed-ended responses, the questionnaire usually contains opportunities for open-ended responses by the expert. Once they have completed the questionnaires, the respondents return them to the researcher, who then analyzes and summarizes the results. Methods used for this analysis are undefined. The role of the researcher is to maintain objectivity. The outcome of the statistical analysis is returned to

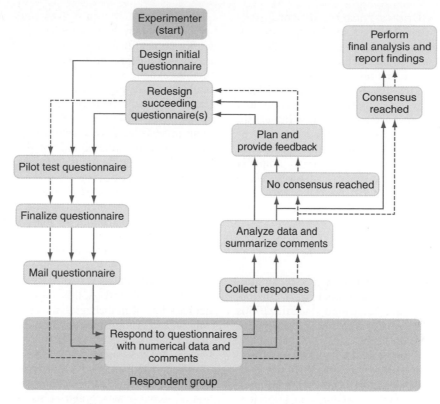

Figure **16-9** Delphi technique sequence model. Multiple arrows indicate repeated cycles of review by experts.

the panel of experts, along with a second questionnaire. Respondents with extreme responses to the first round of questions may be asked to justify their responses. The respondents return the second round of questionnaires to the researcher for analysis. This procedure is repeated until the data reflect a consensus among the panel. Limiting the process to two or three rounds is not a good idea if consensus is the goal. In some studies, true consensus is reached, whereas in others, "majority rules." Some question whether the agreement reached is genuine (Beretta, 1996; Crisp et al., 1997). Couper (1984) developed a model of the Delphi technique, which is presented in Figure 16-9.

Goodman (1987) identified several potential problems that researchers could encounter when using the Delphi technique. There has been no documentation that the responses of "experts" are different from those one would receive from a random sample of subjects. Because the panelists are anonymous, they have no accountability for their responses. Respondents could make hasty, ill-considered judgments because they know that no negative feedback will result. Feedback

on the consensus of the group tends to centralize opinion, and traditional analysis with the use of means and medians may mask the responses of those who are resistant to the consensus. Thus, conclusions could be misleading.

Lindeman (1975) conducted one of the initial studies to determine research priorities in clinical nursing using a Delphi survey. She used a panel of 433 experts, both nurses and non-nurses, with a wide range of interests. The panel was sent four rounds of a 150-item questionnaire. The report, published in *Nursing Research*, had an important influence on the research conducted in nursing for clinical practice.

PROJECTIVE TECHNIQUES

Projective techniques are based on the assumption that an individual's responses to unstructured or ambiguous situations reflect the person's attitudes, desires, personality characteristics, and motives. The technique is most frequently used in psychology and includes techniques such as the Rorschach Inkblot

Test, Machover's Draw-a-Person Test, word association, sentence completion, role-playing, and play techniques. The technique is an indirect measure of data that are unlikely to be obtained directly. Analysis of the data requires that inferences be made about the meaning and is therefore subjective. Many of the tests require extensive training for administration and interpretation and thus have not been used frequently in nursing research. However, with the increased frequency of interdisciplinary research, their use in nursing studies may increase. At present, the technique is used in nursing primarily in studying children (Waltz et al., 1991). Johnson (1990) provided an excellent explanation of the techniques used to interpret children's drawings.

DIARIES

A **diary** is a recording of events over time by an individual to document experiences, feelings, or behavior patterns. Diaries have been used since the 1950s to collect data for research from a variety of populations including children, the acute and chronically ill, pregnant women, and the elderly (Aroian & Wal, 2007). A diary, which allows recording shortly after an event, is thought to be more accurate than obtaining the information through recall during an interview. In addition, the reporting level of incidents is higher, and one tends to capture the participant's perception of situations (McColl, 2004).

The diary technique gives nurse researchers a means to obtain data on topics of particular interest within nursing that have not been accessible by other means. Some potential topics for diary collection include expenses related to a health care event (particularly out-of-pocket expenses), self-care activities (frequency and time required), symptoms of disease, eating behavior, exercise behavior, the child development process, and care provided by family members in a home-care situation. Although diaries have been used primarily with adults, they are also an effective means of collecting data from school-aged children. Butz and Alexander (1991) reported an 88% completion rate in a study of children with asthma, with most children (72.3%) keeping the diary without assistance from their parents.

Health diaries have been used to document health problems, responses to symptoms, and efficacy of responses. Diaries may also be used to determine how people spend their days; this information could be particularly useful in managing the care needs of individuals with chronic illnesses. In experimental studies, diaries may be used to determine subjects' responses to experimental treatments. Two types of health diaries are used: a ledger in which different types of events are recorded, such as the occurrence of a symptom, and a journal in which entries related to specific topics are made daily. Figure 16-10 shows an example of a ledger, and an example of a journal is shown in Figure 16-11. Figure 16-12 shows a sample patient diary.

Date	What symptom did you have?	Did you talk with a family member or friend about the symptom?		Did you talk with a health professional about it?		Did you take any pills or treatments for the symptom?	
		No	Yes	No	Yes	No	Yes, Specify

Figure **16-10** Sample ledger diary.

Validity and reliability have been examined by comparing the results with data obtained through interviews and have been found to be acceptable. Participation in studies using health diaries has been good, and attrition rates are reported as low. Adequate instructions related to recording data in the diary and arranging for pickup of the completed document are critical (Burman, 1995).

Burman (1995) made some recommendations regarding the general use of health diaries.

1. *Critically analyze the phenomenon of interest to ensure that it can be adequately captured using a diary. Infrequent major events, very minor health events or behaviors, and vague symptoms are less likely to be reported than more frequent, definable acute problems. The use of a diary should be evaluated in light of other data collection approaches such as interviews and emailed or mailed surveys, which may lead to higher data quality depending on the specific phenomenon of interest.*
2. *Determine which format—ledger or journal— should be used to decrease participant burden while minimizing missing data. The ledger format may be less burdensome but evaluation of missing data is more complicated.*
3. *Evaluate whether closed- or open-ended questions will result in clearer reporting. Closed-ended questions reduce respondent burden, but may result in overreporting of symptoms.*
4. *Pilot test any new or refined diary with the target population of interest to identify possible problems, to ensure that the phenomenon can be recorded with this approach, and to evaluate the ability of participants to complete diaries. Participation rates in diary studies vary, although those with high incomes and education levels, and better writing skills may be overrepresented. However, diaries have been used successfully with ill and general-community populations.*
5. *Determine the diary period that is necessary to adequately record changes and fluctuations in the phenomenon of interest, balancing this with respondent burden. Typical diary periods are 2 to 4 weeks.*
6. *Provide clear instructions to all participants on the use of a diary before participation begins to enhance data quality. Participants need to know how to use the diaries, what types of events are to be reported, and how to contact the investigator or clinician with questions.*

---

1. Did you have any symptoms today?
   a. NO → go to question 5
   b. YES, Please specify _____

2. Did you talk to a family member about the symptom(s)?
   a. NO
   b. YES

3. Did you talk to a health care professional about the symptom(s)?
   a. NO
   b. YES

4. Did you take any pills for the symptom(s)?
   a. NO → go to question 5
   b. YES, Please specify _____

5. How would you rate your health today?

Excellent _____ Poor

Figure 16-11 Sample journal diary.

The following samples are provided as a guide to keeping your diary. Every day when you write in the diary, please:

1. Record any health problem or problems you had (for example: constipation, skin rash on back, need bandages for surgery wound).

2. For each health problem, list the type of contact and person you contacted outside your home (such as nurse, doctor, social worker, pharmacist, or family member) and the place or agency (name of hospital, agency or facility, for example: Visiting Nurse Association).

3. Check (✓) whether you made the contact by telephone or in person for each contact.

4. Record the date of each contact. If you visited or called the same place at different times list each contact separately.

5. Identify, "yes" or "no," if the visit or telephone call helped you with your health problem.

6. Record the health problem even if you did not contact someone outside your home for help with it.

Sample Patient Diary

What health problem did you have?	What person and place did you contact for this health problem?	What type of contact did you make? Check ✓ one		When did you call/visit? (Record date)	Did you receive the help you needed?	
		Telephone call	Visit		Yes	No
skin irritation on back	Nurse, St. Jude Hospital	✓		Dec. 6, 1980	✓	
needed cold pack for leg pain	Pharmacist Mitchel's Pharmacy		✓	Jan. 6, 1981		✓
difficulty in walking, needed a cane	Counselor, American Cancer Society	✓		Jan. 26, 1981	✓	
feeling depressed	Minister, St. Paul's Church		✓	Jan. 26, 1981	✓	

Figure **16-12** Patient diary reports of home nursing.

7. *Use follow-up procedures during data collection to enhance completion rates. Telephone contacts enhance completion rates. Diaries may be mailed; however, returning diaries through the mail may result in somewhat lower completion rates.*

8. *Plan analysis procedures during diary development or refinement to be sure the data are in the appropriate form for the analyses. Diary data are very dense and rich, carefully prepared plans can minimize problems.* (Burman, 1995, p. 151)

Problems related to the diary method include costs, subject cooperation, quality of the data, conditioning effects on the subject of keeping a diary, and the complexity of data analysis. Costs include interview time, mail and telephone expenses, and remuneration to subjects. Costs are higher than single face-to-face interviews but lower than repeated interviews. Costs are lowest when diaries are used with telephone interviews and highest when diaries are used with repeated face-to-face interviews. Costs are lower when diaries are mailed rather than picked up. Most subject noncooperation occurs in the first month, with only 1% to 2% subject loss after that point. Diary completion rates are higher (80% to 88%) than the completion rates of other data collection methods such as surveys. Picking up the diary increases the completion rate (Butz & Alexander, 1991).

The use of diaries, however, has some disadvantages. Keeping the diary may, in some cases, alter the behavior or events under study. For example, if a person were keeping a diary of the nursing care that he or she was providing to patients, the insight that the person gained from recording the information in the diary might lead to changes in care. Subjects can become more sensitive to items (such as symptoms or problems) reported in the diary, which could result in overreporting. Subjects may also become bored with keeping the diary and become less thorough in recording items, which could result in underreporting (Butz & Alexander, 1991).

Aroian and Wal (2007) investigated the use of a diary for collecting data on symptom experiences in community-dwelling elderly. They found the participants' reporting of symptoms of chronic illness in the diary declined over the 7 days of the study and did not provide additional information that was not obtained from an interview. Arion and Wal (2007, p. 322) have recommended that researchers be very cautious in their selection of data collection methods for the elderly and that the diary might best be used to "focus on new symptoms or how symptoms unfold over time" rather than to record symptoms of chronic illnesses. Thus, there are strengths and weaknesses to the use of diaries in research, and investigators must determine what measurement method will provide the most valid and reliable information to address their study purpose.

SELECTION OF AN EXISTING INSTRUMENT

Selecting an instrument to measure the variables in a study is a critical process in research. The method of measurement must closely fit the conceptual definition of the variable. You may need to conduct an extensive search of the literature to identify appropriate methods of measurement. In many cases, you will find instruments that measure some of the needed elements but not all, or the content may be related to but somehow different from what you need for your study. Instruments found in the literature may have little or no documentation of their validity and reliability.

Beginning researchers often conclude that no appropriate method of measurement exists and that they therefore must develop a tool. At the time, this solution seems to be the most simple, because the researcher has a clear idea of what needs to be measured. You should not use this solution, however, unless all else fails. Tool development is a lengthy process and requires sophisticated research. Using a new instrument in a study without first evaluating its validity and reliability is unacceptable; it is a waste of subject and investigator time.

Thus, for novice researchers developing their first study, it is essential to identify existing instruments to measure your study variables. Jones (2004) developed a flowchart that might help you to select an existing instrument for your study (Figure 16-13). The major steps include (1) identifying an instrument from the literature, (2) determining if the instrument is appropriate for measuring your study variable, and (3) examining the performance of the instrument by evaluating its reliability and validity. These steps are detailed in the following sections.

Locating Existing Instruments

Locating existing measurement methods has become easier in recent years. A relatively new computer database, the Health and Psychological Instruments Online (HAPI), is available in many libraries and can search for instruments that measure a particular concept or for information on a particular instrument. Sometimes a search on Medline or CINAHL might uncover an instrument that might be useful (Roberts & Stone, 2003).

Many reference books have compiled published measurement tools, some that are specific to instruments used in nursing research. Dissertations often contain measurement tools that have never been published, so a review of *Dissertation Abstracts* might be helpful. *Dissertation Abstracts* is now online.

Another important source of recently developed measurement tools is word-of-mouth communication among researchers. Information on tools is often presented at research conferences years before publication. There are often networks of researchers conducting studies on similar nursing phenomena. These researchers are frequently associated with a nursing organization and keep in touch through newsletters, correspondence, telephone, e-mail, computer bulletin boards, and web pages. Thus, questioning available nurse researchers can lead to a previously unknown tool. These researchers can often be reached by telephone, letter, or e-mail and are usually willing to share their tools in return for access to the data to facilitate work on developing validity and reliability information. The Sigma Theta Tau *Directory of Nurse Researchers* provides address and phone information on nurse researchers. In addition, it lists nurse researchers by category according to their area of research.

Evaluating Existing Instruments for Appropriateness and Performance

You may need to examine several instruments to find the one most appropriate for your study. When selecting an instrument for research, carefully consider how the instrument was developed, what the instrument

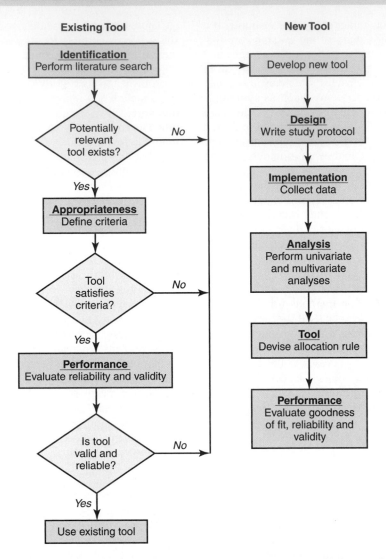

Figure **16-13** Flowchart depicting the identification and assessment of an existing tool and development of a new tool.

measures, and how to administer it. Before you review existing instruments, be sure you have conceptually defined your study variable and are clear on what you desire to measure. You will then need to address the following questions to determine the best instrument for measuring your study variable:

1. Does this instrument measure what you want to measure?
2. Does the instrument reflect your conceptual definition of the variable?
3. Is the instrument well constructed?
4. Does your population resemble populations previously studied with the instrument?
5. Is the readability level of the instrument appropriate for your population?
6. How sensitive is the instrument in detecting small differences in the phenomenon you want to measure (what is the effect size)?
7. What is the process for obtaining, administering, and scoring the instrument? Are there costs associated with the instrument?
8. What skills are required to administer the instrument? Do you have to have training or a particular credential to administer the instrument (Roberts & Stone, 2003)?
9. How are the scores interpreted?

10. What is the time commitment of the subjects and researcher for administration of the instrument?
11. What evidence is available related to the instrument's reliability and validity? Have multiple types of validity been examined (content validity, validity from factor analysis, validity from examining convergence and divergence, or evidence of validity from prediction of concurrent and future events)? Chapter 15 provided a detailed discussion of reliability and validity.

Particular populations may require further assessment to determine their instrumentation requirements. Burnside, Preski, and Hertz (1998) provided an excellent discussion of research instrumentation for elderly subjects. They identified four factors that should be considered when selecting research instruments for use with older adults: fatigue, anxiety, ethnic background, and education.

Assessing Readability Levels of Instruments

The readability level of an instrument is a critical factor when selecting an instrument for a study. Regardless of how valid and reliable the instrument is, you cannot use it effectively in your study if your subjects do not understand the items. Calculating readability is relatively easy and can be performed in about 20 minutes. Many word processing programs and computerized grammar checkers will report the readability level of written material. The Fog formula described in Chapter 15 provides a quick and easy way to assess readability. If the reading level of the instrument is beyond that of your population, you will need to select another instrument for use in your study. Changing the items on an instrument to reduce the reading level can alter the validity and reliability of the instrument.

CONSTRUCTING SCALES

Scale construction is a complex procedure that should not be undertaken lightly. There must be firm evidence of the need for developing another instrument to measure a particular phenomenon important to nursing practice. However, in many cases, measurement methods have not been developed for phenomena of concern to nurse researchers, or measurement tools that have been developed may be poorly constructed and have insufficient evidence of validity to be acceptable for use in studies. It is possible for the researcher to carry out instrument development procedures on an existing scale with inadequate evidence of validity before using it in a study. Neophyte nurse researchers could assist researchers in carrying out some of the field studies required to complete the development of scale validity and reliability.

The procedures for developing a scale have been well defined. The following discussion describes this theory-based process and the mathematical logic underlying it. The theories on which scale construction is most frequently based include classic test theory (Nunnally & Bernstein, 1994), item response theory (Hulin, Drasgow, & Parsons, 1983), multidimensional scaling (Davison, 1983; Kruskal & Wish, 1990), and unfolding theory (Coombs, 1950). Most existing instruments used in nursing research have been developed with classic test theory, which assumes a normal distribution of scores.

Constructing a Scale by Using Classic Test Theory

In classic test theory, the following process is used to construct a scale:

1. *Define the concept.* A scale cannot be constructed to measure a concept until the nature of the concept has been delineated. The more clearly the concept is defined, the easier it is to write items to measure it (Spector, 1992). Concepts are defined through the process of concept analysis, a procedure discussed in Chapters 4 and 7.
2. *Design the scale.* Items should be constructed to reflect the concept as fully as possible. The process of construction will differ somewhat depending on whether the scale is a rating scale, Likert scale, or semantic differential scale. Items previously included in other scales can be used if they have been shown empirically to be good indicators of the concept (Hulin et al., 1983). A blueprint may ensure that all elements of the concept are covered. Each item must be stated clearly and concisely and express only one idea. The reading level of items must be identified and considered in terms of potential respondents. The number of items constructed must be considerably larger than planned for the completed instrument because items will be discarded during the item analysis step of scale construction. Nunnally and Bernstein (1994) suggested developing an item pool at least twice the size of that desired for the final scale.
3. *Review the items.* As items are constructed, it is advisable to ask qualified individuals to review them. Crocker and Algina (1986) recommend asking for feedback in relation to accuracy, appropriateness, or relevance to test specifications;

technical flaws in item construction; grammar; offensiveness or appearance of bias; and level of readability. Revise items according to the critical appraisal.

4. *Conduct preliminary item tryouts.* While items are still in draft form, it is helpful to test them on a limited number of subjects (15 to 30) who represent the target population. Observe the reactions of respondents during testing to note behavior such as long pauses, answer changing, or other indications of confusion about specific items. After testing, a debriefing session must be held during which respondents are invited to comment on items and offer suggestions for improvement. Descriptive and exploratory statistical analyses are performed on data from these tryouts while noting means, response distributions, items left blank, and outliers. Revise items on the basis of this analysis and comments from respondents.

5. *Perform a field test.* Administer all the items in their final draft form to a large sample of subjects who represent the target population. Spector (1992) recommended a sample size of 100 to 200 subjects. However, the sample size needed for the statistical analyses to follow somewhat depends on the number of items. Some recommend including 10 subjects for each item being tested. If the final instrument was expected to have 20 items and 40 items were constructed for the field test, as many as 400 subjects could be required.

6. *Conduct item analyses.* The purpose of item analysis is to identify items that form an internally consistent or reliable scale and eliminate items that do not meet this criterion. Internal reliability implies that all the items are consistently measuring a concept. Before these analyses, negatively worded items must be reverse-scored or given a score as though the item was stated positively. For example, the item might read: I do not believe exercise is important to health with the responses of 1 strongly disagree, 2 disagree, 3 uncertain, 4 agree, and 5 strongly agree. If the subject marked a 1 for strongly disagree, this item would be reversed-scored and given a 5 indicating the subject thinks exercise is very important to health. The analyses examine the extent of intercorrelation among the items. The statistical computer programs currently providing (as a package) the set of statistical procedures needed to perform item analyses are SPSS, SPSS/PC, and SYSTAT.

These packages perform item-item correlations and item-total correlations. In some cases, the value of the item being examined is subtracted from the total score and an item-remainder coefficient is calculated. This latter coefficient is most useful in evaluating items for retention in the scale.

7. *Select items to retain.* Depending on the number of items desired in the final scale, items with the highest coefficients are retained. Alternatively, a criterion value for the coefficient (e.g., 0.40) can be set and all items greater than this value retained. The greater the number of items retained, the smaller the item-remainder coefficients can be and still have an internally consistent scale. After this selection process, a coefficient alpha is calculated for the scale. This value is a direct function of the number of items and the magnitude of intercorrelation. Thus, one can increase the value of a coefficient alpha by increasing the number of items or raise the intercorrelations through inclusion of more highly intercorrelated items. Values of coefficient alphas range from 0 to 1. The alpha value should be at least 0.70 to indicate sufficient internal consistency in a new tool (Nunnally & Bernstein, 1994). An iterative process of removing or replacing items, or both, recalculating item-remainder coefficients, and then recalculating the alpha coefficient is repeated until a satisfactory alpha coefficient is obtained. Deleting poorly correlated items will raise the alpha coefficient, but decreasing the number of items will lower it (Spector, 1992). The initial attempt at scale development may not achieve a sufficiently high coefficient alpha. In this case, additional items will need to be written, more data collected, and the item analysis redone. This scenario is most likely to occur when too few items were developed initially or when many of the initial items were poorly written. It may also be a consequence of attempts to operationalize an inadequately defined concept (Spector, 1992).

8. *Conduct validity studies.* When scale development is judged to be satisfactory, studies must be performed to evaluate the validity of the scale. (Refer to the discussion of validity in Chapter 15.) These studies require the researcher to collect additional data from large samples. As part of this process, scale scores must be correlated with scores on other variables proposed to be related to the concept being put

into operation. Hypotheses must be generated regarding variations in mean values of the scale in different groups. Exploratory and then confirmatory factor analysis (discussed in Chapter 20) is usually performed as part of establishing the validity of the instrument. As many different types of evidence of validity should be collected as possible (Spector, 1992).

9. *Evaluate the reliability of the scale.* Various statistical procedures must be performed to determine the reliability of the scale. These analyses can be performed on the data collected to evaluate validity. (See Chapter 15 for a discussion of the procedures performed to examine reliability.)

10. *Compile norms on the scale.* To determine norms, the scale must be administered to a large sample that is representative of the groups to which the scale is likely to be given. Norms should be acquired for as many diverse groups as possible. Data acquired during validity and reliability studies can be included for this analysis. To obtain the large samples needed for this purpose, many researchers permit others to use their scale with the condition that data from these studies be provided for compiling norms.

11. *Publish the results of development of the scale.* Scales are often not published for a number of years after the initial development because of the length of time required to validate the instrument. Some researchers never publish the results of this work. Studies using the scale are published, but the instrument development process may not be available except by writing to the author. This information needs to be added to the body of knowledge, and colleagues should encourage instrument developers to complete the work and submit it for publication (Lynn, 1989; Norbeck, 1985). Johnson and Rogers (2006) provided a detailed discussion of their development of the Purposeful Action Medication-Taking Questionnaire that might help you to understand the instrument development process. These researchers conducted a psychometric study to develop a questionnaire to measure the adherence to medication treatment by individuals with hypertension.

Constructing a Scale by Using Item Response Theory

Using item response theory to construct a scale proceeds initially in a fashion similar to that of classic test theory. There is an expectation of a well-defined concept

to operationalize. Items are initially written in a manner similar to that previously described, and item try-outs and field testing are also similar. However, the process changes with the initiation of item analysis. The statistical procedures used are more sophisticated and complex than those used in classic test theory. Using data from field testing, item characteristic curves are calculated by using logistic regression models (Hulin et al., 1983). After selecting an appropriate model based on information obtained from the analysis, item parameters are estimated. These parameters are used to select items for the scale. This strategy is used to avoid problems encountered with classic test theory measures.

Scales developed by using classic test theory effectively measure the characteristics of subjects near the mean. The statistical procedures used assume a linear distribution of scale values. Items reflecting responses of subjects closer to the extremes tend to be discarded because of the assumption that scale values should approximate the normal curve. Therefore, scales developed in this manner often do not provide a clear understanding of subjects at the high or low end of values.

One of the purposes of item response theory is to choose items in such a way that estimates of characteristics at each level of the concept being measured are accurate. To accomplish this goal, researchers use maximal likelihood estimates. A curvilinear distribution of scale values is assumed. Rather than choosing items on the basis of the item remainder coefficient, the researcher specifies a test information curve. The scale can be tailored to have a desired measurement accuracy. By comparing a scale developed by classic test theory with one developed from the same items with item response theory, one would find differences in some of the items retained. Biserial correlations would be lower in the scale developed from item response theory than in the scale developed from classic test theory. Item bias is lower in scales developed by using item response theory and occurs when respondents from different subpopulations having the same amount of an underlying trait have different probabilities of responding to an item positively (Hulin et al., 1983).

Constructing a Scale by Using Multidimensional Scaling

Multidimensional scaling is used when the concept being operationalized is actually an abstract construct believed to be represented most accurately by multiple dimensions. The scaling techniques used allow the researcher to uncover the hidden structure in the construct. The analysis techniques use proximities among the measures as input. The outcome of the analysis is a spatial representation, or a geometrical configuration of data points, that reveals the hidden structure. The procedure tends to be used to examine differences in stimuli rather than differences in people. Thus, a researcher might use this method to measure differences in perception of light or pain. Scales developed by using this procedure reveal patterns among items. The procedure is used in the development of rating scales and semantic differentials (Kruskal & Wish, 1990).

Constructing a Scale by Using Unfolding Theory

When a scale is being constructed with the use of unfolding theory, the researchers ask subjects to respond to the items in the rating scale. Next, they ask the subjects to rank the various response options in relation to the response option that they selected for that item. This procedure is followed for each item in the scale. By using this procedure, the underlying continuum for each scale item is "unfolded." As an example, suppose you developed the following item:

My preference for a diet to lose weight is
1. A low-fat diet
2. A low-calorie diet
3. A low-carbohydrate diet
4. A vegetarian diet

You would ask subjects to select their response to the item. You would then ask them to rank the other options according to the proximity to their choice. The subject might choose a low-calorie diet as number 1, a low-carbohydrate diet as number. 2, a low-fat diet as number 3, and a vegetarian diet as number 4. Although the preferences of other subjects would differ, the results can be plotted to reveal patterns of an underlying continuum. Items selected for the scale would be those with evidence of a pattern of responses. Degner (1998) used unfolding to analyze the results of patient responses to the Control Preferences Scale, a measure of consumer preferences about participating in decisions regarding treatment.

TRANSLATING A SCALE TO ANOTHER LANGUAGE

Contrary to expectations, translating an instrument from the original language to a target language is a complex process. By translating a scale, you can compare concepts among respondents of different cultures. The comparison requires that you first infer and then validate that the conceptual meaning in which the scale was developed is the same in both cultures. This process is highly speculative, and conclusions about the similarities of meanings in a measure must be considered tentative (Hulin et al., 1983).

Four types of translations can be performed: pragmatic translations, aesthetic-poetic translations, ethnographic translations, and linguistic translations. Pragmatic translations communicate the content from the source language accurately in the target language. The primary concern is the information conveyed. An example of this type of translation is the use of translated instructions for assembling a computer. Aesthetic-poetic translations evoke moods, feelings, and affect in the target language that are identical to those evoked by the original material. In ethnographic translations, the purpose is to maintain meaning and cultural content. In this case, translators must be familiar with both languages and cultures. Linguistic translations strive to present grammatical forms with equivalent meanings. Translating a scale is generally done in the ethnographic mode (Hulin et al., 1983).

One strategy for translating scales is to translate from the original language to the target language and then back-translate from the target language to the original language by using translators not involved in the original translation. Discrepancies are identified, and the procedure is repeated until troublesome problems are resolved. After this procedure, the two versions are administered to bilingual subjects and scored by standard procedures. The resulting sets of scores are examined to determine the extent to which the two versions yield similar information from the subjects. This procedure assumes that the subjects are equally skilled in both languages. One problem with this strategy is that bilingual subjects may interpret meanings of words differently from monolingual subjects. This difference in interpretation is a serious concern because the target subjects for most cross-cultural research are monolingual (Hulin et al., 1983).

Yu, Lee, and Woo (2004) provided an excellent description of their process of translating the Medical Outcomes Study Social Support Survey (MOS-SSS) from English to Chinese. These researchers used the forward and backward translation process previously discussed, and the steps they took are outlined in the following excerpt.

This translation model includes a cycle of four steps as follows.

Forward translation of the MOS-SSS by a bilingual health professional. The translation process began with forward translation of the original source language (SL) version (English) of the MOS-SSS into the target language (TL) of Chinese by a bilingual native Chinese registered nurse....

Review of the Chinese MOS-SSS by a monolingual reviewer. The Chinese version of the MOS-SSS was then reviewed by a Chinese monolingual reviewer for incomprehensible or ambiguous wordings....

Backward translation of the Chinese MOS-SSS by a bilingual health professional. In this step, the reviewed Chinese version of the MOS-SSS (as discussed in Step 2) was back translated by another bilingual nurse, who was "blinded" to the original English version....

Comparison of the SL version and back-translated version. The researcher, at this stage, compared the back-translated version of the MOS-SSS with its original version for linguistic congruence and cultural relevancy. Items with apparent discrepancies were examined to ascertain whether the problems originated in the forward translation or the backward translation. The error in items resulting from the forward translation had to go through the whole-cycle again from Steps 1 to 4, whereas the latter type of error was subjected to further back translation. This process was repeated until a maximum equivalence between the SL and back-translated versions was achieved. (Yu et al., 2004, pp. 309–310)

In 1997, the Medical Outcomes Trust introduced new translation criteria that are much more comprehensive. The discussion of these criteria is available at www. outcomes-trust.org/bulletin/0797blltn.htm.

Hulin et al. (1983) suggested the use of item response theory procedures to address some of the problems of translation. These procedures can provide direct evidence about the meanings of items in the two languages. Item characteristic curves for an item in the two languages can be compared, as can scale scores in the two languages. This procedure eliminates the need for bilingual samples. It also eliminates the need for the two populations to be equivalent in terms of the distributions of their scores on the trait being measured.

Rather than translating an instrument into each language, Turner, Rogers, Hendershot, Miller, and Thornberry (1996) tested the use of electronic technology involving multilingual audio computer-assisted self-interviewing (Audio-CASI) to enable researchers to include multiple linguistic minorities in nationally representative studies and clinical studies. This system uses electronic translation from one language to another. In the funded project to develop and test the system, a backup phone bank was available to provide multilingual assistance if needed. Whether this strategy will provide equivalent validity of a translated tool is unclear.

SUMMARY

- The measurement approaches used in nursing research include physiological measures, observations, interviews, questionnaires, and scales and some specialized instruments such as Q-sort method, Delphi technique, projective techniques, and diaries.
- Measurements of physiological variables can be either direct or indirect and sometimes require the use of specialized equipment or laboratory analysis.
- To measure observations, every variable is observed in a similar manner in each instance, with careful attention given to training data collectors.
- In structured observational studies, category systems must be developed; and checklists or rating scales are developed from the category systems and used to guide data collection.
- Interviews involve verbal communication between the researcher and the subject, during which the researcher acquires information. Interviewers must be trained in the skills of interviewing, and the interview protocol must be pretested.
- A questionnaire is a printed self-report form designed to elicit information through a subject's written responses. The information obtained through questionnaires is similar to that obtained by interview, but the questions tend to have less depth. An item on a questionnaire usually has two parts: a lead-in question and a response set.
- Scales, another form of self-reporting, are more precise in measuring phenomena than are questionnaires and have been developed to measure psychosocial and physiological variables. The types of scales include the rating scale, Likert scale, semantic differential scale, and the visual analogue scale.
- A rating scale is a crude form of measurement that includes a list of an ordered series of categories of a variable, which are assumed to be based on an underlying continuum. A numerical value is assigned to each category.
- The Likert scale is designed to determine the opinion or attitude of a subject and contains a number of declarative statements with a scale after each statement.
- A semantic differential scale consists of two opposite adjectives with a seven-point scale between them and measures the connotative meaning of a concept to a subject.
- The visual analogue scale, sometimes referred to as magnitude scaling, is a 100-mm line with right-angle stops at each end with bipolar anchors placed

beyond each end of the line. These end anchors must cover the entire range of sensations possible in the phenomenon being measured.

- The Delphi technique measures the judgments of a group of experts, assesses priorities, or makes forecasts. It provides a means for researchers to obtain the opinions of a wide variety of experts across the United States without the need for the experts to meet.
- Projective techniques are based on the assumption that the responses of individuals to unstructured or ambiguous situations reflect their attitudes, desires, personality characteristics, and motives.
- A diary, which allows one to record an experience shortly after an event, is more accurate than obtaining the information through recall at an interview, the reporting level of incidents is higher, and one tends to capture the participant's perception of situations.
- The choice of tools for use in a particular study is a critical decision that will have a major impact on the significance of the study.
- The researcher must first conduct an extensive search for existing tools. Once found, the tools must be carefully evaluated. Tools that are selected for a study need to be described in great detail in the proposal or publication.
- Scale construction is a complex procedure that should not be undertaken lightly. Theories on which scale construction is most frequently based include classic test theory, item response theory, multidimensional scaling, and unfolding theory. Most existing instruments used in nursing research have been developed through the use of classic test theory.
- Translating a scale to another language is a complex process that allows concepts among respondents of different cultures to be compared.

REFERENCES

Adachi, K., Shimada, M., & Usui, A. (2003). The relationship between the parturient's positions and perceptions of labor pain intensity. *Nursing Research, 52*(1), 47–51.

Aroian, K. J., & Wal, J. S. V. (2007). Measuring elders' symptoms with daily diaries and retrospective reports. *Western Journal of Nursing Research, 29*(3), 322–337.

Berdie, D. R., Anderson, J. F., & Niebuhr, M. A. (1986). *Questionnaires: Design and use*. Metuchen, NJ: Scarecrow Press.

Beretta, R. (1996). A critical review of the Delphi technique. *Nurse Researcher, 3*(4), 79–89.

Briggs, C. L. (1986). *Learning how to ask: A sociolinguistic appraisal of the role of the interview in social science research*. Cambridge, England: Cambridge University Press.

Burman, M. E. (1995). Health diaries in nursing research and practice. *Image: Journal of Nursing Scholarship, 27*(2), 147–152.

Burnard, P. (1994). The telephone interview as a data collection method. *Nurse Education Today, 14*(1), 67–72.

Burns, N. (1986). *Research in progress*. Atlanta: American Cancer Society, Texas Division.

Burnside, I., Preski, S., & Hertz, J. E. (1998). Research instrumentation and elderly subjects. *Image: Journal of Nursing Scholarship, 30*(2), 185–190.

Butz, A. M., & Alexander, C. (1991). Use of health diaries with children. *Nursing Research, 40*(1), 59–61.

Chapple, A. (1997). Personal recollections on interviewing GPs and consultants. *Nurse Researcher, 5*(2), 82–91.

Chung, J. W. Y., Ng, W. M. Y., & Wong, T. K. S. (2002). An experimental study on the use of manual pressure to reduce pain in intramuscular injections. *Journal of Clinical Nursing, 11*(4), 457–461.

Converse, J. M., & Presser, S. (1986). *Survey questions: Handcrafting the standardized questionnaire*. Newbury Park, CA: Sage.

Coombs, C. H. (1950). Psychological scaling without a unit of measurement. *Psychological Review, 57*(3), 145–158.

Couper, M. R. (1984). The Delphi technique: Characteristics and sequence model. *Advances in Nursing Science, 7*(1), 72–77.

Cowan, M. J., Heinrich, J., Lucas, M., Sigmon, H., & Hinshaw, A. S. (1993). Integration of biological and nursing sciences: A 10-year plan to enhance research and training. *Research in Nursing & Health, 16*(1), 3–9.

Craig, J. V., & Smyth, R. L. (2007). *The evidence-based practice manual for nurses* (2nd ed.). Edinburgh, Scotland: Churchill Livingstone.

Crisp, J., Pelletier, D., Duffield, C., Adams, A., & Nagy, S. (1997). The Delphi method? *Nursing Research, 46*(2), 116–118.

Crocker, L., & Algina, J. (1986). *Introduction to classical modern test theory*. New York: Holt, Rinehart & Winston.

Davison, M. L. (1983). *Multidimensional scaling*. New York: Wiley.

Degner, L. F. (1998). Preferences to participate in treatment decision making: The adult model. *Journal of Pediatric Oncology Nursing, 15*(3, Suppl 1), 3–9.

DeKeyser, F. G. & Pugh, L. C. (1991). Approaches to physiologic measurement. In C. F. Waltz, O. L. Strickland, & E. R. Lenz (Eds.), *Measurement in nursing research* (2nd ed., pp. 387–412). Philadelphia: F.A. Davis.

Dennis, K. E. (1986). Q methodology: Relevance and application to nursing research. *Advances in Nursing Science, 8*(3), 6–17.

DeVon, H. A., & Zerwic, J. J. (2003). The symptoms of unstable angina: Do women and men differ? *Nursing Research, 52*(2), 108–118.

Dillman, D. (1978). *Mail and telephone surveys: The total design method*. New York: Wiley.

Dillon, J. T. (1990). *The practice of questioning*. New York: Routledge.

Drankiewicz, D., & Dundes, L. (2003). Handwashing among female college students. *American Journal of Infection Control, 31*(2), 67–71.

Dubbert, P. M., White, J. D., Grothe, K. B., O'Jile, J., & Kirchner, K. A. (2006). Physical activity in patients who are severely mentally ill: Feasibility of assessment for clinical and research applications. *Archives of Psychiatric Nursing, 20*(5), 205–209.

Dzurec, L. C., & Coleman, P. A. (1995). A hermeneutic analysis of the process of conducting interviews. *Image: Journal of Nursing Scholarship*, 27(3), 245.

Etris, M. B., Pribble, J., & LaBrecque, J. (1994). Evaluation of two wound measurement methods in a multi-center, controlled study. *Ostomy/Wound Management*, 40(7), 44–48.

Faulkner, M. S., Hathaway, D., & Tolley, B. (2003). Cardiovascular autonomic function in healthy adolescents. *Heart & Lung*, 32(1), 10–22.

Flaskerud, J. H. (1988). Is the Likert scale format culturally biased? *Nursing Research*, 37(3), 185–186.

Fowler, F. J. (1990). *Standardized survey interviewing: Minimizing interviewer-related error*. Newbury Park, CA: Sage.

Fox, J. A., & Tracy, P. E. (1986). *Randomized response: A method for sensitive surveys*. Beverly Hills, CA: Sage.

Gentzkow, G. D. (1995). Methods for measuring size in pressure ulcers. *Advances in Wound Care*, 8(4), 43–45.

Gift, A. G. (1989). Visual analogue scales: Measurement of subjective phenomena. *Nursing Research*, 38(5), 286–288.

Goodman, C. M. (1987). The Delphi technique: A critique. *Journal of Advanced Nursing*, 12(6), 729–734.

Gorden, R. L. (1987). *Interviewing: Strategy, techniques, and tactics*. Chicago: Dorsey Press.

Guinan, M. E., McGuckin-Guinan, M., & Sevareid, A. (1997). Who washes hands after using the bathroom? *American Journal of Infection Control*, 25(5), 424–425.

Guyatt, G. H., Berman, L. B., Townsend, M., Pugsley, S. O., & Chambers, L. W. (1987). A measure of quality of life for clinical trials in chronic lung disease. *Thorax*, 42(11), 773–778.

Hansen, G. L., Sparrow, E. M., Kokate, J. Y., Leland, K. J., & Iaizzo, P. A. (1997). Wound status evaluation using color image processing. *IEEE Transactions on Medical Imaging*, 16(1), 78–86.

Harding, K. G. (1995). Methods for assessing change in ulcer status. *Advances in Wound Care*, 8(4), 37–42.

Harralson, T. L. (2007). Factors influencing delay in seeking treatment for acute ischemic symptoms among lower income, urban women. *Heart & Lung*, 36(2), 96–104.

Holaday, B., & Turner-Henson, A. (1989). Response effects in surveys with school-age children. *Nursing Research*, 38(4), 248–250.

Hulin, C. L., Drasgow, F., & Parsons, C. K. (1983). *Item response theory: Application to psychological measurement*. Homewood, IL: Dow Jones-Irwin.

Im, E., Chee, W., Guevara, E., Liu, Y., Lim, H., Tsai, H., et al., (2007). Gender and ethnic differences in cancer pain experience: A multiethnic survey in the United States. *Nursing Research* 56(5), 296–306.

Johnson, B. H. (1990). Children's drawings as a projective technique. *Pediatric Nursing*, 16(1), 11–17.

Johnson, M. J., & Rogers, S. (2006). Development of the Purposeful Action Medication-Taking Questionnaire. *Western Journal of Nursing Research*, 28(3), 335–351.

Jones, J. M. (2004). Nutritional methodology: Development of a nutritional screening or assessment tool using a multivariate technique. *Nutrition* 20(3), 298–306.

Kapella, M. C., Larson, J. L., Patel, M. K., Covey, M. K., & Berry, J. K. (2006). Subjective fatigue, influencing variables, and consequences in chronic obstructive pulmonary disease. *Nursing Research*, 55(1), 10–17.

Kreman, R., Yates, B. C., Agrawal, S., Fiandt, K., Briner, W., & Shurmur, S. (2006). The effects of motivational interviewing on physiological outcomes. *Applied Nursing Research*, 19(3), 167–170.

Kruskal, J. B., & Wish, M. (1990). *Multidimensional scaling*. Newbury Park, CA: Sage.

Lee, K. A., & Kieckhefer, G. M. (1989). Measuring human responses using visual analogue scales. *Western Journal of Nursing Research*, 11(1), 128–132.

Lindeman, C. A. (1975). Delphi survey of priorities in clinical nursing research. *Nursing Research*, 24(6), 434–441.

Liskay, A. M., Mion, L. C., & Davis, B. R. (1993). Comparison of two devices for wound measurement. *Dermatology Nursing*, 5(6), 437–441.

Lodge, M. (1981). *Magnitude scaling: Quantitative measurement of opinions*. Beverly Hills, CA: Sage.

Luniewski, M., Riegle, J. K., & White, B. (1999). Card sort: An assessment tool for the educational needs of patients with heart failure. *American Journal of Critical Care*, 8(5), 297–302.

Lynn, M. R. (1989). Instrument reliability: How much needs to be published? *Heart & Lung*, 18(4), 421–423.

Malloch, K., & Porter-O'Grady, T. (2006). *Introduction to evidence-based practice in nursing and health care*. Sudbury, MA: Jones & Bartlett.

Marshall, C., & Rossman, G. B. (2006). *Designing qualitative research* (4th ed.). Thousand Oaks, CA: Sage.

McColl, E. (2004). Best practice in symptom assessment: A review. *Gut*, 53(Suppl 4), iv49–54.

McCracken, G. D. (1988). *The long interview*. Newbury Park, CA: Sage.

McKeown, B., & Thomas, D. (1988). *Q methodology*. Newbury Park, CA: Sage.

McLaughlin, P. (1990). *How to interview: The art of asking questions* (2nd ed.). North Vancouver, BC: International Self-Counsel Press.

Melhuish, J. M., Plassman, P., & Harding, K. G. (1994). Circumference, area and volume of the healing wound. *Journal of Wound Care*, 3(8), 380–384.

Melnyk, B. M. (1994). Coping with unplanned childhood hospitalization: Effects of informational interventions on mothers and children. *Nursing Research*, 43(1), 50–55.

Melnyk, B. M., Alpert-Gillis, L. J., Hensel, P. B., Cable-Beiling, R. C., & Rubenstein, J. S. (1997). Helping mothers cope with critically ill child: A pilot test of the COPE intervention. *Research in Nursing & Health*, 20(1), 3–14.

Minnick, A. F., Mion, L. C., Johnson, M. E., Catrambone, C., & Leipzig, R. (2007). Prevalence and variation of physical restraint use in acute care settings in the US. *Journal of Nursing Scholarship*, 39(1), 30–37.

Mishler, E. G. (1986). *Research interviewing: Context and narrative*. Cambridge, MA: Harvard University Press.

Mitchell, M. P. (1998). Nursing education planning: A Delphi study. *Journal of Nursing Education*, 37(7), 305–307.

National Institute of Nursing Research (NINR). (2006). *Strategic plan National Institute of Nursing Research: Areas of research emphasis*. Retrieved November 7, 2007, from www.ninr.nih.gov/AboutNINR/NINRMissionandStrategicPlan.

Norbeck, J. S. (1985). What constitutes a publishable report of instrument development? *Nursing Research*, 34(6), 380–381.

Nunnally, J. C., & Bernstein, I. H. (1994). *Psychometric theory* (3rd ed.). New York: McGraw-Hill.

Osgood, C. E., Suci, G. J., & Tannenbaum, P. H. (1957). *The measurement of meaning*. Urbana, IL: University of Illinois Press.

Paratz, J., & Lipman, J. (2006). Manual hyperinflation caused norepinephrine release. *Heart & Lung*, 35(4), 262–268.

Pope, D. S. (1995). Music, noise, and the human voice in the nurse-patient environment. *Image: Journal of Nursing Scholarship*, 27(4), 291–296.

Pugh, L. C., & DeKeyser, F. G. (1995). Use of physiologic variables in nursing research. *Image: Journal of Nursing Scholarship*, 27(4), 273–276.

Ro, Y., Ha, H., Kim, C., & Yeom, H. (2002). The effects of aromatherapy on pruritus in patients undergoing hemodialysis. *Dermatology Nursing*, 14(4), 231–234, 237–239.

Roberts, W. D., & Stone, P. W. (2003). Ask and expert: How to choose and evaluate a research instrument. *Applied Nursing Research*, 16(1), 70–72.

Rudy, S. F. (1996). Research forum: A review of Delphi surveys conducted to establish research priorities by specialty nursing organizations from 1985 to 1995. *ORL: Head & Neck Nursing*, 14(2), 16–24.

Saris, W. E. (1991). *Computer-assisted interviewing*. Newbury Park, CA: Sage.

Schallom, L., Sona, C., McSweeney, M., & Mazuski, J. (2007). Comparison of forehead and digit oximetry in surgical/trauma patients at risk for decreased peripheral perfusion. *Heart & Lung*, 36(3), 188–194.

Schuman, H. (1981). *Questions and answers in attitude surveys: Experiments on question form, wording, and context*. New York: Academic Press.

Sennott-Miller, L., Murdaugh, C., & Hinshaw, A. S. (1988). Magnitude estimation: Issues and practical applications. *Western Journal of Nursing Research*, 10(4), 414–424.

Shelley, S. I. (1984). *Research methods in nursing and health*. Boston: Little, Brown.

Simpson, S. H. (1989). Use of Q-sort methodology in cross-cultural nutrition and health research. *Nursing Research*, 38(5), 289–290.

Small, L., & Melnyk, B. M. (2006). Early predictors of post-hospital adjustment problems in critically ill young children. *Research in Nursing & Health*, 29(6), 622–635.

Spector, P. E. (1992). *Summated rating scale construction: An introduction*. Newbury Park, CA: Sage.

Sudman, S., & Bradburn, N. (1982). *Asking questions: A practical guide to questionnaire design*. San Francisco: Jossey-Bass.

Tetting, D. W. (1988). Q-sort update. *Western Journal of Nursing Research*, 10(6), 757–765.

Thomas, D. R. (1997). Existing tools: Are they meeting the challenges of pressure ulcer healing? *Advances in Wound Care*, 10(5), 86–90.

Turner, C. F., Rogers, S. M., Hendershot, T. P., Miller, H. G., & Thornberry, J. P. (1996). Improving representation of linguistic minorities in health surveys. *Public Health Reports*, 111(3), 276–279.

Waltz, C. F., Strickland, O. L., & Lenz, E. R. (1991). *Measurement in nursing research*. Philadelphia: F.A. Davis.

Wewers, M. E., & Lowe, N. K. (1990). A critical review of visual analogue scales in the measurement of clinical phenomena. *Research in Nursing & Health*, 13(4), 227–236.

Williams, J. E., Singh, S. J., Sewell, L., Guyatt, G. H., & Morgan, M. D. (2001). Development of a self-report Chronic Respiratory Questionnaire (CRQ-SR). *Thorax*, 56(12), 954–959.

Yu, D. S. F., Lee, D. T. F., & Woo, J. (2004). Issues and challenges of instrument translation. *Western Journal of Nursing Research*, 26(3), 307–320.

Zung, W. W. K. (1965). A self-rating depression scale. *Archives of General Psychiatry*, 12, 63–70.

CHAPTER 17
Collecting and Managing Data

Data collection is one of the most exciting parts of research. After all the planning, writing, and negotiating, you are ready for the real part of research—the action part. There is a sense of euphoria and excitement, an eagerness to start the study. However, before you leap into data collection, spend some time carefully planning this adventure. It may save you difficulties later on as you implement the final steps of the research process. Consider problems you might encounter while collecting data, and develop strategies for addressing them. You must make careful plans for managing data as you collect it. This chapter is divided into three sections to assist you in planning data collection, collecting data, and managing data for quantitative studies. Data collection strategies for qualitative studies are described in Chapter 23.

PLANNING DATA COLLECTION

A data collection plan details how you will implement your study. The plan for collecting data is specific to the study being conducted and requires that you consider some of the more commonplace elements of research. You will need to map out the procedures you will use to collect data, anticipate the time and cost of data collection, develop data collection forms that ease data entry, and prepare a codebook that will help you to identify data to be entered in a database. This extensive planning increases the accuracy of the data collected and the validity of the study findings. The strength of the findings from several studies increases the quality of the research evidence that is available for use in practice (Craig & Smith, 2007; Melnyk & Fineout-Overholt, 2005).

Planning Data Collection Procedures

To plan the process of data collection, you must determine step by step how and in what sequence data will be collected from a single subject. The timing of this process also must be established. For example, how much time will be required to identify potential subjects, explain the study, and obtain consent? How much time is needed for activities such as completing questionnaires or obtaining physiological measures? Next, envision the overall activities that will be occurring during data collection. At what point are subjects assigned to groups? When and how will you implement the study treatment? Will data be collected from more than one subject at a time, or is it necessary to focus attention on one subject at a time? How many subjects per day can be accessed for data given the study design and the setting? It might be helpful to conduct a trial run or even a pilot study by collecting data from three to five subjects to determine the strengths and weaknesses of the data collection plan. You will need a minimum of five subjects if you plan to conduct a pilot study. You might develop a data collection tree or flow diagram to illustrate the process for collecting data in your study. An example is shown in Figure 17-1.

Decision Points

Decision points that occur during data collection must be identified and all options considered. Decisions might include whether potential subjects meet

ENROLLMENT AND SURVEY ADMINISTRATION PROCEDURES

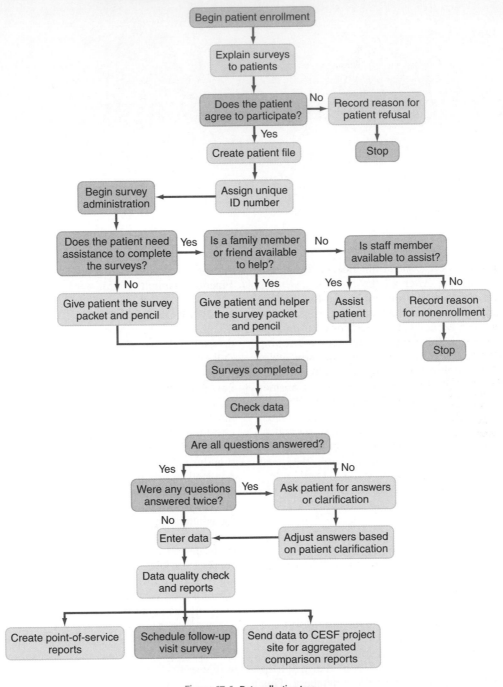

Figure **17-1** Data collection tree.

the sampling criteria, whether a subject understands the information needed to give informed consent, what group the subject will be assigned to, whether the subject comprehends instructions related to providing data, and whether the subject has provided all the data needed. Your data collection tree should indicate each point at which a decision is made.

Consistency

Consistency in data collection across subjects is critical. If more than one person is collecting the data, consistency among data collectors (interrater reliability) is also necessary (see Chapter 15). Identify situations in your study that might interfere with consistency, and develop a plan that will maximize consistency. The specific days and hours of data collection may influence the consistency of the data collected and thus must be carefully considered. For example, the energy level and state of mind of subjects from whom data are gathered in the morning may differ from that of subjects from whom data are gathered in the evening. Visitors are more likely to be present at certain times of day and may interfere with data collection or influence subject responses. Patient care routines vary with the time of day. In some studies, the care recently received or the care currently being provided may alter the data you gather. The subjects you approach on Saturday to participate in the study may differ from the subjects you approach on weekday mornings. Subjects seeking care on Saturday may have a full-time job, whereas those seeking care on weekday mornings may be either unemployed or too ill to work.

You and your research team also must decide who will collect the data. Will the researcher collect all the data, or will data collectors be employed for this purpose? Can data collectors be nurses working in the area? Researchers have experienced difficulties in studies in which they expected nurses providing patient care to also be data collectors. Patient care takes priority over data collection, which may lead to missing data or missed subjects.

If you decide to use data collectors, they must be informed about the research project, familiarized with the instruments to be used, and provided equivalent training in the data collection process. In addition to training, data collectors need written guidelines or protocols that indicate which instruments to use, the order in which to introduce the instruments, how to administer the instruments, and a time frame for the data collection process (Gift, Creasia, & Parker, 1991).

After training, data collectors must be evaluated to determine their consistency in the data collection process. Washington and Moss (1988) suggested that a minimum of 10 subjects must be rated with the complete instrument before interrater reliability can be adequately assessed. The data collectors' interrater reliability is usually assessed intermittently throughout data collection to ensure consistency. Data collectors also must be encouraged to identify and record any problems or variations in the environment that affect the data collection process.

Determine how you will reliably and competently deliver the study treatment. Often researchers develop detailed protocols to guide them in delivering the treatment or intervention, and they train data collectors in this process. Stein, Sargent, and Rafaels (2007) stressed the importance of achieving intervention fidelity in a study, which involves training an individual called an interventionalist to deliver the intervention protocol. To achieve intervention fidelity, the delivery of the intervention must include the core components of adherence and competence. Adherence is the most basic and exists when the interventionalist reliably or consistently implements the behaviors of the intervention protocol. Competence is more complex and focuses on the interventionalist's skill and expertise in delivering the study intervention. For more details on intervention protocol development and implementation, refer to Chapters 11 and 13.

Time Factors

Researchers often underestimate the time required to collect data for a study, which sometimes takes two to three times longer than anticipated. It is helpful to write out a time plan for the data collection period. Conduct a pilot study to refine the data collection process, and determine the time required to collect data from a subject.

Events during the data collection period sometimes are not under the researcher's control. For example, a sudden heavy staff workload may make data collection temporarily difficult or impossible, or the number of potential subjects might be reduced for a period. In some situations, researchers must obtain permission from each subject's physician before they are permitted to collect data on that subject. Activities required to meet this stipulation—such as contacting physicians, explaining the study, and obtaining permission—require extensive time. In some cases, potential subjects are lost before the researcher can obtain the mandatory permission, thus extending the time required to obtain the necessary number of subjects.

Cost Factors

Cost is another consideration when planning a study. Measurement tools—such as Holter monitors, spirometers, infrared thermometers, pulse oximeters, or Glucometers—used in physiological studies may need to be rented, purchased, or obtained from the company manufacturing the equipment. You may need to pay a fee for questionnaires or scales and for analyzing the data. Data collection forms must be typed and duplicated. In some cases, printing costs for materials that are to be distributed during data collection must be factored in, such as teaching materials, questionnaires, or scales. In some studies, postage is an additional expense. There may be costs involved in coding the data for entry into the computer and for conducting data analyses. Consultation with a statistician early in the development of a research project and during data analysis must also be budgeted. You may need to hire a secretary to type the final report, research presentations, or a manuscript for publication.

In addition to these direct costs, there are also indirect costs. The researcher's time is a cost and costs for travel to and from the study site and for meals eaten out while working on the study must be taken into account. You also must estimate the expense of presenting the research project at conferences, and include that cost in the budget. To prevent unexpected expenses from delaying the study, examine all costs in an organized manner during the planning phase of the study. A budget is best developed early in the planning process and revised as plans are modified (see Chapter 28 for a sample budget). Seeking funding for at least part of the study costs can facilitate the conduct of a study (see Chapter 29 on funding for research).

Neophyte researchers have difficulty making reasonable estimates of time and costs related to a study. We advise validating the time and cost estimates with an experienced researcher. If the cost and time factors are prohibitive, simplify your study so that fewer variables are measured, fewer instruments are used. Make the design less complex, and use fewer data collectors. These are serious modifications, however, so you and your team should thoroughly examine the consequences before making such revisions. If time or cost estimates go beyond expectations, you can revise the time schedules and budget with a new projection for completing the study.

Developing Data Collection Forms

Before data collection begins, you may need to develop or modify forms on which to record data. These forms can be used to record demographic data, information from the patient record, observations, or values from physiological measures. The demographic variables commonly collected in nursing studies include age, gender, race, education, income or socioeconomic status, employment status, diagnosis, and marital status. You also might need to collect other data that may be either extraneous or confounding variables such as the subject's physician, stage of illness, length of illness or hospitalization, complications, date of data collection, time of day and day of week of data collection, and any untoward events that occur during the data collection period. In some cases, the length of time required of individual subjects for data collection may be a confounding variable and must be recorded. If it is necessary to contact the subject at a later time, you will need to obtain the subject's address and telephone number, but only with that person's awareness and permission. Names and phone numbers of family members may also be useful if subjects are likely to move or be difficult to contact. Consider the importance of each piece of datum and the amount of the subject's time required to collect it. If the data can be obtained from patient records or any other written sources, you do not need to ask the subject to provide this information; just make sure that the institutional review board (IRB) has authorized your team to collect these data in the study setting. You also need to protect the participant's private health information that is regulated by the Health Insurance Portability and Accountability Act (HIPAA) (available online at www.hhs.gov/ocr/hipaa).

Data collection forms must be designed so that the data are easily recorded and entered into the computer. Decide whether data will be collected in raw form or coded at the time of collection. Coding is the process of transforming data into numerical symbols that can be entered easily into the computer. For example, variables such as gender, ethnicity, and diagnoses can be categorized and given numerical labels. For gender, the male category could be identified by a 1 and the female category by a 2. For the ethnicity variable, the African-American category could be represented by the number 1, Caucasian by a 2, Hispanic by a 3, and Other by a 4.

The coding categories developed for a study must be not only mutually exclusive but also exhaustive, which means that the value for a specific variable fits into only one category, and each observation must fit into a category. For example, the income ranges would not be mutually exclusive or exhaustive if they were categorized in the following way on a demographic questionnaire:

Income Range (Please check the range that most accurately reflects your income.)
___ (1) $30,000 to $35,000
___ (2) $35,000 to $39,000
___ (3) $40,000 to $45,000
___ (4) $45,000 to $50,000
___ (5) $50,000 and more

These categories are not exclusive because they overlap and a subject with a $35,000 income could mark category 1, or category 2, or both. The categories are not exhaustive because a subject may have an income of either $25,000 or $39,500, yet the questionnaire does not contain categories that include each of these incomes. For many items, a code for "Other" should be included for unexpected classifications of variables such as marital status, ethnicity, or diagnosis. The following income ranges are both exclusive and exhaustive and would be appropriate for collecting demographic data from subjects:

Income Range (Please check the range that most accurately reflects your income.)
___ (1) Less than $30,000
___ (2) $30,000 to $39,999
___ (3) $40,000 to $49,999
___ (4) $50,000 to $59,999
___ (5) $60,000 or greater

Data collection forms offer a number of response styles. The person completing the form (subject or data collector) might be asked to check a blank space before or after the words *male* or *female*, to circle the word *male* or *female*, or to write a 1 or a 2 in a blank space before or after the word selected. If codes are used, the meaning of the codes should be indicated on the collection forms so that the individual completing the form will understand them.

Placement of the data on the forms is important, because careful placement makes it easier for users to complete the form and to locate responses for computer entry. Placement of blanks on the left side of the page seems to be most efficient for data entry, but this layout may prove problematic when subjects are completing the forms. The least effective arrangement is when the data are positioned irregularly on the form, because the risk of data being missed during data entry is high. Subjects' names should not be on the data collection forms; only the subject's identification number should appear. The researcher will usually keep a master list of subjects and associated coding numbers, which is stored in a separate location to ensure the subjects' privacy. Often this master list of subjects and codes is kept with the subject consent forms.

Figure 17-2 provides a sample data collection form. It includes four items that could be problematic in terms of coding, data analysis, or both. The blank used to enter Surgical Procedure Performed would lead to problems when it is time to enter the data into a computerized data set. Because multiple surgical procedures could have been performed, developing

DATA COLLECTION FORM

Demographics
____Subject Identification Number
____Age
____Gender
1. Male
2. Female
____Weight (in pounds)
____Height (in inches)
__________Surgical Procedure Performed
_/_/_Surgery Date (Month/Day/Year)
_/_/_Surgery Time (Hour/Minute/AM or PM)
Narcotics Ordered After Surgery________________
____

Narcotic Administration

Date	Time	Narcotic	Dose
1.			
2.			
3.			
4.			
5.			

Instruction on Use of Pain Scale
_/_/_Date (Month/Day/Year)
_/_/_Time (Hour/Minute/AM or PM)
Comments:

_Treatment Group
1. TENS
2. Placebo-TENS
3. No-Treatment Control

Treatment Implemented
_/_/_Date (Month/Day/Year)
_/_/_Time (Hour/Minute/AM or PM)
Comments:

Dressing Change
_/_/_Date (Month/Day/Year)
_/_/_Time (Hour/Minute/AM or PM)
____Hours since surgery
Comments:

Measurement of Pain
____Score on Visual Analogue Pain Scale
_/_/_Date Pain Measured (Month/Day/Year)
_/_/_Time Pain Measured (Hour/Minute/AM or PM)
____Hours since surgery
Comments:

____Data Collector Code
Comments:

Figure 17-2 Example of a data collection form.

codes for the various surgical procedures would be difficult and time consuming. In addition, different words might be used to record the same surgical procedure. It may be necessary to tally the surgical procedures manually. Unless this degree of specification of procedures is important to the study, an alternative would be to develop larger categories of procedures before data collection and place the categories on the data collection form. A category of "Other" might be useful for less commonly performed surgical procedures. This method would require the data collector to make a judgment regarding which category was appropriate for a particular surgical procedure. Another option would be to write in the category code number for a particular surgical procedure after the data collection form is completed but before data entry. Similar problems occur with the items Narcotics Ordered after Surgery and Narcotic Administration. Unless these data are to be used in statistical analyses, it might be better to manually categorize this information for descriptive purposes. If these items are needed for planned statistical procedures, use care to develop appropriate codes. In this study, the researcher might be interested in determining differences in the amount of narcotics administered in a given period in relation to weight and height. Recording the treatment groups on the data collection form may be problematic because the information could influence the data recorded by the data collectors.

Using Electronic Devices for Data Collection

Electronic devices can be used to collect a variety of scale, questionnaire, or physiological data. However, the use of these devices for research may require considerable preparation. You may need to purchase, rent, or borrow the equipment. You also may need to make arrangements with the data collection site or to place measurement scales on special forms.

Scantron Sheets

Scantron sheets are forms that allow subjects to respond to test questions or scale items by using a pencil to bubble in responses. These responses can be entered directly into the computer by optic scanner (Dennis, 1994) and stored into a database for analysis. This practice speeds up the process of entering data and reduces errors related to data entry. However, subjects not familiar with Scantron sheets may be reluctant to use them, and some inaccuracies in data may occur because of subject error. These forms have been used commonly for administering multiple-choice tests to nursing students. Scantrons are best used when subjects cannot be accessed by e-mail or there is

no computer for direct data entry and data must be collected using paper-and-pencil forms.

Teleform

Teleform is a computer software package developed by Cardiff (see www.cardiff.com) that enables researchers to design a form specific to a scale or questionnaire to be used for data collection. Cardiff software has unique features that allow users to develop point-and-click automated forms that can be distributed electronically. Additional features include data accuracy verification, selective data extraction and analysis, digital record signature support, auditing and tracking, print merge applications, and flexible export interfaces (www.cardiff.com/products/teleform/index.html). Training is available at the Cardiff website or in person at locations around the United States. Figure 17-3 shows a Teleform version of the Burns Cancer Belief Scale, which allows data to be scanned and stored in a database. Or this form could be developed and sent to subjects electronically, and the data are collected online and automatically entered into a database. Universities and schools of nursing are purchasing this software, as are some researchers who can purchase it with grant monies. The costs of acquiring the hardware and software are considerably less than the costs of entering data manually.

Im et al. (2007) conducted a multiethnic survey in the United States of the gender and ethnic differences in the cancer pain experience. These researchers administered their questionnaire over the Internet and through a paper-and-pencil format based on the desires of the subjects. The following excerpt describes the data collection procedure for this study.

To administer the Internet questionnaire, a Web site conforming to the Health Insurance Portability and Accountability Act standards, the System Administration, Networking, and Security Institute Federal Bureaus of Investigation recommendations, and the Institutional Review Board policy of the institution where the researchers were affiliated was developed and published on an independent, dedicated Web site server. When potential participants visited the project Web site, informed consent was obtained by asking them to click a button labeled *I agree to participate*. After this, questions on specific diagnoses, cancer therapies, and medications were asked, and the appropriateness of answers was checked automatically through a server-side program; participants were connected automatically to the Internet survey web page if the answers were appropriate.

Upon request, pen-and-pencil questionnaires were provided by mail to the community consultants, who distributed the questionnaires in person only to those who were identified as cancer patients. These questionnaires accompanied hard copies of the same informed consent form included in the Internet format of the questionnaire, and the pen-and-pencil questionnaire included a sentence "Filling out this questionnaire means that you are aged over 18 years old and giving your consent to participate in this survey." After the self-administered questionnaires were completed, community consultants retrieved all except five (these were mailed directly to the research team by the participants) in person at the community settings and mailed them to the research team. Supplementing pen-and-pencil questionnaires was essential to recruit the target number of ethnic minority cancer patients across the nation who did not have access to the Internet but were interested in participating in the study. Among the 276 participants who were recruited through community settings, 246 (49 Hispanics, 6 N-H [non-Hispanic] Whites, 99 N-H African Americans, and 92 N-H Asians) used the pen-and-pencil questionnaires. With an α level of 0.05, there were no statistically significant differences in psychometric properties between the Internet format and the pen-and-pencil format of the questionnaire. More detailed findings on psychometric properties of the Internet and pen-and-pencil format of the questionnaire can be found in the larger study (Im et al., 2006). It took an average of 30-40 minutes for the participants to complete either the Internet format or the pen-and-pencil format of the questionnaire. (Im et al., 2007, pp. 299–300)

Im et al. (2007) maximized their sample size and obtained a more representative sample by giving participants an option to complete their questionnaire on the Internet or via the pen-and-pencil format. The researchers then took steps to ensure that the data collected by the two formats were comparable by testing for significant differences and finding none. The time to complete the Internet and pen-and-pencil questionnaires did not vary. Im et al. (2007) also ensured that the rights of the subjects were protected and an ethical study was conducted.

Computerized Data Collection

With the advent of microcomputers, data collectors can code data directly into a microcomputer at the data collection site. If a computer is used for data collection, a program must be written for entering, cleaning, and storing data. A microcomputer enables users to collect large amounts of data with few errors, which can be readily analyzed with a variety of statistical software packages.

Personal Digital Assistants

Personal digital assistants (PDAs) are small handheld computers that allow the researcher to enter data directly into the computer from observations as they occur or to download data from a larger computer for easy access. Bernhardt et al. (2001) used PDAs to collect survey data and found that participants preferred the PDA to paper-and-pencil surveys. Health care providers are loading programs on their PDAs that facilitate accurate assessment, diagnosis, and pharmacological and nonpharmacological management of patients with a variety of health needs. In addition, PDAs are being used to store patient data from office computers in a form that is easily transportable. Thus, they have easy access to information about patients who call during off hours. These small computers can also be used for research purposes. PDA software is currently available that may help nurse practitioners in busy offices to collect data for research. Multiple nurse practitioners involved in a research project could forward data electronically from PDAs to a central research site for analysis. Care would need to be taken to protect the confidentiality of the data during transmission. Also, PDAs can be misplaced or stolen, thus threatening confidentiality. Researchers need to protect the information on their PDAs with a security code to ensure that no one but themselves can access their PDAs.

Bioinstruments

Advancements in technology have made it possible to interface bioinstruments with computers for data collection. The advantages of using computers for the acquisition and storage of physiological data from bioinstruments are numerous. Harrison (1989) summarized them as follows:

1. *Increased accuracy and reliability are achieved by reducing errors that may occur when manually recording or transcribing physiologic data from patient monitors or other clinical instruments.*
2. *Linking microcomputers with biomedical instruments (e.g., cardiac, respiratory, blood pressure, or oxygen saturation monitors) permits more frequent acquisition and storage of larger amounts of data (e.g., once or more per second) than is practical with manual recording procedures.*
3. *Once established, computerized data acquisition systems save researcher time during both the data collection and analysis phases of research.*

BURNS CANCER BELIEF SCALE

The following items have been selected to help give us a picture of your feelings about cancer. Of course, the response you give may not be true of your feelings for *all* cancer *all* of the time. Try to respond as you feel generally about cancer—not a specific situation. Each line contains opposites of a thought, with 7 choices in between the two words. For example:

Guilty......... ◯ ◯ ◯ ◯ ◯ ◯ ◯ ....Innocent

If you believe cancer is associated with feeling guilty, you would circle the first choice by guilty.

Guilty......... ① ◯ ◯ ◯ ◯ ◯ ◯ ....Innocent

If you believe cancer is associated with feeling very innocent, you would circle the first choice by innocent.

Guilty......... ◯ ◯ ◯ ◯ ◯ ◯ ⑦ ....Innocent

If you believe the feeling is usually somewhere between the two responses, circle the choice you believe most appropriately describes your feelings about cancer and those two choices.

Please circle <u>only one</u> choice. More than one response will be treated as no response at all.

There are no right or wrong answers to these items. Your response simply indicates how *you* feel about cancer.

NOW PLEASE COMPLETE THE FOLLOWING ITEMS:

Hopefulness	◯	◯	◯	◯	◯	◯	◯	Hopelessness
Certain death	◯	◯	◯	◯	◯	◯	◯	Being cured
Helplessness	◯	◯	◯	◯	◯	◯	◯	Control
Painless	◯	◯	◯	◯	◯	◯	◯	Severe constant untreatable pain
Punishment	◯	◯	◯	◯	◯	◯	◯	No punishment
Optimism	◯	◯	◯	◯	◯	◯	◯	Pessimism
No fear	◯	◯	◯	◯	◯	◯	◯	Terror
Unknown	◯	◯	◯	◯	◯	◯	◯	Known

	Cancer Belief Scale	0674454662

Figure **17-3** Teleform of Burns Cancer Belief Scale.

4. *Even though the initial cost of equipment may be high, over the long run computerized data collection systems are less expensive, more efficient, and more reliable than hiring and training multiple human data collectors. (Harrison, 1989, p. 131)*

There are some concerns with the use of computerized bioinstruments, but physiological data are usually best gathered and stored directly into computer databases to ensure accurate, complete data collection. Researchers must make every effort to deal with any problems. The microcomputer and the equipment required to

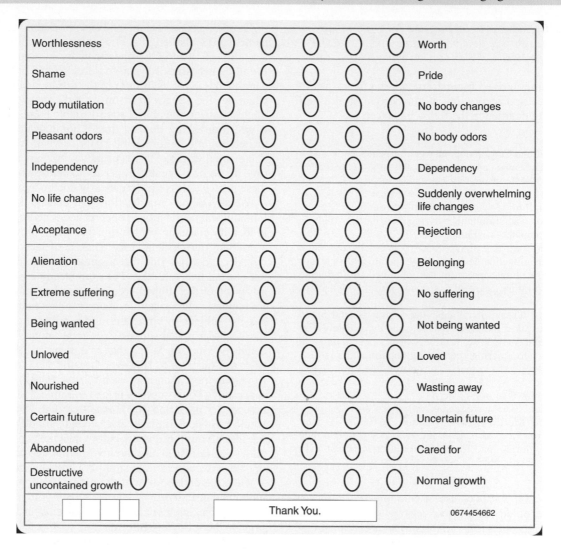

Worthlessness	O O O O O O O	Worth
Shame	O O O O O O O	Pride
Body mutilation	O O O O O O O	No body changes
Pleasant odors	O O O O O O O	No body odors
Independency	O O O O O O O	Dependency
No life changes	O O O O O O O	Suddenly overwhelming life changes
Acceptance	O O O O O O O	Rejection
Alienation	O O O O O O O	Belonging
Extreme suffering	O O O O O O O	No suffering
Being wanted	O O O O O O O	Not being wanted
Unloved	O O O O O O O	Loved
Nourished	O O O O O O O	Wasting away
Certain future	O O O O O O O	Uncertain future
Abandoned	O O O O O O O	Cared for
Destructive uncontained growth	O O O O O O O	Normal growth

Thank You.   0674454662

Figure **17-3** Cont'd

interface it with the bioinstruments take up space in an already crowded clinical setting; when possible, existing equipment should be used to collect data. Purchasing the equipment, setting it up, and installing the software can be time consuming and expensive at the start of the research project. Thus, initial studies will usually require external funding. Another concern is that the nurse researcher will focus on the machine and neglect observing and interacting with the patient. The most serious disadvantage is the possibility of measurement error that can occur with equipment malfunctions and software errors, although regular maintenance and reliability checks of the equipment and software will reduce this problem.

Savian, Paratz, and Davies (2006) conducted a single-blind randomized, crossover study with 14 mechanically ventilated intensive care unit (ICU) patients. The purpose of the study was to determine the effectiveness of

manual hyperinflation (MHI) and ventilator hyperinflation (VHI) on respiratory mechanics (static compliance [C_{st}]), oxygenation (arterial oxygen tension [PaO_2]/fraction of inspired oxygen [FIO_2] ratio), and secretion removal (wet weight of sputum and peak expiratory flow rate [PEFR]) at different levels of PEEP [positive end-expiratory pressure]... a secondary aim was to investigate the hemodynamics (heart rate

[HR], mean arterial pressure [MAP] and meta-bolic response (carbon dioxide output [VCO$_2$]) during MHI and VHI. (Savian et al., 2006, p. 335)

The computerized bioinstruments that were used to collected and record data in the Savian et al. (2006) study are detailed in the following excerpt.

PEFR and CO$_2$ production were measured using a flow and CO$_2$ sensor connected to the patient's airways and to the CO$_2$SMO respiratory mechanics monitor (CO$_2$SMO Plus Model 8000, Novametrix Medical Systems Inc., Wallingford, CN). All information from the CO$_2$SMO monitor was simultaneously recorded in the Analysis Plus computer program.

Static lung compliance was recorded by the static measures function device on the Bennett 7200 ventilator where a plateau pressure was obtained by including an inspiratory pause of 2 seconds into the mandatory breath…

PaO$_2$/FIO$_2$ ratio was calculated from arterial blood samples taken immediately before and immediately after MHI and VHI. Four milliliters of arterial blood were drawn into a syringe containing heparin and analyzed by a blood gas machine (Bayer Australian Limited 865, Pymble, NSW, CAN 000128 714). This procedure was standardized across subjects.

HR and MAP were read directly from the monitoring system (Merlin pressure module M1006A Hewlett Packard, Palo Alto, CA) and recorded every minute before, during, and for 5 minutes after MHI and VHI. (Savian et al., 2006, p. 336)

Savian et al.'s (2006) use of computerized bioinstruments enabled them to collect repeated measures on several physiological variables in an accurate and precise way. The data were collected by sensors and stored in the computer to reduce error and ease data analysis.

Developing a Codebook for Data Definitions

A codebook identifies and defines each variable in your study and includes an abbreviated variable name (often limited to six to eight characters), a descriptive variable label, and the range of possible numerical values for every variable entered in a computer file. Some codebooks also identify the source of each datum, thus linking your codebook with your data collection forms and scales. The codebook keeps you in control and provides a safety net for when you access the data later. Some computer programs, such as SPSS for Windows, allow you to print out your data definitions after setting up a database. Figure 17-4 is an example of data definitions from SPSS for Windows. Another example of coding is presented in Figure 17-5.

Developing a logical method of abbreviating variable names can be challenging. For example, you might use a quality-of-life (QOL) questionnaire in your study. It will be necessary for you to develop an abbreviated variable name for each item in the questionnaire. For example, the fourth item on a QOL questionnaire might be given the abbreviated variable name QOL4. A question asking the last time a home health nurse visited might be abbreviated HHN Lstvisit. Although abbreviated variable names usually seem logical at the time the name is created, it is easy to confuse or forget these names unless they are clearly documented.

We advise that you develop your codebook before initiating data collection. This practice encourages you to identify places in your forms that might prove to be a problem during data entry because of lack of clarity. Also, you may find that a single question contains not one but five variables. For example, an item might ask whether the subject received support from her or his mother, father, sister, brother, or other relatives and ask the subject to circle the number that represents those who provided support. You might think that you could code mother as 1, father as 2, sister as 3, brother as 4, and other as 5. However, because the individual can circle more than one, each relative must be coded separately. Thus, mother is one variable and would be coded 1 if circled and 0 if not circled. The father would be coded similarly as a second variable, and so on. Identifying these items before data collection may allow you to restructure the item on the questionnaire or data collection form to simplify computer entry.

Give the codebook with its data definitions to the individual or individuals who will enter your data into the computer *before initiating data collection*. In addition, provide the following information:

1. Copies of all scales, questionnaires, and data collection forms to be used in the study.
2. Information on the location of every variable on scales, questionnaires, or data collection forms.
3. Information on the statistical package to be used for analysis of the data.
4. Identification of the analyses to be conducted to describe the sample and to address the research purpose and the objectives, questions, or hypotheses.
5. Identification of a statistician to consult with about data analysis.
6. Determination of the database in which the data will be entered.
7. Information related to receiving the data, for example, whether you will deliver the data in batches or wait until all the data have been gathered before delivering it.

Text continued on p. 443

Name	Position
SOCMID1 SOC SIT MID 1 FRIENDS	78

Format: F1
Value   Label
  1   NEVER EXPERIENCED
  2   NO DIFFICULTY
  3   SLIGHT DIFFICULTY
  4   MODERATE DIFFICULTY
  5   GREAT DIFFICULTY
  6   EXTREME DIFFICULTY

Name	Position
SOCMID2 SOC SIT MID 2 SHOPPING	79

Format: F1
Value   Label
  1   NEVER EXPERIENCED
  2   NO DIFFICULTY
  3   SLIGHT DIFFICULTY
  4   MODERATE DIFFICULTY
  5   GREAT DIFFICULTY
  6   EXTREME DIFFICULTY

SOCMID3 SOC SIT MID 3 PUB TRANSPORTATION   80
Format: F1
Value   Label
  1   NEVER EXPERIENCED
  2   NO DIFFICULTY
  3   SLIGHT DIFFICULTY
  4   MODERATE DIFFICULTY
  5   GREAT DIFFICULTY
  6   EXTREME DIFFICULTY

SOCMID5 SOC SIT MID 5 MAKING MEXICAN   82
FRIENDS
Format: F1
Value   Label
  1   NEVER EXPERIENCED
  2   NO DIFFICULTY
  3   SLIGHT DIFFICULTY
  4   MODERATE DIFFICULTY
  5   GREAT DIFFICULTY
  6   EXTREME DIFFICULTY

SOCMID12 SOC SIT MID 12 BEING WITH   89
OLDER MEXICAN PEOPLE
Format: F1
Value   Label
  1   NEVER EXPERIENCED
  2   NO DIFFICULTY
  3   SLIGHT DIFFICULTY
  4   MODERATE DIFFICULTY
  5   GREAT DIFFICULTY
  6   EXTREME DIFFICULTY

Name	Position
SOCMID13 SOC SIT MID 13 MEETING STRANGERS/NEW PEOPLE	90

Format: F1
Value   Label
  1   NEVER EXPERIENCED
  2   NO DIFFICULTY
  3   SLIGHT DIFFICULTY
  4   MODERATE DIFFICULTY
  5   GREAT DIFFICULTY
  6   EXTREME DIFFICULTY

Figure **17-4** Example of data definitions from SPSS for Windows.

(Continued)

20 Feb 96 SPSS for MS WINDOWS Release 6.1   Page 1
——— **SYSFILE INFO** ———

File a:\mxco2.sav
  Created: 25 Jan 96 15:18:39–241 variables and 151 cases

File Type: SPSS Data File

N of Cases: 151
Total # of Defined Variable Elements: 241
Data Are Not Weighted
Data Are Compressed
File Contains Case Data

Variable Information:

Name	Position
STUDY-ID STUDY ID NUMBER	1
Format: F3	

RACE   RACE   2
  Format: F1
  Value Label
    1 white
    2 black
    3 Hispanic
    4 Asian
    5 other

EDUC   EDUCATION   3
  Format: F1
  Value   Label
    1 CURRENTLY ENROLLED IN HIGH SCHOOL
    2 CURRENTLY ENROLLED IN COLLEGE
    3 PREVIOUS COLLEGE WORK
    4 COLLEGE GRADUATE
    5 CURRENTLY ENROLLED GRAD STUDENT

GENDER   GENDER   4
  Format: F1
  Value Label
    1   MALE
    2   FEMALE

AGE   AGE   5
  Format: F1
  Value   Label
    1 16–18 YEARS
    2 19–21 YEARS
    3 22–25 YEARS
    4 26–40 YEARS
    5 41–50 YEARS
    6 51–60 YEARS
    7 OVER 60 YEARS

Name	Position

INCOME   ANNUAL INCOME   6
  Format: F1
  Value Label
    1 <$10,000
    2 $10,000–$19,999
    3 $20,000–$29,999
    4 $30,000–$39,999
    5 $40,000–$49,999
    6 >$50,000

AHEALTH   OVERALL HEALTH STATUS   55
  Format: F1
  Value Label
    1 EXCELLLENT
    2 GOOD
    3 FAIR
    4 POOR

AEXP1   EXPECT PRE 1 EXPECT MEXICANS   56
TO BE FRIENDLY
  Format: F1
  Value Label
    0 NO
    1 YES

AEXP2 EXPECT PRE 2 EXPECT TO USE   57
PUBLIC TRANSPORTATION
  Format: F1
  Value Label
    0 NO
    1 YES

AEXP3   EXPECT PRE 3 EXPECT TO MAKE   58
FRIENDS WITH MEXICANS
  Format: F1
  Value Label
    0 NO
    1 YES

AEXP4   EXPECT PRE 4 EXPECT TO   59
UNDERSTAND MEXICAN HUMOR
  Format: F1
  Value Label
    0 NO
    1 YES

AEXP5   EXPECT PRE 5 EXPECT MEXICANS   60
TO BE POLITE/HELPFUL
  Format: F1
  Value Label
    0 NO
    1 YES

Figure **17-4 Cont'd**

Variable Name	Variable Label	Source	Value Levels	Valid Range	Missing Data	Comments
A1 to A5	Family Apgar	Q2Family Apgar	1=never 2=hardly ever 3=some of the time 4=almost always 5=always	1 – 5	9	Code as is (CAI)
MF3	Mother's feeling, Day 3	Tuesday diary, mother	1=poor 6=good	1 – 6	9	Code 1 to 6 left to right

Figure **17-5** Example of coding.

8. Estimation of the number of subjects to be included in the study.
9. Plan for documenting refusal rate, sample size, and attrition during the study.
10. Plan of the dates for data collection initiation and completion and for data entry.

With this information, the assistant can develop the database in preparation for receiving the data. It will take an average of 16 hours of concentrated work to prepare the database. Approximate dates for completion of the data entry, analyses, or both must be negotiated before beginning data collection. If you have a deadline for completing or presenting your results, such as an upcoming conference, you should share this information with those performing data entry and analysis.

COLLECTING DATA

Data collection is the process of selecting subjects and gathering data from these subjects. The actual steps of collecting the data are specific to each study and depend on the research design and measurement methods. Data may be collected on subjects by observing, testing, measuring, questioning, recording, or any combination of these methods. The researcher is actively involved in this process either by collecting data or by supervising data collectors. You will apply people-management and problem-solving skills constantly as data collection tasks are implemented, kinks in the research plan are resolved, and support systems are used.

Data Collection Tasks

In both quantitative and qualitative research, the investigator performs four tasks during the process of data collection. These tasks are interrelated and occur concurrently rather than in sequence. The tasks are selecting subjects, collecting data in a consistent way,

maintaining research controls as indicated in the study design, and solving problems that threaten to disrupt the study. Selecting subjects is discussed in Chapter 14. Collecting data may involve administering Internet or paper-and-pencil scales; asking subjects to complete data collection forms in person or online; or recording data from observations, patients' records, or health care equipment (Chapter 16 focuses on measurement strategies). Data collection tasks for qualitative studies are discussed in more detail in Chapter 23.

Maintaining Controls

Maintaining consistency and controls during subject selection and data collection protects the integrity or validity of the study. Research controls were built into the design to minimize the influence of intervening forces on the study findings. Maintenance of these controls is essential. They are not natural in a field setting, and letting them slip is easy. In some cases, these controls slip without the researcher realizing it. In addition to maintaining the controls identified in the plan, you must continually watch for previously unidentified extraneous variables that might have an impact on the data being collected. These variables are often specific to a study and tend to become apparent during the data collection period. The extraneous variables identified during data collection must be considered during data analysis and interpretation. These variables also must be noted in the research report to allow future researchers to control them.

Problem Solving

Problems can be perceived either as a frustration or as a challenge. The fact that the problem occurred is not as important as successfully resolving it. Therefore, the final and perhaps most important task of the data collection period may be problem resolution. Little has been written about the problems encountered by nurse researchers. Research reports often read as though everything went smoothly. The implication is that if you are a good researcher, you will have no problems, which is not true. Research journals generally do not provide enough space for the researcher to describe the problems encountered, and inexperienced researchers may get a false impression. A more realistic picture can be obtained through personal discussions with researchers about the process of data collection. Some of the common problems experienced by researchers are discussed in the following section.

Data Collection Problems

Murphy's law (if anything can go wrong, it will, and at the worst possible time) seems to prevail at times in research, just as in other dimensions of life. For example, data collection frequently requires more time than was anticipated, and collecting the data is often more difficult than was expected. Sometimes changes must be made in the way the data are collected, in the specific data collected, or in the timing of data collection. People react to the study in unpredicted ways. Institutional changes may force modifications in the research plan, or unusual or unexpected events may occur. You must be as consistent as possible during the data collection process, but you must also be flexible in dealing with unforeseen problems. Sometimes, sticking with the original plan at all costs is a mistake. Skills in finding ways to resolve problems that will protect the integrity of the study can be critical.

In preparation for data collection, possible problems must be anticipated, and solutions for these problems must be explored. The following discussion describes some of the common problems and concerns and presents possible solutions. Problems that tend to occur with some regularity in studies have been categorized as people problems, researcher problems, institutional problems, and event problems.

People Problems

Nurses cannot place a subject in a laboratory test tube, instill one drop of the independent variable, and then measure the effect. Nursing studies are conducted by examining subjects as they interact with their environments. When research involves people, nothing is completely predictable. People, in their complexity and wholeness, have an impact on all aspects of nursing studies. Researchers, potential subjects, family members of subjects, health professionals, institutional staff, and others ("innocent bystanders") interact within the study situation. You will need to closely observe and evaluate these interactions to determine their impact on your study.

Problems Selecting a Sample. The first step in initiating data collection—selecting a sample—may be the beginning of people problems. You may find that few available people fit your sample criteria or that many of those you approach refuse to participate in the study even though the request seems reasonable. Appropriate subjects, who were numerous a month earlier, seem to have disappeared. Institutional procedures may change, which might make many potential subjects ineligible for participation in the study. You may have to reevaluate the sample criteria or seek additional sources for potential subjects. In research institutions that care for the indigent, patients tend to be reluctant to participate in research. This lack of participation might arise because these patients are frequently exposed to studies, feel manipulated, or misunderstand the research. Patients may feel that they are being used or are afraid that they will be harmed.

Subject Attrition or Mortality. After you have selected a sample, certain problems might cause subject attrition (a loss of subjects from the study). For example, some subjects may agree to participate but then fail to follow through. Some may not complete needed forms and questionnaires or may fill them out incorrectly. To reduce these problems, someone from the research team can supervise the subjects while they complete essential documents. Some subjects may not return for a second interview or may not be home for a scheduled visit. Although you have invested time to collect data from these subjects, their data may have to be excluded from analysis because of incompleteness.

Sometimes subjects must be dropped from the study because of changes in health status. For example, the patient may be transferred out of intensive care where the study is being conducted; the patient's condition may worsen, so he or she may no longer meet sample criteria; or the patient may die. Clinic patients may be transferred to another clinic or be discharged from the service. In the community, subjects may choose to discontinue services, or the limits of third-party reimbursement may force the health care provider to discontinue the services you are studying.

Subject attrition occurs, to some extent, in all studies. One way to deal with this problem is to anticipate the attrition rate and increase the planned number of subjects to ensure that a minimally desired number will complete the study. If subject attrition is higher than expected, consider continuing the data collection process for a longer period of time to achieve an adequate sample size. Sometimes a study might have to be completed with a smaller than expected sample size. If so, the effect of a smaller sample on the power of planned statistical analyses must be considered, because the smaller sample may not be adequate to test the hypotheses and result in a type II error.

An increasing number of researchers are providing important information about subjects' acceptance to participate in a study and attrition during the study to determine if the sample is representative of the study target population. Some published studies include a flow diagram that indicates the number of subjects meeting sample criteria, the potential subjects refusing to participate and their rationale, and the sample size

for the study. If data are collected over time (repeated measures) or the study intervention is implemented over time, subjects will often drop out of a study, and it is important to document the attrition of these subjects. Badger, Segrin, Dorros, Meek, and Lopez (2007) provided a flow diagram that documented the participants' selection, refusal rate, assignment to groups, and attrition over the weeks of data collection (Figure 17-6). The flow diagram clearly identifies important aspects of the sampling process and the rationale

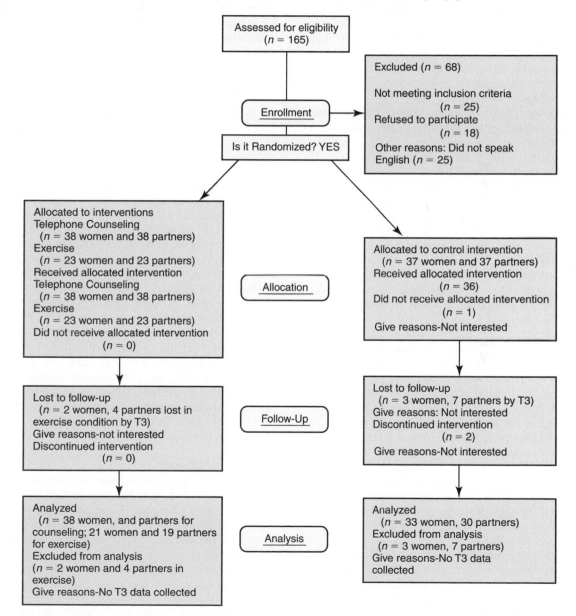

Figure **17-6** Sample selection and allocation.

for the attrition of study subjects. This information enabled these researchers to determine the representativeness of their sample and any potential for bias.

Subject as an Object. The quality of interactions between the researcher and subjects during the study is a critical dimension for maintaining subject participation. When researchers are under pressure to complete a study, people can be treated as objects rather than as subjects. In addition to being unethical, such treatment alters interactions, diminishes the subject's satisfaction, and increases subject mortality. Subjects are scarce resources and must be treated with care. The researcher's treatment of the subject as an object can lead to similar treatment by other health care providers and result in poor quality of care. In this case, participation in the study becomes detrimental to the subject.

External Influences on Subject Responses. People interacting with the subject, the researcher, or both can have an important impact on the data collection process. Family members may not agree to the subject's participation in the study or may not understand the study process. These people will, in most cases, influence the subject's decisions related to the study. Researchers benefit from taking the time to explain the study and to seek the cooperation of family members. Family cooperation is essential when the potential subject is critically ill and unable to give informed consent.

Family members or other patients may also influence the subject's responses to scales or interview questions. In some cases, subjects may ask family members, friends, or other patients to complete study forms for them. The subject may discuss questions on the forms with whomever happens to be in the room, and therefore the questionnaire may not record the subjects' real feelings. If interviews are conducted while other persons are in the room, the subject's responses may depend on his or her need to meet the expectations of other persons. Sometimes, a family member may answer questions addressed verbally to the patient. Thus, the setting in which a questionnaire is completed or an interview is conducted may determine the extent to which the answers are a true reflection of the subject's feelings. If the privacy afforded by the setting varies from one subject to another, the subjects' responses may also vary.

Usually, the most desirable setting for an interview is a private area away from distractions. If it is not possible to arrange for such a setting, the researcher can be present at the time the questionnaire is completed to decrease the influence of others. If the questionnaire is to be completed later or taken home and returned at a later time, the probability of influence by others increases and the return of questionnaires greatly decreases. The impact of this problem on the integrity of the study depends on the nature of the questionnaire.

Passive Resistance. Health professionals and institutional staff working with the subject may affect the data collection process. Some professionals verbalize strong support for the study and yet passively interfere with data collection. For example, nurses providing care may fail to follow the guidelines agreed on for providing the specific care activities being studied, or information needed for the study may be left off patient records. The researcher may not be informed when a potential subject has been admitted, and a physician who has agreed that his or her patients can be study subjects may decide as each patient is admitted that this one is not quite right for the study. In addition, the physician might become unusually unavailable to the researcher.

Nonprofessional staff may not realize the impact of the data collection process on their work patterns until the process begins. The data collection process may violate their beliefs about how care should be provided (and has been provided for the past 20 years). If ignored, their resistance can completely undo a carefully designed study. For example, research on skin care may disrupt a nursing aide's bathing routine, so he or she may continue the normal routine regardless of the study protocol and thereby invalidate the study findings.

Because of the potential impact of these problems, the researcher must maintain open communication and nurture positive relationships with other professionals and staff during data collection. Problems that you and your team recognize early and deal with promptly will have fewer serious consequences than will those that you ignore. However, not all problems can be resolved. Sometimes you may need to seek creative ways to work around an individual or to counter the harmful consequences of passive resistance.

Researcher Problems

Some problems are a consequence of the researcher's interaction with the study situation or lack of skill in data collection techniques. These problems are often difficult to identify because of the researcher's personal involvement. However, their effect on the study can be serious.

Researcher Interactions. The researcher can become so involved in interactions with people involved in the study that data collection on the subject is not completed. Researcher interactions can also interfere with data collection in interview situations.

If you are collecting data while you are surrounded by professionals with whom you interact socially and professionally, it is sometimes difficult to focus completely on the study situation. This lack of attention usually leads to loss of data.

Lack of Skill in Data Collection Techniques. The researcher's skill in using a particular data collection technique can affect the quality of the data collected. A researcher who is unskilled at the beginning of data collection might practice the data collection techniques with the assistance of an experienced researcher. A pilot study to test data collection techniques can be helpful. If data collectors are being used, they also need opportunities to practice data collection techniques before the study is initiated. Sometimes a skill is developed during the course of study; if this is the case, as one's skill increases, the data being collected may change and thereby confound the study findings and threaten the validity of the study. If more than one data collector is used, changes in skill can occur more frequently than if the researcher is the data collector. The skills of data collectors must be evaluated during the study to detect any changes in their data collection techniques.

Researcher Role Conflict. Professional nurses conducting clinical research often experience a conflict between the researcher role and the clinician role during data collection. As a researcher, one is observing and recording events. In some cases, the researcher's involvement in the event, such as providing physical or emotional care to a patient during an interview, could alter the event and thus bias the results. It would be difficult to generalize the findings to other situations in which the researcher was not present to intervene. However, the needs of patients must take precedence over the needs of the study. The dilemma is to determine when the needs of patients are great enough to warrant researcher intervention.

Some patient situations are life threatening—such as respiratory distress and changes in cardiac function—and require immediate action by anyone present. Other patient needs are simple, can be addressed by any nurse available, and are not likely to alter the results of the study. Examples of these interventions include giving the patient a bedpan, informing the nurse of the patient's need for pain medication, or helping the patient to open food containers. These situations seldom cause a dilemma.

Solutions to other situations are not as easy. Suppose, for example, that your study involves examining the emotional responses of patients' family members during and immediately after the patients' operations. Your study includes an experimental group that receives one 30-minute family support session before and during the patients' operations and a control group that receives no support session. Both sets of families are being monitored for 1 week after the surgeries to measure their levels of anxiety and coping strategies. You are currently collecting data on the control group. The data consist of demographic information and scales measuring anxiety and coping. One of the family members is in great distress. After completing the demographic information, she verbally expresses her fears and the lack of support she has received from the nursing staff. Two other subjects from different families hear the expressed distress and concur; they move closer to the conversation and look to you for information and support. In this situation, a supportive response from you is likely to modify the results of the study because these responses are part of the treatment to be provided to the experimental group only. This interaction is likely to narrow the difference between the two groups and thus decrease the possibility that the results will show a significant difference between the two groups. How should you respond? Are you obligated to provide support? To some extent, almost any response will be supportive. One alternative is to provide the needed support and not include these family members in the control group. Another alternative is to recruit the help of a nonprofessional to collect the data from the control group. However, recognize that most people will provide some degree of support in the described situation, even though their skills in supportive techniques may vary.

Other dilemmas include witnessing unethical behavior that interferes with patient care or witnessing subjects' unethical or illegal behavior (Field & Morse, 1985). Try to anticipate these dilemmas before data collection whenever possible. Pilot studies can help you to identify dilemmas likely to occur in a study, and you can build strategies into the design to minimize or avoid them. However, some dilemmas cannot be anticipated, and you must respond to these problems spontaneously. There is no prescribed way to handle difficult dilemmas; each case must be dealt with individually. We recommend discussing unethical and illegal behavior with colleagues, members of ethics committees, or legal advisors. After you have resolved the dilemma, it is wise to reexamine the situation for its effect on study results and consider options in case the situation arises again.

Maintaining Perspective. Data collection includes both joys and frustrations. Researchers must be able to maintain some degree of objectivity during the process and yet not take themselves too seriously (Marshall & Rossman, 2006). A sense of humor is invaluable. You must be able to experience the emotions and then become the rational problem solver. Management skills and mental health are invaluable to a lifetime researcher.

Institutional Problems

Institutions are in a constant state of change. They will not stop changing for the period of a study, and these changes often affect data collection. A nurse who has been most helpful in your study may be promoted or transferred. The unit on which your study is conducted may be reorganized, moved, or closed during the study. An area used for subjects' interviews may be transformed into an office or a storeroom or may be torn down. Patient record forms may be revised, omitting data that you and your team collected. The record room personnel may be reorganizing their files and be temporarily unable to provide needed charts.

These problems are, for the most part, completely outside of the researcher's control. Keep an ear to the internal communication network of the institution for advanced warning of impending changes. Contacts within the institution's administrative decision-making system could warn you about the impact of proposed changes on an ongoing study. However, in many cases, data collection strategies might have to be modified to meet the newly emerging situation. Again, flexibility while maintaining the integrity of the study may be the key to successful data collection. Byers (1995) suggested that in the future the home setting may be more desirable than institutions as a data collection site and that the response rate in this setting is better than that in institutions. The disadvantage is that home visits are time intensive and the subject may not be home at the agreed appointment time.

Event Problems

Unpredictable events can be a source of frustration during a study. Research tools ordered from a testing company may be lost in the mail. The duplicating machine may break down just before 500 data collection forms are to be copied, or a machine to be used in data collection may break down and require 6 weeks for repair. A computer ordered for data collection may not arrive when promised, a tape recorder may jam in the middle of an interview, or after an interview the data collector may discover that he or she had not pushed the record button and there is no recording of the interview. Data collection forms may be misplaced, misfiled, or lost.

Local, national, or world events and nature can also influence subjects' responses to a study. For example, one of our graduate students was examining patients' attitudes toward renal dialysis. She planned to collect data for 6 months. Three months into the data collection process, three patients died as a result of a dialysis machine malfunction in the city where the study was being conducted. The event made national headlines. Obviously, this event could be expected to modify subjects' responses. In attempting to deal with the impact of the event on the study, the graduate student could have modified the study and continued collecting data to examine the impact of news such as this on attitudes. However, the emotional climate of the clinics participating in the study was not conducive to this option. She chose to wait 3 months before collecting additional data and examined the data before and after the event for statistically significant differences in responses. Because she could not find any differences, she could justify using all the data for analysis.

Other less dramatic events can also have an impact on data collection. If data collection for the entire sample is planned for a single time, a snowstorm or a flood may require that the researcher cancel the meeting or clinic. Weather may decrease attendance far below that expected at a support group or series of teaching sessions. A bus strike can disrupt transportation systems to such an extent that subjects can no longer get to the data collection site. A new health agency may open in the city, which may decrease demand for the care activities being studied. Conversely, an external event can also increase attendance at clinics to such an extent that existing resources are stretched and data collection is no longer possible. These events are also outside the researcher's control and are impossible to anticipate. In most cases, however, restructuring the data collection period can salvage the study. To do so, it is necessary to examine all possible alternatives for collecting the study data. In some cases, data collection can simply be rescheduled; in other situations, the changes needed may be more complex.

SERENDIPITY

Serendipity is the accidental discovery of something useful or valuable. During the data collection phase of studies, researchers often become aware of elements or relationships that they had not previously identified. These aspects may be closely related to the study being conducted or have little connection with it. They come from increased awareness and close observation of the study situation. Because the researcher is focused on close observation, other elements in the situation can come into clearer focus and take on new meaning. Like the open context situation discussed in Chapter 4, the researcher's perspective shifts, and new gestalts are formed.

Serendipitous findings are important to the development of new insights in nursing theory. They can be important for understanding the totality of the phenomenon being examined. Additionally, they lead to areas of research that generate new knowledge. Therefore, it is essential to capture these insights as they occur. These events must be carefully recorded, even if their impact or meaning is not understood at the time. Sometimes, when these notes are reexamined at a later time, patterns begin to emerge.

Serendipitous findings can also lead the researcher astray. Sometimes researchers forget the original plan and redirect their attention to the newly discovered dimensions. Although modifying data collection to include data related to the new discovery may be valid, there has not been time to carefully plan a study related to the new findings. Examination of the new data should only be an offshoot of the initial study. Data collected as a result of serendipitous findings can guide future studies and must be included in presentations and publications related to the study. Although the meaning of the discovery may not be understood, sharing the information may lead to insights by researchers studying related phenomena.

HAVING ACCESS TO SUPPORT SYSTEMS

The researcher must have access to individuals or groups who can provide support and consultation during the data collection period. Support systems themselves have been the subject of much study in recent years. In some cases, they can be the source of both stress and support. However, current theorists propose that to be classified as support, the individual or group must enhance the ego strength of the individual. Three dimensions of support have been identified: (1) physical assistance, (2) the provision of money or other concrete needs such as equipment or information, and (3) emotional support. These types of support can usually be obtained from academic committees; from institutions serving as research settings; and from colleagues, friends, and family.

Support of Academic Committees

Although thesis and dissertation committees are basically seen as stern keepers of the sanctity of the research process, they also serve as support systems for neophyte researchers. In fact, committee members must be selected from faculty who are willing and able to provide the needed support. Experienced researchers among faculty are usually more knowledgeable about the types of support needed. Because they are directly involved in research, they tend to be sensitive to the needs of neophyte researchers.

Institutional Support

A support system within the institution where the study is being conducted is also important. Support might come from people serving on the institutional research committee or from nurses working on the unit where the study is to be conducted. These people often have knowledge of how the institution functions, and their closeness to the study can increase their understanding of the problems experienced by the researcher and subjects. Do not overlook their ability to provide useful suggestions and assistance. Your ability to resolve some of the problems encountered during data collection may depend on having someone within the power structure of the institution who can intervene.

Personal Support

In addition to professional support, it is helpful to have at least one significant other with whom one can share the joys, frustrations, and current problems of data collection. A significant other can often serve as a mirror to allow you to see the situation clearly and perhaps more objectively. Through personal support, the researcher can share and release feelings and distance himself or herself from the data collection situation. Alternatives for resolving the problem can then be discussed. Data collection is a demanding, but rewarding, time that increases the confidence and expertise of the neophyte researcher.

MANAGING DATA

When data collection begins, you will have to handle large quantities of data. To avoid a state of total confusion, make careful plans before data collection begins. Plans are needed to keep all data from a single subject together until analysis is begun. Write the subject code number on each form, and check the forms for each subject to ensure that they are all present. Researchers have been known to sort their data by form, such as putting all the scales of one kind together, only to realize afterward that they had failed to code the forms with subject identification numbers first. They then had no idea which scale belonged to which subject, and valuable data were lost.

Allot space needs for storing forms. Purchase file folders, and design a labeling method to allow easy access to data; color coding is often useful. For example, if you are using multiple forms, the subject's demographic sheet could be one color, with different colors for the visual analogue scale; the pain questionnaire;

the physiological data sheet with blood pressure, pulse, and respiration readings; and the interview notes. Use envelopes to hold small pieces of paper or note cards that might fall out of a file folder. Plan to code data and enter them into the computer as soon as possible after data collection to reduce the loss or disorganization of data. If data are collected on a computer, make sure the data are backed up so that they are not lost if the computer fails.

Preparing Data for Computer Entry

Data must be carefully checked and problems corrected before you initiate the data entry phase. The data entry process should be essentially automatic and require no decisions regarding the data. Such simplicity in data entry will reduce the number of data entry errors and markedly decrease the time required for entry. It is not sufficient to establish general rules for those entering data such as "in this case always do X." This action still requires the data enterer to recognize a problem, refer to a general rule, and correct the data before entering them. Anything that alters the rhythm of data entry increases errors. Carefully examine each datum to search for the following problems and resolve them before data entry:

1. *Missing data.* Provide the data if possible or determine the impact of the missing data on your analysis. In some cases, the subject must be excluded from at least some of the analyses, so you must determine what data are essential.
2. *Items in which the subject provided two responses when only one was requested.* For example, if the item asked the subject to mark the most important in a list of 10 items and the subject selected 2, you must decide how to resolve this problem; do not leave the decision to an assistant who is entering the data. On the form, indicate how the datum is to be coded.
3. *Items in which the subject has marked a response between two options.* This problem commonly occurs with Likert-type scales, particularly those using forced choice options. Given four options, the subject places a mark on the line between response 2 and response 3. On the form, indicate how the datum is to be coded (missing data is an option).
4. *Items that ask the subject to write in some information such as occupation or diagnosis.* Such items are a data enterer's nightmare. Develop a list of codes for entering such data. Rather than leaving it up to the assistant to determine which code matches the subject's written response, the researcher should enter this code before turning

the data over for entry. After the data have been checked and needed codes written in, it is prudent to make a copy rather than turning over the only set of your data to an assistant.

Data Entry Period

If you are entering your own data, develop a rhythm to your entry. Avoid distractions while entering data, and limit your data entry periods to 2 hours at a time to reduce errors. Back up the database after each data entry period, and store it on a flash stick or CD-ROM. It is possible for the computer to crash and lose all of your data. If an assistant is entering your data, make yourself as available as possible to respond to questions and address problems. After entry, the data should be checked for accuracy. Data checking is discussed in Chapter 18 in the Preparation of the Data for Analysis section.

Storage and Retrieval of Data

In this time of flash sticks and CD-ROM burners, it is relatively easy to store data. Decide how long you wish to store the data. The original data forms must be stored, as well as the database. There are several reasons to store data. The data can be used for secondary analyses. For example, individuals who are participating in a research program related to a particular research focus may pool data from various studies for access by all members of the group. The data are available to document the validity of your analyses and the published results of your study. Because of nationally publicized incidents of scientific misconduct where researchers invented data from which multiple publications were developed, you are wise to preserve documentation that your data were obtained as you claim. Issues that have been raised include how long data should be stored, the need for institutional policy regarding data storage, and whether graduate students who conduct a study should leave a copy of their data at the university. Thomas (1992) surveyed 153 researchers to determine their responses to these questions. She found that the length of data storage varied greatly, with 29% storing their data 5 years, 31% storing it 10 years, and 21% storing it forever. Most researchers stored their data in their office (84%), and a few used a central location (12%) or a laboratory (4%). The forms of data storage devices preferred were disk (54%), tape (47%), and paper/raw data (32%). Some researchers preferred more than one storage device for their data. The majority of the researchers (86%) indicated that their institutions did not have a policy for data storage, and most graduate students (74%) did not leave a copy of their data at the university.

SUMMARY

- To plan the process of data collection, the researcher must determine step by step how and in what sequence data will be collected and the timing of the process.
- Decision points that occur during data collection must be identified and all options considered.
- The researcher must decide who will collect the data.
- If data collectors are used, they must be informed about the research project, introduced to the instruments, and provided equivalent training in the data collection process. After training, data collectors must be evaluated to determine their consistency.
- Consistency in data collection across subjects is critical, and so is consistency among data collectors if more than one data collector is used.
- The researcher must develop data collection forms so that data can be recorded and entered into the computer more easily.
- A research treatment or intervention must be implemented in a reliable and competent way to promote intervention fidelity in a study. The person implementing the study intervention (an interventionalist) must be trained to ensure adherence and competence in the intervention protocol.
- Data collection involves four tasks: selecting subjects, collecting data in a consistent way, maintaining research controls, and solving problems that threaten to disrupt the study.
- Some of the problems researchers encounter during data collection include problems in selection of a sample, subject mortality, treatment of the subject as an object, external influences on subject responses, passive resistance, researcher interactions, lack of skill in data collection techniques, researcher role conflicts, and maintaining perspective.
- A successive study requires support that is often obtained from academic committees; health care agencies; and personnel, family members, and friends.
- Data collected during a study must be accurately entered in a computer and safely stored.

REFERENCES

Badger, T., Segrin, C., Dorros, S., Meek, P., & Lopez, A. M. (2007). Depression and anxiety in women with breast cancer and their partners. *Nursing Research, 56*(1), 44–53.

Bernhardt, J. M., Strecher, V. J., Bishop, K. R., Potts, P., Madison, E. M., & Thorp, J. (2001). Handheld computer-assisted self-interviews: User comfort level and preferences. *American Journal of Health Behavior, 25*(6), 557–563.

Byers, V. L. (1995). Overview of the data collection process. *Journal of Neuroscience Nursing, 27*(3), 188–193.

Craig, J. V., & Smyth, R. L. (2007). *The evidence-base practice manual for nurses* (2nd ed.). Edinburgh, Scotland: Churchill Livingstone.

Dennis, K. E. (1994). Managing questionnaire data through optical scanning technology. *Nursing Research, 43*(6), 376–378.

Field, P. A., & Morse, J. M. (1985). *Nursing research: The application of qualitative approaches* (pp. 65–90). Rockville MD: Aspen.

Gift, A. G., Creasia, J., & Parker, B. (1991). Utilizing research assistants and maintaining research integrity. *Research in Nursing & Health, 14*(3), 229–233.

Harrison, L. L. (1989). Interfacing bioinstruments with computers for data collection in nursing research. *Research in Nursing & Health, 12*(2), 129–133.

Im, E., Chee, W., Guevara, E., Liu, Y., Lim, H., Tsai, H., et al. (2006). *Cancer pain management: Decision support computer program*. Unpublished manuscript.

Im, E., Chee, W., Guevara, E., Liu, Y., Lim, H., Tsai H., et al. (2007). Gender and ethnic differences in cancer pain experience: A multiethnic survey in the United States. *Nursing Research, 56*(5), 296–306.

Marshall, C., & Rossman, G. B. (2006). *Designing qualitative research* (4th ed.). Thousand Oaks, CA: Sage.

Melnyk, B. M., & Fineout-Overholt, E. (2005). *Evidence-based practice in nursing & healthcare: A guide to best practice*. Philadelphia, Lippincott Williams & Wilkins.

Savian, C., Paratz, J., & Davies, A. (2006). Comparison of the effectiveness of manual and ventilator hyperinflation at different levels of positive end-expiratory pressure in artificially ventilated and intubated intensive care patients. *Heart & Lung, 35*(5), 334–341.

Stein, K. F., Sargent, J. T., & Rafaels, N. (2007). Intervention research: Establishing fidelity of the independent variable in nursing clinical trials. *Nursing Research, 56*(1), 54–62.

Thomas, S. P. (1992). Storage of research data: Why, how, where? *Nursing Research, 41*(5), 309–311.

Washington, C. C., & Moss, M. (1988). Methodology corner: Pragmatic aspects of establishing interrater reliability in research. *Nursing Research, 37*(3), 190–191.

CHAPTER 18
Introduction to Statistical Analysis

Data analysis is probably the most exciting part of research. During this phase, you will finally obtain answers to the questions that initially generated your research activity. Nevertheless, nurses probably experience greater anxiety about this phase of the research process than any other, as they question issues that range from their knowledge about critiquing published studies to their ability to conduct research. To critique a quantitative study, you need to be able to (1) identify the statistical procedures used; (2) judge whether these statistical procedures were appropriate for the hypotheses, questions, or objectives of the study and for the data available for analysis; (3) comprehend the discussion of data analysis results; (4) judge whether the author's interpretation of the results is appropriate; and (5) evaluate the clinical significance of the findings. A neophyte researcher performing a quantitative study is confronted with many critical decisions related to data analysis that require statistical knowledge. To perform statistical analysis of data from a quantitative study, you need to be able to (1) prepare the data for analysis; (2) describe the sample; (3) test the reliability of measures used in the study; (4) perform exploratory analyses of the data; (5) perform analyses guided by the study objectives, questions, or hypotheses; and (6) interpret the results of statistical procedures. Critiquing studies and performing statistical analyses both require an understanding of the statistical theory underlying the process of analysis.

This chapter and the following five will provide you with the information needed to critique the statistical sections of published studies or perform statistical procedures. This chapter introduces the concepts of statistical theory and discusses some of the more pragmatic aspects of quantitative data analysis: the purposes of statistical analysis, the process of performing data analysis, the method for choosing appropriate statistical procedures for a study, and resources for statistical analysis. Chapter 19 explains the use of statistics for descriptive purposes; Chapter 20 discusses the use of statistics to test proposed relationships; Chapter 21 explores the use of statistics for prediction; and Chapter 22 guides you in using statistics to examine causality.

CONCEPTS OF STATISTICAL THEORY

One reason that nurses tend to avoid statistics is that many were taught only the mathematical mechanics of calculating statistical formulas and were given little or no explanation of the logic behind the analysis procedure or the meaning of the results. This mechanical process is usually performed by computer, and information about it offers little assistance to those making statistical decisions or explaining results. We will approach data analysis from the perspective of enhancing your understanding of the meaning underlying statistical analysis. You can then use this understanding either to critique or to perform data analyses.

As is common in many theories, theoretical ideas related to statistics are expressed by unique terminology and logic that is unfamiliar to many. Research ideas (particularly data analysis as expressed in the language of the clinician and the researcher) are perceived by statisticians to be relatively imprecise and vague because they are not expressed in the formal language of the professional statistician. To resolve this language barrier, it is necessary to translate a data analysis plan from the common language (or even general research language) to the language of statisticians. When the analysis is complete, the results must be translated from the language of the statistician back to the language of the researcher and the clinician. Thus, explaining the results is a process of interpretation (Chervany, 1977). Figure 18-1 illustrates this process of translation and interpretation.

The ensuing discussion explains some of the concepts commonly used in statistical theory. The logic of statistical theory is embedded within the explanations of these concepts. The concepts presented include probability theory, decision theory, inference, the theoretical normal curve, sampling distributions, sampling distribution of a statistic, shapes of distributions, standardized scores, confidence intervals, statistics and parameters, samples and populations, estimation of parameters, degrees of freedom, tailedness, type I and type II errors, level of significance, power, clinical significance, parametric and nonparametric statistical analyses, causality, and relationships.

Probability Theory

Probability theory addresses statistical analysis as the likelihood of accurately predicting an event or the extent of a relationship. Nurse researchers might be interested in the probability of a particular nursing outcome in a particular patient care situation. With probability theory, you could determine how much of the variation in your data could be explained by using a particular statistical analysis. In probability theory, the researcher interprets the meaning of statistical results

in light of his or her knowledge of the field of study. A finding that would have little meaning in one field of study might be important in another (Good, 1983). Probability is expressed as a lowercase p, with values expressed as percentages or as a decimal value ranging from 0 to 1. If the exact probability is known to be 0.23, for example, it would be expressed as $p = 0.23$.

Decision Theory and Hypothesis Testing

Decision theory is inductive in nature and is based on assumptions associated with the theoretical normal curve. When using decision theory, one always begins with the assumption that all the groups are members of the same population. This assumption is expressed as a null hypothesis. See Chapter 8 for an explanation of null hypothesis. To test the assumption, a cutoff point is selected before data collection. This cutoff point, referred to as alpha (α), or the level of significance, is the point on the normal curve at which the results of statistical analysis indicate a statistically significant difference between the groups. Decision theory requires that the cutoff point be absolute. Thus, the meaning applied to the statistical results is not based on the researcher's interpretation. Absolute means that even if the value obtained is only a fraction above the cutoff point, the samples are considered to be from the same population and no meaning can be attributed to the differences. Thus, it is inappropriate when using this theory to make a statement that "the findings approached significance at the 0.051 level" if the alpha level was set at 0.05. By decision theory rules, this finding indicates that the groups tested are not significantly different and the null hypothesis is accepted. On the other hand, if the

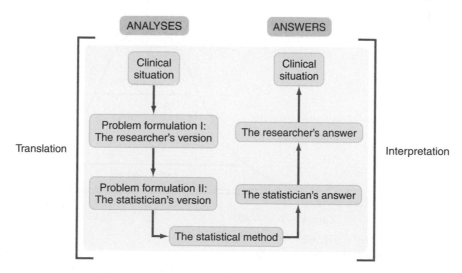

Figure **18-1** Process of translation and interpretation in statistics.

analysis reveals a significant difference of 0.001, this result is not more significant than the 0.05 originally proposed (Slakter, Wu, & Suzuki-Slakter, 1991).

Inference

Statisticians use the term inference or infer in somewhat the same way that a researcher uses the term *generalize*. Inference requires the use of inductive reasoning. One infers from a specific case to a general truth, from a part to the whole, from the concrete to the abstract, from the known to the unknown. When using inferential reasoning, you can never prove things; you can never be certain. However, one of the reasons for the rules that have been established with regard to statistical procedures is to increase the probability that inferences are accurate. Inferences are made cautiously and with great care.

Normal Curve

The theoretical normal curve is an expression of statistical theory. It is a theoretical frequency distribution of all *possible* scores. However, no real distribution exactly fits the normal curve. The idea of the normal curve was developed by an 18-year-old mathematician, Johann Gauss, in 1795, who found that data measured repeatedly in many samples from the same population by using scales based on an underlying continuum can be combined into one large sample. From this large sample, one can develop a more accurate representa-

tion of the pattern of the curve in that population than is possible with only one sample. Surprisingly, in most cases, the curve is similar, regardless of the specific data that have been examined or the population being studied.

This theoretical normal curve is symmetrical and unimodal and has continuous values. The mean, median, and mode (summary statistics) are equal (Figure 18-2). The distribution is completely defined by the mean and standard deviation. The measures in the theoretical distribution have been standardized by using Z scores. These terms are explained further in Chapter 19. Note the Z scores and standard deviation (SD) values indicated in Figure 18-2. The proportion of scores that may be found in a particular area of the normal curve has been identified. In a normal curve, 68% of the scores will be within 1 SD or 1 Z score above or below the mean, 95% will be within 1.96 SD above or below the mean, and more than 99% will be within 2.58 SD above or below the mean. Even when statistics, such as means, come from a population with a skewed (asymmetrical) distribution, the sampling distribution developed from multiple means obtained from that skewed population will tend to fit the pattern of the normal curve. This phenomenon is referred to as the central limit theorem. One requirement for the use of parametric statistical analysis is that the data must be normally distributed—normal meaning that the data approximately fit the normal curve.

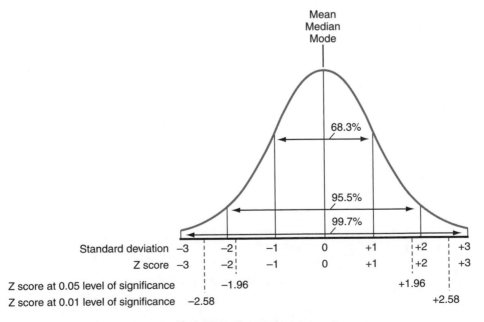

Figure **18-2** The normal curve.

Many statistical measures from skewed samples also fit the normal curve because of the central limit theorem; thus, some statisticians believe that it is justifiable to use parametric statistical analysis even with data from skewed samples if the sample is large enough (Volicer, 1984).

Sampling Distributions

A distribution is the state or manner in which values are arranged within the data set. A sampling distribution is the manner in which statistical values (such as means), obtained from multiple samples of the same population, are distributed within the set of values. The mean of this type of distribution is referred to as the mean of means (μ). Sampling distributions can also be developed from standard deviations. Other values, such as correlations between variables, scores obtained from specific measures, and scores reflecting differences between groups within the population, can yield values that can be used to develop sampling distributions.

The sampling distribution allows us to estimate sampling error. Sampling error is the difference between the sample statistic used to estimate a parameter and the actual, but unknown, value of the parameter. If we know the sampling distribution of a statistic, it allows us to measure the probability of making an incorrect inference. One should never make an inference without being able to calculate the probability of making an incorrect inference.

Sampling Distribution of a Statistic

Just as it is possible to develop distributions of summary statistics within a population, it is possible to develop distributions of inferential statistical outcomes. For example, if you repeatedly obtained two samples of the same size from the same population and tested for differences in the means with a *t*-test, you could develop a sampling distribution from the resulting *t* values by using probability theory. With this approach, you could develop a distribution for samples of many varying sizes. Such a distribution has, in fact, been generated by using *t* values. A table of *t* distribution values is available in Appendix C. Tables have been developed with this strategy to organize the statistical outcomes of many statistical procedures from various sample sizes. Because listing all possible outcomes would require many pages, most tables include only values that have a low probability of occurring in the present theoretical population. These probabilities are expressed as alpha (α), commonly referred to as the level of significance, and as beta (β), the probability of a type II error.

By using the appropriate sampling distribution, you could determine the probability of obtaining a specific statistical result if the two samples you have been studying are really from the same population. Statistical analysis makes an inference that the samples being tested can be considered part of the population from which the sampling distribution was developed. This inference is expressed as a null hypothesis.

The Shapes of Distributions

The shape of the distribution provides important information about the data. The outline of the distribution shape is obtained by using a histogram. Within this outline, the mean, median, mode, and standard deviation can then be graphically illustrated (see Figure 18-2). This visual presentation of combined summary statistics provides insight into the nature of the distribution. As the sample size becomes larger, the shape of the distribution will more accurately reflect the shape of the population from which the sample was taken.

Symmetry

Several terms are used to describe the shape of the curve (and thus the nature of a particular distribution). The shape of a curve is usually discussed in terms of symmetry, skewness, modality, and kurtosis. A *symmetrical curve* is one in which the left side is a mirror image of the right side (Figure 18-3). In these curves, the mean, median, and mode are equal and are the dividing point between the left and right sides of the curve.

Skewness

Any curve that is not symmetrical is referred to as skewed or asymmetrical. Skewness may be exhibited in the curve in a variety of ways (Figure 18-4). A curve

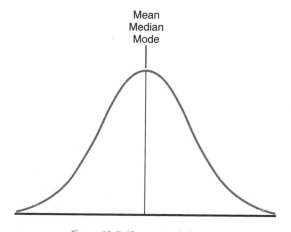

Mean
Median
Mode

Figure **18-3** The symmetrical curve.

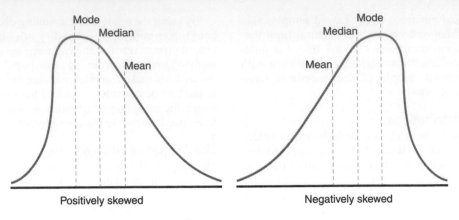

Figure **18-4** **Skewness.**

may be positively skewed, which means that the largest portion of data is below the mean. For example, data on length of enrollment in hospice are positively skewed. Most of the people die within the first 3 weeks of enrollment, whereas increasingly smaller numbers survive as time increases. A curve can also be negatively skewed, which means that the largest portion of data is above the mean. For example, data on the occurrence of chronic illness by age in a population are negatively skewed, with most chronic illnesses occurring in older age groups.

In a *skewed distribution,* the mean, median, and mode are not equal. Skewness interferes with the validity of many statistical analyses; therefore, statistical procedures have been developed to measure the skewness of the distribution of the sample being studied. Few samples will be perfectly symmetrical; however, as the deviation from symmetry increases, the seriousness of the impact on statistical analysis increases. A popular skewness measure is expressed in the following equation:

$$\text{Skewness} = \frac{\Sigma \left(X - \bar{X} \right)^3}{N \left(SD^3 \right)}$$

In this equation, a result of zero indicates a completely symmetrical distribution, a positive number indicates a positively skewed distribution, and a negative number indicates a negatively skewed distribution. Statistical analyses conducted by computer often automatically measure skewness, which is then indicated on the computer printout. Strongly skewed distributions often must be analyzed by nonparametric techniques, which make no assumptions of normally distributed samples. In a positively skewed distribution, the mean is greater than the median, which is

greater than the mode. In a negatively skewed distribution, the mean is less than the median, which is less than the mode. There is no firm rule about when data are sufficiently skewed to require the use of nonparametric techniques. The researcher and the statistician should make this decision jointly.

Modality

Another characteristic of distributions is their modality. Most curves found in practice are unimodal, which means that they have one mode and frequencies progressively decline as they move away from the mode. Symmetrical distributions are usually unimodal. However, curves can also be bimodal (Figure 18-5) or multimodal. When you find a bimodal sample, it usually means that you have not adequately defined your population.

Kurtosis

Another term used to describe the shape of the distribution curve is kurtosis. Kurtosis explains the degree of peakedness of the curve, which is related to the spread of variance of scores. An extremely peaked curve is referred to as leptokurtic, an intermediate degree of kurtosis as mesokurtic, and a relatively flat curve as platykurtic (Figure 18-6). Extreme kurtosis can affect the validity of statistical analysis because the scores

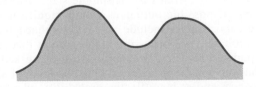

Figure **18-5** **Bimodal distribution.**

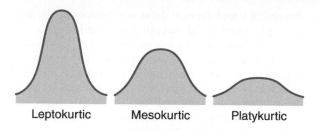

Figure **18-6** Kurtosis.

have little variation. Many computer programs analyze kurtosis before conducting statistical analysis. A common equation used to measure kurtosis is

$$Kurtosis = \frac{\Sigma\left(X - \bar{X}\right)^3}{N\left(SD^4\right)} - 3$$

A kurtosis of zero indicates that the curve is mesokurtic. Values below zero indicate a platykurtic curve (Box, Hunter, & Hunter, 1978). There is no firm rule about when data are sufficiently kurtotic to affect the validity of the statistical procedures. The researcher and the statistician should make this decision jointly.

Standardized Scores

Because of differences in the characteristics of various distributions, comparing a score in one distribution with a score in another distribution is difficult. For example, if you were comparing test scores from two classroom examinations and one test had a high score of 100 and the other had a high score of 70, the scores would be difficult to compare. To facilitate this comparison, a mechanism has been developed to transform raw scores into standard scores. Numbers that make sense only within the framework of the measurements used within a specific study are transformed into numbers (standard scores) that have a more general meaning. Transformation to standard scores makes it easier for those evaluating the numbers to conceptually grasp of the meaning of the score.

A common standardized score is called a Z score. It expresses deviations from the mean (difference scores) in terms of standard deviation units. The equation for a Z score is

$$Z = \frac{\Sigma\left(X - \bar{X}\right)}{SD}$$

A score that falls above the mean will have a positive Z score, whereas a score that falls below the mean will have a negative Z score (see Figure 18-2). The mean expressed as a Z score is zero. The SD of Z scores is 1.

Thus, a Z score of 2 indicates that the score from which it was obtained is 2 SD above the mean. A Z score of −0.5 indicates that the score was 0.5 SD below the mean. The larger the absolute value of the Z score, the less likely the observation is to occur. For example, a Z score of 4 would be extremely unlikely. The cumulative normal distribution expressed in Z scores is provided in Appendix B.

Confidence Intervals

When the probability of including the value of the parameter within the interval estimate is known (as described in Chapter 19), it is referred to as a confidence interval. Calculating the confidence interval involves the use of two formulas to identify the upper and lower ends of the interval. The formula for a 95% confidence interval when sampling from a population with a known standard deviation or from a normal population with a sample size greater than 30 is

$$\bar{X} - 1.96 \; SD \; / \sqrt{N} \qquad \bar{X} + 1.96 \; SD \; / \sqrt{N}$$

If you had a sample with a mean of 40, an SD of 5, and an N of 50, you would be able to calculate a confidence interval:

$$40 - 1.96\left(\frac{5}{\sqrt{50}}\right) = 40 - 1.386 = 38.6$$

$$40 + 1.96\left(\frac{5}{\sqrt{50}}\right) = 40 + 1.386 = 41.4$$

Confidence intervals are usually expressed as "(38.6, 41.4)," with 38.6 being the lower end and 41.4 being the upper end of the interval. Theoretically, we can produce a confidence interval for any parameter of a distribution. It is a generic statistical procedure. For example, confidence intervals can also be developed around correlation coefficients (Glass & Stanley, 1970). Estimation can be used for a single population or for multiple populations. In *estimation,* we are inferring the value of a parameter from sample data and have no preconceived notion of the value of the parameter. In contrast, in *hypothesis testing* we have an a priori theory about the value of the parameter or parameters or some combination of parameters.

Statistics and Parameters, Samples and Populations

Use of the terms *statistic* and *parameter* can be confusing because of the various populations referred to in statistical theory. A statistic ($\bar{x}$) is a numerical value obtained from a sample. A parameter is a true (but unknown) numerical characteristic of a population. For example, μ is the population mean or arithmetic average. The mean of the sampling distribution (mean of samples' means) can also be shown to be equal to μ. Thus, a numerical value that is the mean ($\bar{x}$) of the sample is a statistic; a numerical value that is the mean of the population is a parameter (Barnett, 1982).

Relating a statistic to a parameter requires an inference as one moves from the sample to the sampling distribution and then from the sampling distribution to the population. The population referred to is in one sense real (concrete) and in another sense abstract. These ideas are illustrated as follows:

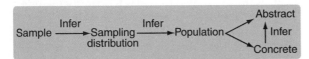

For example, perhaps you are interested in the cholesterol level of women in the United States. Your population is women in the United States. Obviously, you cannot measure the cholesterol level of every woman in the United States; therefore, you select a sample of women from this population. Because you wish your sample to be as representative of the population as possible, you obtain your sample by using random sampling techniques. To determine whether the cholesterol levels in your sample are like those in the population, you must compare the sample with the population. One strategy would be to compare the mean of your sample with the mean of the entire population. Unfortunately, it is highly unlikely that you *know* the mean of the entire population. Therefore, you must make an estimate of the mean of that population. You need to know how good your sample statistics are as estimators of the parameters of the population.

First, you make some assumptions. You assume that the mean scores of cholesterol levels from multiple randomly selected samples of this population would be normally distributed. This assumption implies another assumption: that the cholesterol levels of the population will be distributed according to the theoretical normal curve—that difference scores and standard deviations can be equated to those in the normal curve.

If you assume that the population in your study is normally distributed, you can also assume that this population can be represented by a normal sampling distribution. Thus, you infer from your sample to the sampling distribution, the mathematically developed theoretical population made up of parameters such as the mean of means and the standard error. The parameters of this theoretical population are those measures of the dimensions identified in the sampling distribution. You can then infer from the sampling distribution to the population. You have both a concrete population and an abstract population. The concrete population consists of all those individuals who meet your sampling criteria, whereas the abstract population consists of individuals who will meet your sampling criteria in the future or those groups addressed theoretically by your framework.

Estimation of Parameters

You may use two approaches to estimate the parameters of a population: point estimation and interval estimation.

Point Estimation

A statistic that produces a value as a function of the scores in a sample is called an estimator. Much of inferential statistical analysis involves the use of point estimation to evaluate the fit between the estimator (a statistic) and the population parameter. A point estimate is a single figure that estimates a related figure in the population of interest. The best point estimator of the population mean is the mean of the sample being examined. However, the mean of the sample rarely equals the mean of the population. In addition to the mean, other commonly used estimators include the median, variance, standard deviation, and correlation coefficient.

Interval Estimation

When sampling from a continuous distribution, the probability of the sample mean being exactly equal to the population mean is zero. Therefore, we know that we are going to be in error if we use point estimators. The difference between the sample estimate and the true, but unknown, parameter value is sampling error. The source of sampling error is the fact that we did not count every individual in the population. Sampling error is due to chance and chance alone. It is not due to some flaw in the researcher's methodology. Interval estimation is an attempt to overcome this problem by controlling the initial precision of an estimator. An interval procedure that gives a 95% level of confidence will produce a set of intervals, 95% of which will include the true value of the parameter. Unfortunately, after a sample is drawn and the estimate is calculated, it is not possible to tell whether the interval contains the true value of the parameter.

An interval estimate is a segment of a number line (or range of scores) where the value of the parameter is thought to be. For example, in a sample with a mean of 40 and an SD of 5, one might use the range of scores between 2 SD below the mean to 2 SD above the mean (30 to 50) as the interval estimation. This type of estimation provides a set of scores rather than a single score. However, it is not absolutely certain that the mean of the population lies within that range. Therefore, it is necessary to determine the probability that this interval estimate contains the population mean.

This need to determine probability brings us back to the sampling distribution. We know that 95% of the means in the sampling distribution lie within ±1.96 SD of the mean of means (the population mean). If these scores are converted to Z scores, the unit normal distribution table can be used to determine how many standard deviations out from the mean of means one must go to ensure a specified probability (e.g., 70%, 95%, or 99%) of obtaining an interval estimate that includes the population parameter that is being estimated.

By examining the normal distribution (see Figure 18-2), one finds that 2.5% of the area under the normal curve lies below a Z score of −1.96, or $\mu - (1.96\ SD/\sqrt{N})$, and 2.5% of the area lies above a Z score of 1.96, or $\mu + (1.96\ SD/\sqrt{N})$, where μ is the mean of means, SD is the standard deviation, and N is the sample size. The probability is 0.95 that a randomly selected sample would have a mean within this range. Calculation of confidence intervals is explained in Chapter 19.

Degrees of Freedom

The concept of degrees of freedom (*df*) is a product of statistical theory and is easier to calculate than it is to explain because of the complex mathematics involved to justify the concept. Degrees of freedom involve the freedom of a score's value to vary given the other existing scores' values and the established sum of these scores.

A simple example may begin to explain the concept. Suppose difference scores are obtained from a sample of 4 and the mean is 4. The difference scores are −2, −1, +1, and +2. As with all difference scores, the sum of these scores is 0. As a result, if any three of the difference scores are calculated, the value of the fourth score is not free to vary. Its value will depend on the values of the other three to maintain a mean of 4 and a sum of 0. The degree of freedom in this example is 3 because only three scores are free to vary. In this case and in many other analyses, the degree of freedom is the sample size (N) minus 1 ($N - 1$).

$$df = N - 1$$

In this example, $df = 4 - 1 = 3$ (Roscoe, 1969). In some analyses, determining levels of significance from tables of statistical sampling distributions requires knowledge of the degrees of freedom.

Tailedness

On a normal curve, extremes of statistical values can occur at either end of the curve. Therefore, the 5% of statistical values that are considered statistically significant according to decision theory must be distributed between the two extremes of the curve. The extremes of the curve are referred to as **tails**. If the hypothesis is nondirectional and assumes that an extreme score can occur in either tail, the analysis is referred to as a two-tailed test of significance (Figure 18-7).

In a **one-tailed test of significance**, the hypothesis is directional, and extreme statistical values that occur in a single tail of the curve are of interest. Developing a one-tailed hypothesis requires sufficient knowledge of the variables and their interaction on which to base a one-tailed test. Otherwise, the one-tailed test is inappropriate. This knowledge may be theoretical or from previous research. (Refer to Chapter 8 for formulating hypotheses.) One-tailed tests are uniformly more powerful than **two-tailed tests**, and this fact increases the possibility of rejecting the null hypothesis. In this case, extreme statistical values occurring on the other tail of the curve are not considered significantly different. In Figure 18-8, which is a one-tailed figure, the portion of the curve where statistical values will be considered significant is in the right tail of the curve.

Type I and Type II Errors

According to decision theory, two types of error can occur when making decisions about the meaning of a value obtained from a statistical test: **type I errors** and type II errors. A type I error occurs if the null hypothesis is rejected when, in fact, it is true. This error is possible because even though statistical values in the extreme ends of the tail of the curve are rare, they do

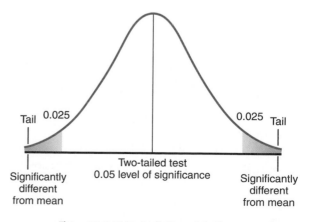

Figure **18-7** The two-tailed test of significance.

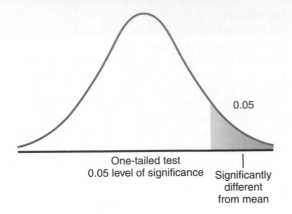

Figure **18-8** The one-tailed test of significance.

occur within the population. In viewing Table 18-1, remember that the null hypothesis states that there is no difference or no association between groups.

The risk of making a type I error is greater with a 0.05 level of significance than with a 0.01 level. As the level of significance becomes more extreme, the risk of a type I error decreases, as illustrated in Figure 18-9. For example, suppose you studied the effect of a treatment in an experimental study consisting of two groups and found that the difference between the two groups was relatively equivalent in magnitude to the standard error. The sampling distribution of the difference between the group means tells you that even if there is no real difference between the groups, a difference as large as or larger than the one you detected would occur by chance about once in every three times. That is, the difference that you found is just what you could expect to occur if the true treatment effect were zero. This statement does not mean that the true difference is zero, but that on the basis of the results of the study you would not be justified in claiming a real

difference between the groups. The data from your samples do not establish a case for the position that a true treatment effect exists.

Suppose, on the other hand, that you find that the difference in your groups is over twice its standard error (Z score >1.96). (Examine the Z scores in Figure 18-2.) A treatment difference of this magnitude would occur by chance less than 1 time in 20, and we say that these results are statistically significant at the 0.05 level. A difference of more than 2.58 times the standard error would occur by chance less than 1 time in 100, and we say that the difference is statistically significant at the 0.01 level. Cox (1958) stated, "Significance tests, from this point of view, measure the adequacy of the data to support the qualitative conclusion that there is a true effect in the direction of the apparent difference" (p.159). Thus, the decision is a judgment and can be in error. The level of statistical significance attained indicates the degree of uncertainty in taking the position that the difference between the two groups is real.

A **type II error** occurs if the null hypothesis is regarded as true when, in fact, it is false. This type of error occurs as a result of some degree of overlap between the values of different populations in some cases, so a value with a greater than 5% probability of being within one population may in fact be within the dimensions of another population (Figure 18-10).

As the risk of a type I error decreases (by setting a more extreme level of significance), the risk of a type II error increases. When the risk of a type II error decreases (by setting a less extreme level of significance), the risk of a type I error increases. It is not possible to decrease both types of error simultaneously without a corresponding increase in sample size. Therefore, the researcher needs to decide which risk poses the greatest threat within a specific study. In nursing research, many studies are conducted with small samples and instruments that are not precise measures of the variables under study. Many nursing situations include multiple variables that interact to lead to differences within populations. However, when one is examining only a few of the interacting variables, small differences can be overlooked and could lead to a false conclusion of no differences between the samples. In this case, the risk of a type II error is a greater concern, and a more lenient level of significance is in order.

As an example of the concerns related to error, consider the following problem. If you were to obtain three samples by using the same methodology, each sample would have a different mean. Yet you need to make a decision to accept or reject the null hypothesis.

TABLE **18-1** Occurrence of Type I and Type II Errors		
	In Reality the Null Hypothesis Is	
Data Analysis Indicates	**True**	**False**
Results significant Null rejected	Type I error	Correct decision (power)
Results not significant Null not rejected	Correct decision	Type II error

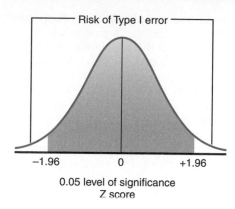 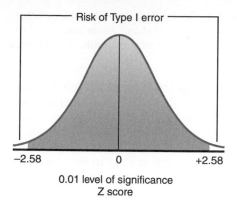

Figure **18-9** Risk of type I error.

The null hypothesis states that the population mean is 50 and that the three samples shown here are all from the same population. Assume that you obtain the following results:

Sample Size	Sample Size
$N = 50$ subjects	$\overline{X} = 52.0$
$N = 50$ subjects	$\overline{X} = 60.5$
$N = 50$ subjects	$\overline{X} = 52.2$

How much evidence would it take to convince you to switch from believing the null hypothesis to believing the alternative hypothesis? Will you choose correctly, or will you make a type I or a type II error?

Level of Significance: Controlling the Risk of a Type I Error

The formal definition of the level of significance (α) is the probability of making a type I error when the null hypothesis is true. The level of significance, developed from decision theory, is the cutoff point used to determine whether the samples being tested are members of the same population or from different populations. The decision criteria are based on the selected level of significance and the sampling distribution of the mean. For this example, we assume that the sampling distribution of the mean is normally distributed. As mentioned previously, 68% of the means from samples in a population will fall within 1SD of the mean of means (μ), 95% will fall within 1.96SD, 99% within 2.58SD, and 99.7% within 3SD. This decision theory explanation of the expected distribution of means is equivalent to the confidence interval explanation described previously. It is simply expressed differently. In keeping with

decision theory, the level of significance sought in a statistical test must be established before conducting the test. In fact, the significance level needs to be established before collecting the data. In nursing studies, the level of significance is usually set at 0.05 or 0.01. However, in preliminary studies, it might be prudent to select a less stringent level of significance, such as 0.10.

If one wishes to predict with a 95% probability of accuracy, the level of significance would be $p \leq 1 - 0.95$, or $p \leq 0.05$. The mathematical symbol $\leq$ means "less than or equal to." Thus, $p \leq 0.05$ means that there is a probability of 5% or less of getting a test statistic at least as extreme as the calculated test statistic if the null hypothesis is true.

In computer analysis, the observed level of significance (p value) obtained from the data is frequently provided on the printout. For example, the actual level of significance might be $p \leq 0.03$ or $p \leq 0.07$. This level of significance should be provided in the research

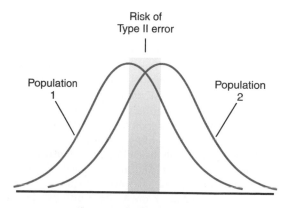

Figure **18-10** Risk of type II error.

report, as well as the level of significance set before the analysis. This practice allows other researchers to make their own judgment of the significance of your findings.

Power: Controlling the Risk of a Type II Error

Power is the probability that a statistical test will detect a significant difference that exists. Often, reported studies failing to reject the null hypothesis (in which power is unlikely to have been examined) will have only a 10% power level to detect a difference if one exists. An 80% power level is desirable. Until recently, the researcher's primary interest was in preventing a type I error. Therefore, great emphasis was placed on the selection of a level of significance but little on power. This point of view is changing as we recognize the seriousness of a type II error in nursing studies.

A type II error occurs when the null hypothesis is not rejected by the study even though a difference actually exists between groups. If the null hypothesis assumes no difference between the groups, the difference score in the measure of the dependent variable between groups would be zero. In a two-sample study, this relationship would be expressed mathematically as $A - B = 0$. The research hypothesis would be stated as $A - B \neq 0$, where $\neq$ means "not equal to." A type II error occurs when the difference score is not zero but is small enough that it is not detected by statistical analysis. In some cases, the difference is negligible and not of interest clinically. However, in other cases, the difference in reality is greater than indicated. This undetected difference is often due to research methodology problems.

Type II errors can occur for three reasons: (1) a stringent level of significance (such as $\alpha = 0.01$), (2) a small sample size, and (3) a small difference in measured effect between the groups. A difference in the measured effect can be due to a number of factors, including large variation in scores on the dependent variable within groups, crude instrumentation that does not measure with precision (e.g., does not detect small changes in the variable and thus leads to a small detectable effect size), confounding or extraneous variables that mask the effects of the variables under study, or any combination of these factors.

You can determine the risk of a type II error through power analysis and modify the study to decrease the risk if necessary. Cohen (1988) has identified four parameters of power: (1) significance level, (2) sample size, (3) effect size, and (4) power (standard of 0.80). If three of the four are known, the fourth can be calculated by using power analysis formulas. Significance level and sample size are fairly straightforward. Effect size is "the degree to which the phenomenon is present in the population, or the degree to which the null hypothesis is false" (Cohen, 1988, pp. 9–10). For example, suppose you were measuring changes in anxiety levels, measured first when the patient is at home and then just before surgery. The effect size would be large if you expected great change in anxiety. If you expected only a small change in the level of anxiety, the effect size would be small.

Small effect sizes require larger samples to detect these small differences. If the power is too low, it may not be worthwhile conducting the study unless a large sample can be obtained because statistical tests are unlikely to detect differences that exist. Deciding to conduct a study in these circumstances is costly in time and money, cannot add to the body of nursing knowledge, and can actually lead to false conclusions. Power analysis can be used to determine the sample size necessary for a particular study (see Chapter 14). Power analysis can be calculated by using a program in the Number Crunchers Statistical System (NCSS) called Power Analysis and Sample Size (PASS). Sample size can also be calculated by a program called Ex-Sample produced by Idea Works, Inc. (Brent, Scott, & Spencer, 1988). Statistical Packages for the Social Sciences (SPSS) for Windows program also now has the capacity to perform power analysis. Yarandi (1994) has provided the commands needed to perform power analysis for comparing two binomial proportions with the Statistical Analysis System (SAS).

The power analysis should be reported in studies that fail to reject the null hypothesis in the results section of the study. If power is high, it strengthens the meaning of the findings. If power is low, the researcher needs to address this issue in the discussion of implications. Modifications in the research methodology that resulted from the use of power analysis also need to be reported.

Clinical Significance

The findings of a study can be statistically significant but may not be clinically significant. For example, one group of patients might have a body temperature 0.1 °F higher than that of another group. Data analysis might indicate that the two groups are statistically significantly different. However, the findings have no clinical significance. In studies it is often important to know the magnitude of the difference between groups. However, a statistical test that indicates significant differences between groups (as in a t-test) provides no information on the magnitude of the difference. The extent of the level of significance (0.01 or 0.0001) tells you nothing about the magnitude of the difference between the groups. These differences can best be determined through descriptive or exploratory analysis of the data (see Chapter 19).

Parametric and Nonparametric Statistical Analysis

The most commonly used type of statistical analysis is parametric statistics. The analysis is referred to as parametric statistical analysis because the findings are inferred to the parameters of a normally distributed population. These approaches to analysis emerged from the work of Fisher and require meeting the following three assumptions before they can justifiably be used: (1) the sample was drawn from a population for which the variance can be calculated. The distribution is usually expected to be normal or approximately normal (Conover, 1971). (2) Because most parametric techniques deal with continuous variables rather than discrete variables, the level of measurement should be at least interval data or ordinal data with an approximately normal distribution. (3) The data can be treated as random samples (Box, Hunter, & Hunter, 1978).

Nonparametric statistical analysis, or distribution-free techniques, can be used in studies that do not meet the first two assumptions. However, the data still need to be treated as random samples. Most nonparametric techniques are not as powerful as their parametric counterparts. In other words, nonparametric techniques are less able to detect differences and have a greater risk of a type II error if the data meet the assumptions of parametric procedures. However, if these assumptions are not met, nonparametric procedures are more powerful. The techniques can be used with cruder forms of measurement than required for parametric analysis. In recent years, there has been greater tolerance in using parametric techniques when some of the assumptions are not met if the analyses are robust to moderate violations of the assumptions. Robust means that the analysis will yield accurate results even if some of the assumptions are violated by the data used for the analysis. However, one needs to think carefully through the consequences of violating the assumptions of a statistical procedure. The assumption that is most frequently violated is that the data were obtained from a random sample. The validity of the results diminishes as the violation of assumptions becomes more extreme.

PRACTICAL ASPECTS OF DATA ANALYSIS
Purposes of Statistical Analysis

Statistics can be used for a variety of purposes, such as to (1) summarize, (2) explore the meaning of deviations in the data, (3) compare or contrast descriptively, (4) test the proposed relationships in a theoretical model, (5) infer that the findings from the sample are indicative of the entire population, (6) examine causality, (7) predict, or (8) infer from the sample to a theoretical model. Statisticians such as John Tukey (1977) divided the role of statistics into two parts: exploratory data analysis and confirmatory data analysis. You can perform exploratory data analysis to obtain a preliminary indication of the nature of the data and to search the data for hidden structure or models. Confirmatory data analysis involves traditional inferential statistics, which you can use to make an inference about a population or a process based on evidence from the study sample.

Process of Data Analysis

The process of quantitative data analysis consists of several stages: (1) preparation of the data for analysis; (2) description of the sample; (3) testing the reliability of measurement; (4) exploratory analysis of the data; (5) confirmatory analysis guided by the hypotheses, questions, or objectives; and (6) post hoc analysis. Although not all of these stages are equally reflected in the final published report of the study, they all contribute to the insight you can gain from analyzing the data. Many novice researchers do not plan the details of data analysis until the data are collected and they are confronted with the analysis task. This research technique is poor and often leads to the collection of unusable data or the failure to collect the data needed to answer the research questions. Plans for data analysis need to be made during development of the methodology.

Preparation of the Data for Analysis

Except in very small studies, computers are almost universally used for data analysis. This use of computers has increased as personal computers (PCs) have become more accessible and easy-to-use data analysis packages have become available. When computers are used for analysis, the first step of the process is entering the data into the computer.

Before entering data into the computer, the computer file that will hold the data needs to be carefully prepared with information from the codebook as described in Chapter 17. The location of each variable in the computer file needs to be identified. Each variable must be labeled in the computer so that the variables involved in a particular analysis will be clearly designated on the computer printouts. Develop a systematic plan for data entry that is designed to reduce errors during the entry phase, and enter data during periods when you have few interruptions. However, entering data for long periods without respite results in fatigue and increases errors. If your data are being stored in a PC hard disk drive, make sure to back up the information each time you enter more data. It is wise to keep a second copy of the data filed at a separate, carefully protected site. If your data are being stored on a mainframe computer, request that a backup be made that you can keep in your possession, or download the data onto a transportable form. After data entry, store the original data in locked files for safekeeping.

Cleaning the Data

Print the data file. When data size allows, cross-check every datum on the printout with the original datum for accuracy. Otherwise, randomly check the accuracy of data points. Correct all errors found in the computer file. Perform a computer analysis of the frequencies of each value of every variable as a second check of the accuracy of the data. Search for values outside the appropriate range of values for that variable. Data that have been scanned into a computer are less likely to have errors but should still be checked. See Chapter 17 for more information on computerizing and cleaning data.

Identifying Missing Data

Identify all missing data points. Determine whether the information can be obtained and entered into the data file. If a large number of subjects have missing data on specific variables, you need to make a judgment regarding the availability of sufficient data to perform analysis with those variables. In some cases, subjects must be excluded from the analysis because of missing essential data.

Transforming Data

In some cases, data must be transformed before initiating data analysis. Items in scales are often arranged so that the locations of the highest values for the item are varied. This arrangement prevents the subject from giving a global response to all items in the scale. To reduce errors, the values on these items need to be entered into the computer exactly as they appear on the data collection form. Values on the items are then reversed by computer commands.

Skewed, or nonlinear, data that do not meet the assumptions of parametric analysis can sometimes be transformed in such a way that the values are expressed in a linear fashion. Various mathematical operations are used for this purpose. Examples of these operations include squaring each value or calculating the square root of each value. These operations may allow the researcher insight into the data that is not evident from the raw data.

Calculated Variables

Sometimes, a variable used in the analysis is not collected but calculated from other variables (a calculated variable). For example, if data are collected on the number of patients on a nursing unit and on the number of nurses on a shift, one might calculate a ratio of nurse to patient for a particular shift. The data will be more accurate if this calculation is performed by computer rather than manually. The results can then be stored in the data file as a variable rather than being recalculated each time the variable is used in an analysis.

Making Data Backups

When the data-cleaning process is complete, backups need to be made again; labeled as the complete, cleaned data set; and carefully stored. Data cleaning is a time-consuming process that you will not wish to repeat unnecessarily.

Description of the Sample

The next step is to obtain as complete a picture of the sample as possible. Begin with frequencies of descriptive variables related to the sample. Calculate measures of central tendency and measures of dispersion relevant to the sample. If the study is composed of more than one sample, comparisons of the various groups need to be performed. Relevant analyses might include examination of age, educational level, health status, gender, ethnicity, or other features for which data are available. If information is available on estimated parameters of the population from previous research or meta-analyses, measures in the present study need to be compared with these estimated parameters. If your samples are not representative of the population or if two groups being compared are not equivalent in ways important to the study, you will need to decide if you are justified in continuing the analysis.

Testing the Reliability of Measurement

Examine the reliability of the methods of measurement used in the study. The reliability of observational measures or physiological measures may have been obtained during the data collection phase but needs to be noted at this point. Additional evaluation of the reliability of these measures may be possible at this point. If you used paper-and-pencil scales in data collection, *alpha coefficients* need to be calculated. The value of the coefficient needs to be compared with values obtained for the instrument in previous studies. If the coefficient is unacceptably low (below 0.7 for a new tool and below 0.8 for an existing tool), you will have to determine if you are justified in performing analysis on data from the instrument.

Exploratory Analysis of the Data

Examine all the data descriptively, with the intent of becoming as familiar as possible with the nature of the data. Neophyte researchers often omit this step and jump immediately into the analysis that was designed to test their hypotheses, questions, or objectives. However, they omit this step at the risk of missing important information in the data and performing analyses on data inappropriate for the analysis. The researcher needs to examine data on each variable by using measures of central tendency and dispersion. Is the data skewed or normally distributed? What is the nature of the variation in the data? Are there outliers with extreme values that seem unlike the rest of the sample? The most valuable insights from a study often come from careful examination of outliers (Tukey, 1977).

In many cases, as a part of exploratory analysis, inferential statistical procedures are used to examine differences and associations within the sample. From an exploratory perspective, these analyses are relevant only to the sample under study. There should be no intent to infer to a population. If group comparisons are made, effect sizes need to be determined for the variables involved in the analyses.

In many nursing studies, the purpose of the study is exploratory analysis. In such studies, it is often found that sample sizes are small, power is low, measurement is crude, and the field of study is relatively new. If treatments are tested, the procedure is approached as a pilot study. The most immediate need is tentative exploration of the phenomena under study. Confirming the findings of these studies will require more rigorously designed studies with much larger samples. Unfortunately, many of these exploratory studies are reported in the literature as confirmatory studies, and attempts are made to infer to larger populations. Because of the unacceptably high risk of a type II error in these studies, negative findings should be viewed with caution.

Using Tables and Graphs for Exploratory Analysis

Although tables and graphs are commonly thought of as a way of presenting the findings of a study, these tools may be even more useful in helping the researcher to become familiar with the data. Tables and graphs need to illustrate the descriptive analyses being performed, even though they will probably never be included in a research report. They are prepared for the sole purpose of helping the researcher to identify patterns in the data and interpret exploratory findings. Visualizing the data in various ways can greatly increase insight regarding the nature of the data.

Confirmatory Analysis

As the name implies, *confirmatory analysis* is performed to confirm expectations regarding the data that are expressed as hypotheses, questions, or objectives. The findings are inferred from the sample to the population. Thus, inferential statistical procedures are used. The design of the study, the methods of measurement, and the sample size must be sufficient for this confirmatory process to be justified. A written analysis plan needs to describe clearly the confirmatory analyses that will be performed to examine each hypothesis, question, or objective. Follow these steps for each analysis used when performing a systematic confirmatory analysis:

1. Identify the level of measurement of the data available for analysis with regard to the research objective, question, or hypothesis.
2. Select a statistical procedure or procedures appropriate for the level of measurement that will respond to the objective, answer the question, or test the hypothesis.
3. Select the level of significance that you will use to interpret the results.
4. Choose a one-tailed or two-tailed test if appropriate to your analysis.
5. Determine the sample size available for the analysis. If several groups will be used in the analysis, identify the size of each group.
6. Evaluate the representativeness of the sample.
7. Determine the risk of a type II error in the analysis by performing a power analysis.
8. Develop dummy tables and graphics to illustrate the methods that you will use to display your results in relation to your hypotheses, questions, or objectives.
9. Determine the degrees of freedom for your analysis.
10. Perform the analysis manually or with a computer.

11. Compare the statistical value obtained with the table value by using the level of significance, tailedness of the test, and degrees of freedom previously identified. If you have performed your analysis on a computer, this information will be provided on the computer printout.
12. Reexamine the analysis to ensure that the procedure was performed with the appropriate variables and that the statistical procedure was correctly specified in the computer program.
13. Interpret the results of the analysis in terms of the hypothesis, question, or objective.
14. Interpret the results in terms of the framework.

Post Hoc Analysis

Post hoc analyses are commonly performed in studies with more than two groups when the analysis indicates that the groups are significantly different but does not identify which groups are different. This situation occurs, for example, in chi-square analyses and in analysis of variance. In other studies, the insights obtained through the planned analyses generate further questions that can be examined with the available data. These analyses may be tangential to the initial purpose of the study but may be fruitful in providing important information and generating questions for further research.

Storing Computer Printouts from Data Analysis

Computer printouts tend to accumulate rapidly during data analysis. Results of data analysis can easily become lost in the mountain of computer paper. These printouts need to be systematically stored to allow easy access later when theses or dissertations are being written or research papers are being prepared for publication. We recommend storing the printouts by time sequence. Most printouts identify the date (and even the hour and minute) that the analysis was performed. Some mainframe computers also assign a job number to each printout, which can be recorded. This feature makes it easy to distinguish earlier analyses from those performed later. Sometimes, printouts can be sorted by variable or by hypothesis and then arranged within these categories by time.

When you are preparing papers that describe your study, the results of each analysis reported in the paper need to be cross-indexed with the computer printout for reference as needed, with the job number, date, time, and page number of the printout listed. In addition, include a printout of the program used for the analysis. As interpretation of the results proceeds and

you attempt to link various findings, you may question some of the results. They may not seem to fit with the rest of the results, or they may not seem logical. You may find that you have failed to include necessary statistical information. When rewriting the paper, you may decide to report results not originally included. The search for a particular data analysis printout can be time consuming and frustrating if the printouts have not been carefully organized. It is easy to lose needed results and have to repeat the analysis.

After you have submitted your paper for publication (or to a thesis or dissertation committee), we recommend storing a copy of the page from the printout for each statistical value reported with the text. This copy needs to provide sufficient detail to allow you to gain access to the entire printout if needed. Thesis and dissertation committees and journal reviewers frequently recommend including additional information related to statistical procedures before acceptance. You often have only a short time frame within which to obtain the information and modify the paper to meet deadlines. Even after a paper has been published, we have had requests from readers for validation of our results. If this request is made months (or years) after the study is complete, finding the information can be a nightmare if you have failed to store your printouts carefully.

RESOURCES FOR STATISTICAL ANALYSIS COMPUTER PROGRAMS

Packaged computer analysis programs such as SPSS, SAS, and Biomedical Data Processing (BMDP) are available on the mainframe computers of many universities. A variety of data analysis packages such as SAS, SPSS, ABSTAT, and NCSS are also available for the PC. Table 18-2 lists sources of data analysis packages for the PC. The emergence of more powerful, high-speed PCs has made it relatively easy to conduct most analyses. Although the mathematical formulas needed to conduct analysis with a packaged program have been written as part of the computer program, you will need to know how to instruct the computer program to perform the selected analysis. Manuals, available for each program, demonstrate how to perform the analyses and provide a detailed discussion of the mathematical logic behind each type of analysis. As the researcher, you need to understand this logic, even though the computer will perform the analysis. For each type of analysis, most manuals suggest up-to-date and comprehensive sources that may help you to further understand the logic of the procedure.

TABLE 18-2 Sources of Data Analysis Packages for the Pc
NCSS (Number Cruncher Statistical System) www.ncss.com SPSS (Statistical Packages for the Social Sciences) http://spss.com SAS (Statistical Analysis System) http://sas.com

Packaged computer programs can perform your data analysis and provide you with the results of the analysis on a computer printout. However, an enormous amount of information is provided on a computer printout, and its meaning can easily be misinterpreted. In addition, computers conduct analysis on whatever data the user provides. If the data entered into the computer are garbage (e.g., numbers from the data are entered incorrectly or data are typed in the wrong columns), the computer output will be garbage. If the data are inappropriate for the particular type of analysis selected, the computer program is often unable to detect that error and will proceed to perform the analysis. The results will be meaningless, and the researcher's conclusions will be completely in error (Hinshaw & Schepp, 1984).

Statistical Assistance

Programmers assist in writing the programs that give commands to the computer to implement the mathematical processes selected. Programmers are skilled in the use of computer languages but are not statisticians; thus, they do not interpret the outcomes of analysis. Computer languages are the messages used to give detailed commands to the computer. Even when packaged programs are being used, a programmer skilled in the use of common software packages can be of great help in selecting the appropriate programs, writing them according to guidelines, and speeding up the debugging process. In universities, computer science students are often available for programming services.

A *statistician* has an educational background that qualifies him or her as an expert in statistical analysis. Statisticians vary in their skill pertaining to specific statistical procedures and usually charge an hourly fee for services. However, some may contract to perform an agreed on analysis for a set fee. Although the extent of need for statistical consultation depends on the educational background of the researcher, most nurse researchers will benefit from statistical consultation. However, the researcher remains the content expert and must be the final authority in interpreting

the meaning of the analyses in terms of the discipline's body of knowledge. Therefore, it is not acceptable to abdicate the total responsibility for data analysis to the statistician. The nurse researcher remains accountable for understanding the statistical procedures used and for interpreting these procedures to various audiences when the results of the study are communicated.

CHOOSING APPROPRIATE STATISTICAL PROCEDURES FOR A STUDY

Multiple factors are involved in determining the suitability of a statistical procedure for a particular study. Some of these factors are related to the nature of the study, some to the nature of the researcher, and others to the nature of statistical theory. Specific factors include (1) the purpose of the study; (2) hypotheses, questions, or objectives; (3) design; (4) level of measurement; (5) previous experience in statistical analysis; (6) statistical knowledge level; (7) availability of statistical consultation; (8) financial resources; and (9) access to computers. Use items 1 to 4 to identify statistical procedures that meet the requirements of the study. Then further narrow your options through the process of elimination based on items 5 through 9.

One approach to selecting an appropriate statistical procedure or judging the appropriateness of an analysis technique for a critique is to use a decision tree. A decision tree directs your choices by gradually narrowing your options through the decisions you make. Two decision trees that have been helpful in selecting statistical procedures are presented in Figures 18-11 and 18-12.

One disadvantage of decision trees is that if you make an incorrect or uninformed decision (guess), you can be led down a path in which you might select an inappropriate statistical procedure for your study. Decision trees are often constrained by space and therefore do not include all the information needed to make an appropriate selection. The most extensive decision tree that we have found is presented in *A Guide for Selecting Statistical Techniques for Analyzing Social Science Data* by Andrews, Klem, Davidson, O'Malley, and Rodgers (1981). The following examples of questions designed to guide the selection or evaluation of statistical procedures were extracted from this book:

1. *How many variables does the problem involve?*
2. *How do you want to treat the variables with respect to the scale of measurement?*

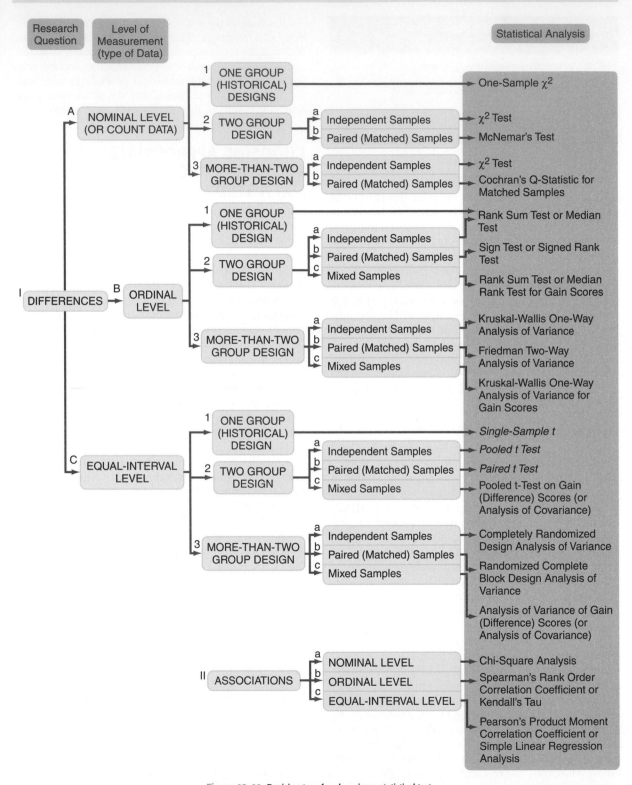

Figure **18-11** Decision tree for choosing a statistical test.

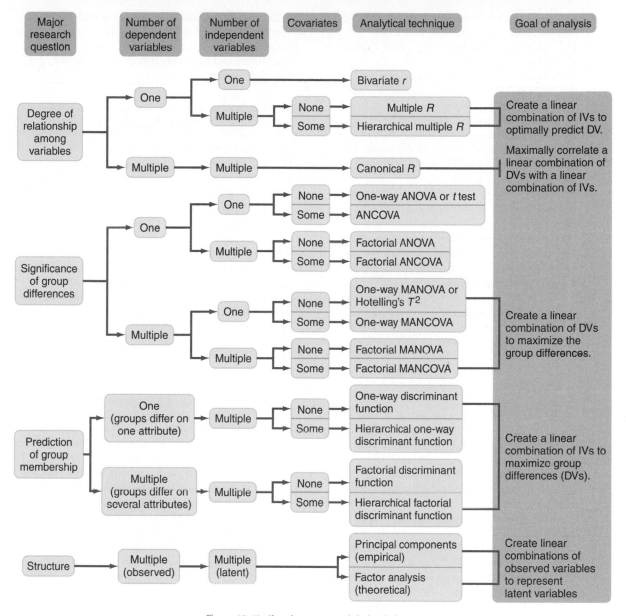

Figure **18-12** Choosing among statistical techniques.

3. What do you want to know about the distribution of the variable?

4. Do you want to treat outlying cases differently from others?

5. What is the form of the distribution?

6. Is a distinction made between a dependent and an independent variable?

7. Do you want to test whether the means of the two variables are equal?

8. Do you want to treat the relationship between variables as linear?

9. How many of the variables are dichotomous?

10. Is the dichotomous variable a collapsing of a continuous variable?

11. *Do you want to treat the ranks of ordered categories as interval scales?*

12. *Do the variables have the same distribution?*

13. *Do you want to treat the ordinal variable as though it were based on an underlying normally distributed interval variable?*

14. *Is the interval variable dependent?*

15. *Do you want a measure of the strength of the relationship between the variables or a test of the statistical significance of differences between groups (Kenny, 1979)?*

16. *Are you willing to assume that an intervally scaled variable is normally distributed in the population?*

17. *Is there more than one dependent variable?*

18. *Do you want to statistically remove the linear effects of one or more covariates from the dependent variable?*

19. *Do you want to treat the relationships among the variables as additive?*

20. *Do you want to analyze patterns existing among variables or among individual cases?*

21. *Do you want to find clusters of variables that are more strongly related to one another than to the remaining variables?*

Each question confronts you with a decision. The decision you make narrows the field of available statistical procedures. Decisions must be made regarding the following:

1. Number of variables (1, 2, more than 2)
2. Type of measurement (nominal, ordinal, interval)
3. Type of variable (independent, dependent, research)
4. Distribution of variable (normal, non-normal)
5. Type of relationship (linear, nonlinear)
6. What you want to measure (strength of relationship, difference between groups)
7. Nature of the groups (equal or unequal in size, matched or unmatched, dependent or independent)
8. Type of analysis (descriptive, classification, methodological, relational, comparison, predicting outcomes, intervention testing, causal modeling, examining changes across time)

As you can see, selecting and evaluating statistical procedures requires that you make a number of judgments regarding the nature of the data and what you want to know. Knowledge of the statistical procedures

and their assumptions is necessary for selecting appropriate procedures. You must weigh the advantages and disadvantages of various statistical options. Access to a statistician can be invaluable in selecting the appropriate procedures.

SUMMARY

- This chapter introduces you to the concepts of statistical theory and discusses some of the more pragmatic aspects of quantitative data analysis: the purposes of statistical analysis, the process of performing data analysis, the choice of the appropriate statistical procedures for a study, and resources for statistical analysis.

- Two types of errors can occur when making decisions about the meaning of a value obtained from a statistical test: type I errors and type II errors.

- A type I error occurs when the researcher concludes that the samples tested are from different populations (the difference between groups is significant) when, in fact, the samples are from the same population (no significant difference between groups).

- A type II error occurs when the researcher concludes that the samples are from the same population when, in fact, they are from different populations.

- The formal definition of the level of significance, or alpha (α), is the probability of making a type I error when the null hypothesis is true.

- The level of significance, developed from decision theory, is the cutoff point used to determine whether the samples being tested are members of the same population or from different populations.

- Power is the probability that a statistical test will detect a significant difference that exists.

- Statistics can be used for a variety of purposes, such as to (1) summarize, (2) explore the meaning of deviations in the data, (3) compare or contrast descriptively, (4) test the proposed relationships in a theoretical model, (5) infer that the findings from the sample are indicative of the entire population, (6) examine causality, (7) predict, or (8) infer from the sample to a theoretical model.

- Quantitative data analysis consists of several stages: (1) preparation of the data for analysis; (2) description of the sample; (3) testing the reliability of measurement; (4) exploratory analysis of the data; (5) confirmatory analysis guided by the hypotheses, questions, or objectives; and (6) post hoc analysis.

REFERENCES

Andrews, F. M., Klem, L., Davidson, T. N., O'Malley, P. M., & Rodgers, W. L. (1981). *A guide for selecting statistical techniques for analyzing social science data* (2nd ed). Ann Arbor, MI: Survey Research Center, Institute for Social Research, University of Michigan.

Barnett, V. (1982). *Comparative statistical inference.* New York: Wiley.

Box, G. E. P., Hunter, W. G., & Hunter, J. S. (1978). S*tatistics for experimenters.* New York: Wiley.

Brent, E. E., Jr., Scott, J. K., & Spencer, J. C. (1988). *Ex-Sample: An expert system to assist in designing sampling plans. User's guide and reference manual*, Version 2.0. Columbia, MO: Idea Works.

Chervany, N. L. (1977). *The logic and practice of statistics.* Written materials provided with a presentation at the Institute of Management Science. Bloomington, MN, December 15.

Cohen, J. (1988). *Statistical power analysis for the behavioral sciences* (2nd ed.). New York: Academic Press.

Conover, W. J. (1971). *Practical nonparametric statistics.* New York: Wiley.

Cox, D. R. (1958). *Planning of experiments.* New York: Wiley.

Glass, G. V., & Stanley, J. C. (1970). *Statistical methods in education and psychology.* Englewood Cliffs, NJ: Prentice-Hall.

Good, I. J. (1983). *Good thinking: The foundations of probability and its applications.* Minneapolis: University of Minnesota Press.

Hinshaw, A. S., & Schepp, K. (1984). Problems in doing nursing research: How to recognize garbage when you see it! *Western Journal of Nursing Research*, 6(1), 126–130.

Kenny, D. A. (1979). *Correlation and causality.* New York: Wiley.

Roscoe, J. T. (1969). *Fundamental research statistics for the behavioral sciences.* New York: Holt, Rinehart & Winston.

Slakter, M. J., Wu, Y. B., & Suzuki-Slakter, N. S. (1991). *, **, and ***, statistical nonsense at the .00000 level. *Nursing Research*, 40(4), 248–249.

Tukey, J. W. (1977). *Exploratory data analysis.* Reading, MA: Addison-Wesley.

Volicer, B. J. (1984). *Multivariate statistics for nursing research.* New York: Grune & Stratton.

Yarandi, H. N. (1994). Using the SAS system to estimate sample size and power for comparing two binomial proportions. *Nursing Research*, 43(2), 124–125.

CHAPTER 19
Using Statistics to Describe Variables

D ata analysis begins with description; this applies to any study in which the data are numerical, including some qualitative studies. Descriptive statistics allow the researcher to organize the data in ways that give meaning and insight and to examine a phenomenon from a variety of angles. The researcher can use descriptive analyses to generate theories and develop hypotheses. For some types of descriptive studies, descriptive statistics will be the only approach to analysis of the data. The selection of statistical tests is dependent upon the level of measurement (nominal, ordinal, interval, or ratio). This chapter describes a number of uses for descriptive analysis: to summarize data, to explore deviations in the data, and to describe patterns across time.

USING STATISTICS TO SUMMARIZE DATA
Frequency Distributions

A frequency distribution is usually the first strategy a researcher uses to organize data for examination. In addition, frequency distributions will allow you to check for errors in coding and computer programming. There are two types of frequency distributions: ungrouped and grouped. In addition to providing a means to display the data, these distributions may influence decisions concerning further data analysis.

Ungrouped Frequency Distribution

Most studies have some categorical data that are presented in the form of an ungrouped frequency distribution. To develop an ungrouped frequency distribution, list all categories of that variable on which

you have data and tally each datum on the listing. For example, suppose you wanted to list the categories of pets in the homes of elderly clients; the groupings might include dogs, cats, birds, and rabbits. A tally of the ungrouped frequencies would have the following appearance:

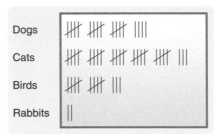

You would then count the tally marks and develop a table to display the results. This approach is generally used on discrete (categorical) rather than continuous data. Data commonly organized in this manner include gender, ethnicity, marital status, and diagnostic category. Continuous data, such as test grades or scores on a data collection instrument, could be organized in this manner as well; however, if the number of possible scores is large, it is difficult to extract meaning from examining the distribution.

Grouped Frequency Distribution

In general, it is best to determine some method of grouping when you are examining continuous variables. Age, for example, is a continuous variable. Many measures taken during data collection are continuous, including income, temperature, vital lung capacity, weight, scale scores, and time. Grouping will require you to make a number of decisions that will be important to the meaning derived from the data.

Any method you use to group data will result in a loss of some information and will change the level of measurement, which will impact how you can use the data. For example, if you are developing a group based on age, a breakdown of under 65/over 65 will provide considerably less information than will groupings that have been separated into 10-year spans. The grouping should be devised to provide the greatest possible meaning in terms of the purpose of the study. If the data are to be compared with data in other studies, groupings should be similar to those of other studies in that field of research.

The first step in developing a grouped frequency distribution is to establish a method of classifying the data. The classes that are developed must be exhaustive: Each datum must fit into one of the identified classes. The classes must be mutually exclusive: each datum can fit into only one of the established classes. A common mistake is to list ranges that contain overlaps. For example, you might have age categories of 40 to 50, 50 to 60, etc. Thus, the age 50 would overlap, allowing the age of 50 to be coded as 40 to 50, 50 to 60, or both. The range of each category must be equivalent. In the case of age, for example, if 10 years is the range, each category must include 10 years of ages. The first and last categories may be open-ended and worded to include all scores above or below a specified point. The precision with which the data will be reported is an important consideration. For example, you may decide to list your data only in whole numbers, or decimals may be used. If you use decimals, you will need to decide at how many decimal places rounding off will be performed.

Percentage Distribution

Percentage distribution indicates the percentage of the sample with scores falling in a specific group, as well as the number of scores in that group. Percentage distributions are particularly useful in comparing the present data with findings from other studies that have varying sample sizes. A cumulative distribution is a type of percentage distribution in which the percentages and frequencies of scores are summed as one moves from the top of the table to the bottom (or the reverse). Thus, the bottom category would have a cumulative frequency equivalent to the sample size and a cumulative percentage of 100 (Table 19-1). Frequency distributions can be displayed as tables, diagrams, or graphs. Four types of illustrations are commonly used: charts, bar graphs, histograms, and frequency polygons. Examples of diagrams and graphs are presented in Chapter 25. Frequency analysis and graphic presentation of the results can be performed on the computer.

Measures of Central Tendency

A measure of central tendency is frequently referred to as an average. Average is a lay term not commonly used in statistics because of its vagueness. Measures of central tendency are the most concise representation of the location of the data. The three measures of central tendency commonly used in statistical analyses are the mode, median (MD), and mean.

Mode

The mode is the numerical value or score that occurs with the greatest frequency; it does not necessarily indicate the center of the data set. To determine the mode, examine an ungrouped frequency distribution of the data. In Table 19-1, the mode is the score of 5, which occurred 14 times in the data set. The mode can be used to describe the most common subject or to identify the value that occurs most frequently on a scale item. The mode is the only appropriate measure of central tendency for nominal data and is used to calculate some nonparametric statistics. Otherwise, it is seldom used in statistical analysis.

TABLE 19-1	Example of a Cumulative Frequency Table			
Score	Frequency	Percentage	Cumulative Frequency (*f*)	Cumulative Percentage
1	4	8	4	8
3	6	12	10	20
4	8	16	18	36
5	14	28	32	64
7	8	16	40	80
8	6	12	46	92
9	4	8	N = 50	100

A data set can have more than one mode. If two modes exist, the data set is referred to as bimodal; a data set that contains more than two modes would be multimodal.

Median

The median (MD) is the score at the exact center of the ungrouped frequency distribution. It is the 50th percentile. You can obtain the MD by rank-ordering the scores. If the number of scores is an uneven number, exactly 50% of the scores are above the MD and 50% are below it. If the number of scores is an even number, the MD is the average of the two middle scores. Thus, the MD may not be an actual score in the data set. It is not considered to be as precise an estimator of the population average when sampling from normal populations (and distributions) as the sample average is. In most cases of skewed distributions, it is actually the preferred choice because in these cases it is a more precise measure of central tendency. An example of a skewed distribution would be "days of hospitalization." The largest incidence would be only a few days with fewer instances occurring as the number of days of hospitalization increase. The MD is not affected by extreme scores in the data (outliers), as is the mean. An example of an outlier could be, in "days of hospitalization," data showing higher numbers of days as follows: 42, 44, 56, 64, 244. The value of 244 is an outlier because it is extremely high in comparison with the other values. The MD is the most appropriate measure of central tendency for ordinal data but is also used for interval and ratio data. It is frequently used in nonparametric analysis.

Mean

The most commonly used measure of central tendency is the mean. The mean is the sum of the scores divided by the number of scores being summed. Thus, like the MD, the mean may not be a member of the data set. The formula for calculating the mean is as follows:

$$\bar{X} = \frac{\Sigma X}{N}$$

where

X = the mean
Σ = sigma (the statistical symbol for the process of summation
X = a single raw score
N = number of scores being entered in the calculation

The mean was calculated for the data provided in Table 19-1 as follows:

$$\bar{X} = \frac{4+18+32+70+56+48+36}{50} = \frac{264}{50} = 5.28$$

The mean is an appropriate measure of central tendency for approximately normally distributed populations with variables measured at the interval or ratio level. This formula is presented repeatedly within more complex formulas of statistical analysis. The mean is sensitive to extreme scores such as outliers.

USING STATISTICS TO EXPLORE DEVIATIONS IN THE DATA

Although the use of summary statistics has been the traditional approach to describing data or describing the characteristics of the sample before inferential statistical analysis, its ability to clarify the nature of data is limited. For example, using measures of central tendency, particularly the mean, to describe the nature of the data obscures the impact of extreme values or deviations in the data. Thus, significant features in the data may be concealed or misrepresented. Often, anomalous, unexpected, problematic data and discrepant patterns are evident but are not regarded as meaningful. Measures of dispersion, such as the modal percentage, range, difference scores, sum of squares (SS), variance, and standard deviation (SD), provide important insight into the nature of the data.

Measures of Dispersion

Measures of dispersion, or variability, are measures of individual differences of the members of the population and sample. They indicate how scores in a sample are dispersed around the mean. These measures provide information about the data that is not available from measures of central tendency. They indicate how different the scores are—the extent to which individual scores deviate from one another. If the individual scores are similar, measures of variability are small and the sample is relatively homogeneous in terms of those scores. Heterogeneity (wide variation in scores) is important in some statistical procedures, such as correlation. Heterogeneity is determined by measures of variability. The measures most commonly used are modal percentage, range, difference scores, SS, variance, and SD.

Modal Percentage

The modal percentage is the only measure of variability appropriate for use with nominal data. It indicates the

TABLE 19-2 Data for Calculation of Mean and Standard Deviation

Score X	Frequency (f)	fX	fX²
1	4	4	4(1) = 4
3	6	18	6(9) = 54
4	8	32	8(16) = 128
5	14	70	14(25) = 350
7	8	56	8(49) = 392
8	6	48	6(64) = 384
9	4	36	4(81) = 324
	N = 50	ΣX = 264	ΣX² = 1636

relationship of the number of data scores represented by the mode to the total number of data scores. To determine the modal percentage, divide the frequency of the modal scores by the total number of scores. For example, in Table 19-2, the mode is 5 because 14 of the subjects scored 5, and the sample size is 50; thus, 14/50 = 0.28. Next, multiply the result of that operation by 100 to convert it to a percentage. In the example, the modal percentage is 28%, which means that 28% of the sample is represented by the mode. The complete calculation would be 14/50(100) = 28%. This strategy allows the present data to be compared with other data sets. Calculate the modal percentage of the data in Table 19-1.

Range
The simplest measure of dispersion is the range. In published studies, range is presented in two ways: (1) the range is the lowest and highest scores, or (2) the range is calculated by subtracting the lowest score from the highest score. The range for the scores in Table 19-2 is 1 and 9 or can be calculated as follows: 9 − 1 = 8 to provide the value of 8 as the range. In this form, the range is a difference score that uses only the two extreme scores for the comparison. Most studies list the low value and the high value as the range. The range is a crude measure, but it is sensitive to outliers. Outliers are subjects with extreme scores that are widely separated from scores of the rest of the subjects. The range is generally reported but is not used in further analyses. The range is not a useful measure for comparing the present data with data from other studies.

Difference Scores
Difference scores are obtained by subtracting the mean from each score. Sometimes a difference score is referred to as a deviation score because it indicates the extent to which a score deviates from the mean. The

difference score is positive when the score is above the mean, and it is negative when the score is below the mean. Difference scores are the basis for many statistical analyses and can be found within many statistical equations. The sum of all difference scores is zero, which makes the sum a useless measure. The formula for difference scores is

$$X - \bar{X}$$

Sum of Squares
A common strategy used to manipulate difference scores in a meaningful way is to square them. These squared scores are then summed. The mathematical symbol for the operation of summing is S. When negative scores are squared, they become positive, and therefore the sum will no longer equal zero. This mathematical maneuver is referred to as the sum of squares (SS). The SS is also the sum of squared deviations. The equation for SS is

$$SS = \Sigma\left(X - \bar{X}\right)^2$$

The larger the value of SS, the greater the variance. (Variance is a measure of dispersion that is the mean or average of the sum of squares.) Because the value of SS depends on the measurement scale used to obtain the original scores, comparison of SS with that obtained in other studies is limited to studies using similar data. SS is a valuable measure of variance and is used in many complex statistical equations. The SS is important because when deviations from the mean are squared, this sum is smaller than the sum of squared deviations from any other value in a sample distribution. This relationship is referred to as the least-squares principle and is important in mathematical manipulations.

Variance
Variance is another measure commonly used in statistical analysis. The equation for variance (V) is

$$V = \frac{\Sigma\left(X - \bar{X}\right)^2}{N-1}$$

As you can see, variance is the mean or average of SS. Again, because the result depends on the measurement scale used, it has no absolute value and can be compared only with data obtained by using similar measures. However, in general, the larger the variance, the larger the dispersion of scores.

Standard Deviation

Standard deviation (SD) is a measure of dispersion that is the square root of the variance. This step is important mathematically because squaring mathematical terms changes them in some important ways. Obtaining the square root reverses this change. The equation for obtaining SD is

$$SD = \sqrt{\frac{\Sigma \left(X - \bar{X} \right)^2}{N-1}}$$

Although this equation clarifies the relationships among difference scores, SS, and variance, using it requires that all these measures in turn be calculated. If SD is being calculated directly by hand (or with the use of a calculator), the following computational equation is easier to use. Data from Table 19-2 were used to calculate the SD:

$$SD = \sqrt{\frac{\Sigma X^2 - (1/N)(\Sigma X)^2}{N-1}}$$

$$SD = \sqrt{\frac{1636 - (1/50)(264)^2}{50-1}}$$

$$SD = \sqrt{\frac{1636 - 1393.92}{49}}$$

$$SD = \sqrt{4.94}$$

$$SD = 2.22$$

Just as the mean is the "average" score, the SD is the "average" difference (deviation) score. SD measures the average deviation of a score from the mean in that particular sample. It indicates the degree of error that would be made if the mean alone were used to interpret the data. SD is an important measure, both for understanding dispersion within a distribution and for interpreting the relationship of a particular score to the distribution. Researchers usually use computers to calculate descriptive statistics (mean, MD, mode, and SD).

Bland and Altman Plots

Bland and Altman plots are used to examine the extent of agreement between two measurement techniques. Generally, they are used to compare a new technique with an established one and have been used primarily with physiological measures. For example, suppose you wanted to compare pulse oximeter values with arterial blood gas values (Figure 19-1). You

can plot the difference between the measures of the two methods against the average of the two methods. Thus, for each pair you would calculate the difference between the two values, as well as the average of the two values. You can then plot these values on a graph, displaying a scatter diagram of the differences plotted against the averages. Three horizontal lines are displayed on the graph to show the mean difference, the mean difference plus 1.96 times the SD of the differences, and the mean difference minus 1.96 times the SD of the differences. The value of 1.96 corresponds to 95% of the areas beneath the curve. The plot reveals the relationship between the differences and the averages, allows you to search for any systematic bias, and identifies outliers. In some cases, two measures may be closely related near the mean but become more divergent as they move away from the mean. This pattern has been the case with measures of pulse oximetry and arterial blood gases (see Figure 19-1). Traditional methods of comparing measures such as correlation procedures will not identify such problems. Interpretation of the results is based on whether the differences are clinically important (Bland & Altman, 1986).

You can also use this analysis technique to examine the repeatability of a single method of measurement. By using the graph, you can examine whether the variability or precision of a method is related to the size of the characteristic being measured. Because the same method is being measured repeatedly, the mean difference should be zero. Use the following formula to calculate a coefficient of repeatability (CR). MedCalc can perform this computation of CR, as follows:

$$CR = 1.96 \times \sqrt{\frac{\Sigma \left(d_2 - d_1 \right)^2}{n-1}}$$

where d is the value of a measure.

USING STATISTICS TO DESCRIBE PATTERNS ACROSS TIME

One of the critical needs in nursing research is to examine patterns across time. Most nursing studies have examined events at a discrete point in time, and yet the practice of nursing requires an understanding of events as they unfold. This knowledge is essential for developing interventions that can have a positive effect on the health and illness trajectories of the patients in our care. Data analysis procedures that hold promise of providing this critical information include plots displaying variations in variables across time and survival analysis.

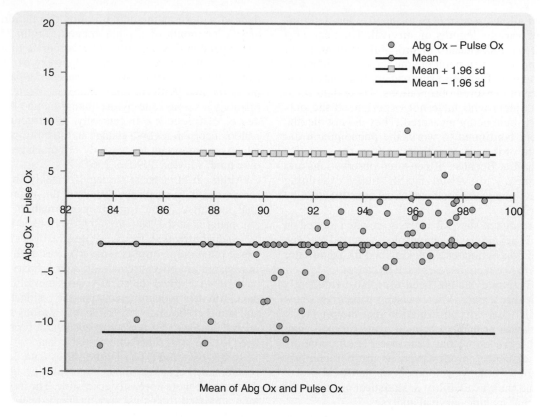

Figure **19-1** Example of a Bland and Altman plot.

Analysis of Case Study Data

In case studies, large volumes of both qualitative and quantitative data are often gathered over a certain period. A clearly identified focus for the analysis is critical. Yin (1994) identified purposes for a case study:

1. To explore situations, such as those in which an intervention is being evaluated, that have no clear set of outcomes
2. To describe the context within which an event or intervention occurred
3. To describe an event or intervention
4. To explain complex causal links
5. To confirm or challenge a theory
6. To represent a unique or extreme case

Data analysis strategies vary depending on the research questions posed. Because multiple sources of data (some qualitative and some quantitative) are usually available for each variable, triangulation strategies are commonly applied in case study analyses. The qualitative data are analyzed by methods described in Chapter 23. A number of analysis approaches are available for examining quantitative data. Some analytical techniques include pattern matching, explanation building, and time-series analysis (Yin, 1994). Pattern matching compares the pattern found in the case study with one that is predicted to occur. Explanation building is an iterative process that builds an explanation of the case. Time-series analysis may involve visual displays of variations in variables across time, which are presented in the form of plots. If more than one subject was included in the study, plots may be used to compare variables across subjects. Any judgments or conclusions that you make during the analyses must be considered carefully. You should clearly link information from the case to each conclusion.

Survival Analysis

Survival analysis is a set of techniques designed to analyze repeated measures from a given time (e.g., beginning of the study, onset of a disease, beginning of a treatment, initiation of a stimulus) until a certain attribute (e.g., death, treatment failure, recurrence of a phenomenon, return to work) occurs. This form of analysis allows researchers to identify the determinants of various lengths of survival. They can also analyze the risk (hazard or probability) of an event occurring at a given point in time for an individual.

A common feature in survival analysis data is the presence of censored observations. These data come from subjects who have not experienced the outcome attribute being measured. They did not die, the treatment continued to work, the phenomenon did not recur, or they were withdrawn from the study for some reason. Because of censored observations and the frequency of skewed data in studies examining such outcomes, common statistical tests may not be appropriate.

The results of survival analysis are often plotted on graphs. For example, you might plot the period between the initiation of cigarette smoking and the occurrence of smoking-related diseases such as cancer.

Survival analysis has been used most frequently in medical research. When a cancer patient asks how long will I live, the information that the physician provides was probably obtained using survival analysis. The procedure has been used less commonly in nursing research. However, its use is increasing because of further development of statistical procedures and their availability in statistical packages for the PC that include survival analyses.

This procedure allows researchers to study many previously unexamined facets of the nursing practice. Possibilities include the effectiveness of various pain relief measures, the consequences of altering the length of breast-feeding, maintenance of weight loss, abstinence from smoking, recurrence of decubitus ulcers, the likelihood of urinary tract infection after catheterization, and the effects of rehospitalization for the same diagnosis within the 60-day period in which Medicare will not provide reimbursement. The researcher could examine variables that are effective in explaining recurrence within various time intervals or the characteristics of various groups who have received different treatments.

Time-Series Analysis

Time-series analysis is a technique designed to analyze changes in a variable across time and thus to uncover a pattern in the data. Multiple measures of the variable collected at equal intervals are required. Interest in these procedures in nursing is growing because of the interest in understanding patterns. For example, the wave-and-field pattern is one of the themes of Martha Rogers's (1986) theory. Pattern is also an important component of Margaret Newman's (1999) nursing theory. Crawford (1982) conceptually

defined pattern as the configuration of relationships among elements of a phenomenon. Taylor (1990) has expanded this definition to incorporate time into the study of patterns and defines pattern as "repetitive, regular, or continuous occurrences of a particular phenomenon. Patterns may increase, decrease, or maintain a stable state by oscillating up and down in degree of frequency. In this way, the structure of a pattern incorporates both change and stability, concepts which are important to the study of human responses over time" (Taylor, 1990, p. 256).

Although the easiest strategy for analyzing time-series data is to graph the raw data, this approach to analysis misses some important information. Important patterns in the data are often overlooked because of residual effects in the data. (Residual is defined as extra, remaining, surplus, unused). Residual effects in research are effects remaining after primary effects have been identified statistically and removed from the data. The data remaining contains the residual effects and can then be analyzed to identify various residual effects. Various statistical procedures have been developed to analyze residual effects in the data.

In the past, analysis of time-series data has been problematic because computer programs designed for this purpose were not easily accessible. The most common approach to analysis was ordinary least-squares multiple regression. However, this approach has been unsatisfactory for the most part. Better approaches to analyzing this type of data are now available. With easier access to computer programs designed to conduct time-series analysis, information in the nursing literature on these approaches has been increasing.

SUMMARY

- Data analysis begins with descriptive statistics in any study in which the data are numerical, including some qualitative studies.
- Descriptive statistics allow the researcher to organize the data in ways that facilitate meaning and insight.
- Three measures of central tendency are the mode, median, and mean.
- The measures of dispersion most commonly used are modal percentage, range, difference scores, sum of squares, variance, and standard deviation.
- One of the critical needs in nursing research is to examine patterns across time.
- Data analysis procedures that hold promise for providing patterns include time series analysis and survival analysis.

REFERENCES

Bland, J. M., & Altman, D. G. (1986). Statistical methods for assessing agreement between two methods of clinical measurement. *Lancet, 1*(8476), 307–310.

Crawford, G. (1982). The concept of pattern in nursing: Conceptual development and measurement. *Advances in Nursing Science, 5*(1), 1–6.

Newman, M. A. (1999). *Health as expanding consciousness.* Sudbury, MA: Jones & Bartlett.

Rogers, M. (1986). Science of unitary human beings. In V. M. Malinski (Ed.), *Exploration on Martha Rogers' science of unitary human beings* (pp. 3–8). Norwalk, CT: Appleton-Century-Crofts.

Taylor, D. (1990). Use of autocorrelation as an analytic strategy for describing pattern and change. *Western Journal of Nursing Research, 12*(2), 254–261.

CHAPTER 20
Using Statistics to Examine Relationships

Correlational analyses identify relationships between or among variables. In addition, the analysis may be used to clarify the relationships among theoretical concepts or assist in identifying causal relationships, which can then be tested by inferential analysis. The researcher should obtain all data for the analysis from a single population from which values are available on all variables to be examined. Data measured at the interval level will provide the best information on the nature of the relationship (i.e., if it is positive or negative). However, analysis procedures are available for most levels of measurement. To prepare for correlational analysis, the researcher plans data collection strategies to maximize the possibility of obtaining the full range of possible values on each variable.

This chapter discusses the use of scatter diagrams before correlational analysis, bipolar correlational analysis, testing the significance of a correlational coefficient, the correlational matrix, spurious correlations, the role of correlation in understanding causality, and multivariate correlational procedures, including factor analysis.

SCATTER DIAGRAMS

Scatter diagrams provide useful preliminary information about the nature of the relationship between variables. The researcher should develop and examine scatter diagrams before performing correlational analysis. Scatter diagrams may be useful for selecting appropriate correlational procedures, but most correlational procedures are useful for examining linear relationships only. A scatter plot can easily identify

nonlinear relationships; if the data are nonlinear, the researcher should select other approaches to analysis (Figure 20-1). In addition, in some cases, data for correlational analysis have been obtained from two distinct populations. If the populations have different values for the variables of interest, the researcher will obtain inaccurate information on relationships among the variables. Differences in values from distinctly different populations are clearly visible on a scatter plot, thus allowing accurate interpretation of correlational results (Figure 20-2).

BIVARIATE CORRELATIONAL ANALYSIS

Bivariate correlation measures the extent (strength and direction) of linear relationship between two vari-

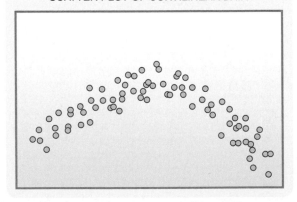

SCATTER PLOT OF CURVILINEAR DATA

Figure **20-1** Scatter plot of curvilinear data.

ables and is performed on data collected from a single sample. Measures of the two variables to be examined must be available for each subject in the data set. Less commonly, data are obtained from two related subjects, such as blood lipid levels in father and son. The statistical analysis techniques used will depend on the type of data available. Correlational techniques are available for all levels of data: nominal (phi, contingency coefficient, Cramer's *V*, and lambda), ordinal (gamma, Kendall's tau, and Somers' *D*), or interval and ratio (Pearson's correlation). Many of the correlational techniques (gamma, Somers' *D*, Kendall's tau, contingency coefficient, phi, and Cramer's *V*) are used in conjunction with contingency tables. Contingency tables are explained further in Chapter 22.

Correlational analysis provides two pieces of information about the data: the nature or direction of the linear relationship (positive or negative) between the two variables and the magnitude (or strength) of the linear relationship. The outcomes of correlational analysis are symmetrical rather than asymmetrical. *Symmetrical* means that the direction of the linear relationship cannot be determined from the analysis. One cannot say from the analysis that variable *A* causes variable *B*.

In a positive linear relationship, the scores being correlated vary together (in the same direction). When one score is high, the other score tends to be high; when one score is low, the other score tends to be low. In a negative linear relationship, when one score is high, the other score tends to be low (for example, height and weight). A negative linear relationship is sometimes referred to as an inverse linear relationship (for example, the number of courses taken at one time and GPA). You can plot these linear relationships as a straight line on a graph. Sometimes, the outcome is not linear, but curvilinear, in which case a linear relationship plot will appear as a curved line rather than a straight one. (At first the relationship is positive, then it becomes negative. An example is memory and age.) Analyses designed to test for linear relationships, such as Pearson's correlation, cannot detect a curvilinear relationship.

Pearson's Product-Moment Correlation Coefficient

Pearson's correlation was the first of the correlation measures developed and is the most commonly used. All other correlation measures have been developed from Pearson's equation and are adaptations designed to control for violation of the assumptions that must be met to use Pearson's equation. These assumptions are as follows:

1. Interval measurement of both variables (e.g., years of education and income)
2. Normal distribution of at least one variable
3. Independence of observational pairs
4. Homoscedasticity

Data that are homoscedastic are evenly dispersed both above and below the regression line, which indicates a linear relationship on a scatter diagram (plot). Homoscedasticity reflects equal variance of both variables. In other words, for every value of x, the distribution of y scores should have equal variability. A regression line is the line that best represents the values of the raw scores plotted on a scatter diagram.

Calculation

Numerous formulas can be used to compute Pearson's *r*. With small samples, Pearson's *r* can be generated fairly easily with a calculator by using the following formula:

$$r = \frac{n(\Sigma XY) - (\Sigma X)(\Sigma Y)}{\sqrt{[n(\Sigma X^2) - (\Sigma X)^2][n(\Sigma Y^2) - (\Sigma Y)^2]}}$$

where

r = Pearson's correlation coefficient
n = Number of paired scores
X = Score of the first variable
Y = Score of the second variable
XY = Product of the two paired scores

An example demonstrates the calculation of Pearson's *r*. Correlation between the two variables of functioning and coping was calculated. The functional variable (variable *X*) was operationalized by using Karnofsky's scale, and a family coping tool was used to

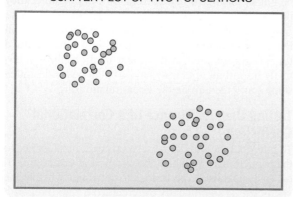

SCATTER PLOT OF TWO POPULATIONS

Figure **20-2** Scatter plot showing data from two different populations.

operationalize coping. Karnofsky's scale ranges from 1 to 10; 1 is normal function, and 10 is moribund (fatal processes progressing rapidly). Nursing diagnosis terminology was used to develop the family coping tool (variable *Y*); scores ranged from 1 to 4, with 1 being effective family coping; 2, ineffective family coping, potential for growth; 3, ineffective family coping, compromised; and 4, ineffective family coping, disabling. Table 20-1 presents the data for these two variables in 10 subjects. Usually, correlations are conducted on larger samples; this example serves only to demonstrate the process of calculating Pearson's *r:*

$$r = \frac{(10)(172)-(55)(26)}{\sqrt{[10(385)-(55)^2][10(80)-(26)^2]}}$$

$$= \frac{1720-1430}{\sqrt{(3850-3025)(800-676)}}$$

$$= \frac{290}{\sqrt{102,300}} = \frac{290}{319.844} = 0.907$$

Interpretation of Results

The outcome of the Pearson product-moment correlation analysis is an *r* value of between −1 and +1. This *r* value indicates the degree of linear relationship between the two variables. A score of zero indicates no linear relationship.

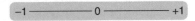

A value of −1 indicates a perfect negative (inverse) correlation. In a negative linear relationship, a high score on one variable is related to a low score on the other variable. A value of +1 indicates a perfect positive linear relationship. In a positive linear relationship,

a high score on one variable is associated with a high score on the other variable. A positive correlation also exists when a low score on one variable is related to a low score on the other variable. A perfect positive or negative correlation is almost nonexistent between variables. As the negative or positive values of *r* approach zero, the strength of the linear relationship decreases. Traditionally, an *r* value of < 0.03 is considered a weak linear relationship, 0.3 to 0.5 is a moderate linear relationship, and > 0.5 is a strong linear relationship. However, this interpretation depends to a great extent on the variables being examined and the situation within which they were observed. Therefore, as a researcher you will need to apply some judgment when interpreting the results. In the example provided, the *r* value was 0.907, which indicates a strong positive linear relationship between the Karnofsky scale and the family coping tool in this sample.

Nursing researchers have tended to disregard weak correlations. However, such tendencies create a serious possibility of ignoring a linear relationship that may have some meaning within nursing knowledge when examined in the context of other variables. This situation is similar to a type II error (failing to reject the null when it is false) and commonly occurs for three reasons. First, many nursing measurements are not powerful enough to detect fine discriminations, and some instruments may not detect extreme scores. In this case, the linear relationship may be stronger than indicated by the crude measures available. Second, correlational studies must have a wide range of variance for linear relationships to be detected. If the study scores are homogeneous or if the sample is small, linear relationships that exist in the population will not show up as clearly in the sample. Third, in many cases, bivariate analysis does not provide a clear picture of the dynamics in the situation. A number of variables can be linked through weak correlations, but together they provide increased insight into situations of interest. Therefore, although one should not overreact to small Pearson coefficients, the information must be recorded for future reference. If the linear relationship is intuitively important, one may have to plan better-designed studies and reexamine the linear relationship.

Testing the Significance of a Correlational Coefficient

To infer that the sample correlation coefficient applies to the population from which the sample was taken, statistical analysis must be performed to determine whether the coefficient is significantly different from zero (no correlation). In other words, we can test the hypothesis that the population Pearson correlation coefficient is 0. The test

TABLE 20-1		Data and Computations for Pearson's R		
Subjects	X	Y	XY	X²	Y²
1	10	4	40	100	16
2	7	3	21	49	9
3	3	2	6	9	4
4	6	3	18	36	9
5	1	1	1	1	1
6	5	2	10	25	4
7	2	2	4	4	4
8	9	4	36	81	16
9	4	1	4	16	1
10	8	4	32	64	16
Sums	55	26	172	385	80

statistic used is the t, distributed according to the t distribution, with $n-2$ degrees of freedom. The formula for calculating the t statistic follows. This formula was used to calculate the t value for the example where $r = 0.907$:

$$t = \frac{r\sqrt{n-2}}{1-r^2} \quad t = \frac{0.907\sqrt{10-2}}{\sqrt{1-(0.907)^2}}$$

$$= \frac{2.565}{\sqrt{1.77}} = \frac{2.565}{0.421} = 6.09$$

where

r = Pearson's product-moment correlation coefficient
n = Sample size of paired scores
$df = n - 2$

The statistical significance of the t obtained from the formula is determined by using the t distribution table in Appendix A. With a small sample, a very high correlation coefficient (r) can be nonsignificant. With a very large sample, the correlation coefficient can be statistically significant when the degree of association is too small to be clinically significant. Therefore, when judging the significance of the coefficient, you must consider both the size of the coefficient and the significance of the t-test. The t value calculated in the example was 6.09, and the df for the sample was 8. This t value was significant at the 0.001 level. If the p value of the t test is significant, then the r value is statistically significant. When reporting the results of a correlation coefficient, both the r value and the p value should be reported.

The r value also must be examined for clinical importance. To do this, square the r value (r^2) to determine the percentage of variance explained by this relationship. The stronger the r value, the greater the variability that is explained for the two variables. If the r value is of at least moderate strength ($r = 0.3$) or high, then the percentage of variance explained is 9% or higher. If the percentage of variance explained is 9% or higher the relationship has potential clinical importance that the researcher must evaluate. Research reports would be strengthened by discussing the statistical significance and clinical importance of an r value (Grove, 2007).

When Pearson's correlation coefficient is squared (r^2), the resulting number is the **percentage of variance** explained by the linear relationship. This is also called the coefficient of determination. In the preceding computation based on data in Table 20-3, $r = 0.907$ and $r^2 = 0.822$. In this case, the linear relationship explains 82% of the variability in the two scores. Except for perfect correlations, r^2 will always be lower than r. This r value

is very high. Results in most nursing studies will be much lower. r^2 is important because it helps correct for sample size issues, for example when large sample sizes are more likely to result in significant correlations.

Correlational Matrix

A **correlational matrix** is obtained by performing bivariate correlational analysis on every pair of variables in the data set. Figure 20-3 shows the appearance of the matrix. On the matrix, the r value and the p value are given for each pair of variables. At a diagonal line through the matrix, the variables are correlated with themselves. Often, these variables are identified in statistical software packages with asterisks. The r value for these correlations is 1.00 and the p value is 0.000 because when a variable is related to itself, the correlation is perfect. Note that to the left and the right of this diagonal, correlations for each pair of variables are repeated. Therefore, one must examine only half the matrix to obtain a full picture of the relationships. Grove (2007) provided a statistical workbook that that can increase your understanding of correlational tables and narrative results that are included in published studies.

When examining the matrix values, you must place weight only on those r values with a p value of 0.05 or smaller. Once these pairs of variables are singled out, you will note variable pairs with an r value sufficiently large to be of interest in terms of the study problem. By examining these pairs of variables, you can gain theoretical insight into the dynamics of the variables within the problem of concern in the study. Of particular interest are pairs of variables that are unexpectedly significantly related. These results can sometimes provide new insight into the research problem.

Spurious Correlations

Spurious correlations are relationships between variables that are not logical. In some cases, these significant relationships are a consequence of chance and have no meaning. When you choose a level of significance of 0.05, 1 in 20 correlations that you perform in a matrix will be significant by chance. Other pairs of variables may be correlated because of the influence of other variables. For example, you might find a positive correlation between the number of deaths on a nursing unit and the number of nurses working on the unit. Clearly, the number of deaths cannot be explained as occurring because of increases in the number of nurses. It is more likely that a third variable (units having patients with more critical conditions) explains the increased number of nurses. In most cases, the "other" variable will remain unknown. You can use reasoning to identify and exclude most of these correlations.

Correlations		AGE	educ12	HIGHER EDUCATION (fill one)	KNIDTOT
AGE	Pearson Correlation Sig. (2-tailed) N	1.000 304	0.090 0.118 304	0.175 0.004 266	−0.119[†] 0.038 304
educt12	Pearson Correlation Sig. (2-tailed) N	0.090 0.118 304	1.000 305	0.390[*] 0.000 267	−0.100 0.080 305
HIGHER EDUCATION (fill one)	Pearson Correlation Sig. (2-tailed) N	−0.175[†] 0.004 266	0.390[*] 0.000 267	1.000 267	−0.096 0.118 267
KNIDTOT	Pearson Correlation Sig. (2-tailed) N	−0.119[†] 0.038 304	−0.100 0.080 305	−0.096 0.118 267	1.000 305

[†] Correlation is significant at the 0.01 level (2-tailed).

[*] Correlation is significant at the 0.05 level (2-tailed).

Figure **20-3** Correlational matrix using SPSS Version 9. *KNIDTOT*, knowledge of infant development by English-speaking Hispanic mothers.

Spearman Rank-Order Correlation Coefficient

The Spearman rank-order correlation coefficient is an adaptation of the Pearson product-moment correlation, discussed later in this chapter. Use this test when the assumptions of Pearson's analysis cannot be met. For example, the data may be ordinal, or the scores may be skewed. (Data might be, for example, placement on test by rank and income level by rank.) (Grove, 2007)

Calculation

The data must be ranked to conduct the analysis. Therefore, if a researcher uses scores from measurement scales to perform the analysis, the scores must be converted to ranks. As with all correlational analyses, each subject in the analysis must have a score (or value) on each of two variables (variable x and variable y). The scores on each variable are ranked separately. Rho is calculated based on difference scores between a subject's ranking on the first and second set of scores. The formula for this calculation is as follows:

$$D = x - y$$

As in most statistical analyses, difference scores are difficult to use directly in equations because negative scores tend to cancel out positive scores; therefore, the scores are squared for use in the analysis. The formula is as follows:

$$\text{rho} = 1 - \frac{6 \Sigma D^2}{N^3 - N}$$

where

Rho = Spearman correlation coefficient (derived from Pearson's r)
D = Difference score between the ranking of a score on variable x and the ranking of a score on variable y
N = Number of paired ranked scores

Interpretation of Results

When you use an equation to analyze data that meet the assumptions of Pearson's correlational analysis, the results are equivalent or slightly lower than Pearson's r, discussed later in this chapter. If the data are skewed, rho has an efficiency of 91% in detecting an existing relationship. The significance of rho must be tested as with any correlation; the formula used is presented in the following equation. The t distribution is presented in Appendix C, and $df = N - 2$.

$$t = \text{rho} \sqrt{\frac{N - 2}{1 - \text{rho}^2}}$$

TABLE 20-2 ■ Ranking of Scores for Calculation of Kendall's Tau

Subject	Score on Variable x	Ranking on Variable x	Score on Variable y	Ranking on Variable y
A	3	3	4	2
B	5	2	2	1
C	6	3	6	3
D	9	4	8	5
E	12	5	7	4

Kendall's Tau

Kendall's tau is a nonparametric measure of correlation used when both variables have been measured at the ordinal level (e.g., strength of evidence and education of researcher). You can use it with very small samples. The statistic tau reflects a ratio of the actual concordance obtained between rankings with the maximal concordance possible. This text uses Marascuilo and McSweeney's (1977) explanation of this analysis technique.

Calculation

To calculate tau, rank the scores on each of the two variables independently. Arrange the paired scores by subject, with the lowest ranking score on variable x at the top of the list and the ranking score on variable y for the same subject in the same row. Table 20-2 presents an example of the ranking of scores for five subjects on variables x and y.

Then compare the relative ranking position between each pair of subjects on variable y, shown in the last column in the table. (It is not necessary to compare rankings on variable x because the data have been arranged in order by rank.) If the comparison is concordant, the ranking of the score below will be higher than the ranking of the score above and is assigned a value of +1. If the comparison is discordant, the ranking of the score below will be lower than the ranking of the score above and is assigned a value of −1. In Table 20-3, the comparisons are identified as concordant (+1) or discordant (−1) for the ranked scores identified in Table 20-1. In this example, the number of discordant pairs is two; the number of concordant pairs is eight. The statistic S is then calculated with the following equation:

$$S = N_c - N_d$$

Example:

$$S = 8 - 2 = 6$$

where

N_c = Number of concordant pairs
N_d = Number of discordant pairs

TABLE 20-3 ■ Calculation of Concordant-Discordant States in Kendall's Tau

Comparison of Subjects	Value for x	Value for y	State
AB	+1	−1	Discordant
AC	+1	+1	Concordant
AD	+1	+1	Concordant
AE	+1	+1	Concordant
BC	+1	+1	Concordant
BD	+1	+1	Concordant
BE	+1	+1	Concordant
CD	+1	+1	Concordant
CE	+1	+1	Concordant
DE	+1	−1	Discordant

At this point, tau is calculated by using the following equation:

$$Tau = \frac{2S}{n(n-1)}$$

$$\text{Example: Tau} = \frac{(2)(6)}{5(5-1)} = 0.6$$

where

$$n = \text{Number of paired scores}$$

Interpretation of Results

If the ranking of values of x is not related to the ranking of values of y, any particular rank ordering of y is just as likely to occur as any other. The sample tau can be used to test the hypothesis that the population tau is 0. The significance of tau can be tested by using the following equation for the Z statistic. The Z statistic was calculated for the previous example.

$$Z = \frac{\text{tau} - \text{mean}}{SD_{\text{tau}}}$$

$$Z = \frac{0.6 - 0}{\sqrt{\dfrac{2(10+5)}{(9)(5)(5-1)}}} = \frac{0.6}{0.408} = 1.47$$

where :

$$\text{mean} = \mu_{\text{tau}} = 0$$

$$SD_{\text{tau}} = \sqrt{\frac{2(2n+5)}{9n(n-1)}}$$

The Z values are approximately normally distributed, and therefore you can use the table of Z scores available in Appendix 2 (available on the Evolve website at http://evolve.elsevier.com/Burns/Practice/). The Z score for the example was 1.47, which is nonsignificant at the $p \le 0.05$ level.

Role of Correlation in Understanding Causality

In any situation involving causality, a relationship will exist between the factors involved in the causal process. Therefore, the first clue to the possibility of a causal link is the existence of a relationship. However, a relationship does not mean causality. For example, blood sugar level may be related to body temperature, however this does not mean that one causes the other. Two variables can be highly correlated but have no causal relationship whatsoever. However, as the strength of a relationship increases, the possibility of a causal link increases. The absence of a relationship precludes the possibility of a causal connection between the two variables being examined, given adequate measurement of the variables and absence of other variables that might mask the relationship. Thus, a correlational study can be the first step in determining the dynamics important to nursing practice within a particular population. Determining these dynamics can allow us to increase our ability to predict and control the situation studied. However, correlation cannot be used to demonstrate causality.

MULTIVARIATE CORRELATIONAL PROCEDURES

Multivariate correlational procedures are more complex analysis techniques that examine linear relationships among three or more variables.

Factor Analysis

Factor analysis examines interrelationships among large numbers of variables and disentangles those relationships to identify clusters of variables that are most closely linked together (factors). Several factors may be identified within a data set. Sample sizes must be large for factor analysis. Nunnally and Bernstein (1994) recommended 10 observations for each variable. Arrindell and van der Ende (1985) suggested that a more reliable determination is a sample size of 20 times the number of factors. You can also perform a power analysis to determine the sample size.

Once the factors have been identified mathematically, the researcher explains why the variables are grouped as they are. Thus, factor analysis aids in the identification of theoretical constructs. Factor analysis is also used to confirm the accuracy of a theoretically developed construct. For example, a theorist might state that the concept "hope" consists of the elements (1) anticipation of the future, (2) belief that things will work out for the best, and (3) optimism. Instruments could be developed to measure these three elements, and factor analysis could be conducted on the data to determine whether subject responses clustered into these three groupings.

Factor analysis is frequently used in the process of developing measurement instruments, particularly those related to psychological variables such as attitudes, beliefs, values, or opinions. The instrument operationalizes a theoretical construct. The method can also be used with physiological data. For example, Woods, Lentz, and Mitchell (1993) identified a large pool of symptoms commonly experienced during the perimenstruum, and daily rating of the severity of these symptoms by subjects was used to identify premenstrual symptom patterns. Testing of the validity of these patterns by factor analysis resulted in the selection of 33 symptoms for classification of women as having a low-severity symptom pattern, a premenstrual syndrome pattern, or a premenstrual magnification pattern. The analysis revealed that these patterns (factors) were consistent across menstrual cycle phases and had internal consistency reliability estimates above 0.70 (Woods, Mitchell, & Lentz, 1995). This work has now been recognized in medicine as well as nursing in defining menstrual difficulties clinically as well as in research. Factor analysis can be used as a data reduction strategy in studies examining large numbers of variables. It can also be used to attempt to sort out meaning from large numbers of items on survey instruments.

The two types of factor analysis are exploratory and confirmatory. **Exploratory factor analysis** is similar to stepwise regression, in which the variance of the first factor is partialed out before analysis on the second factor begins. It is performed when the researcher has few prior expectations about the factor structure. **Confirmatory factor analysis** is more closely related to ordinary least-squares regression analysis or path analysis. It is based on theory and tests a hypothesis about the existing factor structure. In confirmatory factor analysis, the researcher determines the statistical significance of the analysis outcomes and estimates the parameters of the population. Confirmatory factor analysis is usually conducted after the correlation matrix has been examined or after initial development of the factor structure through exploratory factor analysis.

Exploratory Factor Analysis

The first step in exploratory factor analysis is the development of a correlation matrix of the scores for all variables to be included in the factor analysis. The computer program conducting the analysis usually develops this matrix automatically. Although multiple procedures can be used for the actual factor analysis, the procedure described here is the one most commonly reported in the nursing literature.

The second step is a **principal components analysis**, which provides the preliminary information that the researcher needs to make decisions before the final factoring. The computer printout of the principal components analysis will give (1) the eigenvalues, (2) the amount of variance explained by each factor, and (3) the weight for each variable on each factor. Weights (**loadings**) express the extent to which the variable is correlated with the factor. Weightings on the variables from a principal components factor analysis are essentially uninterpretable and are generally disregarded (Nunnally & Bernstein, 1994).

Eigenvalues are the sum of the squared weights for each factor. The researcher examines the eigenvalues to decide how many factors will be included in the factor analysis. To decide the number of factors to include, the researcher determines the minimal amount of variance that must be explained by the factor to add significant meaning. This decision is not straightforward, however, and some have criticized the analysis for being subjective. Several strategies have been proposed for determining the number of factors to be included in a construct. One approach is to select factors that have an eigenvalue of 1.00 or above. Another strategy used is the screen test. *Scree* is a geological term that refers to the debris that collects at the bottom

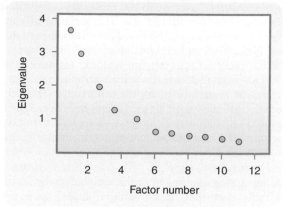

Figure **20-4** Graphed eigenvalues from a factor analysis.

of a rocky slope. This test, which is considered by some to be the most reliable, requires that the eigenvalues be graphed (Figure 20-4).

This graph shows a change in the angle of the slope. A steep drop in value from one factor to the next indicates a large difference score between the two factors and an increase in the amount of variance explained. When the slope begins to become flat, which is an indication of small difference scores between factors, little additional information will be obtained by including more factors. In Figure 20-4, the slope begins to flatten at factor 6; therefore, six factors would be extracted to explain the construct.

The third step in exploratory factor analysis is **factor rotation**. Factor rotation simplifies the factor structure, and the procedure most commonly used is referred to as varimax rotation. In **varimax rotation**, the factors are rotated for the best fit (best factor solution), and the factors are uncorrelated. An **oblique rotation** results in correlated factors.

The process of factor analysis is actually a series of multiple regression analyses (Kim & Mueller, 1978a, 1978b). The equation for a factor could be expressed as

$$F = b_1X_1 + b_2X_2 + b_3X_3 + \ldots + b_kX_k$$

where

F = Factor score
X_k = Original variables from the matrix
b_k = Weights of the individual variables in the factor
(If the scores used are standardized, b is a beta weight.)

In exploratory factor analysis, regression analysis is performed for the first factor. The variance of each variable explained by the first factor is then partialed out. Next, a second regression analysis is performed for the second factor on the residual variance. The variance from that analysis is then partialed out, and a regression is performed for the third factor. This process is continued until all the factors have been developed. The computer printout will include a rotated factor matrix that contains information similar to that in Table 20-4.

Factor Loadings. A factor loading is actually the regression coefficient of the variable on the factor. In Table 20-4, the factor loading indicates the extent to which a single variable is related to the cluster of variables. In variable 1, the factor loading is 0.76 for factor I and 0.27 for factor II. Squaring the factor loadings ($[0.76]^2 = 0.578$, and $[0.27]^2 = 0.073$) gives the amount of variance in variable 1, which explains factors I and II.

Communality. Communality (h^2) is the squared multiple regression coefficient for each variable and closely relates to the R^2 coefficient in regression. Thus, the communality coefficient describes the amount of variance in a single variable that is explained across all the factors in the analysis. To obtain the communality for a variable, sum the squared factor loadings on the variable for each factor. In Table 20-4, the communality coefficient for variable 1 is $(0.76)^2 + (0.27)^2 = 0.65$.

Identifying the Relevant Variables in a Factor. Only variables with factor loadings that indicate that a meaningful portion of the variable's variance is explained within the factor are included as elements of the factor. A cutoff point is selected to identify these variables, with the minimal acceptable cutoff point being 0.30. In Table 20-4, the factor loadings with asterisks indicate the variables that will be included in each factor. In this example, which uses a 0.50 cutoff, variables 1, 2, and 3 would be included in factor I, and variables 4, 5, and 6 would be included in factor II. Ideally, a variable will *load* (have a factor loading above the selected cutoff point) on only one factor. If the variable does have high loadings on two factors, the lowest loading is referred to as a secondary loading. When many secondary loadings occur, it is not considered a clean factoring, and the researcher reexamines the variables included in the analysis. Sometimes, researchers attempt to set the cutoff point high enough to avoid secondary loadings of a variable.

"Naming" the Factor. At this point, the mathematics of the procedure takes a back seat, and the researcher's theoretical reasoning takes over. The researcher examines the variables that have clustered together in a factor and explains that clustering. Variables with high loadings on the factor must be included, even if they do not fit the researcher's preconceived theoretical notions. The purpose is to identify the broad construct of meaning that has caused these particular variables to be so strongly intercorrelated. Naming this construct is an important part of the procedure because naming of the factor provides theoretical meaning.

Factor Scores. After the initial factor analysis, additional studies are conducted to examine changes in the phenomenon in various situations and to determine the relationships of the factors with other concepts. Factor scores are used during data analysis in these additional studies. To obtain factor scores, the variables included in the factor are identified, and the scores on these variables are summed for each subject. Thus, each subject will have a score for each factor in the instrument. Because some variables explain a larger portion of the variance of the factor than others do, additional meaning can be added by multiplying the variable score by the weight (factor loading) of that variable in the factor. In the example in Table 20-4, variable 1 had a factor loading of 0.76 on factor I. If the subject score on variable 1 were 7, the score would be weighted by multiplying the variable score by the factor loading as follows:

$$7 \times 0.76 = 5.32$$

A computer can generate these weighted scores. If studies are to be compared, standardized (Z) scores (for variable scores) and beta weights (for factor

TABLE 20-4	Factor Loading and Variance for Two Factors		
	Factors		
Variable	I	II	h_2
1	0.76*	0.27	0.65
2	0.91*	0.03	0.83
3	0.64*	0.29	0.49
4	0.14	0.67*	0.47
5	0.22	0.59*	0.40
6	0.07	0.77*	0.60
Sum of squared loadings	1.89	1.55	
Variance	0.22	0.13	Total = 0.35

* Indicates the variables to be included in each factor.

loadings) are used. Once analysis is complete, factor scores can be used as independent variables in multiple regression equations.

Ramirez, Tart, and Malecha (2006) used factor analysis to identify treatment competencies of nurse practitioners providing care in emergency rooms. The factor analysis is reported as follows:

Nurse practitioners (NPs) providing care in the emergency department do not have recognized treatment competencies. The purpose of the study was to establish a definition of the NPs in emergency care settings, by examining the treatment competencies. The overall goals of this research project were to perform psychometric testing on the Nurse Practitioner Treatment Competency Instrument (NPTCI) and identify competencies relevant to the NP in the emergency department. The research questions for this study were as follows: What were the internal consistency reliability estimates for the NPTCI as measured by Cronbach's alpha reliability coefficients? What was the construct structure of the NPTCI as evidenced by the factor loading extracted from an orthogonal, rotated, exploratory factor analysis? What items in the NPTCI were relevant to the emergency nurse practitioner? The task analysis branch of the Kane model, "Model-Based Practice Analysis and Test Specifications," is the segment this study used to establish the framework for conceptualization and identification of treatment competencies for NPs in emergency care.

A descriptive postal survey was conducted using a national sample. The data for this study was collected using the NPTCI that examines demographic information related to NP practice and the relevance of specific activities/tasks that are identified by established family and acute care competencies. The instrument was sent to family, acute care, and emergency NPs. The total estimated sample size was 1,778; of the 582 who responded to the questionnaire, 42 were emergency NPs. The NPTCI was found to be reliable and valid using factor analysis and Cronbach's alpha. The factor analysis resulted in 5 factors, which were named 1. Implements clinical treatment plan, 2. Implements holistic treatment plan, 3. Incorporates health promotion, prevention, and education in treatment, 4. Treatment of women and children, and 5. Performance of Invasive procedures as part of treatment plan. Emergency nurse practitioners (ENPs) identified fifteen items on the instrument as not relevant to the ENP role. The items identified were primarily specific invasive procedures and utilizing technology to sustain physiologic function. Two were related to pre- and postpartum assessment. The last item that ENPs indicated as not relevant to their practice was dealing with end-of-life issues. It is not clear why ENPs did not consider this activity relevant to their practice. (Ramirez et al., 2006)

SUMMARY

- Correlational analyses identify relationships between or among variables.
- The purpose of the analysis is also to clarify relationships among theoretical concepts or help to identify potentially causal relationships, which can then be tested by inferential analysis.
- All data for the analysis should have been obtained from a single population from which values are available on all variables to be examined.
- Data measured at the interval or ratio level provide the best information on the nature of the relationship.
- Correlational analysis provides two pieces of information about the data: the nature of a linear relationship (positive or negative) between the two variables and the magnitude (or strength) of the linear relationship.
- The Spearman rho, a nonparametric test, is used when the assumptions of Pearson's analysis cannot be met.
- Kendall's tau is a nonparametric measure of correlation used when both variables have been measured at the ordinal level.
- Pearson's correlation is used when both variables have been measured at the interval or ratio level.
- A correlational matrix is obtained by performing bivariate correlational analysis on every pair of variables in the data set.
- The first clue to the possibility of a causal link is the existence of a relationship, but a relationship does not necessarily mean causality.
- Multivariate correlational procedures are more complex analysis techniques that examine linear relationships among three or more variables.
- Factor analysis examines interrelationships among large numbers of variables and disentangles those relationships to identify clusters of variables that are most closely linked (factors).

REFERENCES

Arrindell, W. A., & van der Ende, J. (1985). An empirical test of the utility of the observations-to-variables ratio in factor and components analysis. *Applied Psychological Measurement, 9*(2), 165–178.

Grove, S. K. (2007). *Statistics for health care research: A practical workbook.* Philadelphia: Saunders.

Kim, J., & Mueller, C. W. (1978a). *Factor analysis: Statistical methods and practical issues.* Beverly Hills, CA: Sage.

Kim, J., & Mueller, C. W. (1978b). *Introduction to factor analysis: What it is and how to do it.* Beverly Hills, CA: Sage.

Marascuilo, L. A., & McSweeney, M. (1977). *Nonparametric and distribution-free methods for the social sciences*. Monterey, CA: Brooks/Cole.

Nunnally, J. C., & Bernstein, I. (1994). *Psychometric theory* (3rd ed.). New York: McGraw-Hill.

Ramirez, E. G., Tart, K., & Malecha, A. (2006). Developing nurse practitioner treatment competencies in emergency care settings. *Advanced Emergency Nursing Journal, 28*(4), 346–359.

Woods, N. F., Lentz, M. J., & Mitchell, E. S. (1993). *Prevalence of perimenstrual symptoms*. Unpublished report to National Center for Nursing Research.

Woods, N. F., Mitchell, E. S., & Lentz, M. J. (1995). Social pathways to premenstrual symptoms. *Research in Nursing & Health, 18*(3), 225–237.

CHAPTER **21**

Using Statistics to Predict

The ability to predict future events is becoming increasingly important in our society. We are interested in predicting who will win the football game, what the weather will be like next week, or what stocks are likely to rise in the near future. In nursing practice, as in the rest of society, the capacity to predict is crucial. For example, we need to predict the length of stay of patients with varying severity of illness, as well as the response of patients with a variety of characteristics to nursing interventions. We need to know what factors play an important role in patients' responses to rehabilitation. One might be interested in knowing what variables were most effective in predicting a student's score on the State Board of Nurse Examiners' Licensure Examination.

The statistical procedure most commonly used for prediction is regression analysis. The purpose of a regression analysis is to predict or explain as much of the variance in the value of a dependent variable as possible. In some cases, the analysis is exploratory, and the focus is prediction. In others, selection of variables is based on a theoretical position, and the purpose is to develop an explanation that confirms the theoretical position.

Predictive analyses are based on probability theory rather than decision theory. Prediction is one approach to examining causal relationships between or among variables. The independent (predictor) variable or variables cause **variation** in the value of the dependent (outcome) variable. The goal is to determine how accurately one can predict the value of an outcome (or dependent) variable based on the value or values of one or more predictor (or independent) variables. This chapter describes some of the more common statistical procedures used for prediction. These procedures include simple linear regression, multiple regression, and discriminant analysis.

SIMPLE LINEAR REGRESSION

Simple linear regression provides a means to estimate the value of a dependent variable based on the value of an independent variable. The regression equation is a mathematical expression of a causal proposition emerging from a theoretical framework. This link between the theoretical statement and the equation should be made clear before the analysis. Simple linear regression is an effort to explain the dynamics within the scatter plot by drawing a straight line (the line of best fit) through the plotted scores. This line is drawn to best explain the linear relationship between two variables. Knowing that linear relationship, we can, with some degree of accuracy, use regression analysis to predict the value of one variable if we know the value of the other variable.

Simple linear regression is a method of determining parameters a and b. When squared deviation values are minimized, variance from the line of best fit is minimized. To understand the mathematical process, recall the algebraic equation for a straight line:

$$y = a + bx$$

In regression analysis, the straight line is usually plotted on a graph, with the horizontal axis representing x (the independent, or predictor, variable) and the vertical axis representing y (the dependent, or predicted, variable). The value represented by the letter a is referred to as the y intercept, or the point where the regression line crosses (or intercepts) the y axis. At this point on the regression line, $x = 0$. The value represented by the letter b is referred to as the slope, or the coefficient of x. The slope determines the direction and angle of the regression line within the graph. The slope expresses the extent to which y changes for every 1-unit change in x. Figure 21-1 is a graph of these points.

In simple, or bivariate, regression, predictions are made in cases with two variables. The score on variable y (dependent variable) is predicted from the same subject's known score on variable x (independent variable). The predicted score (or estimate) is referred to as $\hat{y}$ (expressed y-hat) or occasionally as y' (expressed y-prime).

No single regression line can be used to predict with complete accuracy every y value from every x value. In fact, you could draw an infinite number of lines through the scattered paired values. However, the purpose of the regression equation is to develop the line to allow the highest degree of prediction possible—the line of best fit. The procedure for developing the line of best fit is the method of least squares.

Interpretation of Results

The outcome of analysis is the regression coefficient R. When R *is* squared, it indicates the amount of variance in the data that is explained by the equation. A null regression hypothesis states that the population regression slope is 0, which indicates that there is no useful linear relationship between x and y. (There are regression analyses that test for nonlinear relationships.) The test statistic used to determine the significance of a regression coefficient is t. However, the test uses a different equation than the t-test used to determine significant differences between means. In determining the significance of a regression coefficient, t tends to become larger as b moves farther from zero. However, if the sum of squared deviations from regression is large, the t value will decrease. Small sample sizes also decrease the t value.

In reporting the results of a regression analysis, the equation is expressed with the calculated coefficient values. The R^2 value and the t values are also documented. The format for reporting the results of regression is as follows:

$$\underset{\downarrow}{y\,\text{intercept}} \qquad \underset{\downarrow}{b\,(\text{slope})}$$
$$\hat{y} = 3.45 + 8.72x \qquad R^2 = 0.63$$
$$(2.79)(4.68) \leftarrow t\,\text{value}$$

The figures in parentheses are not always t values. They may be the standard error of the estimate. Therefore, the report must indicate which values are being reported. If t values are being used, the t value that indicates significance should also be reported. A t value equal to or greater than the table value (see Appendix A) indicates significance. Researchers can use these results to develop a graph that illustrates the outcome. Additionally, a table can be developed to indicate the changes that are predicted to occur in the value of y with each increase in the value of x. Names are usually given to identify the variables of x and y. In the example in which the y intercept = 3.45 and $b = 8.72$, a table of x and y values was developed (Table 21-1). These values are graphed in Figure 21-2.

After a regression equation has been developed, the equation is tested against a new sample to determine its accuracy in prediction, a process called *cross-validation*. In some studies, data are collected from a holdout sample obtained at the initial data collection period but not included in the initial regression analysis. The regression equation is then tested against this sample. Some "shrinkage" of R^2 is expected because

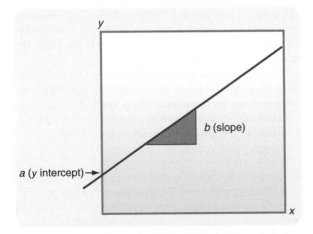

Figure **21-1** Graph of a regression line.

TABLE **21-1** Predicted Values of y from Known Values of x by Regression Analysis	
Value of x	Predicted Value of y
0	3.45 (y intercept)
1	12.17 (y intercept +b)
2	20.89 (+b)
3	29.61 (+b)
4	38.33 (+b)

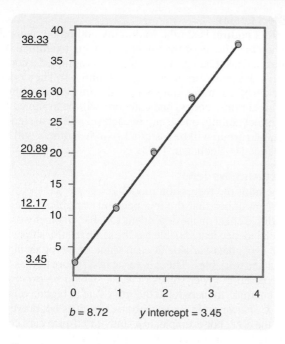

Figure **21-2** Regression line developed from values in Table 21-1.

the equation was generated to best fit the sample from which it was developed. However, an equation is most useful if it maintains its ability to accurately predict across many and varied samples. The first test of an equation against a new sample should use a sample similar to the initial sample.

MULTIPLE REGRESSION

Multiple regression analyses are closely related mathematically to analysis of variance (ANOVA) models (ANOVA is described in Chapter 22); however, their focus is predicting rather than determining differences in groups. ANOVA is based on decision theory, whereas regression analysis is based on probability theory. Multiple regression is an extension of simple linear regression in which more than one independent variable is entered into the analysis. Examples of simple and multiple regression analysis results from published studies are presented in the Grove (2007) statistical workbook. The workbook can expand your understanding of regression analyses and the implications of the findings for practice.

Multicollinearity

Multicollinearity occurs when the independent variables in a multiple regression equation are strongly correlated. In nursing studies, some multicollinearity is inevitable; however, you can minimize multicollinearity by carefully selecting the independent variables. Multicollinearity does not affect predictive power (the capacity of the independent variables to predict values of the dependent variable in that specific sample); rather it causes problems related to generalizability. If multicollinearity is present, the equation will not have predictive validity. The amount of variance explained by each variable in the equation will be inflated. The b values will not remain consistent across samples when cross-validation is performed.

The first step in identifying multicollinearity is to examine the correlations among the independent variables. Therefore, you would perform multiple correlation analyses before conducting the regression analyses. The correlation matrix is carefully examined for evidence of multicollinearity. Most researchers consider multicollinearity to exist if a bivariate correlation is greater than 0.65. However, some researchers use a stronger correlation of 0.80 or greater as an indication of multicollinearity (Schroeder, 1990).

The coefficient of determination (R^2), computed from a matrix of correlation coefficients, provides important information on multicollinearity. This value indicates the degree of linear dependencies among the variables. As the value of the determinant approaches zero, the degree of linear dependency increases. Thus, it is preferable that this R^2 be large. Identifying the extent of multicollinearity is important when selecting regression procedures and interpreting results. Therefore, Schroeder (1990) described additional procedures that researchers use to diagnose the extent of multicollinearity.

The researcher needs to examine the extent of multicollinearity in the data as part of the analysis procedure and should report this information when the study is published. An example from Braden (1990) follows.

A correlation matrix of model variables showed no evidence of multicollinearity in the multiple regression equations used to answer the research questions. Gordon's (1968) criteria of $r \leq 0.65$ for correlation of variables entered in the same equation was used. (p. 44)

Types of Independent Variables Used in Regression Analyses

Variables in a regression equation can take many forms. Traditionally, as with most multivariate analyses, variables are measured at the interval level. However, researchers also use categorical or dichotomous measures (referred to as **dummy variables**), multiplicative terms, and **transformed terms**. A mixture of types of variables may be used in a single regression equation. The following discussion describes the various terms used as variables in regression equations.

Dummy Variables

To use categorical variables in regression analysis, a coding system is developed to represent group membership. Categorical variables of interest in nursing that might be used in regression analysis include gender, income, ethnicity, social status, level of education, and diagnosis. If the variable is dichotomous, such as gender, members of one category are assigned the number 1, and all others are assigned the number 0. In this case, for gender the coding could be

  1 = female
  0 = male

If the categorical variable has three values, two dummy variables are used; for example, social class could be classified as lower class, middle class, or upper class. The first dummy variable (X_1) would be classified as

  1 = lower class
  0 = not lower class

The second dummy variable (X_2) would be classified as

  1 = middle class
  0 = not middle class

The three social classes would then be specified in the equation in the following manner:

  Lower class $X_1 = 1$, $X_2 = 0$
  Middle class $X_1 = 0$, $X_2 = 1$
  Upper class $X_1 = 0$, $X_2 = 0$

When more than three categories define the values of the variable, increased numbers of dummy variables are used. The number of dummy variables is always one less than the number of categories.

Time Coding

Time is commonly expressed in a regression equation as an interval measure. However, in some cases, codes may need to be developed for time periods. In this strategy, time is coded in a categorical form and used as an independent variable. For example, if 5 years of data were available, the following system could be used to provide dummy codes for the time variable:

  −2 = subjects cared for in the first year
  −1 = subjects cared for in the second year
  0 = subjects cared for in the third year
  +1 = subjects cared for in the fourth year
  +2 = subjects cared for in the fifth year

Effect Coding

Effect coding is similar to dummy coding but is used when the effects of treatments are being examined by the analysis. Each group of subjects is assigned a code. The code numbers used are 1, 0, and −1. The codes are assigned in the same way as dummy codes. While using dummy codes, one category will be assigned 0; in effect coding, one group in each set will be assigned −1, one group will be assigned 1, and all others will be assigned 0 (Pedhazur, 1997).

Multiplicative Terms

The multiple regression model $Y = a + b_1X_1 + b_2X_2 + b_3X_3$ assumes that the independent variables have an additive effect on the dependent variable. In other words, each independent variable has the same relationship with the dependent variable at each value of the other independent variables. Thus, if variable X_1 increased as X_2 increased in lower values of X_2, X_1 would be expected to continue to increase at the same rate at higher values of X_2. However, in some analyses, this does not prove to be the case. For example, in a study of hospice care conducted by one of the authors (Burns & Carney, 1986), minutes of care (MC) was used as the dependent variable. Duration (DUR), or number of days of care, and age (AGE) were included as independent variables. When duration was short, minutes of care increased as age increased. However, when duration was long, minutes of care decreased as age increased.

In this situation, better prediction can occur if multiplicative terms are included in the equation. In this case, the regression model takes the following form:

$$Y = a + b_1X_1 + b_2X_2 + b_3X_1X_2$$

The last term ($b_3X_1X_2$) takes the form of a **multiplicative term** and is the product of the first two variables (X_1 multiplied by X_2). This term expresses the joint effect of the two variables. For example, duration (DUR) might be expected to interact with the subject's age (AGE). The third term shows the combined effect of the two variables (DURAGE). The example equation would then be expressed as

$$MC = a + b_1DUR + b_2AGE + b_3DURAGE$$

This procedure is similar to multivariate ANOVA, in which main effects and interaction effects are considered. Main effects are the effects of a single variable. **Interaction effects** are the multiplicative effects of two or more variables.

Transformed Terms

The typical regression model assumes a linear regression in which the relationship between X and Y can be illustrated on a graph as a straight line. However, in some cases, the relationship is not linear but **curvilinear**. A researcher can sometimes demonstrate the fact that the scores are curvilinear by graphing the values. In these cases, deviations from the regression line will be great and predictive power will be low; the F ratio will not be significant, R^2 will be low, and a type II error will result. Adding another independent variable to the equation, a transformation of the original independent variable obtained by squaring the original variable, may accurately express the curvilinear relationship. This strategy improves the predictive capacity of the analysis. An example of a mathematical model that includes a squared independent variable is

$$Y = a + b_1 X + b_2 X^2$$

This equation states that Y is related to both X and X^2 in such a way that changes in Y's values are a function of both X and X^2. The **nonlinearity analysis** can be extended beyond the squared term to add more transformed terms; thus, values such as X^3, X^4, and so on can be included in the equation. Each term adds another curve in the regression line. With this strategy, complicated relationships can be modeled. However, small samples can incorrectly lead to a perfect fit. For these complex equations, the researcher needs a minimum of 30 observations per term (Cohen & Cohen, 1983). If the complex equation provides better prediction, R^2 will increase and the F ratio will be significant.

Many versions of regression analyses are used in a variety of research situations. Some versions have been developed especially for situations in which some of the foregoing assumptions are violated.

The typical multiple regression equation is expressed as

$$Y = a + bX_1 + bX_2 + \dots bX_i$$

The dependent variable (or predicted variable) is represented by Y in the regression equation. The independent variables (or indicators) are represented by X_i in the regression equation. The i indicates the number of independent variables in the equation. The coefficient of the independent variable, b, is a numerical value that indicates the amount of change that occurs in Y for each change in the associated X and can be reported as a b weight (based on raw scores) or a beta weight (based on Z scores).

The outcome of a multiple regression is an R^2 value. For each independent variable, the significance of R^2 is reported, as well as the significance of b. Regression, unlike correlation, is one-way; the

independent variables can predict the values of the dependent variable, but the dependent variable cannot be used to predict the values of the independent variables. If the b value of an independent variable is not significant, that independent variable is not an effective predictor of the dependent variable when that set of independent variables is used. In this case, the researcher may remove variables with nonsignificant coefficients from the equation and repeat the analysis. This action often increases the amount of variance explained by the equation and thus raises the R^2 value. To be effective predictors, independent variables selected for the analysis should have strong correlations with the dependent variable but only weak correlations with other independent variables in the equation.

The significance of an R^2 value is tested with an F test. A significant F value indicates that the regression equation has effectively predicted variation in the dependent variable and that the R^2 value is not a random variation from an R^2 value of zero.

Results

The outcome of regression analysis is referred to as a **prediction equation**. This equation is similar to that described for simple linear regression except that making a prediction is more complex. Consider the following sample equation:

DURATION =

$10.6 + 0.3$ AGE $+ 2.4$ INCOME $+ 3.5$ COPING

$(4.56) \quad (2.78) \qquad (4.43) \qquad\qquad (7.52)$

R2$=0.51$ n $= 350$ F $= 1.832$ p <0.001

If duration were measured as the number of days that the patient received care, the Y intercept would be 10.6 days. (This value is not meaningful apart from the equation.) For each increase of 1 year in age, the patient would receive 0.3 days more of care. For each increase in income level, the patient would receive an additional 2.4 days of care. For each increase in coping ability measured on a scale, the patient would receive an additional 3.5 days of care. In this example, $R^2 = 0.51$, which means that these variables explain 51% of the variance in the duration of care. The regression analysis of variance indicates that the equation is significant at a $p \leq 0.001$ level. The values in parentheses are the standard deviation for that variable.

Relating these findings to real situations requires additional work. First, it is necessary to know how the variables were coded for the analysis; for example, one would need to know the range of scores on the coping scale, the income classifications, and the range of ages in the sample. Possible patient situations would then be proposed, and the duration of care would be predicted for a patient with those particular dimensions of each independent variable. For example, suppose a patient is 64 years of age, in income level 3, and in coping level 5. In this case, the patient's predicted duration would be $10.6 + (64 \times 0.3) + (3 \times 2.4) + (5 \times 3.5)$, or 54.5 days of care.

The results of a regression analysis are not expected to be sample specific. The final outcome of a regression analysis is a model from which values of the independent variables can be used to predict and perhaps explain values of the dependent variable in the population. If so, the analysis can be repeated in other samples with similar results. The equation is expected to have predictive validity. Knapp (1994) has listed the essential elements of a regression analysis that need to be included in a publication.

Lacara et al. (2007), all advanced practice nurses, performed a regression analysis to examine values obtained from blood for point-of-care analysis of glucose levels. Blood was often taken from different sources (e.g., fingerstick, arterial, or central venous catheter). Their objective was to examine the agreement between point-of-care and laboratory glucose values and to judge the accuracy of the point-of-care values. The researchers used a t-test to determine differences in values between each point-of-care source and the laboratory value. They used multiple regression analysis to determine if serum level of carbon dioxide, hematocrit, or mean arterial pressure significantly contributed to the difference in bias and precision for the point-of-care blood sources. They reported their results as follows.

> Mean laboratory glucose level was 135 (SEM 5.3, range 58-265) mg/dL. In point-of-care testing, bias ± precision and root-mean square differences were 2.1 ± 12.3 and 12.35, respectively, for fingerstick blood and 0.6 ± 10.6 and 10.46 for catheter blood. Values for point-of-care and laboratory tests did not differ significantly. (Lacara et al., 2007, p. 336)

Table 21-2 provides results of the multiple regression analysis. The authors also used Bland and Altman plots, described in Chapter 19, to depict the differences between the laboratory glucose value and the point-of-care glucose values (Figure 21-3).

Cross-Validation

To determine the accuracy of the prediction, the predicted values are compared with actual values obtained from a new sample of subjects or values from a sample obtained at the time of the original data collection but held out from the initial analysis. This analysis is conducted on the difference scores between predicted values and the means of actual values. Thus, in the new sample, the number of days of care for all patients 64 years of age, in income level 3, and in coping level 5 is averaged, and the mean is compared with 54.5 days of care. Each possible case within the new sample is compared in this manner. An R^2 is obtained on the new sample and compared with the R^2 of the original sample. In most cases, R^2 will be lower in the new sample, because the original equation was developed to most precisely predict scores in the original sample. This phenomenon is referred to as shrinkage of R^2. Shrinkage of R^2 is greater in small samples and when multicollinearity is great.

DISCRIMINANT ANALYSIS

Discriminant analysis allows the researcher to identify characteristics associated with group membership and to predict group membership. The dependent variable is membership in a particular group. The independent variables (discriminating variables) measure characteristics on which the groups are expected to differ. Discriminant analysis is closely related to both factor analysis and regression analysis. However, in discriminant analysis, the dependent variable values are categorical in form. Each value of the dependent variable is considered a group. When the dependent variable is dichotomous, the researcher performs multiple regression. However, when more than two groups are involved, analysis becomes much more complex. The dependent variable in discriminant analysis is referred to as the *discriminant function*. It is equivalent in many ways to a factor (Edens, 1987).

Two similar data sets are required for complete analysis. The first data set must contain measures on all the variables to be included in the analysis and the group membership of each subject. The purpose of analysis of the first data set is to identify variables that most effectively discriminate between groups. Selection of variables for the analysis is based on the researcher's expectation that they will be effective in this regard. The researcher then tests the variables selected for the discriminant function on a second set of data to determine their effectiveness in predicting group membership (Edens, 1987).

TABLE 21-2 ■ Multiple Regression Analysis of POC and Laboratory Glucose Difference Scores for Three Independent Variables

Independent Variable	Coefficient	SE	P	R^2	Adjusted R^2	Degrees of Freedom	F	P
Dependent Variable: Fingerstick POC Difference Scores for All Patients (n = 49)								
Serum carbon dioxide	−0.409	0.235	0.09					
Hematocrit	−0.523	0.310	0.10					
MAP	0.085	0.107	0.43					
				0.146	0.089	3.45	2.56	0.07
Dependent Variable: Arterial or CVP Catheter POC Difference Scores for All Patients (n = 49)								
Serum carbon dioxide	−0.532	0.175	0.004					
Hematocrit	−0.703	0.231	0.004					
MAP	0.023	0.080	0.77					
				0.353	0.310	3.45	8.17	<0.001
Dependent Variable: Fingerstick POC Difference Scores for Patients with Arterial Catheters (n = 42)								
Serum carbon dioxide	−0.546	0.263	0.04					
Hematocrit	−0.411	0.348	0.24					
MAP	0.099	0.117	0.40					
				0.161	0.095	3.38	2.44	0.08
Dependent Variable: Arterial Catheter POC Difference Scores for Patients with Arterial Catheters (n = 42)								
Serum carbon dioxide	−0.674	0.202	0.002					
Hematocrit	−0.665	0.266	0.02					
MAP	0.054	0.089	0.55					
				0.386	0.337	3.38	7.96	<0.001

CVP, central venous pressure; MAP, mean arterial pressure; POC, point of care.

From Lacara, T., Domagtoy, C., Lickliter, D., Quattrocchi, K. Snipes, L., Kuszaj, J., et al. (2007). Comparison of point-of-care and laboratory glucose analysis in critically ill patients. *American Journal of Critical Care, 16*(4), 341.

SUMMARY

- Predictive analyses are based on probability theory rather than decision theory. Prediction is one approach to examining causal relationships between or among variables.
- The independent (predictor) variable or variables cause variation in the value of the dependent (outcome) variable.
- The purpose of a regression analysis is to predict or explain as much of the variance in the value of the dependent variable as possible.
- Simple linear regression provides a means to estimate the value of a dependent variable based on the value of an independent variable.
- Multiple regression analysis is an extension of simple linear regression in which more than one independent variable is entered into the analysis.

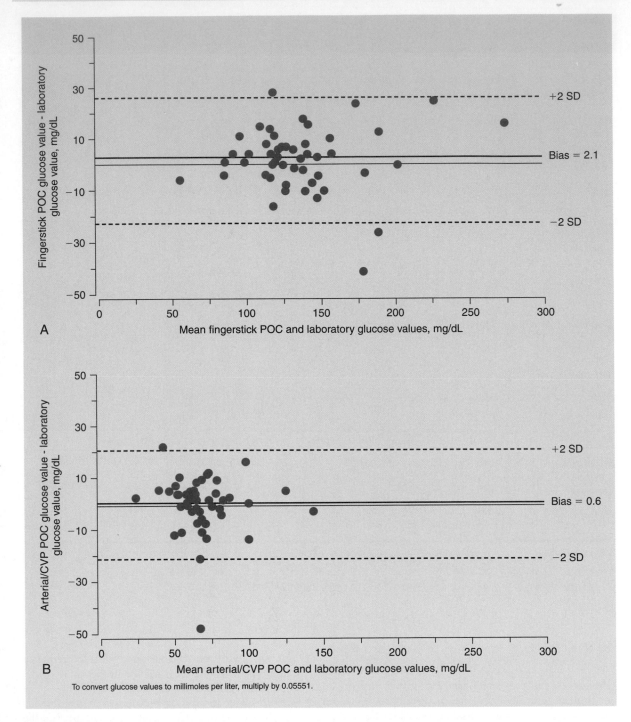

Figure **21-3** Bland and Altman plots depicting the differences between the laboratory glucose value and the point-of-care (POC) glucose values determined with blood from a fingerstick (A) or an arterial or a central venous pressure (CVP) catheter (B) for 49 patients.

- Multicollinearity occurs when the independent variables in a multiple regression equation are strongly correlated.
- The outcome of regression analysis is referred to as a prediction equation. The final outcome of a regression analysis is a model from which values of the independent variables can be used to predict and perhaps explain values of the dependent variable in the population.
- Discriminant analysis allows the researcher to identify characteristics associated with group membership and to predict group membership.

REFERENCES

Braden, C. J. (1990). A test of the self-help model: Learned response to chronic illness experience. *Nursing Research*, *39*(1), 42–47.

Burns, N., & Carney, K. (1986). Patterns of hospice care: The RN role. *Hospice Journal*, *2*(1), 37–62.

Cohen, J., & Cohen, P. (1983). *Applied multiple regression/correlation analysis for the behavioral sciences*. Hillsdale, NJ: Lawrence Erlbaum.

Edens, G. E. (1987). Discriminant analysis. *Nursing Research*, *36*(4), 257–262.

Gordon, R. (1968). Issues in multiple regression. *American Journal of Sociology*, *73*(5), 592–616.

Grove, S. K. (2007). *Statistics for health care research: A practical workbook*. Philadelphia: Saunders.

Knapp, T. R. (1994). Regression analyses: What to report. *Nursing Research*, *43*(3), 187–189.

Lacara, T., Domagtoy, C., Lickliter, D., Quattrocchi, K. Snipes, L., Kuszaj, J., et al. (2007). Comparison of point-of-care and laboratory glucose analysis in critically ill patients. *American Journal of Critical Care*, *16*(4), 336–346.

Pedhazur, E. J. (1997). *Multiple regression in behavioral research*. Philadelphia: Harcourt Brace.

Schroeder, M. A. (1990). Diagnosing and dealing with multicollinearity. *Western Journal of Nursing Research*, *12*(2), 175–187.

CHAPTER 22
Using Statistics to Examine Causality

Causality is a way of knowing that one thing causes another. Statistical procedures that examine causality are critical to the development of nursing science because of their importance in examining the effects of interventions. The statistical procedures in this chapter examine causality by testing for significant differences between or among groups. Statistical procedures are available for nominal, ordinal, and interval data. The procedures vary considerably in their power to detect differences and in their complexity. They are categorized as contingency tables, chi-squares, *t*-tests, and analysis of variance (ANOVA) procedures.

CONTINGENCY TABLES

Contingency tables, or cross-tabulation, allow the researcher to visually compare summary data output related to two variables within the sample. Contingency tables are a useful preliminary strategy for examining large amounts of data. In most cases, the data are in the form of frequencies or percentages. With this strategy, one can compare two or more categories of one variable with two or more categories of a second variable. The simplest version is referred to as a 2 × 2 table (two categories of two variables). Table 22-1 shows an example of a 2 × 2 contingency table from Knafl's (1985) study of how families manage a pediatric hospitalization.

The data are generally referenced in rows and columns. The intersection between the row and column in which a specific numerical value is inserted is referred to as a cell. The upper left cell would be row 1, column 1. In Table 22-1, the cell of row 1, column 1

has the value of 18, the cell of row 1, column 2 has the value of 7, and so on. The output from each row and each column is summed, and the sum is placed at the end of the row or column. In the example, the sum of row 1 is 25, the sum of row 2 is 37, the sum of column 1 is 34, and the sum of column 2 is 28. The percentage of the sample represented by that sum can also be placed at the end of the row or column. The row sums and the column sums total to the same value, which is 62 in the example.

Although researchers commonly use contingency tables to examine nominal or ordinal data, they can be used with grouped frequencies of interval data. However, information about the data will be lost when contingency tables are used to examine interval data. Loss of data usually causes loss of statistical power—that is, the probability of failing to reject a false null hypothesis is greater than if an appropriate parametric procedure could be used. Therefore, it is not generally the technique of choice. A contingency table is sometimes useful when an interval-level measure is being compared with a nominal- or ordinal-level measure.

In some cases, the contingency table is presented and no further analysis is conducted. The table is presented as a form of summary statistics. However, in many cases, a statistical analysis of the relationships or differences between the cell values is performed. The most familiar analysis of cross-tabulated data is use of the chi-square (χ^2) statistic. Chi-square is designed to test for significant differences between cells. Some statisticians prefer to examine chi-square from a probability framework and use it to detect possible relationships (Goodman & Kruskal, 1954, 1959, 1963, 1972).

TABLE 22-1	Relationship between Parents' Reports of Impact on Family Life and Outside Help		
	Parents' Reports		
Outside Help	**Neutral**	**Negative**	**Total**
No*	18	7	25
Yes†	16	21	37
Total	34	28	62

Modified from Knafl, K. A. (1985). How families manage a pediatric hospitalization. *Western Journal of Nursing Research*, 7(2), 163.

$p < 0.05$; $\chi^2 = 4.98$; $df = 1$.

* Includes cases from "Alone" category.

† Combines cases from "Some Help" and "Delegation" categories.

Computer programs are also available to analyze data from cross-tabulation tables (contingency tables). These programs can generate output from chi-square and many correlational techniques and indicate the level of significance for each technique. As the researcher, you should know which statistics are appropriate for your data and how to interpret the outcomes from these multiple analyses. The information presented on each of these tests will guide you in selecting a test and interpreting the findings.

Chi-Square Test of Independence

The chi-square test of independence tests whether the two variables being examined are independent or related. Chi-square is designed to test for differences in frequencies of observed data and compare them with the frequencies that could be expected to occur if the data categories were actually independent of each other. If differences are indicated, the analysis will not identify where these differences exist within the data.

Assumptions

One assumption of the test is that only one datum entry is made for each subject in the sample. Therefore, if repeated measures from the same subject are being used for analysis, such as pretests and posttests, chi-square is not an appropriate test. Another assumption is that for each variable, the categories are mutually exclusive and exhaustive. No cells may have an expected frequency of zero. However, in the actual data, the observed cell frequency may be zero. Until recently, each cell was expected to have a frequency of at least five, but this requirement has been mathematically demonstrated not to be necessary. However, no more than 20% of the cells should have fewer than

five (Conover, 1971). The test is distribution-free, or nonparametric, which means that no assumption has been made of a normal distribution of values in the population from which the sample was taken.

Calculation

The formula is relatively easy to calculate manually and can be used with small samples, which makes it a popular approach to data analysis. The first step in the calculation of chi-square is to categorize the data, record the observed values in a contingency table, and sum the rows and columns. Next, the expected frequencies are calculated for each cell. The expected frequencies are those frequencies that would occur if there were no group differences; these frequencies are calculated from the row and column sums by using the following formula:

$$E = \frac{(Tr)(Tc)}{N}$$

where
E = Expected cell frequency
Tr = Row total for that cell
Tc = Column total for that cell
N = Total number of subjects in the sample

Thus, to obtain the expected frequency for a particular cell, you would multiply the row total by the column total and divide by the sample size. When the expected frequencies have been calculated for all the cells, the sum should be equivalent to the total sample size. Calculations of the expected frequencies for the four cells in Table 22-1 follow; they total 62 (sample size):

Cell 1, 1
$$E = \frac{(25)(34)}{62} = 13.71$$

Cell 1, 2
$$E = \frac{(25)(28)}{62} = 11.29$$

Cell 2, 1
$$E = \frac{(37)(34)}{62} = 20.29$$

Cell 2, 2
$$E = \frac{(37)(28)}{62} = 16.71$$

By using this same example, a contingency table could be constructed of the observed and expected frequencies (Table 22-2). The following formula is then used to calculate the chi-square statistic:

$$\chi^2 = \Sigma \frac{(O-E)^2}{E}$$

TABLE 22-2	Contingency Table of Observed and Expected Frequencies	
	Parents' Reports	
Outside Help	**Neutral**	**Negative**
No	O = 18	O = 7
	E = 13.71	E = 11.29
Yes	O = 16	O = 21
	E = 20.29	E = 16.71

E, expected frequencies; O, observed frequencies.

where
  O = Observed frequency
  E = Expected frequency
Note that the formula includes difference scores between the observed frequency for each cell and the expected frequency for that cell. These difference scores are squared, divided by the expected frequency, and summed for each cell. The chi-square value was calculated by using the observed and expected frequencies in Table 22-2.

$$\chi^2 = \frac{(18-13.71)^2}{13.71} + \frac{(7-11.29)^2}{11.29}$$
$$+ \frac{(16+20.29)^2}{20.29} + \frac{(21-16.71)^2}{16.71} = 4.98$$
$$df = 1; \; p < 0.05$$

With any chi-square analysis, the **degrees of freedom** (df) must be calculated to determine the significance of the value of the statistic. The following formula is used for this calculation:

$$df = (R-1)(C-1)$$

where
  R = Number of rows
  C = Number of columns
In the example presented previously, the chi-square value was 4.98, and df was 1, which was calculated as follows:

$$df = (2-1)(2-1) = 1$$

Interpretation of Results
The chi-square statistic is compared with the chi-square values in the table in Appendix C. The table includes the critical values of chi-square for specific degrees of freedom at selected levels of significance

(usually 0.05 or 0.01). A **critical value** is the value of the statistic that must be obtained to indicate that a difference exists in the two populations represented by the groups under study. If the value of the statistic is equal to or greater than the value identified in the chi-square table, the difference between the two variables is significant. If the statistic remains significant at more extreme probability levels, you will report the largest p value at which significance is achieved. The analysis indicates that there are group differences in the categories of the variable and that those differences are related to changes in the other variable. Although a significant chi-square value indicates difference, the analysis does not reveal the magnitude of the difference. If the statistic is not significant, we cannot conclude that there is a difference in the distribution of the two variables, and they are considered independent (Salkind, 2007).

How one interprets the results depends on the design of the study. If the design is experimental, causality can be considered and the results can be inferred to the associated population. If the design is descriptive, differences identified are associated only with the sample under study. In either case, the differences found are related to differences among all the categories of the first variable and all the categories of the second variable. The specific differences among variables and categories of variables cannot be identified with this analysis. Often, in reported research, the researcher will visually examine the data and discuss differences in the categories of data as though they had been demonstrated to be statistically significantly different. The reader must view these reports with caution. Partitioning, the contingency coefficient C, the phi coefficient, or Cramer's V can be used to examine the data statistically to determine in exactly which categories the differences lie. The last three strategies can also shed some light on the magnitude of the relationship between the variables. These strategies are discussed later in this chapter.

In reporting the results, contingency tables are generally presented only for significant chi-square analyses. The value of the statistic is given, including the df and p values. Data in the contingency table are sufficient to allow other researchers to repeat the chi-square analyses and thus check the accuracy of the analyses.

The chi-square test of independence can be used with two or more groups. In this case, group membership is used as the independent variable. The chi-square statistic is calculated with the same formula as above. If more than two categories of the dependent variable are present, the analysis tests differences in both central tendency and dispersion.

Partitioning of Chi-Square

Partitioning involves breaking up the contingency table into several 2 × 2 tables and conducting chi-square analyses on each table separately. Partitioning can be performed on any contingency table greater than 2 × 2 with more than one degree of freedom. The number of partitions that can be conducted is equivalent to the degrees of freedom. The sum of the chi-square values obtained by partitioning is equal to the original chi-square value. Certain rules must be followed during partitioning to prevent inflating the value of chi-square. The initial partition can include any four cells as long as two values from each variable are used. The next 2 × 2 must compress the first four cells into two cells and include two new cells. This process can continue until no new cells are available. By using this process, it is possible to determine which cells have contributed to the significant differences found.

Phi

The **phi coefficient** (φ) describes relationships in dichotomous, nominal data. It is also used with the chi-square test to determine the location of a difference or differences among cells. Phi is used only with 2 × 2 tables (Table 22-3).

Calculation

If chi-square has been calculated, the following formula can be used to calculate phi. The data presented in Table 22-1 were used to calculate this phi coefficient. The chi-square analysis indicated a significant difference, and the phi coefficient indicated the magnitude of effect:

$$phi = \sqrt{\frac{\chi^2}{N}} \quad phi(\phi) = \sqrt{\frac{4.98}{62}} = \sqrt{0.0803} = 0.238$$

where N is the total frequency of all cells.

TABLE 22-3	Framework for Developing a 2 × 2 Contingency Table		
	Variable X		
Variable Y	**0**	**1**	**Totals**
0	A	B	A + B
1	C	D	C + D
Totals	A + C	B + D	N

Alternatively, phi can be calculated directly from the 2 × 2 table by using the following formula (Salkind, 2007). Again, the data from Table 22-1 are used to calculate the phi coefficient:

$$phi = \frac{AD - BC}{\sqrt{(A+C)(B+D)(A+B)(C+D)}}$$
$$= \frac{(18)(21) - (7)(16)}{\sqrt{(34)(28)(25)(37)}} = 0.283$$

Interpretation of Results

The phi coefficient is similar to Pearson's product moment correlation coefficient (r), except that two dichotomous variables are involved. Phi values range from −1 to +1, with the magnitude of the relationship decreasing as the coefficient nears zero. The results show the strength of the relationship between the two variables.

Cramer's V

Cramer's V is a modification of phi used for contingency tables larger than 2 × 2. It is designed for use with nominal data. The value of the statistic ranges from 0 to 1.

Calculation

The formula can be calculated from the chi-square statistic, and the data presented in Table 22-1 were used to calculate Cramer's V:

$$V = \sqrt{\frac{\chi^2}{N(L-1)}} \quad V = \sqrt{\frac{4.98}{62(7-1)}}$$
$$= \sqrt{0.01334} = 0.115$$

where

L = Smaller of the number of either columns or rows
N = Total frequency of all cells

Contingency Coefficient

The **contingency coefficient (C)** is used with two nominal variables and is the most commonly used of the three chi-square–based measures of association.

Calculation

The contingency coefficient can be calculated with the following formula, which uses the data presented in Table 22-1:

$$C = \sqrt{\frac{\chi^2}{\chi^2 + N}} \qquad C = \sqrt{\frac{4.98}{4.98 + 62}}$$

$$= \sqrt{0.07435} = 0.273$$

The relationship demonstrated by C cannot be interpreted on the same scale as Pearson's r, phi, or Cramer's V because it does not reach an upper limit of 1. The formula does not consider the number of cells, and the upper limit varies with the size of the contingency table. With a 2×2 table, the upper limit is 0.71; with a 3×3 table, the upper limit is 0.82; and with a 4×4 table, the upper limit is 0.87. Contingency coefficients from separate analyses can be compared only if the table sizes are the same.

Lambda

Lambda measures the degree of association (or relationship) between two nominal-level variables. The value of lambda can range from 0 to 1. Two approaches to analysis are possible: asymmetrical and symmetrical. The asymmetrical approach indicates the capacity to predict the value of the dependent variable given the value of the independent variable. Thus, when you use the asymmetrical lambda, it is necessary to specify a dependent and an independent variable. Symmetrical lambda measures the degree of overlap (or association) between the two variables and makes no assumptions regarding which variable is dependent and which is independent (Waltz & Bausell, 1981).

t-TESTS
t-Test for Independent Samples

One of the most common parametric analyses used to test for significant differences between statistical measures of two samples is the *t*-test. The *t*-test uses the standard deviation of the sample to estimate the standard error of the sampling distribution. The ease in calculating line formula is attractive to researchers who wish to conduct their analyses by hand. This test is particularly useful when only small samples are available for analysis. The *t*-test being discussed here is for independent samples.

The *t*-test is frequently misused by researchers who use multiple *t*-tests to examine differences in various aspects of data collected in a study. This practice escalates significance and greatly increases the risk of a type I error. The *t*-test can be used only one time during analysis to examine data from the

two samples in a study. You can use the Bonferroni procedure, which controls for the escalation of significance, if you must perform various *t*-tests on different aspects of the same data. You can easily complete a Bonferroni adjustment by hand; simply divide the overall significance level by the number of tests, and use the resulting number as the significance level for each test. ANOVA is always a viable alternative to the pooled *t*-test and is preferred by many researchers who have become wary of the *t*-test because of its frequent misuse. Mathematically, the two approaches are the same when only two samples are being examined.

Use of the *t*-test involves the following assumptions:
1. Sample means from the population are normally distributed.
2. The dependent variable is measured at the interval level.
3. The two samples have equal variance.
4. All observations within each sample are independent.

The *t*-test is robust to moderate violation of its assumptions. Robustness means that the results of analysis can still be relied on to be accurate when one of the assumptions has been violated. The *t*-test is not robust with respect to the between-samples or within-samples independence assumptions, nor is it robust with respect to an extreme violation of the normality assumption unless the sample sizes are extremely large. Sample groups do not have to be equal for this analysis—the concern is, instead, for equal variance. A variety of *t*-tests have been developed for various types of samples. Independent samples means that the two sets of data were not taken from the same subjects and that the scores in the two groups are *not* related.

Calculation

The t statistic is relatively easy to calculate. The numerator is the difference scores of the means of the two samples. The test uses the pooled standard deviation of the two samples as the denominator, which gives the formula a rather forbidding appearance:

$$t = \frac{\bar{X}_a - \bar{X}_b}{\sqrt{\frac{\Sigma X_a^2 - \frac{(\Sigma X_a)^2}{n_a} + \Sigma X_b^2 - \frac{(\Sigma X_b)^2}{n_b}}{(n_a + n_b - 2)} \left(\frac{1}{n_a} + \frac{1}{n_b}\right)}}$$

$\bar{X}_a$ = Mean of sample 1

$\bar{X}_b$ = Mean of sample 2

n_a = Number of subjects in sample 1

n_b = Number of subjects in sample 2

ΣX_a^2 = Sum of group a squared deviation scores

ΣX_b^2 = Sum of group b squared deviation scores

$$df = n_a + n_b - 2$$

In the following example, the t-test was used to examine the difference between a control group and an experimental group. The independent variable administered to the experimental group was a form of relaxation therapy. The dependent variable was pulse rate. Pulse rates for the experimental and control groups are presented in Table 22-4, along with calculations for the t-test.

$$t = \frac{77 - 70}{\sqrt{\dfrac{71{,}376 - \dfrac{(924)^2}{12} + 58{,}944 - \dfrac{(840)^2}{12}}{(12 + 12 - 2)}\left(\dfrac{1}{12} + \dfrac{1}{12}\right)}}$$

$$= \frac{7}{\sqrt{\dfrac{(71{,}376 - 71{,}148 + 58{,}944 - 58{,}800)(0.1667)}{22}}}$$

$$= \frac{7}{1.679} = 4.169$$

$$df = 12 + 12 - 2 = 22$$

Interpretation of Results

To determine the significance of the t statistic, the researcher must calculate the degrees of freedom. The value of the t statistic is then found in the table for the sampling distribution. If the sample size is 30 or fewer, you can use the t distribution; a table of this distribution can be found in Appendix A. For larger sample sizes, you can use the normal distribution; a table of this distribution is presented in Appendix 2 (available on the Evolve website at http://evolve. elsevier.com/Burns/Practice/). The level of significance and the degrees of freedom are used to identify the critical value of t. This value is then used to obtain the most exact p value possible. The p value is then compared with the significance level. In the example presented in Table 22-4, the calculated $t = 4.169$ and $df = 22$. This t value was significant at the 0.001 level.

Andrus and Clark (2007) conducted a study to determine the effectiveness of having a pharmacist and nurse practitioner run a rural health center. They used a t-test for the following purpose (Table 22-5).

Purpose: Clinical pharmacy interventions and services provided in collaboration with a nurse practitioner in a medically underserved rural health center are described. *Methods:* Data were collected via retrospective chart review of clinical pharmacy notes for all patients referred to the clinical pharmacist from July 2001 through

---

TABLE 22-4 Data and Computations for the t-Test

Pulse Rate (Control Group)

X_a	Frequency (f)	fX_a	X_a^2	fX_a^2
70	1	70	4,900	4,900
72	2	144	5,184	10,368
76	5	380	5,776	28,880
82	3	246	6,724	20,172
84	1	84	7,056	7,056
$n_a = 12$	$\bar{X}_a = 0.77$	$\Sigma X_a = 924$		$\Sigma X_a^2 = 71{,}376$

Pulse Rate (Experimental Group)

X_b	Frequency (f)	fX_b	X_b^2	fX_b^2
64	1	64	4,096	4,096
66	2	132	4,356	8,712
70	5	350	4,900	24,500
72	3	216	5,184	15,552
78	1	78	6,084	6,084
$n_b = 12$	$\bar{X}_b = 70$	$\Sigma X_b = 840$		$\Sigma X_b^2 = 58{,}944$

February 2004. Data collected included demographic information, reasons for referral, duration of follow-up, insurance status, use of medication assistance programs, educational interventions, clinical interventions, and clinical outcomes. Changes in mean low-density-lipoprotein (LDL) cholesterol levels, blood pressures, and glycosylated hemoglobin (HbA[1c]) were analyzed using a paired Student's t test. Smoking cessation, the number of times the international normalized ratio (INR) was in a goal range, and attainment of goal LDL cholesterol, blood pressure, and HbA(1c) levels were also recorded.

Results: Clinical pharmacy interventions were summarized for 101 patients who were seen in 708 patient visits. A mean of 5.6 educational interventions were provided per visit, and a mean of 1.0 clinical intervention occurred per visit. Initiation of new drug therapy or dosage adjustment accounted for 52% of the clinical interventions. A large percentage of patients attained their goals for LDL cholesterol (76%), blood pressure (86%), HbA(1c) (69%), INR (82%), and smoking cessation (43%) during the study period. *Conclusion*: Pharmacotherapy services provided by a clinical pharmacist at a rural nurse practitioner clinic positively affected clinical outcomes and increased patients' attainment rates for LDL cholesterol, systolic and diastolic blood pressures, and HbA(1c). (Andrus & Clark, 2007, p. 294)

t-Tests for Related Samples

When samples are related, the formula used to calculate the *t* statistic is different from the formula just described. Samples may be related because matching has been performed as part of the design or because the scores used in the analysis were obtained from the same subjects under different conditions (e.g., pretest and posttest). This test requires that differences between the paired scores be independent and normally or approximately normally distributed.

Calculation

The following formula assumes that scores in the two samples are in some way correlated (dependent):

$$t = \frac{d}{\sqrt{\dfrac{\Sigma d^2}{n(n-1)}}}$$

where

$\bar{d}$ = Mean difference between the paired scores
Σd^2 = Sum of squared deviation difference scores
n = Number of paired scores
df = $n - 1$

TABLE 22-5	Comparison of Empowerment Scores between Collaborative Governance (Cg) Members and Nonmembers at 1 Year					
Year 1 Variable		Member	N	Mean*	t	P
Opportunity		CG	131	3.46	4.46	0.000‡
		Non-CG	156	3.08		
Information		CG	130	3.15	6.00	0.000‡
		Non-CG	155	2.60		
Support		CG	134	2.99	2.51	0.013†
		Non-CG	158	2.76		
Resources		CG	127	2.70	4.43	0.000‡
		Non-CG	157	2.38		
Job Activity Scale (JAS)		CG	132	2.95	6.91	0.000‡
		Non-CG	156	2.53		
Organizational Relationships Scale (ORS)		CG	133	3.54	4.57	0.000‡
		Non-CG	155	3.19		
Two-Item Empowerment Score		CG	133	3.24	2.03	0.044†
		Non-CG	158	3.00		

From Erickson, J. I., Hamilton, G. A., Jones, D. E., & Ditomassi, M. (2003). The value of collaborative governance/staff empowerment. *Journal of Nursing Administration, 33*(2), 96–104. Full text available in Nursing Collection 2.

CG, Collaborative governance.

* Scale: 1 = low, 5 = high.

† Significant p ≤ 0.05.

‡ Significant p ≤ 0.01.

Interpretation of Results

Results of the analysis are interpreted in the same way as those of the independent *t*-test described previously.

One-Way Analysis of Variance

Although one-way ANOVA is a bivariate analysis, it is more flexible than other analyses in that it can examine data from two or more groups. To accomplish this analysis, the researcher uses group membership as one of the two variables under examination and a dependent variable as the second variable.

ANOVA compares the variance within each group with the variance between groups. The outcome of the analysis is a numerical value for the *F* statistic, which will be used to determine whether the groups are significantly different. The variance within each group is a result of individual scores in the group varying from the group mean and is referred to as the within-group variance. This variance is calculated in the same way as that described in Chapter 19. ANOVA assumes the amount of variation about the mean in each group to be equal. The group means also vary around the grand mean (the mean of the total sample), which is referred to as the between-groups variance. One could assume that if all the samples were drawn from the same population, there would be little difference in these two sources of variance. The variance from within and between the groups explains the total variance in the data. When these two types of variance are combined, they are referred to as the total variance.

Interpretation of Results

The test for ANOVA is always one-tailed. The critical region is in the upper tail of the test. The *F* distribution for determining the level of significance of the *F* statistic can be found in Appendix B. If you are examining only two groups, the location of a significant difference is clear. However, if you are studying more than two groups, it is not possible to determine from the ANOVA exactly where the significant differences lie. One cannot assume that all the groups examined are significantly different. Therefore, post hoc analyses are conducted to determine the location of the differences among groups.

Post Hoc Analyses. One might wonder why a researcher would conduct a test that failed to provide the answer he or she is seeking—namely, where the significant differences were in a data set. It would seem more logical to perform *t*-tests or ANOVAs on the groups in the data set in pairs, thus clearly determining whether a significant difference exists between those two groups. However, when these tests are performed with three groups in the data set, the risk of a type I error increases from 5% to 14%. As the number of groups increases (and with the increase in groups, an increase in the number of comparisons necessary), the risk of a type I error increases strikingly. This type I error, which increases because of escalation of the level of significance, does not occur when one ANOVA is performed that includes all of the groups.

Post hoc tests have been developed specifically to determine the location of differences after ANOVA is performed on analysis of data from more than two groups. These tests were developed to reduce the incidence of a type I error. Frequently used post hoc tests are the Bonferroni procedure, the Newman-Keuls test, the Tukey Honestly Significant Difference (HSD) test, the Scheffe test, and the Dunnett test. When these tests are calculated, the alpha level is reduced in proportion to the number of additional tests required to locate statistically significant differences. As the alpha level decreases, reaching the level of significance becomes increasingly more difficult.

Robbins et al. (2006) conducted an ANOVA in a study examining the effectiveness of a program designed by a pediatric nurse practitioner to reverse the sedentary lifestyle of adolescent girls. The results were reported as follows.

Background: Because physical inactivity poses serious health risks, interventions are urgently needed to reverse the increasingly sedentary lifestyles of adolescent girls.

Objective: The aim of this study was to determine the feasibility of "Girls on the Move," an individually tailored computerized physical activity (PA) program plus nurse counseling intervention, in increasing PA.

Methods: A pretest-posttest control group design was used with 77 racially diverse sedentary girls in Grades 6, 7, and 8 from two middle schools. Each of the instructional grades was randomly assigned to either an intervention or control condition. After completing computerized questionnaires, each girl in the control group received a handout listing the PA recommendations. To encourage PA, each girl in the intervention group received computerized, individually tailored feedback messages based on her responses to the questionnaires, individual counseling from the school's pediatric nurse practitioner (PNP), and telephone calls and mailings from a trained research assistant. At 12 weeks, girls in both groups responded to the questionnaires.

Results: No differences in self-reported PA emerged between the intervention and control groups at Weeks 1 (baseline) and 12 (postintervention). Repeated measures ANOVA showed a significant interaction between group and time for social support for PA, $F(1, 69) = 5.73$, $p = 0.019$, indicating that the intervention group had significantly greater social support across time than did the control group. From baseline to postintervention, social support increased for the intervention group but decreased for the control group.

Discussion: Reasons for the lack of significant differences between the groups on the PA measures were cited. Important information that could inform subsequent studies that test interventions to increase youth PA was acquired from conducting this study. Future efforts to increase PA participation might include this approach for enhancing social support for PA. (Robbins et al., 2006, p. 206)

SUMMARY

- Causality is a way of knowing that one thing causes another.
- Contingency tables (or cross-tabulation) allow the researcher to visually compare summary data output related to two variables within the sample.
- The *t*-test is one of the most commonly used parametric analyses to test for significant differences between statistical measures of two samples.
- ANOVA procedures test for differences between means.
- ANOVA can be used to examine data from more than two groups and compares the variance within each group with the variance between groups.

REFERENCES

Andrus, M. R., & Clark, D. B. (2007). Provision of pharmacotherapy services in a rural nurse practitioner clinic. *American Journal of Health-System Pharmacy, 64*(3), 294–297.

Conover, W. J. (1971). *Practical nonparametric statistics.* New York: Wiley.

Erickson, J. I., Hamilton, G. A., Jones, D. E., & Ditomassi, M. (2003). The value of collaborative governance/staff empowerment. *Journal of Nursing Administration, 33*(2), 96–104.

Goodman, L. A., & Kruskal, W. H. (1954). Measures of association for cross classifications. *Journal of the American Statistical Association, 49,* 732–764.

Goodman, L. A., & Kruskal, W. H. (1959). Measures of association for cross classifications, II: Further discussion and references. *Journal of the American Statistical Association, 54*(285), 123–163.

Goodman, L. A., & Kruskal, W. H. (1963). Measures of association for cross classifications, III: Approximate sampling theory. *Journal of the American Statistical Association, 58*(302), 310–364.

Goodman, L. A., & Kruskal, W. H. (1972). Measures of association for cross classifications, IV: Simplification of asymptotic variances. *Journal of the American Statistical Association, 67*(338), 415–421.

Knafl, K. A. (1985). How families manage a pediatric hospitalization. *Western Journal of Nursing Research, 7*(2), 151–176.

Robbins, L. B., Gretebeck, K. A., Kazanis, A. S., & Pender, N. (2006). Girls on the move program to increase physical activity participation. *Nursing Research, 55*(3), 206–216.

Salkind, N. J. (2007). *Statistics for people who (think they) hate statistics.* Thousand Oaks, CA: Sage.

Volicer, B. J. (1984). *Multivariate statistics for nursing research.* New York: Grune & Stratton.

Waltz, C., & Bausell, R. B. (1981). *Nursing research: Design, statistics and computer analysis.* Philadelphia: F.A. Davis.

CHAPTER **23**

Qualitative Research Methodology

The methodology of qualitative studies is guided by the broad qualitative research paradigm, as well as by a specific philosophical base (see Chapter 4). Strategies for methods of sampling, data gathering, and analyses are not as tightly controlled as those of the quantitative paradigm. Because data analysis begins as data are gathered, insights from early data may suggest fruitful methods of sampling, data gathering, or analyses that were not originally planned. In qualitative studies, the researcher is free to modify the original methodology based on these insights.

This chapter allows you to understand the process and to envision what the experience will be like if you conduct a qualitative study. However, we suggest that you seek additional sources of guidance for understanding the philosophical base you plan to use, as well as the process of collecting and analyzing qualitative data. Developing a mentorship with someone experienced in the type of qualitative analysis you wish to perform is still the most useful approach to learning these skills (Morse, 1997; Sandelowski, 1997).

The steps of the qualitative research process are similar to those used in quantitative research, which include reviewing the literature, developing a framework, developing objectives or questions, and sampling. These aspects of qualitative studies are explored in the chapters that focus on each of these topics. However, researchers conducting a qualitative study use some methods of data collection and analysis that are unique to qualitative research and will be discussed in this chapter. Other methods, similar to quantitative methods, are applied differently in qualitative studies. Because data analysis occurs concurrently with data collection, the researcher is attempting to simultaneously gather the data, manage a growing bulk of collected data, and interpret the meaning of the data. Qualitative analysis techniques use words rather than numbers as the basis of analysis. However, qualitative researchers need the same careful skills in analytical reasoning as those needed for quantitative analysis. In qualitative analysis, reasoning flows from concreteness to increasing abstraction. This reasoning process guides the organization, reduction, and clustering of the findings and leads to theoretical explanations. Even though the researcher may change data collection or analysis strategies during the study, the process is not as spontaneous and impulsive as one might think. The procedures must be carefully planned.

This chapter begins with a description of some of the frequently used approaches for collecting and analyzing qualitative data. Next, research methodologies and designs of specific approaches are presented. These include phenomenology, grounded theory, ethnographical methodology, historical research methodology, philosophical studies, and critical social theory methodology. The chapter ends with a discussion of issues that are important to qualitative research: theoretical frameworks for qualitative studies, researcher-participant relationships, participatory research, reflexivity, auditability, and appraisal of qualitative studies.

DATA COLLECTION METHODS

Because data collection occurs simultaneously with data analysis in qualitative studies, the process is complex. Collecting data is not a mechanical process that can be completely planned before it is initiated.

The researcher as a whole person is totally involved—perceiving, reacting, interacting, reflecting, attaching meaning, and recording. Such is the case whether the study involves observing and participating in social situations, as would occur in phenomenological, grounded theory, ethnographical, or critical social theory research, or whether the study deals with written communications, as might occur in phenomenological, historical, philosophical, or critical social theory studies. For a particular study, the researcher may need to address data collection issues related to relationships between the researcher and the participants, reflections of the researcher on the meanings obtained from the data, and management and reduction of large volumes of data. Methods of gathering data include making unstructured observations, conducting unstructured interviews, observing focus groups, collecting stories, constructing life stories, and interpreting case studies.

Unstructured Observations

Unstructured observation involves spontaneously observing and recording what one sees with a minimum of planning. Although unstructured observations give the observer freedom, there is a risk that the observer may lose objectivity or may not remember all of the details of the event. If possible, the researcher should take notes during the observation periods. If this is not possible, the researcher needs to record the observations soon afterward. You may even find it useful to photograph or videotape the observation period so that you can examine it extensively at a later time (Harrison, 2002; Mullhall, 2002).

Unstructured observations are not unsystematic or sloppy as the term might suggest. Rather, unstructured means that the researcher has few predetermined notions as to what he or she might observe. What notions the researcher does have may change over time as data are collected. As Mulhall (2003) pointed out:

The way people move, dress, interact and use space is very much a part of how particular social settings are constructed. Observation is the key method for collecting data about such matter.... Observers have a great degree of freedom and autonomy regarding what they choose to observe, how they filter that information, and how it is analysed.... Observation also captures the whole social setting in which people function, by recording the context in which they work.... Finally, observation is valuable because it informs about the influence of the physical environment. This aspect of observation is quite

lacking in nursing research. Observations are made of people's behaviour, but data about the physical environment seldom are collected. (pp. 307, 308)

Hamilton and Manias (2007) studied the observational methods of psychiatric nurses and their invisibility in an acute inpatient setting. This excellent study not only gives you as reader a clear understanding of the careful observation conducted during this study, but it also enables you to understand how detailed observation must be in a qualitative study and gives you a chance to think about how you might conduct your own observations. Hamilton and Manias (2007) described their study as follows.

The postmodern approach used in the study was informed by Foucault (1973, 1980, 1995, 1994) and by researchers after him (Fox, 1993; Rhodes, 1991; Silverman, 2005). A postmodern epistemology informed both the positioning of the first author during fieldwork and the emphasis on discourses, power relations and particular concepts in data analysis. A postmodern epistemology informed both the positioning of the first author during fieldwork and the emphasis on discourses, power relations and particular concepts in data analysis. In postmodern ethnography, the ethnographers' power in the portrayal of the field is made explicitly (Alvesson, 2002). Accordingly the first author, an experienced psychiatric nurse, was cast as an objective observer, but as an active participant, recognizing and exposing her own subjectivity in shaping the research. (p. 334)

The study was based in a 44-bed acute psychiatric inpatient unit, on the site of metropolitan acute teaching hospital in Victoria, Australia. Ethics approval was gained from the hospital, in accordance with national guidelines in Australia.

Ethnography has been widely used to study workplaces as subcultures (Silverman, 2005). This study centered on the work of 11 participating psychiatric nurses and the first author, who worked part time as a psychiatric nurse alongside the participants for 18 months. Fieldwork data were generated through: participant observations (180h; 13 individual interviews and two focus groups with the participating psychiatric nurses; transcriptions of their file notes and other documents related to assessment; and the first author's journal that detailed 170h of her work as a registered nurse in the unit. (p. 334)

The ethnography focused on nurses' activities and on nurse-nurse and nurse-patient interactions. The psychiatric nursing experience of the 11 nurses recruited ranged from 2 to 30 years and ages ranged from 28 to 67 years. Six nurses were women, a gender ratio in keeping with the current psychiatric nursing workforce in Australia (Clinton, 2001), which includes a much higher proportion of men than in other specialties of nursing. Nurse participants were positioned as key informants who provided insight into the social life of the unit (Riley & Manias, 2006). Participant observations extended across participants' rostered working shifts, through all days of the week and all three shifts (morning, afternoon and night), in order to attend to a variety of contexts, routines, experiences and practices. (p. 334)

■ *PROCESS OF ANALYSIS*

Central to our analysis of how inpatient psychiatric nurses observed patients were the Foucauldian concepts of the gaze and of discipline, both given form in nurses' discursive practices (Roberts, 2005). Analysis was focused on discursive practices of assessment, understood to be the micro-politics of nurses' language and action (Fox, 1993, p. 161). Everyday nursing practices identified in the fieldwork texts were highlighted as discursive practices when we could show how these practices were imbued with power through social, historical and political conditions, and in the wider context of psychiatric discourse (Irving, 2002). (pp. 334–335)

■ *RESULTS*

We present three identified modes of nurses' observations: nurses' scanning of patients, nurses' obvious and direct probing of patients, and nurses' discreet and hidden observations of patients.

The Nursing Scan

The term *scan* is used here to encompass nurses' frequent sweeping of eyes across rooms, surfaces and spaces of the unit, taking in features and contents of the space as well as impressions of the people occupying it. Nurses relied on their sight, supplemented by other senses to inform the scan. Through scanning, nurses monitored the physical spaces and their objects, commenting on noise, smells and temperature, and noticing and moving hazards. Nurses also scanned for emotional tone in the unit: for potential areas of distress and conflict that might encompass patients, staff and visitors. The nurses' scan took in the demeanour and behaviour of individual patients and groups of patients. Nurses scanned in passing patients' bodies, expressions, movements, gestures and tones of voice...

...nurses' visual observations were supplemented by their tuning into sounds of movement, or 'listening in' to patients talk. Whether in the office or circulating in the unit, nurses were alert to voices and other sounds in the ward environment. Three nurses might all glance or move toward a doorway, in response to a sound such as a heavy footfall, even as they were engaged in other work. Nurses gleaned valuable information about patients through this form of aural surveillance (Riley, 2005), a partner to their visual surveillance. Nurses embraced their scanning role, to the extent that they permitted sounds and conversations

to frequently interrupt their own planned work. They were often drawn away from planned work *to go and see* the event or person at the source of an interruption.

Nurses scanned the unit on arrival, when entering a different area of the unit, or when returning after an absence, such as a tea break. Their scan was brief, capturing the physical and social condition of the unit at that moment. From such activity, details were reported to colleagues, in snatches of conversation and handovers. Nurses exercised the scan both as a baseline form of monitoring and as a prelude to more focused work with individuals and groups of patients, assisting them to determine work priorities and issues for the working shift. (p. 336)

Nurses' Probing Observations of Patients

Nurses focused on patients who were assigned to their care. As they scanned the ward space and occupants, their attention was drawn also to patients who were assigned to other nurses. The probing observation of a patient was a distinctive activity in that nurses stopped circulating, and looked in a more considered way at a patient's body, social interactions and behaviour. From this probing, nurses gleaned clues about the patient's feelings, thoughts and motivations, the patient's ways of interacting, the patient's coping abilities or strengths, as well as evidence of symptoms. On occasions, nurses withdrew after a period of sharp observation, without interrupting the patient's activity or speaking at all... (p. 337)

Through observations, nurses elicited evidence of symptoms and also *absence* of symptoms. Nurses identified evidence of the person 'getting along' in the social sense with other patients, of the person coping with the demands of an activity and even exhibiting prowess in the activity. Nurses' counterbalancing of psychiatric symptoms with a lack of such symptoms, coping and prowess, in the context of unstructured activity, was an element of nurses' assessment. Nurses' accounts of symptoms, based in the behaviour they observed in the unit, were potentially important accounts in the ongoing construction of illness by the treating team. (p. 337)

Nurses' Discreet Observation: Clinical and Civil Surveillance

Nurses' observations of patients in the acute psychiatry unit were shaped substantially by the legal status and admission circumstances of patients, most of whom were detained and treated under the Mental Health Act (1986). The loss of fundamental rights to freedom and choice in psychiatric treatment could cause great offence to patients, many of whom flatly disagreed with the medical diagnosis and bitterly resented being detained and given psychotropic medications.

The ward environment was a place where direct contact with clinicians frequently provoked patients' ire. Since nurses were the group of clinicians in most frequent and close contact with patients, they were attuned to and dealt with patients' rising emotions by avoiding direct discussion about the terms and legitimacy of their hospital admission, including discussion of symptoms, in marked contrast to the probing of psychiatrists or psychologists. Evasion and distraction were common strategies used by nurses, in the moment-to-moment and daily work of maintaining civility and relative calm among inhabitants of the unit, in the face of such a perennial conflict of views.

In the process of examining a patient and with the main aim of not angering the patient, nurses often avoided looking directly at a patient, instead glancing briefly or discreetly…. A feature of surveillance was the nurses' ability to tune in to patient conversations at some distance, or whilst engaged in another conversation themselves. Being the third party to patient's talk gave nurses material from which to construct two valued forms of knowledge: *patients' speech related to mental status* and *patients' coping ability in social situations*. (p. 338)

The authors concluded the following:

Based on an ethnographic study of the assessment practices of 11 psychiatric nurses and the first author in an Australian hospital setting, we found that nurses' observations of patients were rich in situated assessment detail and a powerful strategy for producing civil conduct among patients. While such discreet practice is productive for everyday clinical work, the invisibility of nursing observations undermines the status of acute inpatient psychiatric nurses. Devaluing of tacit practice may encourage experienced nurses to leave inpatient units, at a time when hospitals struggle to address nursing shortages worldwide. We recommend instead that the productive value of diverse and situated practices be investigated and articulated. (p. 331)

Unstructured Interviews

Unstructured interviews are used primarily in descriptive quantitative and qualitative studies. According to market research, in-depth interviews provide more quality data for less money than do focus groups (Palmerino, 1999). However, the interviewer seeks information from a number of individuals, whereas the focus group strategy is designed to obtain the perspective of the normative group, not individual perspectives.

Learning to Interview

Interviewing is a skill. Researchers must give themselves the opportunity to develop this skill before they initiate an interview for a study. A skilled interviewer can elicit higher-quality data than an inexperienced

interviewer. Unskilled interviewers may not know how or when to intervene, when to encourage the participant to continue to elaborate, or when to divert to another subject. The interviewer must know how to handle intrusive questions.

Establishing a Positive Environment for an Interview

When preparing for an interview, establish an environment that encourages a comfortable conversation. If you are going to audio- or videotape the exchange, make sure that the recording equipment is placed unobtrusively. Likewise, using batteries rather than plug-in sources of power tends to be less intrusive. A sensitive microphone will allow you to pick up even faint or distorted voices, thereby increasing your ability to make an accurate transcription later.

Conducting an Effective Interview

For practice, conduct interviews with individuals who meet the sampling criteria. These rehearsals will help you to identify problems before initiating the study. Practice sessions also allow you to determine a realistic time estimate for the interviews.

There are power issues in an interview. As the researcher, you have the power to shape the interview agenda. Participants have the power to choose the level of responses they will provide. You might begin the interview by asking a broad question such as "Describe for me your experience with…" or "Tell me about…" Ideally, the participant will respond as though she or he is telling a story. It is important that the narrative be from the participant's, and not the interviewer's, perspective. Ask your interviewees to speak freely about their experiences.

Once the interview begins, the role of the interviewer is to encourage the subject to continue talking. Nod your head or make sounds that indicate interest. When it seems appropriate, encourage your subject to elaborate further on a particular dimension of the topic (known as probing). Participants may need validation that they are providing the needed information. Some participants may give short answers, so you may need to encourage them to elaborate. The interviewer becomes a detective in his or her search for important information. McEvoy (2001) pointed out that the interviewer is not after factual information. From the perspective of qualitative research, interviews generate socially constructed knowledge. The interviewer influences the interviewee in terms of "how she or he listens, attends, encourages, interrupts, digresses, initiates topics and terminates responses" (p. 51).

Problems with Interviewing

You may encounter some challenges during an interview. Common problems include interruptions such as telephone calls, "stage fright" that often arises when the participant realizes he or she is being recorded, failure to establish a rapport with your subject, verbose participants, and those who tend to wander off the subject. You may need to tactfully guide the interview back to the topic. If the participant is emotionally distressed as a result of the interview, remain with the individual until the participant is able to restore his or her composure. Researchers and interviewers tend to underestimate the amount of time required for an interview. If the participant is hurried, the quality of data is affected.

When the study focuses on families, issues arise regarding which members are interviewed. In some cases, a single member is selected to represent the family. This strategy biases the results because other family members may have different perspectives of the situation. Select two family members and interview each separately. The best strategy, of course, is to interview each member separately, but this requires an inordinate amount of time (Astedt-Kurki, Paavilainen, & Lehti, 2001).

Particular concerns arise when a researcher is interviewing colleagues. The interviewer (an insider) lacks the social distance that facilitates a balanced, objective perspective. Common experiences tend to be taken for granted. Aspects of the social world that should be questioned are overlooked. You may find it difficult to ask questions about sensitive issues of someone in your own social group. However, there are advantages. Because of their unique position, insiders are familiar with the social world and thus can interpret and attach meaning that may elude an outsider. As an insider, you may find that you read between the lines of participants' comments rather than taking them at face value. This capability may be particularly important if the group under study is a minority group or otherwise marginalized (McEvoy, 2001).

From an ethical perspective, interviews tend to be viewed as noninvasive and thus as posing no threat to the interviewee. However, interviews are an invasion of the psyche. For some, this may be therapeutic. However, an interview is capable of producing risks to the health of the participant. Therefore, the interviewer must always avoid inflicting unnecessary harm upon the participant (Munhall, 1991; Sullivan, 1998).

The data you obtain are affected by characteristics of the person being interviewed. These may include age, ethnicity, gender, professional background, educational level, and relative status of interviewer and interviewee, as well as impairments in vision or hearing, speech impediments, fatigue, pain, poor memory, disorientation, emotional state, or language

difficulties. Interviews with children may require special considerations (Deatrick & Ledlie, 2000). In some studies, interviewers may be profoundly affected by participants' stories and may need debriefing. This need may extend to those transcribing the interviews and to researchers analyzing the data. Because of privacy issues, study participants are not able to share their feelings with those who usually provide support and comfort. In these cases, a person or persons should be designated to address these needs (Moyle, 2002; Price, 2002; Sullivan, 1998; Wilmpenny & Gass, 2000).

Berg (1998) has identified the following "ten commandments" of interviewing:

1. *Never begin an interview cold. Remember to spend several minutes chatting and making small talk with the subject. If you are in the subject's home, use what's there for this chatting. Look around the room and ask about such things as photographs, banners, books, and so forth. The idea here is to set the subject at ease and establish a warm and comfortable rapport.*

2. *Remember your purpose. You are conducting an interview in order to obtain information. Try to keep the subject on track, and if you are working with an interview schedule, always have a copy of it in front of you— even though you should have your questions memorized.*

3. *Present a natural front. Because your questions are memorized, you should be able to ask each one as if it had just popped into your head. Be relaxed, affirmative, and as natural as you can.*

4. *Demonstrate aware hearing. Be sure to offer the subjects appropriate nonverbal responses. If they describe something funny, smile. If they tell you something sad, look sad. If they say that something upset them, try to console them. Do not present yourself as uninterested or unaware.*

5. *Think about appearance. Be sure you have dressed appropriately for both the setting and the kind of subject you are working with. Generally, business attire is most appropriate. If you are interviewing children, a more casual appearance may be more effective. Remember to think about how you look to other people.*

6. *Interview in a comfortable place. Be sure that the location of the interview is somewhere the subject feels comfortable. If the*

subject is fearful about being overheard or being seen, your interview may be over before it ever starts.

7. *Don't be satisfied with monosyllabic answers. Be aware when subjects begin giving yes-and-no answers. Answers like these will not offer much information during analysis. When this does occur, be sure to probe with questions such as, "Can you tell me a little bit more about that?" or "What else happened?" Even a simple pause and an uncomfortable silence might yield additional information.*

8. *Be respectful. Be sure the subject feels that he or she is an integral part of your research and that any answer he or she offers is absolutely wonderful. Often subjects will say things like, "You don't really want to know how I feel about that." Assure them that you really do!*

9. *Practice, practice, and practice some more. The only way to actually become proficient at interviewing is to interview. Although this book [Berg, 1998] and other manuals can offer guidelines, it is up to you as a researcher to develop your own repertoire of actions. The best way to accomplish this task is to go out and do interviews.*

10. *Be cordial and appreciative. Remember to thank the subject when you finish, and answer any questions he or she might have about the research. Remember, you are always a research emissary. Other researchers may someday want to interview this subject or gain access to the setting you were in. If you mess things up through inappropriate actions, you may close the door for future researchers. (Berg, 1998, pp. 87–88)*

The following is an abstract of a study on Ph.D.-prepared nurses in the clinical setting (McNett, 2006).

Background: The emergence of new doctoral programs within the nursing discipline has stimulated dialogue regarding the role of the doctorally prepared nurse in the clinical setting. National nursing organizations have cited the need for additional research that would provide information regarding the current practice of doctorally prepared nurses. A review of the literature reveals little published information about the role of PhD nurses in the clinical setting.

A survey from one university in the year 2000 revealed that only 40% of that university's doctoral nursing students planned to seek employment in the academic setting. The remaining 60% were entering the clinical setting. (Munro, 2001) (p. 135)

Purpose: The purpose of this descriptive qualitative study was to investigate how PhD-prepared nurses describe and define their role within the clinical setting.

Methods: Interviews were conducted with 5 PhD nurses who were all employed full time in the clinical setting. Interview notes were recorded, transcribed, and analyzed using qualitative data analysis. Recurrent themes that emerged from the interviews were identified. (p. 134)

Redundancy with participant's responses was seen after interviews with 5 nurses. Given the exploratory nature of this study, the redundancy from participants, and the nature of the findings, it was determined that 5 nurses were sufficient to form a base for the preliminary results reported here. (pp. 135–136)

Interviews were conducted by the principal investigator either in person or via telephone with the participants. The interview began with a series of questions regarding the current title and position of the PhD-prepared nurse, as well as their area of specialty, number of years they have been in their position, and number of years since having earned a PhD. Lastly, the participants were asked to describe their master's degree and from what discipline they had earned their doctoral degrees.

Using an interview schedule of 5 questions, the nurses were then asked to respond to the following statements or questions: (1) Describe your role and responsibilities as a PhD-prepared nurse working in the hospital setting? (2) Compare these roles and responsibilities as a PhD-prepared nurse with a CNS or NP working in this institution who does not have a PhD. (3) What are some of the advantages of having a PhD in your current position? (4) What are some of the obstacles you have encountered in the clinical setting because of your PhD? (5) Tell me a story that best highlights what you consider to be one of your successes as a PhD nurse. (p. 135)

Results: The 2 themes that emerged from the interviews were bridging the research/practice gap and serving as a healthcare leader. All participants spoke to their role in leading, encouraging, or participating in clinical nursing research within their healthcare institutions. Phrases regarding leadership emerged throughout each interview and reflected a number of leadership responsibilities that each participant had within the healthcare environment.

Conclusions: The findings from this qualitative study provide insight into the current role of the PhD-prepared nurse in the clinical setting. This information can be used to guide additional research that might influence the development of future doctoral programs in nursing. (p. 134)

All participants in this study choose to make research a priority within their various hospital roles and responsibilities. All participants are striving to advance nursing science through practice-based research, and all cite the importance of nurses being the principal investigator in these study. This finding is especially significant because 4 of the 5 participants did not hold research or administrative positions within their organizations. Rather, they were employed and practicing as CNSs or NPs with doctoral degrees. This finding differs from that of Sterling and McNally (1999), who found that research did not have such a profound influence on the roles of all of the doctorally prepared nurses that they interviewed. (pp. 137–138)

Focus Groups

Focus groups were designed to obtain the participants' perceptions in a focused area in a setting that is permissive and nonthreatening. One of the assumptions underlying the use of focus groups is that group dynamics can help people to express and clarify their views in ways that are less likely to occur in a one-to-one interview. The group may give a sense of "safety in numbers" to those wary of researchers or those who are anxious.

Focus groups are a relatively recent strategy that was used initially in nursing studies in the late 1980s. However, they have been used in other fields for a long time. The idea of focus groups emerged in the 1920s as an approach for examining the effectiveness of marketing strategies. The concept reemerged during World War II with efforts to determine ways to improve the morale of the troops. The technique serves a variety of purposes in nursing research. It has been used to perform qualitative studies (Twinn, 1998), make policy analyses (Straw & Smith, 1995), assess consumer satisfaction, evaluate the quality of care (Beaudin & Pelletier, 1996), examine the effectiveness of public health programs, assist in professional decision making (Bulmer, 1998; Southern et al., 1999), develop instruments, explore patient care problems and strategies for developing effective interventions, develop education programs (Halloran & Grimes, 1995), and study various patient populations (Disney & May, 1998; Goss, 1998; Quine & Cameron, 1995; Reed & Payton, 1997). It has also been employed as a data collection strategy in participatory research. A focus group study might include from 6 to 50 groups.

The following assumptions underlie focus groups (Morrison & Peoples, 1999):

1. A homogeneous group provides the participants with freedom to express thoughts, feelings, and behaviors candidly.
2. Individuals are important resources of information.
3. People are able to report and verbalize their thoughts and feelings.
4. A group's dynamics can generate authentic information.

5. Group interviews are superior to individual interviews.
6. The facilitator can help people recover forgotten information by focusing the interview.

The effective use of focus groups requires careful planning. Questions that must be addressed include the following:

1. What are the aims of the focus groups?
2. How many focus groups should be assembled?
3. How many individuals should be in each focus group?
4. How will you recruit for the focus groups?
5. Can you locate sufficient people for the focus groups?
6. Are you selecting the right people for the focus groups?
7. Where should the focus groups meet?
8. What skills should the groups' moderators have?
9. How will moderators interact with participants?
10. What questions will the moderators ask?
11. How should the data be analyzed?

Many different communication forms are used in focus groups, including teasing, arguing, joking, anecdotes, and nonverbal approaches such as gesturing, facial expressions, and other body language. Kitzinger (1995, pp. 299–300) has suggested that

> *people's knowledge and attitudes are not entirely encapsulated in reasoned responses to direct questions. Everyday forms of communication may tell us as much, if not more, about what people know or experience. In this sense focus groups reach the parts that other methods cannot reach, revealing dimensions of understanding that often remain untapped by more conventional data collection techniques. (full text available in Health Source Nursing/ Academic edition)*

Recruiting appropriate participants for each of the focus groups is critical, because recruitment is the most common source of failure. Each focus group should include 6 to 10 participants. If there are fewer participants, the discussion tends to be inadequate. In most cases, participants are expected to be unknown to each other. However, when targeting professional groups such as clinical nurses or nurse educators, such anonymity usually is not possible. You may use purposive sampling to seek out individuals known to have the desired expertise. In other cases, you may look for participants through the media, posters, or advertisements. A single contact with an individual who agrees to attend a focus group does not ensure that this person will attend the group session. You will need to make repeated phone calls and remind the candidates by mail. Inform them at the time of consent that you will be calling to remind them of the group and to verify that the phone number they gave you is the best number to call. You may need to offer incentives. Cash payments are, of course, the most effective if the resources are available through funding. Other incentives include refreshments at the focus group meeting, T-shirts, coffee mugs, gift certificates, or coupons. Overrecruiting may be necessary; a good rule is to invite two more potential participants than you need for the group (Morgan, 1995).

Segmentation is the process of sorting participants into focus groups with common characteristics. Selecting participants who are similar to each other in lifestyle or experiences, views, and characteristics facilitates more open discussion. And you can increase the group's validity by conducting multiple focus groups and placing participants with differing characteristics into separate groups. These characteristics might be age, gender, social class, ethnicity, culture, lifestyle, or health status. Strickland (1999) pointed out the problems that could occur if differing cultural groups are included in the same focus group. Communication patterns, roles, relationships, and traditions might interfere with the interactions within the focus group. In some cases, groups may occur naturally such as those who work together. Be cautious about bringing together participants with considerable variation in social standing, education, or authority because some group members may hesitate to participate fully, whereas others may discount the input of those with perceived lower standing (Kitzinger, 1995; Morgan, 1995).

Establish a setting for your focus group that is relaxed. There should be space for participants to sit comfortably in a circle or U-shape and maintain eye contact with all participants. Ensure that the acoustics of the room will allow you to obtain a quality tape recording of the sessions. As with the one-on-one interview discussed earlier, place your tape or video recorders unobtrusively, and use batteries rather than plugging your equipment into a power source as this is less invasive. Use a highly sensitive microphone. However, it may be necessary for the moderator or assistant moderator to take notes when the speaker's voice is soft or when several individuals are speaking at once. Making notes on the dynamics of the group is also useful. Note how group members interact with one another. Sessions will usually last 1 to 2 hours,

although some may extend to an entire afternoon or continue as part of a series of meetings.

It is important for the researcher to clarify the aims of the focus groups and communicate these aims to the moderators and the participants before the group session. Instruct participants that all points of view are valid and helpful and that speakers should not have to defend their positions. Make clear to the group that the facilitator's role is to moderate the discussion, not to contribute. Carefully plan the questions that are to be asked during the focus group, and, if time permits, pilot-test them. Limit the number of questions to those most essential so that sufficient time is left for discussion. You may elect to give participants some of the questions before the group meeting to enable them to give careful thought to their responses. Questions should be posed in such a way that group members can build on the responses of others in the group, raise their own questions, and question each other. Probes can be used to elicit richer details using questions such as "How would that make a difference?" or "What makes you think that?" "Why" questions are not good because they tend to push a participant toward taking a stand and defending it. Then it is difficult to move away from the stand if the group begins moving toward some consensus. The act of questioning or challenging ideas offers a stimulating learning experience for group members. Their thinking may be supported or tested, and participants may be presented with new ways of thinking about a problem (Hollis Openshaw, & Goble, 2002).

A common problem in focus groups is to dive right into the topic of interest to the researcher with little emphasis on the interests of the participants. Early in the session, provide opportunities for participants to express their views on the topic of discussion. Next, proceed with the questions. Use probes if the discussion wanders too far. A good facilitator will weave questions into the discussion naturally. The facilitator's role is to clarify, paraphrase, and reflect back what group members have said. These discussions tend to express group norms, and individual voices of dissent may be stifled. However, when the discussion is on sensitive topics, the group may actively facilitate the discussion because less inhibited members break the ice for those who are more reticent. Participants may also provide group support for expressing feelings, opinions, or experiences. Late in the session, the moderator may encourage group members to go beyond the current discussion or debate and discuss inconsistencies among participants and within their own thinking. The moderator can use disagreements among group members to encourage participants to state their points of view more clearly and provide a rationale for their position (Kitzinger, 1995).

Moderator Role

Selecting effective moderators is as critical as selecting appropriate participants. The moderator must encourage participants to talk about the topic. Sim (1998) pointed out that "the focus group moderator will influence powerfully the process of interaction that takes place, and the way in which the moderator behaves, and the verbal and non-verbal cues that he or she gives to the group, are crucial in this respect" (p. 347). Because expertise in the topic may make participants reluctant to speak, the moderator should make it clear that he or she is there to learn from the group members. In some cases, you will want to include an assistant moderator as well as a moderator. Participants should be encouraged to talk to one another rather than addressing all comments to the moderator. A successful moderator encourages participants to interact with one another, formulates ideas, and draws out cognitive structures not previously articulated. Moderators should remain neutral and nonjudgmental. If the topic is sensitive, moderators need to be able to put participants at ease. To accomplish this goal, use a moderator with characteristics similar to those of the group participants. Extreme dominance or extreme passiveness on the part of the moderator will lead to problems (Kitzinger, 1995; Morgan, 1995; Morrison & Peoples, 1999).

Data Collection

Sim (1998) recommended that the following data be collected:

1. What participants say
2. How participants interact with one another
3. Accurate attribution of quotations to individual group members

Data collection should not interfere with the coordination of the group. The method of data collection should not have reactive effects on the participants.

Berg (1998), citing the work of Reinharz (1992) and Kramer (1983), suggested using a computer group diary as a strategy, combining focus group interviewing and unobtrusive observation to gather information. Participants are given a web site where each individual can enter his or her thoughts. All participants have access to each participant's comments and can enter their own thoughts or respond to comments of others. Thus, these become unguided focus groups in which the discourse is "similar to synergistically created convergence of ideas and experiences" (Berg, 1998, p. 108).

Kelly and Patterson (2006) conducted a study titled "Childhood Nutrition: Perceptions of Caretakers in a Low-Income Urban Setting" in which they used focus groups. The following abstract describes their research.

The incidence of overweight and obese children, especially those from low-income and minority backgrounds, continues to rise. Multiple factors contribute to the rising rates. In order to gain an understanding of factors contributing to obesity in low-income families, a qualitative study was conducted with the purpose of gaining knowledge of low-income urban caretakers' understanding and attitudes regarding children's nutrition. A focused ethnography was used as a means of understanding behavior within the context of a person's cultural environment. The sample was 17 caretakers of children in the 1st–3rd grades. Four focus groups were conducted. Two themes emerged from caretakers' perceptions: knowing the right things children should eat and balancing healthy nutrition with unhealthy choices. Four categories emerged regarding influences on food choices: tradition, finances, time constraints, and role models. Lastly, five barriers and three facilitating factors emerged. Implications of the study findings for school nurses include the need, when implementing healthy eating programs for school children, to gain information from caretakers about their perceptions of childhood nutrition. (p. 345)

Procedure: A semistructured interview guide, based on the health care literature and input from pediatric nurse experts, was used to guide the focus groups. Four focus groups were conducted at an elementary school in a classroom at the end of school hours. The interviews were audiotape-recorded and lasted from 1.5–2 hours. Although there were some challenges to conducting focus groups in this setting (Patterson & Kelly, 2005), participants enthusiastically shared their views and thoughts about the nutrition. Healthy refreshments were served. The same researcher conducted all focus groups. Field notes about observations in classrooms, the cafeteria, and surrounding community were recorded regularly. Data collection continued until saturation was reached. (p. 247)

Collecting Stories

During observation and interviewing, the researcher may record stories shared by participants. Banks-Wallace (1998) described a story as "an event or series of events, encompassed by temporal or spatial boundaries, that are shared with others using an oral medium or sign language. Storytelling is the process or interaction used to share stories. People sharing a story (storytellers) and those listening to a story (storytakers) are the main elements of storytelling" (p. 17). Stories can help researchers to understand a phenomenon of interest. In some qualitative studies, the focus of the research may be the gathering of stories. Gathering of stories can enable health care providers to develop storytelling as a powerful means to increase insight and promote health behavior in clients. For example, Nwoga (1997, 2000) studied how African-American mothers use storytelling to guide their adolescent daughters regarding sexuality. The stories could assist other mothers who are struggling to help their daughters deal with sexuality issues.

Coffey and Atkinson (1996) discussed the importance of capturing stories in qualitative studies.

> The story is an obvious way for social actors, in talking to strangers (e.g., the researcher), to retell key experiences and events. Stories serve a variety of functions. Social actors often remember and order their careers or memories as a series of narrative chronicles, that is, as series of stories marked by key happenings. Similarly, stories and legends are told and retold by members of particular social groups or organizations as a way of passing on a cultural heritage or an organizational culture. Tales of success or tales of key leaders/personalities are familiar genres with which to maintain a collective sense of the culture of an organization. The use of atrocity stories and morality fables is also well documented within organizational and occupational settings. Stories of medical settings are especially well documented (Atkinson, 1992; Dingwall, 1977). Here tales of professional incompetence are used to give warning of "what not to do" and what will happen if you commit mistakes.... Narratives are also a common genre from which to retell or come to terms with particularly sensitive or traumatic times and events. (Coffey & Atkinson, 1996, p. 56)

Mattingly and Lawlor (2000) described their research in which they solicit "illness stories." These authors skillfully guide you in interpreting the process of the story, identifying key turning points as the story progresses.

> During the first interview with Barbara, she told a harrowing story of how she struggled time and time again to get health professionals to find out what was wrong with her little girl. The following extensive excerpt of this first interview gives a powerful picture of this struggle. Since it includes the interviewer's (Cheryl's) questions, it also illustrates the kind of questioning process often required to prompt someone to move from broad descriptions of situations to vivid and fine-grained stories of particular events. (p. 9)

Three people are present in this interview, which takes place in a hospital waiting room. Barbara, the mother, Cheryl, the interviewer, and Rhonda, the ill child. Rhonda, who is just 3 years old at the time, becomes impatient in the way that children do and interrupts, forcing the adults to pay some attention. Barbara is adept at shifting between responding to Rhonda and picking up her narrative train. Cheryl lacks Barbara's easy facility, but tries valiantly to keep Rhonda entertained while listening to Barbara's story. She also tries to keep the tape recorder out of Rhonda's hands who gets curious about how it works. Cheryl has supplied Rhonda with some colored pens and paper since Rhonda loves to draw. (p. 9)

At the stage of the interview excerpted below, Barbara has been remembering the period of several months in which Rhonda has often been violently sick to her stomach, but no doctor has discovered anything the matter. She then remarks:

So on Labor Day (pause) Labor Day, her Dad had her … and he was keeping her till the next morning. So the next morning, at 5 o'clock, he called and said, "Oh she's really vomiting bad." And I said, "Bring her here so I can take her," I said, "I'm taking her to City Hospital." So I said, "Bring her here."

The very way that Barbara has phrased things signals Cheryl that a significant moment is about to be described. A key marker of a story is the location of an event in a specific time. Barbara begins this part of their conversation with specific temporal indicators. Not only Labor Day (a 24-h time period) but even "5 o'clock in the morning." Here is the verbal equivalent of a zoom lens, which moves from a hazy distance to an increasingly sharp focus on one particular moment in time. Barbara is setting the stage and we know that something important is about to happen. A second marker that a significant story is about to unfold is Barbara's narrative strategy of recalling dialogue. She shifts in a "he said, she said" mode in which she not only simulates the remembered phone conversation, supplying actual conversation, but she even shifts her voice to imitate the various characters, namely herself and her estranged husband.

While, upon reading the transcript, it is clear that Barbara is heading in an important direction, at the time Cheryl seems a bit oblivious to these clues and asks a series of distracting questions, which Barbara politely answers.

C: Had you been to City Hospital yet so far?
B: No. "Cause I couldn't …
C: It's a long trip.
B: And plus the job. I figured the pediatrician that I was taking her to, that she's had ever since she was born—that you know, they would handle it, and plus, I was at the kind of job that I couldn't, like, take off, you know, or, you know, I was always stressed that if I take off, you know, that I would lose my job, you know?
C: Yeah.
B: And, especially since I had got separated. You know, I really couldn't afford to take no time, you know.
C: Yeah

But then, tenacious storyteller that she is, when Barbara sees an opening she returns to her story as though she had never been interrupted.

B: So, I was taking her, you know, to a lot of the emergencies and to, you know, X Hospital and Y Hospital, and I was taking her there, but then I started just saying, forget it. [Barbara means here that she finds she is not getting any helpful treatment for Rhonda and gives up on the idea of continually taking her to the doctor's] I started taking her to my ex-husband's place. And so, he didn't bring her home that morning when he called me at 5 o'clock. He brought her home, like, later in the afternoon. But by then, she stopped vomiting, okay? But later on that evening, it started back up. She just, like when she was drinking something, it would, like, just shoot back out across the room. Just like how the Exorcist—

C: Yeah, yeah.

B: You know? And I was, like, really getting, um, crazy, so I had brought her down ... I called Z Hospital, and I told them that my daughter's like, vomiting and having headaches, you know, and um, they said, well um, "Bring her." You know, and then so I brought her to the emergency there. And then, um, I had a little confrontation with the lady in there, okay?

In this passage Barbara begins the shift from general description of her life to specific, vivid storytelling. She begins with an overview of her situation during this time prior to Rhonda's diagnosis in which she speaks about her difficulties in getting time off work and her continual trips to various clinics in the area. But then she switches to a specific highly dramatic incident, which she locates at a specific time, "that morning." Though her account is a bit confusing in detail, it is clear that something much more frightening is going on with Rhonda than has happened before. Barbara uses a graphic image, vomiting like "the Exorcist" to get her message across of what this experience was like for her.

At this point, Cheryl had caught on that this is a pivotal episode in Barbara's illness story. She suspects that Barbara's phrase "little confrontation" is the tip of an iceberg and that much could be learned about Barbara's perspective on what it is like to deal with healthcare professionals if she can get Barbara to tell the story of this "little confrontation." Cheryl also hears in Barbara's voice that, whatever else, this confrontation is not little, is in fact momentous... (p. 10)

Cheryl moves in to facilitate the storytelling, drawing Barbara out and slowing her down by asking her to describe, in graphic detail, what happened in that confrontation. As Barbara answers, Cheryl requests even more specificity. Twice she asks that Barbara remember and repeat the actual words of participants. Barbara responds by telling the study in greater and greater detail and as she shifts to this increasingly vivid portrayal of the dramatic scene, Cheryl only needs to sit back and listen, to murmur and show, through her body, that she is intently following Barbara's story.

C: Tell me about this. Just describe that. What happened?

B: Yeah. That evening, when I brought her um ... the doctor down there in the emergency, she um, came and checked her, and I was telling her, she's really ... she's constantly vomiting and having headaches really bad. And she did her little checking, and she said, "Well, I don't see anything." And we did her urine, and, "I don't see anything." I said, "But I'm not leaving here unless you guys tell me to do something because ..." and then she started, like, getting a little smart on me.

C: Yeah, like what did she say? Just go... just go through this.

B: Okay. She was, like, saying, well, if you don't think that I'm doing my job, then you could just take her to the, um ... I'm gonna make you an appointment and you can take her to the day hospital. I said, "Oh, it's not that I don't think you're doing your job; I just want my daughter to get help." You know, as you understand, I've been taking her everywhere and she still be doing the same thing constantly, over and over. And so then, she got a little upset, so she left ...

C: What did she say?

B: And she went across the hall and ... where her little office was ... when all that time, the door was open, you know, all the time she was seeing patients. But when she left there from talking to me, she went over there and she closed her door, and I guess she was telling the social worker ... because the social worker came down and came in there and talked to me and was asking me, "What's going on? Is there something wrong?" I said, "Yes, there's something wrong." She said, "Well, the doctor feels that you don't think she's doing her job." I said, "So, but why does she have to call the social worker on me?" You know? And then I started feeling like they was, um ... I felt like she thought that I was, like, kind of crazy or did something to my daughter myself. That's the kind of feeling I got. I felt very uncomfortable. I said, "Do you guys call the social worker on all people?" you know? And she ... and I was letting the social worker explain. "No, it's not on all people. It's just when the parents feel that you're not happy with your doctor, and the doctor will call." You know, but then, she kinda calmed me down. You know, I wasn't arguing or I wasn't saying any, you know, bad ... anything ... I just wanted my baby to get help, you know? I didn't want to take her home again and be like she was. You know, she'd done been through it too much.

C: Yeah. (p. 11)

This confrontation is repeated and amplified just 1 week later, in September, when Rhonda is again severely ill and Barbara picks her up from school and rushes her back to City Hospital. Again she has to fight with nurses, doctors and other healthcare workers to get her child seen. Barbara tells the story of this fateful day. She talks to person after person, going from one department in the hospital to another, telling them "that nobody wants to see my baby … I said, 'Nobody wants to see my baby and she's really sick, and I keep getting the run-around.'" She remembers that they tell her, "'Well, Rhonda's appointment is not until the 21st,' you know, 'of October, so you have to wait.' Finally, she gets one "administrative lady" to listen to her and this woman locates Dr. Romburg. "And so he was doing a little history on Rhonda…I said, 'My baby keeps complaining of her headaches.'"

Just then, the doctor has Rhonda walk. Barbara recalls her horror at what happens next. "But she started walking like she couldn't walk by herself anymore you know? And started walking, like, into the wall, you know, to the right. And I said, 'Oh Lord! Something is really going on.'" The doctor then "hurried up and ran and got another doctor…and he told her to walk for him, so she did the same thing for him. So then they went and talked and they came back. They said to me, 'It seems like it's some form of a mass or something, pressing down on her head to give her headaches.' So then I was saying, 'Oh Lord.'" As terrified as Barbara is, there is one phrase this doctor told her, one she repeated several times and in later interviews again, that deeply reassured her. While others had only paid attention to Rhonda's stomach because of her violent vomiting, "Dr Romburg, he said, 'We're gonna start from her head and work our way down.'"

Again, note the contrast of Barbara's wrenching story to the pristine note in the medical chart in which the doctor reports, "Physical examination: looks well but wobbly … has me concerned about mass in head, will schedule CT." No one would know what Barbara endured to get this essential CT scan, which led to Rhonda's diagnosis of a brain tumor just 3 days later.

Rhonda is now 5 years old, still very sick, still receiving treatment, but still alive. (p. 12)

Constructing Life Stories

A life story is designed to reconstruct and interpret the life of an ordinary person. The methodology, which emerged from history, from anthropology, and more recently from phenomenology, has been described by a number of scholars (Bateson, 1989; Bertaux, 1981; Frank, 1979; Gergen & Gergen, 1983; Josselson & Lieblich, 1995; Linde, 1993; Mattingly & Garro, 1994; Polkinghorne, 1988; Sarbin, 1986; Tanner et al., 1993; Ventres, 1994). The life story can be used to clarify the meanings of various states of health, chronic illness, and disability in the lives of patients, their families, and other caregivers. These stories can help us understand the meaning to patients of their health behavior, lifestyles, illnesses, or impairments; the meaning of symptoms; their experiences of treatment; how they adapt; and their hopes and possibilities of reconstructing their lives. Interviews are tape-recorded and transcribed. Notes

from observations may be important, and personal documents such as diaries or historical records may be used. Analysis involves more than just stringing events together; events should be linked in an interpretation through which the researcher can create theoretical sense. Materials are organized and analyzed according to theoretical interests. Constructing a life story often requires a long-term contact and extensive collaboration with the participant (Frank, 1996; Larson & Fanchiang, 1996; Mallinson, Kielhofner, & Mattingly, 1996).

Roesler (2006) provided a life story of Herr Bittner in an article describing a narratological methodology for identifying archetypal story patterns in autobiographical narratives. The article is translated from German.

The following transcript is taken from an autobiographical interview with a person called Herr Bittner. Herr Bittner has been severely physically disabled from birth by spastic cerebral palsy. He has always been totally dependent on external help. In his life story he describes himself as a political person. He was an active member of the political movement of disabled persons fighting for an independent life and for equal rights. Actually he was the first disabled person in Germany who could live outside of any institution through help from young people doing their civil service. In his narrative self-presentation, he lives a life exemplary for all disabled people, always before the eyes of the public. His life is a political fight for equal rights for all disabled people, and the changes in his own life, his growing autonomy and self-respect, mirror the changing attitude in society towards disabled people and their rights. (p. 577)

In his introduction to the actual narrative he argues that physically disabled persons are often mistaken by the public as being also mentally retarded and are discriminated against just because they have physical problems with speaking, with precise pronunciation, or just because they look strange. He now wants to take on the task of showing and proving to the public, again in a way that will be exemplary for all disabled people, that they are at least as intelligent as normal people, and his only possibility of doing so is by showing that he can speak clearly and precisely. With the actual narrative he gives an example of that: (p. 577)

Herr Bittner: … and still today I love to surprise experts. I want to give an example; years ago I have been to a university clinic and then the professor and his whole staff came to my bed and he says, "Now how do you feel, how do we feel today?," that is, in we-form. And then I said, "Professor, I cannot judge how you feel today I just know how I feel." T cha. Then I said, "You actually asked me how we feel" (Laughs) and one hour later an assistant doctor came in and she said "Are you mad, we just

*could not laugh in his presence, and he went out into the
hallway and said what did the guy really mean to say?"
(laughs).*

Unfortunately the transcript cannot show how strongly
his speech is distorted by his spasticity and how he still
tries very hard to speak clearly and exactly. (p. 577)

Case Studies

A case study examines a single unit within the context
of its real-life environment. The unit may be a person,
a family, a nursing unit, or an organization. In the early
twentieth century, the most common nursing study was
a case study. Medical case studies were also common.
Nursing case studies were published in the *American
Journal of Nursing* and initiated a variety of nursing
studies of patient care. As nursing research began to
use more rigorous methods, the case study fell into dis-
repute. However, the importance of information from
case studies is again being recognized. Case studies can
use quantitative, qualitative, or mixed methods of data
collection. It is important for the researcher to consider
the multiple aspects that affect a particular case and to
include this essential information in the plan for data
collection and analysis.

Research questions, as well as the qualitative
method chosen for the study, guide the data collection.
However, as with most qualitative studies, as an understanding of the situation begins to emerge, other questions arise and new data may be gathered to address the
new question. A researcher might want to understand
the multiplicity of factors that affect patient care, all of
the elements that affect the emotional state of a person
with a particular illness, or the factors that affect learning from a particular approach to patient education.
Factors might include the social and political environment in which care is being provided. Thus, identifying
all of the variables to be examined is a critical component to planning the study. Multiple sources of information for as many of the variables as possible give the
study greater validity. This is referred to as data triangulation. A field diary is also useful because insights
can be recorded as they occur. The researcher might
also recognize new variables that need to be examined.
Personal response to events should also be recorded.
If the case is a person, multiple interviews may need to
be conducted, requiring a strong commitment from the
respondent. Documentary evidence is also a valuable
source of details related to the case. Analysis focuses
on providing a rich, in-depth description of the case.
Generalization, as with many qualitative studies, is not
possible. However, comparisons with similar situations
are sometimes possible.

Benderix and Sivberg (2007) provided an example
of a case study.

> The aim of this study was to describe the present and
> past experiences of 14 siblings from five families in
> terms of having a brother or sister with autism and men-
> tal retardation. Personal interviews were conducted with
> the siblings before their brothers or sisters were moved to
> a newly opened group home. Qualitative content analy-
> sis was used for the analysis of the transcribed texts. The
> analysis resulted in seven content categories: precocious
> responsibility, feeling sorry, exposed to frightening behav-
> ior, empathetic feelings, hoping that a group home will be
> a relief, physical violence made siblings feel unsafe and
> anxious, and relations with friends were affected nega-
> tively. The conclusion is that these siblings' experiences
> revealed stressful life conditions. Counseling for the fam-
> ily and for siblings is recommended to help them deal
> with their feelings and problems. For the siblings in these
> five families, a group home was a relevant alternative as
> a temporary or permanent placement for the child with
> autism and mental retardation. (p. 410)

DATA MANAGEMENT AND REDUCTION

Using the Computer for Qualitative Analysis

Traditionally, qualitative data collection and analysis
were performed manually. The researcher recorded the
data on small bits of paper or note cards, which were
then carefully coded, organized, and filed at the end of
a day. Manual analysis requires cross-checking each
bit of data with all the other bits of data on little pieces
of paper. It is easy to lose data in the mass of paper.
Keeping track of connections between various bits of
data requires meticulous record keeping. This method
was developed because it was important for the qualitative researcher to maintain a close link with—or
become immersed in—the data being analyzed.

Some qualitative researchers believe that using
the computer can make analysis of qualitative data
quicker and easier without the researcher losing touch
with the data (Anderson, 1987; Miles & Huberman,
1994; Pateman, 1998; St John & Johnson, 2000; Taft,
1993). Taft has suggested that because of the ease of
coding and recoding, the researcher feels more free
to play with the data and experiment with alternative ways of coding. This freedom fosters analytical
insight and thus facilitates data analysis. Researchers
can also search for codes that tend to occur together.
Also, easy access to the data facilitates team research.
Pateman (1998; full text available in Nursing Collection) suggested that "some would argue that scientific,

mathematically-minded people are more computer literate than those with more artistic, humanistic interests, in which case affinity with computing may have something to do with personal traits.... Some of the ... arguments [by qualitative researchers against using computers] could simply be rationalisation by computer-phobic researchers." However, Taft expressed concern about the dark side of computer technology for qualitative researchers. The researcher may be tempted to study larger samples and sacrifice depth for breadth. Meaningful understanding of the data may also be sacrificed. Sandelowski (1995a) expressed concern that the use of computers will alter the aesthetics of qualitative research and suggested that the key motivation for using computer technology in qualitative research is to legitimize the claim that qualitative researchers are doing science. She stated, "computer technology permits qualitative researchers to have computer printouts of data (with the veneer of objectivity they confer) comparable to their quantitative counterparts whose claims to doing science are often not questioned. Even so-called *soft* data can become *hard* when produced by *hard*ware. Qualitative work can now have the look and feel, or aesthetic features, of science" (p. 205).

The computer can assist researchers in activities such as processing, storage, retrieval, cataloging, and sorting and leaves the analysis activities up to the researcher. Anderson (1987) pointed out that "the computer does not perform the thinking, reviewing, interpretative, and analytic functions that the researcher must do for himself or herself. Rather, the computer makes the researcher more efficient and effective in those high-level functions, and eases some of the tedious 'mindless' tasks that otherwise consume so much time and energy" (pp. 629–630). However, Sandelowski (1995a) has argued that replacing and streamlining the cutting and pasting activities may be seen as desirable by some because they are uncomfortably reminiscent of childhood play. She argued against the claim that machine technology saves human labor and suggested that it may actually increase labor because more data are stored and retrieved and once the data are stored, one has more of a sense that it must all be accounted for in the report of results.

Computer use has several advantages over the more traditional methods of recording and storing data. Multiple copies can be made with ease, and files can be copied onto backup disks and stored at another site without the need for a large amount of storage space. Blocks of data can also be moved around in the file or copied to another file when data are being sorted by category. The same block of data could be inserted within several categories, if desired. At the same time, interviews or descriptions of observations can be kept intact for reference as needed. In addition, most word processing programs can perform sort operations and can search throughout a text file for a selected word or a string of words. Many of these activities can be performed with a traditional word processing program (Burnard, 1998). Files in a word processing program can be transferred to a database spreadsheet such as Excel, dBase, or Lotus 1–2–3 to organize the data into **matrices.**

A number of computer programs have been developed specifically to perform qualitative analyses. Podolefsky and McCarty (1983) described one of the earliest attempts. This program, Computer Assisted Topical Sorting (CATS), allowed users to insert codes, designated as numbers, into a text file. A mainframe text editor gave users the capacity to search for strings of characters such as words or phrases. St John and Johnson (2000) explored the pros and cons of various data analysis software for qualitative research.

Transcribing Interviews

Tape-recorded interviews are generally transcribed word for word. Field and Morse (1985) provided the following instructions for transcribing a tape-recorded interview.

> Pauses are denoted in the transcript with dashes, while series of dots indicate gaps or prolonged pauses. All exclamations, including laughter and expletives, are included. Instruct the typist to type interviews single-spaced with a blank line between speakers. A generous margin on both sides of the page permits the left margin to be used for coding and the researcher's own critique of the interview style, and the right margin to be used for comments regarding the content. ... Start a new paragraph each time a topic is changed. ... Ensure that all pages are numbered sequentially and that each page is coded with the interview number and the informant's number. (Field & Morse, 1985, pp. 97–99)

Sandelowski (1994) indicated that the researcher must choose which features about the interview to preserve in print. These choices directly influence the nature and direction of the analysis. Once the interview has been transcribed, the transcript takes on an independent reality and becomes the researcher's raw data. Sandelowski suggested that the process of transcription alters reality. The text is "many transformations removed from the so-called unadulterated reality it was intended to represent" (p. 312).

She recommended asking the following questions regarding transcription:

1. *Is a transcript necessary to achieve the research goals?*
2. *If a transcription is required, what features of the interview event should be preserved (if at all possible) and what features can be safely ignored?*
3. *What notation system should be used?*
4. *What purposes besides investigator analysis per se will the transcript serve? (Sandelowski, 1994, pp. 312–313)*

Sandelowski pointed out that transcriptions require about 3.5 hours for each 1 hour of interview time. The cost for this work may be $20/hour for an experienced typist.

Hutchinson (2005) has developed an innovative method of data analysis that uses audio-editing software to save selected audio bytes from digital audio recordings. The data are never transcribed but remain in audio form. A database is used to code and manage the linked audio files and generate detailed and summary reports. Although the system is time consuming to set up, it negates the need for expensive and time-intensive transcription of recorded data.

Listen to the tape recordings as soon after the interview as possible. Listen carefully to voice tone, inflection, and pauses of the researcher and the participant, as well as the content. These features may indicate that the topic is very emotional or very important. While you are listening, read the written transcript of the tape. Make notations of your observations on the transcript.

Ayers and Poirier (1996) pointed out that "qualitative analysis results from the recontextualization of chunks of data, always with the caveat that the new context must in some way be faithful to its origins. Narrative data are meaningless without context" (p. 164). Using the reader response theory emerging from the work of Iser (1980) and Kermode (1983), Ayers and Poirier indicated that "the meaning of a text arises from the interaction of the mind (including the personal history) of the reader with the content of the text (which in turn arose from the mind and personal history of the interview respondent)" (p. 164). Reading the text results in an interaction between the mind and personal history of the respondent and the mind and personal history of the researcher. This interaction results in the emergence of a "virtual text," which is the entity being interpreted. Thus, there is no real objective, authentic information from which only one correct interpretation can be made. The text does not explain everything. "Motives, histories, antecedents, and causal links, sometimes entire subplots are left to the reader, to the researcher, to infer" (Ayers & Poirier, 1996, p. 165). The process of **interpretation** occurs in the mind of the reader. The virtual text grows in size and complexity as the researcher reads and rereads. Throughout the process of analysis, the virtual text develops and evolves. Although multiple valid interpretations may occur if different researchers examine the text, all findings must remain trustworthy to the data. This trustworthiness applies to the unspoken meanings emerging from the totality of the data, not just the written words of the text.

Immersion in the Data

Data collected during a qualitative study may be narrative descriptions of observations, transcripts from tape recordings of interviews, entries in the researcher's diary reflecting on the dynamics of the setting, or notes taken while reading written documents. In the initial phases of data analysis, you need to become familiar with the data as you gather them. This process may involve reading and rereading notes and transcripts, recalling observations and experiences, listening to tapes, and viewing videotapes until you have become immersed in the data. Tapes contain more than words; they contain feeling, emphasis, and nonverbal communications. These aspects are at least as important to the communication as the words are. In phenomenology, this immersion in the data is referred to as **dwelling with the data**.

Data Reduction

Because of the volumes of data acquired in a qualitative study, initial efforts at analysis focus on reducing the volume of data so that the researcher can more effectively examine them, a process referred to as **data reduction**. During data reduction, you begin attaching meaning to elements in your data. You will discover classes of things, persons, and events and detect properties that characterize things, persons, and events. You will also note regularities in the setting or the people. These discoveries will lead to classifying elements in your data. In some cases, you may apply the classification scheme used by participants or authors. In other cases, you may wish to construct your own classification scheme.

According to Sandelowski (1995b),

Although data preparation is a distinctive stage in qualitative work where data are put into a form that will permit analysis, a rudimentary kind of analysis often begins when the researcher proofs transcripts against the audiotaped interviews from which they were prepared.

Indeed, the proofing process is often the first time a researcher gets a sense of the interview as a whole; it is, occasionally, the first time investigators will hear something said, even though they conducted the interview. During the proofing process, researchers will often underline key phrases, simply because they make some as yet inchoate impression on them. They may jot down ideas in the margins next to the text that triggered them, just because they do not want to lose some line of thinking. (p. 373)

Data Analysis

The following is a description of some of the techniques qualitative researchers use during the process of data analysis and interpretation. These techniques include coding, reflective remarks, marginal remarks, memoing, and developing propositions.

Codes and Coding

Coding is a means of categorizing. A code is a symbol or abbreviation used to classify words or phrases in the data. Codes may be placed in the data at the time of data collection, when entering data into the computer, or during later examination. Through the selection of categories, or codes, the researcher defines the domain of the study. Therefore, it is important that the codes be consistent with the philosophical base of the study. Organization of data, selection of specific elements of the data for categories, and naming of these categories all reflect the philosophical base used for the study. Later in the study, coding may progress to the development of a taxonomy. For example, you might develop a taxonomy of types of pain, types of patients, or types of patient education. Initial categories should be as broad as possible, but categories should not overlap. As you collect more data in relation to a particular category, you can section the major category into smaller categories.

SmithBattle (2007) described her coding process as follows.

Data consisted of joint and individual tape-recorded interviews that were professionally transcribed. I interviewed the White families, and a master's-prepared Black nurse interviewed the Black families. During third-trimester interviews, teens and grandparents privately described the pregnancy and their expectations, hopes, and fears about the future. At 1, 3, 6, and 9 months, participants were asked in separate interviews to recall recent stressful and meaningful episodes in being a parent or a grandparent, and what they thought, felt, and

did in each situation. Teens were also provided with disposable cameras and a baby book journal in which they wrote about their experiences. Following each postpartum interview, the teen described her photos and shared her journal entries with the interviewer. A family history interview was conducted with grandparents at 6 months. At 9 months, mother and baby were videotaped in routine activities. After viewing the videotape with the interviewer, the mother described her reactions to taped segments. In joint interviews at 3 and 10 months, teens and grandparents described their daily schedules and the care of the baby. Individual and joint interviews were scheduled at family members' convenience and typically lasted less than 1.5 hours. Teens received US$10 for each interview or US$60 for completing the study. Parents were not reimbursed.

Data were analyzed using interpretive strategies. Codes emerged directly from the data and were used to tag interview excerpts that were then moved as a block to case summaries for each family. Summaries were amended as additional interviews were coded. This approach made it possible to condense each family's set of lengthy interviews into one file so that my analyses and interview excerpts could be easily retrieved for subsequent analysis. As cases were analyzed, I searched for patterns in teens' and grandparents' concerns, meanings, practices, and interactions. Cases were then compared to uncover similarities and differences in personal and family concerns, meanings, practices, and interactions. The second interviewer and two additional researchers read selected cases to validate or refine my interpretation. (p. 262)

The types of codes that can be used are descriptive, interpretative, and explanatory. Descriptive codes classify elements of the data by using terms that describe how the researcher is organizing the data. It is the simplest method of classification and is commonly used in the initial stages of data analysis. Descriptive codes remain close to the terms that the participant used during the interview. For example, if you were reading a transcribed interview in which a participant described experiences in the first days after surgery, you might use descriptive codes such as PAIN, MOVING, FEAR, and REST.

Interpretative codes are usually developed later in the data-collecting process as the researcher gains some insight into the processes occurring and begins to move beyond simply sorting statements. The participant's terms are used to attach meanings to these statements. For example, in a study of postoperative experiences, you might begin to recognize that the participant was investing much energy in seeking to relieve symptoms and seeking information about how the health care providers believed that he or she was doing. These might be classified by using interpretative codes of RELIEF and INFO.

Explanatory codes are developed late in the data-collecting process after theoretical ideas from the study have begun to emerge. The explanatory codes are part of the researcher's attempt to unravel the meanings inherent in the situation. These codes connect the data to the emerging theory, and the codes used may be specific to the theory or be more general, such as PATT (pattern), TH (theme), or CL (causal link). Typically, codes will not stay the same throughout the study. Some codes will have to be divided into subclassifications. Other codes may be discontinued because they do not work.

Reflective Remarks

While she or he is recording notes, thoughts or insights often emerge into the researcher's consciousness. These thoughts are generally included within the notes as **reflective remarks** and are separated from the rest of the notes by double parentheses (()). Later, they may need to be extracted and used for memoing (Miles & Huberman, 1994).

Marginal Remarks

As you are reviewing your notes, immediately write down any observations you may have about them. These remarks are usually placed in the right-hand margin of the notes. The remarks often connect the notes with other parts of the data or suggest new interpretations. Reviewing notes can become boring, which is a signal that thinking has ceased. Making **marginal remarks** assists the researcher in "retaining a thoughtful stance" (Miles & Huberman, 1994, p. 65).

Memoing

The researcher develops a memo to record insights or ideas related to notes, transcripts, or codes. **Memos** move the researcher toward theorizing and are conceptual rather than factual. They may link pieces of data together or use a specific piece of data as an example of a conceptual idea. The memo may be written to someone else in the study or may be just a note you make to yourself. The important thing is to value your ideas and get them written down quickly. Whenever an idea emerges, even if it is vague and not well thought out, develop the habit of writing it down immediately. Initially you might feel that the idea is so clear in your mind that you can write it down later. However, you may soon forget the thought and be unable to retrieve it. As you becomes immersed in the data, these ideas will occur at odd times, such as 2 AM, when you are driving, or when you are preparing a meal. Therefore, keep paper and pencil handy. If an idea wakes you up, write it down immediately; it may be gone by morning. Make sure that your memos are dated, titled with the key concept discussed, and connected by codes with the field notes or forms that generated the thoughts (Miles & Huberman, 1994).

Developing Propositions

As the study progresses, relationships among categories, participants, actions, and events will begin to emerge. You will develop hunches about relationships that you can then use to formulate tentative propositions. If the study is being conducted by a team of researchers, everyone involved in the study can participate in the development of propositions. Statements or **propositions** can be written on index cards and sorted into categories or entered into the computer. A working list can then be printed and shared among the researchers to generate further discussion (Miles & Huberman, 1994).

Multimedia Analysis

The purpose of any sort of analysis of transcripts is to ascertain meaning. The type of meaning sought may vary. However, meaning in an interaction is not conveyed totally through the words that are used. The way in which the words were expressed may be critical to the meaning being conveyed. In addition, approximately 70% of communication is nonverbal. As Burnard (1995) wisely pointed out, "often the words used are not particularly relevant or are not 'registered' by the parties involved in a conversation. We do not, after all, usually pick our words very carefully when we speak, nor do we continually 'check each other' to ascertain that understanding has occurred. And yet we do understand one another, most of the time" (full text available in Nursing Collection). In some cases, the words used have little or no meaning. They are used to convey unstated meanings. The meanings are *behind* the words. It may be impossible to capture this meaning by analyzing transcripts. The participant, asked for an exact interpretation of what was meant, may not be able to explain the meaning. Sometimes,

> *words do not convey any meaning at all but instead create a mood.... Sometimes words can be used as "fillers" between pieces of information.... In summary, then, it seems possible that we communicate, using words, in many different ways. First, we may use words precisely and to convey very definite concepts. Second, we may use words to convey or to 'create moods. In this case, we are not conveying particular or precise meanings. Third, it may be that we communicate in chunks of words and phrases. Finally, in this summation, we may note that not everything we*

say is of equal importance—either to ourselves or to the listener. All of these factors make the likelihood of a researcher, using textual data and a method of textual analysis, uncovering the precise meaning of pieces of communication an unlikely scenario. … Transcripts are always post hoc—they always occur after and, sometimes, at some distance from the original interviews. This means that the reader of the transcripts—the researcher—always comes to the transcripts too late. What "really happened" in the interview has been lost. (Burnard, 1995; full text available in Nursing Collection)

One way to address this problem is to use multiple data collection methods. Interviews might be videotaped as well as audiotaped. The researcher might strengthen his or her analysis by simultaneously reviewing video and audio transmissions while reviewing the transcript. Parse (1990) referred to this process as immersion in the data. Multimedia computers are now available in which text, video, graphical media, and sound can be used for such immersion. Burnard (1995) foresees a time when CD-ROM disks might be used to store these multimedia data sets. This type of integrated and triangulated approach to analysis would provide a richer understanding of meaning.

Analysis of Focus Group Data

Historically, content analysis has been used to analyze focus group data. However, data from focus groups are complex in that analysis is required at both the individual level and at the group level, considering interactions among individuals and the group, and making comparisons across groups. It is important to attend to the amount of consensus and interest in topics generated in the discussion. Analysis of deviance and minority opinions is important. Attending to the context within which statements were made is critical to the analysis (Morgan, 1995).

Carey (1995) made the following suggestions regarding analyzing focus group data.

If the unit of analysis is limited to the group, then the evolving interaction of members and the impact on opinions will be unobserved. Because the interaction within the group will affect the data elicited, an appropriate description of the nature of the group dynamics is necessary to incorporate in analysis—for example, heated discussion, a dominant member, little agreement. (p. 488)

It is important in analyzing the data to determine who said what. If only tape-recording is available, this may be a problem. Video recording can help you to obtain this information; if this is not feasible, the cofacilitator can take notes that may provide some information that will help you to make this determination. One useful analysis strategy is to examine all the input of a particular individual and the extent to which this individual's comments influenced the position of other group members. Nonverbal interaction should also be noted. Dominant members of the group may suppress dissonant views that increase the richness of the data. According to Sim (1998):

Certain members of the group may be more assertive or articulate than others, and their views may come to dominate the proceedings; such individuals have been described as "thought leaders." In the process, members of the group who are less articulate may be inhibited from expressing alternative viewpoints. This reflects the tendency of those who find themselves in a minority to acquiesce to the majority view. The effect of this may be that these alternative views are simply not voiced, and those who remain relatively silent are falsely assumed to agree with the prevailing view. Hence, whilst silence may at times indicate agreement, it may also represent an unwillingness to dissent. Skillful questioning by the moderator may assist in distinguishing these two possibilities, and asking participants to write their views down in advance may encourage disclosure from less confident members. This underlies the danger of trying to use the focus group as a measure of consensus…. If a divergence of opinions or perspectives emerges from the data, it is fairly safe to assume that this reflects a corresponding underlying difference of view. However, the converse is not necessarily the case; the absence of diversity in the data does not reliably indicate an underlying consensus. A feeling of consensus or conformity in the data may merely reflect the group dynamics, and say little about the various views held by individual participants. (p. 348)

Generalization from Focus Group Analysis

The common view of focus groups was that they were representative of a target population and thus generalization to the target group was acceptable. However, participants are not obtained using probability sampling, and one is on shaky ground justifying generalization using this argument. The type of person likely to agree to participate in a focus group is probably different from those who decline. The focus group is a carefully constructed environment, with the setting designed to facilitate the group dynamics so that data are generated. The contrived social situation is not a natural one. What a person says in the focus group cannot be assumed to be what the person would say in other settings. Sim (1998) concluded that "it is not clear that any process of analysis can meaningfully separate out from the data the social factors which operate within the context of a focus group—indeed, the very idea of a context-neutral perspective may not even make sense within this sort of epistemological framework" (p. 350). Rather than considering empirical generalization, Sim (1998) recommended theoretical generalization, based on commonalities of the focus group participants with other groups. Different degrees of generalization may be possible based on the extent of commonality.

Displaying Data for Analysis and Presentation

Displays contain highly condensed versions of the outcomes of qualitative research. They are equivalent to the summary tables of statistical outcomes developed in quantitative research and allow the researcher to get the main ideas of the research across succinctly. Strategies for achieving displays are limited only by the researcher's imagination. Some suggested ideas follow. It is relatively easy to develop displays by using computer spreadsheets, graphics programs, or desktop publishing programs. Miles and Huberman (1994) provided helpful guidelines for developing displays of qualitative data. Williamson and Long (2005) described techniques of qualitative data analysis using data displays, including the use of computer packages for making displays.

Critical Incident Chart

In some studies, the researcher, in an effort to gain increased insight into the dynamics of a process, identifies critical incidents occurring in the course of that process. The researcher can then compare these critical incidents in various subgroups of participants. The critical incidents and the subgroups can then be placed in a matrix listing the critical incidents in relation to time. The matrix can make it easier to compare critical incidents in terms of timing and variation across participants or subgroups.

Causal Network

As the data are collected and analyzed, the researcher's understanding of the dynamics involved in the process under study grows. This understanding might be considered a tentative theory. The first tentative theories are vague and poorly pieced together. In some cases, they are altogether wrong. The best way to verify a tentative theory is to share it with others,

particularly informants in the study situation. Informants have their own tentative theories that have never been clearly expressed. The tentative theory needs to be expressed as a map. Developing a good map of the tentative theory is difficult and requires some hard work. The development of a tentative theory and an associated map is presented in Chapter 7.

The validity of predictions developed in a tentative theory must be tested. However, finding effective ways to perform such testing is difficult. Predictions are usually developed near the end of the study. Because the findings are often context specific, the predictions must be tested on the same sample or on a sample that is very similar. One strategy is to predict outcomes expected to occur 6 months after the study has been completed. Six months later, send these predictions to informants who participated in the study. Ask the informants to respond to the accuracy of (1) the predictions and (2) the explanation of why the prediction was expected to occur (Miles & Huberman, 1994).

Cognitive Mapping

Cognitive mapping has been used for analysis and display as an alternative to transcribing taped interview data (Northcott, 1996). The technique might also be used as an adjunct to other approaches to analysis. A cognitive map is a visual representation of the information provided by a participant. It represents the researcher's conceptualizations and interpretations of the participant. The researcher maps the ideas onto a single page, including codes (concepts) and relationships among the codes (similar to the conceptual maps described in Chapter 7), as the researcher listens repeatedly to the taped interview. The interview is not transcribed. The procedure is designed to condense the process of coding, categorizing, and interpreting into one activity. Mapping is performed within 4 days of the interview. For a 45-minute interview, the researcher should allow 3 hours for cognitive mapping. Guidelines for performing cognitive mapping are as follows:

1. Generate field notes immediately after the interview and have them available for the cognitive mapping.
2. Use a large sheet of paper and a black pen (to facilitate photocopying) for the mapping.
3. Listen to the tape without stopping to write comments and rewind the tape.
4. Begin mapping. Start in the center of the paper with a pivotal word (code) and branch out as needed. Listen to the tape repeatedly as you develop the map to ensure that the map accurately reflects the participant's ideas.

5. Consider the data *cognitively*. This process may require formulating codes, establishing relationships (or propositions), and recording nonverbal data. You may need to take breaks to allow time for thought.

6. Keep verbatim quotes from the tape separately and indicate where they emerge on the map.

7. Annotate the map to indicate connections and respondent or researcher input.

8. As a second-level analysis, develop a "macro" map that combines content from all the individual cognitive maps. This map will initiate theory building from the analysis.

Drawing and Verifying Conclusions

Unlike the case in quantitative research, conclusions are formed throughout the data analysis process. Conclusions are similar to the findings in a quantitative study. Miles and Huberman (1994) identified 12 tactics used to draw and verify conclusions.

Counting

Qualitative researchers have tended to avoid any use of numbers. However, when judgments of qualities are made, counting is occurring. The researcher states that a pattern occurs "frequently" or "more often." Something is considered "important" or "significant." These judgments are made in part by counting. If the researcher is counting, it should be recognized and planned. Counting can help researchers see what they have, it can help verify a hypothesis, and it can help keep one intellectually honest. Qualitative researchers work by insight and intuition; however, their conclusions can be wrong. It is easier to see confirming evidence than to see disconfirming evidence. Comparing insights with numbers can be a good method of verification (Miles & Huberman, 1994).

Noting Patterns and Themes

People easily identify patterns, themes, and gestalts from their observations—almost too easily. The difficulty is in seeking real additional evidence of that pattern while remaining open to disconfirming evidence. Any pattern that is identified should be subjected to skepticism—that of the researcher and that of others (Miles & Huberman, 1994).

Seeing Plausibility

Often during analysis, a conclusion is seen as plausible. It seems to fit; it "makes good sense." When asked how one arrived at that point, the researcher may state that it "just feels right." These intuitive feelings are important in both qualitative and quantitative research. However, plausibility cannot stand alone. After plausibility must come systematic analysis. First, intuition occurs and, then, the data are carefully examined to verify the validity of that intuition (Miles & Huberman, 1994).

Clustering

Clustering is the process of sorting elements into categories or groups. It is the first step in inductive theorizing. To cluster objects, people, or behavior into a group, one must first conceptualize them as having similar patterns or characteristics. Clusters, however, like patterns, must be viewed with caution and verified. Alternative ways to cluster may be found that would be more meaningful (Miles & Huberman, 1994).

Making Metaphors

Miles and Huberman (1994) have suggested that qualitative researchers should think and write metaphorically. A metaphor uses figurative language to suggest a likeness or analogy of one kind of idea used in the place of another. Metaphors provide a strong image with a feeling tone that is powerful in communicating meaning. For example, stating rationally and logically that you are in a heavy work situation does not provide the emotional appeal and meaning that you could express by saying, "I am up to my ears in work!" Miles and Huberman also believe that metaphors add meaning to the findings and use the example of a mother's separation anxiety, a phrase "which is less appealing, less suggestive, and less theoretically powerful than the empty nest syndrome" (p. 221). The phrase "empty nest syndrome" communicates images loaded with meaning far beyond that conveyed by the words alone.

Metaphors are also *data-reducing devices* that involve generalizing from the particulars. They are pattern-making devices that place the pattern into a larger context. Metaphors are also effective *decentering devices*. They force the viewer to step back from the mass of particular observations to see the larger picture. Metaphors are also ways of connecting findings to theory. They are what initiates the researcher to think in more general terms. A few suggestions about developing metaphors may be of use: (1) It is unwise to look for metaphors early in the study. (2) To develop metaphors, one must be cognitively playful and move from the denotative to the connotative. Interacting with others in a cognitively playful environment can be useful. (3) Metaphors can be taken too far in terms of meaning; therefore, one must know when to stop.

Splitting Variables

Qualitative research is strongly oriented toward integrating concepts. However, in some cases, researchers must recognize the need for differentiation. They must have the courage to question; Miles and Huberman (1994) have referred to this early integration as premature parsimony. Splitting variables is particularly important during the initial stages of the analysis to allow more detailed examination of the processes that are occurring. It also often occurs with the development of matrices. During theorizing, if the variable does not seem to relate well with the rest of the framework, it may have to be split to allow a more coherent, integrated model to be developed (Miles & Huberman, 1994).

Subsuming Particulars into the General

This process is similar to clustering in that it involves clumping things together. Clustering tends to be intuitive and is similar to coding. Subsuming particulars into the general is a move from the specific and concrete to the abstract and theoretical.

Factoring

The idea of factoring is taken from the quantitative procedure of factor analysis. If you have a list of characteristics, are there general themes within the list that allow you to explain more clearly what is going on? As with factor analysis, when clusters have been identified, they must be named. Factoring can occur at several levels of abstraction in the data. The important consideration is that they make a meaningful difference in clarity (Miles & Huberman, 1994).

Noting Relationships between Variables

Earlier we discussed the development of relationships between variables. However, at this point, it is important to go beyond verifying that a relationship in fact exists; the next step is to explain the relationship. The relationships described in Chapter 7 can be used to describe qualitative findings. Some relationships that might occur are as follows (Miles & Huberman, 1994, p. 257):

1. *A+, B+ (both are high, or both low at the same time)*
2. *A+, B− (A is high, B is low, or vice versa)*
3. *A↑, B↑ (A has increased, and B has increased)*
4. *A↑, B↓ (A has increased, and B has decreased)*
5. *A↑ then→B↑ A↓ (A increased first, then B increased)*
6. *A↑ then → B↑ then A↑ (A increased, then B increased, then A increased some more)*

Finding Intervening Variables

In some cases, the researcher believes that two variables should go together; however, the findings do not verify this thinking. In other cases, two variables are found during data analysis to go together, but their connection cannot be explained. In both these situations, a third variable may be responsible for the confusion. Therefore, the third variable must be identified. The matrices described earlier can help researchers to search for this variable, and the search often requires some careful detective work. Finding an intervening variable is easiest when multiple cases of the two-variable relationship can be examined (Miles & Huberman, 1994).

Building a Logical Chain of Evidence

At first glance, this step would seem to be the same activity described earlier that resulted in the development of a tentative theory; however, this activity assumes the prior development of a tentative theory. Building a logical chain of evidence involves testing that theory. The researcher must go back and carefully trace evidence from the data through development of the tentative theory; the elements, relationships, and propositions of the theory are then tested against new data. The researcher looks for cases that closely fit the theory and for those that clearly do not fit the theory. The theory may then be modified.

This process is referred to as analytical induction and uses two interlocking cycles. The first cycle is enumerative induction, in which a number and variety of instances are collected that verify the model. The second cycle, eliminative induction, requires that the hypothesis be tested against alternatives. The researcher is required to check carefully for limits to generalizability of the theory. The process of constant comparisons used in grounded theory is related to eliminative induction (Miles & Huberman, 1994).

Making Conceptual/Theoretical Coherence

The previous steps have described a gradual move from empirical data to a conceptual overview of the findings. Inferences have been made as the analysis moved from the concrete to the more abstract. The steps then moved from metaphors to interrelationships, then to constructs, and from there to theories. The theory must now be connected with existing theories in the body of knowledge. To accomplish this step, you must become familiar with a wide variety of theories that could explain the current phenomenon. If you can connect the new theory with other theories, it further strengthens the present theoretical explanation (Miles & Huberman, 1994).

Content Analysis

Content analysis is designed to classify the words in a text into a few categories chosen because of their theoretical importance. Because content analysis uses counting, many qualitative researchers do not consider it to be a qualitative analysis technique. Content analysis is frequently used in historical research. It is the primary approach to analysis used by Kalisch and Kalisch (1977); Kalisch, Kalisch, and Belcher (1985); Kalisch, Kalisch, and Young (1983); and Kalisch, Kalisch, and Clinton, J. (1982) in their series of studies examining the image of nursing as reflected in news media and primetime television.

The technique provides a systematic means of measuring the frequency, order, or intensity of the occurrence of words, phrases, or sentences. Initially, the specific characteristics of the content to be measured must be defined, and then the researcher develops rules for identifying and recording these characteristics. The researcher first selects a specific unit of analysis, which may be individual words, word combinations, or themes. This unit of analysis is considered a symbolic entity and often indicates an abstract concept. Downe-Wamboldt (1992, p. 314) pointed out that "content analysis is more than a counting game; it is concerned with meanings, intentions, consequences, and context. To describe the occurrences of words, phrases, or sentences without consideration of the contextual environment of the data is inappropriate and inadequate."

To perform content analysis, text is divided into units of meaning (idea categories). These units are then quantified according to specific rules. Idea categories are constructed and words considered representative of these idea categories are selected; this is a crucial phase of content analysis. In more complex studies, more than one categorizing scheme may be used. One common approach to categorization is the use of a dictionary to identify terms and delineate their meaning (Kelly & Sime, 1990).

In some studies, the researcher is searching for latent meaning within the text. In these studies, the text cannot be analyzed by directly observing or identifying specific terms. The researcher may have to infer meaning by more indirect means, such as by looking for relationships among ideas, reality, and language (Kelly & Sime, 1990).

Narrative Analysis

Narrative analysis is a qualitative means of formally analyzing text including stories. When stories are analyzed, the researcher "unpacks" the structure of the story. A story includes a sequence of events with a beginning, a middle, and an end. Stories have their own logic and are temporal (Coffey & Atkinson, 1996; Denzin, 1989). The structures can also be used to determine how people tell stories, how they give shape to the events that they describe, how they make a point, how they "package" events and react to them, and how they communicate their stories to audiences. The structure used for narrative analysis as identified by Coffey and Atkinson (1996, p. 58) is as follows:

Structure	Question
Abstract	What is this about?
Orientation	Who? What? When? Where?
Complication	Then what happened?
Evaluation	So what?
Result	What finally happened?
Coda	Finish narrative

The abstract initiates the narrative by summarizing the point of the story or by giving a statement of the proposition that the narrative will illustrate. Orientation provides an introduction to the major events central to the story. Complication continues the narrative by describing complications in the event that make it a story; it takes the form "And then what happened?" Evaluation is the point of the narrative, followed by the result, which gives the outcome or resolution of events. The coda ends the story and is a transition point at which talk may revert to other topics.

The narrative analysis can focus on social action embedded in the text or examine the effect of the story. Stories serve a purpose. They may make a point or be moralistic. They may be success stories or may be a reminder of what not to do or how not to be, with guidance on how to avoid the fate described in the story. The purpose of the story can be the starting point for a more extensive narrative analysis. Narrative analysis may examine multiple stories of key life events and gain greater understanding of the impact of these key events; it may help to explain the relationship between social processes and personal lives; and it may be used to elucidate the cultural values, meanings, and personal experiences. Issues related to power, dominance, and opposition can be examined. Through stories, silenced groups can be given voice (Coffey & Atkinson, 1996). You could perform a narrative analysis of Barbara's story under Collecting Stories.

Coding is not used in narrative analysis. Coding breaks data up into separate segments and is not useful in analyzing a story; the researcher can lose the sense that informants are providing an account or narrative of events.

Qualitative researchers may choose to communicate the findings of their study as a story. A story can be a powerful way to make a point. Stories can be presented to readers from a variety of perspectives: chronological order, the order in which the story was originally presented, progressive focusing, focusing only on a critical or key event in the story, describing the plot and characters as one would stage a play, following an analytical framework, providing versions of an event from the stories of several viewers, or presenting the story as one would write a mystery and thus appealing to problem solvers.

Reporting Results

In any qualitative study, the first section of a research report should be a detailed description of the participants, the setting, and observing and experiencing the environment in which the data were gathered. This description should be so vivid that the readers or listeners will feel that they are there with you. To accomplish this goal, the qualitative author must go beyond the skills required for technical writing to creative writing skills. Many qualitative authors suggest that researchers are so eager to get right into the results of data analysis, such as those described in this section, that they pay only brief attention to writing the description. The final part of a qualitative research report should express the theoretical ideas emerging from the data analysis.

RESEARCH METHODOLOGY OF SPECIFIC QUALITATIVE APPROACHES

Historically in qualitative research in nursing, the researcher selected a particular research method for conducting studies. A researcher might spend considerable time becoming familiar with the philosophy and strategies used by that method. These researchers were expected to continue to use this same method throughout their careers. This approach has faded over time and now, qualitative researchers commonly use one method for one study and switch to another method for the next study. In many cases, the researcher will use a mixed collection of strategies from various methods for a study. It is rare now that a study rigidly adheres to a particular method. However, we will present the strategies of each method in their "pure" form as a heuristic.

Phenomenological Research Methods

In phenomenological studies, the researcher can use several strategies for data collection, and it is possible to use combinations of strategies. To conduct these data collection strategies, you will involve your personality and use intuiting. Intuiting is the process of actually looking at the phenomenon. During intuiting, you will focus all awareness and energy on the subject of interest to allow an increase in insight. Thus, this process requires absolute concentration and complete absorption with the experience being studied. Intuiting is a strange idea to those of us in the Western world. It is a more common practice in Eastern thought and is related to meditation practices and the directing of personal energy forces.

Data Collection Strategies

In one data collection strategy, participants are asked to describe verbally their experiences of a phenomenon. These verbal data need to be collected in a relaxed atmosphere, and the respondent must be allowed sufficient time to provide complete description. Alternatively, informants can be asked to provide a written description of their experiences. Ruffing-Rahal (1986) has recommended the use of personal documents, particularly autobiographical accounts, as a source of data.

Another strategy requires that the researcher be more directly involved in the experience. During the participant's experience, the researcher simultaneously observes verbal and nonverbal behavior, the environment, and his or her own responses to the situation. Written notes may be used, or the experience may be tape-recorded or videotaped. When observed behavior is being recorded, the researcher describes rather than evaluates observations.

Several variations may be used to analyze phenomenological data. Porter (1998) clarified the steps of the Husserlian method in Table 23-1. Beck (1994) compared the three methods of Van Kaam, Giorgi, and Colaizzi in Table 23-2. Within nursing, Parse (1990) developed a methodology that is now being used in phenomenological nursing studies.

Van Kaam. Van Kaam (1966) suggested classifying data and ranking the classifications according to the frequency of occurrence. A panel of judges verifies this ranking. The number of categories is then reduced to eliminate overlapping, vague, or intricate categories, and again, agreement of the panel of judges is sought. Hypotheses are developed to explain the categories theoretically, and these hypotheses are tested on a new sample. This process continues until no new categories emerge.

Giorgi. Giorgi (1970) recommended a similar process but prefers to maintain more of the sense of wholeness. Although individual elements of the phenomenon are identified, their importance to the

TABLE 23-1 ■ Husserlian Method	
Step	**Philosophical***
1. Explore the diversity of one's consciousness.	"Each has his place whence he sees the things that are present, and each enjoys accordingly different appearances of the things" (p. 95)
2. Reflect on experiences Choose an experience to study. Develop a phenomenological framework. Specify a research question.	It is through reflection, one of the many spontaneities of consciousness that experiences are "brought under … [the] glance of the Ego [p. 197] [and become] objects for the Ego" (p. 196)
3. Bracket or perform the phenomenological reduction.	"Not a single theorem [should] … be taken from any of the related sciences, nor allowed as premises for phenomenological purposes" (p. 165)
4. Explore the participants' life-world.	Engage in a "thorough inspection, analysis, and description of the life-word as we encounter it" (p. 161)
5. Intuit the structures through descriptive analysis. Perform the eidetic reduction (intuit the principle shared by the facts). Create a taxonomy for the experience: intention, component phenomenon. Create a taxonomy for the context of experience: element, descriptor, and feature.	"We … must strive … to describe faithfully what we really see from our own point of view and after the most earnest consideration" (p. 259) "A living picture of the fruitfulness of phenomenology … can be won only when domain after domain has been actually tramped and the problem-vistas it possesses opened up for all to see" (p. 258)
6. Engage in intersubjective dialogue about the phenomena and contextual features.	To develop a phenomenon fully, two "formations in the constituting of the Thing" (p. 387) are needed: the first formation (reflection, bracketing, and intuiting by the researcher) and the second formation ("the intersubjective identical thing" [p. 387]) to discuss phenomena and "counter-case" (p. 388)
7. Attempt to fill out the phenomena and features. Cycle through reflection, bracketing, and intuiting. Cycle between the first and second formations. Integrate the bracketed material into the analysis.	"The possibility remains of changes in apprehension [but the goal is a] harmonious filling out" (pp. 131, 356) of phenomena
8. Determine uses for the phenomena and features.	"In the end, the conjectures must be redeemed by the real vision of the essential connections" (p. 193)

From Porter, E. J. (1998). On "being inspired" by Husserl's phenomenology: Reflections on Omery's exposition of phenomenology as a method of nursing research. *Advances in Nursing Research, 21*(1), 16–28.

*From Husserl, E., & Gibson, W. R. B. (1962). *Ideas: General introduction to pure phenomenology*, (Trans.). New York: Macmillan (original work published 1913).

phenomenon is not established by the frequency of their occurrence but rather by the intuitive judgment of the researcher. Giorgi considered it important to identify the relationships of the units to each other and to the whole. In Table 23-3, Pallikkathayil and Morgan (1991) illustrated the steps of the Giorgi method of analysis by using examples from their study of suicide attempters.

Colaizzi. Colaizzi (1978) has developed a method that involves observing and analyzing human behavior within its environment to examine experiences that cannot be communicated. This strategy is useful in studying phenomena such as the behavior of preverbal children, subjects with Alzheimer's disease, the combative behavior of an unconscious patient, and the body motion of subjects with new amputations.

Parse. Parse (1990) described a research methodology specific to the man-living-health theory. This methodology involves dialogical engagement, in which the researcher, and respondent participate in an unstructured discussion about a lived experience. The experience is described as an I-Thou intersubjective *being with* the participant during the discussion:

The researcher, in true presence with the participant, engages in a dialogue surfacing the remembered, the now, and the not-yet all at once. Before the dialogue with the participant, the researcher "dwells with" the meaning of the lived experience, centering self in a way to be open to a full discussion of the experience as shared by the participant. The discussion is audio and video tape-recorded (when possible), and the dialogue is transcribed to typed format for the extraction-synthesis process. Extraction-synthesis is a process of moving the descriptions from the language of the participants up the levels of abstraction to the language of science. (Parse, 1990, p. 11)

TABLE 23-2 ■ Comparison of Three Phenomenological Methods

Colaizzi	Giorgi	Van Kaam
1. Read all the subjects' description to acquire a feeling for them.	1. One reads the entire description to get a sense of the whole.	1. Listing and preliminary grouping of descriptive expressions that must be agreed upon by expert judges. Final listing presents percentages of these categories in that particular sample.
2. Return to each protocol and extract significant statements.	2. Researcher discriminates units from the participants' description of the phenomenon being studied. Researcher does this from within a psychological perspective and with a focus on the phenomenon under study.	2. In reduction the researcher reduces the concrete, vague, and overlapping expressions of the participants to more precisely descriptive terms. There again, intersubjective agreement among judges is necessary.
3. Spell out the meaning of each significant statement, known as formulating meanings.	3. Researcher expresses the psychological insight contained in each of the meaning units more directly.	3. Elimination of elements that are not inherent in the phenomenon being studied or that represent a blending of this phenomenon with other phenomena that most frequently accompany it.

4. Organize the formulated meanings into clusters of themes.
  a. Refer these clusters of themes back to the original protocols to validate them.
  b. At this point, discrepancies may be noted among and/or between the various clusters. Researchers must refuse temptation of ignoring data or themes that do not fit.
	4. Researcher synthesizes all the transformed meaning units into a consistent statement regarding the participant's experiences. This is referred to as the structure of the experience and can be expressed on a specific or a general level.	4. A hypothetical identification and description of the phenomenon being studied is written.

5. Results so far are integrated into an exhaustive description of the phenomenon under study.		5. The hypothetical description is applied to randomly selected cases of the sample. If necessary, the hypothesized description is revised. This revised description must be tested again on a new random sample of cases.
6. Formulate the exhaustive description of the investigated phenomenon in as unequivocal a statement of identification as possible.		6. When operations described in previous steps have been carried out successfully, the formerly hypothetical identification of the phenomenon under study may be considered to be a valid identification and description.
7. A final validating step can be achieved by returning to each subject and asking about the findings so far.		

From Beck, C. T. (1994). Reliability and validity issues in phenomenology. *Western Journal of Nursing Research, 16*(3), 254–267.

The researcher contemplates the phenomenon under study while listening to the tape, reading the transcribed dialogue, and viewing the videotape. Thus, the researcher is multisensorily immersed in the data. According to Parse (1990), the details of this process include the following:

1. *Extracting essences from transcribed descriptions (participant's language). An extracted essence is a complete expression of a core idea described by the participant.*
2. *Synthesizing essences (researcher's language). A synthesized essence is an expression of the core idea of the extracted essence conceptualized by the researcher.*
3. *Formulating a proposition from each participant's description. A proposition is a nondirectional statement conceptualized by*

TABLE 23-3 ■ Application of Giorgi's Method of Analysis of Phenomenological Data

Step No.	Theoretical Process	Pragmatic Process Used in Example
One	Reading of the entire disclosure of the phenomenon straight through to obtain a sense of the whole.	Reading and rereading the first three transcripts to look for emerging themes. Establishing the coding process and decision rules for coding.
Two	Rereading the same disclosure again in a purposeful manner to delineate each time that a transition in meaning occurs. This is done with the intention of discovering the essence of the phenomenon under study. The end result is a series of meaning units or themes.	Reading and coding each of the 20 transcripts for themes by each member of the research team. Weekly meetings of the coders to review the coding process and to reach consensus where questions or discrepancies had arisen. Intrarater and interrater reliability was established during this step.
Three	Examining the previously determined meaning units for redundancies, clarification, or elaboration by relating meaning units to each other and to a sense of the whole.	The meaning units or themes were examined and categories were developed that represented a higher level of abstraction. Themes not related to the research questions were categorized appropriately. The result was an extensive listing of data by categories.
Four	Reflecting on the meaning units (still expressed essentially in the language of the subject) and extrapolating the essence of the experience for each subject. Systematic interrogation of each unit is undertaken for what it reveals about the phenomenon under study for each subject. During this process, each unit is transformed into the language of psychological science when relevant.	After reflecting on the categories, such as thoughts, feelings, and responses of the subjects, a narrative capturing the essence of the phenomenon of an encounter with a suicide attempter was formulated for each subject. It was during this time that the true richness of the phenomenological method was realized.
Five	Formalizing a consistent description of the structure of the phenomenon under study across subjects by synthesizing and integrating the insights achieved in the previous steps.	Decisions were made regarding what to accept as the common experience for the phenomenon. Responses offered by 25% or more of the subjects were accepted as the structure of the phenomenon of an encounter with a suicide attempter.

From Pallikkathayil, L., & Morgan, S. A. (1991). Phenomenology as a method for conducting clinical research. *Applied Nursing Research, 4*(4), 197.

the researcher joining the core idea of the synthesized essences from each participant.

4. *Extracting core concepts from the formulated propositions of all participants. An extracted core concept is an idea (written in a phrase) that captures the central meaning of the propositions.*
5. *Synthesizing a structure of the lived experience from the extracted concepts. A synthesized structure is a statement conceptualized by the researcher joining the core concepts. The structure as evolved answers the research question, "What is the structure of this lived experience?" (Parse, 1990, p. 11)*

The results of this analysis are then moved up another level of abstraction to represent the meaning of the lived experience at the level of theory. The findings are interpreted in terms of the principles of the Parse theory.

Outcomes

Findings are often described from the orientation of the participants studied rather than being translated into scientific or theoretical language. For example, the actual words participants use to describe an experience are often used when reporting the findings. The researcher identifies themes found in the data and uses them to develop a structural explanation of the findings.

Descriptions of human experience need to produce a feeling of understanding in the reader. To do so, the author must focus not only on issues related to truth (validity) but also on issues related to beauty (aesthetics). Therefore, the author must communicate in such a way that the reader is presented with both the structure and the texture of the experience (Todres, 1998).

Phenomenological Nursing Study

Bunkers (2007) conducted a phenomenological study titled "The experience of feeling unsure for women at end-of-life." The following is an abstract of the study.

The purpose of this study was to answer the research question, What is the structure of the lived experience of feeling unsure? The participants were 9 women at end-of-life. The Parse research method, a phenomenological-hermeneutic method, was used to discover the structure of feeling unsure. Through the process of extraction-synthesis three core concepts were identified: disquieting apprehensiveness, pressing on, and intimate sorrows. Thus, the lived experience of feeling unsure for these 9 women is disquieting apprehensiveness arising while pressing on with intimate sorrows. The structure provides knowledge about feeling unsure and its connection to health and quality of life. Feeling unsure is discussed in relation to the principles and concepts of human becoming and in relation to how it can inform nursing practice and future research. (p. 56)

Grounded Theory Methodology

Data collection for a grounded theory study is referred to as fieldwork. Participant observation is a commonly used technique. Observation focuses on social interactions within the phenomenon of interest. Interviews may also be conducted to obtain the perceptions of participants. Data are coded in preparation for analysis, which begins with data collection. Stern (1980) and Turner (1981) described the methodology used for grounded theory analysis.

1. *Category development.* Categories derived from the data are identified and named. These categories are then used as codes for data analysis. This process is the beginning stage of the development of a tentative theory.

2. *Category saturation.* Examples of the categories identified are collected until the characteristics of items that fit into the category become clear to the researcher. The researcher then examines all instances of the category in the data to determine whether they fit the emerging pattern of characteristics identified.

3. *Concept development.* The researcher defines the category (now properly referred to as a concept) by using the characteristics verified in step 2.

4. *Search for additional categories.* The researcher continues to examine the data and collect additional data to search for categories that were not immediately obvious but seem to be essential to understand the phenomenon under study.

5. *Category reduction.* Categories, which at this point in the research may have become numerous, are clustered by merging them into higher-order categories.

6. *Search for negative instances of categories.* The researcher continually seeks instances that contradict or otherwise do not fit the characteristics developed to define a category.

7. *Linking of categories.* The researcher seeks to understand relationships among categories. To accomplish this goal, data collection becomes more selective as the researcher seeks to determine conditions under which the concepts occur. The researcher develops hypotheses and tests them with available data or by selecting additional interviews or observations specifically to examine proposed links among the categories. The researcher then develops a narrative of the emerging theory, including the concepts, conceptual definitions, and relationships. She or he rewrites the narrative repeatedly until the emerging theory has been clearly expressed, is logically explained, reflects the data, and is compatible with the knowledge base of nursing. A conceptual map may be provided to clarify the theory (Burns, 1989).

8. *Selective sampling of the literature.* Background and significance of the research question are validated through the literature, and the researcher conducts a brief review of previous research. A more extensive literature review is conducted during the interpretation phase to determine the fit of findings from earlier studies with the present findings and the fit of existing theory with the emerging grounded theory.

9. *Emergence of the core variable.* Through the aforementioned activities, the concept most important to the theory emerges. This concept, or core variable, becomes the central theme or focus of the theory.

10. *Concept modification and integration.* The researcher wraps up the process by finalizing the theory and again comparing it with the data. "As categories and patterns emerge, the researcher must engage in the critical act of challenging the very pattern that seems so apparent. The researcher must search for other, plausible explanations for the data and the linkages among them" (Marshall & Rossman, 1989, p. 119). Sometimes, the fit between the data and the emerging theory is poor. A poor fit can occur when patterns in the data are identified before the researcher can logically fit all the data within the emerging framework. In this case, the relationships proposed among the phenomena may be spurious. Miles and Huberman (1994) have suggested that plausibility is the opiate of the intellectual. If the emerging schema makes good sense and fits with other theorists' explanations of the phenomena, the researcher may lock into it prematurely. Therefore, it is critical to test the schema by rechecking the fit between the emerging theory and the original data.

Zoffmann and Kirkevold (2007) conducted a grounded theory study of relationships and their potential for change developed in difficult type 1 diabetes. The abstract of the study is provided here.

■ *GROUNDED THEORY STUDY*

Few researchers have explored how relationships between patients and providers might change problem solving in clinical practice. The authors used *grounded theory* to study dyads of 11 people with diabetes and poor glycemic control, and 8 nurses interacting in diabetes teams. Relational Potential for Change was identified as a core category that involved three types of relationships. Professionals mostly shifted between less effective relationships characterized by I-you-distant provider dominance and I-you-blurred sympathy. Although rarely seen, a third relationship, I-you-sorted mutuality proved more effective than the others in exploiting the Relational Potential for Change. The three types of relationship differed in (a) scope of problem solving, (b) the roles assigned to the patient and the professionals, (c) use of difficult feelings and different points of view, and (d) quality of knowledge achieved as the basis for problem solving and decision making. The authors discuss implications for practice and further research. (p. 625)

Ethnographical Methodology
Gaining Entrance
One of the critical steps in any study is gaining entry into the area being studied. This step can be particularly sensitive in ethnographical studies. The mechanics of this process may vary greatly, depending on whether you are attempting to gain entrance to another country or into a specific institution. The researcher is responsible for explaining the purposes and methods of the study to those with the power to grant entrance.

Acquiring Informants
To understand the culture, seek out individuals who are willing to interpret the culture for you. These people (usually members of the culture) will not be research subjects in the usual sense of the word, but rather colleagues. You must have the support and confidence of these individuals to complete your research. Therefore, maintaining these relationships is of utmost importance. Not only will the informants answer questions, but they may also help you to formulate the questions because they understand the culture better than you do.

Immersion in the Culture
Ethnographical researchers must become familiar with the culture being studied by living in it (active participation) and by extensive questioning. The process of becoming immersed in the culture involves gaining increasing familiarity with the language, sociocultural norms, traditions, and other social dimensions, including family, communication patterns (verbal and nonverbal), religion, work patterns, and expression of emotion. Immersion also involves the researcher's gradual acceptance into the culture.

Gathering Data (Elicitation Procedures)
The activity of collecting data is referred to as field research and requires taking extensive notes. The quality of these notes will depend on the expertise of the researcher. A skilled researcher experienced in qualitative research techniques will discern more easily what observations need to be noted than will a less experienced researcher or assistant. During observations, you and your research team will be bombarded with information. Intuition plays an important role in determining which data to collect. Although you must be actively involved in the culture you are studying, avoid "going native," which will interfere with both data collection and analysis. In going native, the researcher becomes a part of the culture and loses all objectivity—and with it the ability to observe clearly.

Analysis of Data
Data analysis is essentially the analysis of the field notes and interviews. The notes themselves may be superficial. However, during the process of analysis, you will clarify, extend, and interpret those notes. Abstract thought processes (intuition, introspection, and reasoning, discussed in Chapter 1) are involved in analysis. Interpretations are checked out with the informants. The data are then formed into categories and relationships developed between categories. Patterns of behavior are identified.

Outcomes
The analysis process in ethnography provides detailed descriptions of cultures. These descriptions may be applied to existing theories of cultures. In some cases, the findings may lead to the development of hypotheses, theories, or both. The results are tested by whether another ethnographer, using the findings of the first ethnographical study, can accurately anticipate human behavior in the studied culture. Although the findings are not usually generalized from one culture or subculture to another, a case may be made for some degree of generalization to other similar cultures (Germain, 1986).

Ethnographical Study

Penney and Wellard (2007) conducted an ethnographic study of older consumers' perceptions of participating in their care. The abstract follows.

A study exploring older people's participation in their care in acute hospital settings reveals both consumers' and nurses' views of participation. Using a critical *ethnographic* design, data were collected through participant observation and interviews from consumers in acute care settings who were over 70 years old and nurses who were caring from them. Thematic analysis identified that older people equated participation with being independent. Importantly, consumers highlighted the complexity of the notion of participation when describing situations where they were unable to participate in their own care. The difficulties in communicating with health professionals and an inability to administer their own medications in inpatient settings were identified as barriers to participation. Understanding what consumers believe participation means provides a starting point for developing meaningful partnerships between health professionals and people receiving care. (p. 61)

Historical Research Methodology

The methodology of historical research consists of the following steps: (1) formulating an idea, (2) developing research questions, (3) developing an inventory of sources, (4) clarifying the validity and reliability of data, (5) developing a research outline, and (6) conducting data collection and analysis.

Formulating an Idea

The first step in historical research is selecting a topic. Some appropriate topics for historical research in nursing are "origins, epochs, events treated as units; movements, trends, patterns over stated periods; history of specific agencies or institutions; broad studies of the development of needs for specialized types of nursing; biographies and portrayals of the nurse in literature, art, or drama" (Newton, 1965, p. 20).

As with many types of research, the initial ideas for historical research tend to be broad. Once your initial ideas have been clearly stated and narrowed to a topic that is precisely defined, the time predicted to search for related materials is realistic. In addition to narrowing the topic, it is often important to limit the historical period to be studied. Limiting the period requires a knowledge of the broader social, political, and economic factors that would have an impact on the topic you are studying.

Spend much time extensively reading related literature before making a final decision about the precise topic. For example, Waring (1978) conducted her doctoral dissertation using historical research to examine the idea of the nurse experiencing a "calling" to practice nursing. In the following abstract from that dissertation, she describes the extensive process of developing a precise topic.

Originally my idea was to pursue concepts in the area of Puritan social thought and to relate concepts such as altruism and self-sacrifice to nursing. Two years after the formulation of this first idea, I finally realized that the topic was too broad. Reaching that point was slow and arduous but quite essential to the development of my thinking and the prospectus that developed as an outcome.

When I first began the process, it seemed that I might have to abandon the topic "calling." Now, since the clarification and tightening up of my title and the clarification of my study thesis, I open volumes fearing that I will find yet another reference, once overlooked. It is only recently that I have become convinced that there was a needle in the haystack and that I had indeed found it. (Waring, 1978, pp. 18–19)

In historical research, there frequently is no problem statement. Rather than being defined in a problem statement, the research topic is usually expressed in the title of the study. For example, the title of Waring's dissertation was *American Nursing and the Concept of the Calling*.

Developing Research Questions

After you have clearly defined your topic, identify the questions you will examine during the research process. These questions tend to be more general and analytical than those found in quantitative studies. In the following excerpt, Evans, then a doctoral student, describes the research questions she developed for her historical study.

I propose to study the nursing student. Who was this living person inside the uniform? Where did she come from? What were her experiences as a nursing student? I use the word "experience" in terms of the dictionary definition of "living through." What did she live through? What happened to her and how did she respond, or react, as the case may be? What was her educational program like? We have a pretty good notion of what nurse educators and others thought about the educational program, but what about it from the students' point of view?

What were the functions of rituals and rites of passage such as bed check, morning inspection, and capping?

What kind of person did the nursing student tend to become in order to successfully negotiate studenthood? What are the implications of this in terms of her own personal and professional development and the development of the profession at large? (Evans, 1978, p. 16)

Developing an Inventory of Sources

The next step is to determine whether sources of data for the study exist and are available. Many of the materials needed for historical research are contained within private archives in libraries or are privately owned. One must obtain written permission to gain access to library archives. Private materials are often difficult to ferret out, and when they are discovered, access to them may be a problem. However, Sorensen (1988) believes that the primary problem is the lack of experience of nurse researchers with the use of archival data. Sorensen (1988) and Fairman (1987) have identified the major sources of archival data for historical nursing studies (see Table 4-1). Lusk (1997) also provided an extensive discussion of sources for historical researchers. Lusk suggests that the pleasure of the pursuit for sources should not be underrated. The assistance of a librarian in selecting appropriate indexes is recommended.

Historical materials in nursing, such as letters, memos, handwritten materials, and mementos of significant leaders in nursing, are being discarded because no one recognizes their value. The same is true of materials related to the history of institutions and agencies within which nursing has been involved. Christy (1978, p. 9) observed, "It seems obvious that interest in the preservation of historical materials will only be stimulated if there is a concomitant interest in the value of historical research."

Sometimes, when such material is found, it is in such poor condition that much of the data are unclear or completely lost. In the following excerpt, Christy describes one of her experiences in searching for historical data:

M. Adelaide Nutting and Isabel M. Stewart are two of the greatest leaders we have ever had, and their friends, acquaintances, and former students were persons of tremendous importance to developments in nursing and nursing education throughout the world. Since both of these women were historians, they saved letters, clippings, manuscripts—primary source materials of inestimable value. Their friends were from many walks of life: physicians, lawyers, social workers, philanthropists—supporters and nonsupporters of nursing and nursing interests. Miss Nutting and Miss Stewart crammed these documents into boxes, files, and whatever other receptacles were available and—unfortunately—some of these materials are this very day in those same old boxes.

When I began my research into the Archives in 1966, the files were broken, rusty, and dilapidated. Many of the folders were so old and ill-tended that they fell apart in my hands, the ancient paper crumbled into dust before my eyes. My research was exhilaratingly stimulating, and appallingly depressing at the same time; stimulating due to the gold mine of data available, and depressing as I realized the lack of care provided for such priceless materials. In addition, there was little or no organization, and one had to go through each document, in each drawer, in each file, piece by piece.... The boxes and cartons were worse, for materials bearing absolutely no relationship to each other were simply piled, willy-nilly, one atop the other. Is it any wonder that it took me eighteen months of solid work to get through them? (Christy, 1978, pp. 8–9)

Currently, most historical nursing research has focused on nursing leaders. However, Noel (1988, p. 107) suggested that "women in general are woefully underrepresented in the biographical form." She comments that worthy nurses are those controversial figures who have influenced broad segments of their cultures, although any life well told can help the reader understand and value the individual and his or her contributions. She suggests two prerequisites for selecting a subject: "the biographers' interest, affinity, or fatal fascination for the subject (living or dead) … and the existence and availability of data" (Noel, 1988, p. 107).

Life histories can provide insight into the lives of significant nursing figures. Gathering data for life histories involves collecting the stories and interpretations of the individual being studied. This method allows the individuals to present their views of their lives in their own words. Life histories have been viewed with skepticism because findings are difficult to verify, results are vague, and generalization is limited. In-depth and repeated interviews longitudinally overcome some of these drawbacks, but selective memory of the subject can be problematic. Triangulation of data collection methods and verification with other sources reduce this limitation (Admi, 1995).

Rosenberg (1987) has identified eight areas that are important to examine from a nursing history perspective: (1) history from below—the life of ordinary men and women in nursing, (2) gender and the professions, (3) knowledge and authority, (4) the role of technology, (5) the new institutional history, (6) the hospital as problematic, (7) the nurse as worker, and (8) history as meaning.

There seems to have been no examination of historical patterns of nursing practice. Because so much of nursing knowledge has been transmitted verbally or by role modeling, we as nurses may lose much of the understanding of our roots unless studies are initiated to record them. We have no clear picture of how nursing practice has changed over the years (e.g., when, how, and for what reasons have nursing care patterns changed for individuals experiencing diabetes, cardiovascular disease, surgery, or stroke?). Changes in nursing procedures, such as bed baths, enemas, and the feeding of patients, could be examined. Procedure manuals, policy books, and nurses' notes in patient charts are useful sources for examining changes in nursing practice.

Some possible research questions are as follows:
1. Which nursing practice changes were due to medical actions, and which were nursing innovations?
2. What factors in nursing influence changes in nursing practice?
3. What are the time patterns for changes in practice?
4. Have the time patterns for changes in practice remained fairly consistent, or have they changed over the history of nursing?
5. What has been the influence of levels of education on nursing practice?
6. What has been the influence of advanced nursing practice roles (clinical nurse specialist, nurse practitioner, nurse midwife, nurse anesthetist) on nursing practice?
7. How has the quality of nursing care changed over the past decade? Over the past century?

This type of information might provide greater insight into future directions for nursing practice, research, and theory development. However, to conduct quality historical research, those of us in the process of making history must accept responsibility for preserving the sources.

Historical researchers spend considerable time refining their research questions before they start collecting data. They identify sources of data relevant to the research question. Sources of data are often remote, so the researcher may need to make travel plans to obtain access to the data. In many cases, the researcher must obtain special written permission from the relevant library to obtain access to needed data. The validity and reliability of the data are an important concern in historical research.

Clarifying Validity and Reliability of Data

The validity and reliability concerns in historical research are related to the sources from which data are collected. The most valued source of data is the primary source. A primary source is material most likely to shed true light on the information you are seeking. For example, material written by a person who experienced an event or letters and other mementos saved by the person being studied are primary source material. A secondary source is material written by those who have previously read and summarized the primary source material. History books and textbooks are secondary source materials. Primary sources are considered more valid and reliable than secondary sources:

> *The presumption is that an eyewitness can give a more accurate account of an occurrence than a person not present. If the author was an eyewitness, he is considered a primary source. If the author has been told about the occurrence by someone else, the author is a secondary source. The further the author moves from an eyewitness account, the less reliable are his statements. (Christy, 1975, p. 191)*

Historiographers use primary sources whenever possible.

The historical researcher must consider the validity and reliability of primary sources used in the study. To do so, the researcher uses principles of historical criticism.

One does not merely pick up a copy of Grandmother's diary and gleefully assume that all the things Grandma wrote were the unvarnished facts. Grandmother's glasses may at times have been clouded, at other times rose-colored. The well-prepared researcher will scrutinize, criticize, and analyze the diary before even accepting that Grandma wrote it! Even after the document has been validated, the researcher must make every attempt to uncover bias, prejudice, or just plain exaggeration on Grandmother's part. Healthy skepticism becomes a way of life for the serious historiographer (Christy, 1978, p. 6). Two strategies have been developed to determine the authenticity and accuracy of the source: external and internal criticism.

External criticism determines the validity of source material. The researcher needs to know where, when, why, and by whom a document was written, which may involve verifying the handwriting or determining the age of the paper on which it was written.

Christy (1975) described some difficulties she experienced in establishing the validity of documents:

An interesting problem presented by early nursing leaders was their frugality. Nutting occasionally saved stationery from hotels, resorts, or steamship lines during vacation trips and used it at a later date. This required double checking as to her exact location at the time the letter was written. When she first went to Teachers College in 1907, she still wrote a few letters on Johns Hopkins stationery. I found this practice rather confusing in early stages of research. (Christy, 1975, p. 190)

Internal criticism involves establishing the reliability of the document. The researcher must determine possible biases of the author. To verify the accuracy of a statement, the researcher should have two independent sources that provide the same information. In addition, the researcher should ensure that he or she understands the writer's statements, because words and their meanings change across time and across cultures. It is also possible to read into a document meaning that the author did not originally intend. This shortcoming is most likely to happen when one is seeking a particular meaning. Sometimes, words can be taken out of context (Christy, 1975).

Developing a Research Outline

The research outline is a guide for the broad topics to be examined and also serves as a basis for a filing system for classifying the data collected. For example, you may file data by time period and cross-reference the material for easy access. One piece of data may be filed under several classifications, and you can place a note in one file referring to data stored in another file. The research outline will provide you with a checkpoint during the process of data collection and can be used to help you to identify gaps in the data collection process.

Data Collection

Data collection may require months or years of dedicated searching for pertinent material. Sometimes, one small source may open a door to an entire new field of facts. In addition, data collection has no clear, obvious end. By examining the research outline, the researcher must decide to stop collecting data. Newton (1965) described these facets of data collection.

The search for data takes the researcher into most unexpected nooks and corners and adds facet after facet to the original problem. It may last for months or years or a decade. Days and weeks may be fruitless and endless references may be devoid of pertinent material. Again, one minor reference will open the door to the gold mine of facts. The search becomes more exciting when others know of it and bring possible clues to the investigator. The researcher cultivates persistence, optimism, and patience in his long and sometimes discouraging quest. But one real "find" spurs him on and he continues his search. Added to this skill is the training in the most meticulous recording of data with every detail complete, and the logical classification of the data. (Newton, 1965, p. 23)

Careful attention to note taking is critical. Lusk (1997) provided the following instructions related to note taking:

Note taking begins as the first folder of documents is delivered. Each card or computer entry must clearly identify the archive, the collection, the folder, the file, and the document. References must be correct, for personal integrity, deference to the archivist and other researchers, and for being able to return to the source. In addition to careful note identification, a system of ordering the data by subject greatly facilitates the writing stage; Jensen (1992) suggests using colored pencils or stickers. Kruman (1985) recommends cross-referencing if information is applicable to two subjects.

Whether to take notes on paper, cards, or laptop computers is a matter of personal preference. Paper may be cut into half-sheets and is lighter to carry than cards if notes become extensive. Some researchers use loose-leaf journals, leaving a wide margin for source identification. A computer, used at the discretion of the archivist, may be preferred and some consider it essential for voluminous notes. Hand-held scanners with parallel port interfaces have recently become available for use with laptop computers. Scanners have enormous potential to reduce time and expense, and are safer for fragile documents than photocopiers. Scanners, typically come with text-recognition software to partially automate the note-taking process. Text-based management systems allow users to organize the data following entry. (Lusk, 1997, p. 358)

Analysis of Data

Data analysis involves synthesizing all the data collected. The researcher must sift data and make choices about which to accept and which to reject. Sometimes, interesting data that do not contribute to the questions of the study are difficult to discard. Also, conflicting evidence must be reconciled. For example, if two primary sources give opposite information about an incident, you will need to interpret the differences and determine, as nearly as possible, what actually occurred.

Outcomes

The perspective of the researcher influences interpretations about the outcomes of a historical study inasmuch as competing explanations can be created from the same data set. Evidence for conclusions is always partial because of missing data. Historical interpretation is not about describing the progress of events but about ascribing meaning to them. Thus, the responsibilities of interpreting historical data are great. Lynaugh and Reverby (1987, p. 4) suggested that "historical scholarship is judged on its ability to assemble the best facts and generate the most cogent explanation of a given situation or period."

Developing a Writing Outline

Before proceeding to write the research report, you must decide the most appropriate means of presenting the data. Some options include a biography, a chronology, and a paper organized to focus on issues. If your outline has been well organized and detailed, the writing that follows should flow easily and smoothly.

Writing the Research Report

Historical research reports do not follow the traditional formalized style of much research. The studies are designed to attract the interest of the reader and may appear deceptively simple. An untrained eye may not recognize the extensive work required to write the paper. As Christy explained (1975, p. 192), "The reader is never aware of the painstaking work, the careful attention to detail, nor the arduous pursuit of clues endured by the writer of history. Perhaps that is why so many nurses have failed to recognize historiography as a legitimate research endeavor. It looks so easy."

Example of a Historical Study

Mu and Lin (2007) provided an oral historical study of the development of the discipline of military nursing in Taiwan from 1948 to 1970. The following abstract describes their study.

In an attempt to redress the gap in Chinese nursing and military history, this study aims to provide an understanding of the nature of military nursing development from 1948 to 1970. The National Defense Medical Center (NDMC) was established in 1902 and is recognized as the first military medical school in Chinese history. In 1949, in order to continue her studies, Prof. Fu-I Chao followed the school, when it moved from mainland China to Taiwan. The school's move was a result of the defeat on mainland China of the nationalist government led by Generalissimo Chiang Kai-Shek. The researchers adopted an oral history approach. This consisted of a literature review, the collection of photographs, a review of formal documents and four face-to-face in-depth interviews with Prof. Chao. After data collection, content analysis was performed on the information collected. The study explored the development of the discipline of military nursing in its historical, social, and economic context. Four themes emerged. These were a personal history of experience and growth, the foundation phase of nursing, the developmental phase of nursing, and the historical developments and trends in nursing. Prof. Chao's comments reveal how the students missed their parents and families, the special friendships among them, and the love and care that they received from Chief Mei-Yu Chow and Director Chih-Teh Loo. Tribute is paid to their resilience in the face of hardship, and their industry during the initial development of the nursing profession. The results also provide the suggestions of creating a history of health-care that privileges new meanings about military nursing's past and worth. (p. 117)

Another recently published historical study of significance is Benedict and Georges (2006) study of nurses' involvement in the sterilization experiments of Auschwitz.

The medical experiments conducted on non-consenting prisoners of Nazi concentration camps during World War II necessitated the codification of principles to protect human subjects of research. Auschwitz was the largest and one of the most infamous of the camps and the site of numerous "medical" experiments. This historical study uses primary source documents obtained from archives in England and Germany to describe one type of experiment carried out at Auschwitz—the sterilization experiments. The purpose of these experiments was to perfect a technique in which non-Aryans could be prevented from reproducing while still being able to work as slave laborers. These narratives regarding the sterilization experiments at Auschwitz are remarkable in that they contain previously undocumented information regarding the voluntary and involuntary involvement of nurses. Following these narratives, a discussion of ethics in relation to the Holocaust is presented with a specific focus on the work of Agamben. Implications of the Auschwitz narratives for the application of codes of ethical principles and contemporary nursing are discussed from a postmodernist perspective. (p. 277)

Philosophical Studies

The purpose of philosophical research is to clarify meanings, make values manifest, identify ethics, and study the nature of knowledge (Ellis, 1983). A philosophical researcher is expected to consider a philosophical question from all perspectives by examining conceptual meaning, raising further questions, proposing answers, and suggesting the implications of those answers. The data source for most philosophical studies is written material and verbally expressed ideas relevant to the topic of interest. The researcher critically examines the text or the ideas for flaws in logic. A key element of the analysis is the posing of philosophical questions. The data are then searched for information relevant to the question. Ideas or values implied in the text are an important source of information because many philosophical analyses address abstract topics. The researcher attempts to maintain an objective distance from perspectives in the data so that the logic of the idea can be abstractly examined. Ideas, questions, answers, and consequences are often explored, debated, or both with colleagues during the analysis phase.

Three types of philosophical studies are foundational inquiry, philosophical analyses, and ethical analyses.

Foundational Inquiries Methodology

Foundational inquiries are critical and exploratory. The researcher asks questions that reveal flaws in the logic with which the ideas of the science were developed. These flaws may be ambiguities, discrepancies, or puzzles in the way those within the science speak, think, and act. Generally, those within the science do not see this knowledge as having logic problems. The knowledge questioned could be in the form of ideas, concepts, facts, theories, or even various sorts of experiences and ways of doing things (Manchester, 1986). For example, one might question whether adaptation is a desired outcome of nursing action consistent with nursing's definition of health.

Outcomes. Foundational studies provide critical analyses of ideas and thought within a discipline and thereby facilitate further development of the body of knowledge. The critique of studies within the science is guided by the outcomes of foundational studies and entails the use of five traditional criteria for scientific thinking: accuracy, consistency, scope, simplicity, and fruitfulness (Manchester, 1986).

Example of a Foundational Study. By far, the best-known foundational inquiry in nursing is Carper's (1978) study of the ways of knowing in nursing. This study was her doctoral dissertation, and only a portion of it has been published. In conducting the study, Carper examined nursing textbooks and journals from 1964 to 1974. She identified four ways of knowing in nursing: empirical, aesthetic, personal, and ethical.

Philosophical Research

The primary purpose of philosophical analysis is to examine meaning and to develop theories of meaning. This objective is usually accomplished through concept analysis or linguistic analysis (Rodgers, 1989). Concept analyses have become common exercises for graduate nursing students, although most have not been performed with philosophical research strategies. Many of them have been published and are providing an important addition to the body of knowledge in nursing. One of the best-known analyses, Smith's (1986) idea of health, was performed by philosophical inquiry.

Example of Philosophical Inquiry. Smith searched the literature for fundamental concepts on the nature of health. Regardless of how health was defined, it was considered one extreme on a continuum of health and illness. Health was a relative term. A person was judged healthy when measured against some ideal of health. Who was considered healthy was based on the particular ideal of health being used. Smith identified four models (or ideals) of health: the eudaimonistic model, the adaptive model, the role performance model, and the clinical model. This analysis has proved useful in exploring many issues related to nursing, including differing expectations of clients in relation to their health. An instrument has been developed to put this concept into operation and will allow it to be examined in relation to a number of variables important to nursing (Smith, 1986).

Ethical Analysis

In ethical inquiry, the researcher identifies principles to guide conduct that are based on ethical theories. Problems in ethics are related to obligation, rights, duty, right and wrong, conscience, justice, choice, intention, and responsibility. An analysis using a selected ethical theory is performed. The actions prescribed by the analysis may vary with the ethical theory used. The ideas are submitted to colleagues for critique and debate. Conclusions are associated with rights and duties rather than preferences.

Example of Ethical Analysis. Happ et al. (2007) conducted an ethical analysis of communication with patients related to ethical decision making during prolonged mechanical ventilation. Their abstract follows.

We describe patterns of communication of patients involved in health-related decision making during prolonged mechanical ventilation (PMV). Data were collected using observation, interview, and record review.

Twelve of 30 patients participated in decisions about initiating, withdrawing, and withholding life-sustaining treatment, surgery, artificial feeding, financial/legal issues, discharge care, and daily care procedures. Patient involvement was largely validation or confirmation of what clinicians and families had already decided. Patients' participation was enlisted by clinicians and family members even when the patients did not exhibit full decisional capacity. Patient involvement in health-related decisions during prolonged critical illness is a shared and negotiated process that requires continued empirical study and *ethical analysis*. (p. 361)

Critical Social Theory Methodology

Three means of collecting data for a critical social theory study may be used: verbal or written questions posed to individuals or groups, observation, or use of written documents. Data may be quantitative or qualitative and include numbers and stories. Methods are selected that are expected to yield the most compelling evidence, which is most likely to be a combination of stories and numbers. This strategy may use one of three basic approaches:

1. *Numbers foreground, stories background.* These studies are primarily quantitative with a lesser qualitative focus. Use this approach when the purpose of the study is to influence those in positions of power and the general public who are most likely to be influenced by "hard evidence" (numbers). In this case, stories are used to "put a face" on the numbers so that the intended audience can hear the voices of the participants and consider the meaning of the numbers.
2. *Stories foreground, numbers background.* These studies are primarily qualitative with a lesser quantitative focus. The purpose of these studies is to provide opportunities for researchers and participants to engage in dialogue, reflection, and critique in relation to the phenomenon being studied. Telling a story enables the participants to name their reality and explore strategies for changing that reality. Emphasis is on personal change, growth, and empowerment. However, problems and concerns of individuals do not occur in isolation and are often beyond the control of the individual. Lasting changes must occur on many levels.
3. *Stories and numbers with equal emphasis.* A research program fostering individual empowerment and system change may use a full range of methods and types of data. This approach

might include a combination of standardized instruments and various interview techniques. Use these data to specify a theory, establish the prevalence of a phenomenon, explore the context of a phenomenon, test a nursing intervention, or any combination of these objectives (Berman et al., 1998).

The research process of critical social theory requires that researchers use oppositional thinking to perform a critique of the social situation under study by applying the following four steps: (1) critical examination of the implicit rules and assumptions of the situation under study in a historical, cultural, and political context; (2) use of reflection to identify the conditions that would make uncoerced knowledge and action possible; (3) analysis of the constraints on communication and human action to develop a theoretical framework that uses causal relationships to explain distortions in communications and repression, the theoretical framework is then tested against individual cases (Hedin, 1986); and, finally, (4) participation in dialogue with those oppressed individuals within the social situation. Dialogue raises the collective consciousness and identifies ways to take action against oppressive forces. The action for change must come from the groups and communities rather than from the researcher. The groups and communities must consider "(a) their common interests; (b) the risks they are willing to undergo; (c) the consequences they can expect; and (d) their knowledge of the circumstances of their own lives" (Hedin, 1986, p. 146).

As with most qualitative research methodologies, it is difficult to separate the steps. Dialogue is used both to collect and to interpret the data, and researchers constantly move back and forth between collection and interpretation. Dialogue, which uses some of the techniques of phenomenology, includes conversations between the researcher and persons within the society and requires a relationship of equality and active reciprocity. In addition, by reflection and insight, the researcher dialogues with the data while collecting, analyzing, and interpreting it. "New meanings emerge, and phrases that have always been ignored suddenly come alive and demand explanation" (Thompson, 1987, p. 33). The process "exposes ways in which the self has been formed (or deformed) through the influence of coercive power relations. The work of critical scholarship is to make these power relations transparent, for these relations lose power when they become transparent" (Thompson, 1987, p. 33). Knowledge is created, and this knowledge furthers autonomy and responsibility by enlightening individuals about how they may rationally act to realize their own best interests (Holter, 1988).

Example of a Critical Social Theory Study

Cueto (2004) conducted a critical social theory analysis of the origins of primary health care and selective primary health care in Latin America. The abstract follows.

I present a historical study of the role played by the World Health Organization and UNICEF in the emergence and diffusion of the concept of primary health care during the late 1970s and early 1980s. I have analyzed these organizations' political context, their leaders, the methodologies and technologies associated with the primary health care perspective, and the debates on the meaning of primary health care. These debates led to the development of an alternative, more restricted approach, known as selective primary health care. My study examined library and archival sources; I cite examples from Latin America. (p. 1864)

Feminist Research Methodology

Purpose. The purpose of feminist research is transformational and directed at social structures and social relationships, including logical arguments (Rafael, 1997).

Review of Literature. The review of literature focuses on a search for evidence of the relationship between power and knowledge. For example, who decides what counts as knowledge? How is power produced? What resistance to power exists? Whose interests are silenced, marginalized, or excluded? How open is power to change (Rafael, 1997)?

Participant-Researcher Relationships. The feminist method requires a leveling of the usual power imbalance between researcher and participant. The perspective of participants is considered primary, yet they are assisted in gaining some distance from their views. The method promotes a balance between objectivity and subjectivity (Rafael, 1997).

Methods of Inquiry. Feminist research methods include a broad range of quantitative and qualitative methods. Qualitative methods commonly used in feminist research include narratives, advocacy, oral history, and textual analyses.

Example of Critical Social Theory (Feminist) Study

Ismail, Berman, and Ward-Griffin (2007) conducted a feminist study of dating violence. An abstract is provided here.

Dating violence is a significant public health problem in the lives of young women. Their age, in conjunction with perceived pressures to engage in intimate relationships, makes these women particularly vulnerable to dating violence. The pressures to be in relationships can be intense and therefore may add to young women's willingness to overlook, forgive, or excuse the violence that is occurring. The authors' purposes in this feminist study were to examine the experience of dating violence from young women's perspectives; investigate how contextual factors shape their experiences; examine how health is shaped by these experiences; and explore ways that dating violence is perpetuated and normalized in young women's lives. Findings revealed that family environment and gender are critical in shaping young women's experiences. The participants described a range of physical and emotional health problems and perceived few sources of support. Their efforts to obtain support were often met with skeptical and dismissive attitudes on the part of health care providers and other trusted adults. Recommendations for health care practice, education, and research are presented. (p. 453)

QUALITATIVE RESEARCH ISSUES
Theoretical Frameworks

It has been the position of qualitative researchers that they do not use theoretical frameworks as do quantitative researchers. In some cases, theory was developed as an emerging part of the analysis process. Two recent texts are changing that stance by arguing that atheoretical research is impossible. Flinders and Mills (1993), in their text *Theory and Concepts in Qualitative Research*, first addressed the issue saying, "Few of us now claim that we enter the field tabula rasa, unencumbered by notions of the phenomena we seek to understand" (p. xi). Anfara and Mertz (2006) in their text *Theoretical Frameworks in Qualitative Research*, stated that "no comprehensive discussion of theoretical frameworks exists to assist those engaged in qualitative research" (p. xiii). Their goal is to describe what a theoretical framework is and how it is used in qualitative research as well as the effects it has on the qualitative research process. Each chapter in their text offers the framework of a qualitative researcher as a guide for qualitative researchers as they develop frameworks.

The framework development process for qualitative studies is not unlike that described in Chapter 7 of this text. The role that theory plays in qualitative research will likely differ from that of quantitative research. Some qualitative researchers may refer to a theoretical stance, whereas others may not be quite ready to take the leap to frameworks. Strategies for using frameworks to guide the development of qualitative studies, and in the interpretation of results, are not yet clear. It will be interesting to see how the move to frameworks in qualitative research plays out over the next few years.

Researcher-Participant Relationships

One of the important differences between quantitative and qualitative research is the nature of relationships between the researcher and the individuals being studied. The nature of these relationships has an impact on the data collected and their interpretation. In many qualitative studies, the researcher observes social behavior and may participate in social interactions with those being studied. Four types of participant observation are commonly distinguished: (1) complete participation, in which the observer becomes a member of the group and conceals the researcher role; (2) participant as observer, in which participants are aware of the dual roles of the researcher; (3) observer as participant, in which most of the researcher's time is spent observing and interviewing and less in the participation role; and (4) complete observer, in which the researcher is passive and has no direct social interaction in the setting. You must carefully consider the type(s) of researcher-participant relationships that you will use in your study and specify them when describing your methodology.

In varying degrees, the researcher influences the individuals being studied and, in turn, is influenced by them. The mere presence of the researcher may alter behavior in the setting. Although this involvement is considered a source of bias in quantitative research, qualitative researchers consider it to be a natural and necessary element of the research process. The researcher's personality is a key factor in qualitative research as skills in empathy and intuition are cultivated. You will need to become closely involved in the subject's experience to interpret it. It is necessary to be open to the perceptions of the participants rather than attaching your own meaning to the experience. Individuals being studied often participate in determining research questions, guiding data collection, and interpreting results. Watts (2006) described challenges in feminist research when researching women who do not identify with feminist aims. She discussed the impact the insider researcher role has on "truth telling." She pointed out that there is a fine line between empathy and exploitation. Dickson-Swift, James, Kippen, and Liamputtong (2006) conducted a study examining the blurring of boundaries between the researcher and the participants. Many researchers conducting research in sensitive areas found themselves becoming friends

with the participants. Poor boundary management adds stress to research work. A number of researchers described emotional exhaustion and feeling overwhelmed. The authors recommend that you develop protocols for studies of sensitive areas before initiating the study. Training is also recommended for managing boundary issues before commencing such studies.

The interface between the participant-observer role and the nurse role of the researcher is a concern. Because of the possible impact of the nursing role on the study, Robinson and Thorne (1988) claimed that the nurse researcher has an obligation to explain in the study report the influence that his or her professional perspective had on the process and outcomes of the study. In some studies, the researcher is expected to interact with participants but to stay in the role of researcher and avoid relating to participants as a nurse. Some insist that the nurse researcher must always relate first as a nurse and second as a researcher (Cooper, 1988; Fowler, 1988). Connors (1988) suggested that qualitative researchers must be authentic and engaged as a whole person rather than just as a researcher or as a nurse. Colbourne and Sque (2005) pointed out that nurse researchers, while in the role of qualitative researcher, "may offer the participant a mechanism for reflection, greater self-awareness, finding a voice, obtaining information, and venting repressed emotions." Positive and negative aspects of this therapeutic component are explored along with cautions that the nurse researcher think carefully about the stance taken in the field.

In addition to the role you will take in the relationship, carefully consider the expectations of your study. Munhall (1988) pointed out that ethically, it is essential that the qualitative researcher think through both the aims and the means of the study and determine whether these aims and means are consistent with those of the participants. For example, if your desire as a researcher is to change the behavior of the participants, the participants need to share this goal. During the study, a level of trust develops between the researcher and the participant, who may provide information labeled as secret. Establishing relationships with participants, however, can cause harm. Participant observation requires a close relationship that invades the privacy of the individual. Although participants may experience confidence, commitment, and friendship from the encounter, they may also experience disappointment, perceived betrayal, and desertion as the researcher functions in the researcher role and then leaves (Munhall, 1988). The relationship can also harm the researcher. Cowles (1988) described emotional pain and difficulty sleeping as she collected data from family members of murdered individuals. She frequently required support and opportunities to explore her feelings with colleagues during the process. Draucker (1999) cautioned that little is known about the effects on participants in studies of sexual violence.

Participatory Research

In some qualitative studies, participants partner with the researchers in planning and conducting the study. This is referred to as participatory research. The method began in ethnographical research and is now being used in some quantitative and outcome studies as well.

Participatory research is a strategy designed to include representatives of the community under study as members of the research team. It allows members of the community to have a voice in the way the study is conducted and the results that are disseminated. The strategy also serves as a check on the researchers' biases and makes the scientific community directly accountable to the client communities. Commonly, issues related to imbalances in power between the researchers and the community representatives must be addressed.

In vulnerable populations, suspicion of researchers is prevalent. Many people fear being misused. Establishing and maintaining trust is the ongoing key to success. In a participatory research project, the partnership leads to the researchers and the people being studied being involved in all phases of the research process. Questions of immediate concern to the community may be added to the research program. Through dialogue, the researchers often gain new insights into the problem under study, as well as interventions that might be effective in addressing the problem. Change is one of the primary purposes of the project (Henderson, 1995; Seng, 1998).

Friere, a Brazilian scholar whose ideas were described in Chapter 4, originated participatory research strategies. The methods used to promote social change are those of critical social theory as described in Chapter 4. Participatory studies include a variety of designs, some qualitative, some quantitative, and some a triangulated mix of strategies. Some of the strategies that might be used in a participatory research project were described in more detail in Chapter 13, which describes another new paradigm in research, intervention research.

Mullings et al. (2001) used participatory research methods in their study of reproductive experiences in Harlem. The following quotes from this excellent study on a topic difficult to examine sheds light on how to implement participatory research methods.

We used four approaches for organizing community participation: 1) recruitment of organizations and researchers with longstanding relationships and commitment to the community, 2) development of a community advisory board, 3) community dialogue groups, and 4) community meetings.

The New York Urban League was chosen as the general contractor for the Harlem Birth Right Project because of its long-term links with the Harlem community and its involvement in a number of other health-related projects, including overseeing the Harlem Healthy Start program. In addition, all four principal investigators had long histories of residence, activism, or work in Harlem.

■ *DEVELOPMENT OF A COMMUNITY ADVISORY BOARD*

To involve a broad cross-section of the community, the research team established a 24-member Community Advisory Board (CAB). This Board was composed of Harlem residents, who met quarterly with the researchers throughout the 4-year research period. In constituting the CAB, the researchers attempted to make it representative of the socioeconomic, occupational, gender, religious, age, and ethnic heterogeneity of Central Harlem. To operationalize this, CAB members were recruited from community organizations, unions, youth programs, and service organizations, and participated as individuals and not as representatives of their organizations. Some members were unaffiliated persons encountered in the course of fieldwork. The CAB actively participated in all phases of the research, including designing and facilitating the research (e.g., selection of the research sites, and development of the focus groups and the ethnographic questionnaire), facilitating research contracts and entry into research sites, representing the project at various public functions, serving as resources in the hiring of personnel (e.g., interviewers) from the community, and helping develop strategies for public dissemination of the project objectives and results. Furthermore, the CAB maintained continuous dialogue with the researchers, providing insight into research problems on the basis of their experiences as long-term residents or workers in Harlem.

■ *COMMUNITY DIALOGUE GROUPS*

In addition to the CAB, several Community Dialogue Groups (CDGs) of 5–10 persons each were convened during the active field research to discuss specific issues, such as selection of the sites for intensive ethnographic data collection, selection and recruitment of longitudinal participants, focus group criteria, structure and content of the ethnographic questionnaire, and improved community participation. The CDGs allowed the researchers to involve an even broader group of Harlem residents in the Project, to discuss specific issues in greater depth and to avoid overburdening the CAB members.

■ COMMUNITY MEETINGS

Additional participation was elicited through two general community meetings open to the public, which were held to provide information about the Harlem Birth Right Project and to solicit advice. Moreover, ethnographers provided persons at all participant observation sites and public meetings with detailed explanations about the research.

■ OPERATIONALIZING QUALITATIVE RESEARCH

In collaboration with the CAB and the CDG, the researchers developed an ethnographic research design with four components: participant observation, longitudinal case studies, focus groups, and ethnographic questionnaire. A thorough literature review and pilot fieldwork were conducted over the 6 months prior to initial data collection. Analysis of media reports, archival information, public documents, and academic literature was undertaken throughout the research to situate the Harlem data in a broader social and political context. (Mullings et al., 2001, pp. 86–87)

In this Project, community participation was critical to achieving new theoretical and methodological insights, and assisted in the ways in which material was prepared for presentation to the community. As many proponents have pointed out, community participation has an important role to play in facilitating access, trust, and implementation. But the incorporation of community participation also has real implications for addressing biases in traditional public health and social science research. (Mullings et al., 2001, p. 91)

Reflexivity

Qualitative researchers need to critically think through the dynamic interaction between the self and the data occurring during analysis. This interaction occurs whether the data are communicated person to person or through the written word. The critical thinking used to examine this interaction is referred to as **reflexive thought** or **reflexivity** (Lamb & Huttlinger, 1989). During this process, the researcher explores personal feelings and experiences that may influence the study and integrates this understanding into the study. The process requires a conscious awareness of self.

Drew (1989), in a paper recounting her experience conducting a phenomenological study of caregiving behavior, demonstrated reflexivity as she described the impact of relationships on her study.

A session with a person who had been willing to talk about his or her experiences with caregivers, and who had invested energy into the interview session, often generated for me a sense of doing something worthwhile, as well as a feeling that I would be competent to analyze the transcribed material in a meaningful way. This sense of competency dispelled any doubts about being an intruder. I became relaxed, unself-conscious, and more self-assured. However, an encounter with a person with blunt affect, abrupt answers, and a paucity of responses left me feeling awkward and self-conscious. A sense of doubt about the validity of my project encroached as I attempted to elicit that person's thoughts. At the time, my immediate reaction was to think that I had obtained nothing from these individuals, when in fact, as I was to discover later, the "nothing" was something important that I was as yet unable to see.

It was at the point of discouragement about my interviewing skills that I became aware that I was mentally classifying interviews as either "good" or "bad," depending on my emotional response to the subjects. Good interviews were those in which I felt effective as an interviewer and was able to facilitate the person's recounting of experiences with caregivers. I enjoyed the interaction and felt that we connected on some level that produced meaningful discussion about the topic of relationships between patient and caregiver.

Bad interviews, on the other hand, were those in which I could not seem to get subjects to talk about how they had experienced their caregivers. There seemed to be no questions that I could devise with which to explore feelings, either positive or negative, with them. They gave no indications of awareness of their feelings, or of feelings in others. Whereas the subjects of the good interviews were people I experienced as open, curious, and thoughtful, those of the bad interviews were experienced as distrustful and elicited in me a sense of anxiety and frustration; it seemed I could not get through to them. I felt inadequate as an interviewer and was ready to discard these interviews. Frustration and anxiety arose because I felt that I was not getting the information that I needed for the study.

Subsequently, I discovered that my feelings of frustration and inadequacy were causing me to overlook data and that when I could put them aside, new data that were rich in meaning became apparent. ... This discovery was a powerful experience for me, affecting my approach to subsequent interviews and influencing analysis of data thereafter. (Drew, 1989, pp. 433–434)

In some phenomenological research, this critical thinking leads to bracketing, which researchers use to avoid misinterpreting the phenomenon as the individual experiences it. **Bracketing** is suspending or laying aside what is known about the experience being studied (Oiler, 1982). Researchers using the Husserl interpretation of phenomenology most commonly use bracketing. Other phenomenologists, especially those using Heideggerian phenomenology, do not believe bracketing is possible. However, they do identify beliefs, assumptions, and preconceptions about the research topic, which are put in writing at the beginning of the study for self-reflection and external review. These procedures are intended to facilitate openness and new insight.

Most researchers inexperienced in qualitative research require mentoring in reflexive thought. Part of this mentoring is developing a plan for reflexive thought during the conduct of the study. Dialogue with the mentor(s) during the study about the researcher's experiences and reactions during the study and their implications are also critical. Walsh and Downe (2006), in developing criteria for appraising the quality of qualitative research, developed the following criteria for judging reflexivity. These criteria are especially helpful for students who seem to have difficulty grasping the idea of reflexivity.

Criteria for Judging Reflexivity

Walsh and Downe provide criteria for evaluating the presence and quality of reflexivity in a qualitative study.

> *Discussion of relationship between researcher and participants during fieldwork*
>   *Demonstration of researcher's influence on stages of the research process*
> *Evidence of self-awareness/insight*
>   *Documentation of the effects of the research on researcher*
>   *Evidence of how problems/complications were dealt with (Walsh & Downe, 2006, p. 115)*

Auditability

The larger scientific community has in some cases seriously questioned the credibility of qualitative data analysis. The concerns relate to the inability to replicate the outcomes of a study, even when using the same data set. Miles and Huberman (1994) described the problem as follows.

Most qualitative researchers work alone in the field. Each is a one-person research machine: defining the problem, doing the sampling, designing the instruments, collecting the information, reducing the information, analyzing it, interpreting it, writing it up. A vertical monopoly. And when we read the reports, they are most often heavy on the "what" (the findings, the descriptions) rather than on the "how" (how you got to the "what"). We rarely see information that displays the data—only the conclusions. In most cases, we don't see a procedural account of the analysis, explaining just how the researcher got from 500 pages of field notes to the main conclusions drawn. So we don't know how much confidence we can place in them. Researchers are not being cryptic or obtuse. It's just that they have a slim tradition to guide their analytic moves, and few guidelines for explaining to their colleagues what they did, and how. (Miles & Huberman, 1994, p. 262)

To respond to this concern, some qualitative researchers have attempted to develop strategies by which other researchers, using the same data, can follow the logic of the original researcher and arrive at the same conclusions. Guba and Lincoln (1982) referred to this strategy as auditability.

Auditability requires that the researcher establish decision rules for categorizing data, arriving at ratings, or making judgments. A decision rule might say, for example, that a datum would be placed in a specific category if it met specified criteria. Another decision rule might say that an observed interaction would be considered an instance of an emerging theoretical explanation if it met specific criteria. A record is kept of all decision rules used in the data analysis. All raw data are stored so that they are available for review if requested. As the analysis progresses, the researcher documents the data and the decision rules on which each decision was based and the reasoning that entered into each decision. Thus, evidence is retained to support the study conclusions and the emerging theory and is made available on request (Burns, 1989). Marshall (1984, 1985), however, cautioned against undermining the strengths of qualitative research by overly mechanistic data analysis. Marshall and Rossman (1989, p. 113) expressed concern that efforts to increase validity will "filter out the unusual, the serendipitous—the puzzle that if tended to and pursued would provide a recasting of the entire research endeavor."

If you intend to use auditability strategies, plan for auditability before you begin collecting data, because analysis is initiated at that point. You should include these plans in your research proposal.

Appraisal of Qualitative Studies

Synthesis of studies in preparation for evidence-based practice has, until recently, focused entirely on quantitative research. Qualitative research has been left out of the equation, not considered sufficiently relevant to evidence-based practice to be included.

This decision has serious implications for the contribution of qualitative knowledge to clinical practice. Funding of studies, funding of educational programs, and valuing of qualitative knowledge is determined by the inclusion of these studies in the evidence base for practice. A small group of qualitative scholars have been working to persuade those in decision-making positions to include qualitative research in the studies examined for inclusion in evidence-based practice reports. A book describing their work, *Handbook for Synthesizing Qualitative Research* (Sandelowski & Barroso, 2007), is an excellent guide for qualitative researchers working in the teams to synthesize qualitative studies for inclusion of the evidence base. Of particular interest to a broader group of users, faculty, and students interested in qualitative research is a chapter titled "Appraising Reports of Qualitative Studies." This chapter provides a detailed guide to the appraisal of individual qualitative studies and to the comparative appraisal of qualitative studies. This book takes the art of writing a qualitative research report and the application of findings well beyond auditability to a whole new level of analysis. We recommend it to students, faculty, and researchers who are invested in qualitative research.

SUMMARY

- Qualitative data analysis occurs concurrently with data collection rather than sequentially as is true in quantitative research.
- Methods of data collection include unstructured observations, unstructured interviews, focus groups, collecting stories, constructing life stories, and case studies.
- Some qualitative researchers use the computer for data analysis, whereas others perform their analysis manually.
- Data are often transcribed from tape recordings to typed manuscripts before analyses.
- After the analyses, a variety of methods are used to display data for analyses and presentation, including critical incident charts, causal networks, and cognitive mapping.
- Methods of analyzing the data may include content analysis and narrative analysis.
- Six research methodologies for qualitative studies are described: phenomenological, grounded theory, ethnographical, historical, philosophical, and critical social theory including feminist approaches.
- Although theoretical frameworks have not traditionally been used in qualitative studies, some researchers are beginning to include frameworks in their studies.

- Research-participant relationships are critical to the effective conduct of qualitative studies and are explored in the chapter.
- Participatory research, which began in ethnographical studies, is emerging as an important approach in both qualitative and quantitative studies.
- Reflexivity, in which the qualitative researcher critically thinks through the dynamic interaction between the self and the data, is an important element of qualitative studies.
- Auditability requires the researcher to establish decision rules for categorizing data, arriving at ratings, and making judgments so that another qualitative researcher, using the same data, can follow the logic of the first researcher and arrive at similar conclusions.
- Appraisal of qualitative studies is a newly developing strategy that provides methods to synthesize relevant qualitative studies so that qualitative findings can be included in evidence-based practice documents.

REFERENCES

Admi, H. (1995). The life history: A viable approach to nursing research. *Nursing Research, 44*(3), 186–188.

Alvesson, M. (2002). *Postmodernism and social research.* Buckingham: Open University Press.

Anderson, N. L. R. (1987). Computer-assisted analysis of textual field note data. *Western Journal of Nursing Research, 9*(4), 626–630.

Anfara, V. A. Jr., & Mertz, N. T. (2006). *Theoretical frameworks in qualitative research.* Thousand Oaks, California: Sage.

Astedt-Kurki, P., Paavilainen, E., & Lehti, K. (2001). Methodological issues in interviewing families in family nursing research. *Journal of Advanced Nursing, 35*(2), 288–293.

Atkinson, P. (1992). The ethnography of a medical setting: Reading, writing and rhetoric. *Qualitative Health Research, 2*(4), 451–474.

Ayers, L., & Poirier, S. (1996). Virtual text and the growth of meaning in qualitative analysis. *Research in Nursing & Health, 19*(2), 163–169.

Banks-Wallace, J. (1998). Emancipatory potential of storytelling in a group. *Image: Journal of Nursing Scholarship, 30*(1), 17–21.

Bateson, M. C. (1989). *Composing a life.* New York: Penguin.

Beaudin, C. L., & Pelletier, L. R. (1996). Consumer-based research: Using focus groups as a method for evaluating quality of care. *Journal of Nursing Care Quality, 10*(3), 28–33.

Beck, C. T. (1994). Phenomenology: Its use in nursing research. *International Journal of Nursing Studies, 31*(6), 499–510.

Benderix, Y., & Sivberg, B. (2007). Siblings' experiences of having a brother or sister with autism and mental retardation: A case study of 14 siblings from five families. *Journal of Pediatric Nursing, 22*(5), 410–418.

Benedict, S., & Georges, J. M. (2006). Nurses and the sterilization experiments of Auschwitz: A postmodernist perspective. *Nursing Inquiry, 13*(4), 277–288.

Berg, B. L. (1998). *Qualitative research methods for the social sciences*. Boston: Allyn & Bacon.

Berman, H., Ford-Gilboe, M., & Campbell, J. C. (1998). Combining stories and numbers: A methodologic approach for a critical nursing science. *Advances in Nursing Science, 21*(1), 1–15.

Bertaux, D. (1981). *Biography and society: The life history approach in the social sciences*. Beverly Hills, CA: Sage.

Bulmer, C. (1998). Clinical decisions: Defining meaning through focus groups. *Nursing Standard, 12*(20), 34–36.

Bunkers, S. S. (2007). The experience of feeling unsure for women at end-of-life. *Nursing Science Quarterly, 20*(1), 56–63.

Burnard, P. (1995). Unspoken meanings: Qualitative research and multi-media analysis. *Nurse Researcher, 3*(1), 55–64.

Burnard, P. (1998). Qualitative data analysis: Using a word processor to categorize qualitative data in social science research. *Social Sciences in Health, 4*(1), 55–61.

Burns, N. (1989). Standards for qualitative research. *Nursing Science Quarterly, 2*(1), 44–52.

Carey, M. A. (1995). Comment: Concerns in the analysis of focus group data. *Qualitative Health Research, 5*(4), 487–495.

Carper, B. (1978). Fundamental patterns of knowing in nursing. *Advances in Nursing Science, 1*(1), 13–24.

Christy, T. E. (1975). The methodology of historical research: A brief introduction. *Nursing Research, 24*(3), 189–192.

Christy, T. E. (1978). The hope of history. In M. L. Fitzpatrick (Ed.), *Historical studies in nursing* (pp. 3–11). New York: Teachers College, Columbia University.

Clinton, M. (2001). *Scoping study of the Australian mental health nursing workforce 1999* (No. 0642735204). Canberra: Mental Health and Special Programs Branch Commonwealth Department of Health and Aged Care.

Coffey, A., & Atkinson, P. (1996). *Making sense of qualitative data: Complementary research strategies*. Thousand Oaks, CA: Sage.

Colaizzi, P. (1978). Psychological research as the phenomenologist views it. In R. S. Valle & M. King (Eds.), *Existential phenomenological alternatives for psychology* (pp. 48–71). New York: Oxford University Press.

Colbourne, L., & Sque, M. (2005). The culture of cancer and the therapeutic impact of qualitative research interviews. *Journal of Research in Nursing, 10*(5), 551–567.

Connors, D. D. (1988). A continuum of researcher-participant relationships: An analysis and critique. *Advances in Nursing Science, 10*(4), 32–42.

Cooper, M. C. (1988). Covenantal relationships: Grounding for the nursing ethic. *Advances in Nursing Science, 10*(4), 48–59.

Cowles, K. V. (1988). Issues in qualitative research on sensitive topics. *Western Journal of Nursing Research, 10*(2), 163–179.

Cueto, M. (2004). The origins of primary health care and selective primary health care. *American Journal of Public Health, 94*(11), 1864–1874.

Deatrick, J. A., & Ledlie, S. W. (2000). Qualitative research interviews with children and their families. *Journal of Child and Family Nursing, 3*(2), 152–158.

Denzin, N. K. (1989). *Interpretive interactionism*. Newbury Park, CA: Sage.

Dickson-Swift, V., James, E. L., Kippen, S., & Liamputtong, P. (2006). Blurring boundaries in qualitative health research on sensitive topics. *Qualitative Health Research, 16*(6), 853–871.

Dingwall, R. (1977). Atrocity stories and professional relationships. *Sociology of Work and Occupations, 4*(4), 371–396.

Disney, J. A., & May, K. M. (1998, August). Focus group method for nursing research: Pleasures and pitfalls [7 pp]. *Nursing Research Methods: An Electronic Journal for Nursing Researchers [Online serial], 3.*

Downe-Wamboldt, B. (1992). Content analysis: Method, applications, and issues. *Health Care for Women International, 13*(3), 313–321.

Draucker, C. B. (1999). The emotional impact of sexual violence research on participants. *Archives of Psychiatric Nursing, 13*(4), 161–169.

Drew, N. (1989). The interviewer's experience as data in phenomenological research. *Western Journal of Nursing Research, 11*(4), 431–439.

Ellis, R. (1983). Philosophic inquiry. In H. H. Werley & J. J. Fitzpatrick (Eds.), *Annual review of nursing research* (Vol. I, pp. 211–228). New York: Springer.

Evans, J. C. (1978). Formulating an idea. In M. L. Fitzpatrick (Ed.), *Historical studies in nursing* (pp. 15–17). New York: Teacher's College.

Fairman, J. A. (1987). Sources and references for research in nursing history. *Nursing Research, 36*(1), 56–59.

Field, P. A., & Morse, J. M. (1985). *Nursing research: The application of qualitative approaches*. Rockville, MD: Aspen.

Flinders, D. J., & Mills, G. E. (1993). *Theory and concepts in qualitative research: perspectives from the field*. New York: Teachers College Press.

Foucault, M. (1973). *The birth of the clinic: An archaeology of medical perception* (A. M. S. Smith, Trans.). New York: Vintage Books.

Foucault, M. (1994). Technologies of the Self (R. Hurley & J. Faubion, Trans). In P. Rabinow(Ed.), Ethics: Subjectivity and truth Vol. 1 (pp. 223-251). New York: The New Press.

Foucault, M. (1995). *Discipline and punish: The birth of the prison* (A. Sheridan, Trans.). New York: Vintage.

Foucault, M. (1980). *Power/knowledge: Selected interviews and other writings 1972–1977* (C. Gordon, L. Marshall, J. Mepham, & K. Soper, Trans.). New York: Pantheon Books.

Fowler, M. D. M. (1988). Issues in qualitative research. *Western Journal of Nursing Research, 10*(1), 109–111.

Fox, N. J. (1993). *Postmodernism, sociology and health*. Buckingham: Open University Press.

Frank, G. (1979). Finding the common denominator: A phenomenological critique of life history method. *Ethos, 7*(1), 68–71.

Frank, G. (1996). Life histories in occupational therapy clinical practice. *American Journal of Occupational Therapy, 50*(4), 251–264.

Gergen, K. J., & Gergen, M. M. (1983). Narratives of the self. In T. R. Sarbin & K. E. Scheibe (Eds.), *Studies in social identity* (pp. 254–273). New York: Praeger.

Germain, C. P. H. (1986). Ethnography: The method. In P. L. Munhall & C. J. Oiler (Eds.), *Nursing research: A qualitative perspective* (pp. 147–162). East Norwalk, CT: Appleton-Century-Crofts.

Giorgi, A. (1970). *Psychology as a human science: A phenomenologically based approach*. New York: Harper & Row.

Goss, G. I. (1998). Focus group interviews: A methodology for socially sensitive research. *Clinical Excellence for Nurse Practitioners, 2*(1), 30–34.

Guba, E. G., & Lincoln, Y. S. (1982). *Effective evaluation*. Washington, DC: Jossey-Bass.

Halloran, J. P., & Grimes, D. E. (1995). Application of the focus group methodology to educational program development. *Qualitative Health Research*, *5*(4), 444–453.

Hamilton, B. E., & Manias, E. (2007). Rethinking nurses' observations: Psychiatric nursing skills and invisibility in an acute inpatient setting. *Social Science & Medicine*, *65*(2), 331–343.

Happ, M. B., Swigart, V. A., Tate, J. A., Hoffman, L. A., & Arnold, R. M. (2007). Patient involvement in health-related decisions during prolonged critical illness. *Research in Nursing & Health*, *30*(4), 361–372.

Harrison, B. (2002). Seeing health and illness worlds—Using visual methodologies in a sociology of health and illness: A methodological review. *Sociology of Health & Illness*, *24*(6), 856–872.

Hedin, B. A. (1986). Nursing, education, and emancipation: Applying the critical theoretical approach to nursing research. In P. L. Chinn (Ed.), *Nursing research methodology: Issues and implementation* (pp. 133–146). Rockville, MD: Aspen.

Henderson, D. J. (1995). Consciousness raising in participatory research: Method and methodology for emancipatory nursing inquiry. *Advances in Nursing Science*, *17*(3), 58–69.

Hollis, V., Openshaw, S., & Goble, R. (2002). Conducting focus groups: Purpose and practicalities. *British Journal of Occupational Therapy*, *65*(1), 2–8.

Holter, I. M. (1988). Critical theory: A foundation for the development of nursing theories. *Scholarly Inquiry for Nursing Practice: An International Journal*, *2*(3), 223–232.

Hutchinson, A. M. (2005). Analysing audio-recorded data: Using computer software applications. *Nurse Researcher*, *12*(3), 20–31.

Irving, K. (2002). Governing the conduct of conduct: Are restraints inevitable? *Journal of Advanced Nursing*, *40*(4), 405–512.

Ismail, F., Berman, H., & Ward-Griffin, C. (2007). Dating violence and the health of young women: A feminist narrative study. *Health Care for Women International*, *28*(5), 453–477.

Iser, W. (1980). The reading process: A phenomenological approach. In J. Tompkins (Ed.), *Reader-response criticism* (pp. 118–133). Baltimore: Johns Hopkins University Press.

Jensen, R. (1992). Text management—History and computing. III: Historians, computers and data, applications in research and teaching. *Journal of Interdisciplinary History*, *22*(4), 711–722.

Josselson, R., & Lieblich, A. (Eds.). (1995). *The narrative study of lives: Vol. 3. Interpreting experience*. Newbury Park, CA: Sage.

Kalisch, B. J., & Kalisch, P. A. (1977). An analysis of the sources of physician-nurse conflict. *Journal of Nursing Administration*, *7*(1), 50–57.

Kalisch, B. J., Kalisch, P. A., & Belcher, B. (1985). Forecasting for nursing policy: A news-based image approach. *Nursing Research*, *34*(1), 44–49.

Kalisch, B. J., Kalisch, P. A., & Young, R. L. (1983). Television news coverage of nurse strikes: A resource management perspective. *Nursing Research*, *32*(3), 175–180.

Kalisch, P. A., Kalisch, B. J., & Clinton, J. (1982). The world of nursing on prime time television, 1950 to 1980. *Nursing Research*, *31*(6), 358–363.

Kelly, A. W., & Sime, A. M. (1990). Language as research data: Application of computer content analysis in nursing research. *Advances in Nursing Science*, *12*(3), 32–40.

Kelly, L. E., & Patterson, B. J. (2006). Childhood nutrition: Perceptions of caretakers in a low-income urban setting. *Journal of School Nursing*, *22*(6), 345–351.

Kermode, F. (1983). *The art of telling: Essays on fiction*. New York: Oxford University Press.

Kitzinger, J. (1995). Introducing focus groups. *British Medical Journal*, *311*(7000), 299–302.

Kramer, T. (1983). The diary as a feminist research method. *Newsletter of the Association for Women in Psychology*, Winter, 3–4.

Kruman, M. W. (1985). Historical method: Implications for nursing research. In M. M. Leininger (Ed.), *Qualitative research methods in nursing* (pp. 109–118). New York: Grune & Stratton.

Lamb, G. S., & Huttlinger, K. (1989). Reflexivity in nursing research. *Western Journal of Nursing Research*, *11*(6), 765–772.

Larson, E. A., & Fanchiang, S. C. (1996). Life history and narrative research: Generating a humanistic knowledge base for occupational therapy. *American Journal of Occupational Therapy*, *50*(4), 247–250.

Linde, C. (1993). *Life stories: The creation of coherence*. New York: Oxford University Press.

Lusk, B. (1997). Historical methodology for nursing research. *Image: Journal of Nursing Scholarship*, *29*(4), 355–359.

Lynaugh, J., & Reverby, S. (1987). Thoughts on the nature of history. *Nursing Research*, *36*(1), 4, 69.

Mallinson, T., Kielhofner, G., & Mattingly, C. (1996). Metaphor and meaning in a clinical interview. *American Journal of Occupational Therapy*, *50*(5), 338–346.

Manchester, P. (1986). Analytic philosophy and foundational inquiry: The method. In P. L. Munhall & C. J. Oiler (Eds.), Nursing research: A qualitative perspective (pp. 229–249). East Norwalk, CT: Appleton-Century-Crofts.

Marshall, C. (1984). Elites, bureaucrats, ostriches, and pussycats: Managing research in policy settings. *Anthropology and Education Quarterly*, *15*(3), 235–251.

Marshall, C. (1985). Appropriate criteria of trustworthiness and goodness for qualitative research on education organizations. *Quality and Quantity*, *19*(4), 353–373.

Marshall, C., & Rossman, G. B. (1989). *Designing qualitative research*. Newbury Park, CA: Sage.

Mattingly, C., & Garro, L. (1994). Narrative representations of illness and healing: Introduction. *Social Science and Medicine*, *38*(6), 771–774.

Mattingly, C., & Lawlor, M. (2000). Learning from stories: Narrative interviewing in cross-cultural research. *Scandinavian Journal of Occupational Therapy*, *7*(1), 4–14.

McEvoy, P. (2001). Interviewing colleagues: Addressing the issues of perspective, inquiry and representation. *Nurse Researcher*, *9*(2), 49–59.

McNett, M. M. (2006). The PhD-prepared nurse in the clinical setting. *Clinical Nurse Specialist*, *20*(3), 134–138.

Mental Health Act. (1986). *Victorian Parliament*. Legislative Assembly and Council.

Miles, M. B., & Huberman, A. M. (1994). *Qualitative data analysis: A sourcebook of new methods* (2nd ed.). Beverly Hills, CA: Sage.

Morgan, D. L. (1995). Why things (sometimes) go wrong in focus groups. *Qualitative Health Research*, *5*(4), 516–523.

Morrison, R. S., & Peoples, L. (1999). Using focus group methodology in nursing. *Journal of Continuing Education in Nursing*, *30*(2), 62–65.

Morse, J. M. (1997). Learning to drive from a manual? *Qualitative Health Research*, *7*(2), 181–183.

Moyle, W. (2002). Unstructured interviews: Challenges when participants have a major depressive illness. *Journal of Advanced Nursing*, *39*(3), 266–273.

Mu, P., & Lin, S. (2007). An oral historical study of the development of the discipline of military nursing in Taiwan from 1948 to 1970. *Journal of Nursing Research*, *15*(2), 117–126.

Mulhall, A. (2003). In the field: Notes on observation in qualitative research. *Journal of Advanced Nursing*, *41*(3), 306–313.

Mullings, L., Wali, A., McLean, D., Mitchell, J., Prince, S., Thomas, D. (2001). Qualitative methodologies and community participation in examining reproductive experiences: The Harlem Birth Right Project. *Maternal and Child Health Journal*, *5*(2), 85–93.

Munhall, P. L. (1988). Ethical considerations in qualitative research. *Western Journal of Nursing Research*, *10*(2), 150–162.

Munhall, P. L. (1991). Institutional review of qualitative research proposals: A task of no small consequence. In J. M. Morse (Ed.), *Qualitative nursing research: A contemporary dialogue*. London: Sage.

Munro, B. H. (2001). Doctorally prepared nurses in clinical settings. *Clinical Nurse Specialist*, *15*(5), 197–198.

Newton, M. E. (1965). The case for historical research. *Nursing Research*, *14*(1), 20–26.

Noel, N. L. (1988). Historiography: Biography of "Women Worthies" in nursing history. *Western Journal of Nursing Research*, *10*(1), 106–108.

Northcott, N. (1996). Cognitive mapping: An approach to qualitative data analysis. *NT Research*, *1*(6), 456–464.

Nwoga, I. (1997). *Mother-daughter conversation related to sex-role socialization and adolescent pregnancy*. Unpublished doctoral dissertation, University of Florida, Gainesville.

Nwoga, I. (2000). African American mothers use stories for family sexuality education. *MCN, American Journal of Maternal Child Nursing*, *25*(1), 31–36.

Oiler, C. (1982). The phenomenological approach in nursing research. *Nursing Research*, *31*(3), 178–181.

Pallikkathayil, L., & Morgan, S. A. (1991). Phenomenology as a method for conducting clinical research. *Nursing Research*, *4*(4), 195–200.

Palmerino, M. B. (1999, June 7). Market research: Talk is best when it's one-on-one. Take a quality approach to qualitative research. *Marketing News*, *33*(12), 35.

Parse, R. R. (1990). Health: A personal commitment. *Nursing Science Quarterly*, *3*(3), 136–140.

Pateman, B. (1998). Computer-aided qualitative data analysis: The value of NUD*IST and other programs. *Nurse Researcher*, *5*(3), 77–89.

Patterson, B., & Kelly, L. (2005). Lessons learned: One experience with focus groups in a school setting. *Journal of School Nursing*, *21*(3), 6–11.

Penney, W., & Wellard, S. J. (2007). Hearing what older consumers say about participation in their care. *International Journal of Nursing Practice*, *13*(1), 61–68.

Podolefsky, A., & McCarty, C. (1983). Topical sorting: A technique for computer assisted qualitative data analysis. *American Anthropologist*, *85*(4), 886–890.

Polkinghorne, D. E. (1988). *Narrative knowing and the human sciences*. Albany, NY: State University of New York Press.

Porter, E. J. (1998). On "being inspired" by Husserl's phenomenology: Reflections on Omery's exposition of phenomenology as a method of nursing research. *Advances in Nursing Science*, *21*(1), 16–28.

Price, B. (2002). Laddered questions and qualitative data research interviews. *Journal of Advanced Nursing*, *37*(3), 273–281.

Quine, S., & Cameron, I. (1995). The use of focus groups with the disabled elderly. *Qualitative Health Research*, *5*(4), 454–462.

Rafael, A. R. F. (1997). Advocacy oral history: A research methodology for social activism in nursing; methods of clinical inquiry. *Advances in Nursing Science*, *20*(2), 32–44.

Reed, J., & Payton, V. R. (1997). Focus groups: Issues of analysis and interpretation. *Journal of Advanced Nursing*, *26*(4), 765–771.

Reinharz, S. (1992). *Feminist methods in social research*. New York: Oxford University Press.

Rhodes, L. A. (1991). *Emptying beds: The work of an emergency psychiatric unit*. Berkeley: University of California Press.

Riley, R. (2005). *Snapshots of live theatre: Rethinking the governance of operating room nursing through a discourse analysis of communication processes*. Unpublished Ph.D. thesis, University of Melbourse, Melbourne.

Riley, R. G., & Manias, E. (2006). Governance in operating room nursing: Nurses' knowledge of individual surgeons. *Social Science & Medicine*, *62*(6), 1541–1551.

Roberts, M. (2005). The production of the psychiatric subject: Power, knowledge and Michel Foucault. *Nursing Philosophy*, *6*(1), 33–42.

Robinson, C. A., & Thorne, S. E. (1988). Dilemmas of ethics and validity in qualitative nursing research. *Canadian Journal of Nursing Research*, *20*(1), 65–76.

Rodgers, B. L. (1989). Concepts, analysis and the development of nursing knowledge: The evolutionary cycle. *Journal of Advanced Nursing*, *14*(4), 330–335.

Roesler, C. (2006). A narratological methodology for identifying archetypal story patterns in autobiographical narratives. *Journal of Analytical Psychology*, *51*(4), 574–586.

Rosenberg, C. (1987). Clio and caring: An agenda for American historians and nursing. *Nursing Research*, *36*(1), 67–68.

Ruffing-Rahal, M. A. (1986). Personal documents and nursing theory development. *Advances in Nursing Science*, *8*(3), 50–57.

Sandelowski, M. (1994). Notes on transcription. *Research in Nursing & Health*, *17*(4), 311–314.

Sandelowski, M. (1995a). On the aesthetics of qualitative research. *Image—Journal of Nursing Scholarship*, *27*(3), 205–209.

Sandelowski, M. (1995b). Qualitative analysis: What it is and how to begin. *Research in Nursing & Health*, *18*(4), 371–375.

Sandelowski, M. (1997). "To be of use": Enhancing the utility of qualitative research. *Nursing Outlook*, *45*(3), 125–132.

Sandelowski, M., & Barroso, J. (2007). *Handbook for synthesizing qualitative research*. New York: Springer.

Sarbin, T. R. (Ed.). (1986). *Narrative psychology: The storied nature of human conduct*. New York: Praeger.

Seng, J. S. (1998). Praxis as a conceptual framework for participatory research in nursing. *Advances in Nursing Science*, *20*(4), 37–48.

Silverman, D. (2005). *Doing qualitative research: A practical handbook* (2nd ed). London: Sage.

Sim, J. (1998). Collecting and analyzing qualitative data: Issues raised by the focus group. *Journal of Advanced Nursing, 28*(2), 345–352.

Smith, J. A. (1986). The idea of health: Doing foundational inquiry. In P. L. Munhall & C. J. Oiler (Eds.), *Nursing research: A qualitative perspective* (pp. 251–262). East Norwalk, CT: Appleton-Century-Crofts.

SmithBattle, L. (2007). Learning the baby: An interpretative study of teen mothers. *Journal of Pediatric Nursing, 22*(4), 261–271.

Sorensen, E. S. (1988). Historiography: Archives as sources of treasure in historical research. *Western Journal of Nursing Research, 10*(5), 666–670.

Southern, D. M., Batterham, R. W., Appleby, N. J., Young, D., Dunt, D., & Guibert, R. (1999). The concept mapping method: An alternative to focus group inquiry in general practice. *Australian Family Physician, 28*(Suppl. 1), 35–40.

Sterling, Y., & McNally, J. (1999). Clinical practice of doctorally prepared nurses, *Clinical Nurse Specialist, 13*(6), 296–301.

Stern, P. N. (1980). Grounded theory methodology: Its uses and processes. *Image: Journal of Nursing Scholarship, 12*(1), 20–23.

St John, W., & Johnson, P. (2000). The pros and cons of data analysis software for qualitative research, *Journal of Nursing Scholarship, 32*(4), 393–397.

Straw, R. B., & Smith, M. W. (1995). Potential uses of focus groups in federal policy and program evaluation studies. *Qualitative Health Research, 5*(4), 421–427.

Strickland, C. J. (1999). Conducting focus groups cross-culturally: Experiences with Pacific Northwest Indian people. *Public Health Nursing, 16*(3), 190–197.

Sullivan, K. (1998). Managing the "sensitive" research interview: A personal account. *Nurse Researcher, 6*(2), 72–85.

Taft, L. B. (1993). Computer-assisted qualitative research. *Research in Nursing & Health, 16*(5), 379–383.

Tanner, C. A., Benner, P., Chesla, C., & Gordon, D. R. (1993). The phenomenology of knowing the patient. *Image: Journal of Nursing Scholarship, 25*(4), 273–280.

Thompson, J. L. (1987). Critical scholarship: The critique of domination in nursing. *Advances in Nursing Science, 10*(1), 27–38.

Todres, L. (1998). The qualitative description of human experience: The aesthetic dimension. *Qualitative Health Research, 8*(1), 121–127.

Turner, B. (1981). Some practical aspects of qualitative data analysis: One way of organizing the cognitive processes associated with the generation of grounded theory. *Quality and Quantity, 15*(3), 225–247.

Twinn, S. (1998). An analysis of the effectiveness of focus groups as a method of qualitative data collection with Chinese populations in nursing research. *Journal of Advanced Nursing, 28*(3), 654–661.

Van Kaam, A. L. (1966). *Existential foundations of psychology* (Vol. 3). Pittsburgh, PA: Duquesne University Press.

Ventres, W. (1994). Hearing the patient's story: Exploring physician-patient communication using narrative case reports. *Family Practice Research Journal, 14*(2), 139–147.

Walsh, D., & Downe, S. (2006). Appraising the quality of qualitative research. *Midwifery, 22*(2), 108–119.

Waring, L. M. (1978). Developing the research prospectus. In M. L. Fitzpatrick (Ed.), *Historical studies in nursing* (pp. 18–20). New York: Teachers College.

Watts, J. (2006). "The outsider-within": Dilemmas of qualitative feminist research within a culture of resistance. *Qualitative Research, 6*(3), 385–402.

Williamson, T., & Long, A. F. (2005). Qualitative data analysis using data displays. *Nurse Researcher, 12*(3), 7–19.

Wilmpenny, P., & Gass, J. (2000). Interviewing in phenomenology and grounded theory: Is there a difference? *Journal of Advanced Nursing, 31*(6), 1485–1492.

Zoffmann, V., & Kirkevold, M. (2007). Relationships and their potential for change developed in difficult type 1 diabetes. *Qualitative Health Research, 17*(5), 625–638.

CHAPTER **24**

Interpreting Research Outcomes

When data analysis is complete, there is a feeling that the answers are known and the study is finished. However, the results of statistical analysis alone are inadequate to complete a study. The researcher may know the results, but without careful intellectual examination, these results are of little use to others or to nursing's body of knowledge. To be useful, the evidence from data analysis needs to be carefully examined, organized, and given meaning, and its statistical and clinical significance needs to be assessed. This process is referred to as the interpretation of research outcomes.

Interpretation is the most important part of any study. It requires more critical synthesis and a higher level of thinking than any previous step. Some of the most profound insights of the entire research process occur during interpretation. There is a tendency to rush this important step to finish the study, but it is not a step to be minimized or hurried. The process takes time for reflection. Often times, a researcher becomes too close to the details to be able to see the big picture. At this point, dialogue with colleagues or mentors can add clarity and expand meaning.

Data collection and analysis are action-oriented activities that require more concrete thinking. However, when interpreting the results of the study, one tends to implement abstract thinking, including the creative use of introspection, reasoning, and intuition. In some ways, these last steps in the research process are the most difficult. They require one to synthesize the logic used to develop the research plan, the strategies used in the data collection phase, and the mathematical logic or insight and pattern formation used in data analysis. Evaluating the research process used

in the study, producing meaning from the results, and forecasting the usefulness of the findings are all part of interpretation and require high-level intellectual processes.

Translation is frequently thought of as being synonymous with interpretation. Abstract theoretical statements are sometimes referred to as being translated into more concrete meaning, as, for example, in the operationalization of a variable. Although *translate* and *interpret* are similar words, their meanings have subtle differences. *Translation* means to transform from one language to another or to use terms that can be more easily understood. Interpretation involves explaining the meaning of information. Interpretation seems to include translation and to go beyond it to explore and impart meaning. Thus, in this step of the research process, the researcher translates the results of analysis into findings and then interprets by attaching meaning to the findings.

An example of translation and interpretation is provided in a study of "Predictors of Health-Related Quality of Life 3 months after Traumatic Injury" (Lee, Chaboyer & Wallis, 2008). In the study, data were collected using a telephone survey 3 months after a traumatic injury. The 114 participants were primarily working-age men. One component of the survey measured the physical consequences of the trauma. Statistical results were provided in a table. Translation of these statistical results are reported as follows: "Pain was the most frequently reported symptom; weight and strength loss and fatigue were also reported often in the current study. . . The three higher scoring subscales of the Chinese IPQ-R (Trauma) were Illness coherence, Controllability, and Consequences

(p. 87). Interpretation follows with this statement: "These findings might be because the sample was relatively young and of productive working age. Perhaps these factors indicate that the traumatic injury brought many consequences and had multiple effects on participants' lives. Higher scores on the Illness Coherence and Controllability subscales might also mean that relatively young patients were better able to comprehend their injuries and also consider more ways to control the consequences; however this proposition requires testing" (p. 87).

The process of interpretation includes examining evidence, determining findings, forming conclusions, exploring the significance of the findings, generalizing the findings, considering implications, and suggesting further studies. Each of these activities is discussed in this chapter. The final chapter of theses and dissertations and the final sections of research articles and presentations include the interpretation of research outcomes.

EXAMINING EVIDENCE

The first step in interpretation involves considering all the evidence available that supports or contradicts the validity of results related to the research objectives, questions, or hypotheses. To consider the evidence, one needs first to determine what the evidence is and then gather it together. You will need to carefully consider the impact of each piece of evidence on the validity of the results; then you will synthesize the evidence as a whole to arrive at a final judgment. The process is somewhat like conducting a critical appraisal of your own work. Your temptation is to ignore flaws—certainly not to point them out. However, the honest completion of this process is essential in order to build a body of knowledge. It is a time not for confession, remorse, and apology but rather for thoughtful reflection. As the researcher, you will need to identify the problems and strengths of the study and share them with colleagues at presentations and in publications. They affect the meaning of the results and can serve as guideposts for future researchers.

Evidence from the Research Plan

The initial evidence regarding the validity of the study results is derived from reexamining the research plan. Reexamination requires that the researcher reexplore the logic of the methodology. Analyze the logical links among the problem statement, purpose, research questions, variables, framework design, sample, methods of measurement, and types of analyses. These elements of the study logically link together and are consistent with the research problem. Remember the old adage, a chain is only as strong as its weakest link? This saying is also true of research. Therefore, examine the study needs to identify its weakest links or limitations.

You will then need to examine these limitations in terms of their impact on the results. Could the results, or some of the results, be a consequence of a weakness in the methodology rather than a true test of the hypotheses? Can the research objectives, questions, or hypotheses be answered from the methodology used in the study? Could the results be a consequence of an inappropriate conceptual or operational definition of a variable? Do the research questions clearly emerge from the framework? Can the results be related back to the framework? Are the analyses logically planned to test the questions or hypotheses?

If the types of analyses are inappropriate for examining the research questions, what do the results of analyses mean? For example, if the design failed to control extraneous variables, could some of these variables explain the results, rather than the results being explained by the variables measured and examined through statistical analysis? Was the sample studied a logical group on which to test the hypotheses? The researcher must in this way carefully evaluate each link in the design to determine potential weaknesses. Every link is clearly related to the meaning given to the study results. If the researcher is reviewing a newly completed study and determines that the types of analyses were inappropriate, the analyses, of course, need to be redone. If the study has several weaknesses or breaks in logical links, the findings may need to be seriously questioned.

Evidence from Measurement

One assumption often made in interpreting study results is that the study variables were adequately measured. This adequacy is determined by examining the fit of operational definitions with the framework and through validity and reliability information. Although you should determine the reliability and validity of measurement strategies before using them in your study, you need to reexamine the measures at this point to determine the strength of evidence available from the results. For example, did the scale used to measure anxiety truly reflect the anxiety experienced in the study population? What was the effect size? Were the validity and reliability of instruments examined in the present study? Can this information be used to interpret the results? The validity and reliability of measurement are critical to the validity of results. If the instruments used do not measure the variables as defined conceptually and operationally in the study, the results of analyzed measurement scores mean little.

Scores from measurement instruments without validity and reliability can be used for statistical analyses just as easily as those with validity and reliability. The mathematical formula or the computer cannot detect the difference. The difference is in the meaning attributed to the results, which only researchers, not computers, can detect.

Evidence from the Data Collection Process

Many activities that occur during data collection affect the meaning of study results. Did your study have a high refusal rate for subject participation, or was the attrition high? Was the sample size sufficient? Did strategies for acquiring a sample eliminate important groups whose data would have influenced the results? Did you and your research team achieve intervention fidelity when the treatment was implemented? Did unforeseen events occur during the study that might have changed or had an impact on the data? Were measurement techniques consistent? What impact do inconsistencies have on interpreting results? Sometimes data collection does not proceed as planned. Unforeseen situations alter the collection of data. What were these variations in your study? What impact do they have on interpreting the results? Sometimes someone other than the subject completes data collection forms. Also, variations may occur when scales are administered. For example, an anxiety scale may be given to one subject immediately before a painful procedure and to another subject upon awakening in the morning. Values on these measures cannot be considered comparable. Data integrity also depends on honesty of subjects, which could be compromised by anxiety, time constraints, denial, or other factors not in the direct control of the researcher. The researcher must be on the alert for these subject factors that could compromise the integrity of the data. Values on these measures cannot be considered comparable. These types of differences are seldom reported and sometimes not even recorded. To some extent, only the researcher knows how consistently the measurements were taken. Reporting this information is dependent on the integrity of the researcher (Kerlinger & Lee, 2000; Pyrczak & Bruce, 2005; Stein, Sargent, & Rafaels, 2007).

Evidence from the Data Analysis Process

The process of data analysis is an important factor in evaluating the meaning of results. One important part of this examination is to summarize the study weaknesses related to the data analysis process.

Ask yourself these questions concerning the meaning of your results: How many errors were made while entering the data into the computer? How many subjects have missing data that could affect statistical analyses? Were the analyses accurately calculated? Were statistical assumptions violated? Were the statistics used appropriate for the data? It is best to address these issues initially before analyses are performed and again when completing the analyses and preparing the final report. Researchers should consult with a biostatistician to assure the appropriateness of the data analysis and statistical tests selected. The biostatistician could also be helpful in interpreting the results. Before submitting a paper for publication, we recheck each analysis reported in the paper. We reexamine the analysis statements in the paper (Corty, 2007). Are we correctly interpreting the results of the analysis? Documentation on each statistical value or analysis statement reported in the paper is filed with a copy of the paper. The documentation includes the date of the analysis, the page number of the computer printout showing the results (the printout is stored in a file by date of analysis), the sample size for the analysis, and the number of missing values.

Except in simple studies, data analysis in quantitative studies is usually performed by computer. With prepared statistical analysis programs, multiple analyses can be performed on the data that the researcher does not understand well. To the neophyte researcher, the computer spits out reams of paper with incomprehensible printed information and, in the end, gives a level of significance. The appropriateness of the data and the logic behind the program may remain unknown, but a new researcher may consider the level of significance as absolute "proof" of an important finding.

In gathering evidence for the implications of the study results, it is critical to reexamine the data analysis process. The researcher needs to examine the sufficiency of personal knowledge and proficiency in the analyses used. Reexamine your data for accuracy and completeness. If mathematical operations were performed manually, recheck them for accuracy. Reexamine computer printouts to ensure that no meaningful information has been overlooked. Recheck tables of data for accuracy and clarity.

Evidence from Data Analysis Results

The outcomes of data analysis are the most direct evidence of the results. The researcher has intimate knowledge of the research and needs to evaluate its flaws and strengths carefully when judging the validity of the results. In descriptive and correlational studies, the validity of the results depends on how accurately the variables were measured in selected samples and settings. The value of evidence in any study depends on the amount of variance in the phenomenon explained within the study, a factor that is often not considered when interpreting the results (Tulman & Jacobsen, 1989). In quasi-experimental and experimental studies, in which hypothesized differences in groups are being examined, the differences or lack of differences do not indicate the amount of variance explained. Both differences or lack of differences, and amount of variance explained needs to be reported in all studies and should serve as a basis for interpreting the results (see Chapters 19 through 22 for discussions of methods of identifying the variance explained in an analysis).

Interpretation of results from quasi-experimental and experimental studies is traditionally based on decision theory, with five possible results: (1) significant results that are in keeping with those predicted by the researcher, (2) nonsignificant results, (3) significant results that oppose those predicted by the researcher, (4) mixed results, and (5) unexpected results.

Significant and Predicted Results

Significant results that coincide with the researcher's predictions are the easiest to explain and, unless weaknesses are present, validate the proposed logical links among the elements of the study. These results support the logical links developed by the researcher among the framework, questions, variables, and measurement methods. This outcome is very satisfying to the researcher. However, the researcher needs to consider alternative explanations for the positive findings. What other elements could possibly have led to the significant results?

Nonsignificant Results

Unpredicted nonsignificant or inconclusive results are the most difficult to explain. These results are often referred to as negative results. The negative results could be a true reflection of reality. In this case, the reasoning of the researcher or the theory used by the researcher to develop the hypothesis is in error. If so, the negative findings are an important addition to the body of knowledge. With nonsignificant results, it is important to determine if adequate power of 0.8 or higher was achieved for the data analysis. Thus, the researcher needs to conduct a power analysis to determine if the sample size was adequate to prevent the risk of a type II error. A type II error means that in reality the findings are significant, but, because of weaknesses in the methodology, the significance was not detected.

Negative results could also be due to inappropriate methodology, a deviant sample, problems with internal validity, inadequate measurement, the use of weak statistical techniques, or faulty analysis. Unless these weak links are detected, the reported results could lead to faulty information in the body of knowledge (Angell, 1989). It is easier for the researcher to blame faulty methodology for nonsignificant findings than to find failures in theoretical or logical reasoning. If faulty methodology is blamed, the researcher needs to explain exactly how the breakdown in methodology led to the negative results. Negative results, in any case, do not mean that there are no relationships among the variables or differences between groups; they indicate that the study failed to find any.

Significant and Not Predicted Results

Significant results opposite those predicted, if the results are valid, are an important addition to the body of knowledge. An example would be a study in which the researchers proposed that social support and ego strength were positively related. If the study showed that high social support was related to low ego strength, the result would be the opposite of that predicted. Such results, when verified by other studies, indicate that we were headed in the wrong direction theoretically. Because these types of studies can affect nursing practice, this information is important. Sometimes the researcher believes so strongly in the theory that he or she does not believe the results. The researcher remains convinced that there was a problem in the methodology. Sometimes this belief remains entrenched in the minds of scientists for many years because of the bias that good research supports its hypotheses.

Mixed Results

Mixed results are probably the most common outcome of studies. In this case, one variable may uphold the characteristics predicted whereas another does not, or two dependent measures of the same variable may show opposite results. These differences may be due to methodology problems, such as differing reliability or validity of two methods of measuring variables. Additional study might be indicated. Mixed results may also indicate a need to modify existing theory.

Unexpected Results

Unexpected results are relationships found between variables that were not hypothesized and not predicted from the framework guiding the study. These unexpected results are also called serendipitous results. Most researchers examine as many elements of data as possible in addition to those directed by the research objectives, questions, or hypotheses. They can use these findings to develop or refine theories and to formulate later studies. In addition, serendipitous results are as important as evidence in developing the implications of the study. However, researchers must deal carefully with serendipitous results when considering their meaning, because the study was not designed to examine these results.

Evidence from Previous Studies

The results of the present study should always be examined in light of previous findings. It is important for the researcher to know whether the results are consistent with past research. Consistency in findings across studies is important for developing theories and refining scientific knowledge. Therefore, any inconsistencies need to be explored to determine reasons for the differences. Replication of studies and synthesis of findings from existing studies are critical for the development of empirical knowledge for an evidence-based practice (Craig & Smyth, 2007).

DETERMINING FINDINGS

Findings are developed by evaluating evidence (discussed previously in this chapter) and translating and interpreting study results. Although much of the process of developing findings from results occurs in the mind of the researcher, evidence of such thinking can be found in published research reports. It is important during this process to dialogue with colleagues or mentors to clarify meaning or expand implications of the research findings. The 2003 study of Loescher examines cancer worry in women with hereditary risk factors for breast cancer. Dr. Loescher's excellent study was supported by the National Institutes of Health–National Cancer Institute postdoctoral fellowship and the Oncology Nurses Society Foundation/OrthoBiotech, Inc., Research Fellowship. The article presented here received the 2003 Oncology Nursing Society Excellence in Cancer Nursing Research Award, supported by Schering Oncology/Biotech. Note how Dr. Loescher related her finding to those of previous studies and how she presented her study objectives (aims), results, and findings.

■ *AIM 1*

The first study objective was to "ascertain levels of worry among these women." (Loescher, 2003, p. 768)

Results. The mean total scale score of TACS (the Thoughts About Cancer Scale) was 9.7 (SD = 2.6), suggesting that participants' overall worry about cancer was rarely or never to sometimes. Mean item scores for the six worry items ranged from 1.2 (rarely or never) to 2.3 (sometimes) (Table 24-1). Worry was dichotomized into low worry (scores 6–11) and worry at least sometimes (scores 12–24). The majority of participants (55%–87%) had lower scores for items pertaining to neutral symptoms and breast cancer-specific signs and symptoms. Conversely, most participants (81%–86%) reported higher scores for items concerning general breast cancer worry. (Loescher, 2003, p. 769)

Findings. The main purpose of this study was to investigate cancer worry in women with hereditary risk factors for breast cancer. The mean total worry score as measured by TACS indicated that women in this study sometimes worried about breast cancer. Several other investigators found comparable levels of cancer-specific worry in similar populations (Audrain et al., 1997; Bish et al., 2002; Bowen et al., 1999; Brain et al., 1999; Diefenbach et al., 1999). However, some investigators (Kash et al., 1992; Lloyd et al., 1996) reported higher, almost clinically pathologic levels of worry in high-risk women, whereas others (Leggatt et al., 2000) reported rare cancer worry. These studies of cancer worry did not measure worry in terms of signs and symptoms of cancer or base questionnaire items on qualitative data, so, in that regard, the current study presents new information about cancer worry in high-risk individuals.

The low to moderate levels of worry reported in this study may be explained partially by cognitive determinants of emotion. For example, individuals at risk for a potentially life-threatening disease generally do not worry constantly about this threat because they also are dealing with competing concerns and activities that occur as part of everyday living. Additionally, not worrying constantly could be adaptive in that it prevents overwhelming anxiety (Easterling & Leventhal, 1989; Weinstein, 1988; Weinstein et al., 1986). However, gaining a clearer picture of these assumptions would require asking about worry over time, rather than in a cross-sectional fashion. Although women in this study sometimes worried about developing cancer, the absence of a population-based control group precludes comparisons of worry in high-risk women with women at general population risk.

On average, participants in this study sometimes worried about developing breast cancer and sometimes thought about their own risk for developing breast cancer. These findings reflect results from other studies (Leggatt et al., 2000; Lerman et al., 1994b; McCaul et al., 1998). Many researchers have suggested that this moderate level of worry in women at high risk for breast cancer is the most beneficial—and desired—level for motivating information seeking and practicing recommended risk-reduction behaviors (Bowen et al., 1999; Brain et al., 1999; Lerman et al., 1994a). Higher levels of worry actually may be detrimental to these actions and behaviors (Audrain et al., 1997; Diefenbach et al., 1999).

Although women in this study sometimes thought about breast cancer, an unexpected finding was that when taken individually, neutral symptoms and perceived signs and symptoms of breast cancer did not appear to be worrisome. These findings differed from other studies that reported higher worry for high-risk women experiencing neutral symptoms than for women controls (Cunningham et al., 1998; Easterling & Leventhal, 1989.) One explanation for low symptom-based worry may be that less than half of the sample reported any clinical signs or symptoms, so the cues for worry did not exist. Another untested explanation may be that the women in this study were recruited largely from a dedicated mammography center and cancer-prevention clinics and already were positioned to deal with any cancer signs and symptoms; therefore, these women experienced less worry. (Loescher, 2003, p. 770)

■ *AIM 2*

The second study objective was to "assess correlations of cancer worry, perceived risk of cancer, and clinical signs or symptoms of breast cancer." (Loescher, 2003, p. 768)

Results. The mean total score for absolute risk of developing breast cancer was 51% (SD = 24.8). The mean number of signs and symptoms experienced by the sample was 1.6 (SD = 1.5). Table 24-2 shows individual possible clinical indicators of cancer reported by the sample. Table 24-3 shows correlations of perceived risk and specific clinical indicators of possible breast cancer with cancer worry. (Loescher, 2003, p. 769)

Findings. The nonsignificant correlation of perceived risk with cancer worry was not surprising, given the equivocal nature of this relationship in the literature (Audrain et al., 1997; Cull et al., 2001; Cunningham et al., 1998; Easterling & Leventhal, 1989; Hopwood et al., 1998; Kash et al., 1992; Lerman et al., 1996; Lloyd et al., 1996). The use of one standard risk-assessment question may not have been sufficient to fully characterize risk perception. This problem has been reported previously (Bish et al., 2002; Cull et al., 2001), and future studies of worry should include more sensitive measures of perceived risk.

Previous research reported that the amount and frequency of symptoms (symptom burden) elicited worry about cancer in known at-risk women who perceived that they were at high risk for cancer. However, the equivalent symptom burden in known high-risk women with perceived low risk of cancer did not elicit worry (Easterling & Leventhal, 1989). These results may help to explain why participants in this study worried "sometimes" when the correlation of perceived risk with worry was nonsignificant and total symptom burden was low.

Only one clinical sign, having a breast biopsy, was correlated significantly with cancer worry. Because of the family history of breast cancer, however, this symptom cue would be expected to reactivate a threat cognition (Easterling & Leventhal, 1989). The positive significant correlation of *total* clinical signs of breast cancer with cancer worry suggests that in high-risk women,

a constellation of signs might be more worrisome than occurrence of a single sign or symptom. (Loescher, 2003, pp. 770–771)

■ *AIM 3*

The third study objective was to "evaluate the ability of clinical signs of cancer, age, and family history to predict cancer worry." (Loescher, 2003, p. 768)

Results. Table 24-4 presents the results of a binary logistic regression predicting cancer worry (1 = low worry or 2 = worry sometimes or more). The independent variables in the equation were total signs, age (18–40, 41–50, or 51+), mother's breast cancer history (yes or no), number of sisters with breast cancer, and number of second-degree relatives with breast cancer. This model for high and low concerns about cancer was significant (χ^2 = 12.763, df = 6, p = 0.047). Significant explanatory variables of high worry were total clinical signs of breast cancer and participant age of less than 50 years. (Loescher, 2003, p. 769)

Findings. Women with more clinical breast symptoms were almost 1.5 times more likely to have higher levels of breast cancer worry. This finding was consistent with results of other studies of women at high risk for breast cancer (Audrain et al., 1997; Cunningham et al., 1998.) Informed women at high risk, however, may be more likely to report breast symptoms (Cunningham et al., 1998).

Age was related significantly to cancer worry, and women aged 41–50 were almost four times more likely to have high worry than other women. This age group as an explanatory variable for higher worry scores was expected and reflects the prime age when breast cancer could develop in these women (Lynch & Lynch, 1991). Younger women also may be at the age when their mothers or sisters were diagnosed with breast cancer and become concerned that they may develop cancer as well.

Other reports (Baider et al., 1999; Kash et al., 1992; Lerman et al., 1991; Lloyd et al., 1996; McCaul et al., 1998) found a positive relationship between family history and cancer worry; however, in this study, history of breast cancer in first- or second-degree relatives did not predict worry. Although this finding is difficult to explain, perhaps in this particular group of women, family history, as a stimulus instilling an abstract threat cognition, is so omnipresent that worry diminishes over time and moderate worry becomes stable. (Loescher, 2003, p. 771)

FORMING CONCLUSIONS

Conclusions are derived from the study findings and are a synthesis of findings. Forming conclusions for a study requires a combination of logical reasoning, creative formation of a meaningful whole from pieces of information obtained through data analysis and findings from previous studies, receptivity to subtle clues in the data, and use of an open context in considering alternative explanations of the data.

TABLE 24-1 ⋮▪ Level of Cancer Worry in Women at High Risk for Breast Cancer

Worry Indicator	Total Item Score (Range = 1–4)		Level of Worry			
			Low (Score <12)		At Least Sometimes (Score + 12–24)	
	X	SD	n	%	n	%
General worrying about getting breast cancer	2.2	0.79	39	20	161	81
General thinking about own risk of breast cancer	2.3	0.79	30	15	170	85
Thinking she has cancer every time she feels sick	1.2	0.52	161	81	39	20
Overperforming breast self-examination	1.7	0.84	109	55	91	46
Feeling lumps that cannot be felt by health care provider	1.2	0.51	173	87	27	14
Thinking every ache and pain is cancer	1.2	0.53	169	85	31	16
Total worry	**9.7**	**2.60**	**160**	**80**	**40**	**20**

From Loescher, I. J. (2003). Cancer work in women with hereditary risk factors for breast cancer. *Oncology Nursing Forum, 30*(5), 770

TABLE 24-2 ⋮▪ Possible Clinical Indicators of Breast Cancer Reported by the Sample

Clinical Indicator	n	%
Biopsy of at least one breast lump	64	32
At least one abnormal mammogram	74	37
Lump felt by health care provider	92	46
Lump felt during breast self-examination	85	43

n = 200

From Loescher, I. J. (2003). Cancer work in women with hereditary risk factors for breast cancer. *Oncology Nursing Forum, 30*(5), 770.

TABLE 24-3 ⋮▪ Correlations of Cancer Worry with Perceived Risk and Clinical Signs of Breast Cancer

Breast Cancer Sign	Total Cancer Worry
Perceived absolute risk	−0.900
Had biopsy of at least one lump	0.169
At least one abnormal mammogram or ultrasound	0.112
At least one lump felt by health care provider	0.108
At least one lump felt during breast self-examination	0.123
Total clinical signs	0.171

From Loescher, I. J. (2003). Cancer work in women with hereditary risk factors for breast cancer. *Oncology Nursing Forum, 30*(5), 770.

When forming conclusions, it is important to remember that research never proves anything; rather, research offers support for a position. Proof is a logical part of deductive reasoning, but not of the research process. Therefore, formulation of causal statements is risky. For example, the causal statement that A *causes* B (absolutely, in all situations) cannot be scientifically proved. It is more credible to state conclusions in the form of conditional probabilities that are qualified. For example, it would be more appropriate to state in the study that if A occurred, then B occurred under conditions x, y, and z (Kerlinger & Lee, 2000), or that B had an 80% probability of occurring. Thus, one could conclude that if preoperative teaching was provided, postoperative anxiety would be lowered as long as pain was controlled, complications did not occur, and family contacts were high. Loescher (2003) presented only tentative conclusions that are included in the statement of findings.

The methodology of the study should be examined when drawing conclusions from the findings. In spite of a researcher's higher motives to be objective, subjective

TABLE 24-4 Explanatory Variables for Thoughts about Cancer at Least Sometimes							95% Confidence Interval	
Variable	β	SE	Wald	*df*	*p*	Odds Ratio	Lower	Upper
Total signs of cancer	0.398	0.138	8.275	1	0.004	1.489	1.135	1.953
Age groups								
18–40 years	—	—	—	—	—	1.000	—	—
41–50 years	1.325	0.521	6.476	1	0.011	3.763	1.356	10.445
51+ years	0.487	0.450	1.170	1	0.279	1.627	0.673	3.931
Mother with breast cancer (*n* = 135)	−0.208	0.407	0.262	1	0.608	0.812	0.366	1.802
Sisters with breast cancer (*n* = 79)	0.024	0.051	0.211	1	0.646	1.024	0.926	1.133
Second-degree relatives with breast cancer (*n* = 143)	0.020	0.162	0.015	1	0.903	1.020	0.743	1.400

n = 200

From Loescher, I. J. (2003). Cancer work in women with hereditary risk factors for breast cancer. *Oncology Nursing Forum, 30*(5), 771.

judgments and biases will sometimes creep into the conclusions. As a researcher, you will need to be alert and control subjectivity and biases. Students sometimes want positive findings so much that they will misinterpret statistical results on computer printouts as significant when they are clearly nonsignificant.

Identify the limitations of the study when forming conclusions about the findings. The limitations need to be included in the research report. Loescher (2003) provided the following discussion of limitations:

■ *LIMITATIONS*

Although this study adds to the limited knowledge base of symptom-based cancer worry, this research has additional limitations. Concomitant use of other instruments that assess benign breast problems might present a more complete picture of symptoms and can induce worry. Another limitation was the lack of diversity among participants, particularly regarding ethnicity and educational and socioeconomic levels. However, women who participate in this type of research tend to be white, well educated, and financially secure (Cull et al., 2001). Continued investigations of cancer worry in a less homogenous sample of women at high risk for breast cancer will provide a better understanding of the construct. (Loescher, 2003, p. 771)

One of the risks in developing conclusions in research is going beyond the data, specifically, forming conclusions that the data do not warrant. The most common example is a study that examines relationships between A and B by correlational analysis and then concludes that A causes B. Going beyond the data is due to faulty logic and occurs more frequently in published studies than one would like to believe. Be sure to check the validity of arguments related to conclusions before revealing findings.

EXPLORING THE SIGNIFICANCE OF FINDINGS

The word *significance* is used in two ways in research. Statistical significance is related to quantitative analysis of the results of the study. To be important, the results of quantitative studies that use statistical analysis must be statistically significant. **Statistical significance** means that the results are unlikely to be due to chance. However, statistically significant results are not necessarily important in clinical practice. The results can indicate a real difference that is not necessarily an important difference clinically. For example, Yonkman (1982, p. 356), in reporting results from her study of the effect of cool or heated aerosol on oral temperature, reported that "the statistical tests yielded small values which implied that differences were statistically significant. It is not clear that these differences in temperature are clinically significant."

The **practical significance** of a study is associated with its importance to nursing's body of knowledge. Significance is not a dichotomous characteristic because studies contribute in varying degrees to the body of knowledge. Statistically nonsignificant results can have practical significance. Significance may be associated with the amount of variance explained, control in the study design to eliminate unexplained variance, or detection of statistically significant differences. You and your research team are expected to clarify the significance as much as possible. The areas of significance may be obvious to the researcher who has been immersed in the study but not to a reader or listener. Therefore, always delineate the areas of significance in your research. Determining clinical significance is a judgment based on the researcher's clinical expertise. It is often based, in part, on whether treatment decisions or outcomes would be different in view of the study findings. A clinically significant study should result in altered decisions or actions by the nurse.

A few studies, referred to as landmark studies, become important referent points in the discipline, such as those by Johnson (1972), Lindeman and Van Aernam (1971), Passos and Brand (1966), and Williams (1972). The importance of a study may not become apparent for years after publication. However, some characteristics are associated with the significance of studies. Significant studies make an important difference in people's lives, and the findings have external validity. Therefore, it is possible to generalize the findings far beyond the study sample so that the findings have the potential of affecting large numbers of people. The implications of significant studies go beyond concrete facts to abstractions and lead to the generation of theory or revisions in existing theory. A highly significant study has implications for one or more disciplines in addition to nursing. Others in the discipline accept the study, and it is frequently referenced in the literature. Over a period of time, the significance of a study is measured by the number of studies that it generates.

GENERALIZING THE FINDINGS

Generalization extends the implications of the findings from the sample studied to a larger population or from the situation studied to a larger situation. For example, if the study were conducted on diabetic patients, it may be possible to generalize the findings to persons with other illnesses or to well individuals. Highly controlled experimental studies, which are high in internal validity, tend to be low in generalizability because they tend to have low external validity.

How far can generalizations be made? The answer to this question is debatable. From a narrow perspective, one cannot really generalize from the sample on which the study was done. Any other sample is likely to be different in some way. The conservative position, represented by Kerlinger and Lee (2000),

recommends caution in considering the extent of generalization. Conservatives consider generalization particularly risky if the sample was not randomly selected. According to Kerlinger and Lee (2000), unless special precautions are taken and efforts made, the results of research are frequently not representative and have limited generality. This statement represents the classic sampling theory position. However, as discussed in Chapter 18, generalizations are often made to abstract or theoretical populations. Thus, conclusions need to address applications to theory. Judgments about the reasonableness of generalizing need to address issues related to external validity, as discussed in Chapter 10.

Generalizations based on accumulated evidence from many studies are called empirical generalizations. These generalizations are important for verifying theoretical statements or developing new theories. Empirical generalizations are the base of a science and contribute to scientific conceptualization, which provide a basis for generating evidence-based guidelines to manage specific practice problems (Craig & Smyth, 2007). Nursing currently has limited empirical generalizations.

CONSIDERING IMPLICATIONS

Implications of research findings for nursing are the meanings of conclusions for the body of knowledge, theory, and practice. Implications are based on the conclusions and are more specific than conclusions. They provide specific suggestions for implementing the findings. You will need to consider the areas of nursing for which your study findings would be useful. For example, you might make suggestions about how nursing practice should be modified. If a study indicated that a specific solution was effective in decreasing stomatitis, the suggestion would state that the findings had implications for caring for patients with stomatitis. It would not be sufficient to state that the study had implications for nurses practicing in oncology.

Loescher (2003) suggested the following implications of her findings:

> Worry is an important construct because it may play a critical role in how at-risk women view their vulnerability to cancer and what they do to reduce their risk.... Other studies (Bish et al., 2002; Lerman et al., 1996) found that cancer genetic risk counseling significantly decreased worry. Therefore, nurses should consider including assessments of worry as part of routine data collection for genetic risk counseling. Additionally, by

understanding that some levels of worry (e.g., moderate levels) may be beneficial for high-risk women, nurses can reassure those women that being somewhat worried is not detrimental and even may have positive consequences. Nurses also should be aware that women who exhibit extreme distress require appropriate counseling and support.

This study has further implications for cancer genetic risk counseling in that regardless of the extent of their family histories of cancer, women aged 41–50 with one or more clinical symptoms of breast cancer may have high levels of worry. In this regard, routine assessment of worry and clinical breast symptoms in this age group may be prudent. (Loescher, 2003, pp. 771–772)

Novice researchers have a tendency to go beyond the findings to make recommendations not grounded in evidence. These may represent pre-conceived ideas that color interpretation. Experienced researchers learn to set aside their own notions and focus solely on the evidence as it presents itself. Thus, the novice researcher is wise to seek the council and advice of those more experienced in writing these last sections of the research report. Mentors are critical to learning to think through exactly how far one can go and the best approaches to making statements.

SUGGESTING FURTHER STUDIES

Completing a study and examining its implications should culminate in recommendations for future studies that emerge from the present study and from previous studies in the same area of interest. Suggested studies or recommendations for further study may include replications or repeating the design with a different or larger sample. In every study, the researcher gains knowledge and experience that can be used to design "a better study next time." Formulating recommendations for future studies will stimulate you to define more clearly how to improve your study. From a logical or theoretical point of view, the findings should lead you directly to more hypotheses to further test the framework you are using. Improvements could involve an alternate methodology, a refined measurement tool, changes in sampling criteria, or a different setting.

Loescher (2003) provided the following suggestions for future research:

The relationships among cancer worry, perceived risk, and risk-reducing actions still need further clarification in this population. Additional research is needed to better elucidate the role of neutral and cancer-specific symptoms as cues to worry in individuals at hereditary

risk for cancer. For example, worry levels in younger high-risk women could be ascertained prior to, at the time of, and after their first clinical symptom of breast cancer. More sensitive instruments need to be developed to assess symptoms in high-risk individuals who have not yet had a diagnosis of cancer. Study of the relationship of symptom-based worry with actual preventive behaviors practiced by high-risk women is a logical next step of this research.

Results of this study add to the expanding body of knowledge of cancer worry in women with hereditary risk factors for breast cancer. Continued investigation of cancer worry can lead to studies of interventions specifically targeted toward reducing (or increasing) worry to optimal levels in this high-risk group of women. (Loescher, 2003, pp. 771–772)

SUMMARY

- To be useful, evidence from data analysis needs to be carefully examined, organized, and given meaning; and this process is referred to as interpretation.
- Interpretation includes several intellectual activities, such as examining evidence, forming conclusions, exploring the significance of the findings, generalizing the findings, considering implications, and suggesting further studies.
- The first step in interpretation is considering all of the evidence available that supports or contradicts the validity of the results. Evidence is obtained from a variety of sources, including the research plan, measurement validity and reliability, data collection process, data analysis process, data analysis results, and previous studies.
- The outcomes of data analysis are the most direct evidence available of the results related to the research objectives, questions, or hypotheses.
- Five possible results are (1) significant results that are in keeping with those predicted by the researcher, (2) nonsignificant results, (3) significant results that are opposite those predicted by the researcher, (4) mixed results, and (5) unexpected results.
- Findings are a consequence of evaluating evidence, which includes the findings from previous studies.
- Conclusions are derived from the findings and are a synthesis of the findings.
- Implications are the meanings of study conclusions for the body of knowledge, theory, and practice.
- A study needs to be clinically or practically significant as well as statistically significant, and significance is not a dichotomous characteristic because studies contribute in varying degrees to the body of knowledge.

- Generalization extends the implications of the findings from the sample studied to a larger population.
- Completion of a study and examination of implications should culminate in recommending future studies that emerge from the present study and previous studies.
- Interpretation is a rigorous process requiring critical synthesis, self-analysis, and considerable time. Often, dialogue with a colleague or mentor helps clarify and expand meaning.

REFERENCES

Angell, M. (1989). Negative studies. *New England Journal of Medicine, 321*(7), 464–466.

Audrain, J., Schwartz, M. D., Lerman, C., Hughes, C., Peshkin, B. N., & Biesecker, B. (1997). Psychological distress in women seeking genetic counseling for breast-ovarian cancer risk: The contributions of personality and appraisal. *Annals of Behavioral Medicine, 19*(4), 370–377.

Baider, L., Ever-Hadani, P., & De-Nour, A. K. (1999). Psychological distress in healthy women with familial breast cancer: Like, mother, like daughter? *International Journal of Psychiatry in Medicine, 29*(4), 411–420.

Bish, A., Sutton, S., Jacobs, C., Levene, S., Ramirez, A., & Hodgson, S. (2002). Changes in psychological distress after cancer genetic counseling: A comparison of affected and unaffected women. *British Journal of Cancer, 86*(1), 43–50.

Bowen, D., McTiernan, A., Burke, W., Powers, D., Pruski, J., Durfy, S., et al. (1999). Participation in breast cancer risk counseling among women with a family history. *Cancer Epidemiology, Biomarkers, and Prevention, 8*(7), 581–585.

Brain, K., Norman, P., Gray, J., & Mansel, R. (1999). Anxiety and adherence to breast self-examination in women with a family history of breast cancer. *Psychosomatic Medicine, 61*(2), 181–187.

Corty, E. W. (2007). *Using and interpreting statistics: A practical text for the health, behavioral, and social sciences.* St. Louis, MO: Mosby.

Craig, J. V., & Smyth, R. L. (2007). *The evidence-based practice manual for nurses.* Edinburgh: Churchill Livingstone.

Cull, A., Fry, A., Rush, R., & Steel, C. M. (2001). Cancer risk perceptions and distress among women attending a familial ovarian cancer clinic. *British Journal of Cancer, 84*(5), 594–599.

Cunningham, L. L. C., Andrykowski, M. A., Wilson, J. F., McGrath, P. C., Sloan, D. A., & Keady, D. E. (1998). Physical symptoms, distress, and breast cancer risk perceptions in women with benign breast problems. *Health Psychology, 17*(4), 371–375.

Diefenbach, M. A., Miller, S. M., & Daly, M. B. (1999). Specific worry about breast cancer predicts mammography use in women at risk for breast and ovarian cancer. *Health Psychology, 18*(5), 532–536.

Easterling, D. V., & Leventhal, H. (1989). Contributions of concrete cognition to emotion: Neutral symptoms as elicitors of worry about cancer. *Journal of Applied Psychology, 74*(5), 787–796.

Hopwood, P., Keeling, F., Long, A., Pool, C., Evans, G., & Howell, A. (1998). Psychological support needs for women at high genetic risk of breast cancer: Some preliminary indicators. *Psycho-Oncology, 7*(5), 402–412.

Johnson, J. E. (1972). Effects of structuring patients' expectations on their reactions to threatening events. *Nursing Research, 21*(6), 499–503.

Kash, K., Holland, J. C., Halper, M. S., & Miller, D. G. (1992). Psychological distress and surveillance behaviors of women with a family history of breast cancer. *Journal of the National Cancer Institute, 84*(1), 24–30.

Kerlinger, F. N., & Lee, H. P. (2000). *Foundations of behavioral research* (4th ed.). Fort Worth, TX: Harcourt College.

Lee, B., Chaboyer, W., & Wallis, M. (2008). Predictors of health-related quality of life 3 months after traumatic injury. *Journal of Nursing Scholarship, 40*(1), 83-90.

Leggatt, V., Mackay, J., Marteau, T. M., & Yates, J. R. W. (2000). The psychological impact of a cancer family history questionnaire completed in general practice. *Journal of Medical Genetics, 37*(6), 470–472.

Lerman, C., Daly, M., Masny, A., & Balshem, A. (1994a). Attitudes about genetic testing for breast-ovarian cancer susceptibility. *Journal of Clinical Oncology, 12*(4), 843–850.

Lerman, C., Rimer, B. K., Daly, M., Lustbader, E., Sands, C., Balshem, A., et al. (1994b). Recruiting high risk women into a breast cancer health promotion trial. *Cancer Epidemiology, Biomarkers, and Prevention, 3*(3), 271–276.

Lerman, C., Rimer, B. K., & Engstrom, P. F. (1991). Cancer risk notification: Psychosocial and ethical implications. *Journal of Clinical Oncology, 9*(7), 1275–1282.

Lerman, C., Schwartz, M. D., Miller, S., Daly, M., Sands, C., & Rimer, B. K. (1996). A randomized trial of breast cancer risk counseling: Interacting effects of counseling, educational level, and coping style. *Health Psychology, 15*(2), 75–83.

Lindeman, C. A., & Van Aernam, B. (1971). Nursing intervention with the presurgical patient: The effects of structured and unstructured preoperative teaching. *Nursing Research, 20*(4), 319–332.

Lloyd, S., Watson, S., Waites, B., Meyer, L., Eeles, R., Ebbs, S., et al. (1996). Familial breast cancer: A controlled study of risk perceptions, psychological morbidity, and health beliefs in women attending for genetic counseling. *British Journal of Cancer, 74*(3), 482–487.

Loescher, L. J. (2003). Cancer worry in women with hereditary risk factors for breast cancer. *Oncology Nursing Forum, 30*(5), 767–772.

Lynch, H. T., & Lynch, J. E. (1991). Familial factors and genetic predisposition to cancer: Population studies. *Cancer Detection and Prevention, 15*(1), 49–57.

McCaul, K. D., Branstetter, A. D., O'Donnell, S. M., Jacobsen, K., & Quinlan, K. B. (1998). A descriptive study of breast cancer worry. *Journal of Behavioral Medicine, 21*(6), 565–579.

Passos, J. Y., & Brand, L. M. (1966). Effects of agents used for oral hygiene. *Nursing Research, 15*(3), 196–202.

Pyrczak, F., & Bruce, R. R. (2005). *Writing empirical research reports* (5th ed.). Glendale, CA: Pyrczak.

Stein, K. F., Sargent, J. T., & Rafaels, N. (2007). Intervention research: Establishing fidelity of the independent variable in nursing clinical trials. *Nursing Research, 56*(1), 54-62.

Tulman, L. R., & Jacobsen, B. S. (1989). Goldilocks and variability. *Nursing Research*, *38*(6), 377–379.

Weinstein, N. D. (1988). The precaution adoption process. *Health Psychology*, *7*(4), 355–386.

Weinstein, N. D., Grubb, P. D., & Vautier, J. S. (1986). Increasing automobile seat belt use: An intervention emphasizing risk susceptibility. *Journal of Applied Psychology*, *71*(2), 285–290.

Williams, A. (1972). A study of factors contributing to skin breakdown. *Nursing Research*, *21*(3), 238–243.

Yonkman, C. A. (1982). Cool and heated aerosol and the measurement of oral temperature. *Nursing Research*, *31*(6), 354–357.

CHAPTER **25**

Disseminating Research Findings

Imagine that as a nurse researcher you are conducting a study in which you describe a unique phenomenon, detect a previously unrecognized relationship, or determine the effectiveness of an intervention. This information might make a difference in nursing practice; however, you feel unskilled in presenting the information and overwhelmed by the idea of publishing. You place the study in a drawer with the intent to communicate the findings *someday*. Because of this type of response, many valuable nursing studies are not communicated, and the information is lost. Winslow (1996) believes so strongly in the need to communicate research findings that she views failure to do so as a form of scientific misconduct.

Communicating research findings, the final step in the research process, involves developing a research report and disseminating it through presentations and publications to audiences of nurses, health care professionals, policy makers, and health care consumers. Disseminating study findings provides many advantages for the researcher, the nursing profession, and the consumer of nursing services. By presenting and publishing their findings, researchers advance the knowledge of a discipline, which is essential for providing evidence-based practice. For individual researchers, communicating study findings often leads to professional advancement, personal recognition, and other psychological and financial compensations. These rewards are extremely important for the continuation of research in a discipline. By communicating research findings, the researcher also promotes the critical analysis of previous studies, encourages the replication of studies, and identifies additional research problems. Over time, the findings from many quality studies are synthesized with the ultimate goal of providing evidence-based health care to patients, families, and communities (Craig & Smyth, 2007; Goode, 2000; Melnyk, & Fineout-Overholt, 2005). To facilitate the communication of research findings in nursing, this chapter describes the content of a research report, the audiences for communicating study findings, and the processes for presenting and publishing research reports.

CONTENT OF A RESEARCH REPORT

Both quantitative and qualitative research reports include four major sections or content areas: (1) introduction, (2) methods, (3) results, and (4) discussion of the findings (Boyd & Munhall, 2001; Kerlinger & Lee, 2000; Patton, 2002; Pyrczak & Bruce, 2005; Wolcott, 2001). The type and depth of information included in these sections depend on the study conducted, the intended audiences, and the mechanisms for disseminating the report. For example, theses and dissertations are research reports that are usually developed in depth to demonstrate the student's understanding of the research problem and process to faculty members. Research reports developed for publication in journals are written to communicate study findings efficiently and effectively to nurses and other health care professionals. The methods, results, and discussion sections of qualitative studies are usually more detailed than those of quantitative studies because of the complex data collection and analysis procedures and the comprehensive findings (Boyd & Munhall, 2001; Knafl & Howard, 1984; Patton, 2002).

Quantitative Research Report

This section provides direction to novice researchers writing their initial quantitative research report. To begin, the title of your research report needs to indicate what you have studied and attract the attention of interested readers. The title should be concise and consistent with the study purpose and the research objectives, questions, or hypotheses. Often a title includes the major study variables and population and indicates the type of study conducted but should not include the results or conclusions of a study (Pyrczak & Bruce, 2005). Heo, Moser, Lennie, Zambroski, and Chung (2007, p. 16) provided the following title for their study: "A Comparison of Health-Related Quality of Life between Older Adults with Heart Failure and Healthy Older Adults." This title is concise, states the focus of the study (comparative descriptive), identifies a key study variable (health-related quality of life [HRQOL]), and includes the populations studied (older adults with heart failure and healthy older adults). However, this study is also predictive, and this is not indicated in the study title. The researchers studied additional independent variables (health perception, functional status, physical symptom status, emotional symptom status, and social support) to predict the dependent variable HRQOL in older adults with and without heart failure.

Most research reports also include an abstract that summarizes of the key aspects of the study. An abstract is usually about 200 words long and describes the problem, purpose, framework, methods, sample size, key results, and conclusions (Pyrczak & Bruce, 2005). Later in this chapter we provide details for developing an abstract of a study. Heo et al. (2007) included the following abstract for their study.

Background: Health-related quality of life (HRQOL) in older adults with heart failure may be affected by a variety of variables including, aging. It is important to determine the unique impact of heart failure to more effectively improve HRQOL in this population (problem).

Objective: The purpose of this study was to compare HRQOL and physical, psychologic, clinical, and sociodemographic status in older adults with and without heart failure.

Methods: The HRQOL of 90 older adults with heart failure and 116 healthy older adults was compared. The factors best associated with HRQOL in each group were determined using multiple regression model.

Results: HRQOL was substantially worse among older adults with heart failure than among healthy older adults. Older adults with heart failure had more severe physical and emotional symptoms, poorer functional status, and worse health perceptions. Physical symptom status was the strongest predictor of HRQOL in both groups. In addition, in older adults with heart failure, physical symptom status, age, and anxiety were related to HRQOL.

Conclusions: The poor HRQOL seen in patients with heart failure is not just a reflection of aging. Comprehensive interventions targeted toward the factors that specifically negatively impact HRQOL are essential in older adults with heart failure. (Heo et al., 2007, p. 16)

Heo et al. concisely organized their abstract with headings and clearly indicated the problem (background), sample size (90 older adults with heart failure and 116 healthy older adults), results, and conclusions. The purpose of the study was clearly stated but was listed under the heading "Objective," which might be confusing to readers. The methods for this study lack clarity in this abstract. As a reader, you might be unclear about the type of study design, variables studied, measurement methods, and the data collection process. This abstract has many strengths, but it would have been improved if the authors had clearly labeled the purpose and expanded the methods section.

Following the abstract are the four major sections of a research report: introduction, methods, results, and discussion. Table 25-1 provides an outline of the content covered in each of these sections of a quantitative research report. Heo et al.'s (2007) research report is used as an example when discussing these sections. The complete research article can be accessed through CINAHL or is available online at www.heartandlung.org for registered users.

Introduction

The introduction of a research report discusses the background and significance of the problem; identifies the problem statement and purpose; reviews the relevant empirical and theoretical literature; describes the study framework; and identifies the research objectives, questions, or hypotheses (if applicable). You will have developed this content for the research proposal, and then will summarize it in the final report. Depending on the type of research report, the review of literature and framework might be separate sections or even separate chapters as in a thesis or dissertation. Key content from the introduction of the study by Heo et al. (2007) is presented as an example.

TABLE 25-1 ■■ Outline for a Quantitative Research Report

Introduction

Presentation of the problem: significance, background, and problem statement
Statement of the purpose
Presentation of literature review, including empirical and theoretical literature
Discussion of the framework, including proposition(s) guiding the study
Identification of research objectives, questions, or hypotheses (if applicable)
Identification of conceptual and operational definitions of variables

Methods

Discussion of the research design
Description of the study intervention, intervention protocol, or the process to promote intervention fidelity if and intervention is implemented in the study
Description of the sample (sampling method, sample criteria, refusal or acceptance rate, sample size, sample attrition or retention, and sample characteristics), consent process, and setting
Description of the methods of measurement
Discussion of the data collection process

Results

Description of the data analysis procedures
Organization of results by research objectives, questions, or hypotheses
Presentation of results in tables, figures, and narrative

Discussion

Discussion of major findings
Identification of the limitations
Presentation of conclusions
Identification of the implications for nursing
Recommendations for further research

References

Include only references cited in the text
Use format indicated by the journal guidelines, which is often the APA (2001) format

Despite advances in treatment and care, approximately five million people have heart failure in the United States. The number is increasing each year despite high mortality [significance]. . . .In patients with heart failure, health-related quality of life (HRQOL) is an important outcome that is closely related to clinical outcomes

including rehospitalization and even mortality [background]. . .It is essential to compare these variables and their effects on HRQOL between older adults with and without heart failure to determine the unique impact of heart failure and more effectively improve HRQOL in older adults with heart failure [problem statement].

The purpose of this study was to compare HRQOL between older adults with and without heart failure. The specific aims [objectives] were to (1) compare physical, psychologic, and social variables in older adults with heart failure with those in healthy older adults, and (2) determine the best model predicting HRQOL in each group from among the physical, psychologic, and social variables. (Heo et al., 2007, pp. 16–17)

Review of Literature The review of literature section of a research report documents the current knowledge of the problem investigated. The sources included in the literature review are those that you used to develop your study and interpret the findings. A review of literature can be two or three paragraphs or several pages long. In journal articles, the review of literature is concise and usually includes 15 to 30 sources. Theses and dissertations frequently include an extensive literature review to document the student's knowledge of the research problem. The summary of the literature review clearly identifies what is known, what is not known or the gap in the knowledge base, and the contribution of this study to the current knowledge base. Often the objectives, questions, or hypotheses that were used to direct the study are stated at the end of the literature review. Heo et al. (2007) provided a brief summary of the relevant literature and included what is known and not known about the effects of heart failure on HRQOL. The researchers might have expanded the literature reviewed on the effects of age, health perception, functional status, physical symptom status, emotional symptom status, and social support on HRQOL in individuals with and without heart failure.

Framework A research report needs to include an explicitly identified framework. In this section you will identify and define the major concepts in the framework and describe the relationships among the concepts. You can develop a map or model to clarify the logic within the framework. If a particular proposition or relationship is being tested, that proposition should be clearly stated. Developing a framework map and identifying the proposition(s) examined in a study connect the framework and the research purpose to the objectives, questions, or hypotheses. The concepts in the framework need to be linked to the study variables and are used to conceptually define the variables. Heo et al. (2007, p. 17) clearly identified the framework of their study as the Wilson and Cleary's (1995) HRQOL model that was included in their research report (Figure 25-1). The variables were conceptually and operationally defined and presented in a table that is included later in this chapter.

Methods

The methods section of a research report describes how the study was conducted. This section needs to be concise yet provide sufficient detail for nurses to critically appraise or replicate the study procedures. In this section you will describe the study design, sample, setting, methods of measurement, and data collection process. If the research project included a pilot study, briefly describe the planning, implementation, and results obtained from the pilot study. You will also describe any changes made in the research project based on the pilot study (Pyrczak & Bruce, 2005).

Design   The study design and level of significance (0.05, 0.01, or 0.001) selected are identified in the research report. If your design includes a treatment, your report needs to describe the treatment, including the protocol for implementing the treatment, training of people to implement the protocol or interventionalists, and a discussion of the consistency of administration of the treatment (Santacroce Maccarelli, & Grey, 2004). The reliable and competent implementation of an experimental treatment is referred to in the literature as *intervention fidelity*. Intervention fidelity includes two core components: (1) adherence to the delivery of the prescribed treatment behaviors, ses-

sion, or course and (2) competence in the researcher or interventionalist's skillfulness in delivering the intervention (Stein et al., 2007). Santacroce et al. (2004) and Stein, Sargent, and Rafaels (2007) provided detailed directions to promote intervention fidelity in a variety of quasi-experimental studies and clinical trials.

A complex study design might be presented in a table or figure, such as the examples provided in Chapter 11. Heo et al. (2007, p. 17) implemented a comparative descriptive design to address aim or objective 1 of their study: "(1) compare physical, psychologic, and social variables in older adults with heart failure with those in healthy older adults." They used a predictive design to address objective 2: "(2) determine the best model predicting HRQOL in each group from among the physical, psychologic, and social variables" (Heo et al., 2007, p. 17). Thus, the researchers implemented a combined comparative descriptive and predictive design to accomplish the aims of their study.

Sample and Setting   The research report usually describes the sampling method, criteria for selecting the sample, the sample size, and sample characteristics. It also addresses the use of power analysis to determine sample size and the subject refusal or acceptance rate. The number of subjects completing the study should be provided if it differs from the initial sample size, and the sample attrition or retention rate needs to be addressed. If your subjects were divided into groups (experimental and comparison or control groups), identify the method for assigning subjects to groups and the number of subjects in each group. The protection of subjects' rights and the process of informed consent are also covered briefly. In a published study, the setting is often described in one or two sentences, and agencies are not identified by name unless permission has been obtained. Many researchers present the sample and setting for a study in narrative format; however, some researchers present the characteristics of their sample in a table (see Chapter 14 on sampling). Heo et al. (2007) used the heading "Sample and Setting" to introduce the following description of their sampling process:

Patients hospitalized with an exacerbation of heart failure at one of the three hospitals in a large Midwestern city [setting] were screened during admission for inclusion in the study [sample of convenience]. Patients aged more than 55 years were included. The other inclusion criteria were as follows: (1) a primary diagnosis of heart failure with either preserved or nonpreserved left ventricular systolic function; (2) New York Heart Association

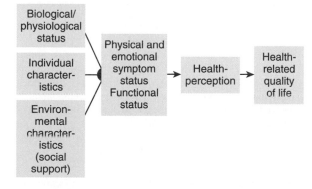

Figure **25-1**   Conceptual framework: Factors affecting health-related quality of life.

(NYHA) functional classification II to IV; (3) discharged home; and (4) living within the greater metropolitan area. Exclusion criteria were as follows: (1) discharged to an extended care facility; (2) referred for hospice or home care; (3) referred to cardiac rehabilitation; or (4) cognitive or psychiatric problems.

Healthy older adults were recruited from three local senior centers [setting] by using flyers and word of mouth [sample of convenience]. Individuals aged more than 55 years were included. Those with the following characteristics were excluded from participation: (1) cognitive or psychiatric problems precluded informed consent; (2) diagnosis of heart disease or heart failure; and (3) other serious chronic illnesses including stroke, chronic lung diseases, and cancer. Older adults with the common comorbidities of hypertension and diabetes were not excluded so individuals with characteristics typical of older adults that are also seen in older adults with heart failure could be included. (Heo et al., 2007, p. 17)

The researchers identified the inclusion and exclusion sample criteria used to determine the target population for the study, older adults with and without heart failure. They also clearly indicated the sample size of 90 older adults with heart failure and 116 healthy older adults, but the sample size would have been strengthened if the researchers had conducted a power analysis. By identifying the refusal and attrition rates for the study, the researchers would have increased the readers' understanding about the representativeness of the sample. The sampling method appeared to be a sample of convenience, but it was not clearly identified. This sampling method increases the potential for sampling error and decreases the ability of the researchers to generalize the study findings.

Methods of Measurement Identifying the methods of measurement operationalizes the variables of a study. Details about the methods of measurement or instruments used in the data collection process are critical if nurses are to critically appraise and replicate a study. Your report needs to describe the information collected by each instrument, the frequency with which the instrument was used in previous research, and any reliability and validity information previously published on the instrument. In addition, your report needs to include the reliability and any further validity development for the current study. If you have used physiological measures, be sure to address their accuracy, precision, selectivity, sensitivity, and sources of error (Kerlinger & Lee, 2000; Pyrczak & Bruce, 2005). In a section titled "Measures," Heo et al. (2007, pp. 17–19) described all of their measurement methods

in detail. Each variable was clearly identified, conceptually defined to link it to the framework, and operationally defined to indicate the measurement methods used. The conceptual and operational definitions (instruments used) were clearly presented in a table (Table 25-2). These researchers provided an excellent link of the framework to the methodology of their study.

Data Collection Process The description of the data collection process in the research report details who collected the data, the procedure for collecting data, and the type and frequency of measurements obtained. In describing who collected the data, your report needs to specify the experience of the data collector and any training provided. If more than one person collected data, describe the precautions taken to ensure consistency (Pyrczak & Bruce, 2005).

Heo et al. (2007) detailed their data collection process in a section of their report titled "Procedure," which is presented in the following excerpt. The data collection process is clear and concise and indicates institutional review board approval, subjects' informed consent, use of trained data collectors, and quality collection of data for each study variable.

■ *PROCEDURE*

Institutional review board approval was obtained for the conduct of this study. Eligible older adults with heart failure were identified by trained nurse research assistants, and those who gave written, informed consent to participate in the study were included. All data on HRQOL, health perception, functional status, physical symptom status, emotional symptom status, biologic/physiologic status, individual characteristics, and environment characteristics (social support) were collected by nurse research assistants after hospital discharge [Table 25-2]. Eligible healthy older adults were identified by investigators among older adults who appeared at three senior centers. Investigators explained the research purpose and procedures, obtained informed consent, and answered participants' questions. All gave written, informed consent. Questionnaires were completed at the senior centers [Table 25-2].

Completion of instruments required 30 to 45 minutes, and trained research nurses were available to assist both older adults with heart failure and healthy older adults. In addition, the instruments were checked to make sure participants did not inadvertently leave any items unanswered. Participants were free to leave items unanswered. (Heo et al., 2007, p. 20)

Results

The results section reveals what you learned from your study and includes the data analysis procedures, the results generated from these analyses, and sometimes

TABLE 25-2 ▪ Variables and Instruments

Variable (Conceptual Definition)	Instrument	
	Older Adults with Heart Failure	Healthy Older Adults
Health-related quality of life (perception of the effects of a clinical condition or its treatment on daily life)	Minnesota Living with Heart Failure	
Health perception (perception of overall health)	One item from SF-36	
Functional status (physical functional impairments in daily activities)	A composite measure from the New York Heart Association functional class	A composite measure from the Duke Activity Status Index
Physical symptom status (dyspnea and fatigue)	A composite measure from Dyspnea and Fatigue Index	A composite measure from two items (dyspnea and fatigue) of the Memorial Symptom Assessment Scale
Emotional symptom status (anxiety and depression)	The subscales (depression and anxiety) of the Brief Symptom Inventory	
Biologic/physiologic status (Number of comorbidities)	Clinical characteristics questionnaire	
Individual characteristic (age and gender)	Demographic questionnaire	
Environmental characteristics (social support)	Marital status and having a confidant by a demographic questionnaire	

From Heo, S., Moser, D. K., Lennie, T. A., Zambroski, C. H., & Chung, M. L. (2007). A comparison of health-related quality of life between older adults with heart failure and healthy older adults. *Heart & Lung, 36*(1), 18.
SF-36, 36-item short form health survey.

the effect size achieved (Kraemer & Thiemann, 1987). The results section is best organized by the research objectives, questions, or hypotheses if stated in the study and, if not, by the study purpose. Heo et al. (2007) provided an excellent description of the analysis techniques used to obtain their results, and they organized their results by characteristics of the sample and the two research aims or objectives.

Data were analyzed using SPSS (Statistical Packages for the Social Sciences) for Windows (version 12.0, SPSS Inc., Chicago, IL). Descriptive statistics including mean, standard deviation, frequency, and percentage were used to present demographic and clinical characteristics. Mann-Whitney *U* test, *t*-test, or chi-square test was used to examine differences in individual characteristics and biologic/physiologic status in older adults with heart failure. To address specific aim [objective] 1, the Mann-Whitney *U* test was used to determine the difference in HRQOL, health perception, functional status, physical and emotional symptom status, and environmental characteristics (social support) because the distribution of each variable in healthy older adults did not show normality. To address specific aim 2, stepwise multiple regression was used to identify variables as a group best associated with HRQOL in each group. A *p* value of less than 0.05 was considered statistically significant. (Heo et al., 2007, p. 20)

Research results can be presented in narrative format and organized into figures and tables. The methods used to present the results depend on the end product of your data analysis and your own preference. When reporting results in a narrative format, include the value of the calculated statistic, the number of degrees of freedom, and probability or *p* value. When reporting nonsignificant results, include the power level for that analysis so that others will be able to evaluate the risk of a type II error (Kraemer & Thiemann, 1987).

The *Publication Manual of the American Psychological Association* (American Psychological Association [APA], 2001) provides direction for citing a variety of statistical results in a research report. For example, the format for reporting chi-square results is χ^2 (degrees of freedom, sample size) = statistical value, *p* value. For example, a chi square value might be presented in the following format in the text of a research report: χ^2 (4, $N = 90$) = 11.14, $p = 0.025$. Statistical values need to be reported with two decimal digits of accuracy; for example, reporting the χ^2 value as 11.14 is more accurate than reporting it as 11.1 (APA, 2001). Heo et al. (2007) presented their results in narrative and table formats. Some of these results are represented in the next section as example tables.

Presentation of Results in Figures and Tables

Figures and tables are used to present a large amount of detailed information concisely and clearly. Researchers use figures and tables to demonstrate relationships, document change over time, and reduce the amount of discussion needed in the text of the report (APA, 2001; Nicol & Pexman, 2003). However, figures and tables are useful only if they are appropriate for the results generated and are well constructed (Wainer, 1984). Table 25-3 provides guidelines for developing accurate and clear figures and tables for a research report. More extensive guidelines and examples for the development of tables and figures for research reports can be found in the *Publication Manual of the American Psychological Association* (APA, 2001) and Nicol and Pexman's books for creating tables (1999) and figures (2003).

TABLE 25-3   Guidelines for Developing Tables and Figures in Research Reports

1. Examine the results obtained from a study, and determine what results are essential to include in the report. Determine which results are best conveyed in figure and table format.
2. Use figures and tables to explain or support only the major points of the report. Using too many figures and tables can overwhelm the rest of the report, but a few receive attention and are effective in conveying the main results. Statistically nonsignificant findings are not usually presented in tables.
3. Keep the figures and tables simple; do not try to convey too much information in a single table. Two simple tables are better than one complex one.
4. Tables and figures should be complete and clear to the reader without referring to the text.
5. Each table and figure needs a clear, brief title.
6. Tables and figures are numbered separately and sequentially in a report. Thus, a report might have a Table 1 and Table 2 and a Figure 1 and Figure 2.
7. The headings, labels, symbols, and abbreviations used in figures and tables need to be appropriate, clear, and easy to read. Any symbols and abbreviations used need to be explained in a note included with the table or figure.
8. Probability values need to be identified with actual p values or with asterisks. If asterisks are used, a single asterisk is used for the least stringent significance level and two or more asterisks for increased stringent significance, such as $*p < 0.05$, $**p < 0.01$, and $***p < 0.001$.
9. Figures and tables need to be referred to in the written text, such as "Table 3 presents…" or "(see Figure 1)." Figures and tables also need to be placed as close as possible to the section of the text where they are discussed (APA, 2001; Nicol & Pexman, 1999, 2003; Pyrczak, 1999; Pyrczak & Bruce, 2005; Wainer, 1984).

Figures Figures or illustrations provide the reader with a picture of the results. Researchers often use computer programs to generate a variety of sophisticated black-and-white and color figures. Some common figures included in nursing research reports are bar graphs and line graphs. Bar graphs can have horizontal or vertical bars that represent the size or amount of the group or variable studied. The bar graph is also a means of comparing one group with another. Jenkins and Ahijevych (2003) conducted a study to describe nursing students' beliefs about cigarette smoking, their own smoking behaviors, as well as their knowledge and use of evidence-based tobacco treatment interventions for patients. The researchers compared the smoking cessation counseling frequency (all, most, some, and none) by smoking status (smoker and nonsmoker) and presented their results in a vertical bar graph (Figure 25-2). The figure indicates that nonsmokers are more likely to counsel patients all of the time about smoking cessation than smokers.

A line graph is developed by joining a series of points with a line and shows how something varies over time. In this type of graph, the horizontal scale is used to measure time, and the vertical scale is used to measure number and quantity (Nicol & Pexman, 2003). A line graph figure needs at least three data points over time on the horizontal axis, and four data points is stronger to show a trend. However, probably no more than 10 data points should be included on a single line on a graph, and there should be no more than four lines per graph. Figure 25-3 is a line

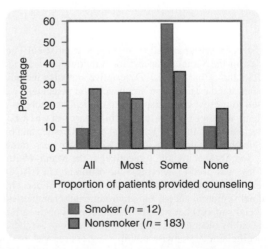

Figure **25-2** Nursing students' self-reported frequency of smoking cessation counseling in percentage by frequency category and student's smoking status (*n* = 195).

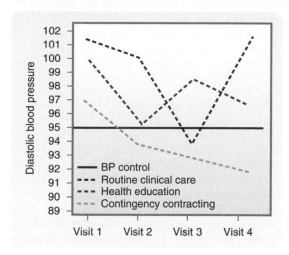

Figure **25-3** Blood pressures by treatment group across four visits.

graph developed by Swain and Steckel (1981, p. 219) to trend the effects of two treatments (health education and contingency contracting) and standard care (routine clinical care) on patients' diastolic blood pressure over four home health visits. Figure 25-3 is well constructed because it includes four data points per line (mean diastolic blood pressures at four visits) and three lines representing the study groups (routine clinical care, health education, and contingency

contracting) being examined for blood pressure differences. The discussion of this graph indicated that blood pressure for the three groups differed significantly ($F = 3.39$, $p < 0.05$), with the contingency contracting group demonstrating the greatest drop in diastolic blood pressure.

Tables Tables are used more frequently in research reports than figures and can be developed to present results from numerous statistical analyses. In tables, the results are presented in columns and rows so that the reader can review them easily. The sample tables included in this section present means, standard deviations, t values, chi-square values (χ^2), Mann-Whitney U values (Z), correlations (r), and regression analysis (R) results. The study variables' means and standard deviations should be included in the published study because of their importance to future research. A variable's mean and standard deviation are essential for (1) providing a basis for comparison across studies, (2) calculating the effect size to determine sample size for future studies, and (3) conducting future meta-analyses (Kraemer & Thiemann, 1987).

Heo et al. (2007) presented the results of their study about HRQOL for older adults with and without heart failure in four tables, and three are included in this chapter. Table 25-4 compares the two groups on individual characteristics (demographic variables) and biological/physiological status. The table includes

TABLE 25-4	Comparison between Older Adults with Heart Failure and Healthy Older Adults in Individual Characteristics and Biological/Physiological Status				
Characteristics	Older Adults with Heart Failure (N = 90) n (%) or M ± SD (Range)	Healthy Older Adults (N = 116) n (%) or M ± SD (Range)	Total (N = 206) n (%) or M ± SD	Statistic	p Value
Age	74.8 ± 8.1 (57-93)	74.2 ± 6.3 (58-92)	74.5 ± 7.1	$t = 0.56$	0.57
Education (y)	11.7 ± 2.6 (3-20)	13.0 ± 2.7 (4-20)	12.4 ± 2.7	$Z = -3.69$	< 0.001
Number of comorbidities	2.3 ± 1.2 (0-5)	1.0 ± 0.9 (0-4)	1.6 ± 1.2	$Z = -7.18$	< 0.001
Sex (male)	48 (53.3)	27 (23.3)	75 (36.4)	$\chi^2 = 18.26$	< 0.001
Marital status					
Married	42 (46.7)	46 (39.7)	88 (42.7)	$\chi^2 = 1.27$	0.74
Divorced/ separated	8 (8.9)	13 (11.2)	21 (10.2)		
Widowed	33 (36.6)	45 (38.8)	78 (37.9)		
Other	7 (7.8)	12 (10.3)	19 (9.2)		
Living arrangements (live alone)	48 (53.3)	61 (52.6)	109 (52.9)	$\chi^2 = 0.01$	0.92

From Heo, S., Moser, D. K., Lennie, T. A., Zambroski, C. H., & Chung, M. L. (2007). A comparison of health-related quality of life between older adults with heart failure and healthy older adults. *Heart & Lung, 36*(1), 19.
SD, Standard deviation.

means and standard deviations (*SDs*) for variables measured at the interval or ratio level (age, education in years, and number of comorbidities) and frequencies and percentages (%) for variables measured at the nominal level (sex, marital status, and living arrangements). The two groups were compared for differences on selected variables using *t*-test (*t*) (variables measured at interval or ratio level), Mann-Whitney *U* (*Z*) (variables measured at ordinal level), and chi-square (χ^2) (variables measured at nominal level). Nonsignificant results ($p > 0.05$) between the two groups on age, marital status, and living arrangements indicate the groups are comparable in these areas. It is expected that the older adults with heart failure would have significantly more comorbidities ($p < 0.001$) than the healthy adults; however, the significant differences for education ($p < 0.001$) and sex ($p < 0.001$) are unexpected. Researchers desire their groups to be comparable on demographic variables, so any differences found between the groups on study variables are less likely to be due to basic demographic differences.

Heo et al. (2007) conducted a Mann-Whitney *U* (*Z*) analysis to address aim or objective 1 to determine differences in two groups for HRQOL, health perception, functional status, physical status, emotional symptoms status (anxiety and depression), and social support (Table 25-5). Older adults with heart failure reported significantly poorer HRQOL, health perceptions,

functional status, physical symptoms status, anxiety, and depression than healthy older adults, with $p < 0.001$. Only social support was not significantly different for the two groups ($p = 0.661$). The results stress the increased needs of individuals with heart failure and the need to develop evidence-based interventions to manage these needs.

McKenna, Maas, and McEniery (1995) examined coronary risk factors before and after percutaneous transluminal coronary angioplasty (PTCA). Table 25-6 presents the results of this study, including descriptive statistics (means, standard deviations, and frequencies) and inferential statistics (*t*-test and chi-square). The *t*-test was used to analyze ratio-level data (serum cholesterol, body mass index, and number of cigarettes per day) and chi-square (χ^2) to analyze nominal data (exercising and smoking habits). In this table, the statistical results are followed by an asterisk, with one asterisk (*) representing results that are significant at $p < 0.05$ and two asterisks (**) representing results significant at $p < 0.001$ (see the key below Table 25-6). McKenna et al. (1995, p. 209) noted that "at post-PTCA follow-up, significant improvements had occurred in mean serum cholesterol levels, mean body mass index, and the number of subjects engaging in regular exercise ($p < 0.001$). … But the frequency of patients smoking after PTCA increased significantly ($p < 0.001$)."

TABLE 25-5	Comparison between Older Adults with Heart Failure and Healthy Older Adults in Health-Related Quality of Life, Health Perception, Functional Status, Physical Symptom Status, Emotional Symptoms Status, and Social Support.			
	Mean ± SD			
Scale	**Older Adults with Heart Failure (N = 90)**	**Healthy Older Adults (N = 116)**	**Statistic**	**p Value**
LHFQ total*	50.8 ± 22.1	14.4 ± 15.9	Z = –9.9	< 0.001
LHFQ physical*	23.1 ± 10.4	7.1 ± 8.1	Z = –9.3	< 0.001
LHFQ emotional*	11.4 ± 7.2	2.3 ± 3.7	Z = –9.1	< 0.001
Health perception*	2.6 ± 0.8	2.1 ± 0.6	Z = –4.9	< 0.001
Functional status*	2.6 ± 0.5	1.7 ± 0.6	Z = –8.6	< 0.001
Physical symptom status†	4.9 ± 2.2	11.0 ± 1.9	Z = –11.8	< 0.001
Emotional symptom status				
Anxiety*	0.9 ± 0.7	0.3 ± 0.5	Z = –6.7	< 0.001
Depression*	1.0 ± 0.8	0.4 ± 0.6	Z = –5.7	< 0.001
Social support†	2.9 ± 0.8	2.8 ± 1.1	Z = –0.4	0.661

From Heo, S., Moser, D. K., Lennie, T. A., Zambroski, C. H., & Chung, M. L. (2007). A comparison of health-related quality of life between older adults with heart failure and healthy older adults. *Heart & Lung, 36*(1), 21.
LHFQ, Minnesota Living with Heart Failure; *SD,* standard deviation.
*Higher scores indicate poor status.
†Higher scores mean better status.

TABLE 25-6 ■ Central Tendency, Variability, and Frequencies with Corresponding Statistics for Risk Factors Pre-PTCA and at Follow-Up

	Descriptive Statistics			
Risk Factor	Pre-PTCA	Follow-up	n	Statistic (Test)
Serum cholesterol	Mean = 240 SD = 47.5	Mean = 222 SD = 39.4	198	$t = 6.24**$
Body mass index	Mean = 26.58 SD = 3.65	Mean = 26.17 SD = 3.61	208	$t = 3.93**$
Currently exercising	$f = 66$ (31.7%)	$f = 135$ (64.9%)	208	$\chi^2 = 38.06**$
Currently smoking	$f = 10$ (4.8%)	$f = 27$ (13.0%)	208	$\chi^2 = 13.80**$
Cigarettes/day	Mean = 9.8 SD = 6.6	Mean = 20.4 SD = 11.9	208	$t = 2.38*$

From McKenna, K. T., Maas, F., & McEniery, P. T. (1995). Coronary risk factor status after percutaneous transluminal coronary angioplasty. *Heart & Lung, 24*(3), 210.
PTCA, Percutaneous transluminal coronary angioplasty; SD, standard deviation.
$*p < 0.05.$
$**p < 0.001.$

Tables are used to identify correlations among variables, and often the table presents a correlational matrix generated from the data analysis. The correlational matrix indicates the correlational values obtained when examining the relationships between variables, two variables at a time (bivariate correlations). The table also includes information about the significance of each correlational value. Evangelista, Doering, and Dracup (2003) conducted a study of the sense of meaning and life purpose from the perspective of women recovering from a heart transplant. One of the questions from their study was "What is the relationship between level of meaning, life purpose, and psychological distress in women after heart transplantation?" (Evangelista et al., 2003, p. 250).

These researchers presented their results in a correlational matrix, shown in Table 25-7. The five variables (meaning, life purpose, anxiety, depression, and hostility) are listed horizontally across the top of the table and vertically down the left side of the table. The relationship of variable 1 Meaning with itself (Meaning) is 1.000. A variable that is correlated with itself results in a perfect positive relationship ($r = 1.000$). Variable 1 Meaning is correlated with variable 2 Life Purpose with $r = 0.353*$. The asterisk (*) indicates that this correlation is significant at $p < 0.05$. Thus, the table identifies the correlational values between the variables and the significance of each of these values. Evangelista et al. (2003) described their table in the text of their article in the following way.

TABLE 25-7 ■ Correlational Matrix for the Key Variables ($N = 33$)

Variable	Meaning	Life Purpose	Anxiety	Depression	Hostility
1. Meaning	1.000				
2. Life Purpose	0.353*	1.000			
3. Anxiety	−0.395*	−0.544†	1.000		
4. Depression	−0.474†	−0.761†	0.719†	1.000	
5. Hostility	−0.313	−0.461†	0.519†	0.796†	1.000

From Evangelista, L. S., Doering, L., & Dracup, K. (2003). Meaning and life purpose: The perspectives of post-transplant women. *Heart & Lung, 32*(4), 253.
$*p < 0.05.$
$†p < 0.001.$

The correlational matrix for the key variables is presented in [Table 25-7]. We observed a correlation between women's sense of meaning and life purpose; higher meaning scores were associated with higher life purpose scores ($p < 0.05$). Meaning was also associated with feelings of anxiety ($p < 0.05$) and depression ($p < 0.001$), but not related to feelings of hostility. On the other hand, perceptions of life purpose were significantly correlated to all 3 mood states ($p < 0.001$); higher levels of life purpose were associated with lower dysphoria [anxiety, depression, and hostility]. (Evangelista et al., 2003, p. 253)

Heo et al. (2007, p. 17) conducted a stepwise regression (R) to address aim or objective 2 in their study "to determine the best model predicting HRQOL in each group from among the physical, psychologic, and social variables." The researchers found "In older adults with heart failure, physical symptom status, age, and one of the emotional symptom status, anxiety, were associated with HRQOL (F [3, 86] = 25.05, p < 0.001)" (Heo et al., 2007, pp. 20–21). The results from the regression analysis are presented in Table 25-8. The table clearly presents the variables included in the regression analysis, the beta (R) result for each variable (physical symptoms status, age, and anxiety), the unique R^2 (percentage of variance of HRQOL explained by each variable), and the accumulated R^2 (0.466 or 46.6% variance explained of HRQOL by the three variables). An analysis of variance (ANOVA) was conducted to determine significance and the result and p value are provided (see Table 25-8).

Discussion

The discussion section ties the other sections of your research report together and gives them meaning. It includes your major findings, limitations of the study, conclusions drawn from the findings, implications of the findings for nursing, and recommendations for further research. Your major findings, which are generated through an interpretation of the results, should be discussed in relation to the research problem; purpose; and objectives, questions, or hypotheses (if applicable). Frequently, a study's findings are compared with the findings from previous research and are linked to the study's framework and the existing theoretical knowledge base. Discussion of the findings also includes the limitations that you identified in the proposal and while conducting the study. For example, a study might have limitations related to sample size, design, or instruments. These limitations influence the generalizability of the findings (Kerlinger & Lee, 2000; Pyrczak & Bruce, 2005).

The research report includes the conclusions or the knowledge generated from the findings. Conclusions are frequently stated in tentative or speculative terms because one study does not produce conclusive findings (Tornquist, Funk, & Champagne, 1989). You might provide a brief rationale for accepting certain conclusions and rejecting others. The conclusions need to be discussed in terms of their implications for nursing knowledge, theory, and practice. Describe how the findings and conclusions might be implemented in specific practice areas. Conclude your research report with recommendations for further research. Identify specific problems that require investigation, and describe procedures for replicating the study. The discussion section of the research report demonstrates the value of conducting the study and stimulates the reader to conduct additional research that is needed to provide evidence-based

TABLE 25-8	Models Best Associated with Health-Related Quality of Life in Older Adults with Heart Failure (N = 90)					
Scale	**Variables**	**Beta**	**Unique R^2**	**Accumulated R^2**	**F**	**p value**
LHFQ	Physical symptom status	−0.501[†]	0.359	0.359	25.050	< 0.001
Total	Age	−0.221[*]	0.071	0.430		
	Anxiety	0.218[*]	0.037	0.466		

LHFQ, Minnesota Living with Heart Failure Questionnaire.

Beta = standardized slope coefficient.

[*]$p < 0.05$.

[†]$p < 0.001$.

From Heo, S., Moser, D. K., Lennie, T. A., Zambroski, C. H., & Misook, L. C. (2007). A comparison of health-related quality of life between older adults with heart failure and healthy older adults. *Heart & Lung, 36*(1), p. 21.

practice (Craig & Smyth, 2007; Melnyk & Fineout-Overholt, 2005).

Heo et al. (2007) linked their study findings with those from previous research, identified the limitations of their study, formed conclusions, indicated areas for future research, and made recommendations for practice. The researchers concluded:

Despite marked differences in physical, psychologic, and HRQOL status between the two groups [healthy older adults and older adults with heart failure] physical symptom status was the variable most strongly related to HRQOL in both groups. Both health care providers and patients who often dismiss negative symptomology as normal signs of aging need to be aware that they are not so appropriate intervention can be undertaken. (Heo et al., 2007, p. 23)

The complete research report for this study can be accessed through CINAHL or is available online at www.heartandlung.org for registered users. We recommend you review the study to increase your understanding of the content and organization of a quantitative research report.

The final aspect of the research report is the reference list, which includes all sources that were cited in the report. Most of the sources in the reference list are relevant studies that provided a knowledge base for conducting the study (O'Neill & Duffey, 2000). These sources need to have complete citations that are recorded in a consistent manner, which is APA format for many nursing journals. The *Publication Manual of the American Psychological Association* (APA, 2001) is in its fifth edition, and Russell and Aud (2002) summarized the key changes that have occurred since the fourth edition. Sources also need to be cited in the text of the report using a consistent format, such as APA (2001). It is also important to follow the format guidelines of the journal the researchers plan to submit their manuscript to for publication.

Qualitative Research Report

Reports for qualitative research are as diverse as the different types of qualitative studies. (The different types of qualitative research are presented in Chapter 4, and results from specific qualitative studies are presented in Chapter 23.) The intent of a qualitative research report is to describe the flexible, dynamic implementation of the research project and the unique, creative findings obtained (Boyd & Munhall, 2001;

Marshall & Rossman, 2006; Munhall, 2001; Patton, 2002). Table 25-9 provides guidelines for developing a qualitative research report. Like the quantitative report, a qualitative research report needs a clear, concise title that identifies the focus of the study. A study by Wright (2003, p. 173) titled "A Phenomenological Exploration of Spirituality among African American Women Recovering from Substance Abuse" is used as an example in presenting the aspects of a qualitative research report.

The abstract for a qualitative research report briefly summarizes the key parts of the study and usually includes the following: (1) aim of the study; (2) evolution of the study; (3) general method of inquiry used (such as phenomenology, grounded theory, ethnography, or historical); (4) brief overview of the method of inquiry applied in the study, including sample, setting, and methods of data collection; (5) brief synopsis of findings; and (6) reflection on the findings (Boyd & Munhall, 2001). Detailed guidelines for developing an abstract for a qualitative study are presented later in this chapter. The abstract for Wright's (2003) study follows.

Spirituality among African American women recovering from substance abuse is a recovery phenomenon: little is known about the individual's experience in this process. The ameliorating effect of spirituality covering a broad range of positive outcomes has been consistent across populations, regardless of gender, race, study design, and religious affiliation. Giorgi's [1985] phenomenological method was used to explore and describe the meaning of spirituality of 15 African American women recovering from substance abuse. The findings are described and discussed relative to the state of the science on spirituality. Implications for substance abuse and recovery practitioners are presented. (Wright, 2003, p. 173)

Wright's abstract (2003) clearly identifies the aim of the study, the type of study conducted (phenomenological), the method used for the investigation (Giorgi), the population (African-American women), and the sample size (15). The abstract might have been expanded to include more detail about the study results and findings. Following the abstract, qualitative research reports usually include four major sections: introduction, methods, results, and discussion. The content included in each of these sections is identified in Table 25-9 and presented next.

TABLE 25-9 ▪ ▪ ▪ Outline for a Qualitative Research Report

Introduction

Identification of the phenomenon to be studied
Identification of the aim or purpose of the study
Identification of the study questions
Identification of the qualitative approach used to conduct the study
Discussion of the significance of the study to nursing
Evolution of the study (sometimes a subheading under the introduction or a separate section)
    Provides a rationale for conducting the study
    Places the study in context historically
    Provides experiential context based on researcher's experience with phenomenon

Methods

Methods of Inquiry: General

Introduction to the specific method (phenomenology, historical, grounded theory, or ethnographical) used to conduct the study
Discussion of the background, philosophy, and assumptions for this method with documentation
Provision of a rationale for choosing this method
Discussion of the general steps, procedures, and outcomes for this method with documentation

Methods of Inquiry: Applied in this Study

Demonstration of the researcher's credentials for conducting a particular type of qualitative study
Description of the sample and setting
Description of the researcher's role
    Entry into the site
    Selection of participants (sample criteria, sampling method, sample size)
    Documentation of ethical considerations: informed consent, confidentiality
    Description of the data collection process, including strengths and weaknesses

Results or Findings of the Inquiry

Description of the data analysis procedures based on the method selected
Presentation of results or findings based on the method used to conduct the study (e.g., experiential themes and the essence of the lived
    experience is provided in a phenomenological study, a theory grounded in study data would be developed with grounded theory
    research, a detailed narrative of a cultural event is developed with ethnographical research, and a detailed description of a historical
    event evolves with historical research)

Discussion

Discussion of findings and relevant literature
Presentation of conclusions and the meanings and understandings developed by the study
Identification of study limitations
Discussion of the relevance of the study
Discussion of the implications for nursing
Recommendations for further research (Boyd & Munhall, 2001; Marshall & Rossman, 2006; Munhall, 2001; Patton, 2002)

References

Include references cited in the report
Use the format indicated by the journal guidelines, which is often the APA (2001) format

Introduction

The introduction section of the report identifies the phenomenon under investigation and specifies the type of qualitative study that was conducted. The study aim or purpose and specific research questions flow from the phenomenon, clarify the study focus, and identify expected outcomes of the investigation. You will use the introduction to describe the significance of the study topic to nursing knowledge and practice, using documentation from the literature. The evolution of the study is described to provide a context for the phenomenon studied. Provide a rationale for conducting the study, and place the study in a historical and an experiential context. The historical context provides a historical basis for the study and situates the study in a period of time. The experiential context presents your involvement in experiencing and understanding the phenomenon under study (Boyd & Munhall, 2001).

Some qualitative studies include a brief literature review in the introduction or a separate section of the report. Other studies include a review of literature only in the discussion of findings. The following text was abstracted from the introduction of Wright's (2003) phenomenological study of spirituality and recovery from substance abuse in African-American women. The complete article can be accessed through CINAHL or found online at www.psychiatricnursing. org for registered users.

Reports in the literature indicate that recovery from substance abuse is a complex multidimensional process that occurs both with and without expert assistance. ... Although studies conducted with women have increased within the last decade, those conducted may not be generalized to African American women. ... Spirituality has often been noted in the healthcare literature to affect recovery. ... Spirituality is considered to be the cornerstone of activities with the African American community (Jackson, 1995). ... A phenomenological understanding of all that spirituality may represent to African American women is relevant to the recovery process from substance abuse. ...

■ *PURPOSE*

A qualitative phenomenological research study was designed to explore the essential elements of the lived experience of spirituality among African American women recovering from substance abuse, and to describe the meanings made of this phenomenon by the person experiencing it. (Wright, 2003, pp. 173–174)

Methods

The methods section includes two parts: general methods of inquiry and the applied or specific methods of inquiry used in the study (see Table 25-9). The general methods section includes the specific qualitative method (such as phenomenology, grounded theory, ethnography, or historical) used to conduct the study and provides a background of that qualitative method. The philosophical basis for and the assumptions of the qualitative method are provided and documented from the current literature. The methodology steps used to conduct a qualitative study vary based on the philosophical

basis of the study, the topic studied, and the experiences of the researcher conducting the study. When developing a report of a qualitative study, you need to discuss the steps of the qualitative method, the procedures, and the outcomes, and provide a rationale for selecting this qualitative method to guide your investigation (Boyd & Munhall, 2001; Marshall & Rossman, 2006). Wright (2003) described the qualitative method used to conduct her investigation in the following way.

■ *METHODS*

Philosophical Perspective. The perspectives of Frankl (1984) provide the conceptual orientation for this study, whereas direction for data analyses was provided by the procedural steps of Giorgi's (1985) method. ... The underpinnings of Frankl's work stresses individual's freedom to transcend suffering and find meaning in life regardless of his circumstances. The substance abuser often looks on his existence as meaningless and without purpose. ... Frankl's (1984) work is based on empirical or phenomenological analysis, which was described as the way in which man understands himself, and how he interprets his own existence [philosophical basis and assumptions for method]. ...

Phenomenology was chosen as the methodology for this study, in that it describes the world as it is experienced before any theories being devised to explain it. The aim of phenomenology in nursing research is to describe the experience of others so that those who care for these individuals may be more empathetic and understanding of the person's experience [method chosen and rationale for using this method]. ...

This study followed the core processes of phenomenology and the four steps outlined in Giorgi's (1985) method, which are as follows: (1) The researcher reads the entire description of the learning situation obtained from the participants to get a sense of the whole statement; (2) next, once a sense of the whole has been grasped, the researcher rereads the same description more slowly with specific intent of discriminating "meaning units" from within a psychological perspective and with a focus on the phenomenon of interest; (3) once the "meaning units" have been delineated, the researcher then goes through all of the "meaning units" and expresses the psychological insight contained in them more directly; ... (4) finally, the researcher synthesizes the transformed meaning units [steps of the method used to analyze data and determine outcomes]. (Wright, 2003, pp. 174–176)

In the applied methods section, you will document your credentials for conducting the study. This documentation is valuable in determining the worth of the study because the researcher serves as a primary data-gathering instrument and the data analyses occur within the reasoning processes of the researcher (Patton, 2002). In the report of your qualitative study, you will describe the site and participants selected for the study. Your unique role as the researcher is also detailed, including training of project staff, entry into the setting, selection of participants, and ethical considerations extended to the participants during data collection and analysis (see Table 25-9).

The data collection process is time consuming and complex. The research report includes a description of the variety of data collection tools used, such as observation guides, open-ended interviews, direct participation, documents, life histories, audiovisual media (photographs, DVDs, videos, or audiotapes), biographies, and diaries (Knafl & Howard, 1984; Leininger, 1985; Patton, 2002). The flexible, dynamic way in which the researcher collects data is described, including the time spent collecting data, how data were recorded, and the amount of data collected. For example, if your data collection involved participant observation, you must describe the number, length, structure, and focus of the observation and participation periods. In addition, you will identify the tools (such as audiotapes or DVDs) for recording the information gained from these periods of observation and participation. Wright (2003) described the methods applied in her study in the following way.

■ *STUDY PARTICIPANTS*

The number of participants was determined by the number of persons required to permit an in-depth exploration and obtain a clear understanding of the phenomenon of interest from various perspectives. This occurred with 15 participants when data saturation was achieved, with no new themes or essences emerging from the participants and the data were repeating. Participants were recruited from a women's shelter with the help of a colleague as contact person, from church support groups within the community by the researcher who made church members aware of the study and the search for participants, and through networking, whereby each participant interviewed suggested the name of a potential new participant [participant selection].

Each participant met the following criteria: over 18 years of age; identified herself as an African American woman; substance free status for at least 1 year; ... and was able to read and write in the English language.

There were 15 participants who ranged from 29 to 49 years of age. ... With respect to abstinence eight participants reported 7–12 years of drug free status, and seven having 15–39 months of substance free status [description of the sample]. ...

■ *PROCEDURE AND DATA COLLECTION*

... The purpose of the study was explained and informed consent obtained. All participants were interviewed in their homes or the shelter with each interview being audiotaped and lasting 45 to 90 minutes. ...

Although Giorgi's (1985) phenomenological analysis does not rely on peer debriefing, to establish qualitative rigor, notes were recorded after each interview regarding the process, feelings, and experiences of the researcher elicited by the interview. In this study during each interview the researcher was genuinely interested in participant's experience and listened honestly to their descriptions. This journaling ensured bracketing or the suspension of presuppositions on the part of the researcher. (Wright, 2003, pp. 176–177)

Results

The results section of the research report includes data analysis procedures and presentation of the findings. The data, in the form of notes, tapes, and other materials from observations and interviews, must be synthesized into meaningful categories or organized into common themes by the researcher. The data analysis procedures (content, symbolic, structural, interactional, philosophical, ethnographical, phenomenological, semantic, historical, inferential, grounded theory, perceptual, and reflexive) are performed during and after the data collection process (Leininger, 1985; Marshall & Rossman, 2006; Miles & Huberman, 1994; Munhall, 2001; Patton, 2002). These analysis procedures and the process for implementing them are described in Wright's (2003) research report.

After each interview was transcribed, the researcher carefully listened to the audiotape to ensure accuracy in the transcription. The narrative of each experience was then analyzed according to Giorgi's (1985) phenomenological method. ... Following this approach, the researcher identified 1669 naïve meaning units in the transcribed interviews. These naïve meaning units were then transformed through the process of reflection and intuitive variation into 631 formulated meaning units or constituents of the essence of spirituality for these recovering women. These essences or themes and supporting theme clusters were then formulated and later discussed in the findings. (Wright, 2003, p. 177)

Present your results in a manner that clarifies for the reader the phenomenon under investigation. These results include gestalts, patterns, and theories that are developed to describe life experiences, cultures, and historical events, which are frequently expressed in narrative format. Sometimes, these theoretical ideas

TABLE 25-10 ■ Major Meaning Units
Major Themes from the Participants' Narratives
1. The absence of spirituality was experienced as abandonment when there was no personal and intimate relationship with God.
2. Spirituality was experienced as surrendering when there was a spiritual awakening.
3. The women recovering from substance abuse experienced spirituality as reconnecting when there was recognition, a realignment, and engagement with God, self, and community.
4. Spirituality was experienced as transformation when the women were able to transcend substance abuse and other difficulties and focus on restoration and growth toward new horizons.
5. Spirituality was experienced as maturation when there was attainment of newness in life.

From Wright, V. L. (2003). A phenomenological exploration of spirituality among African American women recovering from substance abuse. *Archives of Psychiatric Nursing, 17*(4), 177.

are organized into conceptual maps, models, or tables. Researchers often gather additional data or reexamine existing data to verify their theoretical conclusions, and this process is described in the report (Marshall & Rossman, 2006; Miles & Huberman, 1994). Some qualitative study findings lack clarity and quality, which makes it difficult for practitioners to understand and apply them. Some of the problems with qualitative study findings are misuse of quotes and theory, lack of clarity in identifying patterns and themes in the data, and misrepresentation of data and data analysis procedures in the report (Sandelowski & Barroso, 2002). Researchers must clearly and accurately develop their findings and present them in a way that a diverse audience of practitioners and researchers can understand. Wright (2003) presented her study results in tables and narrC

Five major themes were formulated from the narratives [Table 25-10]. Each of these themes has supporting themes that have been extrapolated from the narratives. A typology of the themes and supporting themes [was] created. These themes and supporting theme clusters were not exclusive or isolated experiences but represent aspects of the participants' experiences, which sometimes are interwoven or overlap. Two examples of the themes and supporting themes, are described in [Table 25-11] to provide the reader with information about activities during the process of formulating naïve-meaning units to main themes, which emerged as the essence or meaning structure. Each of the themes is presented with supporting

verbatims to substantiate the researcher's process in identification of themes and for the reader to grasp a full understanding of the participant's experience. (Wright, 2003, pp. 177–178)

Discussion

The discussion section includes conclusions, study limitations, implications for nursing, and recommendations for further research. The conclusions are a synthesis of the study findings and the relevant theoretical and empirical literature. Limitations are often identified and their influence on the formulation of the conclusions is addressed. Conclusions include the study aim and the research questions, which were used to guide the conduct of the study. Implications of the findings for nursing practice and theory development are explored, and suggestions are provided for further research (Boyd & Munhall, 2001; Patton, 2002). Wright (2003) formed conclusions with support from the relevant literature, identified study limitations, and provided implications for practice. She provided limited direction for further research.

> The women spoke of their experience of how they lived in a state of chronic apartness, separated from God and from those who love them. Their attachment to substances usurped God, their desire for love, and their ability to love and trust. ... In this study the women's recovery from substance abuse began when they hit rock bottom, struggled and then let go by surrendering and turning their lives over to God. ...
>
> The study limitations, however, were the researcher having worked in psychiatry and substance abuse for many years observed a difference in the lives of African American women who had incorporated a spiritual belief in their recovery process. Most of the participants were recruited from faith-based women's shelter and church support groups; therefore, it was known that their belief was in God. ...
>
> Only by becoming more knowledgeable about spirituality and the experiences of African American women recovering from substance abuse can nurses become a successful tool in assisting these women in their recovery. (Wright, 2003, pp. 181–184)

Theses and Dissertations

Theses and dissertations are research reports that students develop in depth as part of the requirements for a degree. The content included in a thesis or dissertation depends on the university requirements, the nursing college or school's research guidelines, and the members of the student's research committee. Most theses and dissertations are organized by chapters, and the usual chapters and content for quantitative and outcomes studies are presented in Table 25-12.

TABLE 25-11 ▪ Typology of Major Themes, Meaning Units, and Participant's Description

Themes	Meaning Units (MUs)	Participant's Description
The women recovering from substance abuse experienced the absence of spirituality as abandonment when there was no personal and intimate relationship with God.	MU:1.1. The absence of spirituality was experienced as abandonment when participants recalled feeling as if something was missing from their lives and of being far from God, in the dark, and in bondage.	This participant experienced the absence of spirituality as abandonment by stating, "There was something missing before and I didn't know what it was. It was as if I was searching for something and I had to go through all the hard times to find it. He's shown me the light because I was in the dark."
	MU:1.2. The absence of spirituality was experienced as abandonment when the women related feeling alone and saw separation from God and others because of death or other circumstances as contributing factors.	The participant spoke of abandoning her family: "So at that Christmas dinner all my family ganged up on me and confronted me about my drug use, so I left the dinner. I didn't go to any more family gatherings for about 10 years. I abandoned my family. Even though I was clean, I didn't feel happy. I think after I stopped using, this was the loneliest period of my life. I felt alone, like I had no one in the world."
The women recovering from substance abuse experienced spirituality as surrendering when there was a spiritual awakening.	MU:2.1. The women reported turning their lives and their will over to God, letting go, relinquishing control, and putting the past behind as surrendering.	The woman stated, "I had to learn how to admit that I really don't have all the answers. I surrendered my know-it-all-ism."
	MU:2.2. The women identified struggling, powerlessness, and a total dependency on God as surrendering.	This woman stated, "When I hit 18 months clean I was struggling and I was crying out to everybody. I was showing up for Bible study, I was showing up for church. I was doing all that I could do, but it wasn't enough. I still didn't have what it took on the inside. I had a dependency. I had been praying to the Lord for dependency. I said 'Lord, I want to be totally dependent on you.' So God allowed everything that I had depended on to be gone."

From Wright, V. L. (2003). A phenomenological exploration of spirituality among African American women recovering from substance abuse. *Archives of Psychiatric Nursing, 17*(4), 178.

A thesis or dissertation that involves a qualitative study would include sections or chapters similar to those in Table 25-9.

AUDIENCES FOR COMMUNICATION OF RESEARCH FINDINGS

Before developing a research report, you need to determine *who* will benefit from knowing the findings. The greatest impact on nursing practice can be achieved by communicating nursing research findings to a variety of audiences, including nurses, other health professionals, health care consumers, and policy makers. Nurses, including administrators, educators, practitioners, and researchers, must be aware of research findings for communication in academic programs, for use in practice, and as a basis for conducting additional studies. Other health professionals need to be aware of the knowledge generated by nurse researchers and facilitate the use of that knowledge in the health care system as part of the delivery of evidence-based practice (Craig & Smyth, 2007). Consumers are interested in the outcomes produced by nursing interventions that have been tested through research. Policy makers at the local, state, and federal levels use research findings to generate health policy that will have an impact on consumers, individual practitioners, and the health care system (Brown, 1999).

TABLE 25-12	Outline for Theses and Dissertations of Quantitative Studies
Chapter I	Introduction
	Background and significance of the problem
	Statement of the problem
	Statement of the purpose
Chapter II	Review of Relevant Literature
	Review of relevant theoretical literature
	Review of relevant empirical literature
	Summary
Chapter III	Framework
	Development of a framework
	Identification of proposition(s) to guide the study
	Formulation of objectives, questions, or hypotheses
	Conceptual and operational definition of research variables
	Definition of relevant terms
	Identification of assumptions
Chapter IV	Methods and Procedures
	Identification of the research design
	Description of the intervention, intervention protocol, and or process for promoting intervention fidelity if the study has an intervention
	Description of the population and sample
	Identification of the setting
	Presentation of ethical considerations
	Description of measurement methods
	Description of the data collection process
Chapter V	Results
	Description of data analysis procedures
	Presentation of results
Chapter VI	Discussion
	Presentation of major findings
	Identification of limitations
	Identification of conclusions
	Discussion of the implications for nursing
	Recommendations for further research
References	
Appendices	

TABLE 25-13	Audience and Strategies for Communicating Research
Audience	Strategies for Communicating Research
Nurses— Administrators, Educators, Practitioners, and Researchers	**Oral and Visual Presentations**
	Nursing research conferences
	Professional nursing meetings and conferences
	Collaborative nursing groups
	Thesis and dissertation defenses
	DVD, videotaped, and audiotaped presentations
	Websites
	Written Reports
	Nursing-referred journals
	Nursing books
	Monographs
	Research newsletters
	Theses and dissertations
	Foundation reports
	Electronic databases
Other Health Care Professionals	**Oral and Visual Presentations**
	Professional conferences and meetings
	Interdisciplinary collaboration
	DVD and taped presentations
	Written Reports
	Professional journals and books
	Newsletters
	Foundation reports
	Electronic databases
Policy Makers	**Oral and Visual Presentations**
	Testifying on health problems to state and federal legislators
	Written Reports
	Research reports to legislators
	Research reports to funding agencies

Continued

Strategies for Communicating Research to Different Audiences

Research findings can be communicated through written reports in hard copy or electronic format and by oral and visual presentations. Table 25-13 outlines various strategies for communicating findings to nurses, health care professionals, policy makers, and consumers.

Audience of Nurses

The most common mechanisms nurses use to communicate research findings to their peers are presentations at conferences and meetings. An increasing number of nursing organizations and institutions are sponsoring research conferences. The American

TABLE 25-13 Audience and Strategies for Communicating Research—Cont'd		
	Written Reports Electronic databases AHRQ and NINR reports and presentations to policy makers, practitioners, and consumers	
Health Care Consumers	**Oral and Visual Presentations** Television and radio Community meetings Patient and family teaching	
	Written Reports Newspaper News and popular magazines Electronic databases	

Nurses Association and many of its state associations sponsor annual nursing research conferences. The Western Council of Higher Education for Nursing has sponsored annual research conferences since 1968, and the proceedings from these conferences are published in a volume titled *Communicating Nursing Research Findings.* The members of Sigma Theta Tau, the international honor society for nursing, sponsor international, national, regional, and local research conferences. Specialty organizations, such as the American Association of Critical Care Nurses, the Oncology Nurses' Society, and the Maternal-Child Health Nursing Association, sponsor research meetings and conferences. Many universities and some health care agencies sponsor or cosponsor research conferences. For a variety of reasons, many nurses are unable to attend research conferences. To increase the communication of research findings, conference sponsors provide audiotapes or DVDs of the research presentations. Some sponsors publish abstracts of studies with the conference proceedings or in a specialty journal or make them available electronically on their websites.

The publishing opportunities in nursing continue to escalate—the number of nursing journals published in the United States increased from 22 in 1977 (McCloskey, 1977) to 92 in 1991 (Swanson, McCloskey, & Bodensteiner, 1991). Opportunities to publish research have expanded with the growth of research journals (*Advances in Nursing Science, Applied Nursing Research, Biological Research for Nursing, Clinical Nursing Research, Nursing Research, Qualitative Health Research, Research in Nursing &*

Health, Scholarly Inquiry for Nursing Practice: An International Journal, and *Western Journal of Nursing Research*) and with specialty journals publishing more studies. *Heart & Lung* is now 70% research publications, *Maternal-Child Nursing* is 75% research, and *Journal of Nursing Education* is 80% research (Swanson et al., 1991). The rapidly growing number of peer-reviewed electronic nursing journals also provides opportunities to publish research findings. A number of researchers communicate their findings by publishing books or chapters in books.

Many universities and hospitals publish regular newsletters or monographs that include abstracts or articles about the research conducted by their members. Foundations and federal agencies publish reports of studies that have been conducted or are in progress. The American Nurses' Foundation publishes a newsletter, *Nursing Research Report,* which identifies the studies funded and includes abstracts of these studies. The National Institute for Nursing Research (NINR) publishes reports on its grants, including research project titles, names and addresses of researchers, period of support, a brief description of each project, and publication citations (www.nih.gov/ninr).

Audience of Health Care Professionals and Policy Makers

Nurse researchers communicate their research to other health professionals at meetings and conferences sponsored by such organizations as the American Heart Association, American Public Health Association, American Cancer Society, American Lung Association, National Hospice Organization, and National Rural Health Association. Nurses must believe in the value of their research and present their findings at conferences that attract a variety of health care professionals. Nurse researchers and other health professionals conducting research on the same or similar problems might join together to publish a journal article, a series of articles, a book chapter, or even a book. This type of interdisciplinary collaboration might increase the communication of research findings and the synthesis of research knowledge to promote evidence-based practice.

In 1989, the Agency for Health Care Policy and Research (AHCPR) was established to enhance the quality, appropriateness, and effectiveness of health care services and access to these services. In 1999, the AHCPR was renamed the Agency for Healthcare Research and Quality (AHRQ), which was one of the first organizations to develop and distribute evidence-based guidelines for practice. Recently, the AHRQ implemented the "Evidence-based Practice Centers (EPC) Program that includes the awarding of a 5 year contract to institutions in the United States and Canada to serve as an EPC. The EPCs review all relevant scientific literature on clinical, behavioral, and organization and financing topics to produce evidence reports and technology assessments. These reports are used for informing and developing coverage decisions, quality measures, educational materials and tools, guidelines, and research agendas. The EPCs also conduct research on methodology of systematic reviews" (AHRQ, 2007). The institutions with EPCs and the activities of these centers can be viewed online at www.ahrq. gov/clinic/epc.

Audience of Health Care Consumers

An audience that nurse researchers frequently neglect is the health care consumer. The findings from nursing studies can be communicated rapidly to the public through news releases. A nursing research article published in a local paper has the potential of being picked up by the National Wire Service and published in other papers across the United States. Nurse researchers also need to make their findings available through electronic databases. An increasing amount of health care information is being made available electronically on a variety of websites, but often this information is not based on research. There is a need to provide consumers with evidence-based guidelines and educational materials to assist them in making quality health care decisions.

Nursing research findings could be communicated to consumers by being published in news magazines, such as *Time* and *Newsweek*, or popular women's and health magazines, such as *American Baby* and *Health*. Health articles published for consumer magazines can reach 20,000 to 24 million readers at a time (Jimenez, 1991). Television and radio are other valuable sources for communicating research findings. Currently, the findings from many medical studies are covered through these media; thus, the study findings are reaching many health care consumers and practitioners. Another important method of communicating research findings to consumers is through patient and family teaching. Nursing interventions and practice protocols based on research are more credible to consumers than are unresearched actions, with the ultimate goal being evidence-based practice (Craig & Smyth, 2007).

PRESENTING RESEARCH FINDINGS

Research findings are communicated at conferences and meetings through verbal and poster presentations. With presentations, researchers have an opportunity to share their findings, answer questions about their studies, interact with other interested researchers, and receive immediate feedback on their study. After completion of the research project, the findings are frequently presented at conferences with little delay, whereas when research findings are published, a 1- to 3-year delay in the communication process is typical.

Verbal Presentations

Researchers communicate their findings through verbal presentations at local, national, and international nursing and health care conferences. Presenting findings at a conference requires receiving acceptance as a presenter, developing a research report, delivering the report, and responding to questions.

Receiving Acceptance as a Presenter

Most research conferences require researchers to submit an abstract, and acceptance as a presenter is based on the quality of the abstract. As noted earlier, an abstract is a clear, concise summary of a study that is usually limited to 100 to 250 words (Crosby, 1990; Pyrczak & Bruce, 2005). Nine months to a year before a research conference, the sponsors circulate a call for abstracts. Many research journals and newsletters publish these calls for abstracts, and they are also available electronically. In addition, conference sponsors will e-mail and mail the calls for abstracts to universities, major health care agencies, and known nurse researchers.

The call for abstracts will stipulate the format for the abstract. Frequently, abstracts are limited to one page, single-spaced, and include the content outlined in Table 25-14 or Table 25-15. Table 25-14 includes an outline of the content included in an abstract of a quantitative study, and Table 25-15 includes abstract content for a qualitative study (Boyd & Munhall, 2001). The title of your abstract must create interest, and the body of your abstract "sells" the study to the reviewers. An example of an abstract is presented in Figure 25-4. Writing an abstract requires practice; frequently, a researcher will rewrite an abstract many times until it meets all the criteria outlined by the conference sponsors. Cason, Cason, and Redland (1988) identified six criteria that are often used to rate the quality of an abstract: (1) acceptability of a study for a specific program; (2) overall quality of the work; (3) contribution to nursing scholarship; (4) contribution

TABLE 25-14	Outline for Quantitative Study Abstract

I. Title of the Study

II. Introduction

Statement of the problem and purpose
Identification of the framework

III. Methodology

Design
Sample size
Identification of data analysis methods

IV. Results

Major findings
Conclusions
Implications for nursing
Recommendations for further research

TABLE 25-15	Outline for a Qualitative Study Abstract

I. Title of the Study

II. Introduction

Identification of phenomenon to be studied
Statement of the aim of the study
Identification of the qualitative method used to conduct the study
Evolution of the study (rationale for conducting the study, historical context, and experiential context)

III. Methodology

Discussion of the background, philosophy, and assumptions for the method used to conduct the study
Brief description of the sample, setting, and data collection process

IV. Results

Brief description of data analysis procedures
Major findings
Conclusions
Implications for nursing
Recommendations for further research

to nursing theory and practice; (5) originality of the work; and (6) clarity and completeness of the abstract, according to the content outlined in Tables 25-14 and 25-15. These criteria might assist you in developing and refining your abstract.

Developing a Research Report

The report developed depends on the focus of the conference, the audience, and the time designated for each presentation. Some conferences focus on certain sections of the research report, such as tool development, data collection and analysis, findings, or implications of the findings for nursing practice. However, it is usually important to address the major sections of a research report (introduction, methods, results, and discussion) in a presentation. The content of a presentation varies depending on whether the audience consists of mainly researchers or clinical nurses (Jackle, 1989). If you do not know who your audience is, ask the sponsors of the conference.

Time is probably the most important factor in developing a presentation because many presenters are limited to 12 to 15 minutes, with 5 minutes for questions (Selby, Tornquist, & Finerty, 1989a). As a guideline, you might spend 10% of your time on the introduction, 20% on the methodology, 35% on the results, and 35% on the discussion. Your introduction might include reasons for the study, a brief review of the literature, a simple discussion of the framework, and the research questions or hypotheses. The methodology content includes a brief identification of the design, sampling method, and measurement techniques. The content covered in the results section includes a simple rationale for the analysis methods used and the major statistical results. The presentation concludes with a brief discussion of findings, implications of the findings for nursing practice, and recommendations for future research (Miracle & King, 1994). Most researchers find that the shorter the presentation time, the greater the preparation time needed.

Many researchers develop a typed script of their study for presentation and include visuals such as PowerPoint slides and pictures. The script for the presentation needs to indicate when a visual is to be shown. The information presented on each visual should be limited to eight lines or fewer, with six or fewer words per line. Thus, a single visual should contain information that can be easily read and examined in 30 seconds or a minute (Selby Tornquist, & Finerty, 1989b). Only major points are presented on visuals, so use single words, short phrases, or bulleted points to convey ideas, not complete sentences. Figures such as bar graphs and line graphs usually convey ideas more clearly than tables do

Title: Symptoms of Female Survivors of Child Sexual Abuse

Investigator: Polly A. Hulme

Research indicates that at least 20% of all women have been victims of serious sexual abuse involving unwanted or coerced sexual contact up to the age of 17 years. Women who suffered sexual abuse as children often experience a variety of physical and psychosocial symptoms as adults. Identifying this pattern of symptoms might assist health professionals in recognizing and treating nonreporting survivors of child sexual abuse. The framework of this study is Finkelhor and Browne's (1986) theory of traumagenic dynamics in the impact of child sexual abuse. This theory indicates that child sexual abuse is at the center of the adult survivor's existence and results in four trauma-causing dynamics: traumatic sexualization, betrayal, powerlessness, and stigmatization. These traumagenic dynamics lead to behavioral manifestations that collectively indicate a history of child sexual abuse. The severity of the behavioral manifestations is influenced by the contributing factors or characteristics of the abuse that affect the survivor's life.

The study design was descriptive correlational and the Adult Survivors of Incest (ASI) Questionnaire (Brown & Garrison, 1990) was used to determine the symptoms and contributing factors for 22 adult survivors of child sexual abuse. Six physical symptoms were experienced by 50% of the subjects, and over 75% of the subjects experienced 11 psychosocial symptoms. The number of physical symptoms correlated significantly with other victimizations ($r = 0.59$) and number of psychosocial symptoms ($r = 0.56$). The number of psychosocial symptoms also correlated significantly with other victimizations ($r = 0.40$) and duration of abuse ($r = 0.40$).

The findings suggest that the ASI Questionnaire was effective in identifying patterns of symptoms and contributing factors of adult survivors of child sexual abuse. Additional study is needed to determine the usefulness of this questionnaire in identifying nonreporting survivors in clinical situations (Hulme & Grove, 1994).

Figure 25-4 Example of an abstract.

for presentations. Slides of the research setting, equipment, and researchers collecting data help the audience to visualize the research project. The use of color on a visual can increase the clarity of the information presented and can be appealing to the audience.

Preparing the script and visuals for a presentation is difficult, so enlist the assistance of an experienced researcher and audiovisual expert. Rehearse your presentation with the experienced researcher, and use his or her comments to refine your script, visuals, and presentation style. If your presentation is too long, synthesize your script and provide handouts for important content. PowerPoint slides provide an excellent format for presenting a research report; they include easy-to-read fonts, color, creative background, and visuals or pictures to clarify points. However, consulting an audiovisual expert will ensure that your materials are clear and properly constructed, with the print large enough and dark enough for the audience to read. Once the PowerPoint slides have been developed, view them from the same vantage point as the audience to ensure the visuals are clear.

Delivering a Research Report and Responding to Questions

A novice researcher might attend conferences and examine the presentation style of other researchers. Even though each researcher needs to develop his or her own presentation style, observing others can promote an effective style. The research report can be read from a script, given from an outline, or delivered with slides or transparencies. An effective presentation requires practice. You need to rehearse your presentation several times, with the script, until you are comfortable with the timing, content, and your presentation style. When practicing, use the visuals so that you are comfortable with the equipment. The presentation must be within the time frame designated by conference sponsors. Mathieson (1996) provided some practical advice for the novice presenter.

Some conferences include a presentation by the researcher, a critical appraisal of the study by another researcher, and a question period. When preparing for a presentation, try to anticipate the questions that members of the audience might ask, and rehearse your answers. You could give your presentation to colleagues and ask them to raise questions. If you practice making clear, concise responses to specific questions, you will be less anxious during the actual presentation. When giving a presentation, make notes of the audience's questions, suggestions, or comments because they are often useful when preparing a manuscript for publication or developing the next study.

Poster Sessions

Sometimes, your research will be accepted at a conference not as a presentation but as a poster session. A poster session is a visual presentation of your study.

Before developing a poster, contact the conference sponsors regarding (1) the size limitations or format restrictions for the poster, (2) the size of the poster display area, and (3) the background and potential number of conference participants. A poster usually includes the following content: the title of the study; investigator and institution names; brief abstract; purpose; research objectives, questions, or hypotheses (if applicable); framework; design; sample; instruments; essential data collection procedures; results; conclusions; implications for nursing; and recommendations for further research. For clarity and conciseness, a poster often includes pictures, tables, or figures to communicate the study. Figure 25-5 presents a quality poster developed by Dr. Kathy Daniel, a faculty member at The University of Texas at Arlington and an adult and gerontology nurse practitioner. Dr. Daniel conducted a study with other health care professions to describe the determinants of chronic kidney disease (CKD) progression among indigent elderly. This poster, which was presented at the American Nephrology Society meeting in 2007, has a polished, professional look and presents the key aspects of the study using a balance of text, figures, and color. Conference sponsors often provide boards for displaying posters, so the poster can be easily transported in a tube and rapidly displayed.

A quality poster completely presents a study yet can be comprehended in 5 minutes or less. Bold headings are used for the different parts of the research report, followed by concise narratives. The size of the print on a poster needs to be large enough to be read at 4 to 6 feet (approximately 20 to 30 font size) (Nicol & Pexman, 2003). Poster sessions usually last from 1 to 2 hours; you should remain with your poster during this time. Most researchers provide conference participants with copies of their abstract and other relevant handouts and offer to answer any questions. Websites are available to assist you with research poster development, such as http://ublib.buffalo.edu/libraries/asl/guides/bio/posters.html or www.biology.lsa.umich.edu/research/labs/ktosney/file/PostersHome.html. You can also Google "research poster" or "research poster presentation" and view additional websites to assist you in developing a poster.

Conferences include both quantitative and qualitative research posters. Russell, Gregory, and Gates (1996) reported the results of reviewing qualitative posters at conferences. One-fourth of the posters had too little information; however, many of them had too much information. Narrative content does not lend itself to the crisp presentation required on a poster. Moore, Augspurger, King, & Proffitt (2001, p. 102) noted that an effective poster must have quality in "(a) poster design and layout, (b) poster visuals, (c) poster overall aesthetics, and (d) poster content."

The number of words on a poster of a qualitative study should be kept to a minimum. As stated previously, the size of print should allow viewers to read it easily from 4 to 6 feet. Russell et al. (1996) recommended having color-coordinated sections of the poster with written material provided in matted format. Summary and implications sections are frequently omitted in qualitative posters. This omission is a serious problem, because most viewers search for that content first. Because rich narrative text is so meaningful in qualitative studies, authors are advised to compile a notebook with additional data examples and artwork that viewers can examine. Posters usually take from 10 to 20 hours to develop based on the complexity of the study and the experience of the researcher. Novice researchers usually need more than 20 hours to develop a poster, and posters of qualitative studies often take more time. Some important points in poster development include planning ahead, seeking the assistance of others, and limiting the information on the poster (Moore et al., 2001).

An advantage of a poster session is the opportunity for one-to-one interaction between the researcher and those viewing the poster. At the end of the poster session, individuals interested in a study will frequently stay to speak to the researcher. Have a notepad on hand to record comments and the names and addresses of those conducting similar research. This occasion is an excellent opportunity to begin networking with other researchers involved in the same area of research. Sometimes, conference participants will want study instruments or other items to be mailed, faxed, or e-mailed to them, so it is essential that you keep a record of their names, addresses, fax numbers, e-mail addresses, and requests for information.

PUBLISHING RESEARCH FINDINGS

Presentations are a valuable means of rapidly communicating findings, but their impact is limited. **Published research** findings are permanently recorded in a journal or book and usually reach a larger audience than presentations do (Winslow, 1996). However, the research report developed for a presentation can provide a basis for writing an article for publication. Regrettably, many researchers present their findings at a conference and never submit the paper for publication. Hicks (1995) studied the publishing activities of 500 randomly selected nurses and found that only 10% submitted their studies for publication. Studies with

Determinants of CKD Progression among Indigent Elderly

K. Daniel, PhD, RN, ANP-BC; C. Cason, PhD, RN;
P. Gleason-Wynn, LMSW, PhD; R. Sesso, MD; B. Vicioso, MD

Mildred Wyatt and Ivor P. Wold Center for Geriatric Care, UT Southwestern Medical Center at Dallas, Dallas, TX;
Escola Paulista de Medicina, Sao Paolo, Brazil; and University of Texas at Arlington, Arlington, TX

PURPOSE

To identify variables associated with CKD progression among indigent elders attending a publicly-funded clinic.

SIGNIFICANCE

Although common in the elderly, CKD often goes undetected and untreated. The incidence of ESRD among younger cohorts in the U.S. is declining while incident ESRD in elders continues to rise especially among minority groups.

METHODS

We conducted a retrospective chart review of 134 consecutive patients referred to a dietician who had followed them for at least two years. Demographic and clinical data including medical diagnoses, laboratory parameters, initial consultation time, and medications were collected at two time points: at the time of initial consultation (time 1) and two years later (time 2). Glomerular filtration rate (GFR) was estimated using the Modification of Diet in Renal Disease (MDRD) formula. A rapid decline in GFR was defined as 10/ml/min/l/73m²/year.

CONCLUSIONS

In these mostly minority elderly patients, CKD often went undetected and incident CKD was associated with a rapid decline in GFR.

Our findings emphasize the importance of early detection and management of vascular disease in this cohort.

RESULTS

Sixty-two percent of patients were female, 72% minority. Mean age was 73 but 33% were 75-89 years old and 5% were ≥90 years old. At time 1, only 6% had a CKD chart diagnosis but 22-23% had eGFRs <60 ml/min/l/73m². Among patients with an eGFR <60 at time 1 (group 1), 2% experienced a rapid decline in GFR. In contrast, among patients with eGFR ≥60 ml/min/l/73 m² at time 1 (group 2), 13% experienced a rapid decline in GFR (incident CKD). Compared to those with stable GFRs, those with a rapid decline in GFR were more likely to have incident type 2 diabetes, coronary artery disease and dementia during the 2-year period. Groups 1 and 2 did not differ in age, ethnicity, gender, systolic pressure, diagnoses or medications. Those with eGFR <60 at time 2 had lower BMIs and higher diastolic blood pressures than those with an eGFR ≥60.

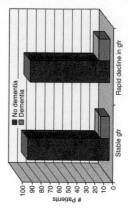

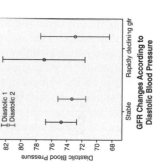

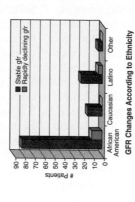

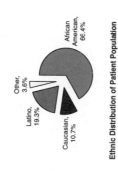

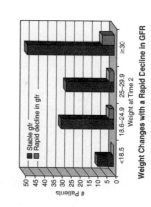

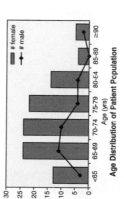

Figure 25-5 Poster of the "Determinants of CKD Progression among Indigent Elderly."

negative findings, such as no significant differences or relationships, are frequently not submitted for presentation or publication. These negative findings can be as important to the development of knowledge as the positive findings, because they direct future research (Angell, 1989).

Publishing research findings is a rewarding experience, but the process demands a great deal of time and energy. The manuscript rejections or requests for major revisions that most authors receive can be discouraging. However, you can take certain steps to increase the probability of having a manuscript accepted for publication. While you are developing your proposal, outline your plans for publishing your study. At this time, you and other members of your research team should discuss and, if possible, determine authorship credit. This issue becomes complex when the research is a collaborative project among individuals from different disciplines. Some researchers develop the entire manuscript and are then faced with the decision of who will be first, second, or third author. There are many ways to determine authorship credit, but the decision should be acceptable to all investigators involved (Nicol & Pexman, 2003). Authorship credit should be given only to those who made substantial contributions to developing and implementing a study and in writing the final report (Duncan, 1999).

Publishing Journal Articles

Developing a manuscript for publication includes the following steps: (1) selecting a journal, (2) developing a query letter, (3) preparing a manuscript, (4) submitting the manuscript for review, and (5) revising the manuscript.

Selecting a Journal

Selecting a journal for publication of your study requires knowledge of the basic requirements of the journal, the journal's refereed status (see the next paragraph), and recent articles published in the journal. Swanson et al. (1991) studied publishing opportunities for nurses by surveying 92 U.S. nursing journals. The authors provided, in table format, the following basic information on each journal: circulation; number of issues published each year; article length; number of copies of the manuscript to be submitted; format for the manuscript; query letter; free reprints; and the percentage of staff-written, unsolicited, and research manuscripts published. The article also reported the number of unsolicited manuscripts received, the number of unsolicited manuscripts published, the number of manuscripts rejected, the percentage of manuscripts accepted, the refereed status, the review process, the time for acceptance, and the time until publication (Swanson et al., 1991, p. 35). Table 25-16 presents some essential publishing information for five research journals included in this survey.

A refereed journal uses referees or expert reviewers to determine whether a manuscript is accepted for publication. In nonrefereed journals, the editor makes the decisions to accept or reject manuscripts, but these decisions are usually made after consultation with a nursing expert (Carnegie, 1975). Most refereed journals require manuscripts to be reviewed anonymously by two or three reviewers. The reviewers are asked to determine the strengths and weaknesses of a manuscript, and their comments or a summary of the comments is sent to the author. Most academic institutions support the refereed system and will recognize only publications that appear in refereed journals.

TABLE 25-16   Publishing Information for Selected Research Journals

Journal	Number of Issues	Query Letter	Refereed	Article Length (Pages)	Format	Copies Required	Acceptance Rate (%)
Advances in Nursing Science	4	Optional	Yes	15–30	APA	3	13
Applied Nursing Research	4	Optional	Yes	8–12	APA	5	48
Nursing Research	6	Preferred	Yes	14–16	APA	3	15
Research in Nursing & Health	6	Optional	Yes	10–15	APA	4	22
Western Journal of Nursing Research	6	Optional	Yes	15	APA	4	20

Adapted from Swanson, E. A., McCloskey, J. C., & Bodensteiner, A. (1991). Publishing opportunities for nurses: A comparison of 92 U.S. journals. *Image: Journal of Nursing Scholarship, 23*(1), 33–38.

The five research journals presented in Table 25-16 are refereed and have the following review process: "Editor receives manuscripts, reviews, and distributes them to experts selected from an established group of reviewers. Decision on the manuscript is based on reviews and mediated by editor" (Swanson et al., 1991, p. 35).

Having a manuscript accepted for publication depends not only on the quality of the manuscript but also on how closely the manuscript matches the goals of the journal (Teijlingen & Hundley, 2002). It is a good idea to review articles recently published in the journal to which you plan to submit a manuscript. This review will let you know whether a research topic has recently been covered and whether the research findings would be of interest to the journal's readers. This selection process will enable you to identify a few journals that would be appropriate for publishing your findings.

Developing a Query Letter

Develop a query letter to determine an editor's interest in reviewing your manuscript. This letter should be no more than one or two pages and usually includes the research problem, a brief discussion of the major findings, the significance of the findings, and the researcher's qualifications for writing the article (Nicol & Pexman, 2003). Address your query letter to the current editor of a journal; frequently, researchers send three or four letters to different journals at the same time. Of the five journals presented in Table 25-16, only *Nursing Research* prefers a query letter; the other research journals indicated that these letters were optional. Some researchers send query letters because the response (positive or negative) enables them to make the final selection of a journal for submitting their manuscript. An example of a query letter is presented in Figure 25-6.

January 31, 2008
Joyce J. Fitzpatrick, PhD, RN, FAAN
Frances Payne Bolton School of Nursing
Case Western Reserve University
10900 Euclid Avenue
Cleveland, OH 44106
E-mail: ANRjournal@hotmail.com

Dear Dr. Fitzpatrick:

An increasing number of nursing studies are focused on interventions to manage clinical problems and improve patient outcomes. A common problem in primary care is chronic low back pain (LBP). I have just completed a study to examine the effects of ice therapy versus heat therapy in the management of patients with chronic LBP.

The framework for this study was the Melzack and Wall gate-control theory of pain. The independent variables, ice and heat therapies, were consistently implemented with structured protocols by nurse research assistants in primary care clinics. The dependent variable, perception of pain, was measured with a visual analog scale and a perception of pain likert scale. The sample included 150 patients with LBP, who were randomly assigned to one of three groups: a comparison group who received standard care but no ice or heat therapy, an experimental group that received ice therapy, and an experimental group that received heat therapy.

An analysis of variance (ANOVA) with post hoc analysis indicated that the patients in the comparison group and heat therapy group perceived their pain to be significantly greater than the perception of pain by the patients receiving ice therapy. The findings suggest that ice therapy is more effective in reducing chronic LBP. Ice therapy is an intervention that can be prescribed and implemented by nurses to reduce patients' perception of pain.

I hope you will consider reviewing this manuscript for possible publication in *Applied Nursing Research*. I look forward to receiving a response from you.

Sincerely,

Susan K. Grove, PhD, RN, ANP-BC, GNP-BC
Professor
School of Nursing, Box 19407
The University of Texas at Arlington
Arlington, TX 76019
E-mail: grove@uta.edu

Figure **25-6** Example of a query letter.

Preparing a Manuscript

A manuscript is written according to the format outlined by the journal. Guidelines for developing a manuscript are usually published in the issue of the journal or on the journal's website. Follow these guidelines explicitly to increase the probability of your manuscript being published. The information provided for authors includes (1) directions for manuscript preparation, (2) discussion of copyright, and (3) guidelines for submission of the manuscript.

Writing research reports for publication requires skills in technical writing that are not used in other types of publication. Technical writing condenses information and is stylistic. The *Publication Manual of the American Psychological Association* (APA, 2001); *A Manual for Writers of Research Papers, Theses, Dissertations* (Turabian, Booth, Colomb, & Williams, 2007); and the *Chicago Manual of Style* (University of Chicago Press Staff, 2003) are considered useful sources for quality technical writing. Most journals will stipulate the format style required for their journal. A quality research report has no punctuation, spelling, or sentence structure errors; confusing words; clichés; jargon; or wordiness. Computer programs have been developed with the capacity to proofread manuscripts for grammar, punctuation, spelling, and sentence structure errors. However, the writer still needs to respond and correct sentences that the computer has identified as problematic.

Knowledge about the author guidelines provided by the journal and a background in technical writing will help you to develop an outline for a proposed manuscript. The brief outlines presented in Tables 25-1 and 25-9 must be expanded in detail to guide the writing of a manuscript. You can use the outline to develop a rough draft of your article, which you will revise numerous times. Present the content of your article logically and concisely under clear headings, and select a title that creates interest and reflects the content. The *Publication Manual of the American Psychological Association* (APA, 2001) provides detailed directions for preparing manuscripts.

Developing a well-written manuscript is difficult. Often, universities and other agencies offer writing seminars to assist students and other investigators in preparing a research report for publication. Some faculty members who chair thesis and dissertation committees will also assist their students in developing an article for publication. In this situation, the faculty member is almost always the second author for the article. The fifth edition of the APA manual (APA, 2001) has a section on how to reduce the content of theses and dissertations for publication.

When you are satisfied with your manuscript, ask one or two colleagues to review it for organization, completeness of content, and writing style. Colleagues' comments can guide you in making any final revisions. The manuscript should be expertly typed according to the journal's specifications; several nursing research journals require an APA (2001) format. The reference list for the manuscript needs to be in a complete and correct format. Computer programs are available with bibliography systems that enable you to compile a consistently formatted reference list in any style you desire. With these programs you can maintain a permanent collection of reference citations. When you need a reference list for a manuscript, you can select the appropriate references from the collection and use the program to print the list. You can also use computer programs to scan your manuscript and create a reference list based on the citations.

Submitting a Manuscript for Review

Guidelines in each journal indicate the name of the editor and the address for manuscript submission. Submit your manuscript to only one journal at a time. You should submit the number of copies of the manuscript requested and the original manuscript, if required. Most journals now encourage researchers to submit their manuscripts electronically, and the editor provides copies for e-mailing to reviewers. When submitting the manuscript, include your complete mailing address, phone number, fax number, and e-mail address. An author usually receives notification of receipt of the manuscript within 1 to 2 days if sent by e-mail and 1 to 2 weeks if sent by regular mail.

Peer Review

Most journals use some form of peer review process to evaluate the quality of manuscripts submitted for publication. The manuscript is usually sent to two or three reviewers with guidelines from the editor for performing the review. In most cases, the review is "blind," which means that the reviewers do not know who the author is and the author does not know who is reviewing the paper. For research papers, the reviewers are asked to evaluate the validity of the study. Broadly, of concern is whether the methodology was adequate to address the research objectives, questions, or hypotheses; whether the findings are trustworthy (for example, if the results were nonsignificant, was a power analysis performed?); whether the discussion is appropriate given the findings; and whether the author discusses the clinical implications of the findings.

Responding to Requests to Revise a Manuscript

After reviewing your manuscript, the journal staff will reach one of four possible decisions: (1) acceptance of the manuscript as submitted, (2) acceptance of the manuscript pending minor revisions, (3) tentative acceptance of the manuscript pending major revisions, and (4) rejection of the manuscript. Accepting a manuscript as submitted is extremely rare. The editor will send you a letter that indicates acceptance of the manuscript and a possible issue of publication.

Most manuscripts are returned for minor or major revisions before they are published. It is regrettable that many of these returned manuscripts are never revised. The author incorrectly interprets the request for revision as a rejection and assumes that the revised manuscript will also be rejected. This assumption is not usually true because revising a manuscript based on reviewers' comments improves the quality of the manuscript. When editors return a manuscript for revision, they include the reviewers' actual comments or a summary of the comments to direct the revision. The researcher must carefully review the comments and make those revisions that improve the quality of the research report without making inaccurate statements about the study. As you revise your manuscript, follow as carefully as possible the recommendations of the reviewers. When the revision is complete, return it with a cover letter explaining exactly how you responded to each recommendation. List each recommendation, and describe your modification. Indicate the page number of your manuscript for that revision. In some cases, you may disagree with the recommendation. If so, in the cover letter, provide rationale for your disagreement and explain how you have chosen to respond to the comment. Do not ignore a recommendation. Sometimes a revised manuscript is returned to the reviewers, yet further modifications are requested in the paper before it is published. Although these experiences are frustrating, they are also opportunities to improve your writing skills and logical development of ideas. Frequently, editors request that the final manuscript be submitted electronically.

An author who receives a rejection feels devastated, but he or she is not alone. All authors, even famous ones, have had their manuscripts rejected (Gay & Edgil, 1989). Manuscripts are rejected for a variety of reasons. Swanson et al. (1991) asked journal editors to rate the frequency of 14 reasons for manuscript rejection. Table 25-17 identifies these reasons and their mean frequencies. "Poorly written" and "poorly developed idea" were the most frequent reasons for rejecting manuscripts. If you receive a rejection notice, give yourself a cooling-off period and then determine why

TABLE 25-17	**Reasons for Manuscript Rejection**
Factor	Mean
Poorly written	3.72
Poorly developed idea	3.62
Not consistent with purpose	3.37
Term paper style	3.28
Methodology problems	3.13
Content undocumented	2.98
Content inaccurate	2.94
Content not important	2.84
Clinically not applicable	2.83
Statistical problems	2.82
Data interpretation problems	2.80
Subject covered recently	2.39
Content scheduled for future	2.11
Too technical	1.66

From Swanson, E. A., McCloskey, J. C., & Bodensteiner, A. (1991). Publishing opportunities for nurses: A comparison of 92 U.S. journals. *Image: Journal of Nursing Scholarship, 23*(1), 38.

the manuscript was rejected. Most manuscripts, especially those that are poorly written, can be revised and submitted to another journal.

Publishing Research Findings in Online Journals

A number of print journals are moving to the Web. These journals continue to provide their traditional print version but also have a website with access to some or all the articles in the printed journal. The number of Web-only online nursing journals is also growing. These online-only journals have some distinct advantages for authors. E-mail links from author to editor to reviewer allow papers to be submitted and sent from editor to reviewer electronically and allow reviewer comments to be sent back to the editor more quickly than usually occurs in print journals. Reviewer comments are sent back to the author by e-mail, after which the article is revised and resubmitted by e-mail, reviewed again, and, if judged satisfactory, accepted for publication. This process is particularly important for international scientific communications. Online journals use "continuous publication," which means that there is no wait for approved articles to be published because the editor does not have to wait until the next issue is scheduled for publication. In fact, the notion of an "issue" is becoming antiquated as a result of electronic publishing. Approved articles are placed online almost immediately, which is important for research reports because it provides more rapid access to recent research findings for other researchers and clinicians interested in facilitating evidence-based practice. The possibilities of dialogue with readers, including other researchers in the same field of study, are great. However, additional work needs to be done to ensure that online publications are secure and that each publication is permanently available with a permanent identifier for citation and linking (Fitzpatrick, 2001).

Not all online journals provide peer review. You may wish to check for information on the peer review process at the online journal website. Peer review is essential to scholars in the university tenure track system. Electronic publishing may result in a more open peer review process. Some journals post a submitted paper for peer review on a secure Internet site accessible only by the editor and reviewers. The review occurs by way of a discussion rather than individual comments. This arrangement provides a measure of quality control in the review process that is missing in the traditional process. Bingham (1999) described the changes in peer review likely to occur because of online journals.

> By creating a more open peer review process, it is possible for reviewers, authors and editors to observe each other's behavior. … This may improve the trust in the system, and the quality of the outcomes. More open review systems widen the educational function of peer review for editors and authors, and extend it to readers for the first time. … Most articles will be reviewed online in a closed forum, then published for review in an open forum, then declared "final." (Bingham, 1999; full-text article available at www.biomednet.com/hmsbeagle/46/cutedge/day1.htm)

Publishing in an online journal has other potential advantages. The constraints on length imposed because of the cost of print publishing do not exist. Multiple tables, figures, graphics, and even streaming audio and video are possibilities with online journals. Animations can be created to assist the reader in visualizing ideas. Links may be established with full-text versions of citations from other online sources. It will be possible to track the number of times that the article has been accessed; this feature will provide the author with additional information, beyond citations of his or her paper, to assess its impact on the scientific community. Forward referencing will allow links to later works, which can be added to the article continuously. The reader will be able to see how the paper influenced later works. Electronic listservs and chat rooms may be available to discuss the paper. All

of these capabilities are not currently available with every online journal. The technology to provide them exists, but there is no free lunch. Most online journals in nursing are free. Online journals with some of these advanced technologies may have to cover their costs by charging subscription fees or by obtaining financing through advertisements (Holoviak & Seitter, 1997; Ludwick & Glazer, 2000; Sparks, 1999).

Because online journals are rapidly emerging, providing a list of websites in this text is not feasible. However, a number of websites maintain a current list of online journals such as www.nursefriendly.com/nursing/linksections/nursingjournals.htm. Another website (www.medscape.com/pages/public/publications) provides a list of and electronic access to the medical journals that are online.

Publishing Research Findings in Books

Some qualitative studies and large, complex quantitative studies are published in books or chapters of books. Publishing a book requires extensive commitment on the part of the researcher. In addition, the researcher must select a publisher and convince the publisher to support the book project. A prospectus must be developed that identifies the proposed content of the book, describes the market for the book, and includes a rationale for publishing the book. The publisher and researcher must negotiate a contract that is mutually acceptable regarding (1) the content and length of the book, (2) the time required to complete the book, (3) the percentage of royalties that the author will receive, and (4) the advances she or he will be offered. The researcher must fulfill the obligations of the contract by producing the proposed book within the time frame agreed on. Publishing a book is a significant accomplishment and an effective, but sometimes slow, means of communicating research findings. Be sure and include all presentations and publications on your vita to document your scholarship activities.

Duplicate Publication in the Nursing Literature

Duplicate publication is the practice of publishing the same article or major portions of the article in two or more print or electronic media without notifying the editors or referencing the other publication in the reference list (Blancett, Flanagin, & Young, 1995; Duncan, 1999). Duplicate publication of studies is a poor practice because it limits the opportunities for publishing new knowledge, artificially inflates the importance of a study topic, clutters the literature with redundant information, rewards researchers for publishing the same content twice, and may violate the copyright law. Blancett et al. (1995) studied the incidence of duplicate publications in the nursing literature. In a sample of 642 articles published by 77 authors over 5 years, 181 of the articles were classified as duplicate publications. Forty-one of the 77 authors published at least one form of duplicate article, and 59 of the duplicate articles did not include a reference to the primary article. Thus, duplicate publications are a serious concern in the nursing literature.

Journals require the submission of an original manuscript or one that has not been previously published, so submitting a manuscript that has been previously published without referencing the duplicate work or notifying the editor of the previous publication is unethical and a form of scientific misconduct (see Chapter 9).

In 1994, the International Academy of Nursing Editors developed guidelines for nurse authors and editors regarding duplicate publications. Both authors and editors have the responsibility to inform readers and reviewers of duplicate publications. Authors must avoid unethical duplication by submitting original manuscripts or by providing full disclosure if portions or the entire manuscript has been previously published. Previous publications must be cited in the text of the manuscript and the reference list. Editors have the responsibility of developing a policy on duplicate publications and informing all authors, reviewers, and readers of this policy. In addition, editors must ensure that readers are informed of duplicate materials by adequate citation of the materials in the article's text and reference list (Yarbro, 1995). Duplicate publications continue to be a problem in the nursing and medical literature. These redundant publications can result in retractions and refusal to accept other manuscripts for publication (Duncan, 1999; International Committee of Medical Journal Editors, 1997).

SUMMARY

- Communicating research findings, the final step in the research process, involves developing a research report and disseminating it through presentations and publications to audiences of nurses, health care professionals, policy makers, and health care consumers.
- Both quantitative and qualitative research reports include four basic sections: (1) introduction, (2) methods, (3) results, and (4) discussion.

- In a quantitative research report, the introduction briefly identifies the problem that was studied and presents an empirical and theoretical basis for the study. The methods section of the report describes how the study was conducted; the results section reveals what was found by conducting the study; and the discussion section includes the study findings, limitations, conclusions, implications for nursing practice, and recommendations for further research.
- In qualitative research, the introduction section identifies the phenomenon under investigation and describes the type of qualitative study that was conducted. The methods section includes both the general and applied methods for the study conducted. The results section of the research report includes the data analysis procedures and presentation of the findings; and the discussion section includes conclusions, limitations, implications for nursing, and recommendations for further research.
- The greatest impact on nursing practice can be achieved by communicating nursing research findings to nurses, other health professionals, policy makers, and health care consumers.
- Research findings are presented at conferences and meetings through verbal and poster presentations of the research report; and the report developed depends on the focus of the conference, the audience, and the time designated for each presentation.
- A poster session is a visual presentation of a study. Conference sponsors guide the development of a poster by providing the following information: (1) size limitations or format restrictions for the poster, (2) the size of the poster display area, and (3) the background and potential number of conference participants.
- Developing a manuscript for publication includes the following steps: (1) selecting a journal, (2) writing a query letter, (3) preparing a manuscript, (4) submitting the manuscript for review, and (5) responding to requests for revision of the manuscript.
- Selecting a journal for publication of a study requires knowledge of the basic requirements of the journal, the journal's refereed status, and recent articles published in the journal.
- An increasing area of concern in publishing is the practice of duplicate publications where the same article or major portions of the article are published in two or more print or electronic media without notifying the editors or referencing the other publication in the reference list.

REFERENCES

Agency for Healthcare Research and Quality (AHRQ). (2007). *Evidence-based practice centers: Synthesizing scientific evidence to improve quality and effectiveness in health care.* Retrieved October 30, 2007, from www.ahrq.gov/clinic/epc.

American Psychological Association. (2001). *Publication manual of the American Psychological Association* (5th ed.). Washington, DC: Author.

Angell, M. (1989). Negative studies. *New England Journal of Medicine, 321*(7), 464–466.

Bingham, C. (1999). The future of medical publishing. *HMS Beagle.* Retrieved January 22, 1999, from www.biomednet.com/hmsbeagle/46/cutedge/day1.htm.

Blancett, S. S., Flanagin, A., & Young, R. K. (1995). Duplicate publication in the nursing literature. *Image: Journal of Nursing Scholarship, 27*(1), 51–56.

Boyd, C. O., & Munhall, P. L. (2001). Qualitative research proposal and report. In P. L. Munhall (Ed.), *Nursing research: A qualitative perspective* (3rd ed., pp. 613–638). Sudbury, MA: Jones & Bartlett.

Brown, S. J. (1999). *Knowledge for health care practice: A guide to using research evidence.* Philadelphia: Saunders.

Carnegie, M. E. (1975). The referee system. *Nursing Research, 24*(4), 243.

Cason, C. L., Cason, G. J., & Redland, A. R. (1988). Peer review of research abstracts. *Image: Journal of Nursing Scholarship, 20*(2), 102–105.

Craig, J. V., & Smyth, R. L. (2007). *The evidence-base practice manual for nurses* (2nd ed.). Edinburgh: Churchill Livingstone.

Crosby, L. J. (1990). The abstract: An important first impression. *Journal of Neuroscience Nursing, 22*(3), 192–194.

Duncan, A. M. (1999). Authorship, dissemination of research findings, and related matters. *Applied Nursing Research, 12*(2), 101–106.

Evangelista, L. S., Doering, L., & Dracup, K. (2003). Meaning and life purpose: The perspectives of post-transplant women. *Heart & Lung, 32*(4), 250–257.

Fitzpatrick, J. J. (2001). Scholarly publishing: Current issues of cost and quality, fueled by the rapid expansion of electronic publishing [Editorial]. Applied Nursing Research, *14*(1), 1–2.

Frankl, V. E. (1984). *Man's search for meaning.* New York: Simon & Schuster.

Gay, J. T., & Edgil, A. E. (1989). When your manuscript is rejected. *Nursing & Healthcare, 10*(8), 459–461.

Giorgi, A. (1985). *Phenomenology and psychological research.* Pittsburgh, PA: Duquesne University Press.

Goode, C. J. (2000). What constitutes the "evidence" in evidence-based practice? *Applied Nursing Research, 13*(4), 222–225.

Heo, S., Moser, D.K., Lennie, T. A., Zambroski, C. H., & Chung, M.L. (2007). A comparison of health-related quality of life between older adults with heart failure and healthy older adults. *Heart & Lung, 36*(1), 16–24.

Hicks, C. (1995). The shortfall in published research: A study of nurses' research publication activities. *Journal of Advanced Nursing, 21*(3), 594–604.

Holoviak, J., & Seitter, K. L. (1997). Transcending the limitations of the printed page. *Journal of Electronic Publishing, 3*(1). Retrieved March 12, 2000, from www.press.umich.edu/jep/033–01/EI.html.

International Committee of Medical Journal Editors. (1997). Uniform requirements for manuscripts submitted to biomedical journals. *Annals of Internal Medicine, 126*(1), 36–47.

Jackle, M. (1989). Presenting research to nurses in clinical practice. *Applied Nursing Research, 2*(4), 191–193.

Jackson, M. S. (1995). Afrocentric treatment of African American women and their children in a residential chemical dependence program. *Journal of Black Studies, 26*(1), 17–30.

Jenkins, K., & Ahijevych, K. (2003). Nursing students' beliefs about smoking, their own smoking behaviors, and use of professional tobacco treatment intervention. *Applied Nursing Research, 16*(3), 164–172.

Jimenez, S. L. M. (1991). Consumer journalism: A unique nursing opportunity. *Image: Journal of Nursing Scholarship, 23*(1), 47–49.

Kerlinger, F. N., & Lee, H. B. (2000). *Foundations of behavioral research* (4th ed.). Fort Worth, TX: Harcourt College Publishers.

Knafl, K. A., & Howard, M. J. (1984). Interpreting and reporting qualitative research. *Research in Nursing & Health, 7*(1), 17–24.

Kraemer, H. C., & Thiemann, S. (1987). *How many subjects? Statistical power analysis in research.* Newbury Park, CA: Sage.

Leininger, M. M. (1985). *Qualitative research methods in nursing.* New York: Grune & Stratton.

Ludwick, R., & Glazer, G. (2000, January 31). Electronic publishing. The movement from print to digital publication. *Online Journal of Issues in Nursing, 5*(5), Manuscript 2. Retrieved March 12, 2000, from www.nursingworld.org/ojin/topic11/tpe112.htm.

Marshall, C., & Rossman, G. B. (2006). *Designing qualitative research* (4th ed.). Thousand Oaks, CA: Sage.

Mathieson, A. (1996). The principles and practice of oral presentation. *Nurse Researcher, 4*(2), 41–54.

McCloskey, J. C. (1977). Publishing opportunities for nurses: A comparison of 65 journals. *Nurse Educator, 11*(4), 4–13.

McKenna, K. T., Maas, F., & McEniery, P. T. (1995). Coronary risk factor status after percutaneous transluminal coronary angioplasty. *Heart & Lung, 24*(3), 207–212.

Melnyk, B. M., & Fineout-Overholt, E. (2005). *Evidence-based practice in nursing & healthcare: A guide to best practice.* Philadelphia: Lippincott Williams & Wilkins.

Miles, M. B., & Huberman, A. M. (1994). *Qualitative data analysis: A sourcebook of new methods* (2nd ed.). Beverly Hills, CA: Sage.

Miracle, V. A., & King, K. C. (1994). Presenting research: Effective paper presentations and impressive poster presentations. *Applied Nursing Research, 7*(3), 147–157.

Moore, L. W., Augspurger, P., King, M. O., & Proffitt, C. (2001). Insights on the poster preparation and presentation process. *Applied Nursing Research, 14*(2), 100–104.

Munhall, P. L. (2001). *Nursing research: A qualitative perspective* (3rd ed.). Sudbury, MA: Jones & Bartlett.

Nicol, A. A., & Pexman, P.M. (1999). *Presenting your findings: A practical guide for creating tables.* Washington, DC: American Psychological Association.

Nicol, A. A., & Pexman, P. M. (2003). *Displaying your findings: A practical guide for creating figures, posters, and presentations.* Washington, DC: American Psychological Association.

O'Neill, A. L., & Duffcy, M. A. (2000). Communication of research and practice knowledge in nursing literature. *Nursing Research, 49*(4), 224–230.

Patton, M. Q. (2002). *Qualitative research & evaluation methods* (3rd ed.). Thousand Oaks, CA: Sage.

Pyrczak, F. (1999). *Evaluating research in academic journals: A practical guide to realistic evaluation.* Los Angeles: Pyrczak.

Pyrczak, F., & Bruce, R. R. (2005). *Writing empirical research reports: A basic guide for students of the social and behavioral sciences* (5th ed.). Glendale, CA: Pyrczak.

Russell, C. L., & Aud, M. A. (2002). Publication manual of the American Psychological Association—5th edition: A review of additions and changes in style requirements. *Nursing Research, 51*(5), 332–335.

Russell, C. K., Gregory, D. M., & Gates, M. F. (1996). Aesthetics and substance in qualitative research posters. *Qualitative Health Research, 6*(4), 542–552.

Sandelowski, M., & Barroso, J. (2002). Finding the findings in qualitative studies. *Journal of Nursing Scholarship, 34*(3), 213–219.

Santacroce, S. J., Maccarelli, L. M., & Grey, M. (2004). Methods: Intervention fidelity. *Nursing Research, 53*(1), 63–66.

Selby, M. L., Tornquist, E. M., & Finerty, E. J. (1989a). How to present your research. Part I: What they didn't teach you in nursing school about planning and organizing the content of your speech. *Nursing Outlook, 37*(4), 172–175.

Selby, M. L., Tornquist, E. M., & Finerty, E. J. (1989b). How to present your research. Part II: The ABCs of creating and using visual aids to enhance your research presentation. *Nursing Outlook, 37*(5), 236–238.

Sparks, S. M. (1999). Electronic publishing and nursing research. *Nursing Research, 48*(1), 50–54.

Stein, K. F., Sargent, J. T., & Rafaels, N. (2007). Intervention research: Establishing fidelity of the independent variable in nursing clinical trials. *Nursing Research, 56*(1), 54–62.

Swain, M. A., & Steckel, S. B. (1981). Influencing adherence among hypertensives. *Research in Nursing & Health, 4*(1), 213–222.

Swanson, E. A., McCloskey, J. C., & Bodensteiner, A. (1991). Publishing opportunities for nurses: A comparison of 92 U.S. journals. *Image: Journal of Nursing Scholarship, 23*(1), 33–38.

Teijlingen, E. V., & Hundley, V. (2002). Methodological issues in nursing research. Getting your paper to the right journal: A case study of an academic paper. *Journal of Advanced Nursing, 37*(6), 506–513.

Tornquist, E. M., Funk, S. G., & Champagne, M. T. (1989). Writing research reports for clinical audiences. *Western Journal of Nursing Research, 11*(5), 576–582.

Turabian, K. L., Booth, W. C., Colomb, G. G., & Williams, J. M. (2007). *A manual for writers of research papers, theses, dissertations: Chicago style for students and researchers* (7th ed.). Chicago: University of Chicago Press.

University of Chicago Press Staff. (2003). *The Chicago manual of style* (15th ed.). Chicago: University of Chicago Press.

Wainer, H. (1984). How to display data badly. *American Statistician, 38*(2), 137–147.

Wilson, I. B., & Cleary, P. D. (1995). Linking clinical variables with health-related quality of life: A conceptual model of patient outcomes. *Journal of the American Medical Association, 273*(1), 59–65.

Winslow, E. H. (1996). Failure to publish research: A form of scientific misconduct? *Heart & Lung, 25*(3), 169–171.

Wolcott, H. F. (2001). *Writing up qualitative research* (2nd ed.). Thousand Oaks, CA: Sage.

Wright, V. L. (2003). A phenomenological exploration of spirituality among African American women recovering from substance abuse. *Archives of Psychiatric Nursing, 17*(4), 173–185.

Yarbro, C. H. (1995). Duplicate publication: Guidelines for nurse authors and editors. *Image: Journal of Nursing Scholarship, 27*(1), 57.

Putting It All Together for Evidence-Based Health Care

CHAPTER 26

Critical Appraisal of Nursing Studies

The nursing profession continues to strive for evidence-based practice, which includes appraising studies critically, synthesizing research findings, and applying sound scientific evidence in practice. Researchers also critically appraise studies in a selected area, develop a systematic review of the current knowledge, and identify areas for future studies. Thus, critically appraising research is essential for evidence-based nursing practice and the conduct of future research. The **critical appraisal of research** involves a systematic, unbiased, careful examination of all aspects of a study to judge the merits, limitations, meaning, and significance. It is based on previous research experience and knowledge of the topic. To conduct a critical appraisal of research, one must possess a background in analysis and the skills in logical reasoning needed to examine the credibility and integrity of a study. This chapter provides a background for critically appraising studies in nursing and other health care disciplines. The critique of research in the nursing profession has evolved over the years as nurses have increased their analysis skills and expertise. The chapter concludes with a description of the critical analysis processes implemented to examine the quality of both quantitative and qualitative research. These processes include unique skills, guidelines, and standards for evaluating different types of research.

EVOLUTION OF CRITICAL APPRAISAL OF RESEARCH IN NURSING

The process for critical appraisal of research has evolved gradually in nursing because until recently only a few nurses have been prepared to conduct comprehensive, scholarly critiques. During the 1940s and 1950s, presentations of nursing research were followed by critiques of the studies. These critiques often focused on the faults or limitations of the studies and tended to be harsh and traumatic for the researcher (Meleis, 1991). As a consequence of these early unpleasant experiences, nurse researchers began to protect and shelter their nurse scientists from the threat of criticism. Public critiques, written or verbal, were rare in the 1960s and 1970s. Those responding to research presentations focused on the strengths of studies, and the limitations were either not mentioned or minimized. Thus, the impact of the limitations on the meaning, validity, and significance of the study was often lost.

Incomplete critiques or the absence of critiques may have served a purpose as nurses gained basic research skills. However, the nursing discipline has moved past this point, and a comprehensive critical appraisal of research is essential to strengthen the scientific investigations needed to provide an evidence-based practice (Brown, 1999; Melnyk & Fineout-Overholt, 2005). As a result of advances in the nursing profession during the 1980s and 1990s, many nurses now have the preparation and expertise to conduct critical appraisals. Nursing research textbooks provide detailed information on the critical appraisal process. Skills in critical appraisal are introduced at the baccalaureate level of nursing education and are expanded at the master's and doctoral levels. Specialty organizations provide workshops on the critical appraisal process to promote the use of scientific evidence in practice.

The critical appraisal of studies is essential for the development and refinement of nursing knowledge. Nurses need these skills to examine the meaning and validity of study findings and to ask searching questions. Was the methodology of a study sound to produce valid findings? Are the findings an accurate reflection of reality? Do they increase our understanding of the nature of phenomena that are important in nursing? Are the findings from the present study consistent with those from previous studies? Can the study be replicated? The answers to these questions require careful examination of the research problem, the theoretical basis of the study, and the study's methodology. Not only must the mechanics of conducting the study be examined, but the abstract and logical reasoning that the researcher used to plan and implement the study must also be evaluated. If the reasoning process used to develop the study has flaws, there are probably flaws in interpreting the meaning of the findings, decreasing the validity of the study.

All studies have flaws, but if all flawed studies were discarded, there would be no scientific knowledge base for practice (Oberst, 1992). In fact, science itself is flawed. Science does not completely or perfectly describe, explain, predict, or control reality. However, improved understanding and an increased ability to predict and control phenomena depend on recognizing the flaws in studies and in science. New studies can then be planned to minimize the flaws or limitations of earlier studies. Thus, a researcher must critically analyze previous studies to determine their limitations and then interpret the study findings in light of those limitations. The limitations can lead to inaccurate data, inaccurate outcomes of analysis, and decreased ability to generalize the findings. You must decide if a study is too flawed to be used in a systematic review of knowledge in an area. Although we recognize that knowledge is not absolute, we need to have confidence in the research evidence synthesized for practice.

All studies have strengths as well as limitations. Recognition of these strengths is also essential to the generation of sound research evidence for practice. If only weaknesses are identified, nurses might discount the value of studies and refuse to invest time in reading and examining research. The continued work of the researcher also depends on recognizing the study's strengths. If no study is good enough, why invest time conducting research? Points of strength in a study, added to points of strength from multiple other studies, slowly build solid research evidence for practice.

When are Critical Appraisals of Research Implemented in Nursing?

In general, research is critically appraised to broaden understanding, summarize knowledge for practice,

and provide a knowledge base for future studies. In addition, critical appraisals are often conducted after verbal presentations of studies, after a published research report, for an abstract section for a conference, for article selection for publication, and for evaluation of research proposals for implementation or funding. Thus, nursing students, practicing nurses, nurse educators, and nurse researchers are all involved in the critical appraisal of research.

Students' Critical Appraisal of Studies

In nursing education, conducting a critical appraisal of a study is often seen as a first step in learning the research process. Part of learning the research process is being able to read and comprehend published research reports. However, conducting a critical appraisal of a study is not a basic skill, and the content presented in previous chapters is essential for implementing this process. Nurses usually acquire basic knowledge of the research process and the critical appraisal process early in the course of their nursing education. More advanced analysis skills are often taught at the master's and doctoral levels. The steps involved in performing a critical appraisal of a study are (1) comprehension, (2) comparison, (3) analysis, (4) evaluation, and (5) conceptual clustering. By critically appraising studies, students expand their analysis skills, strengthen their knowledge base, and increase their use of research evidence in practice.

Critical Appraisal of Research by the Practicing Nurse

Practicing nurses need to critically appraise studies so their practice is based on research evidence and not tradition and trial and error (Melnyk & Fineout-Overholt, 2005). Nursing actions must be updated in response to the current evidence that is generated through research and theory development. Practicing nurses need to design methods for remaining current in their practice areas. Reading research journals or posting current studies at work can increase nurses' awareness of study findings but is not sufficient for critique to occur. Nurses need to question the quality of the studies and the credibility of the findings and share their concerns with other nurses. For example, nurses may form a research journal club in which studies are presented and critically appraised by members of the group (Tibbles & Sanford, 1994). Skills in critical appraisal of research enable the practicing nurse to synthesize the most credible, significant, and appropriate empirical evidence for use in practice (Peat, Mellis, Williams, & Xuan, 2002).

Critical Appraisal of Research by Nurse Educators

Educators critically appraise research to expand their knowledge base and to develop and refine the educational process. The careful analysis of current nursing studies provides a basis for updating curriculum content for use in clinical and classroom settings. Educators act as role models for their students by examining new studies, evaluating the information obtained from research, and indicating what research evidence to use in practice. In addition, educators collaborate in the conduct of studies, which requires a critical appraisal of previous relevant research.

Nurse Researchers' Critical Appraisal of Studies

Nurse researchers critically appraise previous research to plan and implement their next study. Many researchers focus their studies in one area, and they update their knowledge base by critiquing new studies in this area. The outcomes of these appraisals influence the selection of research problems, the development of methodologies, and the interpretations of findings in future studies. The critical appraisal of previous studies for synthesis in the literature review section in a research proposal or report was described in Chapter 6.

Critical Appraisal of Research Presentations and Publications

Critiques following research presentations can assist researchers in identifying the strengths and weaknesses of their studies and generating ideas for further research. Participants listening to study critiques might gain insight into the conduct of research. Experiencing the critical appraisal process can increase the participants' ability to evaluate studies and judge the usefulness of the research evidence for practice.

Currently, at least two nursing research journals, *Scholarly Inquiry for Nursing Practice: An International Journal* and *Western Journal of Nursing Research*, include commentaries after the research articles. In these journals, other researchers critically appraise the authors' studies, and the authors have a chance to respond to these comments. Published critiques of research often increase the reader's understanding of the study and the quality of the study findings. Another, more informal critique of a published study might appear in a letter to the editor. Readers have the opportunity to comment on the strengths and weaknesses of published studies by writing to the journal editor.

Critical Appraisal of Abstracts for Conference Presentations

One of the most difficult types of critical appraisal is examining abstracts. The amount of information available is usually limited because many abstracts are restricted to 100 to 250 words (Pyrczak, 1999). Nevertheless, reviewers must select the best-designed studies with the most significant outcomes for presentation at nursing conferences. This process requires an experienced researcher who needs few cues to determine the quality of a study. Critical appraisal of an abstract usually addresses the following criteria: (1) appropriateness of the study for the program; (2) completeness of the research project; (3) overall quality of the study problem, purpose, framework, methodology, and results; (4) contribution of the study to the nursing knowledge base; (5) contribution of the study to nursing theory; (6) originality of the work (not previously published); (7) implication of the study findings for practice; and (8) clarity, conciseness, and completeness of the abstract (American Psychological Association [APA], 2001; Morse Dellasega, & Doberneck, 1993).

Critical Appraisal of Research Articles for Publication

Nurse researchers who serve as peer reviewers for professional journals evaluate the quality of research papers submitted for publication. The role of these scientists is to ensure that the studies accepted for publication are well designed and contribute to the body of knowledge. Most of these reviews are conducted anonymously so that friendships or reputations do not interfere with the selection process (Tilden, 2002). In most refereed journals (82%), the experts who examine the research report have been selected from an established group of peer reviewers (Swanson, McCloskey, & Bodensteiner, 1991). Their comments or a summary of their comments is sent to the researcher. The editor also uses these comments to make selections for publication. The process for publishing a study was described in Chapter 25.

Critical Appraisal of Research Proposals

Critical appraisals of research proposals are conducted to approve student research projects; to permit data collection in an institution; and to select the best studies for funding by local, state, national, and international organizations and agencies. The process researchers use to seek the approval to conduct a study is presented in Chapter 28. The peer review process in federal funding agencies involves an extremely complex critique. Nurses are involved in this level of research review through the national funding agencies, such as the National Institute of Nursing Research (NINR) and the Agency for

Healthcare Research and Quality (AHRQ). Kim and Felton (1993) identified some of the criteria used to evaluate the quality of a proposal for possible funding, such as the (1) appropriate use of measurement for the types of questions that the research is designed to answer, (2) appropriate use and interpretation of statistical procedures, (3) evaluation of clinical practice and forecasting of the need for nursing or other appropriate interventions, and (4) construction of models to direct the research and interpret the findings. Rudy and Kerr (2000) described audits being done by the National Institutes of Health (NIH) to determine the best studies to receive federal funding. This article included an example audit worksheet with guidelines and questions that focused on the following steps of the research process: purpose, sampling criteria, subjects to be enrolled during the grant period, consent forms, procedures, instruments' reliability and validity, data input, and data analysis. This audit worksheet might assist researchers in developing stronger proposals to submit for NIH funding.

CRITICAL APPRAISAL PROCESS FOR QUANTITATIVE STUDIES

The critical appraisal process for quantitative research includes five steps: (1) comprehension, (2) comparison, (3) analysis, (4) evaluation, and (5) conceptual clustering. Conducting a critical appraisal of a study is a complex mental process that is stimulated by raising questions. The level of critique conducted is influenced by the sophistication of the individual appraising the study (Table 26-1). The initial critical appraisal of research by an undergraduate student often involves only the comprehension step of the process, which includes identification of the steps of the research process in a study. Some baccalaureate programs include more in-depth research courses that incorporate the comparison step of critical appraisal, wherein the quality of the research report is examined using expert sources. A critical appraisal of research conducted by a master's-level student usually involves the steps of comprehension, comparison, analysis, and evaluation. The analysis step involves examining the logical links among the steps of the research process, with evaluation focusing on the overall quality of the study and the credibility and validity of the findings. Conceptual clustering is a complex synthesis of the findings of several studies, and it provides the current, empirical knowledge base for a phenomenon. This critical appraisal step is usually perfected by doctoral students, postdoctoral students, and experienced researchers as they develop systematic reviews of research, meta-analyses, and integrated reviews of research for publication. These summaries of current research evidence are essential to direct practice and conduct future research.

Conducting a critical appraisal of quantitative and qualitative research involves applying some basic guidelines, such as those outlined in Table 26-2. These guidelines stress the importance of examining the expertise of the authors; reviewing the entire study; addressing the study's strengths, weaknesses, and logical links; and evaluating the contribution of the study to nursing practice. These guidelines are linked to the first four steps of the critical appraisal process: comprehension, comparison, analysis, and evaluation. These steps occur in sequence, vary in depth, and presume accomplishment of the preceding steps. However, an individual with critical appraisal experience frequently performs several steps of this process simultaneously.

This section includes the steps of the critical appraisal process and provides relevant questions for each step. These questions are not comprehensive but have been selected as a means for stimulating the logical reasoning necessary for conducting a study review. Persons experienced in the critical appraisal process formulate additional questions as part of their reasoning processes. We cover the comprehension step separately because those new to critical appraisal start with this step. The comparison and analysis steps are covered together because these steps often occur simultaneously in the mind of the person conducting the critical appraisal. Evaluation and conceptual clustering are covered separately because of the increased expertise needed to perform each step.

TABLE 26-1	Educational Level and Expected Level of Expertise in Critical Appraisal of Research
Educational Level	**Expected Level of Expertise in Critical Appraisal of Research**
Baccalaureate	Step I: Comprehension
	Step II: Comparison
Master's	Step III: Analysis
	Step IV: Evaluation
Doctorate or postdoctorate	Step V: Conceptual clustering

TABLE 26-2 ■ Guidelines for Conducting Critical Appraisals of Quantitative and Qualitative Research

1. *Read and evaluate the entire study.* A research appraisal requires identification and examination of all steps of the research process. (Comprehension)
2. *Examine the research, clinical, and educational background of the authors.* The authors need a clinical and scientific background that is appropriate for the study conducted. (Comprehension)
3. *Examine the organization and presentation of the research report.* The title of the research report needs to clearly indicate the focus of the study. The report usually includes an abstract, introduction, methods, results, discussion, and references. The abstract of the study needs to present the purpose of the study clearly and highlight the methodology and major results. The body of the report needs to be complete, concise, clearly presented, and logically organized. The references need to be complete and presented in a consistent format. (Comparison)
4. *Identify the strengths and weaknesses of a study.* All studies have strengths and weaknesses, and you can use the questions in this chapter to facilitate identification of them. Address the quality of the steps of the research process and the logical links among the steps of the process. (Comparison and analysis)
5. *Provide specific examples of the strengths and weaknesses of a study.* These examples provide a rationale and documentation for your critique of the study. (Comparison and analysis)
6. *Be objective and realistic in identifying a study's strengths and weaknesses.* Try not to be overly critical when identifying a study's weaknesses or overly flattering when identifying the strengths.
7. *Suggest modifications for future studies.* Modifications should increase the strengths and decrease the weaknesses in the study.
8. *Evaluate the study.* Indicate the overall quality of the study and its contribution to nursing knowledge. Discuss the consistency of the findings of this study with those of previous research. Discuss the need for further research and the potential to use the findings in practice. (Evaluation)

Step I: Comprehension

Initial attempts to comprehend research articles are often frustrating because the terminology and stylized manner of the report are unfamiliar. **Comprehension** is the first step in the critical appraisal process. It involves understanding the terms and concepts in the report, as well as identifying study elements and grasping the nature, significance, and meaning of these elements. The reviewer demonstrates comprehension as she or he identifies each element or step of the study.

Guidelines for Comprehension

The first step involves reviewing the abstract and reading the study from beginning to end. As you read, address the following questions about the presentation of the study (Brown, 1999; Crookes & Davies, 1998): Does the title clearly identify the focus of the study by including the major study variables and the population? Does the title indicate the type of study conducted—descriptive, correlational, quasi-experimental, or experimental quantitative studies; outcomes studies; or intervention research? Was the abstract clear? Was the writing style of the report clear and concise? Were the different parts of the research report plainly identified? Were relevant terms defined? You might underline the terms you do not understand and determine their meaning from the glossary at the end of this book. Read the article a second time and highlight or underline each step of the quantitative research process. An overview of these steps is presented in Chapter 3. To write a critique of a study, you need to identify each step of the research process concisely and respond briefly to the following guidelines and questions:

I. Introduction
  A. Identify the reference of the article using APA format (APA, 2001).
  B. Describe the qualifications of the authors to conduct the study (such as research expertise, clinical experience, and educational preparation).
  C. Discuss the clarity of the article title (type of study, variables, and population identified).
  D. Discuss the quality of the abstract (includes purpose; highlights design, sample, and intervention [if applicable]; and presents key results).
II. State the problem.
  A. Significance of the problem
  B. Background of the problem
  C. Problem statement
III. State the purpose.
IV. Examine the literature review.
  A. Are relevant previous studies and theories described?
  B. Are the references current? (Number and percentage of sources in the last 10 years and in the last 5 years?)
  C. Are the studies critiqued?
  D. Is a summary provided of the current knowledge (what is known and not known) about the research problem?
V. Examine the study framework or theoretical perspective.

A. Is the framework explicitly expressed or must the reviewer extract the framework from implicit statements in the introduction or literature review?

B. Is the framework based on tentative, substantive, or scientific theory? Provide a rationale for your answer.

C. Does the framework identify, define, and describe the relationships among the concepts of interest? Provide examples of this.

D. Is a map of the framework provided for clarity? If a map is not presented, develop a map that represents the study's framework and describe the map.

E. Link the study variables to the relevant concepts in the map.

F. How is the framework related to nursing's body of knowledge?

VI. List any research objectives, questions, or hypotheses.

VII. Identify and define (conceptually and operationally) the study variables or concepts that were identified in the objectives, questions, or hypotheses. If objectives, questions, or hypotheses are not stated, identify and define the variables in the study purpose and the results section of the study. If conceptual definitions arc not found, identify possible definitions for each major study variable. Indicate which of the following types of variables were included in the study. A study usually includes independent and dependent variables or research variables but not all three types of variables.

A. Independent variables: Identify and define conceptually and operationally.

B. Dependent variables: Identify and define conceptually and operationally.

C. Research variables or concepts: Identify and define conceptually and operationally.

VIII. Identify attribute or demographic variables and other relevant terms.

IX. Identify the research design.

A. Identify the specific design of the study. Draw a model of the design by using the sample design models presented in Chapter 11.

B. Does the study include a treatment or intervention? If so, is the treatment clearly described with a protocol and consistently implemented?

C. If the study has more than one group, how were subjects assigned to groups?

D. Are extraneous variables identified and controlled? Extraneous variables are usually discussed as a part of quasi-experimental and experimental studies.

E. Were pilot study findings used to design this study? If yes, briefly discuss the pilot and the changes made in this study based on the pilot.

X. Describe the sample and setting.

A. Identify inclusion or exclusion sample criteria.

B. Identify the specific type of probability or nonprobability sampling method that was used to obtain the sample. Did the researchers identify the sampling frame for the study?

C. Identify the sample size. Discuss the refusal rate or percentage, and include the rationale for refusal if presented in the article. Discuss the power analysis if this process was used to determine sample size.

D. Identify the characteristics of the sample.

E. Identify the sample mortality or attrition (number and percentage) for the study.

F. Discuss the institutional review board approval. Describe the informed consent process used in the study.

G. Identify the study setting and indicate if it is appropriate for the study purpose.

XI. Identify and describe each measurement strategy used in the study. The table that follows includes the critical information about two measurement methods, the Beck Likert Scale and the physiological instrument to measure blood pressure. Completing this table will allow you to cover essential measurement content for a study.

A. Identify the name of the measurement strategy.

B. Identify the author of each measurement strategy.

C. Identify the type of each measurement strategy (e.g., Likert scale, visual analogue scale, physiological measure).

D. Identify the level of measurement (nominal, ordinal, interval, or ratio) achieved by each measurement method used in the study.

E. Discuss how the instrument was developed.

F. Describe the validity and reliability of each scale for previous studies and this study. If physiological measurement methods were used, discuss their accuracy and precision.

Name of Measurement Method	Author	Type of Measurement Method	Level of Measurement	Development of Measurement Method	Reliability or Precision	Validity or Accuracy
Beck Depression Inventory	Beck	Likert scale	Interval/ratio	Scale developed with depression symptoms from DSM IV (diagnostic statistical manual), review of literature, and review by experts.	Cronbach alpha of 0.82–0.92 from previous research and 0.87 for this study.	Construct validity: content validity obtained from literature review and clinical experience. Reading level sixth grade. Convergent validity with Zung Depression Scale. Factor analysis to document subconcepts. Prediction of future depression episodes. Successive use validity with previous studies and this study.
Omron Blood Pressure Cuff	Health care equipment	Physiological measurement method	Interval/ratio	No details provided in the article but could be obtained from the company.	Recalibration every 50 blood pressure readings to promote precision of measure.	Accuracy of systolic and diastolic pressures ensured to 1 mm mercury by company. Designated steps to take blood pressure followed to promote accuracy.

XII. Describe the procedures for data collection.

XIII. Describe the statistical analyses used.
   A. List the statistical procedures used to describe the sample.
   B. Was the level of significance or alpha identified? If so, indicate what it was (0.05, 0.01, or 0.001).
   C. Complete the following table with the analysis techniques conducted in the study: (1) identify the focus (description, relationships, or differences) for each analysis technique, (2) list the statistical analysis technique performed, (3) list the statistic, (4) provide the specific results, and (5) identify the level of significance or probability achieved by the result.

Purpose of Analysis	Analysis Technique	Statistic	Results	Probability (p)
Description of subjects' pulse rate	Mean Standard deviation Range	$\bar{X}$ SD range	71.52 5.62 58–97	
Difference between males and females on blood pressure	t-test	t	3.75	p = 0.001
Difference between treatment and comparison groups on pounds lost	Analysis of variance	F	427	p = 0.04
Relationship of depression and anxiety for adolescents	Pearson correlation	r	0.46	p = 0.03

XIV. Describe the researcher's interpretation of findings.
   A. Are the findings related back to the study framework? If so, do the findings support the study framework?
   B. Which findings are consistent with those expected?
   C. Which findings were not expected?
   D. Are the findings consistent with previous research findings?

XV. What study limitations did the researcher identify?

XVI. How did the researcher generalize the findings?

XVII. What were the implications of the findings for nursing practice?

XVIII. What suggestions for further study were identified?

XIX. Is the description of the study sufficiently clear for replication?

Step II: Comparison

The next step, comparison, requires knowledge of what each step of the research process should be like. Then the ideal way to conduct the steps of the research process is compared with the actual study steps. During the comparison step, you examine the extent to which the researcher followed the rules for an ideal study. You also need to gain a sense of how clearly the researcher grasped the study situation and expressed it. The clarity of the researchers' explanation of study elements demonstrates their skill in using and expressing ideas that require abstract reasoning.

Step III: Analysis

The analysis step involves examining the logical links connecting one study element with another. For example, the problem needs to provide background and direction for the statement of the purpose. In addition, you need to examine the overall flow of logic in the study. The variables identified in the study purpose need to be consistent with the variables identified in the research objectives, questions, or hypotheses. The variables identified in the research objectives, questions, or hypotheses need to be conceptually defined in light of the study framework. The conceptual definitions provide the basis for the development of operational definitions. The study design and analyses need to be appropriate for the investigation of the study purpose, as well as for the specific objectives, questions, or hypotheses (Ryan-Wenger, 1992).

Most of the limitations in a study result from breaks in logical reasoning. For example, biases caused by sampling and design impair the logical flow from design to interpretation of findings. The previous levels of critical appraisal have addressed concrete aspects of the study. During analysis, the process moves to examining abstract dimensions of the study, which requires greater familiarity with the logic behind the research process and increased skill in abstract reasoning.

Guidelines for Comparison and Analysis

To conduct the steps of comparison and analysis, you need to review Unit II of this text on the research process as well as other research textbooks (Burns & Grove, 2007; Houser, 2008; LoBiondo-Wood & Haber, 2005; Melnyk & Fineout-Overholt, 2005; Nieswiadomy, 2008; Peat et al., 2002; Polit & Beck, 2008). After reviewing several sources on the steps of the research process, compare the elements in the study that you are critically appraising with the criteria established for each element in this textbook or in other sources (Step II: Comparison), and then analyze the logical links among the steps of the study by examining how each step provides a basis for and links with the remaining steps of the research process (Step III: Analysis). The following guidelines will assist you in implementing the steps of comparison and analysis for each step of the research process. Questions relevant to analysis are labeled; all other questions direct comparison of the steps of the study with the ideal presented in research texts. The written critique will be a summary of the *strengths* and *weaknesses* that you noted in the study.

   I. Research problem and purpose
      A. Is the problem sufficiently delimited in scope so it is researchable but not trivial?
      B. Is the problem significant to nursing and clinical practice?
      C. Does the problem have a gender bias and address only the health needs of men to the exclusion of women's health needs (Yam, 1994)?
      D. Does the purpose narrow and clarify the aim of the study?
      E. Was this study feasible to conduct in terms of money commitment; the researchers' expertise; availability of subjects, facilities, and equipment; and ethical considerations?

  II. Review of literature
      A. Is the literature review organized to demonstrate the progressive development of evidence from previous research? (Analysis)
      B. Is a theoretical knowledge base developed for the problem and purpose? (Analysis)
      C. Is a clear, concise summary presented of the current empirical and theoretical knowledge in the area of the study (Stone, 2002)?
      D. Does the literature review summary identify what is known and not known about the research problem and provide direction for the formation of the research purpose? (Analysis)

 III. Study framework
      A. Is the framework presented with clarity? If a model or conceptual map of the framework is present, is it adequate to explain the phenomenon of concern?
      B. Is the framework linked to the research purpose? If not, would another framework fit more logically with the study? (Analysis)
      C. Is the framework related to the body of knowledge in nursing and clinical practice? (Analysis)
      D. If a proposition from a theory is to be tested, is the proposition clearly identified and linked to the study hypotheses? (Analysis and comparison)

 IV. Research objectives, questions, or hypotheses
      A. Are the objectives, questions, or hypotheses expressed clearly?
      B. Are the objectives, questions, or hypotheses logically linked to the research purpose? (Analysis)
      C. Are hypotheses stated to direct the conduct of quasi-experimental and experimental research (Kerlinger & Lee, 2000)?

D. Are the objectives, questions, or hypotheses logically linked to the concepts and relationships (propositions) in the framework? (Analysis)

V. Variables
  A. Are the variables reflective of the concepts identified in the framework? (Analysis)
  B. Are the variables clearly defined (conceptually and operationally) and based on previous research or theories? (Analysis and comparison)
  C. Is the conceptual definition of a variable consistent with the operational definition? (Analysis)

VI. Design
  A. Is the design used in the study the most appropriate design to obtain the needed data?
  B. Does the design provide a means to examine all the objectives, questions, or hypotheses? (Analysis)
  C. Is the treatment clearly described (Brown, 2002)? Is the treatment appropriate for examining the study purpose and hypotheses? Does the study framework explain the links between the treatment (independent variable) and the proposed outcomes (dependent variables) (Sidani & Braden, 1998)? Was a protocol developed to promote consistent implementation of the treatment? Did the researcher monitor implementation of the treatment to ensure consistency (Bowman, Wyman, & Peters, 2002; Santacroce, Maccarelli, & Grey, 2004)? If the treatment was not consistently implemented, what might be the impact on the findings? (Analysis and comparison)
  D. Did the researcher identify the threats to design validity (statistical conclusion validity, internal validity, construct validity, and external validity) and minimize them as much as possible?
  E. Is the design logically linked to the sampling method and statistical analyses? (Analysis)
  F. If more than one group is used, do the groups appear equivalent?
  G. If a treatment was used, were the subjects randomly assigned to the treatment group or were the treatment and comparison group matched? Were the treatment and comparison group assignments appropriate

for the purpose of the study (Bowman et al., 2002)?

VII. Sample, population, and setting
  A. Is the sampling method adequate to produce a representative sample?
  B. What are the potential biases in the sampling method? Are any subjects excluded from the study because of age, socioeconomic status, or race without a sound rationale? (Larson, 1994)
  C. Did the sample include an understudied population, such as the young, elderly, or a minority group (Resnick et al., 2003)?
  D. Were the sampling criteria (inclusion and exclusion) appropriate for the type of study conducted?
  E. Is the sample size sufficient to avoid a type II error? Was a power analysis conducted to determine sample size? If a power analysis was conducted, were the results of the analysis clearly described and used to determine the final sample size? Was the mortality or attrition rate projected in determining the final sample size?
  F. Are the rights of human subjects protected?
  G. Is the setting used in the study typical of clinical settings?
  H. Was the refusal to participate rate a problem? If so, how might this weakness influence the findings? (Analysis)
  I. Was sample mortality or attrition a problem? If so, how might this weakness influence the final sample and the study results and findings? (Analysis)

VIII. Measurements
  A. Do the measurement methods selected for the study adequately measure the study variables? (Analysis)
  B. Are the measurement methods sufficiently sensitive to detect small differences between subjects? Should additional measurement methods have been used to improve the quality of the study outcomes?
  C. Do the measurement methods used in the study have adequate validity and reliability? What additional reliability or validity testing is needed to improve the quality of the measurement methods (Bowman et al., 2002; Roberts & Stone, 2004)?
  D. Respond to the following questions, which are relevant to the measurement approaches used in the study:

1. Scales and questionnaires
   (a) Are the instruments clearly described?
   (b) Are techniques to complete and score the instruments provided?
   (c) Are validity and reliability of the instruments described?
   (d) Did the researcher reexamine the validity and reliability of instruments for the present sample?
   (e) If the instrument was developed for the study, is the instrument development process described?

2. Observation
   (a) Is what is to be observed clearly identified and defined?
   (b) Is interrater reliability described?
   (c) Are the techniques for recording observations described?

3. Interviews
   (a) Do the interview questions address concerns expressed in the research problem? (Analysis)
   (b) Are the interview questions relevant for the research purpose and objectives, questions, or hypotheses? (Analysis)
   (c) Does the design of the questions tend to bias subjects' responses?
   (d) Does the sequence of questions tend to bias subjects' responses?

4. Physiological measures
   (a) Are the physiological measures or instruments clearly described? If appropriate, are the brand names, such as Space Labs or Hewlett-Packard, of the instruments identified?
   (b) Are the accuracy, selectivity, precision, sensitivity, and error of the physiological instruments discussed?
   (c) Are the physiological measures appropriate for the research purpose and objectives, questions, or hypotheses? (Analysis)
   (d) Are the methods for recording data from the physiological measures clearly described? Is the recording of data consistent?

IX. Data collection
   A. Is the data collection process clearly described (Bowman et al., 2002)?
   B. Are the forms used to collect data organized to facilitate computerizing the data?
   C. Is the training of data collectors clearly described and adequate?

   D. Is the data collection process conducted in a consistent manner?
   E. Are the data collection methods ethical?
   F. Do the data collected address the research objectives, questions, or hypotheses? (Analysis)
   G. Did any adverse events occur during data collection, and were these appropriately managed (Bowman et al., 2002)?

X. Data analysis
   A. Are data analysis procedures appropriate for the type of data collected (Corty, 2007)?
   B. Are data analysis procedures clearly described? Did the researcher address any problems with missing data and how this problem was managed?
   C. Do the data analysis techniques address the study purpose and the research objectives, questions, or hypotheses? (Analysis)
   D. Are the results presented in an understandable way by narrative, tables, or figures, or a combination of methods?
   E. Are the statistical analyses logically linked to the design? (Analysis)
   F. Is the sample size sufficient to detect significant differences if they are present? (Analysis)
   G. Was a power analysis conducted for nonsignificant results? (Analysis)
   H. Are the results interpreted appropriately?

XI. Interpretation of findings
   A. Are findings discussed in relation to each objective, question, or hypothesis?
   B. Are various explanations for significant and nonsignificant findings examined?
   C. Are the findings clinically significant (LeFort, 1993; Melnyk & Fineout-Overholt, 2005)?
   D. Are the findings linked to the study framework? (Analysis)
   E. Are the study findings an accurate reflection of reality and valid for use in clinical practice? (Analysis) (Melnyk & Fineout-Overholt, 2005; Peat et al., 2002)
   F. Do the conclusions fit the results from the data analyses? Are the conclusions based on statistically significant and clinically significant results? (Analysis)
   G. Does the study have limitations not identified by the researcher? (Analysis)
   H. Did the researcher generalize the findings appropriately?

I. Were the identified implications for practice appropriate based on the study findings and the findings from previous research? (Analysis)

J. Were quality suggestions made for future research?

Step IV: Evaluation

Evaluation involves determining the meaning, significance, and validity of the study by examining the links between the study process, study findings, and previous studies. The steps of the study are evaluated in light of previous studies, such as an evaluation of present hypotheses based on previous hypotheses, present design based on previous designs, and present methods of measuring variables based on previous methods of measurement. The findings of the present study are also examined in light of the findings of previous studies. Evaluation builds on conclusions reached during the first three stages of the critique and provides the basis for conceptual clustering.

Guidelines for Evaluation

You need to reexamine the findings, conclusions, and implications sections of the study and the researchers' suggestions for further study. Using the following questions as a guide, summarize the *strengths* and *weaknesses* of the study:

1. What rival hypotheses can be suggested for the findings?
2. Do you believe the study findings are valid? How much confidence can be placed in the study findings?
3. To what populations can the findings be generalized?
4. What questions emerge from the findings, and does the researcher identify them?
5. What future research can be envisioned?
6. Could the limitations of the study have been corrected?
7. When the findings are examined in light of previous studies, what is now known and not known about the phenomenon under study?

You need to read previous studies conducted in the area of the research being examined and summarize your responses to the following questions:

1. Are the findings of previous studies used to generate the research problem and purpose?
2. Is the design an advancement over previous designs?
3. Do sampling strategies show an improvement over previous studies? Does the sample selection have the potential for adding diversity to samples previously studied (Larson, 1994)?

4. Does the current research build on previous measurement strategies so that measurement is more precise or more reflective of the variables?
5. How do statistical analyses compare with those used in previous studies?
6. Do the findings build on the findings of previous studies?
7. Is current knowledge in this area identified?
8. Does the author indicate the implication of the findings for practice?

The evaluation of a research report should also include a final discussion of the quality of the report. This discussion should include an expert opinion of the study's contribution to nursing knowledge and the need for additional research in selected areas. You also need to determine if the empirical evidence generated by this study and previous research is ready for use in practice (Whittemore, 2005).

Step V: Conceptual Clustering

The last step of the critique process is conceptual clustering, which involves synthesizing the study findings to determine the current body of knowledge in an area (Pinch, 1995). Until the 1980s, conceptual clustering was seldom addressed in the nursing literature. However, in 1983, the initial volume of the *Annual Review of Nursing Research* was published to provide conceptual clustering of specific phenomena of interest in the areas of nursing practice, nursing care delivery, nursing education, and the profession of nursing (Werley & Fitzpatrick, 1983). These books continue to be published each year and provide integrated reviews of research on a variety of topics relevant to nursing. Conceptual clustering is also evident in the publication of systematic reviews of research and integrative reviews of research in clinical and research journals and on national websites such as www.guideline.gov (Stone, 2002; Whittemore, 2005)

Guidelines for Conceptual Clustering

Through conceptual clustering, current knowledge in an area of study is carefully analyzed, relationships are examined, and the knowledge is summarized and organized theoretically. Conceptual clustering maximizes the meaning attached to research findings, highlights gaps in knowledge, generates new research questions, and provides empirical evidence for use in practice.

I. Process for clustering findings and developing the current knowledge base

A. Is the purpose for reviewing the literature clearly identified? Are specific questions articulated to guide the literature review (Stone, 2002; Whittemore, 2005)?

B. Are protocols developed to guide the literature review?

C. Is a systematic and comprehensive review of the literature conducted (Stone, 2002)?

D. Are the criteria for including studies in the review clearly identified and used appropriately (Whittemore, 2005)?

E. Are the studies systematically critiqued for quality outcomes?

F. Is the process for clustering study findings clearly described? Are the data statistically combined?

G. Is the current knowledge base clearly expressed, including what is known and what is not known?

II. Theoretical organization of the knowledge base

A. Draw a map showing the concepts and relationships found in the studies reviewed in the previous criteria (section I) to detect gaps in understanding relationships. You can also compare this map with current theory in the area of study by asking the following questions:

1. Is the map consistent with current theory?

2. Are there differences in the map that are upheld by well-designed research? If so, modification of existing theory should be considered.

3. Are there concepts and relationships in existing theory that have not been examined in the studies diagrammed in the map? If so, studies should be developed to examine these gaps.

4. Are there conflicting theories within the field of study? Do existing study findings tend to support one of the theories?

5. Are there no existing theories to explain the phenomenon under consideration?

6. Can current research findings be used to begin the development of nursing theory to explain the phenomenon more completely?

III. Moving toward evidence-based practice

A. Is there sufficient confidence in the research evidence for application to practice? If so, develop a systematic review of the research to promote the use of this empirical evidence in practice.

B. What are the benefits and risks of using selected research evidence for patient care?

C. When research evidence is used in practice, what are the outcomes for patients, providers, and health care agencies (Brown, 1999; Doran, 2003)?

Meta-analysis is another form of conceptual clustering that goes beyond critique and integration of research findings to conducting statistical analysis on the outcomes of similar studies (Beck, 1999; Whittemore, 2005). A meta-analysis statistically pools the results from previous studies into a single result or outcome that provides the strongest evidence about a relationship between two variables or concepts or the efficacy of a treatment or intervention (LaValley, 1997). Conducting a quality meta-analysis requires a great deal of rigor in implementing the following steps: (1) developing a protocol to direct conduct of the meta-analysis, (2) locating relevant studies, (3) selecting studies for analysis that meet the criteria in the protocol, (4) conducting statistical analyses, (5) assessing the meta-analysis results, and (6) discussing the relevance of the findings to nursing knowledge and practice (Whittemore, 2005). Chapter 27 discusses the processes for critically appraising meta-analyses and for conducting a meta-analysis to synthesize research evidence for practice.

CRITICAL APPRAISAL PROCESS FOR QUALITATIVE STUDIES

Critical appraisal in qualitative research involves examining the expertise of the researchers, noting the organization and presentation of the report, discussing the strengths and weaknesses of the study, suggesting modifications for future studies, and evaluating the overall quality of the study. Thus, the guidelines in Table 26-2 will help you to critique a qualitative study. However, other standards and skills are also useful for assessing the quality of a qualitative study and the credibility of the study findings (Burns, 1989; Cutcliffe & McKenna, 1999; Patton, 2002). The skills and standards for critically appraising qualitative research are described in the following sections.

Skills Needed to Critically Appraise Qualitative Studies

The skills to critically appraise qualitative studies include (1) context flexibility; (2) inductive reasoning; (3) conceptualization, theoretical modeling, and theory analysis; and (4) transformation of ideas across levels of abstraction (Burns, 1989).

Context Flexibility

Context flexibility is the capacity to switch from one context or worldview to another, to shift perception in order to see things from a different perspective. Each worldview is based on a set of assumptions through which reality is defined. To develop the skills necessary to critique qualitative studies, you must be willing to move from the assumptions of quantitative research to those of qualitative research. This skill is not new in nursing; beginning students are encouraged to see things from the patient's perspective. However, accomplishing this switch of context requires investing time and energy to learn more about the patient and setting aside personal, sometimes strongly held views. It is not necessary for you to become committed to a perspective to follow or apply its logical structure. In fact, all scholarly work requires a willingness and ability to examine and evaluate works from diverse perspectives. For example, analysis of the internal structure of a theory requires this same process.

Inductive Reasoning Skills

Although all research requires skill in both deductive and inductive reasoning, the transformation process used during data analysis in qualitative research is based on inductive reasoning. Individuals conducting a critical appraisal of a qualitative study must be able to exercise skills in inductive reasoning to follow the researcher's logic. This logic is revealed in the systematic move from the concrete descriptions in a particular study to the abstract level of science.

Conceptualization, Theoretical Modeling, and Theory Analysis Skills

Qualitative research is oriented toward theory construction. Therefore, an effective reviewer of qualitative research needs to have skills in conceptualization, theoretical modeling, and theory analysis. The theoretical structure in a qualitative study is developed inductively and is expected to emerge from the data. The reviewer must be able to follow the logical flow of thought of the researcher and be able to analyze and evaluate the adequacy of the resulting theoretical schema, as well as its connection to theory development within the discipline (Patton, 2002).

Transforming Ideas across Levels of Abstraction

Closely associated with the necessity of having skills in theory analysis is the ability to follow the transformation of ideas across several levels of abstraction and to judge the adequacy of the transformation. Whenever you review the literature, organize ideas from the review, and then modify those ideas in the process of developing a summary of the existing body of knowledge, you are involved in the transformation of ideas. Developing a qualitative research report requires

transforming ideas across levels of abstraction. Those examining the report evaluate the adequacy of this transformation process.

Standards for Critical Appraisal of Qualitative Studies

Multiple problems can occur in qualitative studies, as in quantitative studies. However, the problems are likely to be different. Reviewers not only need to know the problems that are likely to occur, but they also must be able to determine the probability that the problem may have occurred in the study being evaluated. A scholarly appraisal includes a balanced evaluation of the study's strengths and limitations. Five standards have been proposed to evaluate qualitative studies: descriptive vividness, methodological congruence, analytical preciseness, theoretical connectedness, and heuristic relevance (Burns, 1989; Johnson, 1999). The following sections describe these standards and the threats to them.

Standard I: Descriptive Vividness

Descriptive vividness, or validity, refers to the clarity and factual accuracy of the researcher's account of the study (Johnson, 1999; Munhall, 2001). The description of the site, the study participants, the experience of collecting the data, and the thinking of the researcher during the process needs to be presented so clearly and accurately that the reader has the sense of personally experiencing the event. Glaser and Strauss (1965) suggested that the researcher should "describe the social world studied so vividly that the reader can almost literally see and hear its people" (p. 9). Because one of the assumptions of qualitative research is that all data are context specific, the evaluator of a study must understand the context of that study. From this description, the reader gets a sense of the data as a whole as they are collected and the reactions of the researcher during the data collection and analysis processes. A contextual understanding of the whole is essential and a prerequisite to your capability to evaluate the study in light of the other four standards.

Threats to Descriptive Vividness

1. The researcher failed to include essential descriptive information.
2. The description in the report lacked clarity, depth, or both.
3. The report lacked factual accuracy in the description of the participants and setting (Johnson, 1999).
4. The description in the report lacked authenticity, credibility, or trustworthiness (Beck, 1993; Patton, 2002).

5. The researcher had inadequate skills in writing descriptive narrative.
6. The researcher demonstrated reluctance to reveal his or her self in the written material (Burns, 1989; Kahn, 1993).

Standard II: Methodological Congruence

Evaluation of methodological congruence requires the reviewer to know the philosophy and the methodological approach that the researcher used. The researcher needs to identify the philosophy and methodological approach and cite sources where the reviewer can obtain further information (Beck, 1994; Munhall, 2001). Methodological excellence has four dimensions: rigor in documentation, procedural rigor, ethical rigor, and auditability.

Rigor in Documentation Rigor in documentation requires the researcher to provide a comprehensive presentation of the following study elements: phenomenon, purpose, research question, justification of the significance of the phenomenon, identification of assumptions, identification of philosophy, researcher credentials, the context, the role of the researcher, ethical implications, sampling and study participants, data-gathering strategies, data analysis strategies, theoretical development, conclusions, implications and suggestions for further study and practice, and a literature review. The reviewer examines the study elements or steps for completeness and clarity and identifies any threats to rigor in documentation.

Threats to Rigor in Documentation
1. The researcher fails to present all elements or steps of the study in the qualitative study report.
2. The researcher fails to present all elements or steps of the study accurately or clearly.

Procedural Rigor Another dimension of methodological congruence is the rigor of the researcher in applying selected procedures for the study. To the extent possible, the researcher needs to make clear the steps taken to ensure that data were accurately recorded and that the data obtained are representative of the data as a whole (Knafl & Howard, 1984; Patton, 2002). All researchers have bias, but reflexivity needs to be used in qualitative studies to reduce bias. Reflexivity is an analytical method in which the "researcher actively engages in critical self reflection about his or her potential biases and predispositions" to reduce their impact on the conduct of the study (Johnson, 1999, p. 103). Methodological congruence can also be promoted by extended fieldwork, where the researcher collects data in the study setting for an extended period to ensure accuracy. When evaluating a qualitative study, examine

the description of the data collection process and the study findings for threats to procedural rigor.

Threats to Procedural Rigor
1. The researcher asked the wrong questions. The questions need to tap the participants' experiences, not their theoretical knowledge of the phenomenon.
2. The questions included terminology from the theoretical orientation of the researcher (Kirk & Miller, 1986; Knaack, 1984).
3. The informant might have misinformed the researcher, for several reasons. The informant might have had an ulterior motive for deceiving the researcher. Some individuals might have been present who inhibit free expression by the informant. The informant might have wanted to impress the researcher by giving the response that seemed the most desirable (Dean & Whyte, 1958).
4. The informant did not observe the details requested or was not able to recall the event and substituted instead what he or she supposed happened (Dean & Whyte, 1958).
5. The researcher placed more weight on data obtained from well-informed, articulate, high-status individuals (an elite bias) than on data from those who were less articulate, obstinate, or of low status (Miles & Huberman, 1994).
6. The presence of the researcher distorted the event being observed.
7. The researcher's involvement with the study participants distorted the data (LeCompte & Goetz, 1982).
8. Atypical events were interpreted as typical.
9. The informants lacked credibility (Becker, 1958).
10. An insufficient amount of data was gathered.
11. An insufficient length of time was spent in the setting gathering the data.
12. The approaches for gaining access to the site, the participants, or both were inappropriate.
13. The researcher failed to keep in-depth field notes.
14. The researcher failed to use reflexivity or critical self-reflection to assess his or her potential biases and predispositions (Patton, 2002).

Ethical Rigor Ethical rigor requires the researcher to recognize and discuss the ethical implications related to the conduct of the study. Consent is obtained from the study participants and documented. The report must indicate that the researcher took action to ensure that the rights of the participants were protected during the consent process, data collection and analysis, and communication of the findings (Munhall, 1999, 2001). Examine the consent process, the data-gathering process, and the results for potential threats to ethical rigor.

Threats to Ethical Rigor

1. The researcher failed to inform the participants of their rights.
2. The researcher failed to obtain consent from the participants.
3. The researcher failed to protect the participants' rights during the conduct of the study.
4. The results of the study were presented in such a way that they revealed the identity of individual participants (Munhall, 2001).

Auditability A fourth dimension of methodological congruence is the rigorous development of a decision trail (Miles & Huberman, 1994; Patton, 2002). Guba and Lincoln (1982) referred to this dimension as auditability. To achieve this end, the researcher must report all decisions involved in the transformation of data to the theoretical schema. This reporting should be in sufficient detail to allow a second researcher, using the original data and the decision trail, to arrive at conclusions similar to those of the original researcher. When critically appraising the study, examine the decision trail for threats to auditability.

Threats to Auditability

1. The description of the data collection process was inadequate.
2. The researcher failed to develop or identify the decision rules for arriving at ratings or judgments.
3. The researcher failed to record the nature of the decisions, the data on which they were based, and the reasoning that entered into the decisions.
4. The evidence for conclusions was not presented (Becker, 1958).
5. Other researchers were unable to arrive at similar conclusions after applying the decision rules to the data.

Standard III: Analytical Preciseness

The analytical process in qualitative research involves a series of transformations during which concrete data are transformed across several levels of abstraction. The outcome of the analysis is a theoretical schema that imparts meaning to the phenomenon under study. The analytical process occurs primarily within the reasoning of the researcher and is frequently poorly described in published reports. Some transformations may occur intuitively. However, analytical preciseness requires that the researcher make intense efforts to identify and record the decision-making processes through which the transformations are made. The processes by which the theoretical schema is cross-checked with data also need to be reported in detail.

Premature patterning may occur before the researcher can logically fit all the data within the emerging schema. Nisbett and Ross (1980) have shown that patterning happens rapidly and is the way that individuals habitually process information. The consequence may be a poor fit between data and the theoretical schema (LeCompte & Goetz, 1982; Sandelowski, 1986). Miles and Huberman (1994) suggested that plausibility is the opiate of the intellectual. If the emerging schema makes sense and fits with other theorists' explanations of the phenomenon, the researcher locks into it. For that reason, it is critical to test the schema by rechecking the fit between the schema and the original data. The participants could be asked to provide feedback on the researcher's interpretations and conclusions to gain additional insight or verification of the theoretical schema proposed (Johnson, 1999). Beck (1993) recommended that the researcher have the "data analysis procedures reviewed by a judge panel to prevent researcher bias and selective inattention" (p. 265). When evaluating a study, examine the decision-making processes and the theoretical schema to detect threats to analytical preciseness.

Threats to Analytical Preciseness

1. The interpretive statements do not correspond with the findings (Parse, Coyne, & Smith, 1985).
2. The categories, themes, or common elements are not logical.
3. The samples are not representative of the class of joint acts referred to by the researcher (Denzin, 1989).
4. The set of categories, themes, or common elements fails to set forth a whole picture.
5. The set of categories, themes, or common elements is not inclusive of data that exist.
6. The data are inappropriately assigned to categories, themes, or common elements.
7. The inclusion and exclusion criteria for categories, themes, or common elements are not consistently followed.
8. The working hypotheses or propositions are not identified or cannot be verified by data.
9. Various sources of evidence fail to provide convergence.
10. The evidence is incongruent.
11. The participants fail to validate findings when appropriate (Johnson, 1999).
12. The conclusions are not data based or do not encompass all the data.
13. The data are made to appear more patterned, regular, or congruent than they actually are (Beck, 1993; Sandelowski, 1986).

Standard IV: Theoretical Connectedness

Theoretical connectedness requires that the theoretical schema developed from the study be clearly expressed, logically consistent, reflective of the data, and compatible with the knowledge base of nursing.

Threats to Theoretical Connectedness
1. The findings are trivialized (Goetz & LeCompte, 1981).
2. The concepts are inadequately refined.
3. The concepts are not validated by data.
4. The set of concepts lacks commonality.
5. The relationships between concepts are not clearly expressed.
6. The proposed relationships between concepts are not validated by data.
7. The working propositions are not validated by data.
8. Data are distorted during development of the theoretical schema (Bruyn, 1966).
9. The theoretical schema fails to yield a meaningful picture of the phenomenon studied.
10. A conceptual framework or map is not derived from the data.

Standard V: Heuristic Relevance

To be of value, the results of a study need heuristic relevance for the reader. This value is reflected in the reader's capacity to recognize the phenomenon described in the study, its theoretical significance, its applicability to nursing practice situations, and its influence on future research activities. The dimensions of heuristic relevance include intuitive recognition, relationship to the existing body of knowledge, and applicability.

Intuitive Recognition Intuitive recognition means that when individuals are confronted with the theoretical schema derived from the data, it has meaning within their personal knowledge base. They immediately recognize the phenomenon being described by the researcher and its relationship to a theoretical perspective in nursing.

Threats to Intuitive Recognition
1. The reader is unable to recognize the phenomenon.
2. The description is not consistent with common meanings.
3. Theoretical connectedness is lacking.

Relationship to the Existing Body of Knowledge
The researcher must review the existing body of knowledge, particularly the nursing theoretical perspective from which the phenomenon was approached, and compare them with the findings of the study. The study should have intersubjectivity with existing theoretical knowledge in nursing and previous research. The researcher should explore reasons for differences with the existing body of knowledge. When critically appraising a study, examine the strength of the link of study findings to the existing knowledge.

Threats to the Relationship to the Existing Body of Knowledge
1. The researcher failed to examine the existing body of knowledge.
2. The process studied was not related to nursing and health.
3. The results lack correspondence with the existing knowledge base in nursing (Parse et al., 1985).

Applicability Nurses need to be able to integrate the findings into their knowledge base and apply them to nursing practice situations. The findings also need to contribute to theory development (Munhall, 2001; Patton, 2002). Examine the discussion section of the research report for threats to applicability.

Threats to Applicability
1. The findings are not significant for the discipline of nursing.
2. The report fails to achieve methodological congruence.
3. The report fails to achieve analytical preciseness.
4. The report fails to achieve theoretical connectedness.

By applying these five standards in critically appraising qualitative studies, you can determine the strengths and weaknesses of a study. A summary of the strengths will indicate adherence to the standards, and a summary of weaknesses will indicate potential threats to the integrity of the study. A final evaluation of the study involves applying the standard of heuristic relevance. This standard is used to determine the quality of the study. It also establishes the usefulness of the study findings for the development and refinement of nursing knowledge and for the provision of evidence-based practice.

SUMMARY

- Critical appraisal of research involves carefully examining all aspects of a study to judge its merits, limitations, meaning, validity, and significance in light of previous research experience, knowledge of the topic, and clinical expertise
- Critical appraisals of research are conducted (1) to summarize evidence for practice, (2) to provide a basis for future research, (3) to evaluate presentations and publications of studies, (4) for abstract section for a conference, (5) to select an article for publication, and (6) to evaluate research proposals for funding and implementation in clinical agencies.

- The critical appraisal process for quantitative research includes the following steps: comprehension, comparison, analysis, evaluation, and conceptual clustering.
- The comprehension step involves understanding the terms and concepts in the report, as well as identifying study elements.
- The comparison step requires knowledge of what each step of the research process should be like and the ideal is compared with the real.
- The analysis step involves examining the logical links connecting one study element with another.
- The evaluation step involves examining the meaning, validity, and significance of the study according to set criteria.
- Conceptual clustering involves generating new questions, developing and refining theory, and synthesizing research for use in practice.
- The critical appraisal process in qualitative research includes the skills of (1) context flexibility; (2) inductive reasoning; (3) conceptualization, theoretical modeling, and theory analysis; and (4) transformation of ideas across levels of abstraction.
- The standards proposed to evaluate qualitative research include descriptive vividness, methodological congruence, analytical preciseness, theoretical connectedness, and heuristic relevance.
- Descriptive vividness means that the site, the study participants, the experience of collecting data, and the thinking of the researcher during the process are presented so clearly that the reader has the sense of personally experiencing the event.
- Methodological congruence has four dimensions: rigor in documentation, procedural rigor, ethical rigor, and auditability.
- Analytical preciseness is essential to perform a series of transformations in which concrete data are transformed across several levels of abstraction.
- Theoretical connectedness requires that the theoretical schema developed from the study be clearly expressed, logically consistent, reflective of the data, and compatible with the knowledge base of nursing.
- Heuristic relevance includes intuitive recognition, a relationship to the existing body of knowledge, and applicability.

REFERENCES

American Psychological Association. (2001). *Publication manual of the American Psychological Association* (5th ed.). Washington, DC: Author.

Beck, C. T. (1993). Qualitative research: The evaluation of its credibility, fittingness, and auditability. *Western Journal of Nursing Research, 15*(2), 263–266.

Beck, C. T. (1994). Reliability and validity issues in phenomenological research. *Western Journal of Nursing Research, 16*(3), 254–267.

Beck, C. T. (1999). Focus on research methods. Facilitating the work of a meta-analyst. *Research in Nursing & Health, 22*(6), 523–530.

Becker, H. S. (1958). Problems of inference and proof in participant observation. *American Sociological Review, 23*(6), 652–660.

Bowman, A., Wyman, J. F., & Peters, J. (2002). Methods. The operations manual: A mechanism for improving the research process. *Nursing Research, 51*(2), 134–138.

Brown, S. J. (1999). *Knowledge for health care practice: A guide to using research evidence.* Philadelphia: Saunders.

Brown, S. J. (2002). Focus on research methods. Nursing intervention studies: A descriptive analysis of issues important to clinicians. *Research in Nursing & Health, 25*(4), 317–327.

Bruyn, S. T. (1966). *The human perspective in sociology.* Englewood Cliffs, NJ: Prentice-Hall.

Burns, N. (1989). Standards for qualitative research. *Nursing Science Quarterly, 2*(1), 44–52.

Burns, N., & Grove, S. K. (2007). *Understanding nursing research* (4th ed.). Philadelphia: Saunders.

Corty, E. W. (2007). *Using and interpreting statistics: A practical text for the health, behavioral, and social sciences.* St. Louis: Mosby.

Crookes, P., & Davies, S. (1998). *Essential skills for reading and applying research in nursing and health care.* Edinburgh, Scotland: Baillière Tindall.

Cutcliffe, J. R., & McKenna, H. P. (1999). Establishing the credibility of qualitative research findings: The plot thickens. *Journal of Advanced Nursing, 30*(2), 374–380.

Dean, J. P., & Whyte, W. F. (1958). How do you know if the informant is telling the truth? *Human Organization, 17*(2), 34–38.

Denzin, N. K. (1989). *The research act* (3rd ed.). New York: McGraw-Hill.

Doran, D. M. (2003). *Nursing-sensitive outcomes: State of the science.* Sudbury, MA: Jones & Bartlett.

Glaser, B., & Strauss, A. L. (1965). Discovery of substantive theory: A basic strategy underlying qualitative research. *American Behavioral Scientist, 8*(1), 5–12.

Goetz, J. P., & LeCompte, M. D. (1981). Ethnographic research and the problem of data reduction. *Anthropology and Education Quarterly, 12*(1), 51–70.

Guba, E. G., & Lincoln, Y. S. (1982). *Effective evaluation.* Washington, DC: Jossey-Bass.

Houser, J. (2008). *Nursing research: Reading, using, and creating evidence.* Sudbury, MA: Jones & Bartlett.

Johnson, R. B. (1999). Examining the validity structure of qualitative research. In F. Pyrczak (Ed.), *Evaluating research in academic journals: A practical guide to realistic evaluation* (pp. 103–108). Los Angeles: Pyrczak.

Kahn, D. L. (1993). Ways of discussing validity in qualitative nursing research. *Western Journal of Nursing Research, 15*(1), 122–126.

Kerlinger, F. N., & Lee, H. B. (2000). *Foundations of behavioral research* (4th ed.). Fort Worth, TX: Harcourt College.

Kim, M. J., & Felton, F. (1993). The current generation of research proposals: Reviewers' viewpoints. *Nursing Research, 42*(2), 118–119.

Kirk, J., & Miller, M. L. (1986). *Reliability and validity in qualitative research*. Beverly Hills, CA: Sage.

Knaack, P. (1984). Phenomenological research. *Western Journal of Nursing Research*, 6(1), 107–114.

Knafl, K. A., & Howard, M. J. (1984). Interpreting and reporting qualitative research. *Research in Nursing & Health*, 7(1), 17–24.

Larson, E. (1994). Exclusion of certain groups from clinical research. *Image: Journal of Nursing Scholarship*, 26(3), 185–190.

LaValley, M. (1997). Methods article: A consumer's guide to meta-analysis. *Arthritis Care and Research*, 10(3), 208–213.

LeCompte, M. D., & Goetz, J. P. (1982). Problems of reliability and validity in ethnographic research. *Review of Educational Research*, 52(1), 31–60.

LeFort, S. M. (1993). The statistical versus clinical significance debate. *Image: Journal of Nursing Scholarship*, 25(1), 57–62.

LoBiondo-Wood, G. L., & Haber, J. (2005). *Nursing research: Methods and critical appraisal for evidence-based practice* (6th ed.). St. Louis: Mosby.

Meleis, A. I. (1991). *Theoretical nursing: Development and progress* (2nd ed.). Philadelphia: Lippincott.

Melnyk, B. M., & Fineout-Overholt, E. (2005). *Evidence-based practice in nursing & healthcare: A guide to best practice*. Philadelphia: Lippincott Williams & Wilkins.

Miles, M. B., & Huberman, A. M. (1994). *Qualitative data analysis: A source book of new methods* (2nd ed.). Beverly Hills, CA: Sage.

Morse, J. M., Dellasega, C., & Doberneck, B. (1993). Evaluating abstracts: Preparing a research conference. *Nursing Research*, 42(5), 308–310.

Munhall, P. L. (1999). Ethical considerations in qualitative research. In P. L. Munhall & C. O. Boyd (Eds.), *Nursing research: A qualitative perspective* (2nd ed.). New York: National League for Nursing.

Munhall, P. L. (2001). *Nursing research: A qualitative perspective* (3rd ed.). Sudbury, MA: Jones & Bartlett.

Nieswiadomy, R. M. (2008). *Foundations of nursing research* (5th ed.). Upper Saddle River, NJ: Pearson Prentice Hall.

Nisbett, R., & Ross, L. (1980). *Human inference: Strategies and shortcomings of social judgment*. Englewood Cliffs, NJ: Prentice-Hall.

Oberst, M. T. (1992). Warning: Believing this report may be hazardous. *Research in Nursing & Health*, 15(2), 91–92.

Parse, R. R., Coyne, A. B., & Smith, M. J. (1985). *Nursing research: Qualitative methods*. Bowie, MD: Brady.

Patton, M. Q. (2002). *Qualitative research and evaluation methods* (3rd ed.). Thousand Oaks, CA: Sage.

Peat, J., Mellis, C., Williams, K., & Xuan, W. (2002). *Health science research: A handbook of quantitative methods*. Thousand Oaks: CA: Sage.

Pinch, W. J. (1995). Synthesis: Implementing a complex process. *Nurse Educator*, 20(1), 34–40.

Polit, D. F., & Beck, C. T. (2008). *Nursing research: Generating and assessing evidence for nursing practice* (8th ed.). Philadelphia: Lippincott Williams & Wilkins.

Pyrczak, F. (1999). *Evaluating research in academic journals: A practical guide to realistic evaluation*. Los Angeles: Pyrczak.

Resnick, B., Concha, B., Burgess, J. G., Fine, M. L., West, L., Baylor, K., et al. (2003). Brief report. Recruitment of older women: Lessons learned from the Baltimore hip studies. *Nursing Research*, 52(4), 270–273.

Roberts, W. D., & Stone, P. W. (2004). Ask an Expert: How to choose and evaluate a research instrument. *Applied Nursing Research*, 16(10), 70–72.

Rudy, E. B., & Kerr, M. E. (2000). Auditing research studies. *Nursing Research*, 49(2), 117–120.

Ryan-Wenger, N. (1992). Guidelines for critique of a research report. *Heart & Lung*, 21(4), 394–401.

Sandelowski, M. (1986). The problem of rigor in qualitative research. *Advances in Nursing Science*, 8(3), 27–37.

Santacroce, S. J., Maccarelli, L. M., & Grey, M. (2004). Methods: Intervention fidelity. *Nursing Research*, 53(1), 63–66.

Sidani, S., & Braden, C. J. (1998). *Evaluation of nursing interventions: A theory-driven approach*. Thousand Oaks, CA: Sage.

Stone, P. W. (2002). What is a systematic review? *Applied Nursing Research*, 15(1), 52–53.

Swanson, E. A., McCloskey, J. C., & Bodensteiner, A. (1991). Publishing opportunities for nurses: A comparison of 92 U. S. journals. *Image: Journal of Nursing Scholarship*, 23(1), 33–38.

Tibbles, L., & Sanford, R. (1994). The research journal club: A mechanism for research utilization. *Clinical Nurse Specialist*, 8(1), 23–26.

Tilden, V. (2002). Peer review: Evidence-based or sacred cow? [Editorial] *Nursing Research*, 51(5), 275.

Werley, H. H., & Fitzpatrick, J. J. (1983). *Annual review of nursing research* (Vol. 1). New York: Springer.

Whittemore, R. (2005). Methods. Combining evidence in nursing research: Methods and implications. *Nursing Research*, 54(1), 56–62.

Yam, M. (1994). Strategies for teaching nursing research: Teaching nursing students to critique research for gender bias. *Western Journal of Nursing Research*, 16(6), 724–727.

CHAPTER **27**

Strategies for Promoting Evidence-Based Nursing Practice

Research evidence has greatly expanded since the 1980s as numerous, quality nursing and medical studies have been conducted and then communicated via publications, television, and the Internet. The expectation of society and the goal of the health care system is the delivery of high-quality health care to patients, families, and communities. To ensure its quality, health care must be based on the best research evidence available. Health care agencies are emphasizing the delivery of evidence-based health care, and nurses and physicians now focus on building an evidence-based practice (EBP). EBP became a major focus for medicine in the early 1990s and for nursing in 2000s. With the implementation of EBP, outcomes have improved for patients, health care providers, and health care agencies (Craig & Smyth, 2007; Institute of Medicine, 2001; Malloch & Porter-O'Grady, 2006; Melnyk & Fineout-Overholt, 2005; Pearson, Field, & Jordan, 2007; Sackett, Straus, Richardson, Rosenberg, & Haynes, 2000).

Evidence-based practice (EBP) is an important theme in this textbook and was defined earlier as the conscientious integration of best research evidence with clinical expertise and patient values and needs in the delivery of quality, cost-effective health care (Craig & Smyth, 2007; Institute of Medicine, 2001; Sackett et al., 2000). A model of EBP is presented in Chapter 1. **Best research evidence** is produced by the conduct and synthesis of numerous, high-quality studies in a health-related area. The concept of best research evidence is introduced in Chapter 2, and the processes for synthesizing research evidence (systematic review,

meta-analysis, integrative review, metasummary, and metasynthesis) are described. This chapter builds on previous EBP discussions to provide you with strategies for implementing best research evidence in your practice and moving the profession of nursing toward EBP. This chapter examines some of the criticisms and benefits related to the development of an EBP for nursing. Guidelines are provided for synthesizing research to determine the best research evidence. Two nursing models developed to facilitate evidence-based practice in health care agencies are introduced. Expert researchers, clinicians, and consumers—through government agencies, professional organizations, and health care agencies—have developed an extensive number of evidence-based guidelines. This chapter offers a framework for reviewing the quality of these evidence-based guidelines and for using them in practice. The chapter concludes with a discussion of the evidence-based practice centers that have been funded by the U.S. government to expand the research evidence generated, synthesized, and developed into evidence-based guidelines for practice.

CRITICISMS AND BENEFITS OF EVIDENCE-BASED PRACTICE IN NURSING

EBP is a goal for the nursing profession and for each practicing nurse. Currently, some nursing interventions are evidence based or supported by research knowledge generated from quality studies. Other areas of nursing practice, however, require additional research. Some nurses readily use research-based interventions, and others are slower to make changes in their practice. This section identifies the criticisms and benefits of EBP to assist you in applying this discipline in your own nursing efforts.

Criticism of Evidence-Based Practice in Nursing

Criticisms of the EBP movement have been both practical and conceptual. This section focuses on some of the constructive criticisms of EBP that need to be considered as nursing moves toward this method of practice. One of the criticisms is that nursing lacks the research evidence for implementing an EBP. EBP requires synthesizing research evidence from randomized controlled trials (RCTs), and these types of studies are limited in nursing. However, the number of RCTs conducted to test nursing interventions has greatly increased in the 2000s. Also, some of the systematic reviews and meta-analyses conducted in nursing indicate there is inadequate research evidence to support using certain nursing interventions in practice (Pearson et al., 2007). Bolton, Donaldson, Rutledge, Bennett, and Brown (2007, p. 123S) conducted a review of "systematic/integrative reviews and meta-analyses on nursing interventions and patient outcomes in acute care settings." Their literature search covered 1999 to 2005 and identified 4000 systematic/integrative reviews and 500 meta-analyses covering seven topics selected by the authors: developmental care of neonates and infants, symptom management, elder care, caregivers, pressure ulcer prevention/treatment, incontinence, and staffing. The authors found limited association between nursing interventions/processes and patient outcomes in acute care settings. Their findings included the following:

> *The strongest evidence was for the use of patient risk-assessment tools and interventions implemented by nurses to prevent patient harm. We observed significant variation in the methods to measure the effect of independent variables (nursing interventions) on patient outcomes. Results indicate the need for more research measuring the effect of specific nursing interventions that may impact acute care patient outcomes. (Bolton et al., 2007, p. 123S)*

Extensive evidence has been generated through nursing research, but there is a need for additional studies focused on determining the effectiveness of nursing interventions on patient outcomes (Bolton et al., 2007;

Craig & Smyth, 2007; Pearson et al., 2007). Identifying the areas where research evidence is lacking is an important first step in developing the evidence needed for practice. Well-designed experimental and quasi-experimental studies are needed to test selected nursing interventions and to use that understanding to generate sound evidence for practice. Nurses also need to be more active in conducting quality syntheses (systematic review, meta-analyses, and integrative reviews) of research evidence in selected areas (Pearson et al., 2007). The next section of this chapter provides guidelines for different types of research synthesis.

Another concern is that the research evidence is generated based on population data and then is applied in practice to individual patients. Sometimes it is difficult to transfer research knowledge to individual patients who respond in unique ways (Biswas et al., 2007). More work is needed to promote the use of evidence-based guidelines with individual patients. Patients who have poor outcomes when managed according to an evidence-based guideline need to be reported and, if possible, their circumstances should be published as a case study.

Best research evidence is generated mainly from quantitative, outcomes, and intervention research methodologies (Craig & Smyth, 2007; Sackett et al., 2000) with limited focus on the contributions of qualitative research and theories. Nurse researchers need to ensure that their studies are linked to theory with an explicit study framework and that theory is used to interpret the findings (Schmelzer, 2007). Qualitative research also makes a contribution to the research evidence in selected areas. Currently, qualitative researchers have developed metasummary and metasynthesis processes to synthesize the findings from qualitative studies (Sandelowski & Barroso, 2007; Whittemore, 2005). The contribution that qualitative research will make to EBP is still evolving.

Another criticism of the EBP movement is that the development of evidence-based guidelines has led to a "cookbook" approach to health care. Health professionals are expected to follow these guidelines in their practice as developed (Pearson et al., 2007). However, the definition of EBP describes it as the conscientious *integration* of best research evidence with clinical expertise and patient values and needs. Thus, the clinician has a major role in determining how the best research evidence will be implemented when caring for an individual patient. For example, a nurse practitioner uses the national evidence-based guidelines for the treatment of patients with hypertension (Joint National Committee on Prevention, Detection, Evaluation, and Treatment of High Blood

Pressure [JNC 7]) but also makes clinical decisions based on the individual patients' needs and values. If the patient has a dry, persistent, irritating cough when taking angiotensin converting enzyme (ACE) inhibitor medications, this type of medication will not be used to manage the patient's high blood pressure if at all possible. If a patient refuses a treatment based on cultural or religious reasons, these reasons will be taken into consideration in developing the patient's treatment plan. Evidence-based guidelines provide the gold standard for managing a particular health condition, but the health care provider and patient individualize the treatment plan (Sackett et al., 2000).

Another criticism is that some health care agencies and administrators do not provide the resources necessary for nurses to implement EBP. Their lack of support might include the following: (1) not providing access to research journals and other sources of synthesized research findings and evidence-based guidelines, (2) limited time to make research-based changes in practice, (3) limited authority to change patient care based on research findings, (4) no funds to support research-based changes for practice, and (5) no rewards for providing evidence-based care to patients and families (McCaughan, Thompson, Cullum, Sheldon, & Thompson, 2002; Parahoo, 2000; Pettengill, Gillies, & Clark, 1994; Retsas, 2000). Some nurses lack the knowledge to implement EBP and need support from expert nurse researchers and clinicians. Clinical agencies could ensure that these resources are provided to practicing nurses to expand their understanding and use of research evidence in practice. The success of EBP is determined by all involved including health care agencies, administrators, nurses, physicians, and other health care professionals. We must all take an active role in ensuring that the health care provided patients and families is based on the best research available.

Benefits of Evidence-Based Practice in Nursing

The benefits of EBP are improved outcomes for patients, providers, and health care agencies. The best research evidence has been synthesized in many areas by teams of expert researchers and clinicians and then used to develop strong evidence-based guidelines for practice. These guidelines indicate the best treatment plan or gold standard for patient care in a selected area to promote quality health outcomes. Health care providers have easy access to numerous evidence-based guidelines to assist them in making their best clinical decisions. These evidence-based guidelines are

communicated by presentations and publications and can be easily accessed online. They help students, novice nurses, and advanced practice nurses (APNs) to provide the best possible care (Kania-Lachance, Best, McDonah, & Ghosh, 2006). Expert APNs access evidence-based guidelines to ensure their patient care is based on the most recent research evidence available. They also use them to manage patients with uncommon conditions. EBP ensures that nurses and other health care professionals are making clinical decisions based on research evidence and not on tradition or trial and error.

Health care agencies are highly supportive of EBP because it promotes quality, cost-effective care for patients and families and meets accreditation requirements. The Joint Commission revised their accreditation criteria in 2002 to emphasize patient care quality achieved through EBP. Approximately 25% of the chief nursing officers (CNOs) identified the movement toward evidence-based nursing practice as their number one priority (Nursing Executive Center, 2005).

Many CNOs and health care agencies are trying either to obtain or to maintain magnet status that documents the excellence of nursing care in an agency. The health care agencies that currently have magnet status can be viewed online at the American Nurses Credentialing Center (ANCC) website at www.nursecredentialing.org/magnet/index.html (ANCC, 2007). The Magnet Status Program, provided through ANCC, recognizes evidence-based practice as a way to improve the quality of patient care and revitalize the nursing environment. Select criteria for magnet status, which require health care agencies to promote the conduct of research and the use of research evidence in practice, are presented next.

■ *FORCE 6: QUALITY CARE*

Research and Evidence-Based Practice

22. Describe how current literature, appropriate to the practice setting, is available, disseminated, and used to change administrative and clinical practices.
23. Discuss the institution's policies and procedures that protect the rights of participants in research protocols. Include evidence of consistent nursing involvement in the governing body responsible for protection of human subjects in research.
24. Provide evidence that research consultants are actively involved in shaping nursing research infrastructure, capacity, and mentorship.
25. Provide a copy of the nursing budget or other sources of funding for the past year, the current year-to-date, and the future projection, highlighting the allocation and utilization of resources for nursing research.

26. Supply documentation of all nursing research activities that are ongoing, including internal validation studies, internal and external research, and participation in surveys completed within the past twelve (12) month period.
27. Provide evidence of education and mentoring activities that have effectively engaged staff nurses in research- and/or evidence-based practice activities.
28. Describe resources available to nursing staff to support participating in nursing research and nursing research utilization activities. (Nursing Executive Center, 2005, p. 15)

In working toward an EBP, nurses are encouraged to embrace the benefits of EBP, to use the evidence-based guidelines available, and to support or participate in the research needed to determine the effectiveness of certain nursing interventions.

GUIDELINES FOR SYNTHESIZING RESEARCH EVIDENCE

Many nurses lack the expertise and confidence to synthesize research evidence in a selected area of nursing. They would benefit from interacting with nurses who have expert skills in conducting research; critically appraising studies; and synthesizing research evidence through systematic reviews, integrative reviews, and meta-analyses. Synthesizing research evidence is best done with at least two and maybe more expert researchers and clinicians. However, novice researchers should also be included in this process to promote their understanding of the synthesis processes implemented to determine the best research evidence in an area. Five different synthesis processes (systematic review, meta-analysis, integrative review, metasummary, and metasynthesis) were introduced in Chapter 2, and the following section provides guidelines to help you understand and participate in these synthesis processes. Numerous research syntheses have been conducted in nursing and medicine, so be sure to search for an existing synthesis of research in an area before undertaking such a project.

Guidelines for Implementing and Evaluating a Systematic Review

A systematic review is a structured, comprehensive synthesis of quantitative studies in a particular health care area to determine the best research evidence available for expert clinicians to use to promote an EBP. Systematic reviews are conducted to synthesis research evidence from numerous, high-quality quantitative studies with similar methodologies, such as RCT (Craig & Smyth, 2007). Systematic reviews are often conducted by a team or panel of experts whose goal is to provide the best research knowledge for evidence-based guidelines. The following steps may help you to conduct a systematic review of research evidence:

1. State objectives and hypotheses that will focus and guide the review.
2. Outline the eligibility criteria that are used to include and exclude studies from the review, such as the types of studies, participants, design, sampling process, interventions, and outcomes to be examined. Construct a table that includes these criteria.
3. Conduct a comprehensive search of the literature for eligible studies. Chapter 6 provides details for searching the literature.
4. Examine each study to determine if it meets the eligibility criteria identified in step 2, and enter all studies into a table and document how each study meets the eligibility criteria. Two or more researchers or clinical experts need to examine the studies to ensure that the eligibility criteria are consistently implemented.
5. Construct a table describing the characteristics of the included studies such as the purpose of the studies, population, sampling method, sample size, sample acceptance and attrition rates, design, intervention (independent variable), dependent variables, measurement methods for each dependent variable, and major results.
6. Critically appraise the methodological quality of the included studies. Two or more experts need to independently review the studies. Chapter 26 provided guidelines that you can use to critically appraise quantitative studies.
7. Extract essential data from the study—at least two or more investigators need to do this to ensure quality extraction of the data. Contact the study investigators if needed to obtain critical data such as means, standard deviations, and inferential statistical results that were not included in the study publication.
8. Analyze the data from the selected studies by conducting a meta-analysis if appropriate.
9. Develop a report that states the objects of the review, criteria for including studies, search process, summary of the characteristics of the studies reviewed, quality of the studies reviewed, and results and conclusions of the review.

These guidelines were adapted from Craig and Smyth's (2007, p. 188) *Evidence-Based Practice*

Manual for Nurses. They also provided the following steps for critically appraising the quality of a systematic review:

1. *Was the purpose [or objectives] of the review clearly stated?*
2. *Did the reviewers report a systematic and comprehensive search strategy to identify relevant studies?*
3. *Were inclusion and exclusion criteria for studies reported and were they appropriate (i.e. was selection bias avoided)?*
4. *Was the quality of included studies assessed appropriately?*
5. *Were the results of the included studies combined systematically and appropriately?*
6. *Were the conclusions supported by the data? (Craig & Smyth, 2007, p. 194)*

The critique of an evidence-based guideline should also include an assessment of how current the guideline is. This leads to the question, how quickly do systematic reviews become out of date? Shojania et al. (2007) conducted a survival analysis on 100 quantitative systematic reviews published from 1995 to 2005 "to estimate the average time to changes in evidence that are sufficiently important to warrant updating systematic reviews" (Shojania et al., 2007, p. 224). They found the average time before a systematic review should be updated was 5.5 years. However, 23% of the reviews signaled a need for updating within 2 years, and 15% needed updating within 1 year. Shojania et al. (2007) stressed that high-quality systematic reviews that were directly relevant to clinical practice require frequent updating to stay current.

The Cochran Collaboration and library include extensive collections of systematic reviews and meta-analyses (www.cochrane.org/); however, a subscription is required to access these reviews. Many University libraries and some health care agency libraries provide access to the Cochran Collaboration and library holdings. A journal titled *Medical Care Research & Review* includes a variety of research syntheses. The Bolton et al. (2007) review introduced earlier identified 4000 systematic/integrative reviews. There are numerous nursing and medical sources of systematic reviews, but it is important for you to know the steps of the systematic review process and be able to critically appraise the quality of the reviews. Only quality, current, systematic reviews provide the best research evidence to support protocols, algorithms, or policies for nursing practice. Chobanian et al. (2003) conducted an excellent systematic review to determine the best research evidence available for assessing, diagnosing, and managing hypertension. This systematic review, which included several meta-analyses and integrative reviews, was used to develop the JNC 7 evidence-based guideline for hypertension. The 2003 systematic review was an update of the review conducted in 1997 that provided the JNC 6 guidelines for the management of hypertension. The JNC 7 evidence-based guideline is presented later in this chapter.

Conducting Meta-Analysis to Synthesize Research Evidence

Meta-analysis statistically pools the results from previous studies into a single quantitative analysis, which then provides the highest level of evidence for an intervention's efficacy (Conn & Rantz, 2003; LaValley, 1997). This approach allows the application of scientific criteria to factors such as sample size, level of significance, and variables examined. Meta-analysis can generate the following: (1) an extremely large, diverse sample that is more representative of the target population than the samples of the individual studies; (2) the determination of the overall significance or probability of pooled data from quality, confirmed studies; and (3) the average effect size determined from several quality studies, which indicates the efficacy of a treatment or intervention or the strength of relationships among the variables (Conn & Rantz, 2003; Craig & Smyth, 2007).

Meta-analyses make it possible for researchers to be objective rather than subjective when evaluating research findings for practice. The strongest evidence for using an intervention in practice is generated from a meta-analysis of multiple, controlled studies. However, the conduct of a meta-analysis depends on the quality, clarity, and completeness of information presented in studies. Beck (1999) provided a list of information that needs to be included in a research report if a meta-analysis is to be conducted (Table 27-1). Craig and Smyth (2007) provided guidelines for conducting a meta-analysis, which includes the following steps:

1. Formulate a research problem and purpose for the meta-analysis.
2. Conduct a comprehensive search of the literature for eligible studies.
3. Evaluate the available data, and, if possible, contact study investigators for missing data identified in Table 27-1.
4. Pool the results for the studies included in the meta-analysis.
5. Conduct a statistical analysis of the data obtained from the studies.
6. Interpret the findings to determine the benefit or harm of an intervention, the effect size or

TABLE 27-1 ░ Recommended Reporting for Authors to Facilitate Meta-Analysis

Demographic variables relevant to population studied
  Age
  Gender
  Marital status
  Ethnicity
  Education
  Socioeconomic status
Methodological characteristics
  Sample size (experimental and control groups)
  Type of sampling
  Research design
  Data collection techniques
  Outcome measurements
  Reliability and validity of instruments
Data analysis
  Name of statistical tests
  Sample size for each statistical test
  Degrees of freedom for each statistical test
  Exact value of each statistical test
  Exact p value for each test statistic
  One- or two-tailed statistical test
  Measures of central tendency (mean, median, and mode)
  Measures of dispersion (SD)
  Post hoc test values of $df > 1$ for F test

strength of the intervention, the magnitude of relationships among study variables, or the sensitivity and specificity of diagnostic tools and relative risk of an outcome in the treatment versus the control group.

7. The effect size for a relationship is the value of the r obtained through the Pearson Product-Moment Correlation analysis. For example, the relationship between anxiety and depression is r = 0.42 = effect size or strength of the relationship. This is a medium effect size and you can see the ranges for the difference effect sizes (small, medium, and large) in Chapter 14.

8. The effect size for an intervention in a study is calculated using the following formula: Mean of the treatment or intervention group minus the mean of the comparison group divided by the standard deviation of the comparison group. For example, a weight loss intervention resulted in a mean weight loss of 4 pounds (standard deviation [SD] = 5) for the treatment group and the comparison group had a mean weight loss of 1 pound (SD = 6).

> Calculation of the Effect Size = $4 - 1 \div 6$
> $= 3 \div 6 = 0.5$

Mahon, Yarcheski, Yarcheski, Cannella, and Hanks (2006) conducted a meta-analysis to determine the predictors for loneliness during adolescence. They clearly stated their study objective, which was "to identify predictors for loneliness in adolescents through a comprehensive review of the literature and to use quantitative meta-analysis to determine the magnitude of the relationships between each predictor and loneliness" (Mahon et al., 2006, p. 308). The investigators reviewed 242 studies that were published or unpublished between 1980 and 2004. Of the studies reviewed, 95 met the inclusion criteria, and the researchers isolated 11 predictors of loneliness. Mahon et al. (2006) identified the following results and conclusions:

> Four predictors (gender, depression, shyness, and self-esteem) had large effect sizes [ES > 0.5], four predictors (social support, social anxiety, maternal expressiveness, and paternal expressiveness) had large medium to medium effect sizes [ES = 0.3-0.5], two predictors (stress and self-disclosure) had low effect sizes [<0.3], and one predictor (age) had a very low effect size. . .
>
> Theories of loneliness served as a framework for interpreting the findings of the meta-analysis. The most powerful predictors can be used in intervention studies aimed at reducing loneliness in adolescents. (Mahon et al., 2006, p. 308)

This meta-analysis has a clearly stated objective or focus and includes a detailed description of the process used to search the literature. Mahon et al. (2006) also recognized five specific criteria that they used for including studies in the meta-analysis. The results identified the magnitude of the relationships among the variables, and the conclusions indicated the current status of the research evidence.

Conducting Integrative Reviews of Research

An integrative review of research includes the identification, analysis, and synthesis of research findings from independent quantitative and sometimes qualitative studies to determine the current knowledge (what is known and not known) in a particular area. An integrative review of research should be held to the same standards of clarity, rigor, and replication as primary research. Thus, an integrative review needs to include the following steps:

1. Formulate the purpose and scope of the integrative review.
2. Develop questions to be answered by the review or hypotheses to be tested.

3. Establish tentative criteria for inclusion and exclusion of studies in the review.
4. Conduct an extensive literature search including primarily research-based articles from a variety of authors.
5. Locate published and unpublished research sources.
6. Develop a questionnaire with which to gather data from the quantitative and qualitative studies.
7. Contact authors for additional data and information as needed.
8. Critically appraise the scientific merit of the studies.
9. Identify rules of inference to be used in data analyses and interpretation.
10. Analyze data from the studies in a systematic fashion.
11. Interpret data with the assistance of others.
12. Report the review as clearly and completely as possible (Dixon-Woods, Fitzpatrick, & Roberts, 2001; Ganong, 1987; Gates, 2002; Stetler et al., 1998).

In the past, most integrative reviews of research have included quantitative studies, but some major contributions can be made to the body of knowledge in a selected area by examining qualitative studies. Dixon-Woods et al. (2001) identified the following contributions to integrative reviews by qualitative studies:

• Identify and refine the question of the review
• Identify the relevant outcomes of interest
• Identify the relevant types of participants and interventions
• Augment the data to be included in a quantitative synthesis
• Provide data for a non-numerical synthesis of research
• Highlight inadequacies in the methods used in quantitative studies
• Explain the findings of a quantitative synthesis
• Assist in the interpretation of the significance and applicability of the review
• Assist in making recommendations to practitioners and planners about implementing the conclusions in the review (Dixon-Woods et al., 2001, p. 126)

It is essential that the integrative reviews of research be published. The *Annual Review of Nursing Research*, books, research journals, and clinical journals provide excellent sources for the publication of integrative reviews. The publication of the integrative review needs to include (1) the purpose and scope of the review, (2) a description of the literature search, (3) a discussion of the adequacy of the number of studies included in the review, (4) criteria used to evaluate the scientific quality of the studies, and (5) a clear presentation of the findings from the review (Gates, 2002; Stetler et al., 1998).

Gage, Everett, and Bullock (2006) conducted an integrative review of the qualitative research on parenting. They summarized their integrative review process in the following abstract.

Purpose: To synthesize and critically analyze parenting research in nursing.

Design: Qualitative, integrative review of nursing research studies about parenting 1993–2004.

Methods: Studies published by nurse researchers in peer-reviewed journals were systematically searched using CINAHL and Medline databases. Data were organized and analyzed with a sample of 17 nursing research studies from core nursing journals.

Findings: The majority of parenting research has been focused on mothers, primarily about parenting children with physical or developmental disabilities. Research about fathers as parents is sparse. Parenting across cultures, parenting in the context of family, and theoretical frameworks for parenting research are not well developed.

Conclusions: The scope of nursing research on parenting is limited. The roles, functions, and contexts of parenting are not well defined. Further research is required to describe parenting and how parenting affects the health of individuals and families. (Gage et al., 2006, p. 56)

Gage et al. (2006) conducted a strong integrative review of the qualitative research on parenting. They formulated a clear purpose for their review and detailed the methods they used to conduct the review. Their conclusions clearly show that the research evidence on parenting is inadequate to be useful in practice. Thus, Gage et al. (2006) provided direction for the future research that is needed in the area of parenting.

Conducting Metasummary and Metasynthesis of Qualitative Research

Qualitative research synthesis is the process and product of systematically reviewing and formally integrating the findings from qualitative studies (Sandelowski & Barroso, 2007). Qualitative research synthesis includes two categories: qualitative metasummary and qualitative metasynthesis. Recently two noted qualitative researchers, Sandelowski and Barroso (2007), published the *Handbook for Synthesizing Qualitative Research* to facilitate the synthesis of qualitative studies. They identified the following guidelines for conducting qualitative research synthesis:

(a) *systematic and comprehensive retrieval of all of the relevant reports of completed qualitative studies in a target domain of empirical inquiry;*

(b) *systematic use of qualitative and quantitative methods to analyze these reports;*

(c) *analytic and interpretive emphasis on the findings in these reports;*

(d) *systematic and appropriately eclectic use of qualitative methods to integrate the findings in these reports; and the*

(e) *use of reflexive accounting practices to optimize the validity of the study procedures and outcomes. (Sandelowski & Barroso, 2007, p. 22)*

Sandelowski and Barroso (2007) provided a detailed description of these steps and explained how to implement them.

MODELS TO PROMOTE EVIDENCE-BASED PRACTICE IN NURSING

EBP is a complex phenomenon that requires the integration of best research evidence with clinical expertise and patient values and needs in the delivery of quality, cost-effective care. Two models have been developed in nursing to promote EBP: the Stetler Model of Research Utilization to Facilitate EBP (Stetler, 2001) and the Iowa Model of Evidence-Based Practice to Promote Quality of Care (Titler et al., 2001). This section explores these two models.

Stetler Model of Research Utilization to Facilitate Evidence-Based Practice

An initial model for research utilization in nursing was developed by Stetler and Marram in 1976 and expanded and refined by Stetler in 1994 and 2001 to promote EBP for nursing. The Stetler (2001) model (Figure 27-1) provides a comprehensive framework to enhance the use of research evidence by nurses to facilitate an EBP. The research evidence can be used at the institutional or individual level. At the institutional level, study findings are synthesized and the knowledge generated is used to develop or refine policy, procedures, protocols, or other formal programs implemented in the institution. Individual nurses, such as practitioners, educators, and policy makers,

summarize research and use the knowledge to influence educational programs, make practice decisions, and have an impact on political decision making. Stetler's model is included in this text to encourage individual nurses and health care institutions to use research evidence to encourage the development of EBP. The following sections briefly describe the five phases of the Stetler model: (1) preparation, (2) validation, (3) comparative evaluation/decision making, (4) translation/application, and (5) evaluation.

Phase I: Preparation
The intent of Stetler's (1994, 2001) model is to make using research evidence in practice a conscious, critical thinking process that is initiated by the user. Thus, the first phase (preparation) involves determining the purpose, focus, and potential outcomes of making an evidence-based change in a clinical agency. The agency's priorities and other external and internal factors that could be influenced by or could influence the proposed practice change need to be examined. Once the purpose of the evidence-based project has been identified and approved by agency individuals or by committee, a detailed search of the literature is conducted to determine the strength of the evidence available for use in practice. The research literature might be reviewed to solve a difficult clinical, managerial, or educational problem; to provide the basis for a policy, standard, algorithm, or protocol; or to prepare for an in-service program or other type of professional presentation.

Phase II: Validation
In the validation phase, the research reports are critically appraised to determine their scientific soundness. If the studies are limited in number, are weak, or both, the findings and conclusions are considered inadequate for use in practice and the process stops. The quality of the research evidence is greatly strengthened if a systematic review, meta-analysis, or integrative review has been conducted in the area where you want to make an evidence-based change. If the research knowledge base is strong in the selected area, a decision must be made regarding the priority of using the evidence in practice by the clinical agency.

Phase III: Comparative Evaluation/Decision Making
Comparative evaluation includes four parts: (1) substantiation of the evidence, (2) fit of the evidence with the health care setting, (3) feasibility of using research findings, and (4) concerns with current practice. Substantiating evidence is produced by replication,

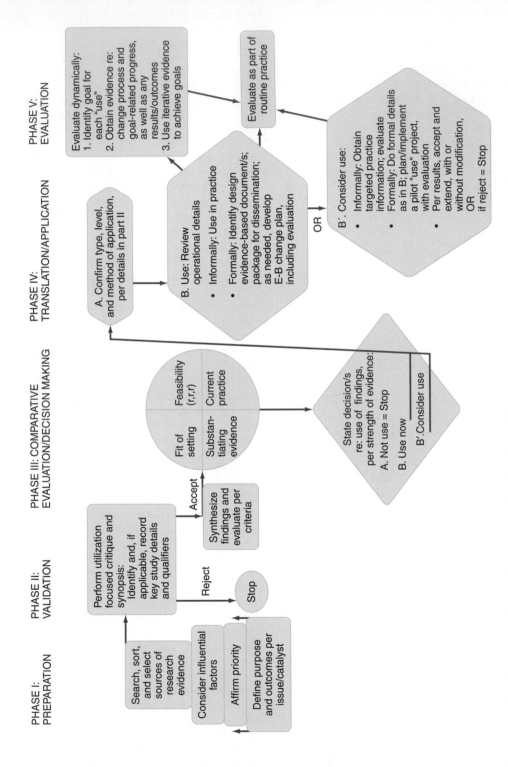

Figure **27-1** The Stetler model, part I: Steps of research utilization to facilitate EBP.

in which consistent, credible findings are obtained from several studies in similar practice settings. The studies generating the strongest research evidence are the RCTs and meta-analyses of RCTs and quasi-experimental studies, which provide extremely strong evidence for making a change in an agency. To determine the fit of the evidence in the clinical agency, the characteristics of the setting are examined to determine the forces that will facilitate or inhibit the evidence-based change such as a policy, protocol, or algorithm for nursing practice. Stetler (2001) believes the feasibility of using research evidence in practice involves examining the three *R*'s related to making changes in practice: (1) potential risks, (2) resources needed, and (3) readiness of those involved. The final comparison involves determining whether the research information provides credible, empirical evidence for making changes in the current practice. Thus, the research evidence needs to document that an intervention increased the quality in current practice by solving practice problems and improving patient outcomes. By conducting phase III, the overall benefits and risks of using the research evidence in a practice setting can be assessed. If the benefits (improved patient physical outcomes or increased patient satisfaction) are much greater than the risks (increased costs or increased nursing time) for the organization, the individual nurse, or both, using the research-based intervention in practice is feasible.

Three types of decisions (decision making) are possible during this phase: (1) to use the research evidence, (2) to consider using the evidence, and (3) to not use the research evidence. The decision to use research knowledge in practice is determined mainly by the strength of the evidence. Depending on the research knowledge to be used in practice, the individual practitioner, hospital unit, or agency might make this decision. Another decision might be to consider using the available research evidence in practice. When a change is complex and involves multiple disciplines, those involved often need additional time to determine how the evidence might be used and what measures will be taken to coordinate the involvement of different health professionals in the change. A final option might be to not use the research evidence in practice because the current evidence is not strong or the risks or costs of change in current practice are too high when compared to the benefits.

Phase IV: Translation/Application
The translation/application phase involves planning for and actually using the research evidence in practice. The translation phase involves determining exactly what knowledge will be used and how that

knowledge will be applied to practice. The use of the research evidence can be cognitive, instrumental, or symbolic. With cognitive application, the research base is a means of modifying a way of thinking or one's appreciation of an issue (Stetler, 1994, 2001). Thus, cognitive application may improve the nurse's understanding of a situation, allow analysis of practice dynamics, or improve problem-solving skills for clinical problems. Instrument application involves using research evidence to support the need for change in nursing interventions or practice protocols. Symbolic or political utilization occurs when information is used to support or change a current policy. The application phase includes the following steps for planned change: (1) assess the situation to be changed, (2) develop a plan for change, and (3) implement the plan. During the application phase, the protocols, policies, procedures, or algorithms developed with research knowledge are implemented in practice (Stetler, 1994, 2001). A pilot project on a single hospital unit might be conducted to implement the change in practice, and the results of this project could be evaluated to determine if the change should be extended throughout the health care agency.

Phase V: Evaluation
The final stage is to evaluate the impact of the research based change on the health care agency, personnel, and patients. The evaluation process can include both formal and informal activities that are conducted by administrators, nurse clinicians, and other health professionals. Informal evaluations might include self-monitoring or discussions with patients, families, peers, and other professionals. Formal evaluations can include case studies, audits, quality assurance, and outcomes research projects. The goal of Stetler's (2001) model is to increase the use of research evidence in nursing to facilitate EBP. This model provides detailed steps to encourage nurses to become change agents and make the necessary improvements in practice based on research evidence.

Iowa Model of Evidence-Based Practice
Nurses have been actively involved in conducting research, synthesizing research evidence, and developing evidence-based guidelines for practice. Thus, nurses have a strong commitment to EBP and can benefit from the direction provided by the Iowa model to expand their research-based practice. The Iowa Model of Evidence-Based Practice provides direction for the development of EBP in a clinical agency. Titler and colleagues initially developed this EBP model in 1994 and revised it in 2001. In a health care agency,

there are triggers that initiate the need for change, and the focus should always be to make changes based on best evidence. These triggers can be problem focused and evolve from risk management data, process improvement data, benchmarking data, financial data, and clinical problems. The triggers can also be knowledge focused, such as new research findings, changes in national agencies or organizational standards and guidelines, an expanded philosophy of care, or questions from the institutional standards committee. The triggers are evaluated and prioritized based on the needs of the clinical agency. If a trigger is considered an agency priority, a group is formed to search for the best evidence to manage the clinical concern (Titler et al., 2001).

In some situations, the research evidence is inadequate to make changes in practice, and additional studies are needed to strengthen the knowledge base. Sometimes the research evidence can be combined with other sources of knowledge (theories, scientific principles, expert opinion, and case reports) to provide fairly strong evidence for developing research-based protocols for practice (Figure 27-2). The strongest evidence is generated from meta-analyses of several controlled clinical trials and systematic reviews that usually include meta-analyses, integrative reviews, and individual studies. Thus, systematic reviews provide the best research evidence for developing evidence-based guidelines. The research-based protocols or evidence-based guidelines would be pilot-tested on a particular unit and then evaluated to determine the impact on patient care. If the outcomes are favorable from the pilot test, the change would be made in practice and monitored over time to determine its impact on the agency environment, staff, costs, and the patient and family (Titler et al., 2001). If an agency strongly supports the use of the Iowa model, implements patient care based on the best research evidence, and monitors changes in practice to ensure quality care, the agency is promoting EBP.

Application of the Iowa Model of Evidence-Based Practice

Preparing to use research evidence in practice raises some important questions. Which research findings are ready for use in clinical practice? What are the most effective strategies for implementing research-based protocols or evidence-based guidelines in a clinical agency? What are the outcomes from using the research evidence in practice? Do the risk management data, process improvement data, benchmarking data, or financial data support making the change in practice based on the research evidence?

Is the research-based change proposed an agency priority?

We suggest that effective strategies for using research evidence in practice will require a multifaceted approach that takes into consideration the evidence available, attitudes of the practicing nurses, the organization's philosophy, and national organizational standards and guidelines. In this section, the steps of the Iowa model (Titler et al., 2001) guide the use of a research-based intervention in a hospital to facilitate EBP. Research knowledge about the effects of heparin flush versus saline flush for irrigating peripheral intravenous (PIV) catheters is evaluated for use in nursing practice. This knowledge is used to develop a research-based protocol for making a change in practice, and outcome measures are identified for determining the effectiveness of this change in practice. Nurses making the switch from heparin flush to saline flush using a research-based protocol are providing evidence-based care (Craig & Smyth, 2007; Pearson et al., 2007; Sackett et al., 2000).

Assemble, Critically Appraise, and Synthesize Research for Use in Practice

The body of nursing research must be assembled and evaluated for scientific merit and clinical relevance, and then the current findings need to be synthesized for use in practice (Conn & Rantz, 2003; Craig & Smyth, 2007; Gates, 2002). All types of research projects—including quantitative, qualitative, outcomes, and intervention studies—need to be evaluated when developing a research knowledge base for use in practice (Doran, 2003; Munhall, 2001; Sidani & Braden, 1998).

Evaluation for Scientific Merit The scientific merit of nursing studies is determined by critically appraising the following aspects of a study: (1) the conceptualization and internal consistency, or the logical links of a study; (2) methodological rigor, or the strength of the design, sample, measurement methods, data collection process, and analysis techniques; (3) the generalizability of the findings, or the representativeness of the sample and setting; and (4) the number of replications (Craig & Smyth, 2007; Malloch & Porter-O'Grady, 2006; Pearson et al., 2007). The steps for critically appraising quantitative and qualitative studies to determine their scientific merit are presented in Chapter 26.

Evaluation of Clinical Relevance The research-based knowledge might be used to solve practice problems, enhance clinical judgment, or measure phenomena in clinical practice. The research knowledge might be used on a single patient care unit, a hospital,

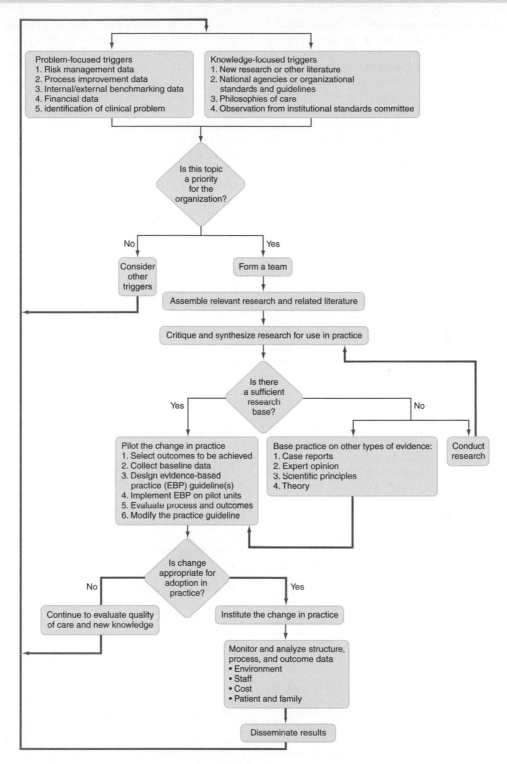

Figure 27-2 The Iowa Model of Evidence-Based Practice to Promote Quality Care.

or all hospitals in a corporation. A cost-benefit analysis can determine the impact of the proposed change on the clinical setting. A practitioner desiring to implement a research-based intervention must assure the agency that the cost in time, energy, and money and any real or potential risks are outweighed by the benefits of the intervention. Nurses lag behind other disciplines in examining the cost of using new research-based interventions in practice. Stone, Curran, and Bakken (2002) suggested five different ways to analyze the costs for using an intervention in practice.

Synthesis of Research Evidence The processes for synthesizing quantitative research evidence include systematic review, meta-analysis, and integrative review, which were described earlier in this chapter. As the researcher you must address this critical question: Is the evidence strong enough to support making a change in practice? For this evidence-based practice project, the objective is to determine the best research evidence available regarding the flushing of a PIV catheter for neonates, children, and adults. The literature was reviewed to determine which is the best flush solution, saline or heparinized saline, for maintaining patency, increasing duration, and decreasing the incidence of phlebitis in PIV catheters. The following section includes a discussion of the research evidence available.

Extensive research was conducted with adults in the 1980s and 1990s to determine if there are significant differences in patency, duration, and incidence of phlebitis for PIV catheters irrigated with saline versus heparin flush. Goode et al. (1991) conducted a meta-analysis "to estimate the effects of heparin flush and saline flush solutions on maintaining patency, preventing phlebitis, and increasing duration of peripheral heparin locks [peripheral venous catheters]" (p. 324). The meta-analysis was conducted on 17 quality studies that are described in Table 27-2. Seven (41%) of the studies were RCTs and 10 (59%) were quasi-experimental (nonrandom) studies, indicating the quality of the studies conducted. The total sample size of the 17 studies was 4,153, and the settings of these studies were a variety of adult medical-surgical and critical care units. The small effect size values (most are less than 0.20) for clotting, phlebitis, and duration indicate that saline flush is as effective as heparin flush in maintaining PIV catheters. Goode et al. (1991) summarized current knowledge on the use of saline versus heparin flushes.

It can be concluded that saline is as effective as heparin in maintaining patency, preventing phlebitis, and increasing duration in peripheral heparin locks. Quality of care can be enhanced by using saline as the flush solution, thereby eliminating problems associated with anticoagulant effects and drug incompatibilities. In addition, an estimated yearly savings of $109,100,000 to $218,200,000 U.S. health care dollars could be attained. (Goode et al., 1991, p. 324)

In 1994, the American Society of Hospital Pharmacists (ASHP) published a therapeutic position statement on the institutional use of 0.9% sodium chloride (saline) flush to maintain patency of PIV catheters versus heparin flush. This is an example of an opinion published by a national organization based on research evidence. This type of evidence provides a basis for making a change in practice, but it is a much weaker form of evidence than the meta-analysis or individual RCTs (see Figure 2-2 in Chapter 2).

Additional research continued to be conducted regarding the best flush solution for PIV catheters. In 1998, Randolph et al. published a systematic review and meta-analysis of RCTs to determine the effectiveness of saline versus heparinized saline as a flush for PIV venous and arterial catheters. These authors concluded that "flushing peripheral venous catheters locked between use with heparinized saline at 10 U/ml [units/milliliter] is no more beneficial than flushing with normal saline" (Randolph, Cook, Gonzales, & Andrew, 1998, p. 969).

Since the late 1990s, research has been conducted to determine the effectiveness of heparinized saline flush versus saline flush in PIV sites in neonates. Only a limited number of studies have been conducted, and the results have been mixed. The Cochran Database included a systematic review of the effect of heparin in prolonging PIV catheter use in neonates. Shah, Ng, and Sinha (2005) developed an abstract of the review, which is presented here.

■ *BACKGROUND*
Peripheral intravenous (PIV) catheters are widely used in modern medical practice. However, mechanical or infectious complications often necessitate their removal and/or replacement. Heparin has been shown to be effective in prolonging the patency of peripheral arterial catheters and central venous catheters, but may result in life threatening complications, especially in preterm neonates.

■ *OBJECTIVES*
The primary objective was to determine the effectiveness of heparin versus placebo or no treatment on duration of PIV catheter patency, defined as number of hours of catheter use. The secondary objectives were to assess the effects of heparin on catheter blockage, phlebitis, or thrombophlebitis, catheter related sepsis, and complications including abnormality of coagulation profile, allergic reactions to heparin, heparin induced thrombocytopenia, intraventricular/intracranial hemorrhage and mortality.

Search Strategy: A literature search was performed using the following databases: MEDLINE (1966–February 2005), EMBASE (1980–February 2005), CINAHL (1982–February 2005), Cochrane Central Register of Controlled Trials (CENTRAL, The Cochrane Library, Issue 1, 2005),

TABLE 27-2 ■ Studies Included in the Meta-Analysis

Study	N	Subjects	Assignment	Heparin Dose (U/cc)	Clotting Effect Size (d_c)	Phlebitis Effect Size (d_p)	Duration Effect Size (d_d)
Ashton et al. 1990	16 exp_c, 16 con_c, 13 exp_p, 14 con_p	Adult critical care	Random, double blind	10	0.3590	-0.1230	
Barrett & Lester, 1990	59 experimental, 50 control	Adult med-surg patients	Nonrandom double-blind crossover	10	-0.1068	-0.4718	
Craig & Anderson, 1991	129 exp. 145 con	Adult med-surg patients	Random double-blind crossover	10	0.0095	-0.0586	
Cyganski et al., 1987	225 exp. 196 con	Adult med-surg patients	Nonrandom	100	0.2510		
Donhan & Denning, 1987	8 exp_c, 4 con_c 7 exp_p, 5 con_p	Adult critical care	Random, double blind	10	0.0000	0.0548	
Dunn & Lenihan, 1987	61 experimental 51 control	Adult patients	Nonrandom	50	-0.2057	-0.2258	
Epperson, 1984	138 exp, 120 con 138 exp, 154 con	Adult med-surg patients	Random, double blind	10 100	-0.1773	-0.1176 -0.1232	
Garrelts et al., 1989	131 exp, 173 con	Adult med-surg patients	Random, double blind	10		0.1057	0.2753
Hamilton et al., 1988	137 exp, 170 con	Adult patients	Random, double blind	100	0.0850	-0.1819	
Holford et al., 1977	39 experimental 140 control	Young adult volunteers	Nonrandom, double blind	3.3, 10, 16.5, 100, 132	0.6545		-0.0604
Kasparek et al., 1988	49 exp. 50 con	Adult med patients	Random, double blind	10	0.3670	-0.5430	
Lombardi et al., 1988	34 experimental 40 control	Pediatric patients (4 wk to 18 yr)	Nonrandom, sequential, double blind	10		-0.2324	0.0000
Miracle et al., 1989	167 exp. 441 con	Adult med-surg patients	Nonrandom	100	-0.0042		
Shearer, 1987	87 exp, 73 con	Med-surg patients	Nonrandom	10	-0.1170	-0.0977	
Spann, 1988	15 experimental 19 control	Adult telemetry step-down	Nonrandom, double blind	10	-0.3163	-0.3252	
Taylor et al., 1989	369 exp, 356 con	Adult med-surg patients	Nonrandom, time series	10	0.0308	0.0288	-0.1472
Tuten & Gueldner, 1991	43 exp, 71 con	Adult med-surg patients	Nonrandom	100	0.0000	0.1662	

From Goode, C. J., Titler, M., Rakel, B., Ones, D. S., Kleiber, C., Small, S., et al. (1991). A meta-analysis of effects of heparin flush and saline flush: Quality and cost implications. *Nursing Research, 40*(6), 325. Used with permission of Lippincott-Raven Publishers, Philadelphia.

and abstracts from annual meetings of the Society for Pediatric Research, American Pediatric Society, and Pediatric Academic Societies published in Pediatric Research (1991–2004). No language restrictions were applied.

Selection Criteria: Randomized or quasi-randomized trials of heparin administered as flush or infusion versus placebo or no treatment were included. Studies, which included a neonatal population and reported on at least one of the outcomes, were included. . .

Main Results: Ten eligible studies were identified. Heparin was administered either as a flush solution, or as an additive to the total parenteral nutrition solution. Five studies reported data on the duration of use of the first catheter. Two of these studies found no statistically significant effect of heparin; two studies showed a statistically significant increase and one study showed a statistically significant decrease in the duration of PIV catheter use in heparin group. The results were not combined for meta-analysis due to significant heterogeneity of the treatment effect (p < 0.01). In addition, there were marked differences between the studies in terms of the methodological quality, the dose, the timing, the route of administration of heparin and the outcomes reported. From a limited number of studies, there were no significant differences between the heparin and the placebo/no treatment groups in the risks of infiltration, phlebitis, and intracranial hemorrhage.

■ AUTHORS' CONCLUSIONS

Implications for practice: The effect of heparin on the duration of peripheral intravenous catheter use varied across the studies. Because of clinical heterogeneity and heterogeneity in treatment effect, recommendations for heparin use in neonates with PIV catheters cannot be made. Implications for research: There are insufficient data concerning the effect of heparin for prolonging PIV catheter use in neonates. Further research on the effectiveness, the optimal dose, and safety of heparin is required. (Shah et al., 2005, Cochrane Database, online)

Sufficiency of the Research Base

The two meta-analyses of controlled clinical trials provide sound scientific evidence for making a change in practice from heparinized saline flush to saline flush for irrigating PIV catheters or heparin locks in adults (Goode et al., 1991; Randolph et al., 1998). Clinical relevance is evident in that the use of saline to flush PIV catheters promotes quality outcomes for the patient (patent heparin lock, fewer problems with anti-coagulant effects, and fewer drug incompatibilities), the nurse (decreased time to flush the catheter and no drug incompatibilities with saline), and the agency (extensive cost savings and quality patient care).

The research knowledge base is extremely strong for making the EBP change from heparin to saline flush to maintain the patency of PIV catheters in adults. This best research evidence continues to support the gold standard of using saline to flush PIV catheters in adults. However, there is need for additional research for the best flush (heparin or saline) to use for maintaining the patency of PIV catheters in neonates and children. The 2005 Cochrane systematic review clearly shows that the research evidence is inadequate to implement in practice regarding the appropriate flush to use with PIV catheters in neonates. The areas for additional research were identified (Shah et al., 2005). Thus, the evidence base for practice is adequate only for adults in the type of flush (saline) to use in irrigating PIV catheters (Goode et al., 1991; Randolph et al., 1998).

Pilot the Change in Practice

The relative advantages of using saline are the improved quality of care and cost savings, clearly documented in the research literature (Goode et al.,

---

TABLE 27-3 ▪▪ Annual Cost Savings from Changing to Saline

Study	Cost Savings	Hospital
Craig & Anderson, 1991	$40,000/year	525-bed tertiary care hospital
Dunn & Lenihan, 1987	$19,000/year	530-bed private hospital
Goode et al., 1991 (this study)	$38,000/year	879-bed tertiary care hospital
Kasparek et al., 1988	$19,000/year	350-bed private hospital
Lombardi et al., 1988	$20,000–$25,000/year	52-bed pediatric unit
Schustek, 1984	$20,000/year	391-bed private hospital
Taylor et al., 1989	$30,000–$40,000/year	216-bed private hospital

From Goode, C. J., Titler, M., Rakel, B., Ones, D. S., Kleiber, C., Small, S., et al. (1991). A meta-analysis of effects of heparin flush and saline flush: Quality and cost implications. *Nursing Research, 40*(6), 325. Used with permission of Lippincott-Raven Publishers, Philadelphia.

1991; Randolph et al., 1998). The cost savings for different sizes of hospitals is summarized in Table 27-3. The compatibility of the change can be determined by identifying the changes that will need to occur in your agency. What changes will the nurses have to make in irrigating PIV catheters with saline? What changes will have to occur in the pharmacy to provide the saline flush? Are the physicians aware of the research in this area? Are the physicians willing to order the use of saline to flush venous catheters?

The change in PIV catheter flush from heparin to saline has minimal complexity. The only thing changed is the flush, so no additional skills, expertise, or time is required by the nurse to make the change. Because saline flush, unlike heparin flush, is compatible with any drug that might be administered through the PIV catheter, the number of potential complications decreases. The change might be started on one unit as a clinical trial and then evaluated. Once the quality of care and cost savings are documented for nurses, physicians, and hospital administrators, the change will probably spread rapidly throughout the institution. Changing heparin flush to saline flush would be relatively simple to implement on a trial basis to demonstrate the positive outcomes for patients, nurses, and the health care agency.

The decision to use saline flush versus heparin flush as an irrigant requires institutional approval, physician approval, and approval of the nurses managing patients' PIV catheters. When a change requires institutional approval, decision making may be distributed through several levels of the organization. Thus, a decision at one level may lead to contact with another official who must approve the action. In keeping with the guidelines of planned change, institutional changes are more likely to be effective if all those affected by the change have a voice in the decision. In your institution, who needs to approve the change? What steps do you need to take to make sure that the change is approved within your institution? Do the physicians support the change? Do the nurses on the units support the change? Who are the leaders in the institution, and can you get them to support the change? Encourage the nurses to make a commitment and take a public stand to make the change, because their commitment increases the probability that the change will be made. Contact the appropriate administrative people and physicians and detail the pros and cons of making the change to saline flush for irrigating PIV catheters. You need to assure physicians and administrators that the change is based on extremely strong research evidence, provides extensive cost savings, and promotes quality patient care. Most physicians are positively influenced by research-based knowledge, and agencies will respond positively to cost savings and research.

Institute the Change in Practice

Implementing a research-based change can be simple or complex, depending on the change. The change might be implemented as indicated in the research literature or may be modified to meet the agency's needs. In some cases, a long time might be spent in planning implementation of the change after the decision is made. In other cases, implementation can begin immediately. Usually, a great deal of support is needed during initial implementation of a change. As with any new activity, unexpected events often occur. Contact with a person experienced in the change (a change agent) can facilitate the process.

The change from heparin flush to saline flush will involve physicians ordering saline for flushing PIV catheters. You will need to speak with the physicians to gain their support for the change. You might convince some key physicians to support the change, and they will convince others. The pharmacy will have to package saline for use as a flush. The nurses will also be provided with information about the change and the rationale for the change. It might be best to implement the change on one nursing unit and give the nurses on this unit an opportunity to design the protocol and plan for implementing the change. The nurses might develop a protocol similar to the one illustrated in Figure 27-3. The protocol must include referencing from the research literature to document that the intervention is evidence based. The evidence-based protocol directs you in preparing for irrigating a PIV catheter, actually irrigating the catheter, and documenting your actions (see Figure 27-3).

Monitor Outcomes

After an evidence-based change has been implemented in practice, nurses and other health professionals need to monitor appropriate outcomes to determine the effectiveness of the change. They need to document that the change has improved the quality of care, decreased the cost of care, saved nursing time, improved access to care, or any combination of these benefits. If the outcomes from the EBP change are positive, nurses, administrators, and physicians will often want to continue implementing the change. Nurses usually seek feedback from those around them. Their peers' reactions to the change in nursing practice will influence its continuation.

You can confirm the effectiveness of the saline flush for PIV catheter irrigation by examining patient care outcomes and cost-benefit ratios. Patient care outcomes

1. Review the medical order for irrigation of the peripheral venous catheter. Order should indicate that the catheter be irrigated with normal saline (0.9% sodium chloride) (Goode et al., 1991; Randolph et al., 1998).

2. Obtain the saline flush from the hospital pharmacy (ASHP, 1994).

3. Wash hands with chlorhexidine, collect equipment for irrigating peripheral venous catheter, and put on gloves.

4. Evaluate the peripheral venous catheter site every 8 hours for complications of phlebitis. The symptoms of phlebitis include the presence of erythema, tenderness, warmth, and a tender or palpable cord (Goode et al., 1991; Randolph et al., 1998).

5. Cleanse the peripheral venous catheter prior to irrigation.

6. Flush the peripheral venous catheter with 1 cc of normal saline every 8 hours if no other medication is being given through the site (Goode et al., 1991; Randolph et al., 1998). Check for loss of catheter patency by noting any resistance in irrigating with 1 cc of saline or by the inability to administer saline solution within 30 seconds (Shoaf & Oliver, 1992).

7. If a patient is receiving IV medication, administer 1 cc of saline, administer the medication, and follow with 1 cc of saline (Goode et al., 1991; Shoaf & Oliver, 1992).

8. Chart the date and time of peripheral venous catheter irrigation and the appearance and patency of the catheter site.

Figure **27-3** Protocol for irrigating peripheral venous catheters in adults.

can be examined by determining the number of clotting and phlebitis complications associated with PIV catheters 1 month before the EBP change and 1 month afterward. If no significant difference is observed, then this outcome supports the use of saline flush. The cost savings can be calculated for 1 month by determining the cost difference between heparin flush and saline flush. This cost difference is then multiplied by the number of saline flushes conducted in 1 month. This cost savings can then be multiplied by 12 months and compared with the cost savings summarized in Table 27-3. Nurses should be given the opportunity to evaluate the change and determine if it has saved nursing time and promoted quality care for managing their patients' PIV catheters. If positive patient and nurse outcomes and cost savings are demonstrated, the health care agency will support and extend the EBP of using saline flush for irrigating PIV catheters.

IMPLEMENTING EVIDENCE-BASED GUIDELINES IN PRACTICE

EBP of nursing and medicine has expanded extensively since the late 1990s. Research knowledge is generated every day that needs to be critically appraised and synthesized to determine the best evidence for use in practice (Craig & Smyth, 2007; Melnyk & Fineout-Overholt, 2005; Pearson et al., 2007). This section discusses the development of evidence-based practice guidelines and provides a model for using evidence-based guidelines in practice. The evidence-based guideline for the assessment, diagnosis, and management of hypertension is provided as an example (Chobanian et al., 2003). The chapter concludes with a discussion of the evidence-based practice centers and their potential to promote EBP in nursing and health care.

Development of Evidence-Based Guidelines

Once a significant health topic or condition has been selected, guidelines are developed to promote effective management of this health condition. Since the 1980s, the Agency for Healthcare Research and Quality (AHRQ) has had a major role in identifying health topics and developing evidence-based guidelines for these topics (www.ahrq.gov). In the late 1980s and early 1990s, a panel or team of experts was often charged with developing the AHRQ's guidelines. The AHRQ solicited the members of the panel, who usually included nationally recognized researchers in the topic area; expert clinicians, such as physicians, nurses, pharmacists, and social workers; health care administrators; policy developers; economists; government representatives; and consumers. The group designated the scope of the guidelines and conducted extensive reviews of the literature including relevant meta-analyses, integrative reviews of research, individual studies, and theories.

The best research evidence available was synthesized to develop recommendations for practice. Most of the evidence-based guidelines included meta-analyses, integrative reviews, and multiple individual studies. The guidelines were examined for their usefulness in clinical practice, their impact on health policy, and their cost-effectiveness (Stone et al., 2002). Often consultants, other researchers, and additional expert clinicians are asked to review the guidelines and provide input. Based on the experts' critique, the AHRQ revised and packaged the guidelines for distribution to health care professionals. Some of the first guidelines focuses on the following health care problems: (1) acute pain management in infants, children, and adolescents; (2) prediction and prevention of pressure ulcers in adults; (3) urinary incontinence in adults; (4) management of functional impairments with cataracts, (5) detection, diagnosis, and treatment of depression; (6) screening, diagnosis, management, and counseling about sickle cell disease; (7) management of cancer pain; (8) diagnosis and treatment of heart failure; (9) low back problems; and (10) otitis media diagnosis and management in children.

Currently, standardized guideline development ranges from a structured process like the one just discussed to a less structured process in which a guideline might be developed by a health care organization, health care plan, or professional organization. The AHRQ initiated the National Guideline Clearinghouse (NGC) in 1998 to store the evidence-based practice guidelines. Initially the NGC had 200 guidelines, but now the collection has expanded to more than 1500 clinical practice guidelines from numerous professional organizations, health care agencies, health care plans, and other groups in the United States and other countries. The NGC is a publicly available database of evidence-based clinical practice guidelines and related documents. It provides Internet users with free online access to guidelines at www.guideline.gov. The NGC is updated weekly with new content that the AHRQ produces in partnership with the American Medical Association (AMA) and the American Association of Health Plans (AAHP) (now the American's Health Insurance Plans). The key components of the NGC and its user-friendly resources can be found on the AHRQ website at www.guideline.gov/about/about. aspx. Some of the critical information on the NGC is provided here so you will know what is available and how to access the NGC resources:

- *Structured abstracts (summaries) about the guideline and its development.*
- *Links to full-text guidelines, where available, and/or ordering information for print copies.*
- *Palm-based PDA Downloads of the Complete NGC Summary for all guidelines represented in the database.*
- *A Guideline Comparison utility that gives users the ability to generate side-by-side comparisons for any combination of two or more guidelines.*
- *Unique guideline comparisons called Guideline Syntheses prepared by NGC staff, compare guidelines covering similar topics, highlighting areas of similarity and difference. NGC Guideline Syntheses often provide a comparison of guidelines developed in different countries, providing insight into commonalities and differences in international health practices.*
- *An electronic forum, NGC-L for exchanging information on clinical practice guidelines, their development, implementation, and use.*
- *An Annotated Bibliography database where users can search for citations for publications and resources about guidelines, including guideline development and methodology, structure, evaluation, and implementation*

Other features include the following:

- *What's New enables users to see what guidelines have been added each week and includes an index of all guidelines in NGC.*
- *NGC Update Service is a weekly electronic mailing of new and updated guidelines posted to the NGC Web site.*
- *Detailed Search enables users to create very specific search queries based on the various attributes found in the NGC Classification Scheme.*
- *NGC Browse permits users to scan for guidelines available on the NGC site by disease/ condition, treatment/intervention, or developing organization.*
- *PDA/Palm List provides users with information regarding the availability of full-text guidelines and/or companion documents available through the guideline developer, that can be downloaded for the handheld computer (Personal Digital Assistant [PDA], Palm, etc.).*
- *Glossary provides definitions of terms used in the standardized abstracts (summaries). (NGC, 2007a, www.guideline.gov/about/about.aspx)*

Criteria for submitting clinical practice guidelines and the application process are provided online. Listed here are the criteria that an evidence-based guideline must meet to be submitted to the NGC:

- *The guideline must contain systematically developed recommendations, strategies, or other information to assist health care decision-making in specific clinical circumstances.*
- *The guideline must have been produced under the auspices of a relevant professional organization (e.g., medical specialty society, government agency, health care organization, or health plan).*
- *The guideline development process must have included a verifiable, systematic literature search and review of existing evidence published in peer-reviewed journals.*
- *The guideline must be current and the most recent version (i.e., developed, reviewed, or revised within the last 5 years). (NGC, 2007a, www.guideline.gov/about/about.aspx)*

The NGC provides varied audiences with an easy-to-use mechanism for obtaining objective, detailed information on clinical practice guidelines. In addition, the NGC provides a list of the guidelines that are in the process of being developed (www.guideline.gov/browse/workqueue.aspx). The audiences that use the NGC are identified as follows:

- *Individual physicians and other clinicians can review and use the NGC in clinical decision-making and patient counseling.*
- *Health care organizations and integrated delivery systems can use information accessible through the NGC to adopt or adapt guidelines for their networks.*
- *Medical specialty and professional societies can use NGC resources in their own guideline development efforts.*
- *Employers and other large purchasers can use information from the NGC to assist them in making health care benefits purchasing decisions.*
- *Educational institutions can incorporate information accessible through the NGC into their curricula and continuing education activities.*
- *State and local governments can use the NGC in their quality assurance and program oversight efforts. (NGC, 2007b, www.ahrq.gov/clinic/ngcfact.htm)*

In addition to the evidence-based guidelines, the AHRQ has developed many tools to assess the quality of care that is provided by the evidence-based guidelines. You can search the AHRQ website (www.qualitytools.ahrq.gov) for an appropriate tool to measure a variable in a research project or to evaluate care in a clinical agency (AHRQ, 2007b).

There are also a variety of professional organizations, health care agencies, universities, and other groups that provide evidence-based guidelines for practice. Some of these websites are identified as follows:

- Academic Center for Evidence-Based Nursing: www.acestar.uthscsa.edu
- Association of Women's Health, Obstetric, and Neonatal Nurse: http://awhonn.org
- Centers for Health Evidence.net: www.cche.net
- CMA InfoBase: http://mdm.ca/cpgsnew/cpgs/index.asp
- Guidelines Advisory Committee: www.gacguidelines.ca
- Guidelines International Network: www.G-I-N.net
- Health Services/Technology Assessment Text (HSTAT): http://hstat.nlm.nih.gov
- HerbMed: Evidence-Based Herbal Database, 1998, Alternative Medicine Foundation: www.herbmed.org
- MD Consult: www.mdconsult.com
- National Association of Neonatal Nurses: www.nann.org
- National Institute for Clinical Excellence (NICE): www.nice.org.uk/catcg2.asp?c=20034
- Oncology Nursing Society: www.ons.org
- PIER—the Physicians' Information and Education Resource (authoritative, evidence-based guidance to improve clinical care; ACP-ASIM members only): http://pier.acponline.org/index.html
- Primary Care Clinical Practice Guidelines: www.medscape.com/pages/editorial/public/pguidelines/index-primarycare
- U.S. Preventive Services Task Force: www.ahrq.gov/clinic/uspstfab.htm

Implementing the JNC 7 Evidence-Based Guideline in Practice

Evidence-based guidelines have become the standards for providing care to patients in the United States and other nations. A few nurses have participated in committees that have developed these evidence-based guidelines, and many advanced practice nurses (nurse practitioners, clinical nurse specialists, nurse midwives, and nurse anesthetists) are using these guidelines in their practices. An evidence-based guideline for the assessment, diagnosis, and management of high blood pressure is provided as an example. This guideline was developed from the seventh report of the Joint National Committee on Prevention, Detection, Evaluation, and Treatment of High Blood Pressure (JNC 7) and was published in the *Journal of the American Medical Association* (Chobanian et al., 2003). The National Heart, Lung, and Blood Institute within the National Institutes of Health (NIH) of Department of Health and Human Services (DHHS) developed educational materials to communicate the specifics of this guideline to promote its use by health care providers. This guideline is presented in Figure 27-4 and provides clinicians with direction for the following: (1) classification of blood pressure as normal,

prehypertension, hypertension stage 1, and hypertension stage 2; (2) conduct of a diagnostic workup of hypertension; (3) assessment of the major cardiovascular disease risk factors; (4) assessment of the identification of causes of hypertension; and (5) treatment of hypertension. An algorithm provides direction for the selection of the most appropriate treatment method(s) for each patient diagnosed with hypertension (U.S. DHHS, NIH, National Heart, Lung, and Blood Institute, 2003).

Advanced practice nurses and registered nurses need to assess the usefulness and quality of each evidence-based guideline before they implement it in their practice. Figure 27-5 presents the Grove Model for Implementing Evidence-Based Guidelines in Practice. In this model, nurses identify a practice problem, search for the best research evidence to manage the problem in their practice, and note that an

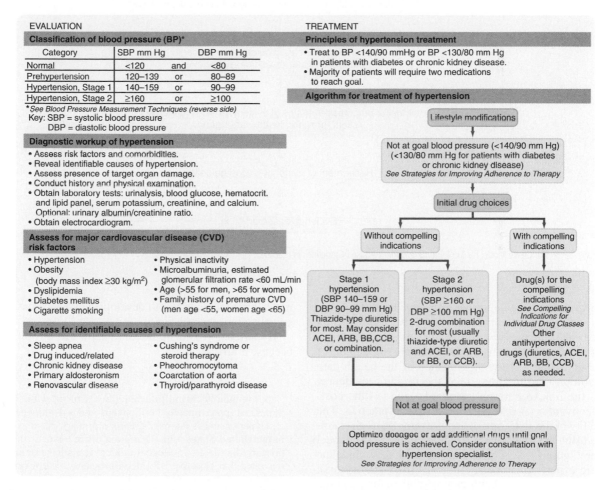

Figure 27-4 Reference card from the seventh report of the Joint National Committee on Prevention, Detection, Evaluation, and Treatment of High Blood Pressure [JNC 7].

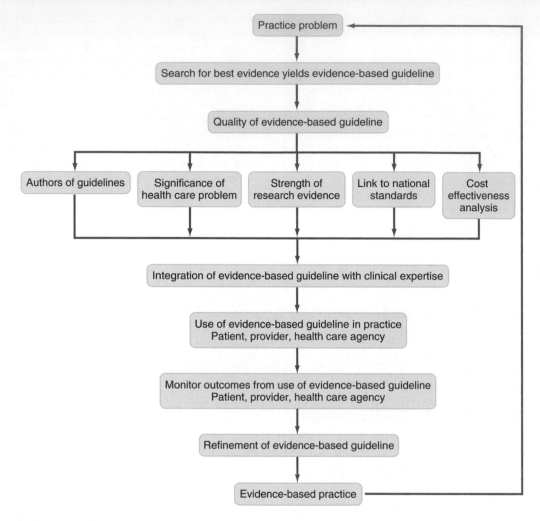

Figure **27-5** The Grove Model for Implementing Evidence-Based Guidelines in Practice.

evidence-based guideline has been developed. The quality and usefulness of the guideline must be assessed by the health care provider before it is used in practice, and that involves examining the following: (1) the authors of the guideline, (2) the significance of the health care problem, (3) the strength of the research evidence, (4) the link to national standards, and (5) the cost-effectiveness of using the guideline in practice. The quality of the JNC 7 guideline is examined as an example using the four criteria identified in the Grove model (see Figure 27-5). The authors of the JNC 7 guideline were expert researchers, clinicians (medical doctors), policy developers, health care administrators, and the National High Blood Pressure Education Program Coordinating Committee. These individuals and com-

mittee have the expertise to develop an evidence-based guideline for hypertension.

Hypertension is a significant health care problem because it affects

approximately 50 million individuals in the United States and approximately 1 billion individuals worldwide. ... Hypertension is the most common primary diagnosis in the United States with 35 million office visits as the primary diagnosis. ... Recent clinical trials have demonstrated that effective BP [blood pressure] control can be achieved in most patients with hypertension, but the majority will require 2 or more antihypertensive drugs. (Chobanian et al., 2003, p. 2562)

The research evidence for the development of the JNC 7 guideline was extremely strong. The JNC 7 report included 81 references; 9 (11%) of the references were meta-analyses and 35 (43%) were randomized controlled trials (experimental studies). Thus, 44 (54%) sources are considered extremely strong research evidence. The other references were strong and included retrospective analyses or case-controlled studies, prospective or cohort studies, cross-sectioned surveys or prevalence studies, and clinical intervention studies (nonrandom) (Chobanian et al., 2003). The JNC 7 provides the national standard for the assessment, diagnosis, and treatment of hypertension. The recommendations from the JNC 7 are supported by DHHS and disseminated through NIH publication no. 03–5231. Use of the JNC 7 guideline in practice is cost-effective because the clinical trials have shown that "antihypertensive therapy has been associated with 35% to 40% mean reductions in stroke incidence; 20% to 25% in myocardial infarction [MI]; and more than 50% in HF [heart failure]" (Chobanian et al., 2003, p. 2562).

The next step is for advanced practice nurses and physicians to use the JNC 7 guideline in their practice (see Figure 27-5). Health care providers can assess the adequacy of the guideline for their practice and modify the hypertension treatments based on the individual health needs and values of their patients. The outcomes for the patient, provider, and health care agency need to be examined. The outcomes would be recorded in the patients' charts and possibly in a database and would include the following: (1) blood pressure readings for patients; (2) incidence of diagnosis of hypertension based on the JNC 7 guidelines; (3) appropriateness of the treatments implemented to manage hypertension; and (4) the incidence of stroke, MI, and HF over 5, 10, 15, and 20 years. The health care agency outcomes include the access to care by patients with hypertension, patient satisfaction with care, and the cost related to diagnosis and treatment of hypertension and the complications of stroke, MI, and HF. This EBP guideline will be refined in the future based on clinical outcomes, outcome studies, and new controlled clinical trials. The use of this evidence-based guideline and additional guidelines promote an EBP for advanced practice nurses and physicians (see Figure 27-5).

Evidence-Based Practice Centers

In 1997, the AHRQ launched its initiative to promote evidence-based practice by establishing 12 evidence-based practice centers (EPCs) in the United States and Canada.

The EPCs develop evidence reports and technology assessments on " topics relevant to clinical, social science/behavioral, economic, and other health care organization and delivery issues—specifically those that are common, expensive, and/or significant for the Medicare and Medicaid populations. With this program, AHRQ became a "science partner" with private and public organizations in their efforts to improve the quality, effectiveness, and appropriateness of health care by synthesizing the evidence and facilitating the translation of evidence-based research findings. Topics are nominated by nonfederal partners such as professional societies, health plans, insurers, employers, and patient groups. (AHRQ, 2007a, www.ahrq.gov/clinic/epc)

Under the EPC Program, the AHRQ awards 5-year contracts to institutions to serve as EPCs. The EPCs review all relevant scientific literature on clinical, behavioral, organizational, and financial topics to produce evidence reports and technology assessments. These reports are used to inform and develop coverage decisions, quality measures, educational materials, and tools, guidelines, and research agendas. The EPCs also conduct research on methodology of systematic reviews. The AHRQ developed the following criteria as the basis for selecting a topic to be managed by an EPC:

- High incidence or prevalence in the general population and in special populations, including women, racial and ethnic minorities, pediatric and elderly populations, and those of low socioeconomic status.
- Significance for the needs of the Medicare, Medicaid, and other Federal health programs.
- High costs associated with a condition, procedure, treatment, or technology, whether due to the number of people needing care, high unit cost of care, or high indirect costs.
- Controversy or uncertainty about the effectiveness or relative effectiveness of available clinical strategies or technologies.
- Impact potential for informing and improving patient or provider decision making.
- Impact potential for reducing clinically significant variations in the prevention, diagnosis, treatment, or management of a disease or condition; in the use of a procedure or technology; or in the health outcomes achieved.
- Availability of scientific data to support the systematic review and analysis of the topic.
- Submission of the nominating organization's plan to incorporate the report into its managerial or policy decision making, as defined above.

• Submission of the nominating organization's plan to disseminate derivative products to its members and plan to measure members' use of these products, and the resultant impact of such use on clinical practice. (AHRQ, 2007a, www.ahrq.gov/clinic/epc)

The AHRQ website (www.ahrq.gov/clinic/epc) provides the names of the EPCs and the focus of each center. This site also provides a link to the evidence-based reports produced by these centers. These EPCs have had an important role in the development of evidence-based guidelines since the 1990s and will continue to make significant contributions to EBP in the future. They are also involved in the development of measurement tools to examine the outcomes from EBP. We hope that the content in this chapter increases your understanding of EBP, the synthesis of best research evidence, and the sources for evidence-based practice guidelines. We encourage you to take an active role in moving nursing toward an EBP that improve outcomes for patients, health care professionals, and health care agencies.

SUMMARY

• Evidence-based practice (EBP) is the conscientious integration of best research evidence with clinical expertise and patient values and needs in the delivery of quality, cost-effective health care. Best research evidence is produced by the conduct and synthesis of numerous, high-quality studies in a health-related area.
• The criticisms and benefits for EBP were described. The benefits of EBP are that the standards for hospital accreditation by the Joint Commission support EBP as does the Magnet Hospital Program managed by the American Nurses' Credentialing Center.
• Guidelines are provided for conducting the research syntheses processes of systematic review, meta-analysis, integrative review, metasummary, and metasynthesis. These synthesis processes are used to determine the best research evidence in a selected area and the quality of the research evidence available for practice.
• Two models have been developed to promote EBP in nursing: the Stetler Model of Research Utilization to Facilitate EBP (Stetler, 2001) and the Iowa Model of Evidence-Based Practice to Promote Quality of Care (Titler et al., 2001).
• The phases of the revised Stetler model are (1) preparation, (2) validation, (3) comparative evaluation/

decision making, (4) translation/application, and (5) evaluation.
• The Iowa model provides guidelines for implementing patient care based on the best research evidence and monitoring changes in practice to ensure quality care. The Iowa model is used to direct the implementation of an EBP protocol for using saline flush versus heparinized saline flush to irrigate intravenous catheters in adults.
• The process for developing evidence-based guidelines was described, and an example of the guideline for assessment, diagnosis, and treatment of hypertension was provided.
• The Grove Model for Implementing Evidence-Based Guidelines in Practice is provided to assist nurses in determining the quality of evidence-based guidelines and the steps for using these guidelines in practice.
• An excellent source for evidence-based guidelines is the National Guideline Clearinghouse that was initiated by the Agency for Healthcare Research and Quality (AHRQ) in 1998.
• Evidence-based practice centers (EPCs), created by the AHRQ in 1997, have had an important role in the conduct of research, development of systematic reviews, and formulation of evidence-based guidelines in selected practice areas.

REFERENCES

Agency for Healthcare Research and Quality (AHRQ). (2007a). *Evidence-based practice centers: Overview.* AHRQ Publication No. 03-P006. Rockville, MD. Retrieved November 25, 2007, from www.ahrq.gov/clinic/epc.
Agency for Healthcare Research and Quality (AHRQ). (2007b). *Research in action: AHRQ tools and resources for better health care.* AHRQ Publication No. 03–0008. Washington, DC: Author. Retrieved November 20, 2007, from www.qualitytools.ahrq.gov.
American Nurses Credentialing Center (ANCC). (2007). *Magnet recognition program.* Silver Springs, MD: Author. Retrieved November 25, 2007, from www.nursecredentialing. org/magnet/index. html.
American Society of Hospital Pharmacists. (1994). ASHP therapeutic position statement on the institutional use of 0.9% sodium chloride injection to maintain patency of peripheral indwelling intermittent infusion devices. *American Journal of Hospital Pharmacy, 51*(12), 1572–1574.
Ashton, J., Gibson, V., & Summers, S. (1990). Effects of heparin versus saline solution on intermittent infusion device irrigation. *Heart & Lung, 19*(6), 608–612.
Barrett, P. J., & Lester, R. L. (1990). Heparin versus saline flush solutions in a small community hospital. *Hospital Pharmacy, 25*(2), 115–118.

Beck, C. T. (1999). Focus on research methods: Facilitating the work of a meta-analyst. *Research in Nursing & Health*, *22*(6), 523–530.

Biswas, R., Umakanth, S., Strumberg, J., Martin, C. M., Hande, M., & Nagra, J. S. (2007). The process of evidence-based medicine and the search for meaning. *Journal of Evaluation in Clinical Practice*, *13*(4), 529–532.

Bolton, L. B., Donaldson, N. E., Rutledge, D. N., Bennett, C., & Brown, D. S. (2007). The impact of nursing interventions: Overview of effective interventions, outcomes, measures, and priorities for future research. *Medical Care Research & Review*, *64*(Suppl. 2), 123S–143S.

Chobanian, A. V., Bakris, G. L., Black, H. R., Cushman, W. C., Green, L. A., Izzo, J. L., et al. (2003). The seventh report of the Joint National Committee on Prevention, Detection, Evaluation, and Treatment of high blood pressure: The JNC 7 report. *Journal of the American Medical Association*, *289*(19), 2560–2572.

Conn, V. S., & Rantz, M. J. (2003). Research methods: Managing primary study quality in meta-analyses. *Research in Nursing & Health*, *26*(4), 322–333.

Craig, F. D., & Anderson, S. R. (1991). *A comparison of normal saline versus heparinized normal saline in the maintenance of intermittent infusion devices*. Unpublished manuscript.

Craig, J. V., & Smyth, R. L. (2007). *The evidence-based practice manual for nurses* (2nd ed.). Edinburgh: Churchill Livingstone.

Cyganski, J. M., Donahue, J. M., & Heaton, J. S. (1987). The case for the heparin flush. *American Journal of Nursing*, *86*(6), 796–797.

Dixon-Woods, M., Fitzpatrick, R., & Roberts, K. (2001). Including qualitative research in systematic reviews: Opportunities and problems. *Journal of Evaluation in Clinical Practice*, *7*(2), 125–133.

Donham, J., & Denning, V. (1987). Heparin vs. saline in maintaining patency in intermittent infusion devices: Pilot study. *Kansas Nurse*, *62*(11), 6–7.

Doran, D. M. (2003). *Nursing-sensitive outcomes: State of the science*. Boston: Jones & Bartlett.

Dunn, D. L., & Lenihan, S. F. (1987). The case for the saline flush. *American Journal of Nursing*, *87*(6), 798–799.

Epperson, E. L. (1984). Efficacy of 0.9% sodium chloride injection with and without heparin for maintaining indwelling intermittent injection sites. *Clinical Pharmacy*, *3*(6), 626–629.

Gage, J. D., Everett, K. D., & Bullock, L. (2006). Integrative review of parenting in nursing research. *Journal of Nursing Scholarship*, *38*(1), 56–62.

Ganong, L. H. (1987). Integrative reviews of nursing research. *Research in Nursing & Health*, *10*(1), 1–11.

Garrelts, J., LaRocca, J., Ast, D., Smith, D. F., & Sweet, D. E. (1989). Comparison of heparin and 0.9% sodium chloride injection in the maintenance of indwelling intermittent I. V. devices. *Clinical Pharmacy*, *8*(1), 34–39.

Gates, S. (2002). Review of methodology of quantitative reviews using meta-analysis in ecology. *Journal of Animal Ecology*, *71*(4), 547–557.

Goode, C. J., Titler, M., Rakel, B., Ones, D. S., Kleiber, C., Small, S., (1991). A meta-analysis of effects of heparin flush and saline flush: Quality and cost implications. *Nursing Research*, *40*(6), 324–330.

Hamilton, R. A., Plis, J. M., Clay, C., & Sylvan, L. (1988). Heparin sodium versus 0.9% sodium chloride injection for maintaining patency of indwelling intermittent infusion devices. *Clinical Pharmacy*, *7*(6), 439–443.

Holford, N. H., Vozeh, S., Coates, P., Porvell, J. R., Thiercelin, J. F., & Upton, R. (1977). More on heparin lock [letter]. *New England Journal of Medicine*, *296*(22), 1300–1301.

Institute of Medicine. (2001). *Crossing the quality chasm: A new health system for the 21st century*. Washington, DC: National Academy Press.

Kania-Lachance, D. M., Best, P. J., McDonah, M. R., & Ghosh, A. K. (2006). Evidence-based practice and the nurse practitioner. *The Nurse Practitioner*, *31*(10), 46–54.

Kasparek, A., Wenger, J., & Feldt, R. (1988). *Comparison of normal versus heparinized saline for flushing or intermittent intravenous infusion devices (pp. 1–18)*. Mercy Medical Center. Cedar Rapids, IA: Unpublished manuscript.

LaValley, M. (1997). Methods article: A consumer's guide to meta-analysis. *Arthritis Care and Research*, *10*(3), 208–213.

Lombardi, T. P., Gunderson, B., Zammett, L. O., Walters, J. K., & Morris, B. A. (1988). Efficacy of 0.9% sodium chloride injection with or without heparin sodium for maintaining patency of intravenous catheters in children. *Clinical Pharmacy*, *7*(11), 832–836.

Mahon, N. E., Yarcheski, A., Yarcheski, T. J., Cannella, B. L., & Hanks, M. M. (2006). A meta-analytic study of predictors for loneliness during adolescence. *Nursing Research*, *55*(5), 308–315.

Malloch, K., & Porter-O'Grady, T. (2006). *Introduction to evidence-based practice in nursing and health care*. Sudbury, MA: Jones & Bartlett.

McCaughan, D., Thompson, C., Cullum, N., Sheldon, T. A., & Thompson, D. R. (2002). Issues and innovations in nursing practice: Acute care nurses' perceptions of barriers to using research information in clinical decision-making. *Journal of Advanced Nursing*, *39*(1), 46–60.

Melnyk, B. M., & Fineout-Overholt, E. (2005). *Evidence-based practice in nursing & healthcare: A guide to best practice*. Philadelphia: Lippincott Williams & Wilkins

Miracle, V., Fangman, B., Kayrouz, P., Kederis, K., & Pursell, L. (1989). Normal saline vs. heparin lock flush solution; One institution's findings. *Kentucky Nurse*, *37*(4), 1, 6–7.

Munhall, P. L. (2001). *Nursing research: A qualitative perspective* (3rd ed.). Sudbury, MA: Jones & Bartlett.

National Guideline Clearinghouse (NGC). (2007a). *About the National Guideline Clearinghouse*. Washington, DC: Agency for Healthcare Research and Quality. Retrieved November 25, 2007, from www.guideline.gov/about/about.aspx.

National Guideline Clearinghouse (NGC). (2007b). *National Guideline Clearinghouse Fact Sheet*. Washington, DC: Agency for Healthcare Research and Quality. Retrieved November 25, 2007, from www.ahrq.gov/clinic/ngcfact.htm.

Nursing Executive Center. (2005). *Evidence-based nursing practice: Instilling rigor into clinical practice*. Washington, DC: The Advisory Board Company

Parahoo, K. (2000). Barriers to, and facilitators of, research utilization among nurses in Northern Ireland. *Journal of Advanced Nursing*, *31*(1), 89–98.

Pearson, A., Field, J., & Jordan, Z. (2007). *Evidence-based clinical practice in nursing and health care: Assimilating research, experience, and expertise.* Oxford: Blackwell.

Pettengill, M. M., Gillies, D. A., & Clark, C. C. (1994). Factors encouraging and discouraging the use of nursing research findings. *Image: Journal of Nursing Scholarship, 26*(2), 143–147.

Randolph, A. G., Cook, D. J., Gonzales, C. A., & Andrew, M. (1998). Benefits of heparin in peripheral venous and arterial catheters: Systematic review and meta-analysis of randomized controlled trials. *British Medical Journal, 316*(7136), 969–975.

Retsas, A. (2000). Barriers to using research evidence in nursing practice. *Journal of Advanced Nursing, 31*(3), 599–606.

Sackett, D. L., Straus, S. E., Richardson, W. S., Rosenberg, W., & Haynes, R. B. (2000). *Evidence-based medicine: How to practice & teach EBM* (2nd ed.). London: Churchill Livingstone.

Sandelowski, M., & Barroso, J. (2007). *Handbook for synthesizing qualitative research.* New York: Springer

Schmelzer, M. (2007). Research in practice column: Where is the theory in evidence-based practice. *Gastroenterology Nursing, 30*(6), 446–448.

Schustek, M. (1984). The cost effective approach to PRN device maintenance. *NITA, 7*(6), 527.

Shah, P. S., Ng, E., & Sinha, A. K. (2005). Heparin for prolonging peripheral intravenous catheter use in neonates. *Cochrane Database of Systematic Reviews,* (4), CD002774.

Shearer, J. (1987). Normal saline flush versus dilute heparin flush. *National Intravenous Therapy Association, 10*(6), 425–427.

Shoaf, J., & Oliver, S. (1992). Efficacy of normal saline injection with and without heparin for maintaining intermittent intravenous site. *Applied Nursing Research, 5*(1), 9–12.

Shojania, K. G., Sampson, M., Ansari, M. T., Ji, J., Doucette, S., & Moher, D. (2007). How quickly do systematic reviews go out of date? Survival analysis. *Annals of Internal Medicine, 147*(4), 224–234.

Sidani, S., & Braden, C. P. (1998). *Evaluating nursing interventions: A theory-driven approach.* Thousand Oaks, CA: Sage.

Spann, J. M. (1988). Efficacy of two flush solutions to maintain catheter patency in heparin locks. *Dissertation Abstracts, 28*(1), 1337125, 1–58. *Dissertation Abstracts International, 42*(4), 1394B (University Microfilms No. 8120152).

Stetler, C. B. (1994). Refinement of the Stetler/Marram model for application of research findings to practice. *Nursing Outlook, 42*(1), 15–25.

Stetler, C. B. (2001). Updating the Stetler Model of Research Utilization to facilitate evidence-based practice. *Nursing Outlook, 49*(6), 272–279.

Stetler, C. B., & Marram, G. (1976). Evaluating research findings for applicability in practice. *Nursing Outlook, 24*(9), 559–563.

Stetler, C. B., Morsi, D., Rucki, S., Broughton, S., Corrigan, B., Fitzgerald, J., (1998). Utilization-focused integrative reviews in a nursing service. *Applied Nursing Research, 11*(4), 195–206.

Stone, P. W., Curran, C. R., & Bakken, S. (2002). Economic evidence for evidence-based practice. *Journal of Nursing Scholarship, 34*(3), 277–282.

Taylor, N., Hutchison, E., Milliken, W., & Larson, E. (1989). Comparison of normal versus heparinized saline for flushing infusion devices. *Journal of Nursing Quality Assurance, 3*(4), 49–55.

Titler, M. G., Kleiber, C., Steelman, V. J., Rakel, B. A., Budreau, G., & Everett, L. Q. (1994). Research-based practice to promote the quality of care. *Nursing Research, 43*(5), 307–313.

Titler, M. G., Kleiber, C., Steelman, V. J., Rakel, B. A., Budreau, G., & Everett, L. Q. (2001). The Iowa Model of Evidence-Based Practice to promote quality care. *Critical Care Nursing Clinics of North America, 13*(4), 497–509.

Tuten, S. H., & Gueldner, S. H. (1991). Efficacy of sodium chloride versus dilute heparin for maintenance of peripheral intermittent intravenous devices. *Applied Nursing Research, 4*(2), 63–71.

U.S. Department of Health and Human Services, National Institutes of Health, National Heart, Lung, and Blood Institute. (2003). *Reference card from the seventh report of the Joint National Committee on Prevention, Detection, Evaluation, and Treatment of High Blood Pressure (JNC 7).* Bethesda, MD: NIH Publication No. 03–5231. Retrieved January 25, 2004, from www.nhlbi.nih.gov/guidelines/hypertension/jnc7card.htm.

Whittemore, R. (2005). Combining evidence in nursing research: Methods and implications. *Nursing Research, 54*(1), 56–62.

UNIT FOUR

Proposing and Seeking Funding for Research

CHAPTER **28**

Writing Research Proposals

With a background in the quantitative, qualitative, and outcomes research methodologies, you are ready to propose a study. A research proposal is a written plan that identifies the major elements of a study, such as the research problem, purpose, and framework, and outlines the methods and procedures to conduct the study. A proposal is a formal way to communicate ideas about a proposed study and to seek approval for conducting the study and funding. To seek approval for the conduct or funding of a study, the researcher submits a research proposal to a selected group for review and, in many situations, verbally defends that proposal. Receiving approval to conduct research has become more complicated because of the increasing complexity of nursing studies, the difficulty involved in recruiting subjects, and rising concerns over legal and ethical issues. In many large hospitals, both the lawyer and the institutional research review committee will evaluate the research proposals. The expanded number of health care studies being conducted has led to conflict among investigators over who has the right to recruit potential research subjects. This chapter focuses on writing a research proposal and seeking approval to conduct a study. Chapter 29 presents the process of seeking funding for research.

WRITING A RESEARCH PROPOSAL

A well-written proposal communicates a significant, carefully planned research project, demonstrates the qualifications of the researcher, and generates support for the project. Conducting research requires precision and rigorous attention to detail. Thus, reviewers often judge a researcher's ability to conduct a study by the quality of the proposal. A quality study proposal is clear, concise, and complete (Dexter, 2000; Tornquist, 1999). Writing a quality proposal involves (1) developing ideas logically, (2) determining the depth or detail of the proposal's content, (3) identifying critical points in the proposal, and (4) developing an aesthetically appealing copy.

Developing Ideas Logically

The ideas in a research proposal must logically build on each other to justify or defend a study, just as a lawyer would logically organize information in the defense of a client. The researcher builds a case to justify why a problem should be studied and proposes the appropriate methodology for conducting the study. Each step in the research proposal builds on the problem statement to give a clear picture of the study and its merit (Brink, 1993; Turabian, Booth, Colomb, & Williams, 2007). Universities, medical centers, federal funding agencies, and grant writing consultants have developed websites to help you and other researchers write successful proposals for quantitative, qualitative, and outcomes research; these sites include www.research.umich.edu/proposals/proposals.html,www.ninr.nih.gov/Training, and www.mayo.edu/research/crtp/resproposal.html. You can use a search engine of your choice, such as Google, and search for proposal guidelines, proposal writing tips, and courses on proposal development for different universities, medical centers, and government agencies. In addition, a variety of publications have been developed to help individuals improve their scientific writing skills (American Psychological Association [APA], 2001;

Dexter, 2000; Pyrczak & Bruce, 2005; Turabian et al., 2007; University of Chicago Press Staff, 2003).

Determining the Depth of a Proposal

The depth of a proposal is determined by guidelines developed by schools of nursing, funding agencies, and institutions where research is conducted. Guidelines provide specific directions for the development of a proposal and should be followed explicitly. Omission or misinterpretation of a guideline is frequently the basis for rejection. In addition to following the guidelines, you need to determine the amount of information necessary to describe each step of your study clearly. The content in a proposal needs to be detailed enough to inform the reader yet concise enough to be interesting and easily reviewed. Often, the guidelines stipulate a page limit, which will determine the depth of the proposal. The relevant content of a research proposal is discussed later in this chapter.

Identifying Critical Points

The key or critical points in a proposal must be evident, even to a hasty reader. You might highlight your critical points with bold or italicized type. Sometimes researchers create headings to emphasize critical content, or they may organize the content into tables or graphs. It is critical in a proposal to detail the background and significance of the research problem, your purpose, your methodology/research design or qualitative method, and your research production plans (data collection and analysis plan, personnel, schedule, and budget) (Tornquist, 1999; Turabian et al., 2007).

Developing an Aesthetically Appealing Copy

An aesthetically appealing copy is typed without spelling, punctuation, or grammatical errors. Even a proposal with excellent content that is poorly typed or formatted will probably not receive the full attention or respect of the reviewer (Dexter, 2000). The format used in typing the proposal should follow the guidelines developed by the reviewer. If no particular format is requested, researchers commonly follow the APA (2001) format. An appealing copy is legible (the print is dark enough to be read) and neatly organized in a folder so that the reviewer can examine it easily.

CONTENT OF A RESEARCH PROPOSAL

The content of a proposal is written with the interest and expertise of the reviewers in mind. Proposals are typically reviewed by faculty, clinical agency members, and representatives of funding institutions. The content of a proposal varies with the reviewer, the guidelines developed for the review, and the type of study (quantitative or qualitative) proposed. This section addresses the content of (1) a student proposal for both quantitative and qualitative studies, (2) condensed research proposals, and (3) preproposals.

Content of a Student Proposal

Student researchers develop proposals to communicate their research projects to the faculty and members of university and agency research review committees. Student proposals are written to satisfy requirements for a degree and are usually developed according to guidelines outlined by the faculty. The faculty member who will be assisting with the research project (the chair of the student's thesis or dissertation committee) generally reviews these guidelines with the student. Each faculty member has a unique way of interpreting and emphasizing aspects of the guidelines. In addition, a student needs to evaluate the faculty member's background regarding a research topic of interest and determine whether a productive working relationship can be developed. Faculty members who are actively involved in their own research have extensive knowledge and expertise that can be helpful to a novice researcher. Both the student and the faculty member benefit when a student becomes involved in an aspect of the faculty's research. This collaborative relationship can lead to the development of essential knowledge for providing evidenced-based nursing practice (Craig & Smyth, 2002; Melnyk & Fineout-Overholt, 2005).

The content of a student proposal usually requires greater detail than does a proposal developed for an agency or funding organization. The proposal is often the first three or four chapters of the student's thesis or dissertation, and the proposed study is discussed in the future tense—that is, what the student *will do* in conducting the research. A student research proposal usually includes a title page, with the title of the proposal, the name of the investigator, and the date, and a table of contents that precede the proposal content.

Content of a Quantitative Research Proposal

A quantitative research proposal usually includes the following chapters or sections: (1) introduction, (2) review of relevant literature, (3) framework, and (4) methods and procedures. Some graduate schools require an in-depth development of these sections, whereas others require a condensed version of the same content. Another approach is that proposals for theses and dissertations be written in a format that can be transformed into a publication. Table 28-1 outlines the content often covered in the chapters of a quantitative research proposal.

TABLE 28-1 ◾ Quantitative Research Proposal Guidelines for Students

Chapter I   Introduction
    A. Background and significance of the problem
    B. Statement of the problem
    C. Statement of the purpose
Chapter II   Review of Relevant Literature
    A. Review of relevant theoretical literature
    B. Review of relevant research
    C. Summary
Chapter III Framework
    A. Development of a framework (Develop a map of the study framework, define concepts in the map, describe relationships or propositions in the map, indicate the focus of the study, and link concepts to study variables)
    B. Formulation of objectives, questions, or hypotheses
    C. Definitions (conceptual and operational) of research variables
    D. Definition of relevant terms
    E. Identification of assumptions
Chapter IV   Methods and Procedures
    A. Description of the research design (Model of the design, strengths and weaknesses of the design, and description of treatment if appropriate)
    B. Identification of the population and sample (Sample size; use of power analysis; sampling criteria; and sampling method, including strengths and weaknesses)
    C. Selection of a setting (Strengths and weaknesses of the setting)
    D. Presentation of ethical considerations (Protection of subjects' right and university and health care agency review processes)
    E. Selection of measurement methods (Reliability, validity, scoring, and level of measurement of the instruments, as well as plans for examining reliability and validity of the instruments, in the present study; precision and accuracy of physiological instruments)
    F. Plan for data collection (Data collection process, training of data collectors if appropriate, schedule, data collection forms, and management of data)
    G. Plan for data analysis (Analysis of demographic data; analyses for research objectives, questions, or hypotheses; level of significance if appropriate; and other analysis techniques)
    H. Identification of limitations (Methodological and theoretical limitations)
    I. Discussion of communication of findings
    J. Presentation of a study budget and timetable
References
Appendixes

Introduction. The introductory chapter identifies the research topic and problem and discusses their significance and background. The significance of the problem addresses its importance in nursing practice and the expected generalizability of the findings. A problem's magnitude is partly determined by the interest of nurses, other health care professionals, policy makers, and health care consumers at the local, state, national, or international level. You can document this interest with sources from the literature. The background describes how the problem was identified and historically links the problem to the nursing practice. Your background information might also include one or two major studies conducted to resolve the problem, some key theoretical ideas related to the problem, and possible solutions to the problem. The background and significance will form the basis for your problem statement, which identifies what is not known and the need for further research. Follow your problem statement with a succinct statement of the research purpose or the goal of the study (Kerlinger & Lee, 2000; Peat, Mellis, Williams, & Xuan, 2002).

Review of Relevant Literature. The review of relevant literature provides an overview of the essential information that will guide you as you develop your study and includes relevant theoretical and empirical literature. The theoretical literature provides a background for defining and interrelating relevant study concepts, whereas the empirical literature includes a summary and critical appraisal of previous studies. Here you will discuss the recommendations made by other researchers, such as changing or expanding a study, in relation to the proposed study. The depth of the literature review varies; it might include only recent studies and theorists' works, or it might be extensive and include a description and critical appraisal of a number of past and current studies and an in-depth discussion of theorists' works. The literature review might be presented in a narrative format or in a pinch table that summarizes relevant studies (see Chapter 6) (Pinch, 1995). The literature review demonstrates that you have a command of the current empirical and theoretical knowledge regarding the proposed problem (Tornquist, 1999).

This chapter concludes with a summary. The summary includes a synthesis of the theoretical literature and findings from previous research that describe the current knowledge of a problem (Pinch, 1995). Gaps in the knowledge base are also identified, with a description of how the proposed study is expected to contribute to the nursing knowledge needed for evidence-based practice.

Framework. A framework provides the basis for generating and refining the research problem and purpose and linking them to the relevant theoretical knowledge in nursing or related fields. The framework includes concepts and relationships among concepts or propositions, which are sometimes represented in a model or a map. The concepts to be studied are conceptually defined and linked to the study variables. If you use another theorist's or researcher's model from a journal article or book, letters documenting permission to use this model from the publisher and the theorist or researcher must be included in your proposal appendices.

In some studies, research objectives, questions, or hypotheses are developed to direct the study. The objectives, questions, or hypotheses evolve from the research purpose and study framework, in particular the proposition(s), and identify the study variables. The variables are conceptually defined to show the link to the framework, and they are operationally defined to describe the procedures for manipulating or measuring the study variables. You also will need to define any relevant terms and to identify assumptions that provide a basis for your study.

Methods and Procedures. The researcher describes the design or general strategy for conducting the study, sometimes including a diagram of the design. Designs for descriptive and correlational studies are flexible and can be unique to the study being conducted. Because of this uniqueness, the descriptions need to include the design's strengths and weaknesses. Presenting a design for quasi-experimental and experimental studies involves (1) describing how the research situation will be structured, (2) detailing the treatment to be implemented, (3) explaining how the effect of the treatment will be measured, (4) specifying the variables to be controlled and the methods for controlling them, (5) identifying uncontrolled extraneous variables and determining their impact on the findings, (6) describing the methods for assigning subjects to the treatment and control groups, and (7) exploring the strengths and weaknesses of a design. The design needs to account for all the objectives, questions, or hypotheses identified in the proposal. If a pilot study is planned, the design should include the procedure for conducting the pilot and for incorporating the results into the proposed study.

Your proposal should identify the target population to which your study findings will be generalized and the accessible population from which the sample will be selected. Outline the criteria you will use to select a study participant or subject, and present the rationale for these criteria. For example, a participant might be selected according to the following criteria: female age 18 to 60 years, hospitalized, and 1 day post–abdominal surgery. The rationale for these criteria might be that the researcher wants to examine the effects of selected pain management interventions on adult females who have recently experienced hospitalization and abdominal surgery. The sampling method and the approximate sample size are discussed in terms of their adequacy and limitations in investigating the research purpose. Usually, a power analysis is conducted to determine an adequate sample size to identify significant relationships and differences in studies.

A proposal includes a description of the proposed study setting, which frequently includes the name of the agency and the structure of the units or sites where the study is to be conducted. The specific setting is often identified in the proposal but not in the final research report. The agency you select should have the potential to generate the type and size of sample required for the study. Thus, your proposal might include the number of individuals who meet the sample criteria and are cared for by the agency in a given period of time. In addition, the structure and activities in the agency need to be able to accommodate the proposed design of the study. If you are not affiliated with this agency, then it would be helpful if you had a letter of support for your study from the agency.

Ethical considerations in a proposal include the rights of the subjects and the rights of the agency where the study is to be conducted. Describe how you plan to protect subjects' rights as well as the risks and potential benefits of your study. Also address the steps you will take to reduce any risks that the study might present. Many agencies require a written consent form, and that form is often included in the appendices of the proposal. With the implementation of the Health Insurance Portability and Accountability Act (HIPAA), health care agencies and providers must have a signed authorization form from patients to release their health information for research (U.S. Department of Health and Human Services [DHHS], 2004) (see Chapter 9 for details). You must also address the risks and potential benefits of the study for the institution (Fullwood, Granger, Bride, & Taylor, 1999). If your study places the agency at risk, outline the steps you will take to reduce or eliminate these risks. It is also necessary for you to state that the proposal will be reviewed by the thesis or dissertation committee, university human rights review committee, and agency research review committee.

Describe the methods you will use to measure study variables, including each instrument's reliability, validity, methods of scoring, and level of measurement. A plan for examining the reliability and validity of the instruments in the present study needs to be addressed. If an instrument has no reported reliability and validity, you may need to conduct a pilot study to examine these qualities. If the intent of the proposed study is to develop an instrument, describe the process of instrument development. If physiological instruments are used, address the instrument's accuracy, precision, sensitivity, selectivity, and error rate. A copy of the interview questions, questionnaires, scales, physiological instruments, or other tools to be used in the study is usually included in the proposal appendices. You must obtain permission from the authors to use copyrighted instruments, and letters documenting that permission has been obtained must be included in the proposal appendices.

The data collection plan clarifies what data are to be collected and the process for collecting the data. In this plan you will identify the data collectors, describe the data collection procedures, and present a schedule for data collection activities. If more than one person will be involved in data collection, it is important to describe methods used to train your data collectors to ensure consistency. The method of recording data is often described, and sample data recording sheets are placed in the proposal appendices. Also discuss any special equipment you will use or develop to collect data for the study, and address data security, including the methods of data storage.

The plan for data analysis identifies the analysis techniques that the researcher will use to summarize the demographic data and answer the research objectives, questions, or hypotheses. The analysis section is best organized by the study objectives, questions, or hypotheses. The analysis techniques identified need to be appropriate for the type of data collected. For example, if an associative hypothesis is developed, correlational analysis is planned. If a researcher plans to determine differences among groups, the analysis techniques might include a t-test or analysis of variance (ANOVA) (Corty, 2007; Kerlinger & Lee, 2000). A level of significance ($\alpha = 0.05, 0.01,$ or 0.001) is also identified. Often, a researcher projects the type of results that will be generated from data analysis. Dummy tables, graphs, and charts can then be developed to present these results and are included in the proposal appendices. The investigator might also project the possible findings for a study. For example, the researcher might consider what support or nonsupport of a proposed hypothesis would mean in light of the study framework and previous research findings. Projecting a study's findings encourages others to logically examine the findings when the study is complete.

The methods and procedures chapter of a proposal usually concludes with a discussion of the study's limitations and a plan for communication of the findings. Both methodological and theoretical limitations are addressed. Methodological limitations might include areas of weakness in the design, sampling method, sample size, measurement tools, data collection procedures, or data analysis techniques, whereas theoretical limitations set boundaries for the generalization of study findings. For example, the accuracy with which the conceptual definitions and relational statements in a theory reflect reality has a direct impact on the generalization of study findings. Theory that has withstood frequent testing through research provides a stronger framework for the interpretation and generalization of findings. A plan is included for communicating the research through presentations and publications to audiences of nurses, other health professionals, policy makers, and health care consumers.

Frequently, a budget and timetable are included in the proposal appendices. The budget projects the expenses for the study, which might include the cost for data collection tools and procedures; special equipment; consultants for data analysis; computer time; travel related to data collection and analysis; typing; copying; and developing, presenting, and publishing the final report. Study budgets requesting external funding for researchers' time include investigators' salaries and secretarial costs. You will need a timetable to direct the steps of your research project and increase the chance that you will complete the project on schedule. A timetable identifies the tasks to be done, who will accomplish these tasks, and when these tasks will be completed. An example proposal for a quantitative study is presented at the end of this chapter.

Content of a Qualitative Research Proposal

A qualitative research proposal might include content similar to that of a quantitative proposal, but the guidelines are unique for the development of knowledge and theories using a variety of qualitative research methods. A qualitative proposal usually includes chapters with the following foci: (1) introduction, (2) research paradigm and general method, (3) applied method of inquiry, and (4) current knowledge, limitations, and plans for communication of the study findings (Boyd & Munhall, 2001; Marshall & Rossman, 2006; Patton, 2002; Sandelowski, Davis, & Harris, 1989). We propose the guidelines in Table 28-2 to assist you in developing a qualitative research proposal.

TABLE 28-2	Qualitative Research Proposal Guidelines for Students
Chapter I	Introduction
	A. Identify the phenomenon to be studied
	B. Identify the study aim or purpose
	C. State the study questions
	D. Describe the evolution of the study
	1. Provide a rationale for conducting the study
	2. Place the study in context historically
	3. Discuss the researcher's experience with phenomenon
	4. Discuss the relevance of the study to nursing
Chapter II	Research Paradigm or General Method for Proposed Study
	A. Identify the type of qualitative research (phenomenological, grounded theory, ethnographic, historical, philosophical inquiry, or critical social theory) to be conducted
	B. Describe the philosophical basis for the research method
	C. Explain the research assumptions
	D. Discuss the general steps, procedures, and outcomes for this method
	E. Translation of concepts or terms
Chapter III	Method of Inquiry: Applied
	A. Demonstrate the researcher's credentials for conducting this qualitative study
	B. Select a site and population
	C. Describe the plan for the researcher's role in the following:
	1. Entry into the site and approval to collect data
	2. Selection of study participants
	3. Ethical considerations
	D. Describe the plan for data collection:
	1. Data to be collected
	2. Procedures for data collection
	3. Procedures for recording data during data collection
	E. Describe the plan for data analysis:
	1. Steps for coding information
	2. Use of specific data analysis procedures advanced in the specific research method (phenomenology, grounded theory, ethnography, historical, philosophical inquiry, or critical social theory)
	3. Steps to be taken to verify the information
Chapter IV	Current Knowledge, Limitations, and Plans for Communication of the Study
	A. Summarize and reference relevant literature as appropriate for the type of qualitative study
	B. Disclose anticipated findings, hypotheses, and hunches
	C. Discuss procedures to remain open to unexpected information
	D. Discuss limitations of the study
	E. Identify plans for communication of findings (Boyd & Munhall, 2001; Marshall & Rossman, 2006; Munhall, 2001; Patton, 2002)
References	Include references cited in the proposal and follow APA (2001) format
Appendixes	Present the study budget and timetable

Introduction. The introduction usually provides a general background for the proposed study by identifying the phenomenon to be investigated and linking this phenomenon to nursing knowledge. The general aim or purpose of the study is identified and indicates the type of qualitative study to be conducted. The study aim is often followed by research questions that direct the investigation (Boyd & Munhall, 2001; Parse, Coyne, & Smith, 1985). For example, an aim for a qualitative study might be to "describe the lived experience of coping with the chronic illness of type 1 diabetes." The research questions would focus on real-world problems and dilemmas, such as the following: How do people cope with a new diagnosis of type 1 diabetes? What is it like to live with the chronic illness of diabetes for 1 year, 2 years, 5 years, and 10 years? What type of support exists for a person with type 1 diabetes? What does it mean to have your diabetes under control? What is the impact of the chronic illness diabetes on the individual and family?

The introduction also includes the evolution of the study and its significance to nursing practice, patients, the health care system, and health policy. The discussion of the evolution of the study often includes how the problem developed (historical context), who or what is affected by the problem, and the researcher's experience with the problem (experiential context) (Boyd & Munhall, 2001). Whenever possible, the significance and evolution of the study aim needs to be documented from the literature. Marshall and Rossman (2006) identified the following questions to assess the significance of a study: (1) Who has an interest in this domain of inquiry? (2) What do we already know about the topic? (3) What has not been answered adequately in previous research and practice? and (4) How will this research add to knowledge, practice, and policy in this area? The introduction section concludes with an overview of the remaining sections that are covered in the proposal.

Research Paradigm and General Methods for the Proposed Study. This section introduces you to the conceptual foundation for the qualitative research method (phenomenological, ethnographic, grounded theory, historical, philosophical inquiry, or critical social theory) selected for the proposed study. The researcher provides a rationale for the qualitative method selected and discusses its ability to generate the knowledge needed in nursing. Qualitative research methods are supported by different paradigms, such as naturalistic, postpositivism, feminism, and postmodernism (Miller, 1997). The investigator introduces the research paradigm and provides the essential elements of philosophy and assumptions of the specific type of qualitative study to be conducted. The philosophy varies for the different types of qualitative research and guides the conduct of the study. For example, a proposal for a phenomenological study might identify the study aim, "to describe the experience of women recovering from substance abuse," discuss the naturalistic paradigm as a basis of understanding for the study, and describe the works of Giorgi (1985) and Frankl (1984) as the philosophical basis for conducting the study (Wright, 2003). Assumptions about the nature of the knowledge and the reality that underlie the type of qualitative research to be conducted are also identified. The assumptions and philosophy provide a theoretical perspective for the study that influences the focus of the study, data collection and analysis, and articulation of the findings.

Method of Inquiry: Applied. Developing and implementing the methodology of qualitative research require a certain expertise that some believe can only be obtained through a mentorship relationship with an experienced qualitative researcher. The role of the researcher and the intricate techniques of data collection and analysis are thought to be best communicated through a one-to-one relationship. Thus, planning the methods of a qualitative study requires knowledge of relevant sources that describe the different qualitative research techniques and procedures (Boyd & Munhall, 2001; Chenitz & Swanson, 1986; Leininger, 1985; Marshall & Rossman, 2006; Miles & Huberman, 1994; Munhall, 2001; Parse et al., 1985; Patton, 2002), in addition to requiring interaction with a qualitative researcher. The proposal needs to reflect the researcher's credentials for conducting the particular type of qualitative study proposed.

Identifying the methods for conducting a qualitative study is a difficult task because the design of the study is still emerging. Unlike quantitative research, in which the design is a fixed blueprint for a study, the design in qualitative research emerges or evolves as the study is conducted. Thus, you must document the logic and appropriateness of the qualitative method and develop a tentative plan for conducting your study. Because this plan is tentative, reserve the right to modify or change the plan as needed during the conduct of the study (Sandelowski et al., 1989). However, the design or plan must be consistent with the study aim and research questions, be well conceived, and address prior criticism, as appropriate (Cohen, Knafl, & Dzurec, 1993). The tentative plan describes the process for selecting a site and population. The site will allow you entry and will include the participants necessary to answer the research aim and questions. For the research question "How do individuals cope with a new diagnosis of type 1 diabetes?" the participants might be identified in hospitals, clinics, practitioners' offices, home care organizations, or rehabilitation facilities, and data collection might be conducted in the participants' homes.

The researcher must gain entry into the setting, develop a rapport with the participants that will facilitate the detailed data collection process, and protect the rights of these participants (Marshall & Rossman, 2006; Sandelowski et al., 1989; U.S. DHHS, 2004). Address the following questions in describing the researcher's role: (1) What is the best setting for the study? (2) How will I ease my entry into the research site? (3) How will I gain access to the participants? (4) What actions will I take to encourage the participants to cooperate? (5) What precautions will I take to protect the rights of the participants and to prevent the setting and the participants from being harmed? You need to describe the process you followed to obtain informed consent and the actions you will use to decrease study risks. The sensitive nature of some qualitative studies increases the risk for participants, which makes ethical concerns and decisions a major focus of the study (Munhall, 2001; Patton, 2002).

The primary data collection techniques used in qualitative research are observation and in-depth interviewing. Observations can range from highly detailed, structured notations of behavior to ambiguous descriptions of behavior or events. The interview can also range from structured, closed-ended questions to unstructured, open-ended questions (Marshall & Rossman, 2006; Munhall, 2001). Address the following questions when describing the proposed data collection process: (1) Who will collect data and provide any training required for the data collectors? (2) What data will be collected? For example, will the data be field notes from memory, audiotapes of interviews, transcripts of conversations, videotapes of events, or examination of existing documents? (3) What techniques or procedures will my research team use to collect the data? For example, if interviews are to be conducted, will I include a list of the proposed questions in the appendix? In historical research, data are collected through an exhaustive review of published and unpublished literature. (4) Where are the identified sources of data located? (5) How much time will I need to collect data? (6) How will my data be recorded and stored?

The methods section also needs to address how you will document the research process. For example, you might keep progress notes during the course of the study. These notes can document the day-to-day activities, methodological events, decision-making procedures, and personal notes about the informants. This information becomes part of the audit trail that you can provide to ensure the quality of the study (Miles & Huberman, 1994; Munhall, 2001; Patton, 2002).

The methods section of the proposal also includes the analysis techniques and the steps for conducting these techniques. In qualitative research, data collection and analysis often occur simultaneously. The data are in the form of notes, tapes, and other material obtained from observation, interviews, and completing questionnaires. Through qualitative analysis techniques, these data are structured and reduced to determine meaning (Miles & Huberman, 1994; Patton, 2002). Determine what strategies you will apply to ensure the credibility, fittingness, and auditability of the findings (Beck, 1993). These qualitative terms relate to the concepts of reliability and validity used in quantitative research and are addressed in Chapters 23 and 26.

Current Knowledge Base, Limitations, and Plans for Communication of the Study. This section of the proposal summarizes and documents all relevant literature that was reviewed for the study. In some

qualitative studies, the researcher reviews the literature before conducting the study. For example, ethnographic research requires a literature review to provide a background for conducting the study, as in quantitative research. Historical research involves a literature review to develop research questions, as does philosophical inquiry to generate philosophical questions. The literature review needs to provide a basis for the aims of the study and clarify how this study will expand nursing knowledge (Boyd & Munhall, 2001; Marshall & Rossman, 2006).

In phenomenological research, grounded theory research, and critical social theory, the literature review is usually conducted toward the end of the research project. The findings from a phenomenological study are compared and combined with findings from the literature to determine current knowledge of the phenomenon. In grounded theory research, the literature is used to explain, support, and extend the theory generated in the study. Study findings obtained through critical social theory are examined in light of the existing literature to determine the current knowledge of a social situation (see Chapter 4).

As the researcher, you will need to describe how the literature reviewed has influenced your proposed research methods. Biases and previous experience with the research problem need to be addressed, as does their potential impact on the proposed study. Often, anticipated findings, hypotheses, and hunches are identified before the study is conducted, followed by a discussion of the procedures that might be used to remain open to new information. You will also need to address the limitations of the study in the context of limitations of similar studies.

Conclude your proposal by describing how you plan to communicate your findings to a variety of audiences through presentations and publications. Often, a realistic budget and timetable are provided in the appendix. A qualitative study budget is similar to a quantitative study budget and includes costs for data collection tools and procedures; consultants for data analysis; travel related to data collection and analysis; typing and copying related to data collection and analysis; and developing, presenting, and publishing the final report. However, the greatest expenditure in qualitative research is usually the researcher's time. Develop a timetable to project how long the study will take; often 2 years or more is designated for data collection and analysis (Marshall & Rossman, 2006; Munhall, 2001; Patton, 2002). You can use your budget and timetable to make decisions regarding funding inasmuch as funding is essential for many qualitative studies.

Some excellent websites have been developed to assist novice researchers in identifying an idea for qualitative study and developing a qualitative research proposal and reports (for example, see www.nova.edu/ssss/QR/qualres.html). The Office of Behavior and Social Sciences Research within the National Institutes of Health (NIH) has developed a website to assist researchers in developing qualitative and quantitative research proposals for funding (see http://grants.nih.gov/grants/writing_application.htm). You can use these websites and other publications to promote the quality of your qualitative research proposal. The quality of a proposal is based on the potential scientific contribution of the research to nursing knowledge; the research paradigm guiding the study; the research methods; and the knowledge, skills, and resources available to the investigators (Cohen et al., 1993; Marshall & Rossman, 2006; Munhall, 2001; Patton, 2002).

Content of a Condensed Proposal

The content of proposals developed for review by clinical agencies and funding institutions is usually a condensed version of the student proposal. However, even though these proposals are condensed, the logical links between components of the study need to be clearly demonstrated. A condensed proposal often includes a statement of the problem and purpose; previous research that has been conducted in the area (usually limited to no more than three to five studies); the framework, variables, design, sample, ethical considerations, and plans for data collection and analysis; and plans for dissemination of findings.

A proposal submitted to a clinical agency needs to identify the specific setting clearly, such as the emergency department or intensive care unit, as well as the projected time span for the study. Members of clinical agencies are particularly interested in the data collection process and involvement of institutional personnel in the study. The researcher will need to identify any expected disruptions in institutional functioning, with plans for preventing these disruptions when possible. The researcher must recognize that anything that slows down or disrupts employee functioning costs the agency money and can interfere with the quality of patient care. By showing that you are aware of these concerns and have proposed ways to minimize their effects, you increase the probability of obtaining approval to conduct your study.

Various companies, corporations, and organizations provide funding for research projects. A proposal developed for these types of funding institutions frequently includes a brief description of the study, the significance of the study to the institution, a timetable, and a budget. Most of these proposals are brief and might contain a one-page summary sheet or abstract at the beginning of the proposal that summarizes the steps of the study. The salient points of the study are included on this page in simple, easy-to-read, nontechnical terminology. Some proposal reviewers for funding institutions are laypersons with no background in research or nursing. An inability to understand the terminology might put the reviewer on the defensive or create a negative reaction, which could lead to disapproval of the study. When a funding institution is examining multiple studies, the summary sheet is often the basis for final decisions. The summary should be concise, informative, and designed to sell the study.

In proposals for both clinical and funding agencies, investigators need to document their research background and supply curriculum vitae if requested. The research review committee for approval of funding will be interested in previous research, research publications, and clinical expertise, especially if a clinical study is proposed. If you are a graduate student, the committee may request the names of the university committee members and verification that your proposal has been approved by the student's thesis or dissertation committee and the university human subjects review committee.

Content of a Preproposal

Sometimes a researcher will send a preproposal or query letter rather than a proposal to a funding institution. A preproposal is a short document of four to five pages plus appendices that explores the funding possibilities for a research project. The parts of the preproposal are logically ordered as follows: "(1) letter of transmittal, (2) proposal for research, (3) personnel, (4) facilities, and (5) budget" (Malasanos, 1976, p. 223). The proposal provides a brief overview of the proposed project, including the research problem, purpose, methodology (brief description), and, most important, a statement of the significance of the work to knowledge in general and the funding institution in particular. By developing a preproposal, researchers are able to determine the agencies interested in funding their study and limit submission of their proposals to only institutions that indicate an interest.

SEEKING APPROVAL FOR A STUDY

Initially, only graduate students developing theses or dissertations and researchers seeking grant money were subject to proposal reviews. However, as a consequence of stricter rules related to the protection of human subjects, most nursing studies are reviewed by at least one research committee. Seeking approval to conduct a study is an action that should be based on knowledge and guided by purpose. Obtaining approval for a study from a research review committee requires understanding the approval process, writing a research proposal for review, and, in many cases, verbally defending the proposal. Little has been written to guide the researcher who is going through the labyrinth of approval mechanisms. This section provides a background for obtaining approval to conduct a study.

Clinical agencies and health care corporations review studies for the following reasons: (1) to evaluate the quality of the study, (2) to ensure that adequate measures are being taken to protect human subjects, and (3) to evaluate the impact of the study on the reviewing institution (Fullwood et al., 1999). What does the researcher hope to result from this institutional review? Most hope to receive approval to collect data at the reviewing institution and to obtain support for the proposed study.

Approval Process

An initial step in seeking approval is to determine exactly what committees in which agencies must grant approval before the study can be conducted. You need to take the initiative to determine the formal approval process rather than assume that you will be told if a formal review system exists. Information on the formal research review system might be obtained from administrative personnel, special projects or grant officers, chairs of institutional review boards (IRBs) in clinical agencies, clinicians who have previously conducted research, and university faculty who are involved in research.

Graduate students usually require approval from their thesis or dissertation committee, the university human subjects review committee, and the agency IRB where the data are to be collected. University faculty conducting research seek approval through the latter two committees. Nurses conducting research in an agency where they are employed must seek approval only at that agency. If the researcher seeks outside funding, additional review committees are involved. Not all studies require full review by the IRB (see Chapter 9 for the types of studies that qualify for exempt or expedited review). However, the IRB, not the researcher, determines the type of review that the study requires for conduct in that agency.

When multiple committees must review a study, sometimes the respective committees agree that the review for the protection of human subjects will be done by only one of the committees, with the findings of that committee generally being accepted by the other committees. For example, if the university human subjects review committee examined and approved a proposal for the protection of human subjects, funding agencies usually recognize that review as sufficient. Reviews in other committees then focus on approval to conduct the study within the institution or decisions to provide study funding.

As part of the approval process, the researcher must determine the agency's policy regarding (1) the use of the clinical facility's name in reporting findings, (2) the presentation and publication of the study, and (3) the authorship of publications. The facility's name is used when presenting or publishing a study only with prior written administrative approval. The researcher may feel freer to report findings that could be interpreted negatively in terms of the institution if the agency is not identified. Some institutions have rules that limit what is presented or published in a study, where it is presented or published, and who is the presenter or author. Before conducting a study, researchers, especially employees of health care agencies, must clarify the rules and regulations of the agency regarding authorship, presentations, and publications. In some cases, recognition of these rules must be included in the proposal if it is to be approved.

Preparing Proposals for Review Committees

The initial proposals for theses and dissertations are often developed as part of a formal class. The faculty members teaching the class provide students with specific proposal guidelines approved by the graduate faculty and assist them in developing their initial proposals. If students elect to conduct a thesis, they ask an appropriate faculty member to serve as chair. With the chair's assistance, the student identifies committee members with expertise in the focus of the proposed study or in conducting research who can work effectively together to refine the final proposal. The number of committee members varies for theses (usually a chair and two members) and dissertations (often a chair and four members) and with the university requirement. This proposal requires approval by the thesis or dissertation committee and the university human rights review committee or IRB.

Conducting research in a clinical agency requires approval by the agency's IRB. This committee has the responsibility to (1) provide researchers with copies of institutional policies and requirements, (2) screen proposals for conducting research in the agency, and (3) assist the researcher with the IRB process (Vessey & Campos, 1992). The approval process policy and proposal guidelines are usually available from the chair of the IRB; and the guidelines should be followed carefully, particularly page limitations. Some committees refuse to review proposals that exceed these limitations. Reviewers on these committees are usually evaluating proposals in addition to other full-time responsibilities, and their time is limited.

Investigators also need to be familiar with the IRB's process for screening proposals. Most agency IRBs screen proposals for (1) scientific merit, (2) protection of human rights, (3) congruence of the study with the agency's research agenda, and (4) impact of the study on patient care (Vessey & Campos, 1992). Researchers need to develop their proposal with these ideas in mind. They also need to determine whether the committee requires specific forms to be completed and submitted with the research proposal. Other important information can be gathered by addressing the following questions: (1) How often does the committee meet? (2) How long before the next meeting? (3) What materials should be submitted before the meeting? (4) When should these materials be submitted? (5) How many copies of the proposal are required? (6) What period of time is usually involved in committee review?

Social and Political Factors

Social and political factors play an important role in obtaining approval to conduct a study. You will need to treat the review process with as much care as development of the study. The dynamics of the relationships among committee members is important to assess. This detail is especially important in the selection of a thesis or dissertation committee to ensure that the members are willing to work together productively. Thorough assessment of the social and political situation in which the study will be reviewed and implemented may be crucial to success of the study.

Clinical agency IRBs may include nurse clinicians who have never conducted research, nurse researchers, and researchers in other disciplines. The reactions of each of these groups to a study could be very different. Sometimes committees are made up primarily of physicians, which is frequently the case in health science centers. Physicians are often not oriented to nursing research methods. The lack of control in nursing studies concerns them, and some believe that the topics of these studies are not important. Sometimes they do not see the nurse researcher as credible because of educational differences, lack of previous experience in research, and few published studies. However, not all physicians view nursing research negatively. Many are strong supporters of nursing research, helpful in suggesting changes in design to strengthen the study, and eager to facilitate access to subjects.

The researcher needs to anticipate potential responses of committee members, prepare the proposal to elicit a favorable response, and consider means of minimizing negative responses. It is wise to meet with the chair of the agency IRB early in the development of a proposal. This meeting could facilitate proposal development, rapport between the researcher and agency personnel, and approval of the research proposal.

In addition to the formal committee approval mechanisms, you will need the tacit approval of the administrative personnel and staff who will be affected in some way by the study. Obtaining informal approval and support often depends on the way in which a person is approached. Demonstrate interest in the institution and the personnel, as well as interest in the research project. The relationships formed with agency personnel should be equal, sharing ones, because these people can often provide ideas and strategies for conducting the study that you may not have considered. The support of agency personnel during data collection can also make the difference between a successful and an unsuccessful study (Fullwood et al., 1999).

Conducting nursing research can benefit the institution, as well as to the researcher. Clinicians have an opportunity to see nursing research in action, which can influence their thinking and clinical practice if the relationship with the researcher is positive. These clinicians may be having their first close contact with a researcher, and interpretation of the researcher's role and the aspects of the study may be necessary. In addition, clinicians tend to be more oriented in the present than researchers are, and they need to see the immediate impact that the study findings can have on nursing practice in their institution. Interactions with researchers might help clinicians see the importance of research in providing evidence-based practice and encourage them to become involved in study activities in the future (Craig & Smyth, 2002). Conducting research and providing evidence-based practice are essential if a hospital is to achieve and maintain magnet status. The award of magnet status from the American Nursing Credentialing Center (ANCC) is prestigious to an institution and validates the excellence in evidence-based nursing care provided by the facility.

Verbal Defense of a Proposal

Graduate students writing theses or dissertations are frequently required to defend their proposal verbally to their university committee members, which is called a thesis or dissertation proposal defense. Most clinical agencies require researchers to meet with the IRB to defend their proposals. In a verbal defense, reviewers can evaluate the researcher as a person, the researcher's knowledge and understanding of the content of the proposal, and his or her ability to reason and provide logical explanations related to the study. And as a researcher, these face-to-face meetings give you opportunity to persuade reluctant committee members to approve your study.

Appearance is important in a personal presentation because it can give an impression of competence or incompetence. These presentations are business-like, with logical and rational interactions, so one should dress in a business-like manner. The committee might perceive individuals who are casually dressed as not valuing the review process.

Nonverbal behaviors are important during the meeting as well, so appearing calm, in control, and confident projects a positive image. Plan and rehearse your presentation to reduce anxiety. Obtain information on the personalities of committee members, their relationships with each other, the vested interests of each member, and their areas of expertise, as this can increase your confidence and provide a sense of control. It is important to arrive at the meeting early, assess the environment for the meeting, and carefully select a seat. Because you are the presenter, all members of the committee need to be able to see you. However, selecting a seat on one side of a table with all the committee members on the other side could make you feel uncomfortable and simulate an interrogation rather than a scholarly interaction. Sitting at the side of a table rather than at the head might be a strategic move to elicit support.

The verbal defense usually begins with a brief presentation of the study. Your presentation needs to be carefully planned, timed, and rehearsed. Salient points should be highlighted, which you can accomplish with the use of audiovisuals. After the presentation the reviewers will ask questions, so be prepared to defend or justify the methods and procedures used in your study. Sometimes it is beneficial to practice responding to questions related to the study with a friend; this rehearsal will help you to determine the best way to defend your ideas without appearing defensive. When the meeting ends, thank the members of the committee for their time. If the committee did not make a decision regarding the study during the meeting, ask when the decision will be made.

Revising a Proposal

Reviewers sometimes suggest changes in a proposal; however, some of these changes may benefit the institution, but not the study. Remain receptive to the suggestions, explore with the committee the impact of the changes on the proposed study, and try to resolve the conflict. If the conflict cannot be resolved, you might need to find another setting.

Many times reviewers make valuable suggestions that might improve the quality of a study or facilitate the data collection process. Revision of the proposal is often based on these suggestions before the study is implemented. Sometimes a study requires revision while it is being conducted because of problems with data collection tools or subjects' participation. However, if clinical agency personnel or representatives of funding institutions have approved a proposal, the researcher needs to examine the situation seriously before making major changes in the study.

Before revising a proposal, address three questions: (1) What needs to be changed? (2) Why is the change necessary? (3) How will the change affect implementation of the study and the study findings? Students need to seek advice from the faculty before revising their studies. Sometimes it is beneficial for seasoned researchers to discuss their proposed study changes with other researchers or agency personnel for suggestions and additional viewpoints.

If a revision is necessary, revise your proposal and discuss the change with members of the IRB in the agency where the study is being conducted. The committee members might indicate that the investigators can proceed with the study or that they will have to seek approval for the revised proposal. If a study is funded, the study changes must be discussed with the representatives of the funding agency. The funding agency has the power to approve or disapprove the changes. However, realistic changes that are clearly described and backed with a rationale will probably be approved.

SAMPLE QUANTITATIVE RESEARCH PROPOSAL

The following proposal of a quantitative study will help you to prepare your first research proposal. The proposal was developed by a thesis student to conduct a quasi-experimental study (Ulbrich, 1995). The content of this proposal is brief and does not include the detail normally presented in a thesis or dissertation. The example provides ideas regarding the content areas that would be covered in developing a proposal for a quantitative study.

■ TITLE: THE EFFECT OF OPERATOR TECHNIQUE ON TYMPANIC MEMBRANE THERMOMETRY

■ INVESTIGATOR: SHERRI L. ULBRICH

■ CHAPTER 1

Introduction

Temperatures are used to monitor and diagnose infection, inflammation, neoplasia, neurological insults, hypothermia, hyperthermia, and metabolic disorders (Wolff, 1988). Accurate assessment of the body's thermal responses can provide information that results in prompt treatment and may prevent further injury, especially in acute care settings. The tympanic thermometer assesses body temperature by measuring the infrared radiation emitted from the tympanic membrane. Clinical studies have shown the tympanic thermometer to be extremely useful when compared with oral and rectal thermometers (Terndrup, 1992). However, some experts doubt the thermometer's ability to detect fever and others note cases of large differences between tympanic and other core temperature routes (Zinder & Terndrup, 1991). Consequently, some health care providers are skeptical about tympanic measurements and adoption in the clinical setting has been delayed.

Some of the skepticism arises from inconsistent measurements and unanswered questions about the technique to be used with tympanic thermometers. Though technique is critical in producing accurate measurements of all vital signs including temperature, little is known about how to best use the tympanic thermometer. Information regarding the operation of this device from the manufacturer and clinical studies is conflicting. In addition, many sources fail to give specific descriptions of operator techniques or only make limited comparisons of these techniques. Currently, few tympanic thermometer technique studies have been conducted on adults (Erickson & Meyer, 1994). If a single, accurate technique for taking tympanic temperatures could be determined, patients and health care providers might benefit from the many advantages of this safe, efficient, and less invasive temperature device. Thus, the purpose of this study is to examine the effects of operator techniques on the measurement of tympanic temperatures in adult critical care patients. This information can be used to develop a research-based protocol, expand the knowledge base about tympanic thermometry, and help meet the demand for better assessment of temperature in critically ill patients.

■ CHAPTER 2

Review of Relevant Literature

Temperature measurement is an important nursing assessment, especially in critically ill patients. Changes in temperature are physiological cues, when accurately assessed, which can lead to prompt, effective treatment (Bruce & Grove, 1991; Holtzclaw, 1992). Temperature can be measured by many routes and instruments. The specifications for the development of tympanic thermometers were congruent with the principles and theories in physics, engineering (Fraden, 1991), and physiology.

Research has shown that tympanic thermometers are accurate in healthy and ill patients of all ages in a variety of clinical and hospital settings, except in the cases of inconsistent or poor operator technique (Terndrup, 1992), exposure to low or high ambient temperatures within 20 minutes of measurement (Doyle, Zehner, & Terndrup, 1992; Zehner & Terndrup, 1991), and near complete occlusion of the tympanic membrane by cerumen or severe scarring (Pransky, 1991). Having otitis media, small or moderate amounts of cerumen, and small ear canals in children do not cause significant differences in temperature. Studies have shown tympanic temperatures to be at least as accurate as oral and rectal temperatures and much more accurate than axillary temperatures (Erickson & Yount, 1991; Schmitz, Bair, Falk, & Levine, 1995). However, tympanic temperatures are not as accurate as bladder or pulmonary artery temperatures (Erickson & Meyer, 1994; Milewski, Ferguson, & Terndrup, 1991; Nierman, 1991; Summers, 1991), especially in detecting fever (Zinder & Terndrup, 1991). Tympanic thermometers are also less invasive and more time and cost efficient (Alexander & Kelly, 1991a); do not transmit infectious agents among patients (Livornese et al., 1992); preserve the patient's modesty; and produce minimal discomfort (Alexander & Kelly, 1991b).

The effect of operator technique on tympanic measurements needs to be investigated carefully. Determining the optimal technique could reduce erroneous and inconsistent measurements in future research and clinical practice (Erickson & Meyer, 1994; Erickson & Woo, 1994; Guthrie & Keunke, 1992; Pransky, 1991). Three elements in tympanic measurement technique have been identified: (1) an eartug to straighten the auditory canal; (2) aiming at the tympanic membrane; and (3) making a snug seal. Additional research is needed that provides control of extraneous variables, use of a core reference temperature, and use of consistent and meaningful analyses for comparison. Multiple techniques have not been previously studied to identify the aspects of technique or combination of techniques that are essential for obtaining the most accurate tympanic temperature measurement. The current study is proposed to expand the knowledge base related to the effects of operator technique on tympanic temperature measurements in critically ill adults. The information obtained from this study can assist nurses in comparing tympanic temperatures with those obtained through bladder or other core temperature routes. (To promote concise coverage of this proposal, only a summary of the theoretical and empirical literature was provided.)

■ CHAPTER 3

Framework

Thermometry is the science of temperature measurement (Schooley, 1986) and provides the framework for this study. As shown in Figure 28-1, a linear path of unimpeded heat transfer between the heat source and the thermometer system response results in a temperature measurement under ideal conditions of thermometry. However, in reality, physiological, mechanical, and environmental factors, as well as instrumental error must be controlled or manipulated to facilitate the transfer of heat and ensure accuracy of the measurement. The extent to which each of these complex factors affects the transfer of heat and temperature measurement has not yet been fully determined. The extent to which operator technique can effectively manipulate or control these factors and influence the transfer of heat to promote optimal accuracy of the thermometer is also unknown.

In this study, the heat sources are the tympanic membrane and urinary bladder. Bladder temperature will be used as the reference core temperature and represents the ideal, accurate temperature measurement. The difference between tympanic temperatures measured using different operator techniques and the accepted standard of measured bladder temperature is the dependent variable in this study. Heat transfer between the heat sources and the thermometer system response occurred by radiation with the tympanic thermometer and conduction with the bladder thermometer. Operator technique is shown in boldface type because it is the concept that

represents the independent variables in this study. The three components of operator technique are otoscopic eartug, aim, and seal when using tympanic thermometers. Combinations of these components are the independent variables and will be used to provide additional control over physiological and mechanical factors and thus influence the transfer of heat and subsequently, the temperature measurement.

Hypothesis

There is no clinically important difference in tympanic temperature measurements using four operator techniques: (1) an otoscopic eartug with aim and seal, (2) an otoscopic eartug and seal without aim, (3) aim and seal without otoscopic eartug, and (4) seal without otoscopic eartug or aim when compared with bladder temperatures taken in critically ill adults.

Definitions of Independent Variables
Operator Techniques for Tympanic Temperatures
Conceptual Definition. Operator techniques are actions used by persons when taking temperatures that affect the physiological and mechanical factors and subsequently influence heat transfer and tympanic temperature measurement.

Operational Definitions. Each of the combined techniques for taking tympanic temperatures listed in the hypothesis is considered to be a single independent variable. The separate elements of each technique are operationally defined as follows:

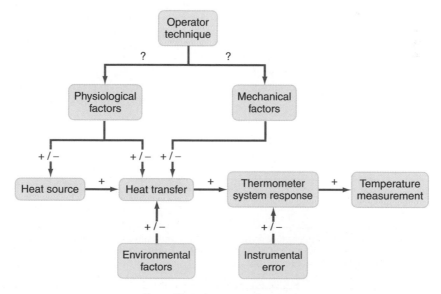

Figure 28-1 Thermometry framework.

Otoscopic eartug is the manipulation of the cartilaginous outer portion of the ear by grasping the auricle firmly but gently, pulling it upward, back, and slightly out in order to straighten the elliptical S-shaped outer canal and improve the view of the lower ear canal and tympanic membrane (Bates, 1983; Erickson & Meyer, 1994).

Aim is aligning the warmest area of the tympanic membrane, the anterior, inferior third, with the tympanic thermometer sensor tip by holding the device level while directing the tip of the probe at the midpoint between the ear and the outer canthus of the eye on the opposite side (Terndrup, 1992).

Seal is leaving no space between the walls of the auditory canal and the covered probe tip by placing the probe tip in the opening of the ear canal and applying gentle but firm pressure to seal the canal from ambient air (Erickson & Yount, 1991).

Definitions of the Dependent Variables
Bladder Temperature
Conceptual Definition. Bladder temperature is the approximation of core body heat reflected in the amount of heat in the bladder (Erickson & Meyer, 1994).

Operational Definition. Bladder temperature is the numerical measurement of heat in the bladder as detected by Bard thermocath and displayed by Bard and Hewlett Packard monitors using a Fahrenheit scale to the nearest tenth of a degree.

Tympanic Temperature
Conceptual Definition. Tympanic temperature is the amount of heat from the tympanic membrane as detected in the auditory canal. This temperature is used as an indicator of core temperature because of its proximity and shared common blood supply with the hypothalamic thermoregulatory center (Fraden, 1991).

Operational Definition. Tympanic temperature is the numerical measurement of temperature as determined and displayed by the infrared tympanic thermometer Genius 3000A Model using the Fahrenheit scale to the nearest tenth of a degree.

Attribute Variables
The attribute or demographic variables of this study are age; race; gender; admitting diagnosis to the intensive care unit (ICU); other significant diagnoses or complications; temperature changes in the previous four hours; history of carotid artery disease, stroke, head trauma, or cranial surgery; cranial turban dressing; and type of supplemental oxygenation.

Relevant Terms
Adult is a person over the age of 18 years.

Intensive care is a part of the hospital that deals specifically with life-threatening health problems.

Assumptions
1. Temperature measurement is important in patient care.
2. Accurately measuring temperature is an important nursing responsibility.
3. The optimal thermometer is accurate, precise, safe, efficient, and noninvasive.

■ CHAPTER 4
Methods and Procedures
This chapter identifies the design, setting, sample, methods of measurement, data collection and analysis plan, and limitations for this proposed study. For conciseness, the key ideas of these sections are presented but not in the detail that usually is included in a thesis.

Design
This study's design is quasi-experimental and includes multiple treatments with nonequivalent dependent variables (see Figure 28-2). An attempt will be made to control the carryover effect of the treatments by changing treatment order for each subject (Burns & Grove, 2005). Efforts will be made to control the extraneous variables of environmental temperature, condition of the ear and tympanic membrane, age, activity level, and diurnal

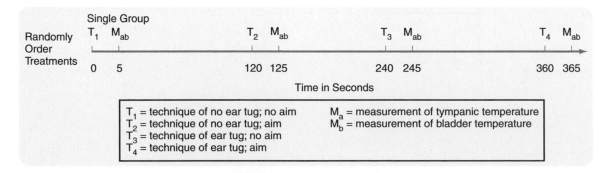

Figure **28-2** Multiple treatments with nonequivalent dependent variables design.

effects. A plan was developed for controlling and/or recording essential information regarding each of these extraneous variables.

A protocol was developed to ensure the consistent implementation of the four treatments: tug with aim, tug without aim, aim without tug, and no tug and no aim (see Appendix 28-A). The seal is considered essential and will be achieved with all four treatments. The investigator will implement all treatments and obtain and record all measurements according to protocol to ensure consistency. A pilot study will be conducted on five subjects to assess the technique administration, determine the adequacy of the treatment protocol, and discover problems in data collection. Any problems noted in the design and data collection process for the study will be examined and modified as needed.

Setting and Sample

The data will be collected in the ICU of two recently merged, fully accredited, and licensed metropolitan hospitals in north central Texas. The strengths and weaknesses of these units are described. The target population is adult ICU patients who meet the sample criteria and consent to participate in the study. The sample criteria are nonexclusive to gender, ethnic background, diagnosis, or hospital treatment plan. The sample inclusion criteria consist of: (1) being a patient in the ICU, (2) being an adult over 18 years of age, (3) having a Bard Urotrack thermocatheter in place and functioning, (4) having no significant scarring or inflammation of the tympanic membrane, (5) having no bleeding or drainage from the tympanic membrane or ear canal, (6) having no obvious occlusion of the ear canal with cerumen, (7) having not been given antipyretics within the previous three hours, (8) having no exposure to extreme temperatures of 35°C within the past two hours, (9) having not been on a heating or cooling blanket within the past two hours, and (10) having a bladder temperature in the range of 96.0–102.0° F or 35.6–38.9° C. The sample size was calculated using a power analysis with a standard power of 0.8, effect size of 0.4, and alpha of 0.05. It was determined that a minimum of 73 subjects will be needed for this study. A nonprobability sample of convenience will be used. However, the design is strengthened by a random selection of right or left ear and a random ordering of treatments. The strengths and weaknesses of this sampling method are described.

Measurement Methods

The tympanic temperatures will be measured using the single First Temp Genius Model 3000A thermometer. This thermometer is equipped with a unique "Peak Select System" that internally records and analyzes 32 separate measurements from the incoming radiation, and displays the average of the highest two readings. The precision, accuracy, sensitivity, and potential error of this thermometer are described.

Bladder temperatures will be measured using Bard Urotrack Foley Catheters, model number 890216/18 sizes 16–18 French, manufactured by Bard Urologic Division of Covington, Georgia. These modified transurethral indwelling Foley catheters, like standard catheters, are made from hydrogel-coated latex tubes with a five milliliter balloon encircling the catheter just below the tip to anchor the catheter in place within the bladder. ... The precision, accuracy, sensitivity, and potential error for this catheter are described.

Plan for Data Collection

The treatments will be implemented and data will be collected by the investigator using the protocol outlined in Appendix 28-A. Data will be recorded on the data collection form developed for this study (see Appendix 28-B). The investigator will note the consistency of the treatment implementation and the data collection process. When the protocol is not followed consistently, this will be recorded (Egan, Snyder, & Burns, 1992). A complete plan for the data collection process is outlined in Appendix 28-C. Raw data and consent forms will be stored in a locked file drawer in the investigator's house for five years.

Ethical Considerations

Permission to conduct this study will be obtained from the investigator's thesis committee, the Human Rights Review Committee for The University of Texas at Arlington, and the hospital's Institutional Review Board. In addition, verbal approval will be obtained from the ICU managers and the primary physicians of the subjects. Subjects will be provided essential information for informed consent and will sign a consent form (see Appendix 28-D). The benefit-risk ratio was assessed for this study, indicating minimal risk and important benefits.

Data Analysis

Data will be input and analyzed by the researcher using Mystat, a software package developed by Munro (1997). All raw data entered in the computer will be checked for errors. Demographic data will be analyzed with frequencies, percents, means, standard deviations, and ranges and presented in a table (see [Appendix 28-E]). The hypothesis will provide direction for the analysis of study data. Means, standard deviations, and ranges will be calculated on the bladder and tympanic temperatures for the four treatments of tug with aim, tug without aim, aim without tug, and no tug and no aim. The Bland-Altman method will be used to compare bladder and tympanic temperatures for each operator technique. Researchers have begun to use this method rather than conventional statistics such as Pearson's product-moment correlations or tests of statistical differences. Bland and Altman (1986) have suggested that conventional statistics are inappropriate when an established method of measurement, such as bladder temperature, is compared to a new method of measurement, such as tympanic temperature. The results will be presented in graphs.

TABLE 28-3   Study Timetable

Task to be Performed	Performer of Task	Completion of Task
1. Complete proposal and forms	Researcher	First through sixth months
2. Defend and revise proposal	Researcher	Seventh month
3. Review board approvals	Researcher	Eighth month
4. Equipment gathering and training	Researcher	Eighth month
5. Assemble data collection packets	Researcher	Eighth month
6. Establish potential subject notification with personnel at clinical agency	Researcher	Eighth month
7. Pilot study	Researcher	Ninth month
8. Analyze pilot data and revise	Researcher	Ninth month
9. Data collection	Researcher	Tenth and eleventh months
10. Analyze data	Researcher	Twelfth month
11. Interpret results	Researcher	Twelfth month
12. Final defense	Researcher	Twelfth month
13. Communicate findings	Researcher	2–3 years

From Ulbrich, S. L. (1995). *The effect of operator technique on tympanic membrane thermometry*. Unpublished master's thesis, University of Texas at Arlington.

Methodological Limitations

The limitations of this study include that (1) the extraneous variables of environmental and core body temperatures will not be completely controlled, (2) nonrandom sample will limit generalizability, and (3) estimation of core body temperature by the bladder thermometer is not quite as accurate as the pulmonary artery catheter, although they correlate at $r = 0.99$ (Erickson & Meyer, 1994).

Communication of Findings

The study findings will be presented to the thesis committee, hospital research committee, ICU nurses and managers, and the manufacturer of the equipment. In addition, an abstract of the study will be submitted for possible presentation of the research at a national critical care meeting. The study will be submitted for publication in a clinical journal such as *Heart & Lung* or *American Journal of Critical Care*. A study timetable and budget have been developed to direct this project and are presented in Tables [28-3] and [28-4]. (Ulbrich, 1995)

TABLE 28-4   Study Budget

Budget Items	Cost per Item	Total Cost
1. Printing costs	1500 pages @ 0.05/page	75.00
2. Consultant costs	Provided by the Center for Nursing Research	0.00
3. Statistical software		50.00
4. Genius II tympanic thermometer and probe covers	Provided by Sherwood Medical	0.00
5. Bard calibration plug	Provided by Bard Urologic Division	0.00
6. Travel costs		150.00
7. Supplies		80.00
8. Communication costs		100.00
	Total	455.00

From Ulbrich, S. L. (1995). *The effect of operator technique on tympanic membrane thermometry*. Unpublished master's thesis, University of Texas at Arlington.

APPENDIX 28-A **Data Collection Protocol**

1. After consent is signed, the data collection form with the corresponding ID No. will be taken to the nursing station.
2. Place the room thermometer in the subject's room.
3. Questions one through ten will be answered by the researcher from information contained within the chart. All demographic questions will be completed prior to experimental data collection.
4. Enter the subject's room, ask any additional questions, and review the procedure if this is appropriate.
5. Record the room temperature from the thermometer left earlier.
6. Place the data collection form, otoscope, tympanic thermometer, and stopwatch on the same side of the patient as the ear selected for intervention.
7. Perform the brief otoscopic examination by gently retracting the subject's ear and inserting the otoscope into the external canal.
8. Note on the data collection form any large amount of cerumen, presence of any trauma, drainage, significant scarring, or severe inflammation. If any of these conditions are present, explain to the subject reasons for exclusion from the study and notify the nursing staff of the findings.
9. Insert the Bard calibration plug into the Urotrack monitor for calibration if applicable.
10. Record the time of day when data collection began.
11. Review the selected treatment order.
12. Remove the tympanic thermometer from its base and place a disposable cover on the probe tip.
13. Manipulate the ear and insert the probe in the exact manner outlined below for the first technique.
    T1 (tug: aim)—Gently grasp the superior aspect of the pinna and retract the ear in an upward, outward, and backward motion. Maintain this position and insert the covered tip of the probe, aiming at the point between the bridge of the nose and outer canthus of the eye on the opposite side of the head. Apply gentle pressure with the probe tip to seal the canal.

T2 (tug: no aim)—Gently grasp the superior aspect of the pinna and retract the ear in an upward, outward, and backward motion. Maintain this position and insert the covered tip of the probe, directing it toward the opposite ear or along the mid-frontal plane of the head. Apply gentle pressure with the probe tip to seal the ear canal.

T3 (no tug: aim)—Steady the subject's head by placing a hand over the temporal area. Insert the covered probe tip, aiming at the point between the bridge of the nose and outer canthus of the eye on the opposite side of the head. Apply gentle pressure with the probe tip to seal the ear canal.

T4 (no tug: no aim)—Steady the subject's head by placing a hand over the temporal area. Insert the covered tip of the probe, directing it at the opposite ear or the probe along the mid-frontal plane of the head. Apply gentle pressure with the probe tip to seal the ear canal.

14. Press the SCAN button on the thermometer.
15. Remove the thermometer, release the ear, and dispose of the probe tip cover.
16. Begin the 2-minute interval timer on the stopwatch.
17. Record the temperature in the appropriate blank on the data collection form.
18. Immediately read the bladder temperature from the thermocath monitor.
19. Record the bladder temperature in the appropriate blank on the data collection form.
20. Allow the 2 minutes to pass.
21. Repeat steps 12–20 for each of the remaining techniques in the order on the data collection form.
22. Record the time that data collection ended.
23. Thank the subject (if appropriate) for participation in the study. Answer any questions or address any concerns.
24. Review the data collection sheet for completeness.
25. Gather the equipment and leave the data collection area.

From Ulbrich, S. L. (1995). *The effect of operator technique on tympanic membrane thermometry.* Unpublished master's thesis, University of Texas at Arlington.

APPENDIX 28-B   **Data Collection Form**

ID No. _____   Date: _____

Demographic Data

A. Age _____   B. Gender   _____ (1) female   _____ (2) male

C. Race _____ (1) Caucasian   _____ (2) Asian   _____ (3) American Indian

      _____ (4) African American   _____ (5) Hispanic   _____ (6) Other

D. Unit _____ (1) CCU   _____ (2) MICU   _____ (3) SICU   _____ (4) NICU

E. Campus

F. Admitting/major diagnosis: _____

G. Other significant diagnoses: _____

H. Supplemental oxygen   _____ (1) NC   _____ (2) vent   _____ (3) FM

                               _____ (4) FT   _____ (5) other   _____ (6) none

I. Turban cranial dressing   _____ (1) yes   _____ (2) no

J. Hx _____ (1) carotid artery disease   _____ (2) cerebral vascular accident

     _____ (3) major head trauma   _____ (4) cranial surgery

     _____ (5) none

K. Most recent temperature _____ F   Time taken _____

L. Room temperature _____ F

Experimental Data

M. Ear_____ (1) right   _____ (2) left

N. Noted upon aural exam   _____ (1) large amount of cerumen   _____ (2) trauma

                             _____ (3) significant scarring   _____ (4) drainage

                             _____ (5) significant inflammation   _____ (6) hair

                             _____ (7) other

Time data collection began _____

Treatment Order	Tympanic Temp.	Bladder Temp

Time data collection ended _____

O. Data collection & treatments followed the protocol _____ (1) yes _____ (2) no _____ (3) partial

Explain, if partial _____

Comments:

_____

_____

_____

_____

From Ulbrich, S. L. (1995). *The effect of operator technique on tympanic membrane thermometry.* Unpublished master's thesis, University of Texas at Arlington.

APPENDIX 28-C **Data Collection Plan**

1. Locate potential subjects by making a daily phone call or visit to the intensive care units. Potential subjects might also be located by asking staff to notify the researcher by telephone of patients with bladder thermocatheters. The phone number of the researcher is already in the list of numbers in each unit.
2. Assess potential subjects in person using the sample criteria. This information can be gathered from the chart or staff. Timing should be considered in this step to avoid the hours near midnight to 3:00 AM and 6:00 AM to 8:00 AM or when nursing activities can be anticipated (timed dressing changes, scheduled procedures, etc.).
3. If all sample criteria are met, pursue consent to participate from the patient or legal representative.
4. Place the signed consent form in a folder to be kept with the researcher until it can be secured in the safe. Give one copy to the subject and place another in the chart.
5. Gather and record the demographic data from the chart or staff.
6. Follow the specific procedures outlined in the protocol (see [Appendix 28-B]) to implement the procedures and gather the experimental data.
7. Review forms for completeness.
8. Thank the staff and patient (if appropriate) for their participation and assistance.
9. Initiate the entire process with any additional subjects.
10. Gather equipment and return to the office.
11. File and secure all consent and data collection forms.
12. Repeat steps 1–11 until at least 30 subjects are recruited and data are collected.

From Ulbrich, S. L. (1995). *The effect of operator technique on tympanic membrane thermometry*, pp. 70–71. Unpublished master's thesis, University of Texas at Arlington.

APPENDIX 28-D **Consent Form**

Study Title: The Effect of Operator Technique on Tympanic Membrane Thermometry
Investigator: Sherri L. Ulbrich R.N., B.S.N., CCRN
Subject ID No. _____ **Hospital No.** _____ **Protocol No.** _____

You are invited to be in a research study to determine how different techniques used by nurses in taking tympanic temperatures affect the accuracy of these thermometers in adult patients in the intensive care unit. Over the next four months about 70 participants will be chosen in this nontherapeutic study without regard for race, gender, or socioeconomic status. Since you are already a patient in the intensive care unit and have a special bladder catheter to monitor your temperature, you have been selected as a possible participant. As a benefit, your temperature will be monitored closely and will provide information that might enable nurses to better assess the temperatures of their patients in the future.

The study and its procedures have been approved by the appropriate people and review boards at the University of Texas at Arlington and the hospital. If you were to participate in the study the specially trained researcher would (1) complete a demographic data sheet, (2) perform a brief ear (otoscopic) examination, (3) take a series of tympanic temperatures using different techniques to straighten the ear canal (similar to an ear examination) and aim the instrument, and (4) record the temperature from the special catheter you already have in place. The risk associated with this study is the possibility of injury to the ear canal and/or tympanic membrane. Neither has ever occurred in previous studies. Also, this risk is no greater than with the routine measurement of your temperature with the thermometer that is currently used throughout the hospital. You will be excluded from the study if any abnormalities are found during the ear examination to avoid this risk. Participation in this study will take approximately 10 minutes. You are free to ask any questions about the study or about being a subject and you may call the investigator at (817) 273-2276 if you have further questions.

Continued

APPENDIX 28-D   **Consent Form—cont'd**

Your participation in this study is voluntary: You are under no obligation to participate. You have the right to withdraw at any time and the care you receive and your relationship with the health care team will not be affected. Neither you nor the hospital will be charged or incur any expense or compensation for your participation. Although your physician is not an investigator, he or she will be informed of your participation.

The study data will be coded so they will not be linked to your name. Your identity will not be revealed while the study is being conducted, except to the doc-

tors and nurses caring for you, or when the study is reported or published. All study data will be collected by the researcher, stored in a secure place, and will not be shared without your permission. A copy of the consent form will be given to you.

I have read this consent form and voluntarily consent to participate in this study. I understand that I am to rely on the investigator for information regarding the nature and purpose of the research study, the risks involved in the research study, and the possibility of complications, and I have been given an opportunity to discuss these with the investigator.

Subject's Signature   Date

I have explained this study to the above subject and have sought his/her understanding for informed consent.

Legally Authorized Representative   Date

Investigator's Signature   Date

From Ulbrich, S. L. (1995). *The effect of operator technique on tympanic membrane thermometry*, pp. 81–82. Unpublished master's thesis, University of Texas at Arlington.

APPENDIX 28-E   **Dummy Table ro Present Sample Characteristics**

Demographic Variables	Sample Statistics* $N = 60$	
	M (*SD*)	Range
Age		
Most Recent Temperature		
Room Temperature		
	Frequency	Percent
Gender		
Male		
Female		
Race		
Caucasian		
African American		
Asian		
Hispanic		
American Indian		
Other		

Continued

APPENDIX 28-E   **Dummy Table ro Present Sample Characteristics—cont'd**

	Frequency	Percent
Unit		
CCU		
MICU		
SICU		
NICU		
Primary Diagnosis		
XXXXXXXX		
XXXXXXXX		
XXXXXXXX		
XXXXXXXX		
Other Significant Diagnoses		
XXXXXXXX		
XXXXXXXX		
XXXXXXXX		
XXXXXXXX		
Mechanically Ventilated		
Turban-Type Cranial Dressing		
History of:		
Carotid artery disease		
Cerebral vascular accident		
Major head trauma		
Cranial surgery		

From Ulbrich, S. L. (1995). *The effect of operator technique on tympanic membrane thermometry*. Unpublished master's thesis, University of Texas at Arlington.

*Only selected statistics are used to analyze each variable.

SUMMARY

- This chapter focuses on writing a research proposal and seeking approval to conduct a study.
- A research proposal is a written plan that identifies the major elements of a study, such as the problem, purpose, and framework, and outlines the methods and procedures to conduct a study.
- Writing a quality proposal involves (1) developing the ideas logically, (2) determining the depth or detail of the proposal content, (3) identifying the critical points in the proposal, and (4) developing an aesthetically appealing copy.
- A quantitative research proposal usually has four chapters or sections: (1) introduction, (2) review of relevant literature, (3) framework, and (4) methods and procedures.
- A qualitative research proposal generally includes the following chapters or sections: (1) introduction; (2) research paradigm and general method; (3) applied method of inquiry; and (4) current knowledge, limitations, and plans to communicate the study.
- Most clinical agencies and funding institutions require a condensed proposal, which usually includes a problem, a purpose, previous research conducted in the area, a framework, variables, design, sample, ethical considerations, plan for data collection and analysis, and plan for dissemination of findings.
- Sometimes a researcher will send a preproposal or query letter to a funding institution rather than a proposal; and the parts of the preproposal are logically ordered as follows: (1) letter of transmittal, (2) proposal for research, (3) personnel, (4) facilities, and (5) budget.
- Seeking approval for the conduct or funding of a study is a process that involves submission of a proposal to a selected group for review and, in many situations, verbally defending that proposal.
- Research proposals are reviewed to (1) evaluate the quality of the study, (2) ensure that adequate measures are being taken to protect human subjects, and (3) evaluate the impact of conducting the study on the reviewing institution.
- Proposals sometimes require revision before or during the implementation of a study; and if a change is

necessary, the researcher needs to discuss the change with the members of the university and clinical agency IRBs and the funding agency.

• The chapter concludes with an example of a brief quantitative research proposal of a quasi-experimental study (Ulbrich, 1995).

REFERENCES

Alexander, D., & Kelly, B. (1991a). Cost effectiveness of tympanic thermometry in the pediatric office setting. *Clinical Pediatrics*, *30*(4 Suppl.), 57–59.

Alexander, D., & Kelly, B. (1991b). Responses of children, parents, and nurses to tympanic thermometry in the pediatric office. *Clinical Pediatrics*, *30*(4 Suppl.), 53–56.

American Psychological Association. (2001). *Publication manual of the American Psychological Association* (5th ed.). Washington, DC: Author.

Bates, B. (1983). *A guide to physical examination* (3rd ed.). Philadelphia: Lippincott.

Beck, C. T. (1993). Qualitative research: The evaluation of its credibility, fittingness, and auditability. *Western Journal of Nursing Research*, *15*(2), 263–266.

Bland, J. M., & Altman, D. G. (1986). Statistical methods for assessing agreement between two methods of clinical measurement. *Lancet*, *1*(8476), 307–310.

Boyd, C. O., & Munhall, P. L. (2001). Qualitative research proposal and report. In P. L. Munhall (Ed.), *Nursing research: A qualitative perspective* (3rd ed., pp. 613–638). Sudbury, MA: Jones & Bartlett.

Brink, H. (1993). Academic nurse leaders' interpretation of concepts and priorities related to the examination of scientific short papers, dissertations and theses: Part 1. *Curationis*, *16*(3), 62–67.

Bruce, J. L., & Grove, S. K. (1991). Fever: Pathology and treatment. *Critical Care Nurse*, *12*(1), 40–49.

Burns, N., & Grove, S. K. (2005). *The practice of nursing research: Conduct, critique, and utilization* (5th ed.). Philadelphia: Saunders.

Chenitz, W. C., & Swanson, J. M. (1986). *From practice to grounded theory: Qualitative research in nursing*. Menlo Park, CA: Addison-Wesley.

Cohen, M. Z., Knafl, K., & Dzurec, L. C. (1993). Grant writing for qualitative research. *Image: Journal of Nursing Scholarship*, *25*(2), 151–156.

Corty, E. W. (2007). *Using and interpreting statistics: A practical text for the health, behavioral, and social sciences*. St. Louis: Mosby.

Craig, J. V., & Smyth, R. L. (2002). *The evidence-base practice manual for nurses*. Edinburgh: Churchill Livingstone.

Dexter, P. (2000). Tips for scholarly writing in nursing. *Journal of Professional Nursing*, *16*(1), 6–12.

Doyle, F., Zehner, W. J., & Terndrup, T. E. (1992). The effect of ambient temperature on tympanic and oral temperatures. *American Journal of Emergency Medicine*, *10*(4), 285–289.

Egan, E. C., Snyder, M., & Burns, K. R. (1992). Intervention studies in nursing: Is the effect due to the independent variable? *Nursing Outlook*, *40*(4), 187–190.

Erickson, R. S., & Meyer, L. T. (1994). Accuracy of infrared ear thermometry and other temperature methods in adults. *American Journal of Critical Care*, *3*(1), 40–54.

Erickson, R. S., & Woo, T. M. (1994). Accuracy of ear thermometry and traditional temperature methods in young children. *Heart & Lung*, *23*(3), 181–195.

Erickson, R. S., & Yount, S. T. (1991). Comparison of tympanic and oral temperatures in surgical patients. *Nursing Research*, *40*(2), 90–93.

Fraden, J. (1991). Noncontact temperature measurements in medicine. In D. L. Wise (Ed.), *Bioinstrumentation and biosensors* (pp. 511–549). New York: Marcel Dekker.

Frankl, V. E. (1984). *Man's search for meaning*. New York: Simon & Schuster.

Fullwood, J., Granger, B. B., Bride, W., & Taylor, M. C. (1999). Heart center nursing research: A team effort. *Progress in Cardiovascular Nursing*, *14*(1), 25–29.

Giorgi, A. (1985). *Phenomenology and psychological research*. Pittsburgh: Duquesne University Press.

Guthrie, K. A., & Keunke, N. E. (1992). *Tympanic-based core temperature measurement in relation to thermometer and technique*. Unpublished master's thesis, Oregon Health Sciences University, Portland.

Holtzclaw, B. J. (1992). The febrile response in critical care: State of the science. *Heart & Lung*, *21*(5), 482–501.

Kerlinger, F. N., & Lee, H. B. (2000). *Foundations of behavioral research* (4th ed.). Fort Worth, TX: Harcourt College Publishers.

Leininger, M. M. (1985). *Qualitative research methods in nursing*. Orlando: Grune & Stratton.

Livornese, L. L., Dias, S., Samuel, C., Romanowski, B., Taylor, S., May, P., (1992). Hospital acquired infection with vancomycin-resistant Enterococcus faecium transmitted by electronic thermometers. *Annals of Internal Medicine*, *117*(2), 112–116.

Malasanos, L. J. (1976). What is the preproposal? What are its component parts? Is it an effective instrument in assessing funding potential of research ideas? *Nursing Research, 25*(3), 223–224.

Marshall, C., & Rossman, G. B. (2006). *Designing qualitative research* (4th ed.). Thousand Oaks, CA: Sage.

Melnyk, B. M., & Fineout-Overholt, E. (2005). *Evidence-based practice in nursing & healthcare: A guide to best practice*. Philadelphia: Lippincott Williams & Wilkins.

Miles, M. B., & Huberman, A. M. (1994). *Qualitative data analysis* (2nd ed). Thousand Oaks, CA: Sage.

Milewski, A., Ferguson, K. L., & Terndrup, T. E. (1991). Comparison of pulmonary artery, rectal, and tympanic membrane temperatures in adult intensive care patients. *Clinical Pediatrics*, *30*(4 Suppl.), 13–16.

Miller, S. (1997). Multiple paradigms for nursing. In S. E. Thorne & V. E. Hayes (Eds.), *Nursing praxis: Knowledge and action* (pp. 140–156). Thousand Oaks, CA: Sage.

Munhall, P. L. (2001). *Nursing research: A qualitative perspective* (3rd ed.). Sudbury, MA: Jones & Bartlett.

Munro, B. H. (1997). *Statistical methods for health care research* (3rd ed.). Philadelphia: Lippincott.

Nierman, D. M. (1991). Core temperature measurement in the intensive care unit. *Critical Care Medicine*, *19*(6), 818–823.

Parse, R. R., Coyne, A. B., & Smith, M. J. (1985). *Nursing research: Qualitative methods*. Bowie, MD: Brady.

Patton, M. Q. (2002). *Qualitative research and evaluation methods* (3rd ed.). Thousand Oaks, CA: Sage.

Peat, J. K., Mellis, C., Williams, K., & Xuan, W. (2002). *Health science research: A handbook of quantitative methods*. Thousand Oaks, CA: Sage.

Pinch, W. J. (1995). Synthesis: Implementing a complex process. *Nurse Educator*, *20*(1), 34–40.

Pransky, S. M. (1991). The impact of technique and conditions of the tympanic membrane upon infrared tympanic thermometry. *Clinical Pediatrics*, *30*(4 Suppl.), 50–51.

Pyrczak, F., & Bruce, R. R. (2005). *Writing empirical research reports: A basic guide for students of the social and behavioral sciences* (5th ed.). Glendale, CA: Pyrczak.

Sandelowski, M., Davis, D. H., & Harris, B. G. (1989). Artful design: Writing the proposal for research in the naturalist paradigm. *Research in Nursing & Health*, *12*(2), 77–84.

Schmitz, T., Bair, N., Falk, M., & Levine, C. (1995). A comparison of five methods of temperature measurement in febrile intensive care patients. *American Journal of Critical Care*, *4*(4), 286–292.

Schooley, J. F. (1986). *Thermometry*. Boca Raton, FL: CRC Press.

Summers, S. (1991). Axillary, tympanic, and esophageal measurement: Descriptive comparisons in postanesthesia patients. *Journal of Post Anesthesia Nursing*, *6*(6), 420–425.

Terndrup, T. E. (1992). An appraisal of temperature assessment by infrared emission detection tympanic thermometry. *Annals of Emergency Medicine*, *21*(12), 1483–1492.

Tornquist, E. M. (1999). *From proposal to publication: An informal guide to writing about nursing research* (2nd ed.). Menlo Park, CA: Addison-Wesley.

Turabian, K. L., Booth, W. C., Colomb, G. G., & Williams, J. M. (2007). *A manual for writers of research papers, theses, dissertations, seventh edition: Chicago style for students and researchers*. Chicago: University of Chicago Press.

Ulbrich, S. L. (1995). *The effect of operator technique on tympanic membrane thermometry*. Unpublished master's thesis. University of Texas at Arlington.

University of Chicago Press Staff. (2003). *The Chicago manual of style* (15th ed.). Chicago: University of Chicago Press.

U.S. Department of Health and Human Services. (2004, July 1). Information for covered entities and researchers on authorizations for research uses or disclosures of protected health information. HIPAA Privacy Rule: Information for Researchers. Retrieved October 25, 2007, from http://privacyruleandresearch.nih.gov/authorization.asp.

Vessey, J. A., & Campos, R. G. (1992). Commentary: The role of nursing research committee. *Nursing Research*, *41*(4), 247–249.

Wolff, S. M. (1988). The febrile patient. In J. B. Wyngaarden & L. H. Smith (Eds.), *Cecil textbook of medicine* (18th ed., vol. 2, pp. 1524–1525). Philadelphia: Saunders.

Wright, V. L. (2003). A phenomenological exploration of spirituality among African American women recovering from substance abuse. *Archives of Psychiatric Nursing*, *17*(4), 173–185.

Zehner, W. J., & Terndrup, T. E. (1991). The impact of moderate temperature variance on the relationship between oral, rectal, and tympanic membrane temperatures. *Clinical Pediatrics*, *30*(4 Suppl.), 61–64.

CHAPTER 29
Seeking Funding for Research

Seeking funding for research is important, both for the researcher and for the profession. Well-designed studies can be expensive. As the control of variance and the complexity of the design increase, the cost of the study tends to increase. By obtaining funding, the researcher can conduct a complex, well-designed study. Funding also indicates that others have reviewed the study and recognize its scientific and social merit. In fact, the scientific credibility of the profession is related to the quality of studies conducted by its researchers. Thus, scientific credibility and funding for research are interrelated.

The profession of nursing has invested a great deal of energy in increasing the sources of funding and amount of money available for nursing research. Each award of funding enhances the status of the researcher and increases the possibilities of greater funding for later studies. In addition, funding provides practical advantages. For example, funding may reimburse part or all of the researcher's salary and therefore release the researcher from other responsibilities, allowing the researcher to devote time to conducting the study. Funding provides you with the resources to hire research assistants and study coordinators to facilitate careful data collection and enhance your productivity. Thus, skills in seeking funding for research are as important as skills in the conduct of research.

PURPOSES FOR SEEKING RESEARCH FUNDING

Two general types of grants are sought in nursing: developmental (or program) grants and research grants. Developmental grant proposals are written to obtain funding for the development of new programs in nursing, such as a program designed to teach nurses to provide a new type of nursing care or to implement a new approach to patient care. Although these programs may involve evaluation, they seldom involve research. For example, the effectiveness of a new approach to patient care may be evaluated, but the findings can seldom be generalized beyond the unit or institution in which the patient care was provided. The emphasis is on implementing the new approach to care, not on conducting research. Research grants provide funding specifically to conduct a study. Although the two types of grant proposals have similarities, they also have important differences in writing techniques and flow of ideas, as well as content. This chapter focuses on seeking funding for research.

The researcher may have one of two purposes for seeking research funding. First, the funding may allow the researcher to conduct a single study that is of immediate concern or interest. This situation is most common among nursing students who are preparing theses and dissertations. However, nurses in clinical practice may also develop an interest in a single study that has emerged from their clinical situation. Except in unusual circumstances, the person seeking funding for a single study, such as a master's thesis, needs to consider sources of small amounts of money. In most cases, this type of funding will not reimburse for salary and will pay only a portion of the cost of the study. Sources of funding are likely to be those described in the section titled Conducting Research on a Shoestring. These funds may pay for the cost of purchasing or printing instruments, postage, research assistants' salaries, travel to data collection sites, computer analysis, the services of a statistician, or any combination of these expenses. If the researcher's experience is a positive one, further studies may be conducted later in his or her career. Thus, these small grants can be steppingstones to larger grants, such as funding for a master's thesis, predoctoral studies in preparation for the doctoral dissertation or funding for the dissertation research. Graduates from doctoral studies in nursing are now moving into post-doctoral studies that prepare them for a career as a researcher. At this point in their career, they seek funding for their post doctoral research in preparation for developing the skills required to obtain the large federal grants needed to fund a career as a nurse researcher and/or a university professor.

An individual planning to continue research activities throughout a career needs to plan a strategy for progressively seeking more extensive funding of research activities. It is unrealistic, even in a university setting, to expect to obtain the time and money needed to conduct full-time research without external funding. An aspiring career researcher needs to be willing to invest the time and energy to develop grantsmanship skills. The researcher must also develop a goal to obtain funding for that portion of time that it seems desirable to commit to research activities. The researcher should discuss this goal with administrative personnel.

An aspiring career researcher needs to initiate a program of research in a specific area of study and seek funding in this area. For example, if your research interest is to promote health in rural areas, you need to plan a series of studies that focus on promoting rural health. Even more desirable is an interdisciplinary team committed to a research program. Funding agencies are usually more supportive of researchers who focus their efforts in one area of study and are members of an interdisciplinary team. Each study conducted within this area will increase the researcher's database and familiarity with the area. Research designs can be built on previous studies. This base of previous research and knowledge greatly increases the probability of receiving further funding. Publication of the studies will also increase the credibility of the researcher.

WAYS TO LEARN GRANTSMANSHIP

Grantsmanship is not an innate skill; it must be learned. Learning the process requires a commitment of both time and energy. However, the rewards can be great. Strategies used to learn grantsmanship are described in the following sections and are listed in order of increasing time commitment, involvement, and level of expertise needed. These strategies are attending grantsmanship courses, developing a reference group, joining research

organizations, participating on research committees or review panels, networking, assisting a researcher, and obtaining a mentor.

Attending Grantsmanship Courses
Some universities offer elective courses on grantsmanship. Continuing education programs or professional conferences sometimes offer topics related to grantsmanship. The content of these sessions may include the process of grant writing, techniques for obtaining grant funds, and sources of grant funds. In some cases, representatives of funding agencies are invited to explain funding procedures. This information is useful for developing skill in writing proposals.

Developing a Reference Group
A reference group consists of individuals who share common values, ways of thinking, activities, or any combination of these traits. These individuals become a reference group when a person identifies with the group, takes on group values and behavior, and evaluates his or her own values and behavior in relation to those of the group. A new researcher moving into grantsmanship may therefore need to switch from a reference group that views research and grant writing to be either over their heads or not worth their time to a group that values this activity. From this group will come the support and feedback necessary to develop grant-writing skills.

Joining Research Organizations
Research organizations are another source of support and new information for grant writing. Regional nursing research associations, located across the United States and internationally, provide many resources useful to the neophyte researcher.

Regional Research Associations
Eastern Nursing Research Society
   www.enrs-go.org
Southern Nursing Research Society
   www.snrs.org
   e-mail: info@snrs.org
Midwest Nursing Research Society
   www.mnrs.org
   e-mail: info@mnrs.org
Western Institute of Nursing
   www.ohsu.edu/son-win
   e-mail: win@ohsu.edu

International Nursing Research Associations
Royal Windsor Society for Nurse Researchers
   www.angelfire.com/on/researchnurses/

Australia—National Health and Medical Research
Council
www.nhmrc.gov.au/
Canada—Canadian Institutes of Health Research
www.cihr-irsc.gc.ca/e/193.html
France—Association of Nursing Research
www.arsi.asso.fr
Germany—German Nursing Association, Agnes Karll
Institute for Nursing Research
www.dbfk.de/english.html
Japan—Japanese Nursing Association
www.nurse.or.jp/jna/english/index.html
The Netherlands—Netherlands Institute for Primary
Care
www.nivel.nl
New Zealand—Health Research Council
www.hrc.govt.nz
Norway—Norwegian Nurses Association
www.nosf.no
Scotland—Nursing Research Initiative for Scotland
(NRIS)
www.nris.gcal.ac.uk
United Kingdom—Research and Development
Coordination Centre
www.man.ac.uk/rcn/rs/index.htm

Other Sources of Support and Information
American Nurses Foundation
www.nursingworld.org/anf
Sigma Theta Tau Honor Society of Nursing
www.nursingsociety.org
International Institute for Qualitative Methodology
www.uofaweb.ualberta.ca/iiqm
Virginia Henderson Library—Registry of Nursing
Knowledge
www.nursinglibrary.org/portal/main.aspx
National Institute for Nursing Research
www.ninr.nih.gov
Agency for Healthcare Research and Quality
(AHRQ)—Nursing Research
www.ahcpr.gov/about/nursing
The Grantsmanship Center
www.tgci.com
University of Washington Research Funding Service
http://healthlinks.washington.edu/rfs/gw/funda-
mentals.html
Winning Grant Proposals Online
www.tgcigrantproposals.com
The Scientist—How to Wow a Study Section:
A Grantsmanship Lesson
www.mountain-research.org/grantsmanship.htm
The Foundation Center
http://cnl.foundationcenter.org/

The Internet's Nursing Resource—Nursing Research—
Funding Information
www.wwnurse.com/nursing/research-funding.
shtml
Canadian International Nurse Researcher Database
(CINRD)
www.causn.org/Databases/international_nurse_
researcher_database.htm
By searching these websites, you will find calls for proposals to which you can respond, help in writing grant proposals, nurse researchers who are interested in the same area of research, and information on nursing meetings where you can present your findings and interact with other researchers. There is a strong interest in promoting international interaction among researchers, including sharing research ideas and conducting multisite research projects. In addition to these sources, specialty nursing organizations have research groups for members interested in conducting studies related to a particular nursing specialty.

Serving on Research Committees
Research committees and institutional review boards exist in many health care and professional organizations. Through membership on these committees, contacts with researchers can be made. Also, many research committees are involved in reviewing proposals for the funding of small grants or granting approval to collect data in an institution. Reviewing proposals and making decisions about funding help researchers become better able to critique and revise their own proposals before submitting them for review.

Networking
Networking is a process of developing channels of communication among people with common interests throughout the country. Contacts may be made by computer networks, mail, telephone, or arrangements to meet in groups. Through this process, nurses interested in a particular area of study can maintain contacts made at meetings by exchanging addresses and telephone numbers. These contacts provide opportunities for brainstorming, sharing ideas and problems, and discussing grant-writing opportunities. In some cases, it is possible to write a grant to include members of a network in various parts of the country. When a proposal is being developed, the network, which may become a reference group, can provide feedback at various stages of development of the proposal.

Assisting a Researcher
Volunteering to assist with the activities of another researcher is an excellent way to learn research and

grantsmanship. Graduate students can gain this experience by becoming graduate research assistants. Assisting in grant writing and reading proposals that have been funded can be particularly helpful. Examining proposals that have been rejected can also be useful if the comments of the review committee are available. The criticisms of the review committee point out the weaknesses of the study and therefore clarify the reasons why the proposal was rejected. Examining these comments on the proposal can increase your insight as a new grant writer and prepare you for similar experiences. However, some researchers are sensitive about these criticisms and may be reluctant to share them. If an experienced researcher is willing, it is enlightening to hear his or her perceptions and opinions about the criticisms.

Obtaining a Mentor

Learning effective means of acquiring funding is difficult. Much of the information needed is transmitted verbally, requires actual participation in grant-writing activities, and is best learned in a mentor relationship. A **mentor** is a person who is more experienced professionally and willing to "teach the ropes" to a less experienced professional. Modeling is an important part of the mentoring process. This type of relationship requires a willingness by both professionals to invest time and energy. A mentor relationship has characteristics of both a teacher-learner relationship and a close friendship. Each must have an affinity for the other, from which a close working relationship can be developed. The relationship usually continues for a long time period. However, mentorship is not well developed in nursing, and nurses who have this opportunity should consider themselves fortunate. Byrne and Keefe (2002) presented an excellent discussion of the need for mentoring new researchers in their paper "Building Research Competence in Nursing through Mentoring." They pointed out emphatically that "when scholarly productivity with funded research is the desired outcome, intense involvement of a protégé with an expert researcher is essential" (p. 391).

Becoming a Funded Researcher

Many of us, as neophyte researchers, have had the fantasy of writing a grant proposal to the federal government or a large foundation for our first study and suddenly achieving "stardom" (100% of our salary and everything needed to conduct the ultimate study, including a laptop, a secretary, and multiple graduate research assistants). Unfortunately, in reality this scenario seldom occurs for an inexperienced researcher.

A new researcher is usually caught in a catch-22 situation: one needs to be an experienced researcher to get funded; however, one needs funding to get the release time needed to conduct research. One way of resolving this dilemma is to design initial studies that can realistically be done without release time and with little or no funding. This approach requires a commitment to put in extra hours of work, which is often unrewarded, monetarily or socially. However, these types of studies, when well carried out and published, will provide the credibility one needs to begin the process toward major grant funding.

The following guidance is included in "Jump Start: What to Do Before Writing a Grant Proposal" (Reif-Lehrer, 1998b):

Although having a good idea is vital for successfully writing a grant proposal ... there are other things that will help you get funded: a good reputation in your field, a solid research group, good preliminary data, and good collaborators whose skills and knowledge complement your own. ... It's good to start building your reputation early. First, make it your business to find out how academia (and your institution) really works. It is true to some extent that what matters is not just what you know, but also who you know. Try to enlist your mentor to help you make your way up the academic career ladder, but don't rely just on her or him. Build relationships with other senior faculty members who are willing to help you attain your goals. The best people in your field often have the most up-to-date information about what is going on. Don't be afraid to approach these people. Talk to them, learn from them, and "repay" them by mentoring younger people when you reach the appropriate stage of your own career. Build networks with peers in your department, in other departments, and at other universities. Learn how to get the most out of professional meetings. As a graduate student, I found attendance at my first meeting exhausting. I went to ten-minute and one-hour talks all day, every day, for all five days. When I told my research director how I spent the time, he looked me in the eye and said, "It's not what you learn at the talks, it's what you learn in the hallways that's most important." Nonetheless, it's important to give good talks at meetings because a large part of your reputation comes from your publications and the talks you give—at professional meetings and when you present seminars at your own and other institutions. Scientists who learn good communications skills early in their education have a substantial professional advantage. (Reif-Lehrer, 1998b, pp. 1–2)

You can increase your productivity by getting people around you to help you achieve your goal. Bear in mind that colleagues, administrators, and support staff are more likely to help people who are kind, generous, pleasant, and helpful than those who are selfish, surly, and demanding. Prima donnas may fare well superficially and for a while. But they tend not to do well in the long run—and even when they do, they are often not well liked. Good public relations skills are a great asset, in science as in many other professions. It rarely hurts to become known as a kind patient person who shares, helps others, and is a good mentor. (Reif-Lehrer, 1998b, p. 3)

Conducting Research on a Shoestring

Ideas for studies often begin in grandiose ways. You envision the ideal study and follow all the rules in the textbooks and in research courses. However, when you determine what is needed in time and money to conduct this wonderful study, you find your resources sadly lacking. This discovery should not lead you to give up the idea of conducting research. Rather, take stock of your resources to determine exactly what can realistically be done and then modify your study to meet existing constraints. The modified study must remain good science but be scaled down to an achievable level. Downscaling might involve studying only one aspect of the original study, decreasing the number of variables examined, or limiting the study to a single site. In many cases, a minimal amount of money is needed to conduct small studies. This project can be the pilot study that is essential to attract larger amounts of research funding.

The next step is to determine potential sources for small amounts of research money. In some cases, management in the employing institution can supply limited funding for research activities if a good case is presented for the usefulness of the study to the institution. In many universities, funds are available for intramural grants, which you can obtain competitively by submitting a brief proposal to a university committee. Some nursing organizations also have money available for research activities. For example, Sigma Theta Tau, the international honor society for nurses, provides small grants for nursing research that can be obtained through submission to international, national, regional, or local review committees. Another source is local agencies, such as the American Cancer Society and the American Heart Association. Although grants from the national offices of these organizations require sophisticated research, local or state levels of the

organization may have small amounts of funds available for studies in the organization's area of interest.

Private individuals who are locally active in philanthropy may be willing to provide financial assistance for a small study in an area appealing to them. You will need to know whom to approach and how and when to make the approach to increase the probability of successful funding. Sometimes this requires knowing someone who knows someone who might be willing to provide financial support. Acquiring funds from private individuals also requires more assertiveness than needed for other approaches to funding.

Requests for funding need not be limited to a single source. If you need a larger amount of money than one source can supply, seek funds from one source for a specific research need and from another source for another research need. Also, one source may be able to provide funds for a small segment of time; you can then approach another source to seek funding for another phase of the study. You can also combine these two strategies.

Seeking funding from local sources is less demanding in terms of formality and length of the proposal than is the case with other types of grants. Often, the process is informal and may require only a two-or three-page description of the study. The important thing is to know what funds are available and how to apply for them. Some of these funds go unused each year because nurses are not aware of their existence or think that they are unlikely to be successful in obtaining the money. This unused money leads granting agencies or potential granting agencies to conclude that nurses do not need more money for research.

Small grants are also available nationally. The American Nurses' Foundation and Sigma Theta Tau award a number of grants for less than $5000 on a yearly basis. The grants are competitive and awarded to new investigators with promising ideas, and receiving funding from these organizations is held in high regard. Information regarding these grants is available from the American Nurses' Foundation. Several federal granting agencies also provide small grants through the Public Health Service. These grants usually limit the amount of money requested to $50,000 to $75,000. Information regarding small grants can be obtained from the *Federal Register,* which is available in local libraries and online at www.gpoaccess.gov/fr/index.html.

Small grants do more than just provide the funds necessary to conduct the research. They are the first step in being recognized as a credible researcher and in being considered for more substantial grants for later studies. Receipt of these grants and your role in the grant need to be listed on curricula vitae or biographical sketches as an indication of first-level recognition as a researcher.

Seeking Funding From Specialty Practice Nursing Organizations

Many of the specialty practice nursing organizations provide support for studies relevant to their specialty, including nurse practitioner groups. These organizations often provide guidance to budding new researchers who need assistance in beginning the process of planning and seeking funding for research. To determine the resources provided by a particular nursing organization, search their website or contact the organization by e-mail, letter, or phone.

Seeking Funding from Industries

Industries are becoming a good source of funding for nursing studies, particularly if one of their products is involved in the study. For example, if a particular type of equipment is being used during an experimental treatment, the industry that developed the equipment might be willing to provide equipment for the study or may be willing to partially fund the study. If a comparison study examining outcomes of one type of dressing versus another is to be conducted, the company that produces one of the products might provide the product and/or fund the study. Some industries are particular supportive of nurses, or recognize that it is nurses who use their products and perhaps influence decisions related to selection of particular brands of products. The ethics of seeking such funding should be carefully considered, since there is sometimes a risk that the researcher might not be unbiased in interpreting study results.

Obtaining Foundation Grants

Identifying Potentially Interested Foundations

Many foundations in the United States provide funding for research, but the problem is to determine which foundations have interests in a particular field of study. Priorities for funding tend to change annually. Once you have identified these foundations, you must determine the characteristics of the foundation, select the appropriate foundations, send query letters, prepare a proposal, and, if possible, make a personal visit to the foundation. Several publications list foundations and their interests. A computerized information system, the Sponsored Programs Information Network (SPIN), can also assist you in locating the most appropriate

funding sources to support your research interests. The database contains approximately 2000 programs that provide information on federal agencies, private foundations, and corporate foundations. Many universities and research institutions have access to SPIN.

Determining Foundation Characteristics

After you have identified these foundations, gather funding information from each one. A foundation might fund only studies by female researchers, or it may be interested only in studies of low-income groups. A foundation may fund only studies being conducted in a specific geographical region. The average amount of money awarded for a single grant and the ranges of awards need to be determined for each foundation. If the average award of a particular foundation is $2500 and if $30,000 is needed, that foundation is not the most desirable source of funds. However, if you have never been funded previously and the project could be conducted with less money, you could combine an application to that foundation with applications to other foundations to obtain the funds needed. The book most useful in determining this information is *The Foundation Directory*, which is available online at http://fconline.fdncenter.org.

Verifying Institutional Support

Grant awards are most commonly made to institutions rather than to individuals. Therefore, it is important to determine the willingness of the institution to receive the grant and support the study. This willingness needs to be documented in the proposal. Supporting the study involves appropriateness of the study topic; adequacy of facilities and services; availability of space needed for the study; contributions that the institution is willing to make to the study, such as staff time, equipment, or data processing; and provision for overseeing the rights of human subjects.

Sending Query Letters

The next step is to send a query letter to foundations that might be interested in the planned study. Address the letter to the director or head of the appropriate office by name rather than to an impersonal title such as "Dear Director." Names of directors are available in a number of reference books, on the organization's website, or can be obtained by calling the organization's switchboard. Your letter needs to reflect spontaneity and enthusiasm for the study, and the opening paragraph should explain why you are sending the letter to that particular foundation. Your query letter should include a succinct description of your proposed study, an explanation of why the study is important, an indication of who will conduct the study, a description of the required facilities, and the estimated duration and cost of the study. Your qualifications for conducting the study need to be made clear. This is no time to be modest about credentials or past achievements. Inquire about the foundation's interest in the topic and information regarding how to apply for funds. If a personal visit is possible, close your letter with a request for an appointment.

Preparing Proposals

When preparing the proposal, carefully follow the foundation's guidelines for an application. In some cases, funding is sought from several sources. For example, funding requests may be submitted to an agency of the federal government, a nonprofit volunteer agency, and several private foundations. You may be tempted to send each source the same proposal rather than rewriting it to meet specific guidelines. However, this tactic can be counterproductive because your proposal will not focus on the interests of each foundation and will not be in the format requested by the foundation, which may lead to it being rejected. Developing a proposal is described in Chapter 28.

The foundation may agree to grant you a personal visit. Although the visit may be informal in a social context, foundation representatives will tend to ask hard, searching questions about the study and planned use of the funding. In a way, this interaction is similar to talking to a banker about a loan. Representatives of the foundation will ask questions geared to helping them to determine the following: Is the study feasible? Is the institution willing to provide sufficient support to permit the study to be completed? Is the researcher using all available resources? Have other sources of funding been sought? Has the researcher examined anticipated costs in detail and been realistic? What are the benefits of conducting the study? Who will benefit, and how? Is the researcher likely to complete the study? Are the findings likely to be published? If the written proposal has not been submitted, the visit is an appropriate time to submit it. Additional information or notes prepared for the visit can be left with foundation representatives for consideration as the decision is made.

OBTAINING FEDERAL GRANTS

The largest source of grant monies is the federal government—so much so that, in effect, the federal government influences what is studied and what is not. Funding can be requested from multiple divisions of the government. Information on funding agencies can be obtained from a document compiled by the federal government, *The Catalog of Federal Domestic Assistance*, which is available online at www.cfda.gov. The National Institutes of Health (NIH), particularly the National Institute for Nursing Research, are particularly interested in receiving nursing proposals, as is the Agency for Healthcare Research and Quality (AHRQ). Each agency has areas of focus and priorities for funding that change yearly. It is important to know this information and prepare proposals within these areas to obtain funding. This information is available online at www.grants.gov, a searchable listing of all federal research funding opportunities.

Two approaches can be used to seek federal funding for research. As the researcher, you can identify a significant problem, develop a study to examine it, and submit a proposal for the study to the appropriate federal funding agency. Alternatively, an agency within the federal government can identify a significant problem, develop a plan by which the problem can be studied, and publish a request for proposals (RFP) or a request for applications (RFA) from researchers.

Reif-Lehrer (1998b) provided excellent guidance for researchers who are seeking federal funding:

> *To get funding from a major government agency today you need a reasonable amount of good preliminary data. These data must indicate to the reviewers that you can wisely and expediently carry out the project, that the experiments are feasible, and that the data obtained are likely to move the field ahead in some substantive way. (Reif-Lehrer, 1998b, p. 4)*

Researcher-Initiated Proposals

If the study is researcher initiated, it is useful for the researcher to contact an official within the government agency early in the planning process to inform the agency of the intent to submit a proposal. Each agency has established dates, usually three times a year, when proposals are reviewed. You will need to start preparing your proposal months ahead of this deadline, and some agencies are willing to provide assistance and feedback to the researcher during development of the proposal. This assistance may occur through e-mail, telephone conversations, or feedback on a draft of the proposal.

Early in the process of planning a study for which you intend to seek federal funding, it is wise to determine what studies on your topic of interest have previously been funded and what funded studies are currently in process. This information is available on CRISP (Computer Retrieval of Information on

Scientific Products). This information is available at the following government website: http://crisp. cit.nih.gov.According to the website information: "The database, maintained by the Office of Extramural Research at the National Institutes of Health, includes projects funded by the National Institutes of Health (NIH), Substance Abuse and Mental Health Services (SAMHSA), Health Resources and Services Administration (HRSA), Food and Drug Administration (FDA), Centers for Disease Control and Prevention (CDCP), Agency for Health Care Research and Quality (AHRQ), and Office of Assistant Secretary of Health (OASH). Users, including the public, can use the CRISP interface to search for scientific concepts, emerging trends and techniques, or identify specific projects and/or investigators."

Reviewing proposals that have been funded by that agency can be helpful. Although the agency cannot provide these proposals, researchers can sometimes obtain them by contacting the principal investigator (PI) of the study personally. In some cases, the researcher may travel to Washington to meet with an agency representative. This type of contact allows the researcher to modify the proposal to fit more closely within agency guidelines, thus increasing the probability of funding. In many cases, proposals will fit within the interests of more than one government agency at the time of submission. It is permissible and perhaps desirable to request that the proposal be assigned to two agencies within the Public Health Service.

Requests for Proposals

An RFP is published in the *Federal Register* and usually has a deadline date that is only a few weeks after publication. Therefore, the researcher needs to have a good background in the field of study and be able to write a proposal quickly. Because a number of researchers will be responding to the same RFP and only one or a few proposals will be approved, these proposals are competitive. The agency staff will not be able to provide the same type of feedback as occurs in researcher-initiated proposals. The agency needs to be informed that a proposal is being submitted. Some questions that require clarification about elements of the RFP can be answered; however, other questions cannot be answered because the proposals are competitive and answering might give one researcher an advantage over others. An RFP allows a wide range of creativity in developing a study design to examine the problem of concern.

Requests for Applications

An RFA is similar to an RFP except that with an RFA, the government agency not only identifies the problem of concern but also describes the design of the study. An RFA is a contract for which researchers bid. A carefully written proposal is still required and needs to follow the RFA in detail. After funding, federal agency staff maintains much more control and supervision over the process of the study than is the case with an RFP.

Developing a Proposal

One of the quickest ways to get help in writing a research proposal is to do a Google search using the terms "Writing Research Grants" and "Writing Research Proposals." Many of the universities have Web-based assistance available, as do the government agencies. Another strategy is to do an electronic search of bookstores for the most recent sources. One recent book of interest is *Writing the NIH Grant Proposal: A Step-by-Step Guide* by William Gerin (2006). Others include *Research Proposals: A Guide by Success* by Thomas E. Ogden and Israel A. Goldberg (2002), *Proposal Writing* by Soraya M. Coley and Cynthia A. Scheinberg (2000), and *Developing Effective Research Proposals* by Keith F. Punch (2006). A book that has received rave reviews is Susan Golden's (1997) *Secrets of Successful Grantsmanship: A Guerrilla Guide to Raising Money*. Another book useful for the beginner is Beverly Browning's (2005) *Grant Writing for Dummies*. A considerable number of books on grantsmanship are available in libraries and bookstores to fit the needs of researchers in various stages of their career.

Set aside sufficient time to carefully develop your proposal, including rewriting the text several times. Writing your first proposal on a tight deadline is not wise. We recommend that you plan on 6 to 12 months for proposal development from the point of early development of your research ideas. Contact the agency to obtain written guidelines, and follow them rigidly. Strictly adhere to the page limitations and type sizes requested. Reif-Lehrer (1998a) pointed out that

> the best writing can't turn a bad idea into a good grant proposal, but bad writing can turn a good idea into an unfunded proposal.... A good proposal idea must also tweak the reviewers' imagination.... Investigators must energetically convey their enthusiasm and sense of excitement about their work and the new research directions they are planning. If the researcher can concretely and clearly describe what is known, and then present a logical leap forward into the unknown, there is great potential for capturing the reviewers' interest. (pp. 1–2)

Input from colleagues can be invaluable in refining your ideas. You need individuals whose opinions you trust and who will go beyond telling you globally how magnificent your proposal is. Seek individuals who have experience in grant writing and are willing to critique your proposal thoroughly and point out its flaws. After you have used their feedback to revise the proposal, contact a nationally known expert in your research field who will agree to examine your proposal critically. Be prepared to pay a consultant fee for this service.

Neophytes are least willing to request a critique by colleagues and experts. There is almost a desire to write the proposal in secrecy, submit it quietly, and wait for the letter from the funding agency. That way, if you fail, no one will know about it. If others do know that a proposal is being developed, another strategy is often used. The author furiously writes up to the very last possible deadline and then, in exhaustion, proclaims that there is no time for review before it is submitted. Both these strategies almost guarantee that the proposal will be rejected. Remember, the critiques of your friends and the expert you have sought are unlikely to be as devastating as that of reviewers at the funding agency. Moreover, you have a chance to make changes after your friends review it. Most, if not all, proposals to the federal government must be submitted online.

Electronic Submission of Grant Proposals

The National Institutes of Health Office of Extramural Research provides a Grants website (http://grants.nih.gov/grants/grants_process.htm) that provides a detailed explanation of their electronic grant application process. They provide step-by-step instructions: planning your application, writing your application, how to apply, receipt and referral, peer review process, grant award, and award management. You use an electronic form to write your proposal, submit your proposal electronically, communicate with the agency by e-mail, and the results of the review are sent to you by e-mail. The time required to complete the process is a minimum of one year. The AHRQ electronic process is described at their website: www.ahrq.gov/path/egrants.htm.

The Federal Grant Review Process

After submission, a grant is assigned to a study section for scientific evaluation. The study sections have no alignment with the funding agency. Thus, staff in the agencies have no influence on the committee's work of judging the scientific merit of the proposal. The proposal is given to two or more researchers from the study section who are considered qualified to evaluate the proposal. These scientists prepare a written critique of the study. The proposal is then sent to all the members of the study section. Each member may have 50 to 100 proposals to read in a 1- to 2-month period. A meeting of the full study section is then held. Those who critiqued the proposal discuss each application, and other members comment or ask questions. A majority vote determines whether the proposal is approved, disapproved, or deferred.

Approved proposals are assigned a numerical score used to develop a priority rating. A study that is approved is not necessarily funded. The PI will be notified at this point whether the study was approved. At a later time, approved studies are further examined to determine actual funding. Funding begins with the proposal that has the highest rank order and continues until available funds are depleted. This process can take 6 months or longer. Because of this process, researchers may not receive the money to initiate a grant for up to a year after submitting the proposal.

Often, researcher-initiated proposals are rejected (or approved but not funded) after the first submission. The critique of the scientific committee, called a summary statement, is available to the researcher via his or her eCommons account. Frequently, the agency staff will encourage the researcher to rewrite the proposal with guidance from comments and resubmit it to the same agency. The probability of funding is often greater the second time if the researcher has followed the suggestions.

Review of RFPs or RFAs is slightly different. These applications first go through technical (scientific) evaluation. Proposals that pass the technical review are then evaluated from the standpoint of cost. After the financial review, the contracting officer may negotiate levels of funding with the proposal writers. Funding decisions are based on the identification of well-designed proposals that offer the best financial advantage to the government (White, 1975).

Rejected Grant Proposals

The researcher's reaction to a rejected proposal is usually anger and then depression. The frustrated researcher may abandon the proposal, stuff it in a bottom drawer somewhere, and forgot it. There seems to be no way to avoid the anger and depression after a rejection because of the amount of emotion and time invested in writing it. However, after a few weeks it is advisable to examine the rejection letter again. The comments can be useful in rewriting the proposal for resubmission. The learning experience of rewriting the proposal and evaluating the comments will also provide a background for seeking funding for another study.

A skilled grant writer will have approximately one proposal funded for every five submitted. The average is far less than this. Thus, the researcher needs to be committed to submitting proposals repeatedly to achieve grant funding.

GRANT MANAGEMENT

Receiving notice that a grant proposal has been funded is one of the highlights in a researcher's career and warrants a celebration. However, when the euphoria begins to fade and reality sets in, you will need to make careful plans for implementing the study. To avoid problems, you need to consider managing the budget, hiring and training research personnel, maintaining the promised timetable, and coordinating activities of the study. In addition to the suggestions given in the following sections, Selby-Harrington, Donat, and Hibbard (1994) provided some excellent guidance in grant management from their experience as PIs of a federally funded grant.

Managing the Budget

Although the supporting institution is ultimately responsible for dispensing and controlling grant monies, the PI is also responsible for keeping track of budget expenditures and making decisions about how the money is to be spent. If this grant is the first one received, a PI who has no previous administrative experience may need some initial guidance in how to keep records and make reasonable budget decisions. If funding is through a federal agency, the PI will be required to provide interim reports, as well as updates on the progress of the study.

Training Research Personnel

When a new grant is initiated, set aside time to interview, hire, and train grant personnel. The personnel who will be involved in data collection need to learn the process, and then data collection needs to be refined to ensure that each data collector is consistent with the other data collectors. This process helps ensure interrater reliability. The PI needs to set aside time to oversee the work of personnel hired for the grant.

Maintaining the Study Schedule

The timetable submitted with the proposal needs to be adhered to whenever possible, which requires careful planning. Otherwise, other work activities are likely to take precedence and delay the grant work. Unexpected events do happen; however, careful planning can minimize their impact. The PI needs to constantly refer back to the timetable to evaluate progress. If the project falls behind schedule, action needs to be taken to return to the original schedule or to readjust the timetable. Keeping on schedule will be a plus when it is time to apply for the next grant.

Coordinating Activities

During a large study with several investigators and other grant personnel, coordinating activities can be a problem. Arrange meetings of all grant workers at intervals to share ideas and solve problems. Keep records of the discussions at these meetings. These actions can lead to a more smoothly functioning team.

Submitting Reports

Federal grants require the submission of interim reports according to preset deadlines. The notice of grant award sent as a PDF (Portable Document Format) document via e-mail will include guidelines for the content of the reports, which will consist of a description of grant activities. Set aside time to prepare the report, which usually requires compiling figures and tables. In addition to the written reports, it is often useful to maintain contact with the appropriate staff at the federal agency.

PLANNING YOUR NEXT GRANT

The researcher should not wait until funding from the first grant has ended to begin seeking funds for a second study because of the length of time required to obtain funding. In fact, it may be wise to have several ongoing studies in various stages of implementation. For example, you could be planning a study, collecting data on a second study, analyzing data on a third study, and writing papers for publication on a fourth study. A full-time researcher could have completed one funded study, be in the last year of funding for a second study, be in the first year of funding for a third study, and be seeking funding for a fourth study. This scenario may sound unrealistic, but with planning, it is not. This strategy not only provides continuous funding for research activities but also facilitates a rhythm of research that prevents time pressures and makes use of lulls in activity in a particular study. To increase the ease of obtaining funding, the studies need to be within the same area of research, each building on previous studies.

SUMMARY

- To receive funding, researchers need to learn grantsmanship skills.
- Writing a grant proposal for funding requires a commitment to putting in extra hours of work.
- The first studies are usually conducted on a shoestring budget. Researchers can seek larger sums of money by writing for foundation grants.
- The largest source of grant monies is the federal government.
- The researcher can identify a significant problem, develop a study to examine it, and submit a proposal for the study to an appropriate federal funding agency.
- Alternatively, someone within the federal government can identify a significant problem, develop a plan through which the problem can be studied, and publish an RFP or an RFA from researchers.
- When a grant proposal is funded, it is a time for the researcher to celebrate. However, the researcher then needs to make careful plans for implementing the study.
- The PI is responsible for keeping up with the budget, training research personnel, maintaining the schedule, and coordinating activities.
- Federal grants also require the submission of interim reports.
- A researcher should not wait until funding from the first grant has ended to begin seeking funds for a second study (and then a third and then a fourth).

REFERENCES

Browning, B. A. (2005). *Grant writing for dummies*. Somerset, NJ: Wiley.

Byrne, M. W., & Keefe, M. R. (2002). Building research competence in nursing through mentoring. *Journal of Nursing Scholarship*, *34*(4), 391–396.

Reif-Lehrer, L. (1998a, May 1). Going for the gold. *HMS Beagle (online), issue 29*. Retrieved May 26, 2008, from www.indiana.edu/~gradgrnt/pubs/Going%20For%20The%20Gold.pdf.

Reif-Lehrer, L. (1998b, June 26). Jump start: What to do before writing a grant proposal. *HMS Beagle, issue 33*.

Selby-Harrington, M. L., Donat, P. L. M., & Hibbard, H. D (1994). Research grant implementation: Staff development as a tool to accomplish research activities. *Applied Nursing Research*, *7*(1), 38–46.

APPENDIX A

Percentage Points of Student's *t* Distribution

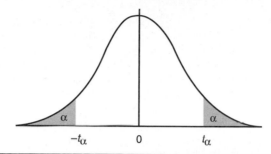

df	α 0.25 2α 0.50	0.20 0.40	0.15 0.30	0.10 0.20	0.05 0.10	0.025 0.05	0.01 0.02	0.005 0.01	0.0005 0.001
1	1.000	1.376	1.963	3.078	6.314	12.706	31.821	63.657	636.619
2	0.816	1.061	1.386	1.886	2.920	4.303	6.965	9.925	31.598
3	0.765	0.978	1.250	1.638	2.353	3.182	4.541	5.841	12.924
4	0.741	0.941	1.190	1.533	2.132	2.776	3.747	4.604	8.610
5	0.727	0.920	1.156	1.476	2.015	2.571	3.365	4.032	6.869
6	0.718	0.906	1.134	1.440	1.943	2.447	3.143	3.707	5.959
7	0.711	0.896	1.119	1.415	1.895	2.365	2.998	3.499	5.408
8	0.706	0.889	1.108	1.397	1.860	2.306	2.896	3.355	5.041
9	0.703	0.883	1.100	1.383	1.833	2.262	2.821	3.250	4.781
10	0.700	0.879	1.093	1.372	1.812	2.228	2.764	3.169	4.587
11	0.697	0.876	1.088	1.363	1.796	2.201	2.718	3.106	4.437
12	0.695	0.873	1.083	1.356	1.782	2.179	2.681	3.055	4.318
13	0.694	0.870	1.079	1.350	1.771	2.160	2.650	3.012	4.221
14	0.692	0.868	1.076	1.345	1.761	2.145	2.624	2.977	4.140
15	0.691	0.866	1.074	1.341	1.753	2.131	2.602	2.947	4.073
16	0.690	0.865	1.071	1.337	1.746	2.120	2.583	2.921	4.015
17	0.689	0.863	1.069	1.333	1.740	2.110	2.567	2.898	3.965
18	0.688	0.862	1.067	1.330	1.734	2.101	2.552	2.878	3.922
19	0.688	0.861	1.066	1.328	1.729	2.093	2.539	2.861	3.883
20	0.687	0.860	1.064	1.325	1.725	2.086	2.528	2.845	3.850
21	0.686	0.859	1.063	1.323	1.721	2.080	2.518	2.831	3.819
22	0.686	0.858	1.061	1.321	1.717	2.074	2.508	2.819	3.792
23	0.685	0.858	1.060	1.319	1.714	2.069	2.500	2.807	3.767
24	0.685	0.857	1.059	1.318	1.711	2.064	2.492	2.797	3.745
25	0.684	0.856	1.058	1.316	1.708	2.060	2.458	2.787	3.725
26	0.684	0.856	1.058	1.315	1.706	2.056	2.479	2.779	3.707
27	0.684	0.855	1.057	1.314	1.703	2.052	2.473	2.771	3.690
28	0.683	0.855	1.056	1.313	1.701	2.048	2.467	2.763	3.674
29	0.683	0.854	1.055	1.311	1.699	2.045	2.462	2.756	3.659
30	0.683	0.854	1.055	1.310	1.697	2.042	2.457	2.750	3.646
40	0.681	0.851	1.050	1.303	1.684	2.021	2.423	2.704	3.551
60	0.679	0.848	1.046	1.296	1.671	2.000	2.390	2.660	3.460
120	0.677	0.845	1.041	1.289	1.658	1.980	2.358	2.617	3.373
∞	0.674	0.842	1.036	1.282	1.645	1.960	2.326	2.576	3.291

This table is taken from Table III p. 46 of *Statistical Tables for Biological Agricultural and Medical Research* (6th ed.), by R. A. Fisher and F. Yates, 1974, published by Longman Group UK Ltd., London. By permission of the authors and publisher.

APPENDIX B

Percentage Points of the F Distribution

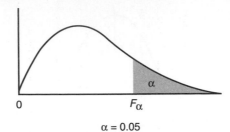

$\alpha = 0.05$

Degrees of Freedom

V_1

V_2	1	2	3	4	5	6	7	8	9
1	161.4	199.5	215.7	224.6	230.2	234.0	236.8	238.9	240.5
2	18.51	19.00	19.16	19.25	19.30	19.33	19.35	19.37	19.38
3	10.13	9.55	9.28	9.12	9.01	8.94	8.89	8.85	8.81
4	7.71	6.94	6.59	6.39	6.26	6.16	6.09	6.04	6.00
5	6.61	5.79	5.41	5.19	5.05	4.95	4.88	4.82	4.77
6	5.99	5.14	4.76	4.53	4.39	4.28	4.21	4.15	4.10
7	5.59	4.74	4.35	4.12	3.97	3.87	3.79	3.73	3.68
8	5.32	4.46	4.07	3.84	3.69	3.58	3.50	3.44	3.39
9	5.12	4.26	3.86	3.63	3.48	3.37	3.29	3.23	3.18
10	4.96	4.10	3.71	3.48	3.33	3.22	3.14	3.07	3.02
11	4.84	3.98	3.59	3.36	3.20	3.09	3.01	2.95	2.90
12	4.75	3.89	3.49	3.26	3.11	3.00	2.91	2.85	2.80
13	4.67	3.81	3.41	3.18	3.03	2.92	2.83	2.77	2.71
14	4.60	3.74	3.34	3.11	2.96	2.85	2.76	2.70	2.65
15	4.54	3.68	3.29	3.06	2.90	2.79	2.71	2.64	2.59
16	4.49	3.63	3.24	3.01	2.85	2.74	2.66	2.59	2.54
17	4.45	3.59	3.20	2.96	2.81	2.70	2.61	2.55	2.49
18	4.41	3.55	3.16	2.93	2.77	2.66	2.58	2.51	2.46
19	4.38	3.52	3.13	2.90	2.74	2.63	2.54	2.48	2.42
20	4.35	3.49	3.10	2.87	2.71	2.60	2.51	2.45	2.39
21	4.32	3.47	3.07	2.84	2.68	2.57	2.49	2.42	2.37
22	4.30	3.44	3.05	2.82	2.66	2.55	2.46	2.40	2.34
23	4.28	3.42	3.03	2.80	2.64	2.53	2.44	2.37	2.32
24	4.26	3.40	3.01	2.78	2.62	2.51	2.42	2.36	2.30
25	4.24	3.39	2.99	2.76	2.60	2.49	2.40	2.34	2.28
26	4.23	3.37	2.98	2.74	2.59	2.47	2.39	2.32	2.27
27	4.21	3.35	2.96	2.73	2.57	2.46	2.37	2.31	2.25
28	4.20	3.34	2.95	2.71	2.56	2.45	2.36	2.29	2.24
29	4.18	3.33	2.93	2.70	2.55	2.43	2.35	2.28	2.22
30	4.17	3.32	2.92	2.69	2.53	2.42	2.33	2.27	2.21
40	4.08	3.23	2.84	2.61	2.45	2.34	2.25	2.18	2.12
60	4.00	3.15	2.76	2.53	2.37	2.25	2.17	2.10	2.04
120	3.92	3.07	2.68	2.45	2.29	2.17	2.09	2.02	1.96
∞	3.84	3.00	2.60	2.37	2.21	2.10	2.01	1.94	1.88

Continued

APPENDIX B—Cont'd

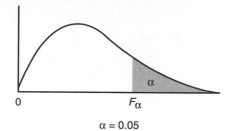

$\alpha = 0.05$

V₁

10	12	15	20	24	30	40	60	120	∞	V₂
241.9	243.9	245.9	248.0	249.1	250.1	251.1	252.2	253.3	254.3	1
19.40	19.41	19.43	19.45	19.45	19.46	19.47	19.48	19.49	19.50	2
8.79	8.74	8.70	8.66	8.64	8.62	8.59	8.57	8.55	8.53	3
5.96	5.91	5.86	5.80	5.77	5.75	5.72	5.69	5.66	5.63	4
4.74	4.68	4.62	4.56	4.53	4.50	4.46	4.43	4.40	4.36	5
4.06	4.00	3.94	3.87	3.84	3.81	3.77	3.74	3.70	3.67	6
3.64	3.57	3.51	3.44	3.41	3.38	3.34	3.30	3.27	3.23	7
3.35	3.28	3.22	3.15	3.12	3.08	3.04	3.01	2.97	2.93	8
3.14	3.07	3.01	2.94	2.90	2.86	2.83	2.79	2.75	2.71	9
2.98	2.91	2.85	2.77	2.74	2.70	2.66	2.62	2.58	2.54	10
2.85	2.79	2.72	2.65	2.61	2.57	2.53	2.49	2.45	2.40	11
2.75	2.69	2.62	2.54	2.51	2.47	2.43	2.38	2.34	2.30	12
2.67	2.60	2.53	2.46	2.42	2.38	2.34	2.30	2.25	2.21	13
2.60	2.53	2.46	2.39	2.35	2.31	2.27	2.22	2.18	2.13	14
2.54	2.48	2.40	2.33	2.29	2.25	2.20	2.16	2.11	2.07	15
2.49	2.42	2.35	2.28	2.24	2.19	2.15	2.11	2.06	2.01	16
2.45	2.38	2.31	2.23	2.19	2.15	2.10	2.06	2.01	1.96	17
2.41	2.34	2.27	2.19	2.15	2.11	2.06	2.02	1.97	1.92	18
2.38	2.31	2.23	2.16	2.11	2.07	2.03	1.98	1.93	1.88	19
2.35	2.28	2.20	2.12	2.08	2.04	1.99	1.95	1.90	1.84	20
2.32	2.25	2.18	2.10	2.05	2.01	1.96	1.92	1.87	1.81	21
2.30	2.23	2.15	2.07	2.03	1.98	1.94	1.89	1.84	1.78	22
2.27	2.20	2.13	2.05	2.01	1.96	1.91	1.86	1.81	1.76	23
2.25	2.18	2.11	2.03	1.98	1.94	1.89	1.84	1.79	1.73	24
2.24	2.16	2.09	2.01	1.96	1.92	1.87	1.82	1.77	1.71	25
2.22	2.15	2.07	1.99	1.95	1.90	1.85	1.80	1.75	1.69	26
2.20	2.13	2.06	1.97	1.93	1.88	1.84	1.79	1.73	1.67	27
2.19	2.12	2.04	1.96	1.91	1.87	1.82	1.77	1.71	1.65	28
2.18	2.10	2.03	1.94	1.90	1.85	1.81	1.75	1.70	1.64	29
2.16	2.09	2.01	1.93	1.89	1.84	1.79	1.74	1.68	1.62	30
2.08	2.00	1.92	1.84	1.79	1.74	1.69	1.64	1.58	1.51	40
1.99	1.92	1.84	1.75	1.70	1.65	1.59	1.53	1.47	1.39	60
1.91	1.83	1.75	1.66	1.61	1.55	1.50	1.43	1.35	1.25	120
1.83	1.75	1.67	1.57	1.52	1.46	1.39	1.32	1.22	1.00	∞

APPENDIX B—Cont'd

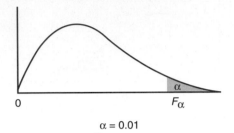

$\alpha = 0.01$

Degrees of Freedom

$$V_1$$

V_2	1	2	3	4	5	6	7	8	9
1	4052	4999.5	5403	5625	5764	5859	5928	5982	6022
2	98.50	99.00	99.17	99.25	99.30	99.33	99.36	99.37	99.39
3	34.12	30.82	29.46	28.71	28.24	27.91	27.67	27.49	27.35
4	21.20	18.00	16.69	15.98	15.52	15.21	14.98	14.80	14.66
5	16.26	13.27	12.06	11.39	10.97	10.67	10.46	10.29	10.16
6	13.75	10.92	9.78	9.15	8.75	8.47	8.26	8.10	7.98
7	12.25	9.55	8.45	7.85	7.46	7.19	6.99	6.84	6.72
8	11.26	8.65	7.59	7.01	6.63	6.37	6.18	6.03	5.91
9	10.56	8.02	6.99	6.42	6.06	5.80	5.61	5.47	5.35
10	10.04	7.56	6.55	5.99	5.64	5.39	5.20	5.06	4.94
11	9.65	7.21	6.22	5.67	5.32	5.07	4.89	4.74	4.63
12	9.33	6.93	5.95	5.41	5.06	4.82	4.64	4.50	4.39
13	9.07	6.70	5.74	5.21	4.86	4.62	4.44	4.30	4.19
14	8.86	6.51	5.56	5.04	4.69	4.46	4.28	4.14	4.03
15	8.68	6.36	5.42	4.89	4.56	4.32	4.14	4.00	3.89
16	8.53	6.23	5.29	4.77	4.44	4.20	4.03	3.89	3.78
17	8.40	6.11	5.18	4.67	4.34	4.10	3.93	3.79	3.68
18	8.29	6.01	5.09	4.58	4.25	4.01	3.84	3.71	3.60
19	8.18	5.93	5.01	4.50	4.17	3.94	3.77	3.63	3.52
20	8.10	5.85	4.94	4.43	4.10	3.87	3.70	3.56	3.46
21	8.02	5.78	4.87	4.37	4.04	3.81	3.64	3.51	3.40
22	7.95	5.72	4.82	4.31	3.99	3.76	3.59	3.45	3.35
23	7.88	5.66	4.76	4.26	3.94	3.71	3.54	3.41	3.30
24	7.82	5.61	4.72	4.22	3.90	3.67	3.50	3.36	3.26
25	7.77	5.57	4.68	4.18	3.85	3.63	3.46	3.32	3.22
26	7.72	5.53	4.64	4.14	3.82	3.59	3.42	3.29	3.19
27	7.68	5.49	4.60	4.11	3.78	3.56	3.39	3.26	3.15
28	7.64	5.45	4.57	4.07	3.75	3.53	3.36	3.23	2.12
29	7.60	5.42	4.54	4.04	3.73	3.50	3.33	3.20	3.09
30	7.56	5.39	4.51	4.02	3.70	3.47	3.30	3.17	3.07
40	7.31	5.18	4.31	3.83	3.51	3.29	3.12	2.99	2.89
60	7.08	4.98	4.13	3.65	3.34	3.12	2.95	2.82	2.72
120	6.85	4.79	3.95	3.48	3.17	2.96	2.79	2.66	2.56
∞	6.63	4.61	3.78	3.32	3.02	2.80	2.64	2.51	2.41

Continued

APPENDIX B—Cont'd

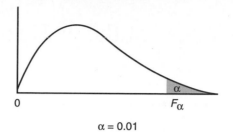

$\alpha = 0.01$

V_1

10	12	15	20	24	30	40	60	120	∞	V_2
6056	6106	6157	6209	6235	6261	6287	6313	6339	6366	1
99.40	99.42	99.43	99.45	99.46	99.47	99.47	99.48	99.49	99.50	2
27.23	27.05	26.87	26.69	26.60	26.50	26.41	26.32	26.22	26.13	3
14.55	14.37	14.20	14.02	13.93	13.84	13.75	13.65	13.56	13.46	4
10.05	9.89	9.72	9.55	9.47	9.38	9.29	9.20	9.11	9.02	5
7.87	7.72	7.56	7.40	7.31	7.23	7.14	7.06	6.97	6.88	6
6.62	6.47	6.31	6.16	6.07	5.99	5.91	5.82	5.74	5.65	7
5.81	5.67	5.52	5.36	5.28	5.20	5.12	5.03	4.95	4.86	8
5.26	5.11	4.96	4.81	4.73	4.65	4.57	4.48	4.40	4.31	9
4.85	4.71	4.56	4.41	4.33	4.25	4.17	4.08	4.00	3.91	10
4.54	4.40	4.25	4.10	4.02	3.94	3.86	3.78	3.69	3.60	11
4.30	4.16	4.01	3.86	3.78	3.70	3.62	3.54	3.45	3.36	12
4.10	3.96	3.82	3.66	3.59	3.51	3.43	3.34	3.25	3.17	13
3.94	3.80	3.66	3.51	3.43	3.35	3.27	3.18	3.09	3.00	14
3.80	3.67	3.52	3.37	3.29	3.21	3.13	3.05	2.96	2.87	15
3.69	3.55	3.41	3.26	3.18	3.10	3.02	2.93	2.84	2.75	16
3.59	3.46	3.31	3.16	3.08	3.00	2.92	2.83	2.75	2.65	17
3.51	3.37	3.23	3.08	3.00	2.92	2.84	2.75	2.66	2.57	18
3.43	3.30	3.15	3.00	2.92	2.84	2.76	2.67	2.58	2.49	19
3.37	3.23	3.09	2.94	2.86	2.78	2.69	2.61	2.52	2.42	20
3.31	3.17	3.03	2.88	2.80	2.72	2.64	2.55	2.46	2.36	21
3.26	3.12	2.98	2.83	2.75	2.67	2.58	2.50	2.40	2.31	22
3.21	3.07	2.93	2.78	2.70	2.62	2.54	2.45	2.35	2.26	23
3.17	3.03	2.89	2.74	2.66	2.58	2.49	2.40	2.31	2.21	24
3.13	2.99	2.85	2.70	2.62	2.54	2.45	2.36	2.27	2.17	25
3.09	2.96	2.81	2.66	2.58	2.50	2.42	2.33	2.23	2.13	26
3.06	2.93	2.78	2.63	2.55	2.47	2.38	2.29	2.20	2.10	27
3.03	2.90	2.75	2.60	2.52	2.44	2.35	2.26	2.17	2.06	28
3.00	2.87	2.73	2.57	2.49	2.41	2.33	2.23	2.14	2.03	29
2.98	2.84	2.70	2.55	2.47	2.39	2.30	2.21	2.11	2.01	30
2.80	2.66	2.52	2.37	2.29	2.20	2.11	2.02	1.92	1.80	40
2.63	2.50	2.35	2.20	2.12	2.03	1.94	1.84	1.73	1.60	60
2.47	2.34	2.19	2.03	1.95	1.86	1.76	1.66	1.53	1.38	120
2.32	2.18	2.04	1.88	1.79	1.70	1.59	1.47	1.32	1.00	∞

From "Tables of Percentage Points of the Inverted Beta (F) Distribution," by M. Merrington and C. M. Thompson, 1943, *Biometrika* 33(1), pp. 73–78.

APPENDIX C

Critical Values of the χ^2 Distribution

df	$P_{0.5}$	P_{01}	$P_{02.5}$	P_{05}	P_{10}	P_{90}	P_{95}	$P_{97.5}$	P_{99}	$P_{99.5}$
1	0.000039	0.00016	0.00098	0.0039	0.0158	2.71	3.84	5.02	6.63	7.88
2	0.0100	0.0201	0.0506	0.1026	0.2107	4.61	5.99	7.38	9.21	10.60
3	0.0717	0.115	0.216	0.352	0.584	6.25	7.81	9.35	11.34	12.84
4	0.207	0.297	0.484	0.711	1.064	7.78	9.49	11.14	13.28	14.86
5	0.412	0.554	0.831	1.15	1.61	9.24	11.07	12.83	15.09	16.75
6	0.676	0.872	1.24	1.64	2.20	10.64	12.59	14.45	16.81	18.55
7	0.989	1.24	1.69	2.17	2.83	12.02	14.07	16.01	18.48	20.28
8	1.34	1.65	2.18	2.73	3.49	13.36	15.51	17.53	20.09	21.96
9	1.73	2.09	2.70	3.33	4.17	14.68	16.92	19.02	21.67	23.59
10	2.16	2.56	3.25	3.94	4.87	15.99	18.31	20.48	23.21	25.19
11	2.60	3.05	3.82	4.57	5.58	17.28	19.68	21.92	24.73	26.76
12	3.07	3.57	4.40	5.23	6.30	18.55	21.03	23.34	26.22	28.30
13	3.57	4.11	5.01	5.89	7.04	19.81	22.36	24.74	27.69	29.82
14	4.07	4.66	5.63	6.57	7.79	21.06	23.68	26.12	29.14	31.32
15	4.60	5.23	6.26	7.26	8.55	22.31	25.00	27.49	30.58	32.80
16	5.14	5.81	6.91	7.96	9.31	23.54	26.30	28.85	32.00	34.27
18	6.26	7.01	8.23	9.39	10.86	25.99	28.87	31.53	34.81	37.16
20	7.43	8.26	9.59	10.85	12.44	28.41	31.41	34.17	37.57	40.00
24	9.89	10.86	12.40	13.85	15.66	33.20	36.42	39.36	42.98	45.56
30	13.79	14.95	16.79	18.49	20.60	40.26	42.77	46.98	50.98	53.67
40	20.71	22.16	24.43	26.51	29.05	51.81	55.76	59.34	63.69	66.77
60	35.33	37.48	40.48	43.19	46.46	74.40	79.08	83.30	88.38	91.95
120	83.85	86.92	91.58	95.70	100.62	140.23	146.57	152.21	158.95	163.64

From *Introduction to Statistical Analysis* (3rd ed.), by W. J. Dixon and F. J. Massey, Jr, 1969, New York: McGraw-Hill.

APPENDIX D

Statistical Power Tables (Δ = Effect Size)

Master Table

5% Level, One-Tailed Test

Δ	99	95	90	80	Power 70	60	50	40	30	20	10
0.01	157695	108215	85634	61823	47055	36031	27055	19363	12555	6453	1321
0.02	39417	27050	21405	15454	11763	9007	6764	4841	3139	1614	331
0.03	17514	12019	9511	6867	5227	4003	3006	2152	1396	718	148
0.04	9848	6578	5348	3861	2939	2251	1691	1210	785	404	84
0.05	6299	4323	3421	2470	1881	1440	1082	775	503	259	54
0.06	4372	3000	2375	1715	1305	1000	751	538	349	180	38
0.07	3209	2203	1744	1259	959	734	552	395	257	133	29
0.08	2455	1685	1334	963	734	562	422	303	197	102	23
0.09	1938	1330	1053	761	579	444	334	239	156	81	18
0.10	1568	1076	852	616	469	359	270	194	126	66	15
0.11	1294	889	704	508	387	297	223	160	104	54	13
0.12	1086	746	590	427	325	249	188	135	88	46	11
0.13	924	635	503	363	277	212	160	115	75	39	10
0.14	796	546	433	313	238	183	138	99	65	34	*
0.15	692	475	376	272	207	159	120	86	56	30	*
0.16	607	417	330	239	182	140	105	76	50	27	*
0.17	537	369	292	211	161	124	93	67	44	24	*
0.18	478	328	260	188	144	110	83	60	39	21	*
0.19	428	294	233	169	129	99	75	54	35	19	*
0.20	385	265	210	152	116	89	67	49	32	17	*
0.22	317	218	173	125	96	74	56	40	27	15	*
0.24	265	182	144	105	80	62	47	34	23	12	*
0.26	224	154	122	89	68	52	40	29	19	11	*
0.28	192	132	105	76	58	45	34	25	17	10	*
0.30	166	114	91	66	51	39	30	22	15	*	*
0.32	145	100	79	58	44	34	26	19	13	*	*
0.34	127	88	70	51	39	30	23	17	12	*	*
0.36	113	78	62	45	35	27	20	15	10	*	*
0.38	100	69	55	40	31	24	18	14	*	*	*
0.40	89	62	49	36	28	21	16	12	*	*	*
0.45	69	48	38	28	21	17	13	10	*	*	*
0.50	54	37	30	22	17	13	10	*	*	*	*
0.55	43	30	24	17	14	11	*	*	*	*	*
0.60	34	24	19	14	11	*	*	*	*	*	*
0.65	28	19	16	12	*	*	*	*	*	*	*
0.70	23	16	13	10	*	*	*	*	*	*	*
0.75	18	13	10	*	*	*	*	*	*	*	*
0.80	15	10	*	*	*	*	*	*	*	*	*
0.85	12	*	*	*	*	*	*	*	*	*	*
0.90	*	*	*	*	*	*	*	*	*	*	*

Continued

APPENDIX D—Cont'd

Master Table

1% Level, One-Tailed Test

Δ	99	95	90	80	Power 70	60	50	40	30	20	10
0.01	216463	157695	130162	100355	81264	66545	54117	42972	32469	22044	10917
0.02	54106	39417	32535	25085	2031	16634	13528	10742	8117	5511	2730
0.03	24040	17514	14456	11146	9026	7391	6011	4773	3607	2449	1214
0.04	13517	9848	8128	6267	5075	4156	3380	2684	2029	1378	683
0.05	8646	6299	5200	4009	3247	2659	2163	1718	1298	882	437
0.06	6000	4372	3609	2783	2254	1846	1501	1192	901	612	304
0.07	4405	3209	2649	2043	1655	1355	1102	876	662	450	224
0.08	3369	2455	2027	1563	1266	1037	843	670	507	344	171
0.09	2660	1938	1600	1234	999	819	666	529	400	272	136
0.10	2152	1568	1295	998	809	663	539	428	324	220	110
0.11	1776	1294	1069	824	668	547	445	354	268	182	91
0.12	1490	1086	897	692	560	459	374	297	225	153	77
0.13	1268	924	763	589	477	391	318	253	191	130	65
0.14	1092	796	657	507	411	337	274	218	165	112	56
0.15	949	692	571	441	357	293	238	190	144	98	49
0.16	833	607	501	387	314	257	209	166	126	86	43
0.17	736	537	443	342	277	277	185	147	112	76	39
0.18	655	478	395	305	247	202	165	131	100	68	34
0.19	587	428	353	273	221	181	148	118	89	61	31
0.20	528	385	318	246	199	163	133	106	81	55	29
0.22	434	317	262	202	164	135	110	87	66	46	24
0.24	363	265	219	169	137	113	92	73	56	38	21
0.26	307	224	185	143	116	95	78	62	47	33	18
0.28	263	192	159	123	100	82	67	53	41	29	16
0.30	227	166	137	106	86	71	58	46	35	25	14
0.32	198	145	120	93	75	62	51	41	31	22	12
0.34	174	127	105	82	66	55	45	36	28	20	11
0.36	154	113	93	72	59	48	40	32	25	18	10
0.38	137	100	83	64	52	43	35	29	22	16	*
0.40	122	89	74	57	47	39	32	26	20	15	*
0.45	94	69	57	44	36	30	25	20	16	12	*
0.50	73	54	45	35	29	24	20	16	13	*	*
0.55	58	43	36	28	23	19	16	13	11	*	*
0.60	47	34	29	23	19	16	13	11	*	*	*
0.65	38	28	23	18	15	13	11	*	*	*	*
0.70	30	23	19	15	12	11	*	*	*	*	*
0.75	25	18	15	12	10	*	*	*	*	*	*
0.80	20	15	12	10	*	*	*	*	*	*	*
0.85	16	12	10	*	*	*	*	*	*	*	*
0.90	12	*	*	*	*	*	*	*	*	*	*

APPENDIX D—Cont'd

Master Table

5% Level, Two-Tailed Test

Δ	Power 99	95	90	80	70	60	50	40	30	20	10
0.01	183714	129940	105069	78485	61718	48986	38414	29125	20609	12508	4604
0.02	45920	32480	26263	19618	15428	12245	9603	7281	5152	3127	1152
0.03	20403	14431	11669	8717	6855	5441	4267	3236	2290	1390	513
0.04	11472	8115	6562	4902	3855	3060	2400	1820	1288	782	289
0.05	7338	5191	4197	3136	2466	1958	1536	1165	824	501	185
0.06	5093	3602	2913	2177	1712	1359	1066	809	573	348	129
0.07	3739	2645	2139	1598	1257	998	783	594	421	256	95
0.08	2860	2023	1636	1223	962	764	599	455	322	196	73
0.09	2257	1597	1292	965	759	603	473	359	255	155	58
0.10	1826	1292	1045	781	615	488	383	291	206	126	47
0.11	1508	1067	863	645	507	403	316	240	170	104	39
0.12	1265	895	724	541	426	338	266	202	143	88	33
0.13	1076	762	616	461	363	288	226	172	122	75	29
0.14	927	656	531	397	312	248	195	148	105	64	25
0.15	806	570	461	345	272	216	170	129	92	56	22
0.16	707	500	405	303	238	190	149	113	81	50	20
0.17	625	442	358	268	211	168	132	100	71	44	18
0.18	556	394	319	238	188	149	117	89	64	39	16
0.19	498	353	286	214	168	134	105	80	57	35	15
0.20	449	318	257	192	152	121	95	72	52	32	13
0.22	369	261	212	158	125	99	78	60	43	27	11
0.24	308	218	177	133	105	83	66	50	36	23	10
0.26	261	185	150	112	89	71	56	43	31	20	*
0.28	223	159	128	96	76	61	48	37	27	17	*
0.30	193	137	111	83	66	53	42	32	23	15	*
0.32	169	120	97	73	58	46	36	28	21	13	*
0.34	148	105	85	64	51	41	32	25	18	12	*
0.36	131	93	75	57	45	36	29	22	16	11	*
0.38	116	83	67	51	40	32	26	20	15	10	*
0.40	104	74	60	45	36	29	23	18	13	*	*
0.45	80	57	46	35	28	22	18	14	11	*	*
0.50	62	45	36	27	22	18	14	11	*	*	*
0.55	50	35	29	22	18	14	12	*	*	*	*
0.60	40	29	23	18	14	12	10	*	*	*	*
0.65	32	23	19	15	12	10	*	*	*	*	*
0.70	26	19	15	12	10	*	*	*	*	*	*
0.75	21	15	13	10	*	*	*	*	*	*	*
0.80	17	12	10	*	*	*	*	*	*	*	*
0.85	13	10	*	*	*	*	*	*	*	*	*
0.90	10	*	*	*	*	*	*	*	*	*	*

Continued

APPENDIX D—Cont'd

Master Table

1% Level, Two-Tailed Test

					Power						
Δ	99	95	90	80	70	60	50	40	30	20	10
0.01	240299	178131	148785	116783	96109	80039	66346	53937	42082	30074	16752
0.02	60064	44525	37190	29191	24024	20007	16584	13483	10520	7518	4188
0.03	26687	19783	16524	12970	10674	8890	7369	5991	4675	3341	1862
0.04	15005	11123	9291	7293	6002	4999	4144	3369	2629	1879	1047
0.05	9598	7115	5943	4665	3840	3198	2651	2155	1682	1202	670
0.06	6661	4938	4125	3238	2665	2220	1840	1496	1168	835	466
0.07	4890	3625	3028	2377	1957	1630	1351	1099	858	613	342
0.08	3740	2773	2316	1819	1497	1247	1034	841	656	469	262
0.09	2952	2189	1829	1436	1182	984	816	664	518	371	207
0.10	2389	1771	1480	1162	956	797	661	537	420	300	168
0.11	1972	1462	1221	959	789	658	545	444	346	248	139
0.12	1654	1227	1025	805	663	552	458	372	291	208	117
0.13	1407	1044	872	685	564	470	390	317	248	177	100
0.14	1212	898	751	590	485	405	336	273	213	153	86
0.15	1054	781	653	513	422	352	292	238	186	133	75
0.16	924	685	573	450	371	309	256	209	163	117	66
0.17	817	606	506	398	328	273	227	185	144	104	58
0.18	727	539	451	354	292	243	202	164	129	92	52
0.19	651	483	404	317	261	218	181	147	115	83	47
0.20	586	435	364	286	235	196	163	133	104	75	42
0.22	482	358	299	235	194	162	134	109	86	62	35
0.24	403	299	250	196	162	135	112	92	72	52	30
0.26	341	253	212	166	137	115	95	78	61	44	26
0.28	292	217	181	143	118	98	82	67	52	38	23
0.30	252	187	157	123	102	85	71	58	45	33	20
0.32	220	163	137	108	89	74	62	51	40	30	18
0.34	193	144	120	95	78	65	54	45	35	26	15
0.36	171	127	106	84	69	58	48	39	31	24	15
0.38	152	113	94	74	62	52	43	35	29	21	13
0.40	135	101	84	67	55	46	38	32	26	19	12
0.45	104	77	65	51	42	36	30	25	20	15	10
0.50	81	61	51	40	33	28	24	20	16	12	*
0.55	64	48	40	32	27	23	19	16	13	10	*
0.60	52	39	32	26	22	19	16	15	11	*	*
0.65	41	31	27	21	18	15	13	11	*	*	*
0.70	33	25	22	17	15	13	11	*	*	*	*
0.75	27	21	17	14	12	10	*	*	*	*	*
0.80	22	17	14	11	*	*	*	*	*	*	*
0.85	17	13	11	*	*	*	*	*	*	*	*
0.90	13	10	*	*	*	*	*	*	*	*	*

From *How Many Subjects: Statistical Power Analysis in Research,* by H. C. Kraemer and S. Thiemann, 1987, Newbury Park, CA: Sage. Reprinted by permission of Sage Publications, Inc.

GLOSSARY

A

absolute zero point

Point at which a value of zero indicates the absence of the property being measured. Ratio-level measurements, such as weight scales, vital signs, and laboratory values, have an absolute zero point.

abstract

Clear, concise summary of a study, usually limited to 100 to 250 words.

abstract thinking

Oriented toward the development of an idea without application to or association with a particular instance, and independent of time and space. Abstract thinkers tend to look for meaning, patterns, relationships, and philosophical implications.

abstract thought processes

Enable both science and theories to be blended into a cohesive body of knowledge, guided by a philosophical framework and applied to clinical practice.

academic library

Located within institutions of higher learning and containing numerous resources for researchers.

acceptance rate

Number or percentage of the subjects who agree to participate in a study. The percentage is calculated by dividing the number of subjects agreeing to participate by the number of subjects approached. For example, if 100 subjects are approached and 90 agree to participate, the acceptance rate is 90% (90 ÷ 100 = 90%).

access to care

The extent to which health care is available to an individual, family, or group, which is an important outcome measured in outcomes research.

accessible population

Portion of a target population to which the researcher has reasonable access.

accidental or convenience sampling

Nonprobability sampling technique in which subjects are included in the study because they happened to be in the right place at the right time. Available subjects are simply entered into the study until the desired sample size is reached.

accuracy in physiological measures

Comparable to validity in that it addresses the extent to which the instrument measured the domain that is defined in the study.

accuracy of a screening test

Test used to confirm a diagnosis is evaluated in terms of its ability to correctly assess the presence or absence of a disease or condition as compared with a gold standard.

across-method triangulation

Combining research methods or strategies from two or more research traditions in the same study.

adaptation

The ability to cope or adjust to life events. Nursing theorist (Roy) uses this term to indicate the health of a person, and the focus of health care is to promote adaptation.

administrative databases

Databases with standardized sets of data for enormous numbers of patients and providers that are created by insurance companies, government agencies, and others not directly involved in providing patient care.

adoption

Full acceptance of the innovation or new evidence-based intervention, and implementation of the ideas in practice.

Agency for Healthcare Research and Quality (AHRQ)

Federal government agency created in 1989 to carry out research, demonstration projects, evidence-based guideline development, training, and research dissemination activities with respect to health care services and systems. Focus of this agency is to promote evidence-based health care; see the website for details at www.ahrq.gov. AHRQ was previously named Agency for Health Care Policy and Research, with a name change in 1999.

alpha (α)

Level of significance or cutoff point used to determine whether the samples being tested are members of the same population (nonsignificant) or different populations (significant); alpha is commonly set at 0.05, 0.01, or 0.001. Alpha is also the probability of making a type I error.

alternate-forms reliability

Also referred to as *parallel forms reliability*, which involves comparing the equivalence of two versions of the same paper-and-pencil instruments.

analogue situations

Situations useful for testing prototypes or primitive designs in intervention research where actors play roles in the intervention and follow the steps of the intervention prescribed by the prototype to determine its adequacy.

analysis of covariance (ANCOVA)

Statistical procedure designed to reduce the error term (or variance within groups) by partialing out the variance resulting from a confounding variable by performing regression analysis before performing analysis of variance (ANOVA).

analysis of sources

Process of determining the value of a source for a particular study. The source is critically appraised and then compared with other studies to determine the existing body of knowledge in relation to the research problem.

analysis of variance (ANOVA)

Statistical technique used to examine differences among two or more groups by comparing the variability between the groups with the variability within the groups.

analysis step of critical appraisal

Determining the strengths and limitations of the logical links connecting one study element with another.

analysis triangulation

Using two or more analysis techniques to analyze the same set of data for the purpose of validation.

analytical induction

Qualitative research technique that includes enumerative induction, in which a number and variety of instances are collected that verify the model, and eliminative induction, which requires that the hypothesis be tested against alternatives.

analytical preciseness

Performing a series of transformations during which concrete data are transformed across several levels of abstractions to develop a theoretical schema that imparts meaning to the phenomenon under study.

anonymity

Subject's identity cannot be linked, even by the researcher, with his or her individual responses.

applied or practical research

Scientific investigations conducted to generate knowledge that will directly influence or improve practice.

ascendance to an open context

Ability to see depth and complexity within the phenomenon examined and a greater capacity for insight than with the sedimented view. Requires deconstructing sedimented views and reconstructing another view.

assent

A child's affirmative agreement to participate in research.

associative hypothesis

Identifies or predicts the relationship between or among variables that occur or exist together in the real world. It is usually developed to guide a correlational study.

associative relationship

Identifies concepts that occur or exist together in the real world; thus, when one concept changes, the other concept changes. These relationships are part of theory and can be tested through research.

assumptions

Statements taken for granted or considered true, even though they have not been scientifically tested.

asymmetrical relationship

If A occurs (or changes), then B will occur (or change), but there may be no indication that if B occurs (or changes), A will occur (or change); A – B.

auditability

Rigorous development of a decision trail that is reported in sufficient detail to allow a second qualitative researcher, using the original data and the decision trail, to arrive at conclusions similar to those of the original qualitative researcher.

authority

Person with expertise and power who is able to influence opinion and behavior.

autonomous agents

Potential subjects informed about a proposed study can voluntarily choose to participate or not participate.

autoregressive integrated moving average (ARIMA) model
This model is an equation or series of equations that explain a naturally occurring process; it is the most commonly used time-series analysis model in nursing.

average
A lay term used to describe the mean of a set of data. The mean is a statistical analysis technique used to determine the numerical center of interval and ratio data

B

background for a research problem
Part of the research problem that indicates what is known or the key research that has been done in the problem area to be studied.

backward stepwise regression analysis
Type of stepwise regression analysis in which all the independent variables are initially included in the analysis. Then, one variable at a time is removed from the equation, and the effect of that removal on R^2 is evaluated.

bar graphs
Figures or illustrations that provide a picture of the results from a study. These graphs can be horizontal or vertical bars that represent the size or amount of the group or variable studied.

basic or pure research
Scientific investigations for the pursuit of knowledge for knowledge's sake or for the pleasure of learning and finding truth.

being
A term in phenomenological research where a person's experiences of the world are unique to that person.

being-in-time
Term from phenomenological research that indicates that a person experiences life situations within the framework of time, and the past and the future influence the now and thus are part of being-in-time.

beneficence, principle of
Encourages the researcher to do good and, above all, to do no harm.

benefit-risk ratio
Researchers and reviewers of research weigh potential benefits and risks in a study to promote the conduct of ethical research.

benefits
The potential positive outcomes that are predicted to occur with the conduct of a study.

best interest standard
In determining whether an individual should participate in a study, the researcher needs to do what is best for the individual on the basis of balancing risks and benefits in a study.

best research evidence
The strongest empirical knowledge available that is generated from the synthesis of quality study findings to address a practice problem.

beta weights
Part of the calculations of regression analysis to develop a predictive formula.

between-group variance
Variance of the group means around the grand mean (the mean of the total sample) that is examined in analysis of variance (ANOVA).

between-method triangulation
See *across-method triangulation.*

bias
Any influence or action in a study that distorts the findings or slants them away from the true or expected.

biased coin design
Technique used to randomly assign subjects to groups where selection of the group to which a particular subject will be assigned is biased in favor of groups that have smaller sample sizes at the point of the assignment of that subject.

bibliographical database
Database that consists of citations relevant to a specific discipline or may be a broad collection of citations from a variety of disciplines.

bimodal
Distribution of scores from a study has two modes (or most frequently occurring scores), which usually means that the researcher has not adequately defined the study population.

bivariate analysis
Statistical procedures that involve comparison of summary values from two groups of the same variable or from two variables within a single group.

bivariate correlation
Analysis techniques that measure the extent of the linear relationship between two variables.

Bland and Altman plot
Analysis technique for examining the extent of agreement between two physiological measurement techniques. Generally used to compare a new technique with an established one.

blinding in a study design

Structure of a design where either the patient or those providing care to the patient are unaware of whether the patient is in the experimental or the control group.

blocking

Part of the randomized block design, where the subjects are rank ordered in relation to the blocking variable to control the effects of this variable, thus improving the validity of study findings.

body of knowledge

Information, principles, theories, and empirical evidence that are organized by the beliefs accepted in a discipline at a given time.

Bonferroni procedure

Parametric analysis technique that controls for escalation of significance and can be used if various *t*-tests must be performed on different aspects of the same data.

borrowing

Appropriation and use of knowledge from other disciplines to guide nursing practice.

bracketing

Qualitative research technique of suspending or laying aside what is known about an experience being studied.

breach of confidentiality

Accidental or direct action that allows an unauthorized person to have access to raw study data or subject identity information.

C

canonical correlation

Extension of multiple regression with more than one dependent variable.

care maps

Type of map developed in intervention research of the intervention theory that illustrates the elements of the intervention and the causal links among them, and the map should show all the causal pathways described in the intervention theory.

carryover effect

Application of one treatment can influence the response to following treatments.

case study

Type of descriptive study that includes a case study design.

case study design

A design that guides the intensive exploration of a single unit of study, such as a person, family, group, community, or institution.

causal connection

The link between the independent variable (cause) and the dependent variable (outcome or effect) that is examined in quasi-experimental, experimental, and intervention research.

causal explanation

The description or explanation of the effect(s) of the independent variable (cause or intervention) on the dependent variable (outcome).

causal hypothesis or relationship

Relationship between two variables in which one variable (independent variable) is thought to cause or determine the presence of the other variable (dependent variable). Some causal hypotheses include more than one independent or dependent variable.

causality

Includes three conditions: (1) must be a strong relationship between the proposed cause and effect, (2) proposed cause must precede the effect in time, and (3) cause has to be present whenever the effect occurs.

cell

Intersection between the row and column in a table where a specific numerical value is inserted.

central limit theorem

States that even when statistics, such as means, come from a population with a skewed (asymmetrical) distribution, the sampling distribution developed from multiple means obtained from that skewed population will tend to fit the pattern of the normal curve.

change agent

Professional outside a system who enters the system to promote implementation of research evidence in practice to move an agency toward evidence-based practice.

checklist

Technique or type of measurement method for indicating whether a behavior occurred during a study.

chi-square test of independence (χ^2)

Used to analyze nominal data to determine significant differences between observed frequencies within the data and frequencies that were expected.

chronology

Type of unstructured observation that provides a detailed description of an individual's behavior in a natural environment.

citation

Act of quoting a source, using it as an example, or presenting it as support for a position taken.

citation search indexes

Link citations on the basis of the references at the end of articles.

cleaning data

Checking raw data to determine errors in data recording, coding, or entry.

clinical databases

Databases of patient, provider, and health care agency information that are developed by health care agencies and sometimes providers to document care delivery and outcomes.

clinical decision analysis

Systematic method of describing clinical problems, identifying possible diagnostic and management courses of action, assessing the probability and value of the various outcomes, and then calculating the optimal course of action.

clinical expertise

Includes a practitioner's knowledge, skills, and past experience in accurately assessing, diagnosing, and managing an individual's health needs.

clinical guidelines

Standardized, current national and international guidelines for the assessment, diagnosis, and management of patient conditions that are developed by clinical guideline panels or professional groups to improve the outcomes of care and promote evidence-based health care (see www.guideline.gov).

clinical judgment

The use of clinical expertise to make sound decisions in the provision of evidence-based health care.

clinical pathways

Critical pathways or guidelines developed by health care agencies to define the expected care activities and outcomes of care in specific patient care situations. These pathways are developed based on previous research, agency data, and clinical experience.

clinical trial

A study conducted to determine the effect of a selected intervention (such as a drug or medical procedure) on identified patient outcomes using a structured experimental design. Produces a strong type of research evidence that can be synthesized with other study findings to determine the current best research evidence in a practice area.

cluster sampling

A sampling frame is developed that includes a list of all the states, cities, institutions, or organizations (clusters) that could be used in a study, and a randomized sample is drawn from this list. Cluster sampling is used when it is not possible to use simple random sampling or the individual elements of the population are unknown, and this prevents development of the sampling frame.

clustering

Qualitative analysis technique of sorting elements into categories or groups to look for patterns.

Cochran Q test

Nonparametric test that is an extension of the McNemar test for two related or dependent samples.

codebook

Identifies and defines each variable in a study and includes an abbreviated variable name, a descriptive variable label, and the range of possible numerical values of every variable entered into a computer file.

coding

Process of transforming qualitative data into numerical symbols that can be computerized.

coefficient of determination (R^2)

Computed from a matrix of correlation coefficients and provides important information on multicollinearity. This value indicates the degree of linear dependencies among the variables.

coercion

Overt threat of harm or excessive reward intentionally presented by one person to another to obtain compliance, such as offering subjects a large sum of money to participate in a dangerous research project.

cognitive anthropology

New approach in ethnographic research where culture is viewed as an adaptive system that is in the minds of the people and is expressed in the language or semantic system of the group.

cognitive application of research

Research-based knowledge is used to affect a person's way of thinking, approaching, and observing situations.

cognitive mapping

Qualitative analysis technique that is a visual representation of the information obtained from the participant, and the ideas are mapped including codes (concepts) and relationships among the codes.

cohorts
Samples in time-dimensional studies within the field of epidemiology.

co-investigators
Two or more professionals conducting a study, whose salaries might be paid partially or in full by grant funding.

communality
The squared multiple regression coefficient for each variable that describes the amount of variance in a single variable that is explained across all the factors in factor analysis.

communicating research findings
Developing a research report and disseminating it through presentations and publications to a variety of audiences.

comparative descriptive design
Used to describe differences in variables in two or more groups in a natural setting.

comparative experimental design
Less rigorous experimental design in which random sampling is difficult if not impossible. These studies include convenience samples with random assignment to groups.

comparison group
This group is not selected using random sampling and usually does not receive a treatment. There are four types of comparison groups: (1) groups that receive no treatment, (2) groups that receive a placebo treatment, (3) groups that receive standard or usual health care, and (4) groups that receive a second experimental treatment or a different treatment dose for comparison with the first experimental treatment.

comparison step of critical appraisal
Ideal for each step of the research process is compared with the real steps in a study.

complete IRB review
Extensive review by an institutional review board (IRB) for studies with greater than minimal risk.

complete observer
The researcher is passive and has no direct social interaction in the setting.

complete participation
The researcher becomes a member of the group and conceals the researcher role.

complex hypothesis
Predicts the relationship (associative or causal) among three or more variables; thus, the hypothesis could include two (or more) independent and two (or more) dependent variables.

complex search of the literature
Search of the literature that combines two or more concepts or synonyms in one search.

comprehending a source
Involves reading the entire source carefully and focusing on understanding the major concepts and the logical flow of ideas within the source.

comprehension step of critical appraisal
Understanding the terms in a research report; identifying study elements; and grasping the nature, significance, and meaning of these elements.

computer searches
Conducted to scan the citations in different databases and identify sources relevant to a research problem.

computerized database
Structured compilation of information that can be scanned, retrieved, and analyzed by computer and can be used for decisions, reports, and research.

concept
Term that abstractly describes and names an object or phenomenon, thus providing it with a separate identity or meaning.

concept analysis
Strategy through which a set of attributes or characteristics essential to the connotative meaning or conceptual definition of a concept are identified.

concept derivation
Process of extracting and defining concepts from theories in other disciplines. May require a concept analysis that examines the use of the concept in the nursing literature, compares the results with the existing conceptual definition, and if the two are different, modifies the definition to be consistent with nursing usage.

concept synthesis
Process of describing and naming a previously unrecognized concept.

conceptual clustering step of critical appraisal
Current knowledge in an area of study is carefully analyzed, summarized, and organized theoretically to maximize the meaning attached to research findings, highlight gaps in the knowledge base,

generate research questions, and provide knowledge for use in practice.

conceptual definition

Provides a variable or concept with connotative (abstract, comprehensive, theoretical) meaning and is established through concept analysis, concept derivation, or concept synthesis.

conceptual map

Strategy for expressing a framework of a study that diagrammatically shows the interrelationships of the concepts and statements.

conceptual model

Set of highly abstract, related constructs that broadly explains phenomena of interest, expresses assumptions, and reflects a philosophical stance.

conclusions

Synthesis and clarification of the meaning of study findings.

concrete thinking

Thinking that is oriented toward and limited by tangible things or events observed and experienced in reality.

concurrent relationship

Relationship in which both variables and concepts occur simultaneously.

condensed proposal

A brief or shorten proposal developed for review by clinical agencies and funding institutions.

confidence interval

Range in which the value of the population parameter is estimated to be.

confidentiality

Management of private data in research so that subjects' identities are not linked with their responses.

confirmatory data analysis

Use of inferential statistics to confirm expectations regarding the data that are expressed as hypotheses.

confirmatory factor analysis

Closely related to ordinary least-squares regression analysis or path analysis and based on theory and testing a hypothesis about the existing factor structure.

confirmatory regression analysis

Regression analysis procedures designed to confirm or support a theoretically proposed set of variables.

confirmatory studies

Conducted only after a large body of knowledge has been generated with exploratory studies and are expected to have large samples and to use random sampling techniques.

confounding variables

Variables that have the potential to affect the outcome of a study, which are recognized before the study is initiated but that cannot be controlled, or variables not recognized until the study is in process.

connecting findings

Linking findings together in a meaningful way to determine conclusions from a study.

consensus knowledge building

Outcomes design that requires critique and synthesis of an extensive international search of the literature on the topic of concern, including unpublished studies, studies in progress, dissertations, and theses.

consent form

Written form, tape recording, or videotape used to document a subject's agreement to participate in a study.

construct validity

Examines the fit between conceptual and operational definitions of variables and determines whether the instrument actually measures the theoretical construct that it purports to measure.

constructs

Concepts at very high levels of abstraction that have general meanings.

consultants

People hired for specific tasks during a study, such as assistance with data analysis.

content analysis

Qualitative analysis technique used to classify words in a text into a few categories chosen because of their theoretical importance.

content-related validity evidence

Examines the extent to which the method of measurement includes all the major elements relevant to the construct being measured. Evidence for content-related validity is obtained from the literature, representatives of the relevant populations, and content experts.

context

The body, the world, and the concerns unique to each person within which that person can be understood. Philosophical element of qualitative research.

context flexibility

Capacity to switch from one context or worldview to another in order to shift perception, to see things from a different perspective.

contextual variables

Factors that could influence the implementation of an intervention and thus the outcomes of the study, or could directly influence the study outcomes.

contingency coefficient (C)

Statistical test that is used with two nominal variables and is the most commonly used of the chi-square–based measures of association.

contingency tables

Cross-tabulation tables that allow visual comparison of summary data output related to two variables within a sample.

contingent relationship

Occurs only if a third variable or concept is present.

control

Imposing of rules by the researcher to decrease the possibility of error and increase the probability that the study's findings are an accurate reflection of reality.

control group

Group of elements or subjects not exposed to the experimental treatment. The term *control group* is used in studies with random sampling methods.

convenience sampling

See *accidental or convenience sampling.*

convergent validity

Type of measurement validity obtained by using two instruments to measure the same variable, such as depression, and correlating the results from these instruments. Evidence of validity from examining convergence is achieved if the data from the two instruments have a moderate to strong positive correlation.

correlational analysis

Statistical procedure conducted to determine the direction (positive or negative) and magnitude (or strength) of the relationship between two variables.

correlational coefficient

Indicates the degree of relationship between two variables; coefficients range in value from [+]1.00 (perfect positive relationship) to 0.00 (no relationship) to −1.00 (perfect negative or inverse relationship).

correlational matrix

A table of the bivariate correlations of every pair of variables in a data set. Along the diagonal through the matrix the variables are correlated with themselves, with the left and right sides of the table being mirror images of each other.

correlational research

Systematic investigation of relationships between two or more variables to explain the type (positive or negative) and strength of relationships in the world and not to examine cause and effect.

correlational study designs

Variety of study designs developed to examine relationships among variables.

cost-benefit analysis

Analysis technique used in outcomes research that examines the costs and benefits of alternative ways of using resources as assessed in monetary terms and the use that produces the greatest net benefit.

cost-effectiveness analysis

Type of outcomes research in which costs and benefits are compared for different ways of accomplishing a clinical goal, such as diagnosing a condition, treating an illness, or providing a service. The goal of cost-effectiveness analyses is to identify the strategy that provides the most value for the money.

costs of care

The expenses encountered in the delivery of health care that are considered an important outcome of care and are often examined in outcomes research. Costs are a measure of the actual use of resources rather than the price charged.

counterbalancing

Various treatments are administered in random order rather than being provided consistently in the same sequence.

covert data collection

Occurs when subjects are unaware that research data are being collected.

Cramer's *V*

Analysis technique for nominal data that is a modification of phi for contingency tables larger than 2×2.

criterion-referenced testing

Comparison of a subject's score with a criterion of achievement that includes the definition of target behaviors. When the subject has mastered the behaviors, he or she is considered proficient in these behaviors, such as being proficient in the behaviors of a nurse practitioner.

critical appraisal of research

Systematic, unbiased, careful examination of all aspects of a study to judge the merits, limitations, meaning, and significance based on previous research experience and knowledge of the topic.

critical appraisal process for qualitative research
Examination of the quality of a qualitative study using the five standards: descriptive vividness, methodological congruence, analytical preciseness, theoretical connectedness, and heuristic relevance.

critical appraisal process for quantitative research
Examination of the quality of a quantitative study using the five steps of comprehension, comparison, analysis, evaluation, and conceptual clustering.

critical cases
Cases that make a point clearly or are extremely important in understanding the purpose of the study and are identified through purposive sampling.

critical pathways
See *clinical pathways*.

critical social theory
Qualitative research methodology guided by critical social theory; the researcher seeks to understand how people communicate and develop symbolic meanings in a society.

critical value
In quantitative data analysis, it is the value at which statistical significance is achieved in a study.

crossover or counterbalanced design
Includes the administration of more than one treatment to each subject, and the treatments are provided sequentially rather than concurrently; comparisons are then made of the effects of the different treatments on the same subject.

cross-sectional designs
Used to examine groups of subjects in various stages of development simultaneously with the intent of inferring trends over time.

cultural immersion
Used in ethnographic research for gaining increased familiarity with such things as language, sociocultural norms, and traditions in a culture.

curvilinear relationship
The relationship between two variables varies depending on the relative values of the variables. The graph of the relationship is a curved line rather than a straight one.

cutoff point
In factor analysis, variables' factor loading must be at least 0.30 to explain a meaningful portion of the variance within a factor, and these variables are included as elements of the factor.

D

data
(plural) Pieces of information that are collected during a study (singular: datum).

data analysis
Conducted to reduce, organize, and give meaning to data.

data coding sheet
A sheet for organizing and recording data for rapid entry into a computer.

data collection
Precise, systematic gathering of information relevant to the research purpose or the specific objectives, questions, or hypotheses of a study.

data collection forms
Forms developed or modified for a study to use for recording demographic data, information from patient records, observations, or values from physiological measures.

data collection plan
Details how a study will be implemented.

data reduction
Technique for analyzing qualitative data that focuses on decreasing the volume of data to facilitate examination.

data triangulation
Collection of data from multiple sources in the same study.

data use agreement
Limits how the data set for a study may be used and how it will be protected to meet the Health Insurance Portability and Accountability Act (HIPAA) requirements.

database
See *computerized database*.

datum
Single piece of information collected for research.

debriefing
Complete disclosure of the study purpose and results at the end of a study.

deception
Misinforming subjects for research purposes.

decision making
Cognitive process of assessing a situation and deciding on a course of action, which is important for conducting research and providing health care.

decision theory
Theory that is inductive in nature and based on assumptions associated with the theoretical normal curve. The theory is applied when testing for differences

between groups, with the expectation that all of the groups are members of the same population.

decision trail

See *auditability*.

Declaration of Helsinki

Ethical code based on the Nuremberg Code that differentiated therapeutic from nontherapeutic research.

deconstructing the sedimented views

Rigorous qualitative research requires that the researcher ascend to an open context and be willing to continue to let go of sedimented views, which involves the process of remaining open to new views. (See *sedimented view* and *open context*.)

deductive reasoning

Reasoning from the general to the specific, or from a general premise to a particular situation.

degrees of freedom (*df*)

Freedom of a score's value to vary given the other existing scores' values and the established sum of these scores ($df = N - 1$).

de-identifying health data

Involves removing the 18 elements that could be used to identify an individual or his or her relatives, employer, or household members, and this term is part of the Health Insurance Portability and Accountability Act (HIPAA).

Delphi technique

Method of measuring the judgments of a group of experts for assessing priorities or making forecasts.

demographic or attribute variables

Specific variables such as age, gender, and ethnicity that are collected in a study to describe the sample.

denotative definition

Dictionary definition of a word.

dependent groups

Groups in which the subjects or observations selected for data collection are in some way related to the selection of other subjects or observations. For example, if subjects serve as their own control by using the pretest as a control, the observations (and therefore the groups) are dependent. Use of twins in a study or matching subjects on a selected variable, such as medical diagnosis or age, results in dependent groups.

dependent variable

Response, behavior, or outcome that is predicted and measured in research; changes in the dependent variable are presumed to be caused by the independent variable.

description

Involves identifying and understanding the nature and attributes of nursing phenomena and sometimes the relationships among these phenomena. This is an outcome of research.

descriptive codes

Terms used to organize and classify qualitative data.

descriptive correlational design

Used to describe variables and examine relationships that exist in a study situation.

descriptive design

Used to identify a phenomenon of interest, identify variables within the phenomenon, develop conceptual and operational definitions of variables, and describe variables in a study situation.

descriptive mode

Qualitative mode of nursing inquiry within grounded theory that provides rich detail and must precede all the other modes.

descriptive research

Provides an accurate portrayal or account of the characteristics of a particular individual, event, or group in real-life situations for the purpose of discovering new meaning, describing what exists, determining the frequency with which something occurs, and categorizing information.

descriptive statistics

Summary statistics that allow the researcher to organize the data in ways that give meaning and facilitate insight, such as frequency distributions and measures of central tendency and dispersion.

descriptive study designs

Variety of designs developed to gain more information about characteristics within a particular field of study and to provide a picture of situations as they naturally happen.

descriptive theory

Describes the causal process occurring in intervention research.

descriptive vividness

Description of the site, subjects, experience of collecting data, and the researcher's thoughts during the qualitative research process that is presented so clearly that the reader has the sense of personally experiencing the event.

design

Blueprint for conducting a study that maximizes control over factors that could interfere with the validity of the findings.

deterministic relationship

Causal statement of what always occurs in a particular situation, such as a scientific law.

developmental grant proposals

Proposals written to obtain funding for the development of a new program in a discipline.

deviation score

Difference score, which is obtained by subtracting the mean from each score, indicates the extent to which a score deviates from the mean.

dialectic reasoning

Involves the holistic perspective, in which the whole is greater than the sum of the parts, and examining factors that are opposites and making sense of them by merging them into a single unit or idea that is greater than either alone.

diary

Record of events kept by a subject over time that is collected and analyzed by a researcher.

difference scores

See *deviation score.*

diminished autonomy

Subjects with decreased ability to voluntarily give informed consent because of legal or mental incompetence, terminal illness, or confinement to an institution.

direct application

Occurs when an innovation or a new intervention is used exactly as it was developed in practice.

direct costs

Specific costs for materials and equipment to conduct a study that are identified in a grant proposal.

direct measurement

Measurement object and measurement strategies are specific and straightforward, such as those for measuring the concrete variables of height, weight, or temperature.

direction of a relationship

The direction of a relationship can be positive or negative. With a positive relationship, the two variables change in the same direction (increase or decrease together). With a negative relationship, the variables change in opposite directions; thus, as one variable increases, the other decreases.

directional hypothesis

States the specific nature of the interaction or relationship between two or more variables.

disadvantaged groups

Groups of individuals who are considered vulnerable or at risk based on economic status, gender, or ethnicity.

discovery mode

Qualitative mode of nursing inquiry within grounded theory that leads to the identification of patterns in life experiences of individuals and relates the patterns to one another to develop substantive theory.

discriminant analysis

Designed to allow the researcher to identify characteristics associated with group membership and to predict group membership.

dismantling strategy

A technique used in outcomes or intervention research to break a complex intervention into smaller facets to determine the impact of the different facets of the intervention on the study outcomes.

disproportionate sampling

In stratification, when each stratum has an equivalent number of subjects in the sample, versus each stratum having a number of subjects in proportion to its occurrence in the population, which is proportionate sampling.

dissemination of research findings

Diffusion or communication of research findings by presentations and publications to a variety of audiences, such as nurses, other health professionals, policy developers, and consumers.

dissertation

Extensive, usually original, research project that is completed as the final requirement for a doctoral degree.

distribution

Spread of scores in a study or database.

divergent validity

Type of measurement validity obtained by finding an instrument that measures the opposite of the concept or variable being studied and correlating the data collected with an instrument that measures the concept or variable studied. For example, the focus of a study might be to measure hope, and one instrument would measure hope and another instrument would measure despair.

double-blinding in a study design

Structure of a design where neither the patient nor the caregivers are aware of the group (experimental or control) to which the patient is assigned during a study.

dummy variables

Categorical or dichotomous variables used in regression analysis.

duplicate publication

Practice of publishing the same article or major portions of the article in two or more print or electronic media without notifying the editors or referencing the other publication in the reference list.

duration of an intervention

The time required to deliver a treatment in a study, which includes examining the time for each individual treatment and the total time the treatment is delivered during the study.

dwelling with the data

Immersion in the data as part of the process of data management and reduction in phenomenology.

E

effect coding

Used in multiple regression analysis and is similar to dummy coding but is used when the effects of the treatments are being examined by the analysis.

effect size

Degree to which the phenomenon is present in the population or to which the null hypothesis is false.

eigenvalues

Numerical values generated with factor analysis that are the sum of the squared weights for each factor.

electronic journals

Journals that are published only in electronic form and can be accessed from Internet commercial websites.

electronic mail (e-mail)

Allows a computer user to rapidly exchange messages, computer files, data, and research reports with others by the Internet.

element of a study

Person (subject), event, behavior, or any other single unit of a study.

eligibility criteria

See *sampling criteria.*

eliminative induction

Qualitative data analysis technique that is part of a process referred to as *analytic induction* and requires that the hypothesis generated from the analysis be tested against alternatives.

embodied

Heideggerian phenomenologist's belief that the person is a self within a body; thus the person is referred to as embodied.

emergent fit mode

Qualitative mode of nursing inquiry within grounded theory that is used to refine substantive theory after it has been developed.

emic approach

Anthropological research approach of studying behavior from within the culture.

empirical generalization

Statements that have been repeatedly tested through research and have not been disproved. Scientific theories have empirical generalizations.

empirical literature

Includes relevant studies published in journals, in books, and online, as well as unpublished studies, such as master's theses and doctoral dissertations.

empirical world

Experienced through our senses and is the concrete portion of our existence.

endogenous variables

Variables whose variations are explained within the theoretical model as part of a study with a model-testing design.

enumerative induction

Qualitative data analysis technique that is part of a process referred to as *analytic induction* in which a number and variety of instances must be collected to verify a model that was developed from the research process.

environmental variable

Type of extraneous variable related to the setting in which a study is conducted.

equivalence

Type of reliability testing that involves comparing two versions of the same paper-and-pencil instrument or two observers measuring the same event.

error score

Amount of random error in the measurement process.

errors in physiological measures

Sources of erroneous measurement with physiological instruments that include environment, user, subject, machine, and interpretation error.

escalates significance

During analysis of study data, there is an increased identification of significant findings that might not be an accurate reflection of reality and might be a type I error (saying something is significant when it is not). For example, performing multiple *t*-tests to analyze study data can cause an increase or escalation of significant findings and an increased incidence of type I error.

estimator

Statistic that produces a value as a function of the scores in a sample. Much of inferential statistical analysis involves the use of point estimation to evaluate the fit between the estimator (a statistic) and the population parameter.

ethical analyses

Analysis conducted in ethical inquiry by using a selected ethical theory to perform it.

ethical inquiry

Intellectual analysis of ethical problems related to obligation, rights, duty, right and wrong, conscience, justice, choice, intention, and responsibility to obtain desirable, rational ends.

ethical principles

Principles of respect for persons, beneficence, and justice relevant to the conduct of research.

ethical rigor

Requires recognition and discussion by the researcher of the ethical implications related to the conduct of a qualitative study.

ethnographic research

Qualitative research methodology developed within the discipline of anthropology for investigating cultures that involves collection, description, and analysis of data to develop a theory of cultural behavior.

ethnonursing research

Emerged from Leininger's theory of transcultural nursing and focuses mainly on observing and documenting interactions with people to determine how daily life conditions and patterns are influencing human care, health, and nursing care practices.

ethnoscientific

Type of ethnographic research that focuses on the ideas, beliefs, and knowledge that a group holds that are expressed in language; may address aspects such as symbolic referents, the network of social relations, and the beliefs reflected in social and political institutions.

etic approach

Anthropological research approach of studying behavior from outside the culture and examining similarities and differences across cultures.

evaluation step of critical appraisal

Examining the meaning and significance of a study according to set criteria and comparing it with previous studies conducted in the area.

event-partitioning designs

Merger of the longitudinal and trend designs to increase sample size and avoid the effects of history on the validity of findings.

event-time matrix

Qualitative analysis technique that can facilitate comparisons of events occurring in different sites during particular time periods.

evidence-based practice (EBP)

Conscientious integration of best research evidence with clinical expertise and patient values and needs in the delivery of quality, cost-effective health care.

evidence-based practice centers

Universities and health care agencies identified by the Agency for Healthcare Research and Quality (AHRQ) as centers for the conduct, communication, and synthesis of research knowledge in selected areas to promote evidence-based health care.

evidence-based practice guidelines

Rigorous, explicit clinical guidelines developed based on the best research evidence available (such as findings from meta-analyses, integrative reviews of research, and extensive clinical trials); supported by consensus from recognized national experts; and affirmed by outcomes obtained by clinicians.

examining evidence

Critical appraisal of research findings with the synthesis of this empirical knowledge to promote evidence-based practice.

exclusion sampling criteria

Sampling requirements identified by the researcher that eliminate or exclude an element or subject from being in a sample. Exclusion criteria are exceptions to the inclusion sampling criteria.

execution errors

Errors that occur because of a defect in the data collection procedure.

exempt from review

Studies that have no apparent risks for the research subjects are often designated as exempt from or not requiring institutional review.

existence statement

Declares that a given concept exists or that a given relationship occurs.

exogenous variables
Those within the theoretical model that are caused by factors from outside the model; these variables are examined in a study with a model-testing design.

expedited IRB review
Review process for studies that have some risk, but the risks are minimal or no greater than those ordinarily encountered in daily life or during the performance of routine physical or psychological examinations.

experimental group
Subjects who are exposed to the experimental treatment or intervention.

experimental research
Objective, systematic, controlled investigation to examine probability and causality among selected independent and dependent variables for the purpose of predicting and controlling phenomena.

experimental study designs
Designs that provide the greatest amount of control possible to examine causality more closely.

experimenter expectancy
Researcher's belief or projection of the outcome of a study.

explanation
Achieved when research clarifies the relationships among phenomena and identifies why certain events occur.

explanatory codes
Developed late in the data collection process after theoretical ideas from the qualitative study have begun to emerge.

exploratory data analysis
Examining the data descriptively to become as familiar as possible with the nature of the data and to search for hidden structures and models.

exploratory factor analysis
Similar to stepwise regression, in which the variance of the first factor is partialed out before analysis is begun on the second factor. It is performed when the researcher has few prior expectations about the factor structure.

exploratory regression analysis
Used when the researcher may not have sufficient information to determine which independent variables are effective predictors of the dependent variable; thus, many variables may be entered into the analysis simultaneously. This type is the most commonly used regression analysis strategy in nursing studies.

exploratory studies
Designed to increase the knowledge of a field of study and are not intended for generalization to large populations. Exploratory studies provide the basis for confirmatory studies.

external criticism
Method of determining the validity of source materials in historical research that involves knowing where, when, why, and by whom a document was written.

external validity
Extent to which study findings can be generalized beyond the sample used in the study.

extraneous variables
Exist in all studies and can affect the measurement of study variables and the relationships among these variables.

F

***F* statistic**
Value or result obtained from conducting a type of analysis of variance.

fabrication in research
Type of misconduct in research that involves making up study results and recording or reporting them.

face validity
Verifies that the instrument looked like or gave the appearance of measuring the content desired for a study.

factor analysis
Analysis that examines interrelationships among large numbers of variables and disentangles those relationships to identify clusters of variables that are most closely linked together. Two types of factor analysis are exploratory and confirmatory factor analysis.

factor loading
The regression coefficient for the variable on the factor determined by factor analysis.

factor rotation
Aspect of factor analysis in which the factors are mathematically adjusted or rotated to reduce the factor structure and clarify the meaning.

factor scores
Variables included in a factor are identified, and the scores on these variables are summed for each subject; thus, each subject will have a score for each factor in the instrument.

factorial analysis of variance

Mathematically, the analysis technique is simply a specialized version of multiple regression; a number of types of factorial ANOVAs have been developed to analyze data from specific experimental designs.

factorial design

Study design that includes two or more different characteristics, treatments, or events that are independently varied within a study.

factors

Clusters of variables that are most closely linked together in factor analysis.

fair treatment

Ethical principle that promotes fair selection and treatment of subjects during the course of a study.

false negative

Result of a diagnostic or screening test that indicates a disease is not present when it is.

false positive

Result of a diagnostic or screening test that indicates a disease is present when it is not.

falsification of research

Type of research misconduct that involves manipulating research materials, equipment, or processes, or changing or omitting data or results such that the research is not accurately represented in the research record.

fatigue effect

When a subject becomes tired or bored with a study, which can affect the findings from the study.

feasibility of a study

Determined by examining the time and money commitment; the researcher's expertise; availability of subjects, facility, and equipment; cooperation of others; and the study's ethical considerations.

feminist research

Research methodology thought to have emerged from critical social theory and is focused on women's experiences and the validity of women's perceptions as the "truth" for them.

field research

Activity of collecting the data that requires taking extensive notes in ethnographic research.

field test

Tests or studies are conducted in clinical settings in which the intervention will typically be implemented in intervention research.

fieldwork

Data collection process for a grounded theory study.

findings

Translated and interpreted results from a study.

fishing

Conducting multiple statistical analyses of relationships or differences searching for significant study findings that can increase the risk for type I error.

focus groups

Groups that are designed to obtain participants' perceptions in a specific (or focused) area in a setting that is permissive and nonthreatening.

forced choice

Response set for items in a scale that have an even number of choices, such as four or six, where the respondents cannot choose an uncertain or neutral response and must indicate support for or against the topic measured.

forward stepwise regression analysis

Type of stepwise regression analysis in which the independent variables are entered into the analysis one at a time and an analysis is made of the effect of including that variable on R^2.

foundational inquiry

Qualitative research method used to examine the foundations for a science, such as studies that provide analysis of the structure of a science and the process of thinking about and valuing certain phenomena held in common by the science. Debates related to quantitative and qualitative research methods emerge from foundational inquiries.

framework

The abstract, logical structure of meaning that guides development of the study and enables the researcher to link the findings to the body of knowledge for nursing.

fraudulent publications

There is documentation or testimony from coauthors that the publication did not reflect what had actually been done.

frequency distribution

Statistical procedure that involves listing all possible measures of a variable and tallying each datum on the listing. The two types of frequency distributions are ungrouped and grouped.

Friedman two-way analysis of variance by ranks

Nonparametric test used with matched samples or in repeated measures to determine differences between samples.

full-text reprint services
Service that provides on request the complete article content (narrative, tables, figures, and references) as it appeared in the professional journal.

G

general proposition
Highly abstract statement of the relationship between two or more concepts that is found in a conceptual model.

generalization
Extends the implications of the findings from the sample that was studied to the larger population or from the situation studied to a larger situation.

geographical analyses
Used to examine variations in health status, health services, patterns of care, or patterns of use by geographical area.

gestalt
Organization of knowledge about a particular phenomenon into a cluster of linked ideas. The clustering and interrelatedness enhance the meaning of the ideas.

going native
In ethnographic research, when the researcher becomes part of the culture and loses all objectivity and, with it, the ability to observe clearly.

gold standard
Most accurate means of currently diagnosing a particular disease and serves as a basis for comparison with newly developed diagnostic or screening tests.

grand mean
In analysis of variance, scores from all groups are combined and summed, and the mean or average is obtained for all scores.

grant
Research funding from private or public institutions to support the conduct of a study.

grantsmanship
Expertise and skill in successfully developing proposals to obtain funding for selected studies.

grounded theory research
Qualitative, inductive research technique based on symbolic interaction theory that is conducted to discover what problems exist in a social scene and the processes persons use to handle them. The research process involves formulation, testing, and redevelopment of propositions until a theory is developed.

Grove Model for Implementing Evidence-Based Guidelines in Practice
Model developed by one of the textbook authors (Grove) to promote the use of national, standardized evidence-based guidelines in clinical practice.

H

Hawthorne effect
Psychological response in which subjects change their behavior simply because they are subjects in a study, not because of the research treatment.

heterogeneity
Researcher's attempt to obtain subjects with a wide variety of characteristics to reduce the risk of bias in studies not using random sampling.

heuristic relevance
Standard for evaluating a qualitative study in which the study's intuitive recognition, relationship to the existing body of knowledge, and applicability are examined.

hierarchical statement sets
Composed of a specific proposition and a hypothesis or research question. If a conceptual model is included in the framework, the set may also include a general proposition.

highly controlled settings
Artificially constructed environments that are developed for the sole purpose of conducting research, such as laboratories, experimental centers, and research medical units.

HIPAA Privacy Rule
Federal regulations implemented in 2003 to protect an individual's health information. The HIPAA Privacy Rule affects not only the health care environment but also the research conducted in this environment.

historical research
Qualitative research method that includes a narrative description or analysis of events that occurred in the remote or recent past.

historiography
The research methodology used for conducting historical research.

history effect
Event that is not related to the planned study but occurs during the time of the study and could influence the responses of subjects to the treatment.

homogeneity
Degree to which objects are similar or a form of equivalence, such as limiting subjects to only one level of

an extraneous variable to reduce its impact on the study findings.

homogeneity reliability
Type of reliability testing used with paper-and-pencil tests that addresses the correlation of various items within the instrument.

homoscedastic
Data are evenly dispersed both above and below the regression line, which indicates a linear relationship on a scatter diagram (plot).

horizontal axis
This is the *x* axis in a scatterplot or graph of a regression line.

human rights
Claims and demands that have been justified in the eyes of an individual or by the consensus of a group of individuals and are protected in research.

hypothesis
Formal statement of the expected relationship(s) between two or more variables in a specified population.

hypothesis guessing
Occurs when subjects within a study guess the hypothesis of the researcher.

hypothetical population
A population that cannot be defined according to sampling theory rules, which require a list of all members of the population.

I

illustrations
Figures used to provide a picture of the results from studies. The most common figures used in research presentations and publications are bar and line graphs.

immersed in the culture
Involves gaining increasing familiarity with such things as language, sociocultural norms, traditions, communication patterns, religion, work patterns, and expression of emotion in a selected culture.

immersion in the data
Initial phase of qualitative data analysis where researchers become very familiar with the data by reading and rereading notes and transcripts, recalling observations and experiences, listening to tapes, and viewing videotapes.

implications of research findings for nursing
Meaning of research conclusions for the body of knowledge, theory, and practice in nursing.

inclusion sampling criteria
Sampling requirements identified by the researcher that must be present for the element or subject to be included in the sample.

incomplete disclosure
Subjects are not completely informed about the purpose of a study because that knowledge might alter the subjects' actions. After the study, the subjects must be debriefed about the complete purpose of the study and the findings.

independent groups
Groups in which the selection of one subject is totally unrelated to the selection of other subjects. An example is when subjects are randomly selected and assigned to the treatment and control groups.

independent samples
See *independent groups*.

independent variable
Treatment, intervention, or experimental activity that is manipulated or varied by the researcher to create an effect on the dependent variable.

index
Provides assistance in identifying journal articles and other publications relevant to a topic of interest.

indirect costs
Expenses related to a research project but not specifically part of the implementation of the steps of the study, such as salaries for researchers and data collectors. Grants that fund indirect costs provide researchers greater freedom to conduct studies.

indirect measurement
Used with abstract concepts; the concepts are not measured directly, but instead, indicators or attributes of the concepts are used to represent the abstraction, such as a perception of pain scale to measure chronic pain.

individually identifiable health information (IIHI)
Any information collected from an individual, including demographic information, that is created or received by health care providers, a health plan, or a health care clearinghouse and is related to the past, present, or future physical or mental health or condition of an individual and identifies the individual.

inductive reasoning
Reasoning from the specific to the general in which particular instances are observed and then combined into a larger whole or general statement.

inference

Use of inductive reasoning to move from a specific case to a general truth. Thus, statistics are used to infer from the specific study results to a general statement about the larger population.

inferential statistics

Statistics designed to allow inference from a sample statistic to a population parameter; commonly used to test hypotheses of similarities and differences in subsets of the sample under study.

inferred causality

Cause-and-effect relationship is identified from numerous studies conducted over time to determine risk factors or causal factors in selected situations.

information-rich cases

Cases selected during the purposive sampling process from which qualitative researchers can learn a great deal about the central focus of their study.

informed consent

Prospective subject's agreement to voluntarily participate in a study, which is reached after the subject assimilates essential information about the study.

inherent variability

Data can be naturally expected to have a few random observations included in the extreme ends of the tails.

innovation

An idea, a practice, or an object that is perceived as new by an individual or other unit of adoption.

innovators

Individuals who actively seek out new ideas and are often the ones most likely to promote the use of best research evidence in practice or to conduct research.

institutional review

Process of examining studies for ethical concerns by a committee of peers to determine if the study can be conducted in a selected agency.

institutional review board (IRB)

Committee that reviews research to ensure that the investigator is conducting the research ethically. Universities, hospital corporations, and many managed care centers have IRBs to promote the conduct of ethical research and to protect the rights of prospective subjects at their institutions.

instrumentation

A component of measurement that involves the application of specific rules to develop a measurement device or instrument.

integrative review of research

Conducted to identify, analyze, and synthesize the results from independent studies to determine the current knowledge (what is known and not known) in a particular area.

integrity of an intervention

The extent to which the intervention is implemented as it was designed in intervention research.

intensity of an intervention

Defines the amount of each activity that must be given and the frequency with which each activity is implemented in an intervention within intervention research.

interaction effects

Influence on the design validity by the interaction of different facets of the study such as selection of subjects and treatment, setting and treatment, or history and treatment.

interaction of different treatments

Is a threat to construct validity and occurs when subjects receive more than one treatment in a study.

intercept

The point where the regression line crosses (or intercepts) the y-axis and is represented by the letter a.

interdisciplinary teams

Variety of health professionals, such as nurses, physicians, and social workers, who work collaboratively to deliver health care based on the needs of patients and families.

interlibrary loan department

Department that locates books and articles in other libraries and provides the sources within a designated time.

internal consistency

Maintaining the integrity of the different steps of the research process, such as sample selection, measurement of study variables, implementation of study treatment, and data collection.

internal criticism

Involves examination of the reliability of historical documents.

internal validity

Extent to which the effects detected in the study are a true reflection of reality rather than being the result of the effects of extraneous variables.

interpretation of research outcomes

Involves examining the results of data analysis, forming conclusions, considering the implications for nursing, exploring the significance of the findings, generalizing the findings, and suggesting further studies.

interpretive codes
Organizational system developed late in the qualitative data collection and analysis process as the researcher gains some insight into the processes occurring.

interpretive reliability
Assesses the extent to which each judge assigns the same category to a given unit of data.

interrater reliability
Degree of consistency between two raters who are independently assigning ratings to a variable or attribute being investigated.

interrupted time-series designs
Designs similar to descriptive time designs except that a treatment is applied at some point in the observations.

interval data
Numerical information collected during a study that has equal distances between intervals of the data and also follows the rules of mutually exclusive categories, exhaustive categories, and rank ordering, which influences the type of statistical analyses that can be conducted.

interval estimate
Researcher identifies a range of values on a number line where the population parameter is thought to be.

interval-scale measurement
Interval scales have equal numerical distances between intervals of the scale in addition to following rules of mutually exclusive categories, exhaustive categories, and rank ordering, such as temperature.

intervening variable
Mediating variable that can affect the occurrence, strength, or direction of a relationship.

intervention effectiveness
The extent to which the treatment produces the outcome desired or predicted in the study hypothesis.

intervention fidelity
Reliable and competent implementation of an experimental treatment that includes two core components: (1) adherence to the delivery of the prescribed treatment behaviors, session, or course, and (2) competence in the researcher or interventionalist's skillfulness in delivery of the intervention.

intervention mode
Qualitative mode of nursing inquiry within grounded theory that is used to test the relationships in the substantive theory developed as part of the study.

intervention research
New methodology for investigating the effectiveness of a nursing intervention in achieving the desired outcome or outcomes in a natural setting.

intervention taxonomy
An organized categorization of all interventions performed by nurses.

intervention theory
This theory includes a careful description of the problem that the intervention will address, intervening actions that must be implemented to address the problem, moderating variables that might change the impact of the intervention, mediating variables that might alter the effect of the intervention, and expected outcomes of the intervention.

interventionist
In intervention research, a person who has been formally prepared to provide a particular intervention and is accountable for the fidelity of the intervention.

interventions
Treatments, therapies, procedures, or actions implemented by researchers to determine their outcomes in a study, and if effective, are implemented by health care professionals to and with patients, in a particular situation, to move the patients' conditions toward desired health outcomes that are beneficial to them.

interviews
Structured or unstructured verbal communication between the researcher and subject during which information is obtained for a study.

introspection
Process of turning your attention inward toward your own thoughts to provide increased awareness and understanding of the flow and interplay of feelings and ideas.

intuiting
Process of actually looking at the phenomenon in qualitative research; the individual focuses all awareness and energy on the subject of interest.

intuition
Insight or understanding of a situation or event as a whole that usually cannot be logically explained.

intuitive recognition
When individuals are confronted with the theoretical schema derived from the data of a qualitative study, it has meaning within their personal knowledge base.

invasion of privacy
When private information is shared without an individual's knowledge or against his or her will.

inverse linear relationship
Indicates that as one variable or concept changes, the other variable or concept changes in the opposite direction; also referred to as a *negative linear relationship*.

investigator triangulation
Exists when two or more research-trained investigators with divergent backgrounds explore the same phenomenon.

Iowa Model of Evidence-Based Practice
Model developed in 1994 and revised in 2001 by Titler and colleagues to promote evidence-based practice in clinical agencies.

J

justice, principle of
States that human subjects should be treated fairly.

K

Kendall's tau
Nonparametric test to determine the correlation among variables used when both variables have been measured at least at the ordinal level.

key informants
Participants in qualitative studies that provide quality information during the conduct of the study.

keywords
Major concepts or variables that must be included in your literature search. Keywords or terms can be identified by determining the concepts relevant to your study, the populations of particular interest in your study, interventions to be implemented, and measurement methods to be used in the study, or possible outcomes for the study.

knowledge
Essential content or body of information for a discipline that is acquired through traditions, authority, borrowing, trial and error, personal experience, role-modeling and mentorship, intuition, reasoning, and research.

knowledge utilization
Process of disseminating and using research-generated information to make an impact on or a change in the existing practices in society.

Kolmogorov-Smirnov two-sample test
Nonparametric test used to determine whether two independent samples have been drawn from the same population.

Kruskal-Wallis test
Most powerful nonparametric analysis technique for examining three independent groups for differences.

kurtosis
Degree of peakedness (platykurtic, mesokurtic, or leptokurtic) of the curve shape that is related to the spread or variance of scores.

L

lack of intervention integrity
A discrepancy between what was planned and what was actually delivered of an intervention or treatment in intervention research.

lambda
Nonparametric analysis technique that measures the degree of association (or relationship) between two nominal-level variables.

landmark studies
Major projects that generate knowledge that influences a discipline and sometimes society in general, and marks an important stage of development or a turning point in a field of research.

latent transition analysis (LTA)
Outcomes research strategy used in situations in which stages or categories of recovery have been defined and transitions across stages can be identified. To use this analysis method, each member of the population is placed in a single category or stage for a given point of time.

least-squares principle
The fact that when deviations from the mean are squared, the sum is smaller than the sum of squared deviations from any other value in a sampling distribution.

legally authorized representative
Individual or other body authorized under applicable law to consent on behalf of a prospective subject to the subject's participation in the procedures involved in the research.

leptokurtic

Term used to describe an extremely peaked-shape distribution of a curve, which means that the scores in the distribution are similar and have limited variance.

level of significance

See *alpha (α)*.

levels of measurement

The rules for assigning numbers to objects so that a hierarchy in measurement was established, and the levels of measurement from lower to higher are nominal, ordinal, interval, and ratio.

library resources

Includes library personnel, interlibrary loan department, circulation department, reference department, audiovisual department, computer search department, and photocopy services.

life story

Narrative analysis designed to reconstruct and interpret the life of an ordinary person. This methodology emerged from history, anthropology, and more recently from phenomenology.

Likert scale

Instrument designed to determine the opinion or attitude of a subject; it contains a number of declarative statements with a scale after each statement.

limitations

Theoretical and methodological restrictions or weaknesses in a study that may decrease the generalizability of the findings.

line graphs

Figures or illustrations that are used to represent the results from studies. Often line graphs are used to show changes in different groups over time.

line of best fit

The use of a regression equation to develop the line that allows the highest degree of prediction possible in a predictive correlational study where independent variables are used to predict the dependent variable.

linear relationship

Relationship between two variables or concepts will remain consistent regardless of the values of each of the variables or concepts

literature review

See *review of relevant literature*.

literature search

Systematic and explicit approach to the identification, retrieval, and bibliographical management of independent studies (usually drawn from published sources) for the purpose of locating information on a topic, synthesizing conclusions, identifying areas for future study, and developing guidelines for clinical practice.

logic

Science that involves valid ways of relating ideas to promote human understanding; includes abstract and concrete thinking and logistic, inductive, and deductive reasoning.

logical chain of evidence

Qualitative data analysis technique where the researcher goes back and carefully traces the evidence from the data through development of the tentative theory; the elements, relationships, and propositions of the theory are then tested against new data.

logical positivism

Branch of philosophy that operates on strict rules of logic, truth, laws, axioms, and predictions. Quantitative research emerged from logical positivism.

logistic reasoning

Used to break the whole into parts that can be carefully examined, as can the relationships among the parts; one can understand the whole by examining the parts.

longitudinal designs

Panel designs used to examine changes in the same subjects over an extended period.

low statistical power

When the strength or power of a study to detect relationships between variables of differences between groups is below the acceptable standard power (0.8) needed to conduct a study. Low statistical power increases the likelihood of a type II error.

M

manipulation

Implementation or controlled movement of a treatment or an independent variable in a study to determine its effect on the study-dependent variable.

Mann-Whitney *U* test

Used to analyze ordinal data with 95% of the power of the *t*-test to detect differences between groups of normally distributed populations.

manual search

Involves examining the catalogue, indexes, abstracts, and bibliographies for relevant sources.

map

See *conceptual map*.

marginal remarks

Qualitative data analysis technique of recording key ideas or observations in the margins of a transcript or file of study data.

matching

Technique used when an experimental subject is randomly selected and a subject similar in relation to important extraneous variables is randomly selected for inclusion in the control or comparison group. This process results in dependent or related groups.

maturation effect

Unplanned and unrecognized changes experienced during a study, such as subjects growing older, wiser, stronger, hungrier, or more tired, that can influence the findings of a study.

McNemar test

Nonparametric test in which a 2×2 table is used to analyze changes that occur in dichotomous variables.

mean

Value obtained by summing all the scores and dividing that total by the number of scores being summed.

mean of means (μ)

Statistical value or mean obtained by analyzing the means from many samples obtained from the same population.

measurement

Process of assigning numbers to objects, events, or situations in accord with some rule.

measurement error

Difference between what exists in reality and what is measured by a research instrument.

measures of central tendency

Statistical procedures (mode, median, and mean) for determining the center of a distribution of scores.

measures of dispersion

Statistical procedures (range, difference scores, sum of squares, variance, and standard deviation) for examining how scores vary or are dispersed around the mean.

median

Score at the exact center of the ungrouped frequency distribution.

mediating processes

A transformational process that occurs as a series of changes in participants and mediator variables after initiation of the intervention in intervention research.

mediator variables

Variables that bring about the effects of the intervention after it has occurred and thus influence the outcomes of an intervention study.

Medical Treatment Effectiveness Program (MEDTEP)

Major research effort initiated by the Agency for Healthcare Research and Quality (AHRQ) that was implemented to improve the effectiveness and appropriateness of medical practice.

memo

Developed by the researcher to record insights or ideas related to notes, transcripts, or codes during qualitative data analysis.

mentee

The protégé who is guided by a mentor in the mentorship process.

mentor

Someone who serves as a teacher, sponsor, guide, exemplar, or counselor for a novice or protégé. For example, an expert nurse serves as a guide or role model for a novice nurse or mentee.

mentorship

Intense form of role-modeling in which an expert nurse serves as a teacher, sponsor, guide, exemplar, and counselor for a novice nurse.

mesokurtic

Term that describes a normal curve with an intermediate degree of kurtosis and intermediate variance of scores.

meta-analysis

Involves the statistical pooling of the results from several previous studies into a single quantitative analysis that provides one of the highest levels of evidence for an intervention's efficacy.

meta-analysis design

Merging of findings from several completed studies to determine what is known about a particular phenomenon.

metasummary, qualitative

Synthesis or summing of findings across qualitative reports to determine the current knowledge in an area.

metasynthesis, qualitative

Synthesis of qualitative studies that provides a fully integrated, novel description or explanation of a target event or experience versus a summary view of that event or experience. Metasynthesis requires more complex, integrative thought in developing a new perspective or theory based on the findings of previous qualitative studies.

method of least squares

Procedure in regression analysis for developing the line of best fit.

methodological congruence

Standard for evaluating qualitative research in which documentation rigor, procedural rigor, ethical rigor, and auditability of the study are examined.

methodological designs

Used to develop the validity and reliability of instruments to measure research concepts and variables.

methodological limitations

Restrictions or weaknesses in the study design that limit the credibility of the findings and the population to which the findings can be generalized.

methodological triangulation

Use of two or more research methods or procedures in a study, such as different designs, instruments, and data collection procedures, usually from both quantitative and qualitative research.

metric ordinal scale

Scales that have unequal intervals; when used to collect data during a study result in ordinal data.

micromediation

Examines causal connections at the level of small particles such as atoms and is part of multicausality theory.

middle range theories

Theories that are less abstract and address more specific phenomena than grand theories and are directly applicable to practice and focus on explanation and implementation.

minimal risk

Risk of harm anticipated in the proposed research is not greater, with regard to probability and magnitude, than that ordinarily encountered in daily life or during the performance of routine physical or psychological examinations.

mixed results

Study results included a combination of significant and nonsignificant outcomes, which are probably the most common results from studies.

modal percentage

Appropriate for nominal data and indicates the relationship of the number of data scores represented by the mode to the total number of data scores.

mode

Numerical value or score that occurs with the greatest frequency in a distribution; however, it does not necessarily indicate the center of the data set.

model-testing designs

Used to test the accuracy of a hypothesized causal model or map.

moderator variable

Variable that occurs with the intervention (independent variable) and alters the causal relationship between the intervention and outcomes. It includes characteristics of the subjects and the person implementing the intervention.

molar

Causal laws related to large and complex objects that are part of the theory of multicausality.

monographs

Books, booklets of conference proceedings, or pamphlets, which are usually written once and may be updated with a new edition.

mono-method bias

More than one measure of a variable is used in a study, but all measures use the same method of recording, such as using two paper-and-pencil scales to measure depression in a study.

mono-operation bias

Occurs when only one method of measurement is used to measure a variable or concept in a study, such as the use of one paper-and-pencil scale to measure chronic pain.

mortality or attrition

Subjects drop out of a study before completion, which creates a threat to the study's internal validity. Sometimes referred to as sample mortality or attrition.

multicausality

Recognition that a number of interrelating variables can be involved in causing a particular effect.

multicollinearity

Occurs when the independent variables in a regression equation are strongly correlated.

multicomponent treatments, effects of

Occur when a set of treatments are combined to manage a patient problem. Outcomes research designs have been developed to examine the effects of these treatment programs, and some of these designs include treatment package strategy, comparative treatment strategy, dismantling strategy, constructive strategy, factorial ANOVA design, fractional factorial designs, dose-response designs, response surface methodology, and mediational analysis.

multidimensional scaling
A measurement method that was developed to examine many aspects or elements of a concept or variable.

multilevel analysis
Used in epidemiology to study how environmental factors and individual attributes and behavior interact to influence individual-level health behavior and disease risk.

multimethod-multitrait technique
When a variety of data collection methods, such as interview and observation, are used and different measurement methods are used for each concept in a study.

multimodal
A distribution of scores that has more than two modes or most frequently occurring scores.

multiple regression analysis
Extension of simple linear regression with more than one independent variable entered into the analysis.

multiple triangulation
Use of two or more types of triangulation (theoretical, data, methodological, investigator, and analysis) in a study.

multistage cluster sampling
Type of cluster sampling when the random selection of the sample continues through several stages.

multivariate analysis techniques
Used to analyze data from complex research projects with more than two study variables. Techniques included in text are multiple regression, factorial analysis of variance, analysis of covariance, factor analysis, discriminant analysis, canonical correlation, structural equation modeling, time-series analysis, clinical trials, and survival analysis.

N

narrative analysis
Qualitative means of formally analyzing text including stories.

natural settings
Field settings or uncontrolled, real-life settings where research is conducted, such as subjects' homes, worksites, and schools.

necessary relationship
One variable or concept must occur for the second variable or concept to occur.

negative likelihood ratio
Ratio of true-negative results to false-negative results and is calculated as follows: Negative likelihood ratio = 100% − Sensitivity ÷ Specificity.

negative linear relationship
See *inverse linear relationship.*

negative results
Unpredicted nonsignificant or inclusive results from a study that are often the most difficult to explain.

nested design
Design that allows the researcher to consider the effect of variables that are found only at some levels of the independent variables being studied.

nested variables
Variables found only at certain levels of the independent variable, such as gender, race, socioeconomic status, and education.

network sampling
Nonprobability sampling method that includes a snowballing technique that takes advantage of social networks and the fact that friends tend to hold characteristics in common. Subjects meeting the sample criteria are asked to assist in locating others with similar characteristics.

networking
Process of developing channels of communication between people with common research interests throughout the country.

nominal data
Lowest level of data that can only be organized into categories that are exclusive and exhaustive, but the categories cannot be compared or rank ordered and can only be analyzed by the lowest level of statistical analyses.

nominal-scale measurement
Lowest level of measurement that is used when data can be organized into categories that are exclusive and exhaustive, but the categories cannot be compared or rank ordered, such as gender, race, marital status, and diagnoses.

nondirectional hypothesis
States that a relationship exists but does not predict the exact nature of the relationship.

nonequivalent control group designs
Designs in which the control group is not selected by random means, such as the one-group posttest-only design, posttest-only design with nonequivalent groups, and one-group pretest–posttest design.

nonparametric statistical analysis

Statistical techniques used when the assumptions of parametric statistics are not met, and most commonly used to analyze nominal- and ordinal-level data.

nonprobability sampling

Not every element of the population has an opportunity for selection in the sample, such as convenience (accidental) sampling, quota sampling, purposive sampling, and network sampling.

nonrandom sampling

See *nonprobability sampling.*

nonsignificant results

Negative results or results contrary to the researcher's hypotheses that can be an accurate reflection of reality or can be caused by study weaknesses. Also see *negative results.*

nontherapeutic research

Research conducted to generate knowledge for a discipline and in which the results from the study might benefit future patients but will probably not benefit those acting as research subjects.

normal curve

A symmetrical, unimodal bell-shaped curve that is a theoretical distribution of all possible scores, but no real distribution exactly fits the normal curve.

normally distributed

Data points that follow the spread or distribution of a normal curve.

norm-referenced testing

Test performance standards that have been carefully developed over years with large, representative samples by using standardized tests with extensive reliability and validity.

norms

Expected behavior patterns within a social system that affect the diffusion of innovations or new interventions in practice.

null hypothesis

States that there is no relationship between the variables being studied; a statistical hypothesis used for statistical testing and interpreting statistical outcomes.

Nuremberg Code

Ethical code of conduct to guide investigators when conducting research.

Nursing Care Report Card

Evaluation of hospital nursing care using 10 indicators (2 structure indicators, 2 process indicators, and 6 outcome indicators). This report card could facilitate benchmarking or setting a desired standard that would allow comparisons of hospitals in terms of their nursing care quality.

nursing interventions

Deliberative cognitive, physical, or verbal activities performed with or on behalf of individuals and their families that are directed toward accomplishing particular therapeutic objectives relative to individuals' health and well-being.

nursing research

Scientific process that validates and refines existing knowledge and generates new knowledge that directly and indirectly influences the delivery of evidence-based nursing practice.

nursing-sensitive patient outcomes

Patient outcomes that are influenced by or associated with nursing.

O

oblique rotation

Type of rotation in factor analysis used to accomplish the best fit (best-factor solution) and in which the factors are allowed to be correlated.

observational measurement

Use of structured and unstructured observation to measure study variables.

observed level of significance

The actual level of significance that is achieved or observed in a study.

observed score

Actual score or value obtained for a subject on a measurement tool.

observer as participant

Researcher's time is spent mainly observing and interviewing subjects and less in the participation role.

one-group posttest-only design

Preexperimental design with numerous threats to validity that is inadequate for making causal references.

one-group pretest-posttest design

Quasi-experimental design where the pretest scores serve as the comparison group and the posttest scores after the treatment serve as the experimental group.

one-tailed test of significance

Analysis used with directional hypotheses in which extreme statistical values of interest are thought to occur in a single tail of the curve.

open context

Requires deconstructing a sedimented view to allow one to see the depth and complexity within the phenomenon being examined in qualitative research.

operational definition

Description of how variables or concepts will be measured or manipulated in a study.

operational reasoning

Involves identification and discrimination among many alternatives or viewpoints and focuses on the process of debating alternatives.

operationalizing a variable or concept

Development of the conceptual definition of a concept or variable to link it to the study framework and the operational definition of a concept or variable so it can be measured or manipulated in a study.

operator

Permits grouping of ideas, selection of places to search in a database record, and ways to show relationships within a database record, sentence, or paragraph. The most common operators include Boolean, locational, and positional.

operator, Boolean

The three words AND, OR, and NOT are used with your identified concepts in conducting searches of databases.

operator, locational

Search operator that identifies terms in specific areas or fields of a record, such as article title, author, and journal name.

operator, positional

Search operator used to look for requested terms within certain distance of one another. Common positional operators are NEAR, WITH, and ADJ.

opportunity costs

Lost opportunities that the patient, family member, or others experience. For example, a family member might have been able to earn more money if he or she had not had to stay home and care for a chronically ill child.

ordinal data

Data that can be ranked, but the intervals between the ranked data are not necessarily equal, such as military ranks. This level of data is analyzed by nonparametric statistical techniques.

ordinal-scale level

Measurement that yields data that can be ranked, but the intervals between the ranked data are not necessarily equal, such as levels of coping.

outcomes of care

The dependent variables or clinical results of health care that are measured to determine the impact of the process of care management techniques. The outcomes from the Medical Outcomes Study Framework include clinical end points, functional status, general well-being, and satisfaction with care.

outcomes research

Important scientific methodology that was developed to examine the end results of patient care. The strategies used in outcomes research are a departure from traditional scientific endeavors and incorporate evaluation research, epidemiology, and economic theory perspectives.

outliers

Extreme scores or values in a set of data that are exceptions to the overall findings.

out-of-pocket costs

Those expenses incurred by the patient or family or both that are not reimbursable by the insurance company; they might include costs of buying supplies, dressings, selected medications, or special foods.

P

paradigm

Particular way of viewing a phenomenon in the world.

parallel-forms reliability

See *alternate-forms reliability.*

parameter

Measure or numerical value of a population.

parametric statistical analyses

Statistical techniques used when three assumptions are met: (1) the sample was drawn from a population for which the variance can be calculated, and the distribution is expected to be normal or approximately normal; (2) the level of measurement should be interval or ratio with an approximately normal distribution; and (3) the data can be treated as though it were obtained from random samples.

paraphrasing

Involves expressing clearly and concisely the ideas of an author in your own words.

partially controlled setting

Environment that the researcher manipulates or modifies in some way when it is used as a setting for a study.

participant as observer

Special form of observation in which researchers immerse themselves in the setting so they can hear, see, and experience the reality as the participants do. However, the participants are aware of the dual roles of the researcher (participant and observer).

participants

Individuals who participate in qualitative research.

participatory research

Strategy that includes representatives from all groups that will be affected by the change (stakeholders) as collaborators. This strategy facilitates a broad base of support for new interventions for the target population, the professional community, and the general public.

path coefficient

Effect of the independent variable on the dependent variable that is determined through path analysis.

patient outcomes research teams (PORTs)

Large-scale, multifaceted, and multidisciplinary projects initiated by the AHRQ that were designed to examine the outcomes and cost of current practice patterns, identify the best treatment strategy, and test methods for reducing inappropriate variations.

pattern

Analysis of qualitative data to determine the trends and links among the facets of the data that can become the meaningful findings from the study. Researchers need to spend extensive time analyzing qualitative data to prevent prematurely identifying patterns, themes, and gestalts.

Pearson's product-moment correlation coefficient (r)

Parametric test used to determine the relationship between two variables.

percentage of variance

Amount of variability explained by a linear relationship; the value is obtained by squaring Pearson's correlation coefficient (r). For example, if an $r = 0.5$ in a study, the percentage of variance explained is $r^2 = 0.25$ or 25%.

periodicals

Subset of serials with predictable publication dates, such as journals, that are published over time and are numbered sequentially for the years published.

permission to participate in a study

Agreement of parents or guardians to the participation of their child or ward in research.

personal experience

Gaining knowledge by being personally involved in an event, situation, or circumstance. Benner described five levels of experience in the development of clinical knowledge and expertise: (1) novice, (2) advanced beginner, (3) competent, (4) proficient, and (5) expert.

phenomenological research

Inductive, descriptive qualitative methodology developed from phenomenological philosophy for the purpose of describing experiences as they are lived by the study participants.

phi coefficient (φ)

Analysis technique to determine relationships or differences in dichotomous, nominal data.

philosophical analysis

Qualitative research method that uses concept or linguistic analysis to examine meaning and develop theories of meaning in philosophical inquiry.

philosophical inquiry

Qualitative research method using intellectual analysis to clarify meanings, make values manifested, identify ethics, and study the nature of knowledge. Types of philosophical inquiry covered in this text are foundational inquiry, philosophical analysis, and ethical analysis.

philosophical research

See *philosophical inquiry.*

philosophy

Broad, global explanation of the world that gives meaning to the world of nursing and provides a framework within which thinking, knowing, and doing occur.

physiological measures

Techniques used to measure physiological variables either directly or indirectly, such as techniques to measure heart rate or mean arterial pressure.

pilot study

Smaller version of a proposed study conducted to develop or refine the methodology, such as the treatment, instrument, or data collection process.

pink sheet

Letter indicating rejection of a research grant proposal and a critique by the scientific committee that reviewed the proposal.

plagiarism

Type of research misconduct that involves the appropriation of another person's ideas, processes, results, or words without giving appropriate credit, including those obtained through confidential review of others' research proposals and manuscripts.

platykurtic

Term that indicates a relatively flat curve with the scores having large variance among them.

point estimate

Single figure that estimates a related figure in the population of interest.

population

All elements (individuals, objects, events, or substances) that meet the sample criteria for inclusion in a study; sometimes referred to as a *target population.*

population-based studies

Important type of outcomes research that involves studying health conditions in the context of the community rather than the context of the medical system.

population parameter

A true but unknown numerical characteristic of a population. Parameters of the population are estimated with statistics.

population studies

Studies that target the entire population.

positive likelihood ratio

Likelihood ratio calculated to determine the likelihood that a positive test result is a true positive and a negative test result is a true negative. Positive Likelihood Ratio = Sensitivity ÷ (100% − Specificity).

positive linear relationship

Indicates that as one variable changes (value of the variable increases or decreases), the second variable will also change in the same direction.

post hoc analyses

Statistical tests developed specifically to determine the location of differences in studies with more than two groups, such as when ANOVA results are significant in a study that has three or more groups. Frequently used post hoc tests are Bonferroni's procedure, the Newman-Keuls test, the Tukey HSD test, the Scheffé test, and Dunnett's test.

poster session

Visual presentation of a study by using pictures, tables, and illustrations on a display board.

posttest-only design with comparison group

Preexperimental design conducted to examine the difference between the experimental group that receives a treatment and the comparison groups that does not.

potential markets

Possible situations or sites where interventions tested through intervention research might be sold and delivered.

power

Probability that a statistical test will detect a significant difference or relationship that exists, which is the capacity to correctly reject a null hypothesis. Standard power of 0.8 is used to conduct power analysis to determine the sample size for a study.

power analysis

Used to determine the risk of a type II error so that the study can be modified to decrease the risk, if necessary. Conducting a power analysis involves alpha, effect size, and standard power of 0.8 to determine the sample size for a study.

practical significance

Associated with its importance to the body of knowledge that applies to nursing and is sometimes referred to as clinical significance.

practice effect

Occurs when subjects improve as they become more familiar with the experimental protocol.

practice pattern profiling

Epidemiological technique used in outcomes research that focuses on patterns of care rather than individual occurrences of care.

practice styles

Particular ways to implement health care that affect health outcomes and are examined in outcomes research. Practice styles are part of the construct process of care from Donabedian's theory of health care.

practice-based research networks

Group of practices focused on patient care that are affiliated in order to analyze their clinical practices in communities.

precision

Accuracy with which the population parameters have been estimated within a study. Also used to describe the degree of consistency or reproducibility of measurements with physiological instruments.

prediction

Ability to estimate the probability of a specific outcome in a given situation that can be achieved through research.

prediction equation

Outcome of regression analysis where a formula or equation is developed to predict a dependent variable.

predictive design

Developed to predict the value of the dependent variable based on values obtained from the independent variables; one approach to examining causal relationships between variables.

predictive validity

Type of construct instrument validity where future performance or attitudes are proposed or predicted based on an instrument's scores—for example, measuring health-related behaviors with an instrument to predict future health status of individuals.

preference clinical trials (PCTs)

Studies in which patients choose among all treatments available rather than being randomized into a study group.

premature parsimony

A weakness in qualitative data analysis where the researcher reduces and summarizes study findings or develops a theory without adequate collection and analysis of essential data.

premise

Statement that identifies the proposed relationship between two or more variables or concepts.

preproposal

Short document (four to five pages plus appendices) written to explore the funding possibilities for a research project.

prescribed behaviors

Behaviors that are elements of the interventions implemented in intervention research.

prescriptive theory

Specifies what must be done to achieve the desired effects, including (1) the components, intensity, and duration required; (2) the human and material resources needed; and (3) the procedures to be followed to produce the desired outcomes.

presentations

The sharing of research findings verbally by delivering a research report and responding to questions, or by displaying a poster of a study at a conference or meeting.

pretest and posttest design with a comparison group

Type of quasi-experimental design frequently implemented to determine the effect of a treatment by comparing the experimental group (treatment group) with the comparison group.

pretest-posttest control group design

Classic experimental design where two randomized groups—one receiving the experimental treatment and one receiving no treatment, a placebo treatment, or usual or standard care—are examined for differences to determine the impact of a treatment.

primary prevention studies

Specially designed studies that attempt to measure things that do not happen. Changes in a community are examined and inferred to be a consequence of the effectiveness of the prevention program (treatment).

primary source

Source that is written by the person who originated or is responsible for generating the ideas published.

primary theoretical source

Source that is written by the theorist who developed the theory or conceptual content.

primordial cell

Concept from Donabedian's framework that is the physical-physiological function of the individual patient being cared for by the individual practitioner.

principal component analysis

Second step in exploratory factor analysis that provides preliminary information that the researcher needs so that decisions can be made before the final factoring.

principal investigator (PI)

In a research grant, the individual who will have primary responsibility for administering the grant and interacting with the funding agency.

privacy

The freedom an individual has to determine the time, extent, and general circumstances under which private information will be shared with or withheld from others.

probability sampling method

Random sampling techniques in which each member (element) in the population should have a greater than zero opportunity to be selected for the sample; examples include simple random sampling, stratified random sampling, cluster sampling, and systematic sampling.

probability statement

Expresses the likelihood that something will happen in a given situation and addresses relative rather than absolute causality.

probability theory

Theory that addresses relative rather than absolute causality. Thus, from a probability perspective, a cause will not produce a specific effect each time that particular cause occurs, but the probability value indicates how frequently the effect might occur with the cause.

probing

Technique interviewers use to obtain more information in a specific area of the interview.

problem statement

Single statement that follows the significance and background of a problem and identifies the gap in the knowledge base needed for practice.

problematic reasoning

Involves identifying a problem, selecting solutions to the problem, and resolving the problem.

procedural rigor

In critical appraisal of qualitative studies, the standard of methodological congruence includes procedural rigor that involve examining a study for the researcher's detail in applying selected procedures or steps of a qualitative study.

process of care

Construct that includes mechanisms for delivering health care, and is one of three constructs (structure, process, and outcomes of care) in Donabedian's theory of health care.

process-outcome matrix

Qualitative analysis technique that allows the researcher to trace the processes that led to differing outcomes.

project team

The members of a research group or team that are conducting a study.

projective technique

Method of measuring individuals' responses to unstructured or ambiguous situations as a means of describing attitudes, personality characteristics, and motives of the individuals; an example is the Rorschach inkblot test.

proportionate sampling

In stratification, each stratum should have numbers of subjects selected in proportion to their occurrence in the population.

proposal, research

Written plan identifying the major elements of a study, such as the problem, purpose, and framework, and outlining the methods to conduct the study; a formal way to communicate ideas about a proposed study to receive approval to conduct the study and to seek funding.

proposition

Abstract statement that further clarifies the relationship between two concepts.

proscribed behaviors

Actions that interventionalists may not do or say during an intervention study.

prospective cohort study

Epidemiological study in which a group of people are identified who are at risk for experiencing a particular event.

protection from discomfort and harm

This is a right of research subjects based on the ethical principle of beneficence, which holds that one should do good and, above all, do no harm. The levels of discomfort and harm are (1) no anticipated effects, (2) temporary discomfort, (3) unusual levels of temporary discomfort, (4) risk of permanent damage, and (5) certainty of permanent damage.

prototype

Primitive design that has evolved to the point that it can be tested clinically. Guided by intervention theory, a prototype includes establishing and selecting a mode of delivery of the intervention.

providers of care

Individuals responsible for delivering care, such as nurse practitioners and physicians, who are part of the structure of care of Donabedian's theory of health care.

published research

Studies that are permanently recorded in hard copies of journals or books or are posted online for readers to access.

purposive sampling

Judgmental or selective sampling method that involves conscious selection by the researcher of certain subjects or elements to include in a study. Purposive sampling is a type of nonprobability sampling.

Q

Q-sort methodology

Technique of comparative rating in which a subject sorts cards with statements on them into designated piles (usually 7–10 piles in the distribution of a normal curve) that might range from best to worst.

qualitative research

Systematic, interactive, subjective approach used to describe life experiences and give them meaning.

qualitative research proposal

A document developed by a researcher of a proposed qualitative study that often includes an introduction, philosophical base, and methodology for conducting the study.

qualitative research report

Report developed to describe the flexible, dynamic implementation of the research project and the unique, creative findings. The report usually includes introduction, methods, results, and discussion sections.

qualitative research synthesis

Process and product of systematically reviewing and formally integrating the findings from qualitative studies. Qualitative research synthesis includes two categories: metasummary and metasynthesis.

quality improvement

Outcome examined to determine the impact of a selected intervention on patient health status.

quality of life

Patient's perception of his or her health status and life that is measured in outcomes research.

quantitative research

Formal, objective, systematic study process to describe and test relationships and to examine cause-and-effect interactions among variables.

quantitative research proposal

A document developed by a researcher of a proposed quantitative study that often includes the introduction, review of the literature, framework, and methodology proposed for the study.

quantitative research report

Report that includes introduction, methods, results, and discussion of findings for a quantitative study.

quasi-experimental research

Type of quantitative research conducted to explain relationships, clarify why certain events happen, and examine causality between selected independent and dependent variables.

quasi-experimental study designs

Designs with limited control that were developed to provide alternative means for examining causality in situations not conducive to experimental controls.

query letter

Letter sent to an editor of a journal to determine interest in publishing an article, or a letter sent to a funding agency to determine interest in funding a study.

questionable publication

Publication in which no coauthor could produce the original data or no coauthor had personally observed or performed each phase of the research or participated in the research publication.

questionnaire

Printed self-report form designed to elicit information that can be obtained through written responses of the subject.

quota sampling

Nonprobability convenience sampling technique with an added strategy to ensure the inclusion of subject types likely to be underrepresented in the convenience sample, such as women, minority groups, and the undereducated.

R

random assignment to groups

Procedure used to assign subjects to treatment or comparison groups in which the subjects have an equal opportunity to be assigned to either group.

random error

Error that causes individuals' observed scores to vary haphazardly around their true score.

random sampling methods

See *probability sampling method.*

random variation

Expected difference in values that occurs when one examines different subjects from the same sample.

randomization

From a sampling theory point of view, each individual in the population should have a greater than zero opportunity to be selected for a sample, which is achieved by random sampling. The methods of assigning subjects to groups can also be random and promote randomization in the final study groups.

randomized blocking design

Experimental design in which the researcher includes subjects with various levels of an extraneous variable in the sample but controls the numbers of subjects at each level of the variable and their random assignment to groups within the study.

randomized clinical trials

Classic means of examining the effects of various treatments in which the effects of a treatment are examined by comparing the treatment group with the no-treatment group.

range

Simplest measure of dispersion, obtained by subtracting the lowest score from the highest score or just identifying the lowest and highest scores in a distribution of scores.

rating scales

Crudest form of measure using scaling techniques; ratings are chosen from an ordered series of categories of a variable assumed to be based on an underlying continuum—for example, rating acute pain on a scale from 1 to 10, with 1 being minimal pain and 10 being extreme pain.

ratio-level measurement

Highest measurement form that meets all the rules of other forms of measure: mutually exclusive categories, exhaustive categories, rank ordering, equal spacing between intervals, and a continuum of values; also has an absolute zero, such as weight.

readability

Is the degree of difficulty in reading and comprehending text that can be determined by a readability formula such as the Fog Index. The readability of a scale can influence the reliability and validity of a scale used in a study.

reasoning

Processing and organizing ideas to reach conclusions; examples include problematic, operational, dialectic, and logistic.

recommendations for future studies

Ideas that emerged from the present study and previous studies in the same area that provide directions for future studies.

reconstructing new ideas or views

In qualitative research, researchers examine many dimensions of the area being studied and form new ideas, while recognizing that the present reconstructing of ideas is only one of many possible ways of organizing data.

recruiting subjects

The process of obtaining subjects or participants for a study that includes identifying potential subjects, approaching them to participate in the study, and gaining their acceptance to participate.

refereed journal

Uses referees or expert reviewers to determine whether a manuscript will be accepted for publication.

reference group

Group of individuals that comprise the standard against which individual subjects' scores are compared.

referencing

Comparing a subject's score against a standard; used in norm-referenced and criterion-referenced testing.

reflexive remarks

Thoughts or insights that often emerge into the consciousness of the researchers while they are analyzing qualitative data and recording notes. These thoughts are generally included with the notes and are separated from the rest of the notes by double parentheses (( )).

reflexive thought

Critically thinking through the dynamic interaction between self and the data during the analysis of qualitative data. During this process, the researcher explores personal feelings and experiences that may influence the study and integrates this understanding into the study.

reflexivity

See *reflexive thought*.

refusal rate

Percentage of potential subjects who decide not to participate in a study. The refusal rate is calculated by dividing the number refusing to participate by the number of potential subjects approached. For example, if 100 subjects are approached and 15 refuse to participate, the refusal rate is $15 \div 100 = 0.15 = 15\%$.

regression coefficient R

Statistic for regression analysis.

regression equation

See *prediction equation*.

regression line

Line that best represents the values of the raw scores plotted on a scatter diagram. The procedure for developing the line of best fit is the method of least squares.

reinvention

Adopters such as nurses modify the innovation or evidence-based intervention to meet their own needs and for use in their practice.

relational statement

Declares that a relationship or link of some kind (positive or negative) exists between two or more concepts. Relational statements are also called propositions in theory and become the focus of testing in quantitative research.

relationship

See *relational statement.*

relative risk

Type of risk associated with conducting any diagnostic and screening test for determining the health problems of patients.

relevant literature

Sources that are pertinent or highly important in providing the in-depth knowledge needed to make changes in practice or to study a selected problem.

reliability

Represents the consistency of the measure obtained. (Also see *reliability testing.*)

reliability testing

Measure of the amount of random error in the measurement technique. Reliability testing of measurement methods focuses on the following three aspects of reliability: stability, equivalence, and homogeneity.

reliable measure

A measurement method used in research that provides consistent data from subjects.

replication

Reproducing or repeating a study to determine whether similar findings will be obtained.

replication, approximate

Operational replication that involves repeating the original study under similar conditions and following the methods as closely as possible.

replication, concurrent

Involves collection of data for the original study and simultaneous replication of the data to provide a check of the reliability of the original study. Confirmation of the original study findings through replication is part of the original study's design.

replication, exact

Involves precise or exact duplication of the initial researcher's study to confirm the original findings.

replication, systematic

Constructive replication that is done under distinctly new conditions in which the researchers conducting the replication do not follow the design or methods of the original researchers; instead, the second investigative team begins with a similar problem statement but formulates new means to verify the first investigator's findings.

representativeness of the sample

Sample must be like the population in as many ways as possible.

request for applications (RFA)

Similar to an RFP except that the government agency not only identifies the problem of concern but also describes the design of the study. Researchers bid for this contract.

request for proposals (RFP)

Federal Register publishes opportunities for funding that usually have deadlines that are only a few weeks after the publication, and researchers need to have a strong background in the area of concern to submit a proposal.

research

Diligent, systematic inquiry or investigation to validate and refine existing knowledge and generate new knowledge.

research benefit

Something of health-related, psychosocial, or other value to an individual research subject, or something that will contribute to the acquisition of generalizable knowledge. Assessing research benefits is part of the ethical process of balancing benefits and risks for a study.

research design

See *design.*

research grant

Funding awarded specifically for conducting a study.

research hypothesis

Alternative hypothesis to the null hypothesis, stating that there is a relationship between two or more variables.

research methodology

The process or plan for conducting the specific steps of the study.

research misconduct

Fabrication, falsification, or plagiarism in processing, performing, or reviewing research, or in reporting research results; it does not include honest error or differences in opinion.

research objectives

Clear, concise, declarative statements that are expressed to direct a study and are focused on identification and description of variables or determination of the relationships among variables, or both.

research problem

Area of concern where there is a gap in the knowledge base needed for nursing practice. Research is conducted to generate essential knowledge to address the practice concern, with the ultimate goal of providing evidence-based nursing care.

research proposal

See *proposal, research.*

research purpose

Concise, clear statement of the specific goal or aim of the study that is generated from the problem.

research questions

Concise, interrogative statements developed to direct studies that are focused on description of variables, examination of relationships among variables, determination of differences between two or more groups, and prediction of dependent variable using independent variables.

research topics

Concepts or broad problem areas that indicate the foci of essential research knowledge needed to provide evidence-based nursing practice. Research topics include numerous potential research problems.

research tradition

Program of research that is important for building a body of knowledge related to the phenomena explained by a particular conceptual model.

research utilization

Process of synthesizing, disseminating, and using research-generated knowledge to make an impact on or a change in the existing practices in society.

research variables or concepts

Qualities, properties, or characteristics identified in the research purpose and objectives or questions that are observed or measured in a study. Research variables or concepts are often used in qualitative studies or descriptive and correlational quantitative studies, where the intent is to observe or measure variables as they exist in a natural setting without the implementation of a treatment.

researcher-participant relationships

In qualitative research, the specific interactions between the researcher and the study participants to accomplish the purpose of the study.

residual variables

Type of variable in a model testing design that indicates the effect of unmeasured variables not included in the model. These variables explain some of the variance found in the data but not the variance within the model.

respect for persons, principle of

Indicates that persons have the right to self-determination and the freedom to participate or not participate in research.

response set

Parameters within which the question or item is to be answered in a questionnaire.

response surface

The plotted figure constructed when several interventions are constructed that represent a number of combinations or differing levels of strength of each component and the outcome is plotted for each combination.

response surface methodology

In intervention research using this methodology, the dose response can be applied to more than one dimension of a treatment.

results

Outcomes from data analysis that are generated for each research objective, question, or hypothesis.

retaining subjects

Specific actions taken by the researcher to retain subjects in a study and to prevent their attrition, which provides a more representative sample for the study and decreases the threats to design validity.

retrospective cohort study

An epidemiological study in which a group of people are identified who have experienced a particular event, such as a study focused on examining occupational exposure to chemicals.

retrospective study

Epidemiological study in which a group of people are identified who have experienced a particular event—for example, studying occupational exposure to chemicals to determine cause-and-effect relationships.

review of relevant literature

Analysis and synthesis of research sources to generate a picture of what is known and not known about a particular situation or research problem.

right to self-determination

See *self-determination, right to.*

rigor

Striving for excellence in research through the use of discipline, scrupulous adherence to detail, and strict accuracy.

rigor in documentation

Standard for critiquing qualitative research that involves clear, concise presentation of the study elements by the researcher.

rival hypothesis

Alternate explanation of cause in a study.

robustness

Analysis procedure that will yield accurate results even if some of the assumptions are violated by the data being analyzed.

role-modeling

Learning by imitating the behavior of an exemplar or role model.

S

sample

Subset of the population that is selected for a study.

sample characteristics

Description of the research subjects obtained by analyzing data acquired from the measurement of the demographic variables (e.g., age, gender, ethnicity, medical diagnoses).

sample mortality or attrition

See *mortality or attrition.*

sample size

Number of subjects or participants recruited and consenting to take part in a study.

sampling

Includes selecting groups of people, events, behaviors, or other elements with which to conduct a study.

sampling criteria

List of the characteristics essential for membership in the target population. Sampling criteria include both inclusion and exclusion criteria.

sampling distribution

Determined by using statistical values (such as means) of many samples obtained from the same population.

sampling error

Difference between a sample statistic used to estimate a population parameter and the actual but unknown value of the parameter.

sampling frame

Listing of every member of the population with membership defined by the sampling criteria.

sampling method

Process of selecting a group of people, events, behaviors, or other elements that are representative of the population being studied; includes probability and nonprobability methods.

sampling plan

Describes the strategies that will be used to obtain a sample for a study and may include either probability or nonprobability sampling methods.

saturation of data

In qualitative research, data saturation occurs when additional sampling provides no new information, only redundancy of previous collected data.

scale

Self-report form of measurement composed of several items that are thought to measure the construct being studied, in which the subject responds to each item on the continuum or scale provided, such as a pain perception scale or state anxiety scale.

scatter diagrams

Figures that provide useful preliminary information about the nature of the relationship between variables that should be developed and examined before performing correlational analysis.

science

Coherent body of knowledge composed of research findings, tested theories, scientific principles, and laws for a discipline.

scientific community

Cohesive group of scholars within a discipline who stimulate the creation of new research ideas and the development of innovative methodologies to conduct research.

scientific method

Incorporates all procedures that scientists have used, currently use, or may use in the future to pursue knowledge, such as quantitative, qualitative, outcomes, and intervention research.

scientific misconduct

See *research misconduct.*

scientific theory

Theory with valid and reliable methods of measuring each concept and relational statements that have been repeatedly tested through research and demonstrated to be valid.

search fields

Fields that indicate the various pieces of information provided about an article by the bibliographical database.

secondary analysis design

Involves studying data previously collected in another study, but different methods of organization of the data and different statistical analyses are used to reexamine the data.

secondary loading

In factor analysis, the lowest loading for a variable when it has high loadings on two factors. When many secondary loadings occur, the factoring is not considered clean.

secondary source
Source that summarizes or quotes content from primary sources.

sedimented view
Seeing things from the perspective of a specific frame of reference, worldview, or theory that gives a sense of certainty, security, and control.

seeking approval to conduct a study
Process that involves submission of a research proposal to a selected group for review and often verbally defending that proposal.

selection effect
Addresses the process by which subjects are chosen to take part in a study and how subjects are grouped within a study.

selectivity in physiological measures
Element of accuracy that involves the ability to identify the signal under study correctly to distinguish it from other signals.

self-determination, right to
Based on the ethical principle of respect for persons, which states that humans are capable of controlling their own destiny. The right to self-determination is violated through the use of coercion, covert data collection, and deception in the research process.

semantic differential scale
Instrument that consists of two opposite adjectives with a seven-point scale between them. The subject selects one point on the scale that best describes his or her view of the concept being examined on the opposite adjectives.

seminal study
First study that prompted the initiation of a field of research.

sensitivity of physiological measures
Related to the amount of change of a parameter that can be measured precisely.

sensitivity of screening or diagnostic test
Refers to the accuracy of a screening or diagnostic test and is the proportion of patients with the disease who have a positive test result or true positive.

sequential relationship
Relationship in which one concept occurs later than the other.

serendipity
Accidental discovery of something valuable or useful during the conduct of a study.

serials
Literature published over time or in multiple volumes; serials do not necessarily have a predictable publication date.

setting
Location for conducting research, such as a natural, partially controlled, or highly controlled setting.

shrinkage of R^2
In regression analysis, a smaller R^2 is calculated on a new sample than on the original sample since the equation developed most precisely fits the original study sample. The shrinkage of R^2 is greatest with small samples and when multicollinearity is great.

sign test
Nonparametric analysis technique developed for data that are difficult to assign numerical values to but can be ranked on some dimension.

significance of a problem
Part of the research problem that indicates the importance of the problem to nursing and to the health of individuals, families, and communities.

significant results
Results that are in keeping with those identified by the researcher.

simple hypothesis
Predicts the relationship (associative or causal) between two variables.

simple linear regression
Parametric analysis technique that provides a means to estimate the value of a dependent variable based on the value of an independent variable.

simple random sampling
Elements are selected at random from the sampling frame for inclusion in a study. Each study element has a probability greater than zero of being selected for inclusion in the study.

skewness
A curve that is asymmetrical (positively or negatively skewed) because of an asymmetrical distribution of scores from a study.

skimming a source
Quick review of a source to gain a broad overview of the content.

slope

Determines the direction and angle of the regression line within the graph. The value is represented by the letter *b*.

small area analyses

Geographical analyses used to examine variations in health status, health services, patterns of care, or patterns of use by geographical areas.

Spearman rank-order correlation coefficient

Nonparametric analysis technique for ordinal data that is an adaptation of the Pearson's product-moment correlation used to examine relationships among variables in a study.

specific propositions

Statements found in theories that are at a moderate level of abstraction and provide the basis for the generation of hypotheses to guide a study.

specificity of a screening or diagnostic test

Proportion of patients without disease who have a negative test result or true negative. Specificity indicates the accuracy of a screening or diagnostic test.

split-half reliability

Used to determine the homogeneity of an instrument's items; the items are split in half, and a correlational procedure is performed between the two halves.

stability

Aspect of reliability testing that is concerned with the consistency of repeated measures.

stakeholders

All the groups that will be affected by a change.

standard deviation (SD)

Measure of dispersion that is calculated by taking the square root of the variance.

standard of care

The national designation of the type of care that patients should receive from health care agencies and providers.

standard scores

Used to express deviations from the mean (difference scores) in terms of standard deviation units, such as *Z* scores, where the mean is 0 and the standard deviation is 1.

statement synthesis

The researcher develops statements proposing specific relationships among the concepts being studied. This step is a part of developing a framework for a study.

statistic

Numerical value obtained from a sample that is used to estimate the parameters of a population.

statistical conclusion validity

Concerned with whether the conclusions about relationships and differences drawn from statistical analyses are an accurate reflection of reality.

statistical hypothesis

See *null hypothesis.*

statistical regression

Movement or regression of extreme scores toward the mean in studies using a pretest-posttest design.

statistical significance

Results are unlikely to be due to chance; thus, there is a difference between groups, or there is a significant relationship between variables.

stepwise regression analysis

Type of exploratory regression analysis in which the independent variables are entered into or removed from the analysis one at a time.

Stetler model

Model developed by Stetler that provides a comprehensive framework to enhance the use of research findings by nurses to facilitate evidence-based practice.

story

An event or series of events that are encompassed by temporal or spatial boundaries and are a source of data in qualitative research.

storytakers

Researchers who receive the information communicated by storytellers.

storytelling

Qualitative data collection technique where an event or series of events, encompassed by temporal or spatial boundaries, are shared with others using an oral medium or sign language.

stratification

Used in a design so that subjects are distributed throughout the sample by using sampling techniques similar to those used in blocking, but the purpose of the procedure is even distribution throughout the sample.

stratified random sampling

Used when the researcher knows some of the variables in the population, which are critical to achieving representativeness. These identified variables are used to divide the sample into strata or groups.

strength of a relationship
Amount of variation explained by the relationship.

structural equation analysis
Analysis technique designed to test theories.

structured interviews
Use of strategies that give the researcher an increasing amount of control over the content of the interview.

structured observation
Clearly identifying what is to be observed and precisely defining how the observations are to be made, recorded, and coded.

study validity
Measure of the truth or accuracy of a claim that is an important concern throughout the research process.

subjects of care
Individuals participating in a study.

substantive theory
Theory of social process developed by the discovery mode to explain a particular social world.

substitutable relationship
Relationship in which a similar concept can be substituted for the first concept and the second concept will occur.

substituted judgment
In the ethical conduct of research, it is a standard concerned with determining the course of action that incompetent individuals would take if they were capable of making a choice.

substruction
See *theoretical substruction*.

sufficient relationship
States that when the first variable or concept occurs, the second will occur regardless of the presence or absence of other factors.

sum of squares
Mathematical manipulation involving summing the squares of the difference scores that is used as part of the analysis process for calculating the standard deviation.

summary statistics
See *descriptive statistics*.

support systems
Individuals or groups in research or health care that provide the continued assistance needed to promote success.

survey
Data collection technique in which questionnaires or personal interviews are used to gather data about an identified population.

survival analysis
Set of techniques designed to analyze repeated measures from a given time (e.g., the beginning of the study, the onset of a disease, the beginning of a treatment) until a certain event (e.g., death, treatment failure, recurrence of the phenomenon) occurs.

symbolic meanings
In qualitative data analysis, the meaning attached to particular ideas or clusters of data.

symmetrical relationship
Complex relationship that consists of two statements: If A occurs (or changes), B will occur (or change); if B occurs (or changes), A will occur (or change); $A \leftrightarrow B$.

symmetry
See *symmetrical relationship*.

synthesis of sources
Clustering and interrelating ideas from several sources to form a gestalt or new, complete picture of what is known and not known in an area.

systematic bias or variation
Consequence of selecting subjects whose measurement values are different or vary in some way from the population.

systematic error
Measurement error that is not random but occurs consistently, such as a scale that inaccurately weighs subjects 3 pounds heavier than they are.

systematic review
Structured, comprehensive synthesis of quantitative studies in a particular health care area to determine the best research evidence available for expert clinicians to use to promote an evidence-based practice.

systematic sampling
Conducted when an ordered list of all members of the population is available and involves selecting every *k*th individual on the list, starting from a point that is selected randomly.

T

tables
Presentation of the results of a study in columns and rows for easy review by the reader.

tails
Extremes of the normal curve where significant statistical values can be found.

target population
Group of individuals who meet the sampling criteria and to which the study findings will be generalized.

tendency statement
Deterministic relationship that describes what always happens in the absence of interfering conditions.

tentative theory
Theory that is newly proposed, has had minimal exposure to critique by the discipline, and has had little testing.

testable hypothesis
Contains variables that are measurable or can be manipulated in the real world.

test-retest reliability
Determination of the stability or consistency of a measurement technique by correlating the scores obtained from repeated measures.

themes
In qualitative data analysis, the theoretical relationships that emerge after researchers have spent extensive time examining the data.

theoretical connectedness
Theoretical schema developed from a qualitative study is clearly expressed, logically consistent, reflective of the data, and compatible with nursing's knowledge base.

theoretical limitations
Weaknesses in the study framework and conceptual and operational definitions that restrict abstract generalization of the findings.

theoretical literature
Includes concept analyses, maps, theories, and conceptual frameworks that support a selected research problem and purpose.

theoretical sampling
Often used in grounded theory research to advance the development of a theory throughout the research process. The researcher gathers data from any individual or group that can provide relevant data for theory generation.

theoretical substruction
Process in which the framework of a published study is separated into component parts to evaluate the logical consistency of the theoretical system and the interaction of the framework with the study methodology.

theoretical triangulation
Use of two or more frameworks or theoretical perspectives in the same study, with development of hypotheses based on the different theoretical perspectives and tested on the same data set.

theory
Consists of an integrated set of defined concepts, existence statements, and relational statements that present a view of a phenomenon and can be used to describe, explain, predict, or control that phenomenon.

therapeutic research
Research that provides the patient an opportunity to receive an experimental treatment that might have beneficial results.

thesis
Research project completed by a master's student as part of the requirements for a master's degree.

time lag
Span of time between the generation of new knowledge through research and the use of this knowledge in practice.

time-dimensional designs
Designs used to examine the sequence and patterns of change, growth, or trends across time.

time-series analysis
Technique designed to analyze changes in a variable across time and thus to uncover a pattern in the data.

total variance
The sum of the within-group variance and the between-group variance is determined by conducting analysis of variance (ANOVA).

traditions
Truths or beliefs that are based on customs and past trends, and provide a way of acquiring knowledge.

transformation of ideas
Movement of ideas across levels of abstraction to determine the existing knowledge base in an area of study.

transformed terms
Conducted in regression analysis to more accurately express the curvilinear relationship between variables.

translation/application
Involves transforming from one language to another to facilitate understanding, and is part of the process of interpreting research outcomes where results are translated and interpreted into findings.

treatment
Independent variable that is manipulated in a study to produce an effect on the dependent variable. The treatment or independent variable is usually detailed

in a protocol to ensure consistent implementation in the study.

treatment diffusion

Occurs when the control group subjects communicate with the experimental subjects and are exposed to aspects of the study treatment.

treatment matching designs

Outcomes research design to compare the relative effectiveness of various treatments.

treatment standardization

Process of ensuring that the research treatment is applied consistently each time the treatment is administered.

trend designs

Designs used to examine changes in the general population in relation to a particular phenomenon.

trial and error

An approach with unknown outcomes that is used in a situation of uncertainty when other sources of knowledge are unavailable.

triangulation

Use of two or more theories, methods, data sources, investigators, or analysis methods in a study. Usually involves combining qualitative and quantitative research methodologies.

true experiment

See *experimental research*.

true negative

Result of a diagnostic or screening test that indicates accurately when a disease is not present.

true positive

Result of a diagnostic or screening test that indicates accurate identification of the presence of a disease.

true score

Score that would be obtained if there were no error in measurement, but some measurement error always occurs.

***t*-test**

A parametric analysis technique used to determine significant differences between measures of two samples; *t*-test analysis techniques exist for dependent and independent groups.

two-tailed test of significance

Type of analysis used for a nondirectional hypothesis in which the researcher assumes that an extreme score can occur in either tail.

type I error

Occurs when the researcher concludes that the samples tested are from different populations (the dif-ference between groups is significant) when, in fact, the samples are from the same population (the difference between groups is not significant). The null hypothesis is rejected when it is true.

type II error

Occurs when the researcher concludes that there is no significant difference between the samples examined when, in fact, a difference exists. The null hypothesis is regarded as true when it is false.

type III error

Type of error encountered in intervention research, where there is a risk of asking the wrong question or a question that does not address the problem of concern.

U

unexpected results

Relationships found between variables or differences between groups that were not hypothesized or predicted from the framework guiding the study.

unimodal

Distribution of scores in a sample has one mode or most frequently occurring score.

unitizing reliability

Extent to which each judge (data collector, coder, researcher) consistently identifies the same units within the data as appropriate for coding.

unstructured interviews

Initiated with a broad question, and subjects are usually encouraged to elaborate on particular dimensions of a topic.

unstructured observations

Involve spontaneously observing and recording what is seen with a minimum of planning.

V

validity from factor analysis

The use of factor analysis to add to the construct validity of a multi-item scale. The factor analysis is used to determine the underlying structure of the scale, and the factors identified need to be consistent with the subconcepts that make up the concept measured by the scale.

validity, design

Strength of a design to produce accurate results, which is determined by examining statistical conclusion validity, internal validity, construct validity, and external validity.

validity, instrument

Determining the extent to which the instrument actually reflects the abstract construct being examined.

validity, study

Measure of the truth or accuracy of a claim; an important concern throughout the research process.

variables

Qualities, properties, or characteristics of persons, things, or situations that change or vary and are manipulated, measured, or controlled in research.

variance

Measure of dispersion that is the mean or average of the sum of squares.

variance analysis

Outcomes research strategy to track individual and group variance from a specific critical pathway. The goal is to decrease preventable variance in process, thus helping patients and their families achieve optimal outcomes.

variation

The spread or varying of scores obtained in a study that are reflective of patients in the real world.

varimax rotation

Type of rotation in factor analysis used to accomplish the best fit (best-factor solution) when the factors are uncorrelated.

verbal presentation

The communication of a research report at a professional conference or meeting.

vertical axis

The y axis in a graph of a regression line or scatterplot.

visual analogue scale

A line 100 mm in length with right-angle stops at each end on which subjects are asked to record their response to a study variable. Also referred to as magnitude scale.

voluntary consent

Prospective subject has decided to take part in a study of his or her own volition without coercion or any undue influence.

W

Wald-Wolfowitz runs test

Nonparametric analysis technique used to determine differences between two populations.

Wilcoxon matched-pairs signed-ranks test

Nonparametric analysis technique used to examine changes that occur in pretest-posttest measures or matched-pairs measures.

within-group variance

Variance that results when individual scores in a group vary from the group mean.

within-method triangulation

Use of both quantitative and qualitative research strategies in conducting a study but within one method, such as using only data triangulation in the study or using only theoretical triangulation in the study.

Y

y **intercept**

Point where the regression line crosses (or intercepts) the *y*-axis. At this point on the regression line; $x = 0$.

Z

Z **scores**

Standardized scores developed from the normal curve.

ILLUSTRATION CREDITS

Chapter 2

2-1, Adapted from Maxine E. Loomis, Ph.D., R.N., C.S., F.A.A.N., unpublished work, 1989, by American Nurses Association [1989]. *Education for participation in nursing research.* Kansas City, MO: American Nurses Association.

Chapter 3

3-2, 3-3, From Hulme, P.A. & Grove, S.K. (1994). Symptoms of female survivors of sexual abuse. *Issues in Mental Health Nursing, 15*(5). Reproduced with permission. All rights reserved. **3-4,** From Artinian, N.T. et al. (2007). Effects of nurse-managed telemonitoring on blood pressure at 12-month follow-up among urban African Americans. *Nursing Research, 56*(5): 313.

Chapter 5

5-1, From Frenn, M., Malin, S., & Bansal, N.K. (2003). Stage-based interventions for low-fat diet with middle school students. *Journal of Pediatric Nursing, 18*(1): 37.

Chapter 7

7-3, Redrawn from Artinian, B.M. (1982). Conceptual mapping: Development of the strategy. *Western Journal of Nursing Research, 4*(4): 385; **7-4,** redrawn from Kamphuis C.B, van Lenthe, F.J., Giskes, K., Brug, J., & Mackenback, J.P. (2007). Perceived environmental determinants of physical activity and fruit and vegetable consumption among high and low socioeconomic groups in the Netherlands. *Health & Place, 13*(2): 495; **7-5,** from Lenz, E.R., Pugh, L.C., Milligan, R.A., Gift, A., & Suppe, F. (1997). The middle-range theory of unpleasant symptoms: An update. *Advances in Nursing Science, 19*(3): 17, ©1997 by Lippincott Williams & Wilkins; from article by Hoffman, A.J., Given, B.A., von Eye, A., Gift, A.G., & Given, C.W. (2007). Relationships among pain, fatigue, insomnia, and gender in persons with lung cancer. *Oncology Nursing Forum, 34*(4): 787; **7-6,** from Pollock, S.E. (1993). Adaptation to chronic illness: A program of research for testing nursing theory. *Nursing Science Quarterly, 6*(2): 87; **7-7,** from Levesque, L. (1998). Empirical verification of a theoretical model derived from the Roy adaptation model: Findings from five studies. *Nursing Science Quarterly, 11*(1): 33.

Chapter 8

8-1, From Jennings-Dozier, K. (1999). Predicting intentions to obtain a Papanicolaou [Pap] smear among African American and Latina women: Testing the theory of planned behaviour. *Nursing Research, 48*(4): 200; **8-2,** from Artinian, N.T., Washington, O.G., & Templin, T.N. (2001). Effects of home telemonitoring and community-based monitoring on blood pressure control in urban African Americans: A pilot study. *Heart & Lung, 30*(3): 197.

Chapter 9

9-3, From U.S. Department of Health and Human Services. (2004, April). HIPAA authorizations for research. *HIPAA Privacy Rule: Information for researchers.* Retrieved October 1, 2007, from http://privacyruleandresearch.nih.gov/authorization.asp.

Chapter 12

12-1, From Donabedian A. (1987). Some basic issues in evaluating the quality of health care. In L.K. Rinke (Ed): *Outcome Measures in Home Care* [Vol. 1, pp. 3–28], New York: National League for Nursing; **12-2,** from American Medical Association, Copyright 1989, *Journal of the American Medical Association, 262*, pp. 925–930; **12-4,** from Lange L.L. & Jacox A. (1993). Using large databases in nursing and health policy research. *Journal of Professional Nursing, 9*(4): 204; **12-5,** from Keeler E.B. (1994). Decision analysis and cost-effectiveness analysis in women's health care. *Clinical Obstetrics and Gynecology, 37*(1): 208.

Chapter 16

16-1, From Waltz, C.F., Strickland, O.L., & Lentz, E.R. (1991). *Measurement in Nursing Research* (p. 389), Philadelphia: F.A. Davis; **16-2,** Courtesy of Respiratory and Monitoring Solutions of Covidien, Boulder, CO; **16-4,** reprinted with the permission of Life's End Institute: Missoula Demonstration Project, Inc., 320 East Main Street, Missoula, MT 59802, 406-728-1613, info@lifes-end.org; and from Hockenberry MJ, Wilson D, Winkelstein ML (2005): *Wong's Essentials of Pediatric Nursing,* ed 7, St. Louis, Mosby,

p. 1259. Used with permission. © Mosby; **16-6,** from Zung, W.W.K. (1965). A self-rating depression scale. *Archives of General Psychiatry, 12*: 63-70; **16-9,** from Couper MR (1984). The Delphi technique: Characteristics and sequence model. *Advances in Nursing Science, 7*(1): 75; **16-10,** from Burman M.E. (1995). Health diaries in nursing research and practice. *Image–Journal of Nursing Scholarship, 27*(2): 148; **16-11,** from Burman M.E. (1995). Health diaries in nursing research and practice. *Image–Journal of Nursing Scholarship, 27*(2): 148; **16-12,** from Oleske, D.M., Heinze, S., & Otte, D.M. (1990). The diary as a means of understanding the quality of life of persons with cancer receiving home nursing care. *Cancer Nursing, 13*(3): 161; **16-13,** from Jones, J.M. (2004). Nutritional methodology: Development of a nutritional screening or assessment tool using a multivariate technique. *Nutrition, 20*(3): 299.

Chapter 17

17-1, From Alles, P. (1995). CESF Medical Outcomes Research Project: Implementing outcomes research in a clinical setting. *Wisconsin Medical Journal, 94*(1): 27–31; **17-5,** from Lobo, M.L. (1993). Code books–A critical link in the research process. *Western Journal of Nursing Research, 15*(3): 380; **17-6,** from Badger, T., Segrin, C., Dorros, S., Meek, P., & Lopez, A.M. (2007). Depression and anxiety in women with breast cancer and their partners. *Nursing Research, 56*(1): 47.

Chapter 21

21-3, From Lacara, T., Domagtoy, C., Lickliter, D., Quattrocchi, K. Snipes, L., Kuszaj, J. et al. (2007). Comparison of point-of-care and laboratory glucose analysis in critically ill patients. *American Journal of Critical Care, 16*(4): 340.

Chapter 25

25-1, From Heo, S., Moser, D.K., Lennie, T.A., Zambroski, C.H., & Misook, L.C. (2007). A comparison of health-related quality of life between older adults with heart failure and healthy older adults. *Heart & Lung, 36*(1): 17; **25-2,** from Jenkins, K. & Ahijevych, K. (2003). Nursing students' beliefs about smoking, their own smoking behaviors, and use of professional tobacco treatment intervention. *Applied Nursing Research, 16*(3): 169; **25-3,** from Swain, M.A. & Steckel, S.B. (1981) Influencing adherence among hypertensives. *Research in Nursing & Health, 4*(1): 219. Copyright © 1981, John Wiley & Sons. Reprinted by permission of John Wiley & Sons, Inc.; **25-5,** developed by Kathy Daniel, MS, APRN-BC, with the assistance of Heather Stieglitz, PhD; presented with permission of Ms. Daniel.

Chapter 27

27-1, From Stetler, C.B. (2001). Updating the Stetler Model of Research Utilization to facilitate evidence-based practice. *Nursing Outlook, 49*(6): 276; **27-2,** from Titler, M.G. et al. (2001). The Iowa model of evidence-based practice to promote quality care. *Critical Care Nursing Clinics of North America, 13*(4): 500; **27-3,** source: American Society of Hospital Pharmacists. (1994). ASHP therapeutic position statement on the institutional use of 0.9% sodium chloride injection to maintain patency of peripheral indewelling intermittent infusion devices. *American Journal of Hospital Pharmacy, 51*(12): 1572–1574; Goode, C.J., Titler, M., Rakel, B., Ones, D.S., Kleiber, C., Small, S. et al. (1991). A meta-analysis of effects of heparin flush and saline flush: Quality and cost implications. *Nursing Research, 40*(6): 324–330; Randolph, A.G., Cook, D.J., Gonzales, C.A., Andrew, M. (1998). Benefits of heparin in peripheral venous and arterial catheters: Systematic review and meta-analysis of randomized controlled trials. *British Medical Journal, 316*(7136): 969–975; Shoaf, J. & Oliver, S. (1992). Efficacy of normal saline injection with and without heparin for maintaining intermittent intravenous site. *Applied Nursing Research, 5*(1): 9–12; **27-4,** from U.S. Department of Health and Human Services, National Institutes of health, National Heart, Lung, and Blood Institute (2003). Reference card from the seventh report of the Joint National Committee on Prevention, Detection, Evaluation, and Treatment of High Blood Pressure (JNC 7). Bethesda, MD: NIH Publication No. 03-5231. Retrieved December 4, 2007 from www.nhlbi.nih.gov/guidelines/hypertension/jnc7card.htm.

Chapter 28

28-1, 28-2, From Ulbrich, S.L. (1995). *The effect of operator technique on tympanic membrane thermometry.* Unpublished master's thesis, University of Texas at Arlington.

INDEX

A

Abbreviated source, 101
Absolute zero point, 375–376
Abstract, 102
 critical appraisal of, 600
 definition of, 583
 outline for
  qualitative study, 584*t*
  quantitative study, 584*t*
Abstract concept, 177
 multiple measures of, 374*f*
 as qualitative study focus, 178
Abstraction, 610
Abstract thinking, 4, 94
Abstract thought process, 4–7
Acceptance rate, 347
Accessible population, 344*f*
 definition of, 343–344
Accession number, 101
Accidental sampling, 353–354
Accuracy
 of physiological measurement, 388
 of screening test, 390
Acquired immunodeficiency syndrome
  (AIDS)
 coping interventions for, 257
 research for, 194
Acute care nurse practitioners, care
  from, 242
Acute Care Setting Report Card, 289
Acute myocardial infarction (AMI), 12
Adaptation
 chronic illness study, 153
 conceptual models for, 135
 encouraging appropriate, 339
Advanced practice nurse (APN)
 evidence-based practice and, 2
 intervention versus outcome, 292
 outcomes classification, 292
 outcomes research and, 291–293
 role of, 4

Advanced Practice Registered Nurses'
  Research Network (APRNet), 293
Advances in Nursing Science, 19
Advisory Council on Performance
  Measurement, 290
Aesthetic-poetic translation, 424
African American
 hypertension in, 12*f*
 smoking in, 69
 TM program for BP in, 34, 36,
  46, 47*f*
Agency for Health Care Policy and
  Research (AHCPR), 21,
  287–288
Agency for Healthcare Research and
  Quality (AHRQ), 75
Agency for Health Services Research
  (AHSR)
 health services, effectiveness of,
  286–287
 Medical Outcomes Study (MOS),
  286–287
 small area analysis, 286
Aggregate, 281–282
Alpha coefficient value, 379,
  462–463
Alternate-forms reliability, 378
American Association of Colleges of
  Nursing, 21
American Association of Critical Care
  Nurses (AACN), 74–75
American Nurses Association (ANA)
 APN, types of, 291–292
 community-based non-acute care
  indicators, 290, 290*f*
 nursing, definition of, 2
 Nursing Care Report Card, 289
 nursing functions and activities, 18
 nursing-sensitive quality
  indicators, 290
 research conferences by, 18–19

American Organization of Nurse
  Executives (AONE), 75
*American Psychological Association,
  Publication Manual of*, 569–570
Analogue test, 333
Analysis
 of change, 308–309
 of content, 528
 in critical appraisal, 605
 of improvement, 309
 multilevel, 310
 narrative, 528–529
 survival, 475–476
 time-series, 476
Analysis of variance (ANOVA), 361
 one-way, 505–506
Analysis triangulation, 232
Analytical induction, 527
Analytical preciseness, in qualitative
  research, 612–613
Analytical variability, 389
Animal subject, 214
Annual Review of Nursing Research,
  20, 115
Anonymity, 196, 202
Anxiety, learning and, 132
Anxiety, measurement of, 373–374
Appalachian adult, preventative health
  services for, 243
Applicability
 Katz activities of daily living (ADL)
  scale, 307*t*
 as outcomes assessment instrument,
  306*t*
Applied research, 34
Approximate replication, 72
Articles
 critical appraisal of, 600
 See also Journal articles
Ascendance to an open context, 53
Assent, 191

Page numbers followed by *f* indicates illustrations; *b* indicates boxes, and *t* indicates tables.

Subject error, 389
Subject heading, 102
Subjects of care, 281–282
Substantive theory, 56, 144
  framework construction from, 151–152
Substitutable relationship, 134
Subsuming particles into the general, 527
Subtraction design, 337
Sudden Infant Death Syndrome
  (SIDS), 243
Sufficient relationship, 134
Summary, 112–113
Summated scale, 410
Sum of squares (SS), 473
Support system
  academic committee as, 447
  institution as, 447
  personal, 447
  for researcher, 447
Survey, 245
Survival analysis, 475–476
Symmetrical curve, 453, 453f
Symmetry, 133
Systematic bias
  definition of, 346
  random sampling and, 349
Systematic error
  conceptualization of, 373f
  true score and, 372
  validity and, 381
Systematic replication, 72
Systematic review, 27–28
  implementing and evaluating, 619 620
  sources for, 620
Systematic sampling, 352–353
Systematic variation
  occurrence of, 347
  as sampling error, 346–348

T

Table
  development of, 571–574
  example of, 571t
Tailedness, 457
Target population, 344f
  definition of, 343–344
Taxonomy, 322
Teleform
  of Burns Cancer Belief Scale, 436f
  features of, 434–435
Telemonitoring
  applied research using, 34

Telemonitoring   (cont'd)
  effects of, 47f
  intervention study using, 36
  quasi-experimental study using, 46–48
Telemonitoring (TM) program, 34
Telephone interview, 306–307
Tendency statement, 134
Tentative theory, 144–145
Terminally ill, research on, 194
Test-retest reliability, 377–378
Textbook, 323
Theme, 115
  formulating from narratives, 579, 580t
  identification of, 526
Theoretical coherence, 527–528
Theoretical connectedness, in
  qualitative research, 613
Theoretical limitation, 41
Theoretical literature, 93
  discussion of, 111
Theoretical sampling, 356–357
Theoretical substruction
  framework, critical analysis of, 153–155
  performance of, 154
Theoretical triangulation, 231–232
Theory, 8, 39
  construction of, 610
  definition of, 139–145
  in nursing, 136t
  of planned behavior, 169f
  research problems and, 73
  testing, 169
  types of, 140
  of unpleasant symptoms, 151f
Theory of caring, 55–56
Theory of humanistic nursing, 55–56
Therapeutic nursing intervention, 249–250
Therapeutic research, 185
Thesis, 93, 579–580
  outline for, 581t
  as research report, 579–580
  See also Study, seeking approval for
Threats
  designs to reduce, 226
  to interrupted time-series designs,
    260
  to statistical conclusion validity,
    221
Time
  for data collection, 431
  patterns across, 474–476
  physiological measurements across, 400
Time coding, 492

Time-dimensional design,
  239–244
Time-series analysis, 476
Title, 101
Tolerability, 269
Tradition, 8–9
Transcription, 523–524
Transcription error, 389
Transformation, of ideas, 610
Transformed term, 492–493
Translation
  forward/backward, 424–425
  interpretation and, 552
  of scale to another language, 424
  strategy for, 424
  types of, 424
Traumatic brain injury (TMI),
  depression and, 354
Treatment
  compensatory equalization and
    rivalry of, 223
  control of, 227
  diffusion or imitation of, 223
  history and, 226
  removed, pretest and posttest designs
    with, 258–259, 259f
  reversed, pretest and posttest designs
    with, 259–260, 260f
  selection and, 225–226
  setting and, 226
  tolerability of, 269
  two-treatment design, 257, 258f
Treatment matching, 336
Treatment mechanism trial (TM trial),
  269
Treatment partitioning
  cohort designs with, 243
  cross-sectional study with, 244f
  longitudinal design with, 244f
Treatment standardization, 222
Trend design
  example of, 242f
  purpose of, 242–243
Trial and error, 9
Triangulation
  pros and cons of, 232–234
  types of, 230–234
True experiment
  problems with, 318–319
True measurement score, 372
True negative, 390
True positive, 390
Truncation, 246

Methods of Statistical Data Analyses for Quantitative Nursing Research: Quick Access Chart

		Bivariate Data Analyses	
		Two Samples	Three or More Samples
Independent Groups Two Variables	Nominal Data	Chi-square, p. 499 Phi, p. 501 Cramer's *V*, p. 501 Contingency Coefficient, p. 501 Lambda, p. 502	Chi-square, p. 499
	Ordinal Data	Spearman Rank-Order Correlation Coefficient, p. 482 Kendall's Tau, p. 483	
	Interval or Ratio Data	*t*-Test for Independent Samples, p. 502 Pearson's Product-Moment Correlation Coefficient, p. 479 Analysis of Variance, p. 505 Simple Linear Regression, p. 489	Analysis of Variance, p. 505 Multiple Regression, p. 491